Children's Speech
An Evidence-Based Approach to Assessment and Intervention

Sharynne McLeod

Charles Sturt University, Australia

Elise Baker

The University of Sydney, Australia

Boston Columbus Hoboken Indianapolis New York San Francisco
Amsterdam Cape Town Dubai London Madrid Milan Munich Paris Montreal Toronto
Delhi Mexico City São Paulo Sydney Hong Kong Seoul Singapore Taipei Tokyo

Editorial Director: Kevin Davis
Executive Editor: Julie Peters
Program Manager: Megan Moffo
Editorial Assistant: Maria Feliberty
Executive Product Marketing Manager: Christopher Barry
Executive Field Marketing Manager: Krista Clark
Procurement Specialist: Deidra Smith
Cover Design: Melissa Welch, Studio Montage
Cover Art: Fotolia/Pavla Zakova
Media Producer: Michael Goncalves
Editorial Production and Composition Services: Lumina Datamatics, Inc.
Full-Service Project Manager: Doug Bell, Raja Natesan
Printer/Binder: LSC Communications
Cover Printer: LSC Communications
Text Font: Stone Serif ITC Pro 9/11

Credits and acknowledgments borrowed from other sources and reproduced, with permission, in the textbook appear on the appropriate page within text.

Feature Icon Credits: Checkmark Icon (Application): 4zevar/Fotolia; Globe Icon (Multicultural Insights): vladvm50/Fotolia; Handprint Icon (Children's Insights): PiXXart Photography/Fotolia; Chat Icon (Comment): DigiClack/Fotolia.

Preface page credit: Image Elise Baker: © The University of Sydney/Louise Cooper.

Library of Congress Cataloging-in-Publication Data
Names: McLeod, Sharynne, author. | Baker, Elise author.
Title: Children's speech : an evidence-based approach to assessment and
    intervention / Sharynne McLeod, Elise Baker.
Description: Boston: Pearson, 2017. | Includes bibliographical references and
    index.
Identifiers: LCCN 2016006775| ISBN 9780132755962 (alk. paper) | ISBN 0132755963
    (alk. paper)
Subjects: LCSH: Speech therapy for children. | Speech disorders in children.
Classification: LCC RJ496.S7 M392 2016 | DDC 618.92/85506–dc23 LC record available at
http://lccn.loc.gov/2016006775

7

ISBN-10:   0-132-75596-3
ISBN-13: 978-0-132-75596-2

eText
ISBN-10:   0-13-420527-8
ISBN-13: 978-0-13-420527-4

PEARSON

Brief Contents

Preface   xiii

About the Authors   xvii

Acknowledgments   xix

Chapter 1   *Children with Speech Sound Disorders*   1

Chapter 2   *Classification, Causes, and Co-occurrence*   37

Chapter 3   *Articulatory Foundations of Speech*   60

Chapter 4   *Transcription of Speech*   84

Chapter 5   *Theoretical Foundations of Children's Speech*   134

Chapter 6   *Children's Speech Acquisition*   175

Chapter 7   *Assessment Preparation, Purpose, and Types*   220

Chapter 8   *Assessment of Children's Speech*   244

Chapter 9   *Analysis of Children's Speech*   288

Chapter 10   *Goal Setting*   340

Chapter 11   *Intervention Principles and Plans*   372

Chapter 12   *Intervention Procedures and Evaluation*   412

Chapter 13   *Phonological Intervention Approaches*   434

Chapter 14   *Articulatory and Motor Speech Intervention Approaches*   483

Chapter 15   *Evidence-Based Practice in Practice*   520

Chapter 16   *Individual Children with Speech Sound Disorders: Case Studies*   541

Glossary   570

References   583

Index   622

Contents

Preface   xiii

About the Authors   xvii

Acknowledgments   xix

Chapter 1   Children with Speech Sound Disorders   1

Overview   2

Defining SSD   4

Prevalence and Impact   9

Prevalence of Communication Disorders   10
Prevalence of children with SSD   10 / Proportion of children with SSD on SLPs' caseloads   13

Natural History and Long-Term Manifestation of SSD   14
Natural history of SSD   15 / Manifestation of SSD in late childhood   15 /
Manifestation of SSD in adolescence and adulthood   16

Impact and Outcomes of Childhood SSD   17
Longitudinal studies of the impact and outcomes of SSD on children's lives   17 / Impact of SSD on
children's lives   19 / Educational impact of SSD   20 / Occupational impact of SSD   23 /
Impact of SSD on children's families   23

Risk and Protective Factors for SSD   26

Evidence-Based Practice   33
Steps involved in clinical decision-making   35

Chapter summary   36

Suggested reading   36

Application of knowledge from Chapter 1   36

Chapter 2   Classification, Causes, and Co-occurrence   37

Overview   38

Types of SSD in Children   38
Speech sound disorders: Phonology   40 / Speech sound disorders: Motor speech   41

Classification Systems of Children with SSD   46
Speech Disorders Classification System (Shriberg, 1980; 2010a)   46 / Differential Diagnosis System
(Dodd, 1995a, 2005, 2013)   48 / Psycholinguistic Framework (Stackhouse & Wells, 1997)   48 /
International Classification of Functioning, Disability and Health – Children and Youth Version
(ICF-CY) (WHO, 2007)   50

SSD of Known and Unknown Origins   51
SSD of known origins   52

Co-occurrence of SSD with Other Types of Communication Impairment   56
Co-occurrence of SSD and language impairment   57 / Co-occurrence of SSD and literacy
difficulties   57 / Co-occurrence of SSD and oromotor difficulties   57 / Co-occurrence of SSD and
voice difficulties   58 / Co-occurrence of SSD and stuttering   58

Chapter summary   59

Suggested reading   59

Application of knowledge from Chapter 2   59

Chapter 3 *Articulatory Foundations of Speech 60*

Overview 61

Anatomical Structures for Speech Production and Perception 61

Structures Involved in Speech Production 61
Tongue 63 / Lips 67 / Teeth 68 / Mandible 70 / Hard palate 71 / Soft palate (Velum) 73 / Nose 74 / Pharynx 75 / Larynx 76 / The respiratory system 77

Structures Involved in Speech Detection 78
Ear 78

Additional Anatomical Structures That Support Perception and Production of Speech 81
The neurological system 81

Chapter summary 83

Suggested reading 83

Application of knowledge from Chapter 3 83

Chapter 4 *Transcription of Speech 84*

Overview 85

Transcription of Speech 85
International Phonetic Alphabet (IPA) 88 / Pulmonic consonant chart 90 / Non-pulmonic consonant chart 95 / Other symbols chart 96 / Diacritics chart 97 / Vowel chart 98 / Suprasegmentals chart 103 / Tones and word accents chart 105

Extensions to the IPA 105

Phonotactics 106
Consonant clusters 106 / Syllable shapes and word positions 107

Understanding English Consonants Using Knowledge of Anatomy and Auditory Transcription 108
Sagittal diagrams of English consonants 109 / Transverse diagrams of English consonants 109 / Bilabial plosives /p, b/ 110 / Alveolar plosives /t, d/ 111 / Velar Plosives /k, g/ 114 / Nasal consonants /m, n, ŋ/ 115 / Labiodental fricatives /f, v/ 116 / Dental fricatives /θ, ð/ 116 / Alveolar fricatives /s, z/ 117 / Postalveolar fricatives /ʃ, ʒ/ 120 / Glottal fricative /h/ 121 / Alveolar approximant /ɹ/ 121 / Palatal approximant /j/ 123 / Alveolar lateral approximant /l/ 123 / Labiovelar approximant /w/ 123 / Affricates /ʧ, ʤ/ 124

Chapter summary 125

Suggested reading 125

Application of knowledge from Chapter 4 125

Appendix 4-1. Transcription decision-making tree 126

Appendix 4-2. Inventory of consonants for 25 languages and dialects 127

Appendix 4-3. Extensions to the International Phonetic Alphabet 132

Appendix 4-4. Voice quality symbols 133

Chapter 5 *Theoretical Foundations of Children's Speech 134*

Overview 135

Phonology—What Is It? 135
Theoretical concepts: Phones, phonemes, allophones, and minimal pairs 136 / Theoretical concepts: Features 138 / Theoretical concepts: Naturalness, markedness, and implicational relationships 145 / Theoretical concepts: Phonotactics 145 / Theoretical concepts: Sonority 146

Phonological Theories 148

Classic Theories of Phonology 148
Generative phonology, underlying and surface representations, and rules 148 / Natural phonology and phonological processes 151

Contemporary theories of phonology 159
Nonlinear phonology (based on Bernhardt & Stemberger, 2000 159 / Optimality theory (based on Dinnsen & Gierut, 2008) 162 / Representation-based accounts of SSD in children 164

Speech Perception   165
   How do we perceive speech?   166 / The theoretical relevance of speech perception for children with
   SSD   167

Speech Production   168
   Phonological planning, motor planning, motor programming, and motor execution   168 /
   Theories and models of speech production   170

Chapter summary   173

Suggested reading   173

Application of knowledge from Chapter 5   174

Chapter 6   *Children's Speech Acquisition*   175

Overview   176

Part 1: Important Issues When Considering Children's Speech Acquisition   177

Typical versus Acceptable Speech Acquisition   178
   Factors influencing typical speech acquisition   179

Theories of Child Development That Have Influenced Our Understanding
of Speech Acquisition   185
   Jean Piaget   185 / Lev Vygotsky   186 / Urie Bronfenbrenner   186

Methodological Issues in Studying Speech Acquisition   187
   Diary studies   188 / Cross-sectional studies   188 / Longitudinal studies   189
   Comparative studies   189 / Summary of Part 1   190

Part 2: Typical Speech Acquisition for English-Speaking Children   191

Speech Acquisition for English-Speaking Infants and Toddlers from Birth to 2 Years   191
   Oral mechanism   192 / Perception   192 / Crying, vocalization, and
   babbling   193 / Intelligibility   194 / Phonetic inventory   194 / Syllable and word shape inventory   195 / Age of acquisition of consonants, consonant clusters, and vowels   196 / Percentage of
   consonants, consonant clusters, and vowels correct   196 / Common mismatches   198 / Phonological processes   199 / Syllable structure   199 / Prosody   199 / Metalinguistic skills   200

Speech Acquisition for English-Speaking Preschoolers from 3 to 5 Years   200
   Oral mechanism   200 / Intelligibility   201 / Phonetic inventory   201 / Syllable and word shape
   inventory   202 / Age of acquisition of consonants, consonant clusters, and vowels   202 / Percentage of consonants, consonant clusters, and vowels correct   205 / Common mismatches   205 /
   Phonological processes   206 / Prosody   207 / Phonological awareness   208

Speech Acquisition for English-Speaking School-Aged Children from 6 Years   208
   Oral mechanism   208 / Intelligibility   210 / Phonetic inventory   210 / Syllable and word shape
   inventory   210 / Age of acquisition of consonants, consonant clusters, and vowels   210 / Percentage of consonants, consonant clusters, and vowels correct   211 / Prosody   212 / Phonological
   awareness and literacy   212

Part 3: Typical Speech Acquisition for All Children   212
   Intelligibility   212 / Phonetic inventory   213 / Syllable and word shape inventory   213 /
   Mastery of consonants and vowels   214 / Percentage of consonants, consonant clusters, and
   vowels correct   214 / Common mismatches   215 / Phonological processes   215 / Prosody   215

Chapter summary   216

Recommended reading   216

Application of knowledge from Chapter 6   216

Appendix 6-1. Summary of studies of English-speaking children's speech acquisition   217

Chapter 7   *Assessment Preparation, Purpose, and Types*   220

Overview   221

Typical Assessments for Children with Suspected SSD   221

Preparation   221
   The most important assessment tool: The SLP   222 / Child-friendly assessments   225 /
   Family-centered and family-friendly assessments   227 / Assessment contexts   227 /
   Collaboration with other professionals   228

Referral and Background Information   228
Case history information   229 / Documenting family history of speech, language, and communication difficulties   229 / Documenting children's language use and proficiency   230 / Learning from those who know the child the best: Parents, grandparents, teachers, siblings, and friends   232

Purposes of Assessment   233
Descriptive assessments   234 / Diagnostic assessments   235 / Intervention planning   235 / Outcome measurement   235

Types of Assessments   236
Standardized assessments   236 / Informal assessments   237 / Norm-referenced assessments   238 / Criterion-referenced assessments   238 / Screening assessments   239 / Static assessments   240 / Dynamic assessments   241 / Response to intervention   242

Chapter summary   242

Suggested reading   243

Application of knowledge from Chapter 7   243

Chapter 8   *Assessment of Children's Speech   244*

Overview   245

Components of Children's Speech Assessments   245

Assessment of Intelligibility   245
Rating scales that quantify perceptions of intelligibility   246 / Single-word measures that quantify intelligible phonetic contrasts   247 / Connected speech measures that quantify word and syllable identification   248 / Assessment of acceptability and comprehensibility   249

Assessment of Speech Production: Elements   250
Consonants   250 / Consonant clusters   252 / Vowels and diphthongs   253 / Polysyllables   255 / Prosody   256 / Tones   257

Assessment of Speech Production: Methods   257
Single-word speech assessments   258 / Single-word testing for young children   260 / Connected speech assessments   261 / Single-word versus connected speech assessments   264 / Assessment of stimulability   264 / Assessment of inconsistency and variability   265

Assessment of Oral Structure and Function   265

Assessment of Speech Perception   267
Auditory discrimination tasks   267 / Auditory lexical discrimination tasks   268

Assessment of Hearing   269

Assessment of Phonological Processing   269
Phonological access   269 / Phonological working memory: Nonword repetition tasks   270 / Phonological awareness   270

Assessment of Emergent Literacy, Early Literacy, and Conventional Literacy Skills   271

Assessment of Psychosocial Aspects   272

Assessment of Children's Communicative Participation   273
Assessment of children's views of their speech within educational and social contexts   273

Language, Voice, and Fluency Assessments   275

Using the ICF-CY Framework to Scaffold Assessment Planning   276

Strategic Assessments Suited to Children with Different Types of SSD   277

Assessments for Children with Suspected Phonological Impairment   278
Assessments for children with suspected inconsistent speech disorder   279 / Assessments for children with suspected articulation impairment   279 / Assessments for children with suspected CAS   279 / Assessments for children with suspected childhood dysarthria   280 / Assessment of SSD for child with craniofacial anomalies   281 / Assessment of SSD for child with hearing loss   282

Differential Diagnosis and Prognostic Statements   283

Chapter summary   283

Suggested reading   284

Application of knowledge from Chapter 8   284

Appendix 8-1. Assessment plan   285

Appendix 8-2. Assessment plan for Luke   286

Chapter 9   *Analysis of Children's Speech   288*

Overview   289

Traditional Articulation Analysis: Substitution, Omission, Distortion, Addition (SODA)   289
   When and how do I use traditional SODA analysis?   291

Differentiating Phonemic (Phonological) from Phonetic (Articulation) Errors   292

Independent and Relational Phonological Analyses   292

Children's independent and relational phonological analysis (CHIRPA)   295
   Independent phonological analysis   296 / Relational phonological analysis   301

Speech Measures   319
   Measures of segments   319 / Measures of whole words   320

Instrumental Analyses of Children's Speech   324
   Acoustic Analysis of Children's Speech   326 / Electropalatography (EPG)   329 / Ultrasound   331

Chapter summary   332

Suggested reading   332

Application of knowledge from Chapter 9   333

Appendix 9-1. Children's Independent and Relational Phonological Analysis (CHIRPA) Template   334

Appendix 9-2. Children's Independent and Relational Phonological Analysis (CHIRPA) Template: Worked example for Luke (4;3 years)   337

Chapter 10   *Goal Setting   340*

Overview   341

What Are Intervention Goals?   341

Identifying Goals for Children with SSD from Different Perspectives   341

Operationally Defined Goals   344

Goal Frameworks and Hierarchies   346

Generalization   348
   Stimulus generalization   348 / Response generalization   348

Approaches to Goal Setting for Children with SSD   350

Goal Setting for Children with Phonological Impairment: The Importance of the Target   350
   Traditional developmental approach   350 / Complexity approach to target selection   351 / Cycles approach to target selection   356 / Systemic (functional) approach to target selection   358 / Constraint-based nonlinear approach to target selection   360 / Neuro-network approach to target selection   362

Goal Setting for Children with Articulation Impairment   363
   Goal setting for children with inconsistent speech disorder   364 / Goal setting for children with CAS   364 / Goal setting for children with childhood dysarthria   367

Goal Setting Considerations for Children with Highly Unintelligible Speech   367

Goal Attack Strategies   368

Chapter summary   369

Suggested reading   370

Application of knowledge from Chapter 10   370

Appendix 10-1. Goal identification template   371

Chapter 11   *Intervention Principles and Plans   372*

Overview   373

What Is Intervention?   373
   Intervention Principles, Plans, and Procedures   373

Principles of Intervention   375
   Principles of intervention: Phonology   375 / Principles of intervention: Speech perception   376 / Principles of intervention: Motor learning   376 / Principles of intervention: Cognition and meta-awareness   385 / Principles of intervention: Behavioral learning   387 / Principles of intervention: Neurological experience   391

Intervention Plans   392
> Models of intervention practice: Therapist-centered, parent-as-therapist aide, family-centered, and family-friendly practice   393 / Management plans   393 / Session plans   395 / Service delivery options   396

Progress and Discharge Planning   402
> Short-term goal criteria: When do I move on to a new goal?   402 / Long-term goals: When is a child discharged from intervention?   402

Chapter summary   403

Suggested reading   403

Application of knowledge from Chapter 11   404

Appendix 11-1. Speech Sound Disorder Management Plan   405

Appendix 11-2. Speech Sound Disorder Intervention Session Plan   408

Chapter 12   *Intervention Procedures and Evaluation   412*

Overview   413

Intervention Procedures   413
> The teaching and learning moment   413 / Stimuli, resources, materials, and activities   420

Evaluating Intervention   422
> Why do I have to collect data?   422 / How do you evaluate intervention?   423

A Framework for Problem-Solving Slow Progress   429

Chapter summary   432

Suggested reading   433

Application of knowledge from Chapter 12   433

Chapter 13   *Phonological Intervention Approaches   434*

Overview   435

Principles of Phonological Intervention in Practice   436

Minimal Pair Approach   437
> Historical background   437 / Theoretical background   437 / Procedure   437 / Evidence   439 / Children suited to the minimal pair approach   440 / Resources for conducting minimal pair intervention   440 / Minimal pairs for children who speak languages other than English   440

Maximal Oppositions and Treatment of the Empty Set   444
> Historical background   444 / Theoretical background   444 / Procedure   444 / Evidence   445 / Children suited to maximal oppositions and treatment of the empty set approaches   446

Multiple Oppositions   447
> Historical background   447 / Theoretical background   447 / Procedure   447 / Evidence   449 / Children suited to the multiple oppositions approach   449 / Resources for conducting multiple oppositions intervention   449

Metaphon   450
> Historical background   450 / Theoretical background   450 / Procedure   451 / Children suited to the metaphon approach   452 / Evidence   452 / Resources for conducting Metaphon intervention   452

Cycles   453
> Historical background   453 / Theoretical background   453 / Procedure   453 / Children suited to the cycles approach   454 / Evidence   454 / Resources for conducting the cycles approach   455

Speech Perception Intervention   456
> Historical background   456 / Theoretical background   457 / Procedure   458 / Children suited to speech perception intervention   458 / Evidence   458 / Resources for speech perception intervention   459

Intervention for Concomitant Phonology and Morphosyntax Difficulties   459
> Historical background   459 / Theoretical background   460 / Procedure   460 / Children suited to the intervention for concomitant phonology and morphosyntax   461 / Evidence   461 / Resources for conducting intervention for concomitant phonology and morphosyntax difficulties   462

Stimulability Intervention 462
Historical background 462 / Theoretical background 462 / Procedure 463 / Children suited to the stimulability approach 463 / Evidence 463 / Resources for conducting stimulability intervention 464

Intervention for Inconsistent Speech Disorder 464
Core vocabulary: Intervention for inconsistent speech disorder 464

Brief Overview of Other Approaches for Managing Phonological Impairment in Children 467

Aligning Phonological Target Selection Approaches with Phonological Intervention Approaches 468

Phonological Intervention for Children Who Are Late Talkers 469
Goals and intervention strategies to use with infants and toddlers at risk of or showing early signs of SSD 470

Phonological Intervention for Multilingual Children 472

Addressing the Risk of Literacy Difficulties in Preschoolers with Phonological Impairment 476
Resources for emergent literacy intervention with children with phonological impairment 477

Chapter summary 477

Suggested reading 478

Application of knowledge from Chapter 13 478

Appendix 13-1. Core Vocabulary Words That May Be Relevant for Working with Children Who Speak Cantonese 479

Appendix 13-2. Core Vocabulary Words That May Be Relevant for Working with Children Who Speak Vietnamese 480

Appendix 13-3. Core Vocabulary Words That May Be Relevant for Working with Children Who Speak Spanish 482

Chapter 14 *Articulatory and Motor Speech Intervention Approaches 483*

Overview 484

Historical Perspectives on Articulation and Motor Speech Interventions 485

Intervention for Articulation Impairment 486
Traditional articulation intervention for articulation impairment 486 / Concurrent treatment: Articulation intervention based on principles of motor learning 493 / Articulation intervention using instrumental feedback: Ultrasound, electropalatography, and spectrography 496

Intervention for Childhood Apraxia of Speech (CAS) 500
Dynamic temporal and tactile cueing (DTTC): Intervention for CAS 500 / Commercial intervention programs for CAS 505 / Rapid syllable transition treatment (ReST): Intervention for dysprosody in CAS 506 / Prompts for restructuring oral muscular phonetic targets (PROMPT): Intervention for motor speech disorders 509 / Integrated phonological awareness intervention for CAS 511

Intervention for Childhood Dysarthria 513
Systems approach: Intervention for childhood dysarthria 513 / Using augmentative and alternative communication (AAC) to improve speech and/or enhance activity and participation for children with severe motor speech disorders 516

Chapter summary 518

Suggested reading 518

Application of knowledge from Chapter 14 519

Chapter 15 *Evidence-Based Practice in Practice 520*

Overview 521

What Is Evidence-Based Practice (EBP)? 521

Integrating External Published Evidence with the Reality of Clinical Practice and Client Factors, Values, and Preferences 522
Step 1: Generate a PICO clinical question 522 / Step 2: Find external evidence relevant to the question 523 / Step 3: Critically evaluate the external evidence 525 / Step 4: Evaluate the

internal evidence from your clinical practice   528 / Step 5: Evaluate the internal evidence with respect to child and family factors, values, and preferences   530 / Step 6: Make a decision by integrating the evidence   531 / Step 7: Evaluate the outcomes of the decision   532 / Summarizing the importance of EBP   532

Ethical Guidelines for Clinical Practice   533

Policies Affecting Clinical Practice   533
International conventions and frameworks   534 / National policies and laws   536

Associations That Support SLPs' Clinical Practice and Continuing Education   536
Speech-Language pathology position and policy papers   538

Chapter summary   540

Suggested reading   540

Application of knowledge from Chapter 15   540

Chapter 16   *Individual Children with Speech Sound Disorders: Case Studies   541*

Overview   542

Luke (4;3 years): Phonological Impairment   542
Luke: Case history   542 / Luke: Assessment results   543 / Adapting Luke's case study for different dialects   546 / Intervention studies of children who have phonological impairment   547

Susie (7;4 years): Articulation Impairment—Lateral Lisp   554
Susie: Case history   554 / Susie: Assessment results   554 / Intervention Studies of children who have an articulation impairment involving rhotics or sibilants   554

Jarrod (7;0 years): Inconsistent Speech Disorder   555
Jarrod: Case history   555 / Jarrod: Assessment results   555 / Published intervention studies of children who have inconsistent speech disorder   559

Michael (4;2 years): Childhood Apraxia of Speech (CAS)   559
Michael: Case history   560 / Michael: Assessment results   560 / Intervention studies of children who have CAS   563

Lian (14;2 years): Childhood Dysarthria   563
Lian: Case history   563 / Lian: Assessment results   563 / Intervention studies of children who have childhood dysarthria   567

Chapter summary   569

Suggested reading   569

Application of knowledge from Chapter 16   569

Glossary   570

References   583

Index   622

Preface

Children's Speech: An Evidence-Based Approach to Assessment and Intervention is about children and a common communication difficulty—speech sound disorders. This book distills the world's research on speech sound disorders across the areas of speech acquisition, assessment, analysis, diagnosis, and intervention. It combines foundational knowledge and scientific evidence with practical knowledge to prepare speech-language pathologists (SLPs) to work with children and their families.

Our inspiration for this book stems from our passion for research to be accessible to students, clinicians, and faculty without compromising on academic rigor. It is based on our strong conviction that good clinical decisions are grounded in knowledge of empirical evidence underscored by theory and principles. It also comes from our desire for SLPs to work holistically with children and appreciate the impact that speech sound disorders can have on children's day-to-day activities and participation.

This book was shaped by the children and families we have worked with as SLPs, the students we have taught as university educators, and the children we have raised as parents. It is written for students and professionals of speech-language pathology, speech pathology, speech and language therapy, logopedics, and phoniatrics. This book may also be of interest to linguists, phoneticians, educators, audiologists, psychologists, physicians, doctors, and others who work with children with speech sound disorders. To this end, we hope the joy and inspiration we have experienced over many years in our various professional and personal roles translates to you across the text. We hope we instill in you a deep respect for empirical research, a passion to see every child as a unique individual, and a sense of excitement about the opportunity to make a difference in the lives of children and their families. As you read the pages of this text, we also hope you are inspired to think carefully and critically about the clinical decisions you make when working with children with speech sound disorders.

TEXT PHILOSOPHY AND ORGANIZATION

The content for this book was guided by two frameworks: evidence-based practice (EBP) (Dollaghan, 2007; Sackett, Rosenberg, Muir Gray, Hayes, & Richardson, 1996) and the International Classification of Functioning, Disability and Health—Children and Youth (ICF-CY) (World Health Organization, 2007). We use these two frameworks because we believe they help guide the successful management of speech sound disorders in children.

We have adopted Dollaghan's (2007) conceptualization of E^3BP. As part of E^3BP, you will learn that SLPs use expertise to make clinical decisions based on three sources of evidence: evidence from empirical research, evidence from day-to-day clinical practice, and evidence from client characteristics, values, and preferences. To this end, we provide you with comprehensive reviews of historical and current-day empirical research that underpins SLPs' clinical decisions. We do not try to simplify knowledge, but instead provide a breadth of views (that are sometimes conflicting) from different parts of the world so that you can make the best decision for each child and family you work with. We consider how you can generate and use your own evidence from clinical practice to guide clinical decisions. We also include detailed case-based data for five children, representing five different types of speech sound disorders: phonological impairment, articulation impairment, inconsistent speech disorder, childhood apraxia of speech, and childhood dysarthria. This information is included in the final chapter of this book (Chapter 16) as a resource for you to refer to as you learn about assessment, analysis, goal setting, intervention principles, plans, procedures, and approaches. These case studies will help you learn how to engage in EBP.

We have adopted the ICF-CY (World Health Organization, 2007) because it provides you with a way of thinking not only about the body structure (e.g., mouth, ears, and brain) and function (e.g., articulation, auditory perception, cognition), but the impact of an impairment on a child's activities and participation, the environmental barriers and facilitators, and personal factors relevant to individual children, such as age, gender, race, social background, education, and past and current experience.

We organized this text such that foundation knowledge is provided first. The foundation knowledge covers important topics such as children with speech sound disorders (Chapter 1), types of speech sound disorders (Chapter 2), anatomical structures (Chapter 3), articulation and transcription (Chapter 4), theoretical foundations of speech (Chapter 5), and speech acquisition (Chapter 6). Foundation knowledge is followed by practical, evidence-based knowledge that mirrors the stages of contact when working with children with speech sound disorders. These chapters address assessment (Chapters 7 and 8), analysis (Chapter 9), goal setting (Chapter 10), intervention principles and plans (Chapter 11), intervention procedures (Chapter 12), phonological interventions (Chapter 13), motor speech interventions (Chapter 14), and the conduct of EBP (Chapter 15). Case-based data is provided in Chapter 16. We deliberately organized the text in this way to help you appreciate the unfolding nature of the professional relationship between SLPs and children with speech sound disorders.

This is an international book. It not only includes information about English-speaking children and SLPs who live in the United States, it also includes information about English-speaking children and SLPs in countries such as Canada, the United Kingdom, Ireland, Australia, and New Zealand. Importantly, this book also goes beyond English, including information about the excellent work being undertaken by SLPs and researchers who speak Cantonese, French, German, Icelandic, Portuguese, Spanish, Swedish, Turkish, Vietnamese, and many other languages across the globe. Embedded within the book is a respect for cultural and linguistic diversity and the need to learn from children, families, and professionals who are multilingual or monolingual in languages other than English. We hope that you learn from the international speech-language pathology profession, and the children with speech sound disorders who are found across the world and speak many languages.

PEDAGOGICAL ELEMENTS

This book includes a range of unique pedagogical elements to facilitate your learning. Each chapter begins with a list of clearly specified **learning objectives**, **key words**, and an **overview** of the chapter. Each chapter ends with a concluding **summary**, **recommended reading**, **case application**, and **study questions**.

Throughout each chapter we include four types of boxes:

 Comments: These boxes provide insights from our own clinical experience, observations about controversies in the field, or commentary about a particular issue.

 Applications: These boxes provide you with an opportunity to stop reading and apply what you have learned. We encourage you to complete the application boxes—they will provide you an opportunity to develop a practical skill (e.g., analyze a speech sample, make a decision about an assessment result). The application boxes will also help you reflect on what you have learned and highlight what you need to learn more about in order to work with children with speech sound disorders and their families.

 Children's insights: These boxes offer unique insights into what children think, do, draw, and say about their lives and living with speech sound disorders, and what they think about receiving speech-language pathology services. These boxes are designed to assist readers to engage in the lives of children with speech sound disorders and become reflective, compassionate clinicians. Listen to what children have to say. Consider children's insights so that you are ready to listen to the children you will work with.

Multicultural insights: These boxes provide you with knowledge, awareness, and confidence to with work with children and families from cultures different to your own.

These boxes remind you that you see the world and the children you work with through your own cultural lens and that as a communication specialist you need to be adept at understanding, respecting, and working with children from diverse cultures and linguistic backgrounds.

To conclude, the title of the book, *Children's Speech: An Evidence-Based Approach to Assessment and Intervention*, does not include terms such as speech sound disorders, articulation and phonological impairment, and other terms that focus on a problem. We have taken a person-first philosophy, foregrounding children and their ability to communicate and participate in society as the overarching focus of this book. We hope that your passion for making a difference in children's lives is fuelled by reading *Children's Speech: An Evidence-Based Approach to Assessment and Intervention*.

> Ui mai koe ki ahau he aha te mea nui o te ao,
> Māku e kī atu he tangata, he tangata, he tangata! (Māori proverb)

> *Ask me what is the greatest thing in the world, I will reply:*
> *It is people, it is people, it is people!*

About the Authors

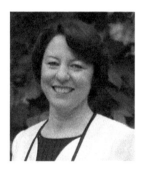

Sharynne McLeod, Ph.D., ASHA Fellow, Life Member SPA, CPSP /ʃæɹən məklæɔd/
Charles Sturt University, Australia

Sharynne McLeod is a speech-language pathologist and professor of speech and language acquisition at Charles Sturt University. She is an elected Fellow of the American Speech-Language-Hearing Association (ASHA) and a Life Member of Speech Pathology Australia. She is a board member of the International Association of Logopedics and Phoniatrics (IALP), Vice President of the International Clinical Linguistics and Phonetics Association (ICPLA), and was editor of the *International Journal of Speech-Language Pathology* (IJSLP), 2005–2013. She has received a Diversity Champion award from ASHA, an Australian Government Citation for Outstanding Contributions to Student Learning for her "sustained dedication, innovation and enthusiasm in university teaching that has had local, national and international impact," and teaching excellence awards from The University of Sydney and Charles Sturt University. Her coauthored books include *The International Guide to Speech Acquisition* (Cengage), *Interventions for Speech Sound Disorders in Children* (Paul H. Brookes), *Speech Sounds* (Plural), *Introduction to Speech, Language, and Literacy* (Oxford University Press), *Listening to Children and Young People with Speech, Language, and Communication Needs* (J&R Press), *Multilingual Aspects of Speech Sound Disorders in Children* (Multilingual Matters), and *Working with Families in Speech-Language Pathology* (Plural).

Professor McLeod's research focuses on monolingual and multilingual children's speech acquisition across the world. She applies the International Classification of Functioning, Disability and Health—Children and Youth (ICF-CY) (World Health Organization, 2007) to children with speech sound disorders, and she is listed as the only individual in Australia to have contributed to the development of the ICF-CY (WHO, 2007). Her research foregrounds the right of everyone (particularly children) to participate in society. Professor McLeod also researches the prevalence and impact of childhood speech sound disorders and links this to policy and service delivery issues. Professor McLeod has been topic chair and invited speaker at many ASHA conventions and has presented her research at conferences, professional associations, and universities in Australia, Canada, Greece, Hong Kong, Iceland, Ireland, Italy, Jamaica, New Zealand, Norway, Sweden, Turkey, Vietnam, the United Kingdom (England, Northern Ireland, Scotland), the United States, and Zambia. Additionally, she has visited and worked with children and families in Belgium, Fiji, France, Germany, Japan, and Tonga.

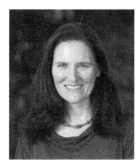

Elise Baker, Ph.D., CPSP /əliːs bæɪkɐ/
The University of Sydney, Australia

Elise Baker is a speech-language pathologist and senior lecturer with The University of Sydney. She is involved in the education and training of undergraduate and graduate speech-language pathology students, the supervision of graduate research students, and continuing education for qualified speech-language pathologists in her main area of interest: speech sound disorders in children. Dr. Baker has received awards for her excellence in teaching from The University of Sydney. She was the 2013 National Tour Speaker for Speech Pathology Australia and has served as a topic chair and invited speaker at ASHA conventions. Dr. Baker is passionate about knowledge translation and the importance of partnerships between speech-language pathologists and researchers in fostering knowledge generation, dissemination, and implementation. She nurtures this passion through service on the steering committee of a large, evidence-based practice network of practicing speech-language pathologists. Dr. Baker's research focuses on intervention for speech sound disorders in children, innovative service delivery solutions for children with speech sound disorder, speech-language pathologists' methods of practice with children who have speech sound disorders, and the conduct of evidence-based practice.

Acknowledgments

Children's Speech: An Evidence-Based Approach to Assessment and Intervention has evolved over 20 years as we have worked with and learned from children and their families, our students, and colleagues around the world. We express gratitude and appreciation to all of these people who have shaped our understanding of ways to make a difference in the lives of children with speech sound disorders. In particular we would like to thank the anonymous reviewers and name the following people who have provided advice on specific chapters: Martin J. Ball, Kirrie Ballard, Caroline Bowen, Mark Cordato, Kathryn Crowe, Barbara Dodd, Leah Fabiano-Smith, David Fitzsimons, Brian A. Goldstein, Anne Hesketh, Lê Thị Thanh Xuân, Sarah Masso, Jane McCormack, Elizabeth Murray, Amelia Paterson, Ben Phạm (Phạm Thị Bền), Carol Kit Sum To, Sarah Verdon, A. Lynn Williams, and Yvonne Wren. We also thank students from Charles Sturt University (Bathurst and Albury, Australia), The University of Sydney (Sydney, Australia), Temple University (Philadelphia, PA), East Tennessee State University (Johnson City, TN), and Phạm Ngọc Thạch University of Medicine (supported by the Trinh Foundation in Ho Chi Minh City, Viet Nam), who have provided feedback on our teaching and explanations of the evidence underpinning our work with children and their families. Thanks also go to the children and adults who have allowed us to include their photographs, drawings, and insights, including Emily and Alex Wray, and Ookeditse Phaswana. Finally and most importantly, we acknowledge the constant support and encouragement of our families. Sharynne thanks David, Brendon, and Jessica. Elise thanks Michael, Harrison, and Adelaide.

1

Children with Speech Sound Disorders

KEY WORDS

Speech sound disorders (SSD)

Prevalence, natural history

Longitudinal studies: Templin Longitudinal Study, Ottawa Language Study, Cleveland Family Speech and Language Study

Impact of SSD: educational, social, occupational

Risk and protective factors: child factors (sex, pre- and postnatal factors, oral sucking habits, psychosocial behaviors and temperament, minority status, race, and languages spoken), parent factors (family history of speech and language problems, maternal and paternal education level), family factors (socioeconomic status, family size and birth order)

Evidence-based practice: research evidence, clinical expertise, client values and preferences

LEARNING OBJECTIVES

1. Define the term *speech sound disorders* (SSD).

2. Outline the prevalence of SSD and the proportion of children with SSD on SLPs' caseloads.

3. Document the natural history of SSD and describe longitudinal studies of children with SSD.

4. Describe the impact of SSD from the perspectives of children, their parents, teachers, adults, and society.

5. List the risk and protective factors associated with SSD of unknown origin.

6. Provide a brief description of the components of evidence-based practice.

OVERVIEW

Children are important. They are the future of our world. They also contribute and belong to our communities now, before they grow up. Children need to communicate successfully to form relationships and interact with people within their family, school, and communities. Children's ability to communicate successfully also forms their foundation to learn to read, write, find employment, and contribute to society. Within a few short years, most children learn to speak intelligibly, pronouncing the consonants, vowels, and words that are appropriate for the languages and dialects that they are exposed to so that they can be competent communicators. However, some children have difficulty learning to speak. This book is about these children.

Children with speech sound disorders (SSD) have speech difficulties compared with their peers and include:

- those who have difficulty producing one or two speech sounds;
- those who have difficulty organizing and producing groups of speech sounds;
- those who have extremely unintelligible speech;
- those who have difficulty producing multisyllabic words such as *ambulance* and *hippopotamus*;
- those who have difficulty perceiving differences between speech sounds; and
- those who have difficulty with prosody (stress, rhythm, intonation) and tones.

These children often present with difficulties that are more complex than we first assume. For example, sometimes children can't use sounds in words that match the adult pronunciation (e.g., children may pronounce the /θ/ in *thing* /θɪŋ/ as [f] in *fing* [fɪŋ]) but can use these same sounds in words that do not match the adult pronunciation (e.g., pronounce the /s/ in *sing* /sɪŋ/ as [θ] in *thing* [θɪŋ]). Therefore, their difficulties do not necessarily arise from their inability to articulate sounds, but to perceive and organize sounds in their minds.

Children's ability to participate within the communities in which they belong is impacted by SSD. The extent of this impact may depend on the severity and nature of the SSD as well as the environmental and personal factors specific to the child. Figure 1-1 shows six drawings created by different preschool children with SSD after being asked to draw themselves talking to someone (McLeod, Harrison, Holliday, McCormack, & McAllister, 2010). These drawings demonstrate that the children are aware of the importance of mouths (row 1), ears (row 2), and proximity to one another (row 3) during communication. In most of the drawings, the children have drawn themselves as happy. Some indicated that they needed people with "listening ears" to be able to be understood (cf. McCormack, McLeod, McAllister, & Harrison, 2010). The final drawing in Figure 1-1 demonstrates one child's isolation and withdrawal from social situations. He indicated that he had to draw himself alone because "they don't let me play," possibly due to his SSD. Difficulties with speech production may impact children's socialization and literacy (McCormack, McLeod, McAllister, & Harrison, 2009). Difficulties with speech production may resolve in childhood, particularly after intervention; however, difficulties may continue into later childhood and adulthood (Law, Boyle, Harris, Harkness, & Nye, 1998), and may impact the ability to gain employment (Ruben, 2000).

This book draws on the principles of evidence-based practice to assist you to incorporate the research data with information about children and their families into your own clinical practice. Children with SSD form a large portion of the caseload of typical pediatric speech-language pathologists (SLPs), so it is likely that you will encounter many children with SSD in your practice. Indeed, in a US study of 6,624 pre-K students enrolled in speech-language pathology services across 25 states, 74.7% of students were receiving services for "articulation/intelligibility" (Mullen & Schooling, 2010). We will discuss the prevalence of children with SSD in greater detail later in this chapter; however, even these data demonstrate that as an SLP it is very likely that you will assess and provide intervention for many children with SSD.

FIGURE 1-1 Preschool children with speech sound disorders drawing themselves talking to someone

Notice the mouths (row 1), ears (row 2), and proximity to one another (row 3).

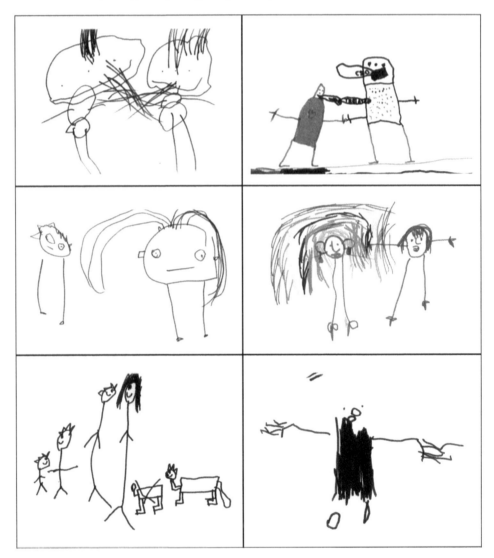

Source: Used by permission from Sharynne McLeod. Copyright 2012 by S. McLeod, L. McAllister, J. McCormack, & L. J. Harrison.

COMMENT: *Reasons for knowing about children with SSD*

Understanding the population of children with SSD provides ways to:

- characterize features of SSD;
- explain SSD to parents and teachers;
- predict children at risk of having an SSD;
- design appropriate assessment and intervention strategies; and
- ultimately work towards the prevention of SSD (Shriberg & Kwiatkowski, 1994).

■ ■

 APPLICATION: *Introducing Luke (4 years, 3 months)*

Throughout almost every chapter of this book we consider case descriptions of five children with SSD: Luke (4;3 years), Susie (7;4 years), Jarrod (7;0 years), Michael (4;2 years), and Lian (14;2 years). The full case studies are provided in Chapter 16. As a way of introducing the field of SSD to you and helping you remember that you are learning about children (and not just a difficulty that children can have), read the overview to Chapter 16 and Luke's case history. Write a reflection about Luke's case history. What did you learn about Luke? Write down your questions. What are some terms that you don't yet understand? Compare your written reflection with a peer. You will learn more about Luke and the other four children as you read through the pages of this book and complete application exercises.

Read more about Luke (4;3 years), Susie (7;4 years), Jarrod (7;0 years), Michael (4;2 years), and Lian (14;2 years) in Chapter 16.

DEFINING SSD

Communication can be divided into the domains of speech, language, voice, fluency, and hearing (see Figure 1-2). Difficulties with communication can manifest as SSD, language disorders, voice disorders, stuttering, or hearing impairment. Some children have difficulties in one of these domains; others have difficulties across these domains. Successful communication is mediated by the communicative environment (e.g., listener characteristics and attitudes, language(s) spoken, level of background noise) that is shown in Figure 1-2 as surrounding the elements of communication.

SSD is a subcategory of communication impairment. According to the International Expert Panel on Multilingual Children's Speech (2012):

> Children with speech sound disorders can have any combination of difficulties with **perception**, **articulation/motor production**, and/or **phonological representation** of speech segments (consonants and vowels), **phonotactics** (syllable and word shapes), and **prosody** (lexical and grammatical tones, rhythm, stress, and intonation) that may impact speech **intelligibility** and **acceptability** . . . speech sound disorders is used as an umbrella term for the full range of speech sound difficulties of both known (e.g., Down syndrome, cleft lip and palate) and presently unknown origin. (International Expert Panel on Multilingual Children's Speech, 2012, p. 1, emphasis added).

FIGURE 1-2   **Components of communication**

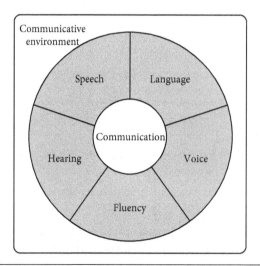

This definition is comprehensive and inclusive, so it will be used within the current book; however, it is important to note that other authors have slightly different definitions. For example, Bowen (2015) stated, "Children with SSD have gaps and simplifications in their speech sound systems that can make what they say difficult to understand . . . the children's speech difficulties can encompass a mixture of phonetic (articulatory), phonemic (phonological or cognitive-linguistic), structural (craniofacial or syndromic), perceptual, or neuromotor bases" (p. 3). Lewis et al. (2006) included a statement about severity in their definition of SSD: "a significant delay in the acquisition of articulate speech sounds" (p. 1294).

The *Diagnostic and Statistical Manual of Mental Disorders* (DSM-5) also includes a definition of SSD that may be used by SLPs, particularly when coding children's areas of difficulty for health and insurance reporting. DSM-5 was developed by the American Psychiatric Association (2013) in consultation with mental health and medical professionals and members of the public. The American Speech-Language-Hearing Association also provided advice to the American Psychiatric Association on categories relating to communication. The fifth edition includes the term "speech sound disorder," replacing the term "phonological disorder" that was used in the fourth edition (DSM-IV, American Psychiatric Association, 2000), in concert with the trends within the speech-language pathology profession. According to the DSM-5 there are a number of components to the classification of SSD:

1. Persistent difficulty with speech sound production that interferes with speech intelligibility or prevents verbal communication of messages.
2. The disturbance causes limitations in effective communication that interfere with social participation, academic achievement or occupational performance, individually or in any combination.
3. Onset of symptoms is in the early developmental period.
4. The difficulties are not attributable to congenital or acquired conditions such as cerebral palsy, cleft palate, deafness or hearing loss, TBI [traumatic brain injury], or other medical or neurological conditions (American Psychiatric Association, 2013, p. 44).

There is one important difference between the DSM-5 definition of SSD and the definition used in this book. Within the current book children with SSD of known origins (e.g., cerebral palsy, cleft palate) are included in the definition of children with SSD; in the DSM-5 they are not.

Another international organization has included SSD in their most recent classification system. The World Health Organization has included SSD in the beta draft of the International Statistical Classification of Diseases and Related Health Problems 11th Revision (ICD-11 Beta Draft, World Health Organization, 2015a, to be finalized in 2017). ICD-11 has included "7A10 developmental speech sound disorder," replacing "F80.0 Specific speech articulation disorder" that was used in ICD-10 (World Health Organization, 2015b). This revision of the ICD-11 was developed in consultation with SLPs from around the world. The revised definition is:

Developmental speech sound disorder is characterized by difficulties in the acquisition, production and perception of speech that result in errors of pronunciation, either in number or types of speech errors made or the overall quality of speech production, that are outside the limits of normal variation expected for age and level of intellectual functioning and result in reduced intelligibility and significantly affect communication. The errors in pronunciation arise during the early developmental period and cannot be explained by social, cultural, and other environmental variations (e.g., regional dialects). The speech errors are not directly attributable to a hearing impairment or to a structural or neurological abnormality. (World Health Organization, 2015a)

As with the DSM-5, the ICD-11 definition aligns closely with the definition used in this book. However, it does not include children with SSD of known origins (e.g., cerebral palsy, cleft palate), whereas these children are included in the definition of children with SSD in the current book.

Over the past century there have been many terms that have been used to describe the difficulties of children with SSD, including **articulation**, **phonological** or **speech**

delay, **disorder**, **impairment**, or **difficulty**. To assist your reading of other texts and journal articles, Table 1-1 provides a summary of some of the terms that have been used within the speech-language pathology literature that are synonymous with SSD. It should be noted that authors use some of these terms to refer to specific subgroups of children with SSD, while other terms are broad-based and refer to all children who have difficulty with speech sounds. Sometimes authors include difficulties with **voice** and **stuttering (fluency)** under the label of speech disorders; however, in this book voice and stuttering are not included. The word *sound* has been inserted in the middle of the term SSD to avoid confusion with information about speech disorders that includes voice and stuttering (fluency). You will learn more about the different types of SSD addressed in this book in Chapter 2.

COMMENT: *A simple representation of SSD*

Children with SSD can have difficulty with:

■ phonological representation and mental organization of speech [MIND];

■ motor production/articulation of speech [MOUTH];

■ perception of speech [EARS]; and

■ intelligibility and acceptability of speech [ENVIRONMENT].

APPLICATION: *Listen to a child with SSD*

At this early stage within the book, it is useful to consider a child with SSD. Jarrod is a 7-year-old child who had a severe SSD and is profiled as a case study in Chapter 16. A scientific forum within the *International Journal of Speech-Language Pathology*[1] was based around Jarrod (McLeod, 2006a). Within the scientific forum, a range of different assessments was undertaken (we will learn more about speech assessments in Chapter 8), then international experts considered his speech and results from assessments and generated intervention plans (we will learn about how to set goals in Chapter 10). The researchers' overarching goals for Jarrod were similar and included increasing his intelligibility and literacy skills. However, the specific goals differed and included ability to produce weak syllables (Bernhardt, Stemberger, & Major, 2006), correct tongue placement for /t, d/ using electropalatography (Müller, Ball, & Rutter, 2006), to produce /spɹ-/consonant clusters (Morrisette, Farris, & Gierut, 2006), to produce final consonants (Hodson, 2006), and to reduce inconsistency in production of words (Dodd, Holm, Crosbie, & McIntosh, 2006). A full comparison of the goals is provided in McLeod (2006a). One group of researchers worked with Jarrod using the Core Vocabulary approach and demonstrated improved speech outcomes (Crosbie, Pine, Holm, & Dodd, 2006). You will learn about a range of different intervention strategies in Chapters 13 and 14. You can see short videos of Jarrod talking and undertaking speech and oromotor assessments within the supplementary material attached to the editorial at the Taylor & Francis Online website.[2] For example, the video showing Jarrod engaging in conversational speech includes Jarrod's description of a movie he had enjoyed. Can you understand his speech? Could the assessor understand his speech? Did he use strategies to make himself better understood? This example of Jarrod shows you the range of information you are going to learn about in this book.

Read more about Jarrod (7;0 years), a boy with inconsistent speech disorder, in Chapter 16 (Case 3).

[1]http://www.tandfonline.com/toc/iasl19/8/3#.Vq6yVLQWpXs
[2]http://www.tandfonline.com/doi/suppl/10.1080/14417040600861086#tabModule

TABLE 1-1 Examples of terminology used within speech-language pathology literature to describe children with SSD

Category	Terms used in this book	Term	Authors who have used this term
Overarching terms	Speech sound disorders (SSD)	Speech sound disorders (SSD)	Lewis et al. (2015); Shriberg (2010a); Sices, Taylor, Freebairn, Hansen, & Lewis (2007); Smit (2004)
		Speech disorders	Williams (2003); Shriberg (2010a)
		Speech impairment	Dodd & Gillon (2001); Leitão & Fletcher (2004); McCormack et al. (2009); Roulstone, Miller, Wren, & Peters (2009)
		Speech disability	Broomfield & Dodd (2004a)
		Speech delay	Broomfield & Dodd (2004b); Shriberg, Tomblin, & McSweeny (1999)
		Speech difficulties	Wren, McLeod, White, Miller, & Roulstone (2013)
		Speech production difficulty	Beitchman et al. (1986a)
		Persistent speech disorder (PSD)[1]	Wren, Roulstone, & Miller (2012); Carrigg, Baker, Parry, & Ballard (2015); Wren (2015)
		Severe and persisting speech difficulties (SPSD)[1]	Newbold, Stackhouse, & Wells (2013)
		Persistent primary speech sound disorders[1]	Cleland, Scobbie, & Wrench (2015)
		Articulation/phonology disorder (APD)	Gibbon (1999); Shriberg, Tomblin, & McSweeny (1999)
		Developmental phonological disorders (DPD)[2]	Rvachew & Brosseau-Lapré (2012); Shriberg (1993)
		Childhood speech disorder	Keating, Turrell, & Ozanne (2001)
		Child speech disorders	Shriberg, Tomblin, & McSweeny (1999)
Phonology	Phonological impairment	Phonological delay	Broomfield & Dodd (2004b)
		Phonological disorder	Smit (2004); Sunderland (2004)
		Phonologically based speech sound disorders	Oliveira, Lousada, & Jesus (2015); Lousada, Jesus, Hall, & Joffe (2014)
		Consistent deviant phonological disorder	Broomfield & Dodd (2004b)
		Functional phonological disorders	Gierut (1998); Gierut & Morrisette (2010)
		Protracted phonological development	Bernhardt, Másdóttir, Stemberger, Leonhardt, & Hansson (2015); Hack, Marinova-Todd & Bernhardt (2012)
	Inconsistent speech disorder	Inconsistent deviant phonological disorder	Broomfield & Dodd (2004b); Peña-Brookes & Hegde (2015)
		Inconsistent phonological disorder	Dodd (2014)
		Inconsistent speech disorder	Dodd, Holm, Crosbie, & McIntosh (2006)

(Continued)

TABLE 1-1	*Continued*		

Category	Terms used in this book	Term	Authors who have used this term
		Inconsistent deviant speech disorder	Bradford & Dodd (1996); Dodd (2005)
Motor speech	Motor speech disorders	Motor speech disorders	Maas et al. (2008); Mitchell (1995); Strand (2003); Weismer (2006)
		Motor speech disorders not otherwise specified	Shriberg, Fourakis et al. (2010a)
	Articulation impairment	Articulation delay	Broen, Strange, Doyle, & Heller (1983)
		Articulation disorder	Broomfield & Dodd (2004b); Sunderland (2004)
		Functional articulation disorder	Shriberg, Tomblin, & McSweeny (1999)
		Residual error	Shriberg, Austin, Lewis, McSweeny, & Wilson (1997b); Smit (2004)
		Residual /ɹ/ misarticulation	Hitchcock & McAllister (2015)
		Speech errors (SE-/s/ and SD-/ɹ/)	Shriberg, Lohmeier, Strand, & Jakielski (2012); Vick et al. (2014)
		Common clinical distortions	Shriberg (1993); Wren, McLeod, White, Miller, & Roulstone (2013)
		Phonetic disorder	Hewlett (1985)
	Childhood apraxia of speech (CAS)	Childhood apraxia of speech (CAS)	Ballard, Robin, McCabe, & McDonald (2010); Morgan & Vogel (2008a); Murray, McCabe, Heard, & Ballard (2015); Shriberg, Potter, & Strand (2011); Teverovsky, Bickel, & Feldman (2009)
		Developmental dyspraxia	Hall (1992); McCabe, Rosenthal, & McLeod (1998)
		Developmental apraxia of speech	Blakeley (2001)
		Developmental verbal dyspraxia	Adegbola, Cox, Bradshaw, Hafler, Gimelbrant, & Chess (2015); Royal College of Speech and Language Therapists (2011); Stackhouse (1992); Stackhouse & Snowling (1992a, b)
	Childhood dysarthria	Dysarthria	Enderby (2014); Morgan & Vogel (2008b); Pennington, Miller, & Robson (2009); Oommen & McCarthy (2014)
		Developmental dysarthria	Hodge (2010)
		Childhood dysarthria	Levy (2014); Murdoch (1998)
		Pediatric dysarthria	Levy, Ramig, & Camarata (2012)

[1]Persistent speech disorder is included here as an overarching term for speech difficulties that is persistent beyond approximately 8 years. It is not intended as an overarching term for a speech disorder at any age.

[2]Developmental phonological disorders (DPD) is included as an overarching term in keeping with use by Rvachew and Brosseau-Lapré (2012) and Shriberg (1993).

> **COMMENT:** *Historical changes in terminology*
>
> Terminology surrounding SSD can be confusing. Not only do different authors use different terms, but the same authors may use a different term to mean the same group of children depending whose theoretical frameworks underpin the particular paper they are writing, the country their paper was published in (e.g., US versus UK), or whether they were writing in the 1900s or 2000s. Over time, the terminology to describe children's speech difficulties has changed (Bowen, 2009). Historically, all children were described as having articulation delay/disorder/impairment; that is, difficulty producing consonants and vowels. Then it was realized that children produced patterns of errors; for example, some children deleted all final consonants from words. So, many children did not have a simple articulation delay/disorder/impairment, but a phonological delay/disorder/impairment that required an appreciation of children's phonological knowledge. The introduction of phonology introduced a dichotomy in the categorization of children's speech difficulties. In the 1980s and 1990s, the term **articulation disorder** was classified as a subset of a speech disorder and **phonological disorder** was considered a subset of a language disorder. More recently, the field has appreciated the complexity of children's speech difficulties. The overarching term **SSD** has been adopted to encompass both articulation and phonology.

The term SSD has been selected to be used within this book because it is an umbrella term for the full range of speech sound difficulties; it is theoretically neutral, and accessible to an international audience. The American Speech-Language-Hearing Association has adopted the use of the term (e.g., ASHA, 2004), and Shriberg (2010a) describes the importance of this consensus:

> The American Speech-Language-Hearing Association's recent adoption of the term *speech sound disorders* (SSD) is a welcome solution to the constraints associated with the *articulation disorders versus phonological disorders* dichotomy of the past three decades. The term SSD provides a theory-neutral cover term for researchers and clinicians who may, as I do, view SSD as a complex neurodevelopmental disorder. The term *childhood* (or in medical contexts, *pediatric*) *speech sound disorders*, which parallels *childhood language disorders*, unifies the study of speech sound disorders of both known (e.g., Down syndrome, cleft palate) and presently unknown origin. (Shriberg, 2010a, p. 2)

In Chapter 2 you will learn more about different types of SSD, and how there are other ways to classify children with SSD, depending on the purpose of classification.

PREVALENCE AND IMPACT

The next section of this chapter addresses the number of children with SSD, and the impact of SSD on children's lives: now when they are children, and into the future as they move through adolescence into adulthood. You will learn about the life histories of children with SSD including some research on the likely outcomes with and without intervention. This information will be useful as you talk with children and families about the possible impact of SSD on their educational, social, and occupational outcomes. This information will also be useful when you advocate to governments, departments, and managers for additional funding, staffing, and resources, since you will learn about the high prevalence of children with SSD in communities, schools, and SLP clinics. While this chapter presents information from published research, it is important to remember that every child is unique. Personal and environmental factors, including their context, background, and support structures, will influence each child's outcome. Use this information to promote optimistic futures for children with SSD.

PREVALENCE OF COMMUNICATION DISORDERS

Communication (including speech and language) is more frequently identified as an area of learning need than almost any other area for children. When advocating for SLP services it is useful to have comparative data about the prevalence of a wide range of learning needs, including communication disorders. The prevalence of nine areas of learning need was identified by teachers within a large school district (37 primary schools and 7 secondary schools) (McLeod & McKinnon, 2007). There were 14,514 students in the first year of data collection (wave 1) and 14,533 students two years later (wave 2). Overall 5,309 (36.57%) students were identified as having some area of learning need in the first year and 4,845 (33.33%) students were identified two years later. Specifically, the areas of learning need (in order) were:

- specific learning difficulty (17.93% in wave 1; 19.10% in wave 2);
- **communication disorder (13.04%; 12.40%);**
- English as a second or other language (9.16%; 5.80%);
- behavioral/emotional difficulty (8.16%; 6.10%);
- early achiever/advanced learner (7.30%; 5.50%);
- physical/medical disability (1.52%; 1.40%);
- intellectual disability (1.38%; 1.20%);
- hearing impairment (0.96%; 0.80%); and
- visual impairment (0.16%; 0.30%) (McLeod & McKinnon, 2007).

In a follow-up study, presence of a communication disorder was the most important predictive factor that students required a high level of support at school (McLeod & McKinnon, 2010).

In another study, parents and educators were asked to indicate any area(s) of concern for 1,205 four- to five-year-old children from a list of eight areas (McLeod, Crowe, White, et al., 2015). They could indicate *yes, a little,* or *no concern,* and their answers for *yes* and *a little* were combined. The most common area of concern was "talking and making speech sounds" (expressive speech and language skills). The parents' and educators' responses for each of the eight areas was as follows:

- **expressive speech and language skills** (parents = 35.1%; educators = 36.8%)
- behavior (parents = 23.4%; educators = 18.5%)
- social-emotional skills (parents = 22.6%; educators = 18.4%)
- school readiness (parents = 19.0%; educators = 15.0%)
- **receptive language** (parents = 15.4%; educators = 21.6%)
- self-help skills (parents = 14.6%; educators = 12.5%)
- fine motor skills (parents = 10.5%; educators = 11.9%)
- gross motor skills (parents = 8.7%; educators = 6.8%)

These two studies demonstrate the high prevalence of speech and language disorders compared with other areas of learning need. Indeed, in a systematic review of literature regarding prevalence of children with primary speech and language impairment, the authors found that speech and language impairment was a "high prevalence condition" (Law, Boyle, Harris, Harkness, & Nye, 2000, p. 179).

■ Prevalence of children with SSD

In their systematic review, Law and colleagues (2000) indicated that the range of prevalence of SSD was 2.30 to 24.60% (i.e., for "speech delay only" [p. 172] without co-occurring language impairment). They also indicated that there was a range of 2.28 to 6.68% (median prevalence of 5.95%) for combined "speech and/or language delay" (p. 170). Law et al. (2000) indicated that prevalence rates for SSD varied more widely than prevalence rates for language delay.

Table 1-2 provides a summary of literature from around the world regarding the prevalence of children with SSD. Wherever possible, data have been separated for SSD only versus speech and language impairment. Here are the results for the reported prevalence for SSD (listed in order from lowest to highest): 1.06% (McKinnon, McLeod, & Reilly, 2007), 1.4% "speech disability" (Paul, Desai & Thorburn, 1992, p. 8), 1.5% (Stewart & Taylor,

TABLE 1-2	A summary of studies examining prevalence of children with SSD (+/– concomitant disorders)

Study	Prevalence	Area(s) considered	Number of participants	Age range	Country	Methodology employed
Beitchman, Nair, Clegg, & Patel (1986a)	6.4% speech only, 4.56% speech and language, 8.04% language only	Speech, language, voice, fluency	1,655	5 years	Canada	Direct assessment
Eadie, Morgan, Ukoumunne, Ttofari Eecen, Wake, & Reilly (2015)	3.4% speech sound disorder	Speech	1,494	4 years	Australia	Direct assessment
Harasty & Reed (1994)	15.3% articulation/phonology impairment, 20.6% language impairment, 5.3% voice, 1.8% stuttering	Speech, language, voice, stuttering	437	Grades K–6	Australia	Direct assessment
Jessup, Ward, Cahill, & Keating (2008)	8.7% isolated speech impairment, 14.3% speech and language impairment, 18.2% isolated language impairment	Speech and language	308	5;4–6;10	Australia	Direct assessment
Keating, Turrell, & Ozanne (2001)	1.7% overall, 7.4% males aged 5 years	Talking, producing sounds, and stuttering	12,388	0 to 14 years	Australia	Parent report during face-to-face interview
Kirkpatrick & Ward (1984)	4.6% articulation errors	Speech	2,251	Grades K–6	Australia	Direct assessment
McKinnon, McLeod, & Reilly (2007)	1.06% speech-sound disorders, 0.33% stuttering, 0.12% voice	Speech-sound disorders, stuttering, voice	10,425	5 to 12 years	Australia	Teacher report followed by direct assessment
McLeod & Harrison (2009)	12.0% had concerns about their child being understood by others, 6.0% had concerns about their child being understood by their family	Speech, language, voice, stuttering	4,983	4 to 5 years	Australia	Parent report
Paul, Desai, & Thorburn (1992)	1.4% speech disability	Speech	5,468	2 to 9 years	Jamaica	Assessed by a physician and a psychologist
Peckham (1973)	10–13% had "some degree of speech impairment," 2.5% "had been seen by a speech therapist"	Speech	15,496	7 years	UK	Teacher, doctor, and parent report + repetition of 6 sentences

(Continued)

TABLE 1-2	*Continued*					
Study	Prevalence	Area(s) considered	Number of participants	Age range	Country	Methodology employed
Roulstone, Miller, Wren, & Peters (2009)	18% "speech impaired"[1]	Speech	741	8 years	UK	Direct assessment
Shriberg, Tomblin, & McSweeny (1999)	3.8% "speech delay"	Speech	1,328	6 years	US	Direct assessment
Stewart & Taylor (1986)	1.5% speech, 2.6% language, and 1.4% hearing	Speech	719	3 to 5 years	US ("urban preschool black population")	Screening + direct assessment
Tuomi & Ivanoff (1977)	20.5% articulation (24.6% in kindergarten, 16.5% in grade 1), 6.7% language	Articulation and language	900	5 to 6 years	Canada	
Warr-Leeper, McShea, & Leeper (1979)	17% had "inadequate speech, voice or fluency" (of the 17%, 37% had "inadequate articulation," 6% had "inadequate articulation and voice," 48% had "inadequate voice," and 0.9% had "inadequate fluency")	Articulation, voice, fluency	107 children	Grades 6–8	US	Direct assessment (screening)
Wren, Roulstone, & Miller (2012)	7.9% had common clinical distortions, 3.6% had persistent speech disorder, and 1.9% had non-persistent speech disorder (total = 13.4%)	Speech	7,390	8 years	UK	Direct assessment (single word, connected speech, nonword repetition)
Wren, McLeod, White, Miller, & Roulstone, (2013)	7.9% had common clinical distortions and 5.5% had "speech difficulties" (e.g., substitutions, distortions, cluster reduction) (total = 13.4%)	Speech	7,390	8 years	UK	Direct assessment (single word, connected speech, nonword repetition)

[1]Roulstone et al. (2009) used the definition of Shriberg, Austin, Lewis, McSweeny, and Wilson (1997) that included children with speech delay and questionable residual errors (QRE).

1986), 3.4% (Eadie, Morgan, Ukoumunne, Ttofari Eecen, Wake, & Reilly, 2015), 3.6% "persistent speech disorder" (Wren, Roulstone, & Miller, 2012, p. 1), 3.8% "speech delay" (Shriberg, Tomblin, & McSweeny, 1999, p. 1461), 4.6% "articulation errors" (Kirkpatrick & Ward, 1984, p. 55), 5.5% "speech difficulties" (Wren, McLeod, White, Miller, & Roulstone, 2013, p. 53), 6.4% (Beitchman, Nair, Clegg, & Patel, 1986a), 8.7% "isolated speech impairment" (Jessup et al., 2008, p. 364), 10–13% (Peckham, 1973), 12.0% parental concerns about their child "being understood by others" (McLeod & Harrison, 2009, p. 1225), 13.4% "atypical speech" (Wren et al., 2013, p. 53), 15.3% (Harasty & Reed, 1994), 18% "speech impaired" (Roulstone et al., 2009, p. 381), 20.5% (Tuomi & Ivanoff, 1977). As can be seen in Table 1-2, data regarding the prevalence of SSD vary widely (cf. Law et al., 2000). Some of the reasons for this variability include:

- **Age range:** some studies included children in a narrow age range (e.g., Beitchman et al., 1986a, studied 1,655 five-year-olds; Wren et al., 2013, studied 7,390 eight-year-olds), whereas others included a wide age range (e.g., Keating, Turrell, & Ozanne, 2001, studied 12,388 children aged 0–14 years). Prevalence rates typically were higher for younger children.
- **Data collection methods:** some studies used direct assessment with standardized speech sampling tools. For example, Beitchman et al. (1986a) used the Photo Articulation Test (Pendergast et al., 1969), Eadie et al. (2015) used the Goldman-Fristoe Test of Articulation (Goldman & Fristoe, 2000), and Shriberg et al. (1999) used connected speech and the Word Articulation subtest of the Test of Language Development–2: Primary (Newcomer & Hammill, 1988). Others used parent and teacher report (McLeod & Harrison, 2009).
- **Definition of SSD:** definition of SSD influences whether children's speech is reported in "absolute rather than developmental terms" (Law et al., 2000, p. 172). That is, whether errors are identified after comparison with developmental norms. It is possible that prevalence rates may be lower after comparison with developmental norms.
- **Sampling:** some studies relied on population sampling techniques across a country or state (county, province) (McLeod & Harrison, 2009; Wren et al., 2013), others used a probability sample (e.g., Beitchman et al., 1986a; Tuomi & Ivanoff, 1977), others sampled an entire school district (e.g., McKinnon, McLeod, & Reilly, 2007), and others relied on children within identified schools (e.g., Harasty & Reed, 1994). Prevalence rates are more representative of a population if they include the entire population.
- **Cut-point on a standardized test:** studies that have used standardized speech sampling tools have varied in the cut-point used to determine the presence of SSD. For instance, Eadie et al. (2015) used a cut-point of ≤ 10th percentile. Beitchman et al. (1986a) used the 16th percentile (equivalent to 1 standard deviation below the mean).

When considering the prevalence of children with SSD, it is useful to make comparisons with other areas of reported difficulty. Overall, the data within Table 1-2 can be used to demonstrate that many children have difficulty producing speech sounds, and require speech-language pathology services.

■ Proportion of children with SSD on SLPs' caseloads

Data regarding the number of children on SLPs' caseloads can be used to advocate for services for children with SSD, since throughout the world there is evidence that children with SSD constitute a high proportion of SLPs' caseloads. Here are some data from the United States that demonstrate the large number of children with primary speech or language disorders, and how many of those have SSD:

- 24.1% (1,460,583) of all children with disabilities aged 3–21 years received services in the US public schools for primary speech or language disorders (U.S. Department of Education, 2005).
- 74.7% of pre-K students enrolled in speech-language pathology services received services for "articulation/intelligibility" in a study of 6,624 pre-K students across 25 states (Mullen & Schooling, 2010, p. 51).
- The majority of 14,852 school students across 37 US states who were receiving speech-language pathology services were receiving services for "speech sound production" (Mullen & Schooling, 2010, p. 48):
  - 55.8% of students in grades K–3,
  - 51.7% of students in grades 4–6, and
  - 22.4% of students in grades 7–12 (Mullen & Schooling, 2010).

> **COMMENT:** *Are all eligible children receiving services?*
>
> Tomblin (2010) encouraged SLPs to look beyond the clinic when considering the number of children who have speech and language difficulties. He stated, "It is quite possible that not all children with SLI [specific language impairment] are clinically identified and served within our service delivery systems. In such circumstances, there is the potential for systematic factors to influence which children do or do not find their way to clinical service" (p. 108). In a population study of 4,983 Australian preschool children, parents and teachers reported that speech-language pathology services had been accessed by 14.5% of children and that an additional 2.2% indicated that they needed but could not access SLP services (McLeod & Harrison, 2009). A follow-up community (non-clinical) study was undertaken to assess 4- to 5-year-old children whose parents indicated that their children had difficulty talking and making speech sounds (McLeod, Harrison, McAllister, & McCormack, 2013). Of the children who were diagnosed during the research as having SSD, parents reported that only 38.5% had contact with an SLP. That is, 61.5% of preschool children identified with SSD during the research had not had a previous speech-language pathology assessment or intervention. McLeod et al. (2013) indicated that "children with SSD whose parents had made contact with an SLP typically had a more severe SSD at the impairment level and greater concerns about the impact of their speech skills on their children's socialization and participation" (p. 517). It is possible that there are children within your own communities that may benefit from, but have not accessed, speech-language pathology services.

In the United Kingdom, the number of referrals to SLP services in the Middlesbrough Primary Care Trust was examined by Broomfield and Dodd (2004a). Of the 1,100 children referred for SLP services,

- 29.1% had "speech difficulties" (p. 303), the most common area of difficulty;
- 20.4% had receptive language difficulties;
- 16.9% had expressive language difficulties;
- 5.3% had dysfluency; and
- 2.0% had voice or nasality disruption.

The majority of referrals were for children aged 2–6 years, and more males than females were referred. From the data above, it is clear that children with SSD form a large portion of the caseloads of SLPs.

Another source of evidence for the high proportion of children with SSD on pediatric caseloads comes from studies where SLPs have been asked to estimate the proportion of children with SSD on their caseloads. In the United States, Brumbaugh and Smit (2013) surveyed 489 pediatric SLPs, and 52% indicated that children with SSD constituted half or more of their caseloads. In the United Kingdom, "Nearly half the respondents said that children with phonological problems were more than 40% of their caseload" (Joffe & Pring, 2008, p. 159). In an Australian study of 231 SLPs, children with SSD constituted between 10 and 39% (35.5%) or between 40 and 70% (35.5%) of their caseloads (McLeod & Baker, 2014). In another Australian survey, 93.1% of 257 SLPs reported that children with SSD were on their caseloads (Westerveld & Claessen, 2014). Similarly in the Netherlands, 90% of 85 SLPs had children with SSD on their caseloads (Priester, Post, & Goorhuis-Brouwer, 2009). In Portugal 88 SLPs reported that they had more children with articulation or phonological disorders on their caseloads than children with childhood apraxia of speech (CAS) (Oliveira, Lousada, & Jesus, 2015).

NATURAL HISTORY AND LONG-TERM MANIFESTATION OF SSD

Do all children with SSD need intervention? How do we differentiate late bloomers from children with persistent SSD? These questions can be answered (in part) by considering studies of natural history.

■ Natural history of SSD

Natural history research examines the progression of a condition (disorder, disease, etc.), typically without intervention. Since many children with SSD receive intervention, there are few studies that describe the natural history of SSD. In their systematic review, Law, Boyle, Harris, Harkness, and Nye (2000) identified three studies that examined the natural history of children with SSD (i.e., without language impairment) and met their review criteria (Bralley & Stoudt, 1977; Felsenfeld, Broen, & McGue, 1992; Renfrew & Geary, 1973). They summarized the outcomes for these three studies and indicated that the median persistence was 50% (range = 22–54%)—that is, a median of 50% of children with SSD continue to have difficulties if they do not receive intervention. The finding that there are two possible paths is consistent with the work of Gruber (1999), who studied 24 children with speech delay. He proposed that children in Path A were more likely to normalize over time and "correct productions increased" as "errors of deletion, substitution, and omission declined" (p. 448). Children in Path B were less likely to normalize over time since "common clinical distortions increased as deletions and substitutions decreased" (p. 448).

Since the review of Law et al. (2000), there have been two studies of natural history conducted by Roulstone and colleagues in the United Kingdom. Roulstone, Peters, Glogowska, and Enderby (2003) considered the natural history of 69 preschool-aged children (including 12 with SSD only, and no concomitant language difficulties) over a 12-month period. The children were not provided with intervention by an SLP over the 12-month period. After 12 months, 58.3% of the children with SSD-only improved so that they would not be classified on assessment as requiring intervention. Fewer children improved if they had general/receptive language difficulties (19.4%) or expressive language difficulties (28.6%). The authors indicated that some of the children who had improved on assessment were still considered to require intervention by their parents and by the therapist, who considered the children's communicative functioning using the Therapy Outcome Measure disability scale (Enderby & John, 1997). These findings lead the authors to conclude that it may be appropriate for some children to be monitored, rather than receive immediate intervention, but that parents' wishes should be taken into consideration (Roulstone et al., 2003).

In another study Roulstone, Miller, Wren, and Peters (2009) considered the natural history of 741 children who were assessed at ages 2, 5, and 8 years to consider whether they had "speech impairment . . . which impact(s) on the intelligibility of a child's spoken output irrespective of the origin" (p. 384). When 8 years old, there were 609 controls (those who had no speech errors), and 132 (18%) cases who made errors on velars, fricatives, liquids, postvocalic consonants, or consonant clusters during a picture description task. The strongest predictor of having ongoing speech errors when 8 years old was the proportion of speech errors when 5 years old, with the odds ratio increasing between 21 and 44% for every 10% rise in the proportion of errors. There were more males than females in the group of 8-year-old children with speech impairment, with 51% of controls and 60% of cases being males. Some (12%) of the control children and 28% of the case children had a previous speech-language pathology assessment; however, the number of children who had intervention was unknown (Roulstone et al., 2009).

To summarize, there are few natural history studies of children with SSD. Of those that have been published, there is evidence that some children will improve without intervention; however, at least half of young children with SSD will not improve and will require intervention. Children who have concomitant language impairment, or produce distortions, may be less likely to demonstrate speech improvements without intervention. However, SLPs also should consider children and parents' concerns when recommending commencing and ending intervention.

■ Manifestation of SSD in late childhood

School-aged children with SSD can have difficulties with speech production, reading, writing, and spelling (Anthony et al., 2011; Bird, Bishop, & Freeman, 1995; Bishop & Adams, 1990; Foy & Mann, 2012; Larrivee & Catts, 1999; Nathan, Stackhouse, Goulandris, & Snowling, 2004a; Raitano, Pennington, Tunick, Boada, & Shriberg, 2004; Teverovsky et al., 2009) (see Chapter 2). By 8 to 9 years of age, children's speech skills should be similar to adults' speech (see Chapter 6); although there are a few areas where typically developing children may continue to have difficulty (e.g., appropriate use of lexical stress). Wren and colleagues documented the speech characteristics of 7,390 eight-year-old children from the United Kingdom (Wren, Roulstone, & Miller, 2012). They identified four groups of children: 86.7% had typical speech, 7.9% made errors on /s/ and /ɹ/ and were described as producing common clinical distortions (CCD) (Shriberg, 1993), 3.6% had persistent speech disorder (PSD), and 1.9% had non-persistent speech disorder (non-PSD) since they did not make enough errors to be categorized with PSD and did not make significantly more errors than children in the control group (Wren et al., 2012). In a follow-up study, Wren, McLeod, White, Miller, and Roulstone (2013) described the speech of 402 children with "speech difficulties" (those in the PSD and non-PSD groups in the previous study). During the single-word task, the 8-year-old children with speech difficulties produced substitutions and distortions. During the connected speech task, these children had problems producing some vowels correctly, omitted single consonants and consonant clusters, and had difficulty producing the correct stress patterns. During nonword repetition tasks they were more likely to produce distorted consonants as well as most of the patterns outlined for the connected speech task. Similar findings were reported for the 25 eight-year-old participants in the lifespan database of Shriberg, Austin, et al. (1997b). Just over half (*n* = 14) had normal or normalized speech acquisition (NSA); seven only produced common clinical distortions (CCD), three had normalized speech acquisition/speech delay (NSA/SD) (i.e., omission or substitution errors on one or two consonants), and one had speech delay. In another study, Shriberg, Gruber, and Kwiatkowski (1994) studied 10 children with SSD over 7 years. They indicated that while there were individual differences across children, word-position, and sampling mode (single word versus connected speech), there were also some patterns of errors. Early-8 consonants (e.g., /m, b, n, w/) were more often omitted, the middle-8 consonants (e.g., /k, g, f, v/) were more often omitted and substituted, and the late-8 consonants (e.g., /s, z, l, ɹ/) were more often distorted. Overall, these studies demonstrate that some children who are 8 years or older do not have adult-like speech, and may benefit from continued intervention and support.

■ Manifestation of SSD in adolescence and adulthood

The manifestation of SSD changes through childhood and becomes more subtle in adolescents and adults. The majority of residual articulation errors displayed by adolescents and adults with histories of SSD include "dentalized fricatives, lateralized fricatives, derhotacized /ɹ/, or uncommon distortions" (Shriberg, 1993, p. 115) and phonological simplification processes such as cluster reduction, depalatalization, and final consonant deletion (Felsenfeld, Broen, & McGue, 1992) (these terms will be explained in Chapter 5). Even though SSD may not be immediately evident in adulthood, individuals with histories of SSD may display subtle difficulties on tasks that stress the phonological system as in polysyllabic words (e.g., *statistics*, *ambulance*), tongue twisters, and difficult articulatory

COMMENT: *International Phonetic Alphabet conventions used in this book*

Within this book, we use slashes / / to surround the transcription of the target (adult-like) production and square brackets [ ] to surround the transcription of the child's actual speech production. We do not use diacritics unless they are necessary to highlight differences in pronunciation. So, if a child produces *fee* as *pea*, we would write this as /fi/ → [pi]. Chapter 4 provides a lot more detail about transcription.

The English letter "r" is an alveolar approximant and is transcribed with the symbol /ɹ/ using the International Phonetic Alphabet (IPA). Some English-language SLP texts use /r/ instead of this /ɹ/ symbol; however, the IPA /r/ refers to the alveolar trill found in languages such as Spanish and Icelandic. To differentiate these two consonants, this book will use /ɹ/ for the alveolar approximant (as used in English) and /r/ as the alveolar trill (as used in Spanish).

sequences (Lewis & Freebairn, 1992; Lewis et al., 2007). Additionally, adolescents and adults with histories of SSD can have difficulties with literacy, including spelling and reading (Leitão & Fletcher, 2004; Lewis & Freebairn, 1992; Lewis, Freebairn, & Taylor, 2000a; Lewis et al., 2015; Stackhouse & Snowling, 1992a).

IMPACT AND OUTCOMES OF CHILDHOOD SSD

Children with SSD are creative and resilient. Children with SSD can make friends, attend school, become literate, gain employment, and live happy lives. Although there are few published examples of success stories of people who had SSD as a child, we encourage you to think of adults who do not articulate speech sounds correctly. It is likely that they had SSD as children and may have received speech-language pathology. Some examples of successful public figures are described in "Successful Adults Who May Have Had SSD as Children."

There have been a number of studies that have described the impact of SSD on children's lives, as children and into adulthood. These studies are valuable to SLPs for understanding the breadth and longevity of impact of SSD, advocating for children with SSD, talking with families about potential long-term outcomes, and considering holistic intervention practices. First, we will consider some longitudinal studies that have followed the same cohort of children into adolescence and adulthood.

◼ Longitudinal studies of the impact and outcomes of SSD on children's lives

Three key longitudinal studies have considered long-term impact and outcomes for children with SSD compared with children who did not have SSD.

Templin Longitudinal Study

The first longitudinal study that we will consider is by Susan Felsenfeld and colleagues, who reported a 28-year follow-up of children with and without SSD in the United States (Felsenfeld, Broen, & McGue, 1992, 1994; Felsenfeld, McGue, & Broen, 1995). They recontacted children involved in Mildred Templin's (Templin, 1966) study of childhood speech and language acquisition when they were 32 to 34 years old. They tested "24 adults with a documented history of moderately severe phonological disorder that persisted at

COMMENT: Successful adults who may have had SSD as children

David Sedaris, Barbara Walters, Jonathan Ross, and Francesca Martinez are all successful adults who (may) have had SSD as children. David Sedaris, the US comedian and author, wrote a chapter in his book titled *Me Talk Pretty One Day* describing his speech-language pathology sessions for a lisp and his ingenious methods to eliminate words beginning with /s/ from his vocabulary as a school student (Sedaris, 2000).[1] Barbara Walters, a US television presenter, has had a highly successful career and has written a book titled *How to Talk with Practically Anybody About Practically Anything* (Walters, 1970). An SLP would describe her speech as using [w] for /ɹ/. Jonathan Ross, a successful English radio and television presenter, also has difficulty pronouncing /ɹ/ (including within his own name). Francesca Martinez is a comedian who has cerebral palsy and dysarthria and describes herself as "being wobbly." There was an interesting interview between Jonathan Ross and Francesca Martinez in which they discussed their "speech impediments."[2]

[1]https://www.nytimes.com/books/first/s/sedaris-me.html
[2]https://www.youtube.com/watch?v=EmDkL6iwhnk

least through the end of first grade and 28 adults from the same birth cohort and schools who were known to have had at least average articulation skills over the same period" (Felsenfeld, Broen, & McGue, 1992, p. 1114). On testing, the adults with histories of SSD were intelligible and had fewer speech errors than they had as children; however, they scored more poorly on tests of articulation and receptive and expressive language than the adults who had typical speech as children. The adults with histories of SSD were more likely to produce errors on /ɪ, s, z/, use phonological processes (e.g., cluster reduction, depalatization, and final consonant deletion), and demonstrate differences in prosody (e.g., rate, stress, voice quality) (Felsenfeld et al., 1992). The authors reported that the two groups did not differ on tests of emotional adjustment in adulthood, with no significant differences in introversion or anxiety. The adults with histories of SSD completed fewer years of education, received lower grades, and required more remedial education than those with no history of SSD (Felsenfeld, Broen, & McGue, 1994). Adults in both groups were likely to be employed; however, the adults with histories of SSD were more likely to have semiskilled or unskilled jobs than the controls or their siblings of the same gender. All of the participants were satisfied with their educational and occupational outcomes (Felsenfeld et al., 1994). The next phase of research involved testing the sons and daughters of the adults in the study (Felsenfeld, McGue, & Broen, 1995). Of the 24 adults with a history of SSD, 42 of their children participated (aged 3;0–13;2 years), and of the 28 adults with no history of SSD, 41 children participated (aged 3;0–14;11 years). For the children whose parents had a history of SSD: 60% had typical speech development, 17% had normalized speech (e.g., after intervention), 14% had speech delay, and 9% had residual errors. For the children whose parents did not have a history of SSD: 93% had typical speech development, 5% had questionable speech delay, and 2% had speech delay. The children of those with a history of SSD produced significantly more errors on tests of articulation and expressive language than those with typically developing parents, and were significantly more likely to have had intervention for SSD (33% versus 0%). These studies show the long-term impact of SSD on speech, education, occupation, and the next generation of children.

Ottawa Language Study

The Ottawa Language Study is another important longitudinal study of the outcomes of having childhood SSD (with or without associated language impairment). The study was undertaken by Beitchman and colleagues in Canada. We already mentioned the first phase of this study in our discussion of the prevalence of children with SSD (Beitchman et al., 1986a) (see Table 1-2). The longitudinal stage of the Ottawa Language Study involved over 200 participants who were identified when they were 5 years old, then followed at 12 years (Beitchman, Hood, & Inglis, 1990; Beitchman et al., 1986b; Beitchman et al., 1994; Beitchman et al., 1996a, 1996b), 19 years (Beitchman et al., 2001; Johnson et al., 1999), and 25 years of age (Johnson, Beitchman, & Brownlie, 2010). The authors indicated that similar findings occurred across the study, so we will discuss the findings at the 20-year follow-up when they were 25 years old. At age 25 there were 244 participants. When these participants were 5 years old, 132 had typical speech and language development (control), 37 had speech impairment only (SSD), and 75 had language impairment (although it was possible that some of these participants also had SSD). When they were 25 years old, there was no significant difference between the three groups regarding whether they were married or in a permanent relationship, or the number of children they had. Overall educational attainment was significantly higher for participants in the control and speech-only groups than the language group. High school had been completed by 92% of participants in the control group, 92% of participants in the speech-only group, and 76% of those in the language group. An undergraduate degree had been completed by 32% of the control group, 27% of the speech-only group, and only 3% of the language group. There was no significant difference between the number of people in full- or part-time jobs (82% of the control group, 76% of the speech-only group, and 76% of the language group), although there was a significant difference in the socioeconomic status of the occupations, with the language group scoring significantly lower than the other two groups. There was no significant difference between the three groups for quality of life ratings. The authors concluded that children with language disorders were more likely to have reduced educational and occupational outcomes than those in the control and speech-only groups. They indicated that the outcomes of those in the speech-only group were different from previous studies because (1) this group did not include children with concomitant language, fluency, or voice disorders, (2) testing did not include spontaneous speech productions, and (3) the study was based on a community rather than clinical sample, so the children were likely to have had less severe SSD (Johnson, Beitchman, & Brownlie, 2010).

Cleveland Family Speech and Language Study

The Cleveland Family Speech and Language Study is the largest longitudinal study to date that has specifically considered children with SSD. It was undertaken by Lewis and colleagues in the United States (Lewis, Freebairn, & Taylor, 2000a, b, c; Lewis et al., 2015). Lewis and colleagues recruited 316 children: 170 four- to six-year-old children with SSD who were receiving speech-language pathology services and 146 of their siblings who did not have SSD or language impairment (Lewis, Freebairn, & Taylor, 2000a, b). The children were followed up at school age (Lewis, Freebairn, & Taylor, 2000c) and at adolescence (when 11 to 18 years old) (Lewis et al., 2015). Additionally, their parents' speech and language skills were assessed (Lewis et al., 2007). Lewis et al. (2015) provided a nuanced approach to understanding these 316 adolescents' outcomes, dividing them into four groups:

- Adolescents with no SSD ($n = 137$) were the siblings of children with SSD, who continued to have no SSD into adolescence. This group performed better than all other groups on tests of vocabulary, reading, and spelling.
- Adolescents with resolved SSD ($n = 105$) were children (and some siblings) who had SSD in early childhood that had resolved by adolescence. Lewis et al. suggested that their lower reading and spelling scores in adolescence (compared with adolescents with no SSD) may have been related to poorer phonological memory possibly due to concomitant language impairment identified in a number of the participants in early childhood.
- Adolescents with low scores on the multisyllabic word repetition task ($n = 33$) had SSD in early childhood. By adolescence their conversational speech contained no errors, but they had difficulty producing polysyllabic words.
- Adolescents with persistent SSD ($n = 41$) had difficulty with polysyllabic words and produced errors in conversational speech. Speech errors included distortion of /s, z, ɹ, l/, substitution errors, phonological processes (e.g., cluster reduction), and abnormal voice, prosody, and fluency. This group had poorer outcomes than the other groups for nonword repetition, vocabulary, reading, and spelling.

Across the groups, gender (being male), lower socioeconomic status, and lower nonverbal cognition mediated the long-term consequences of SSD in early childhood.

■ Impact of SSD on children's lives

The previous section described longitudinal evidence of the impact SSD in childhood can have on the person as an adolescent or adult. It is also important to consider what it is like to be a child with SSD. Listening to children's perspectives about their own lives requires a range of creative strategies, since we are listening to children who have difficulties communicating. A book titled *Listening to Children and Young People With Speech, Language and Communication Needs* (Roulstone & McLeod, 2011) outlined issues to consider including: using child-friendly techniques (e.g., drawing, collage, film, play, and group activities), respecting silence, being aware of the disproportionate power between adults and children, and gaining children's assent (as well as parental consent) to participate.

When listening to children, it is important to be aware that "adults and children do not always share the same world view" (Corsaro, 1976, p. 195). For example, preschool children with SSD may not be aware that their speech is different from others, and may attribute communication breakdown to their communicative partners' difficulties. In a study of 13 preschool children with SSD, McCormack et al. (2010) found that most of the children felt "happy" when asked the question "How do you feel about the way you talk?" A number of these preschool children indicated that their communicative partners had difficulty listening (and did not attribute communication breakdowns to their own speech).

In a related study, preschool children drew large ears on their communicative partners to indicate that listening was important in order to be understood (see Figure 1-1, row 2). The communicative partners in McCormack et al. (2010) also accepted responsibility for the communication breakdown; for example, one mother said, ". . . I'll say 'Can you say it slowly? Mom doesn't understand'" (p. 385).

Studies of school-aged children with SSD have indicated they enjoy being in familiar environments such as at home with family and they also enjoy undertaking nonverbal activities (Markham, Van Laar, Gibbard, & Dean, 2009; McLeod, Daniel, & Barr, 2006, 2013). However, when in public contexts, they have expressed embarrassment, frustration, and sadness about their SSD (Markham et al., 2009; McLeod, Daniel, & Barr, 2013; Owen, Hayett, & Roulstone, 2004). For example, Figure 1-3 shows two contrastive pictures drawn by Luke, an 8-year-old boy with severe SSD. He drew one picture with a large happy mouth and tongue and said, "I like doing anything like art"; then, when asked how he felt about his talking, he drew himself with a large sad mouth (McLeod et al., 2006). Luke's mother indicated, "I know his behavior problems are due to his speech frustration, they always have been" (McLeod, Daniel, & Barr, 2013, p. 76). This quote exemplifies findings from other studies that children with SSD and significant others in their lives (e.g., parents, teachers) also express frustration and embarrassment at the breakdown of communication (Markham et al., 2009; McCormack et al., 2010; McLeod, Daniel, & Barr, 2006, 2013; Owen et al., 2004).

A systematic review to consider factors associated with childhood SSD using the International Classification of Functioning, Disability and Health – Children and Youth Version (ICF-CY) (WHO, 2007) was undertaken by McCormack et al. (2009). Associated limitations and restrictions on participation that were identified in the review can be grouped under three headings: educational, social, and occupational impact. Each will be considered next.

■ Educational impact of SSD

Having SSD can be associated with educational difficulties. Learning to read, spell, and write can pose difficulties for children with SSD. Literacy difficulties affect between 30 and 77% of children with SSD (Anthony et al., 2011), and difficulties with learning to read have been a focus of research on the impact of SSD (Bird et al., 1995; Bishop & Adams, 1990; Foy & Mann, 2012; Larrivee & Catts, 1999; Nathan et al., 2004a; Raitano et al., 2004). Learning

FIGURE 1-3   **Illustrations by Luke, aged 8 years with speech sound disorder**

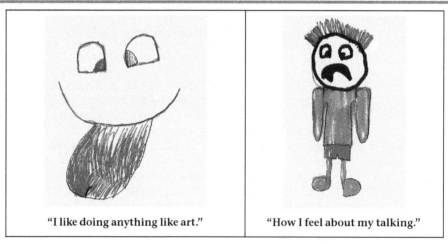

| "I like doing anything like art." | "How I feel about my talking." |

Source: From Using Children's Drawings to Listen to How Children Feel About Their Speech, S. McLeod, G. Daniel, & J. Barr, 2006, *Proceedings of the 2005 Speech Pathology Australia National Conference*, p. 41. Copyright © 2006 by Speech Pathology Australia.

> **COMMENT:** *Children are the people of today*
>
> "Children are not the people of tomorrow, but are people of today. They have a right to be taken seriously, and to be treated with tenderness and respect. They should be allowed to grow into whoever they were meant to be—the unknown person inside each of them is our hope for the future" (Korczak, 1929/2009, p. 7). The writings of Janusz Korczak were influential in the development of the United Nations Convention on the Rights of the Child (UNCRC) (UNICEF, 1989). Here are two of the articles from the UNCRC that have influenced the way we (as authors of this book) undertake research with children and may influence the way you interact with children as an SLP:
>
> > *Article 12: Parties shall assure to the child who is capable of forming his or her own views the right to express those views freely in all matters affecting the child, the views of the child being given due weight in accordance with the age and maturity of the child.*
> >
> > *Article 13: The child shall have the right to freedom of expression; this right shall include freedom to seek, receive and impart information and ideas of all kinds, regardless of frontiers, either orally, in writing or in print, in the form of art, or through any other media of the child's choice. (UNICEF, 1989, p. 4)*

to write also poses a problem for children with childhood apraxia of speech (CAS) according to 49% of parents of 192 children (Teverovsky et al., 2009). In contrast, Bishop and Clarkson (2003) indicated that 7- to 13-year-old children with SSD did not have difficulty with writing, whereas children with speech and language difficulties were "functionally illiterate" (p. 231). Children with a history of speech and language impairment in preschool have been found to have difficulty with mathematical thinking when 6 to 7 years old (Harrison, McLeod, Berthelsen, & Walker, 2009; Nathan, Stackhouse, Goulandris, & Snowling, 2004b) and 8 to 9 years old (McCormack, Harrison, McLeod & McAllister, 2011). There are also studies demonstrating that children with SSD are more likely than their typically developing peers to require remedial education (Felsenfeld, Broen, & McGue, 1994), are more likely to drop out of school (Robertson, Harding, & Morrison, 1998), are more likely to complete vocational education rather than complete school (Snowling, Adams, Bishop, & Stothard, 2001), and are less likely to attend university (Felsenfeld, Broen, & McGue, 1994).

Social impact of SSD

Children with SSD may experience associated difficulties with social interactions (Markham & Dean, 2006; Markham et al., 2009; McCormack et al., 2010; McLeod, Daniel, & Barr, 2013). For example, in a study of 29 school-aged children with speech and/or language impairment, participants indicated that friendships were central to their quality of life (Markham et al., 2009). The authors wrote, "Group discussions revealed a universal desire to make and maintain friendships but also a common difficulty in doing so" (Markham et al., 2009, p. 760). In another study, 8- to 9-year-old children were asked about their social interactions and enjoyment of school in a large study of 1,041 children who were identified as having difficulties talking and making speech sounds when 4 to 5 years old (McCormack, Harrison, McLeod, & McAllister, 2011). These children reported poorer peer relationships, significantly more instances of bullying, lower self-esteem, and less enjoyment of school than 3,288 eight- to nine-year-old typically developing children from the same sample (McCormack et al., 2011). Sweeting and West (2001) asked 2,237 eleven-v-old Scottish children whether they had been bullied or teased. The authors found that "39 per cent and 30 per cent of those with speech and reading difficulties respectively were teased/bullied weekly or more, compared with around 15 per cent overall" (p. 234). To add to this, the factors that correlated with bullying and teasing were additive for children who had a disability (including speech, hearing or vision) were overweight, were perceived to be less attractive or were less capable academically. Children were less likely to be bullied or teased about their race, social class, or sex (Sweeting & West, 2001). A study comparing the conversational interactions of 3- to 5-year-old children demonstrated that children with typical speech and language were most likely to be spoken to in peer interactions, while children with SSD and those who spoke English as a second language were more likely to be avoided in peer conversations, were more likely to initiate conversations with adults (rather than peers), and were more likely to produce shorter utterances (Rice, Sell, & Hadley, 1991).

The attitudes of people towards those with SSD also have a social impact on children and their families. Cambra stated, "during the building of self-concept, one's self-perception is influenced by the attitudes and levels of acceptance of significant individuals in one's immediate environment and in society as a whole" (Cambra, 1996, p. 24), yet many health professionals do not typically consider the attitudes of others towards the children and families they work with (Rosenbaum, 2007). Numerous studies have been undertaken over many years to consider the attitudes of children, adolescents, and adults regarding SSD. Regardless of the age group, most studies provide evidence of more negative attitudes towards people with SSD (even with mild articulation errors) than those with typically developing speech. For example, Hall (1991) examined the attitudes of 348 fourth- and sixth-grade children after watching videos of six children: a boy and girl with typical speech, a boy and girl with /s/ and /z/ errors, and a boy and girl with errors producing /ɹ/. The children with speech errors were rated more negatively than the children with typical speech, and the sixth-grade children gave lower ratings than the fourth-grade children overall. However, not all studies provide conclusive evidence for the social impact of SSD (Freeman & Sonnega, 1956). There is evidence from the Netherlands that while children with SSD are regarded less favorably that those with typical speech, children who stutter or who have voice disorders are regarded less favorably than children with SSD (De Nil & Brutten, 1990).

School teachers have reported the impact of SSD (Bennett & Runyan, 1982; Overby, Carrell, & Bernthal, 2007; Ruscello, Toth, & Stutler, 1983). In a study of 48 second-grade teachers, 58.3% rated children with SSD as having increased risk of academic, social, and behavioral difficulties compared with children with typical speech (Overby et al., 2007). In another study, 66% of 282 educators believed that communication disorders have an adverse effect on educational performance, with 43.9% indicating that children with SSD had increased risk of academic and social difficulties compared with 26.9% for children with language impairment (Bennett & Runyan, 1982). Teachers have reported low confidence and competence for working with children with SSD and other communication disorders (McLeod & McKinnon, 2010; Sadler, 2005). Training has been found to increase teachers' accuracy of perceptions of the ability of children with communication disorders (Ebert & Prelock, 1994).

The attitudes of people towards those with SSD continue to impact into adolescence and adulthood (Allard & Williams, 2008; McKinnon, Hess, & Landry, 1986; Williams & Dietrich, 1996). Studies of adolescents have shown negative attitudes towards peers with mild SSD, including the production of [w] for /ɹ/ (Silverman & Falk, 1992; Silverman & Paulus, 1989). Adults have indicated that males with interdental productions of /s/ and /z/ have lower ratings on speaking ability, intelligence, education, masculinity, and friendship than those with typical speech (Mowrer, Wahl, & Doolan, 1978). Eighty adults from Brazil with residual SSD on /s/ or the alveolar flap were asked about the impact of SSD, and reported that they received negative reactions about their speech (17.5%) and that their speech affected their work (18.8%) and their social life (13.8%) (Veríssimo, Van Borsel, & de Britto Pereira, 2012). There is evidence that people from different cultures (English-speaking North American, Chinese, Southeast Asian, Hispanic) hold different beliefs from one another about the emotional health and capacity for self-improvement of the speech of people with SSD, cleft palate, stuttering, and hearing loss (Bebout & Arthur, 1992). For example, people in their study who were born outside of North America were more likely to consider those with disordered speech as "emotionally disturbed" (p. 49) and that they could improve their speech if they "tried hard" (Bebout & Arthur, 1992, p. 49). These findings indicate that the attitudes of people surrounding those with SSD are an important consideration within assessment and intervention.

Occupational impact of SSD

Having SSD can be associated with difficulties acquiring and keeping a job, particularly since a majority of occupations this century require skilled communication rather than manual labor (Ruben, 2000). A powerful statement reinforcing the importance of communicative competence in adulthood was made by Ruben (2000), who stated: ". . . people with speech disorders . . . have the greatest rate of unemployment—67.4% for those who have difficulty in speaking understandably and 75.6% for those who are unable to speak understandably" (p. 243). Potential difficulties with acquiring a job were highlighted in a study by Allard and Williams (2008) where 455 adults compared an audio recording of a person with an articulation disorder (interdental lisp on /s/) and a person with typical speech. There was a significant difference between the perceived employability of the two, with lower ratings for the person with an interdental lisp. As discussed earlier, Felsenfeld et al. (1994) found that adults with histories of SSD were more likely to be employed in semiskilled or unskilled jobs compared with others of the same gender (siblings and people with typical speech), although they were equally satisfied with their employment. Workplace discrimination for adults with SSD was documented by Mitchell, McMahon, and McKee (2005), who considered 1,637 allegations of employment discrimination for people with "speech impairment." When compared with those with vision or orthopedic difficulties, adults with speech impairment were more likely to report allegations related to harassment and hiring. Negative attitudes by employers have also been documented for people with cleft lip and palate (Chan, McPherson, & Whitehill, 2006; Scheuerle, Guilford, & Garcia, 1982). Further studies of occupational outcomes for adults with histories of SSD would be beneficial.

Impact of SSD on children's families

As you will learn later in this book, SLPs often integrate family-centered and family-friendly practices during assessment and invention for children (Crais, Roy, & Free, 2006; Watts Pappas, McLeod, McAllister, & McKinnon, 2008). It is helpful to consider literature about the impact of a child's SSD on the lives of families, to factor this into assessment and invention practices, and to advocate for additional family-centered (in addition to child-centered) support if required.

Impact of SSD on parents' lives

The impact of SSD extends beyond children to parents of children with SSD. Three studies from Germany have provided insights into the impact of SSD on parents' lives,

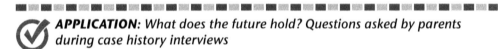

APPLICATION: *What does the future hold? Questions asked by parents during case history interviews*

Use the following questions to enact a role-play scenario involving five hypothetical parents and a speech-language pathologist. Have the speech-language pathologist respond to the following questions asked by the parents. Assume that each parent has a preschool child recently identified with SSD.

1. "Will my child's younger brothers and sisters have the same problem?"
2. "Jenny seems to be so quiet lately. She's withdrawing from her friends at preschool. Why is this happening? What can I do to help?"
3. "I'm reluctant to send Peter (4;2 years) to preschool. I don't know if it would be too hard for him to make friends. He's so difficult to understand. What do you think? Should I send him to preschool?"
4. "I think Dianne (4;7 years) will grow out of her speech problem. I know you have said that there is a problem, but is therapy really necessary at this age?"
5. "What does the future hold for David (who is 3;6 years old)? His speech is so difficult to understand."

documenting quality of life and stigmatization. First, Rudolph, Kummer, Eysholdt, and Rosanowski (2005) found that there were poorer ratings of health-related quality of life amongst 91 mothers of children with SSD in comparison to mothers of healthy children (children without SSD) on six of the eight scales: physical functioning, general health, vitality, social functioning, role physical, and role emotional. The two areas in which poorer scores were not found in comparison to the control group were bodily pain and mental health. The areas of reduced quality of life restricted the mothers' daily activities, and these findings were not found to be influenced by the severity of their child's SSD or their child's age (Rudolph et al., 2005). In contrast, a study by Weigl, Rudolph, Eysholdt, and Rosanowski (2005) found that amongst 50 mothers of children over 12 months of age with cleft lip and palate, quality of life was not significantly altered in comparison with a control group of mothers of children without cleft lip and palate. Macharey and Von Suchodoletz (2008) explored parental perception of the stigmatization of 362 children with speech and language disorders. Almost half (49.7%) of parents reported that negative labeling of their child (e.g., "Think my child is stupid," p. 259) had occurred in various social environments including around other children, other adults, and family members. Further, 30.2% of parents had felt stigmatized by family members or other adults (e.g., "Think we as parents are responsible for our child's developmental problems," p. 259). The findings of this study emphasize the need for a holistic approach to the management of SSD in children, as the impact may be far-reaching, impacting not only children's socialization but also their parents' feelings of stigmatization.

Being a parent of a child with SSD has been described as a "battle." McCormack, McAllister, McLeod, and Harrison (2012) considered the longitudinal experience of two mothers of children with SSD at the time their children were young men. Three themes were used to summarize the experience of living with SSD: knowing, having, and doing. A phenomenological framework was used to describe how these three themes impacted parents across their child's life. It was found that "knowing" about their child's SSD started from early childhood and continued throughout their life, while the battles of "having" SSD and "doing" something about it began during childhood and continued into adulthood and included battles to ensure their children received appropriate services. Different life circumstances lead to different experiences of being a parent to a child with SSD. One mother reported battling with SSD in all three areas, whereas the second mother reported that life challenges (in this instance the death of another child) seemed to outweigh the battles that her other child's SSD presented. The perceived impact of having a child with an SSD is an important consideration for clinical practice when planning and providing services for children and their families.

Some of the battles of parents of children with SSD can be understood through considering a study of parental perceptions of speech-language pathology service delivery for children with speech and language disorders (Ruggero, McCabe, Ballard, & Munro, 2012). Ruggero et al. (2012) found that parents' wishes (and recommendations from the literature) did not align with the reality of service delivery. Many children had to wait for over 6 months to receive services. Long waiting periods can impact the effectiveness of early intervention and lead to a lack of parental satisfaction regarding the services their children receive. Parents reported that they did not always feel they had input into decisions made about their child's speech therapy (e.g., regarding taking breaks or being discharged from therapy). Of parents whose children had been discharged from therapy, 60% reported that they felt the discharge was inappropriate as they held concerns for their child's future or felt that their child had been discharged from intervention without sufficient gains being made. This high level of dissatisfaction from parents around discharge emphasizes the need to effectively communicate with parents around service delivery issues in order to ensure that parents' voices are heard and that the SLP is working in partnership with parents to achieve the best possible outcomes for children with SSD. Each of these studies confirms the need to listen to parents and consider the impact of SSD on their lives.

Impact of SSD on siblings' lives

In a study of SLPs' typical practices for children with SSD, siblings and grandparents were identified as usually or sometimes being involved during assessment and intervention sessions (McLeod & Baker, 2014). To date there is no research that has specifically considered

CHILDREN'S INSIGHTS: *What siblings know*

Siblings of children with SSD have a lot of insights about their brother or sister with SSD, particularly if they are attending the same school. Often, siblings see each other more often and in more contexts than their parents do. Here are some comments from siblings of children with SSD (Barr, McLeod, & Daniel, 2008; McLeod, Daniel & Barr, 2013), cerebral palsy, hearing loss, and other disabilities (Barr & McLeod, 2010):

Being siblings
- "He's usually a quiet child—but when he's around his brothers and he's feeling in his element he's not so quiet" (Mother) (McLeod, Daniel, & Barr, 2013, p. 76).

Observing others' reactions
- ". . . my brother is treated like some sort of baby and people think that he can't understand things, but he can when he has enough time to take in the sentences" (Barr & McLeod, 2010, p. 166).

Supporting their sibling
- "When [my brother] started school I couldn't scrape him off. I couldn't . . . He would follow me around everywhere, everywhere, everywhere I tell you! . . . After a while he slowly and slowly made friends. I started off actually making him friends, like I got him, took him up to his class, found a kid inside his class that was outside the door and I asked him if he'd play with my little brother so he'd get off my back and stop asking me" (Barr, McLeod, & Daniel, 2008, p. 28).

Feelings
- "I cry about it sometimes like because I know that it [my brother's SSD] has to be fixed" (Barr, McLeod, & Daniel, 2008, p. 28).

Thinking about the future
- ". . . it [brother's SSD] stresses Mom as well 'cause she doesn't want him to be like this when he gets older and neither do I" (Barr, McLeod, & Daniel, 2008, p. 28).

the role of grandparents in the lives of children with SSD; however, there is some interesting research that outlines the roles and issues of being a sibling of a child with SSD and other areas of need.

Siblings have additional roles, responsibilities, and concerns when they are a sibling of a child with a disability (Burke, 2004; McHugh, 2003; Moore, Howard, & McLaughlin, 2002; Naylor & Prescott, 2004; Pit-ten Cate & Loots, 2000). For example, Barr and McLeod (2010) coded 676 contributions to an Internet support site for children who had a sibling with one or more of a range of disabilities. They identified three overarching themes written from siblings' perspectives: "(1) strangers stare and have negative attitudes towards my sibling with a disability; (2) peers don't understand what it's like to be me, use certain words that upset me, say nasty things and tease me about my brother/sister; (3) although my family loves me, they don't have a lot of time for me, our plans are often disrupted, and they give me a lot of responsibility" (p. 162). While it may be easy to dismiss these findings by saying that children with SSD may have fewer overt needs (e.g., they rarely need assistance with feeding) and may not have a disability that is visible (although the disability may be visible if they are in a wheelchair due to cerebral palsy or if they have a cochlear implant), there are reports that siblings of children with SSD share similar concerns to other siblings of children with disabilities. A study of six siblings of children with SSD and 15 significant others in their lives was titled "Cavalry on the Hill" (Barr et al.,

2008), since one mother described that her daughter was available whenever needed for her twin brother who had speech and language impairment. This phrase summed up the comments by many others in the study. Barr et al. (2008) revealed that the siblings were asked to act as interpreters for their brother or sister with SSD due to unintelligible speech. This occurred at home, at school, and within the community (e.g., at the store). One sibling was taken out of his own class to go to his brother's class in order to interpret what his brother with SSD said to the teacher. The siblings also expressed jealousy, resentment, worry, and concern towards their brother or sister with SSD. One older sibling said that she tried to go everywhere with her brother in case someone did not understand what he was saying, and would worry about her brother's future. Many parents indicated that the siblings felt that their brothers or sisters with SSD received more attention, including the time spent at speech-language pathology sessions and undertaking homework set by the SLP. The parent-child relationship was impacted as siblings were required to take on parent-like roles for their brothers or sisters with SSD, particularly in the school setting. In contrast, when at home, the children were described as having a typical sibling relationship where they would interact, play games, and communicate without their brother's or sister's SSD having too much impact. One sibling described her brother in the following way: "He's a cool kid. Like he's fun to hang out and stuff when he's not being naughty. Like, me and him have fun together" (Barr et al., 2008, p. 23). Another study by McLeod, Daniel, and Barr (2013) confirmed that children with SSD felt safe and supported amongst their siblings and parents compared with their feelings in public contexts. The title of this paper included a pertinent quote from another mother: "When he's around his brothers . . . he's not so quiet" (McLeod, Daniel, & Barr, 2013, p. 70). These studies provide insights into the important roles siblings play with children with SSD and the impact that being a sibling can have on their own lives.

Throughout this section on the impact of childhood SSD, it is clear that the impact not only manifests in childhood, but it extends to adolescence and adulthood for many people. The impact can be far-reaching and lifelong, extending into educational, social, and occupational contexts and beyond the child to siblings and parents. As we will learn next, when undertaking evidence-based practice, the values and preferences of the child/client/patient should be considered. This section on the impact of childhood SSD can inform your understanding of the complexities of life with SSD.

RISK AND PROTECTIVE FACTORS FOR SSD

Despite there being currently no known cause for the majority of children with SSD, a number of risk and protective factors have been identified in large-scale population studies of children. An understanding of risk and protective factors for SSD enables SLPs to identify children who may be at risk for later SSD and to put into place factors that protect children from developing more severe SSD. It is important to remember that a risk is not the same as a predictor; that is, even though a child may have an increased risk of having SSD due to the presence of a risk factor, he or she may not eventually have an SSD. Risk and protective factors for SSD can be intrinsic to the child, parent, family, or community. Table 1-3 summarizes risk and protective factors that have been identified in the literature. Some studies have considered children only with SSD (Campbell et al., 2003; Felsenfeld & Plomin, 1997; Fox, Dodd, & Howard, 2002; Hauner, Shriberg, Kwiatkowski, & Allen, 2005; To, Cheung, & McLeod, 2013a, b), while others have considered children with both speech and language impairment (D'Odorico, Majorano, Fasolo, Salerni, & Suttora, 2011; Harrison & McLeod, 2010; Lyytinen et al., 2001; Tomblin, Hardy, & Hein, 1991; Weindrich, Jennen-Steinmetz, Laucht, Esser, & Schmidt, 2000; Yliherva, Olsén, Mäki-Torkko, Koiranen, & Järvelin, 2001). As can be seen, there is not always a clear delineation as to whether a factor is a risk, protective, both, or neither. Some of the reasons for differences between the findings include the differing age of the children studied, the size or nature of the sample, differences in the outcome being tested, and the range and number of predictors and covariates included in the analysis (Harrison & McLeod, 2010). Let us consider each of the factors that have been identified as a potential risk or protective factor for SSD.

| TABLE 1-3 | Significant and non-significant risk and protective factors for SSD* identified in the literature | | | |

Identified risk factors	Significant risk factor	Not a significant risk factor	Significant protective factor
Child factors			
Male sex	Campbell et al. (2003); Harrison & McLeod (2010); Keating, Turrell & Ozanne (2001); Tomblin et al. (1991); To et al. (2013a)	—	—
Prenatal factors	Fox et al. (2002)	—	—
Postnatal factors	D'Odorico et al. (2011); Fox et al. (2002); Weindrich et al. (2000); Yliherva et al. (2001)	Harrison & McLeod (2010)	—
Multiple birth	—	Harrison & McLeod (2010)	—
Medical conditions	—	Campbell et al. (2003); Fox et al. (2002); Harrison & McLeod (2010)	—
Hearing status	Harrison & McLeod (2010); Yliherva et al. (2001)	—	—
Oral sucking habits	Fox et al. (2002)	—	—
Intelligence	—	Felsenfeld & Plomin (1997)	—
Temperament	Harrison & McLeod (2010) (reactivity); Hauner et al. (2005)	—	Harrison & McLeod (2010) (persistence)
Parent factors			
Family history of speech and language problems	Campbell et al. (2003); Felsenfeld & Plomin (1997); Fox et al. (2002); Lyytinen et al. (2001); Tomblin et al. (1991)	—	—
Languages spoken and proficiency in home language	—	—	Harrison & McLeod (2010)
Minority status or race	—	Campbell et al. (2003)	—
Educational level of mother (M) and/or father (F)	Campbell et al. (2003) (M); Tomblin et al. (1991) (F); To et al. (2013b) (M); Weindrich et al. (2000) (M/F); Yliherva et al. (2001) (M)	To et al. (2013b) (F); Tomblin et al. (1991) (M)	—
Family factors			
Socioeconomic factors (SES)	To et al. (2013b) (income)	Campbell et al. (2003); Harrison & McLeod (2010)	—
Family size (including birth order)	Harrison & McLeod (2010) (older siblings); Tomblin et al. (1991); Yliherva et al. (2001)	Harrison & McLeod (2010) (younger siblings); To et al. (2013b) (number of siblings)	—
Home learning activities	—	Felsenfeld & Plomin (1997); Harrison & McLeod (2010)	—

*The following studies considered children with SSD: Campbell et al. (2003); Fox et al. (2002); Felsenfeld & Plomin (1997) Hauner et al. (2005); To, Cheung, & McLeod (2013a, b); The other studies considered children with speech *and* language impairment: Harrison & McLeod (2010); Lyytinen et al. (2001); Tomblin et al. (1991); Weindrich et al. (2000); Yliherva al. (2001).

> **COMMENT:** *Typical characteristics of children referred for SSD*
>
> The typical profile of a child referred for SSD in many English-speaking speech-language pathology clinics is a preschool-aged boy with a positive family history of speech and language impairment (Shriberg & Kwiatkowski, 1994). Evidence for this typical profile includes that:
>
> ■ The average age of referral for children with SSD is 4;3 years (Shriberg & Kwiatkowski, 1994).
>
> ■ The ratio of boys to girls with SSD is approximately 2:1 (Lewis, Ekelman, & Aram, 1989; McKinnon, McLeod, & Reilly, 2007).
>
> ■ A child who was male with a family history of speech and language difficulties and low maternal education was 7.71 times as likely to have an SSD as a child without any of these factors (Campbell et al., 2003).
>
> Speaking more than one language (e.g., English and Spanish) is not a cause of SSD (Hambly, Wren, McLeod, & Roulstone, 2013).

Child factors: Sex

Most studies indicate that being female is slightly protective for speech acquisition performance and being male increases the risk of having SSD. To put it another way, girls are (slightly) more likely to acquire speech sounds earlier than boys, and boys are more likely to have SSD. Hyde and Linn (1988) conducted a meta-analysis of 165 studies regarding the relationship between sex and verbal ability. Overall, the review indicated that females exhibited a slight superiority in performance (effect size was 0.11, meaning that females were 0.11 times more likely to score higher than males on verbal ability tasks). Speech production ability had the largest effect size (effect size was 0.33) for female superiority over other variables, including reading comprehension and vocabulary. Within the speech sound acquisition literature, most studies documenting the age of acquisition of speech sounds similarly demonstrate a slight advantage for females (Kenney & Prather, 1986; Smit, Hand, Freilinger, Bernthal, & Bird, 1990; To, Cheung, & McLeod, 2013a); however, there are a few studies that show different results for different ages (Dodd, Holm, Hua, & Crosbie, 2003; Poole, 1934). For example, Dodd et al. (2003) studied speech acquisition in 684 children and found no gender differences for children aged 3;0–5;5; however, at ages 5;6–6;11 girls acquired interdental fricatives and consonant clusters before the boys.

There is consistent evidence for being male as a risk factor for SSD (Campbell et al., 2003; Felsenfeld et al., 1995; Harrison & McLeod, 2010; Law et al., 1998; Lewis et al., 1989; Tomblin et al., 1991). For example, Campbell et al. (2003) indicated that the odds ratio of being male was 2.19; that is, boys were 2.19 times more likely to be identified as having SSD than girls in their study of 639 three-year-old children. Shriberg, Tomblin, and McSweeny (1999) reported the ratio of males to females with SSD ("speech delay") was 1.5:1 in their study of 7,218 six-year-old children. McKinnon et al. (2007) reported the ratio of males to females with SSD was 2.85:1 in their study of 10,425 students across the first 7 years of formal schooling. Correspondence between male sex and SSD was an early impetus for genetic research into communication impairments (Shriberg, Tomblin, & McSweeny, 1999).

Child factors: Pre- and postnatal factors

Some studies show that pre- and postnatal factors are risk factors for SSD, whereas others show no impact. To date, few studies have considered the relationship between prenatal factors and the risk of SSD. One study that has considered this relationship was conducted by Fox, Dodd, and Howard (2002), who studied 113 children living in Germany (65 children with SSD and 48 who were typically developing). They reported that the mothers of 11% of children with SSD had complications during pregnancy including extreme stress, maternal infections, and medications that could cause damage to the fetus during pregnancy. They found a higher incidence of perinatal factors in children with inconsistent speech disorder when compared with other types of SSD. Some studies have shown that postnatal factors pose a risk factor for SSD (Fox et al., 2002; Weindrich et al., 2000; Yliherva et al., 2001). For example, Fox et al. (2002) reported that 15% of children with SSD had birth difficulties. They indicated that the following were significant predictors of SSD: "forceps or ventouse delivery, induced delivery because the infant was overdue, complications such as umbilical cord prolapse, infections, preterm birth, and post-partum resuscitation" (p. 122), and they found a 9.35 odds ratio for perinatal birth factors and 13.13 odds ratio for birth risk factors associated with SSD. That is, children identified with SSD were 13.13 times more likely to have birth risk factors than those in the control group. Low birth weight was identified as a risk factor for phonological development in 24 pre-term Italian children compared with 15 full-term children studied longitudinally (D'Odorico et al., 2011). In contrast, Tomblin et al. (1991) indicated that birth events such as "infections, low birth weight, breathing difficulty, ototoxic drugs, feeding problems, transfusions, and birth defects" (p. 1101) were not significant predictors of speech and language impairment. Similarly, Harrison and McLeod (2010) found that being born prematurely, having a low birth weight, and admission to a neonatal intensive care unit were not associated with parental concern about expressive speech and language skills in 4- to 5-year-old children.

Child factors: Hearing

Hearing loss has been identified as a risk factor for general speech and language difficulties in large epidemiological studies (e.g., Campbell et al., 2003; Harrison & McLeod, 2010; Paradise et al., 2001). Identification of hearing loss in a child who is older than 6 months of age increases the likelihood that the child will have difficulties with speech and language development (Yoshinaga-Itano, Sedey, Coulter, & Mehl, 1998). The association between ongoing ear infections, hearing loss, and SSD is addressed in Chapter 2.

Child factors: Oral sucking habits

Limited research has been conducted to consider the impact of oral sucking habits on children's speech. Some of the findings have also been contradictory. Fox et al. (2002) reported oral habits such as excessive bottle use (i.e., use of a bottle as a pacifier outside of feeding times), pacifier (dummy) use, and thumb sucking for more than 24 months was more likely in the group of children with SSD than their control group; however, only excessive bottle usage was significant between children with SSD and the control group. Tomblin, Smith, and Zhang (1997) demonstrated that being breastfed for less than 9 months was associated with an increased risk of speech and language impairment, whereas Harrison and McLeod (2010) found that being breastfed for less than 9 months was not associated with identified speech and language concern in 4- to 5-year-old children. In a study of the oral sucking habits of 128 preschoolers in Chile, Barbosa et al. (2009) reported that nonnutritive sucking (including pacifiers and digit sucking) for 3 years or more can have a negative effect on children's speech acquisition. By contrast, Shotts, McDaniel, and Neeley (2008) did not find an association between duration of pacifier use and performance on a standardized speech assessment in 68 children with normal hearing and no family history of SSD or cognitive difficulties.

Child factors: Psychosocial behaviors and temperament

There are no definitive personality traits of children with SSD. However, Shriberg and Kwiatkowski (1994) found that 60% of the 178 children they studied demonstrated some psychosocial behaviors such as shyness, speech avoidance, immaturity, need for external reinforcement, and oversensitivity. Later, Hauner et al. (2005) found that "approach-related or withdrawal-related negative affect, negative emotionality or mood, and decreased task persistence or attention" (p. 635) were associated with increased severity of SSD. Lewis et al. (2012) considered 412 children enrolled in a longitudinal study of SSD and concluded that the "children with moderate-severe SSD had higher ratings on the inattention and hyperactive/impulsivity scales than children with no SSD" (p. 247); however, presence of language impairment was more predictive than severity of SSD for symptoms of attention-deficit/hyperactivity disorder (ADHD).

COMMENT: *The pacifier debate*

Pacifiers (dummies) are controversial and recommendations for and against their use are disputed. For instance, pacifier use has been associated with reduced risk of sudden infant death syndrome (SIDS) (e.g., Horne et al., 2014), quicker transition to oral feeding in premature infants (e.g., Yildiz & Arikan, 2012), and reduced infant pain during painful procedures (e.g., Carbajal, Chauvet, Couderc, & Olivier-Martin, 1999). However, pacifier use has been associated with increased risk of ear infections (e.g., Rovers et al., 2008), gastrointestinal infections and diarrhea (e.g., Orimadegun & Obokon, 2015), oral candida (a type of yeast infection) (e.g., Comina et al., 2006), and malocclusion including overjet, open bite, and cross bite (e.g., Drane, 1996; Moimaz et al., 2014). Pacifier use in newborns is thought to lead to nipple confusion and/or reduced opportunities for breastfeeding and subsequently shorter duration of breastfeeding; however, not all research supports a link between pacifier use and breastfeeding duration (e.g., Jaafar, Jahanfar, Angolkar, & Ho, 2012; Zimmerman & Thompson, 2015). Niedenthal et al. (2012) explored possible associations between pacifier use and children's emotional development. They found that school-age boys who frequently used pacifiers at home during the day as a toddler had poorer facial mimicry (an ability considered important in emotional development). They also discovered that longer duration of pacifier use predicted lower emotional intelligence in young adult males (Niedenthal et al., 2012).

 APPLICATION: *To use or not use a pacifier*

Conduct a debate with a group of peers for and against pacifier use. Ensure your debate is informed by the latest research evidence.

Children's temperament (emotional and behavioral traits) has been associated with speech and language acquisition and disorder (Conture, Kelly, & Walden, 2013). Although, the association between psychosocial traits, temperament, speech, and language is not clear: "The question of directionality of effect remains—that is, do temperamental variables lead (a)typical language behavior, does (a)typical language behavior lead to temperament or do they bi-directionally influence one another?" (Conture et al., 2013, p. 133). For example, Harrison and McLeod (2010) conducted a large study of 4,983 preschool children to examine 31 risk and protective factors that were linked with parental concern about their children's speech and language competence. Three of the nine consistent significant risk and protective factors related to the three different temperament types: reactivity (e.g., inhibition and fearfulness in novel situations), persistence (e.g., task completion), and sociability (e.g., shyness) (from the Short Temperament Scale for Children; Sanson, Prior, Garino, Oberklaid, & Sewell, 1987). Having a more reactive temperament was a consistent risk factor and having a more persistent and more sociable temperament were consistent protective factors regarding identification of speech and language difficulties.

Child factors: Minority status, race, and languages spoken

There is no evidence to indicate that the race or language spoken by children and their families increases the risk of having SSD. For example, Campbell et al. (2003) indicated that identification as African-American was not found to be a significant risk factor for SSD for 3-year-old children in the United States. Harrison and McLeod (2010) found that 4- to 5-year-old Australian children who lived in homes where languages other than English were spoken were less likely (protective factor) to be identified by their parents as having difficulty talking and making speech sounds than those who lived in monolingual English-speaking households. Historically, there was a belief that speaking more than one language may increase difficulties with speech and language, but much of this research focused on abilities using the dominant language of the country rather than on all of the languages spoken by the children. As Paradis (2007) stated,

> In the first half of the 20th century it was commonly thought that bilingualism in early childhood was detrimental to children's linguistic and intellectual development, but an established body of research since that time has shown that bilingualism either has neutral or enhancing effects on children's cognitive development. (p. 551)

More recent research has not focused on bilingual children's use of English (or the dominant language of the country they live in). Instead, there has been a focus on research that documents children's speech sound capacity in:

- both languages (e.g., Spanish and English: Fabiano-Smith & Goldstein, 2010a; Goldstein, Fabiano, & Washington, 2005; Cantonese and Putonghua/Mandarin: Law & So, 2006);
- their dominant (minority) language (e.g., Samoan spoken in New Zealand: Ballard & Farao, 2008); or
- the dominant language while accounting for dialect (e.g., African-American English: Pearson, Velleman, Bryant, & Charko, 2009; Chinese-influenced Malaysian English: Phoon, Abdullah, & Maclagan, 2012; Australian Aboriginal English: Toohill, McLeod, & McCormack, 2012).

A systematic review of 66 studies documented speech acquisition of typically developing children and those with SSD in over 20 languages (Hambly, Wren, McLeod, & Roulstone, 2013). The review concluded that there was a complex picture of the rate of acquisition of phonemes, with some studies showing no difference in the rate of acquisition, some showing slower acquisition, and some showing accelerated acquisition compared with monolingual English peers. Typically bilingual children showed a different pattern of development to monolingual peers, and most studies provided evidence of transfer between languages but the amount of transfer varied.

Parent factors: Family history of speech and language problems

There is consistent evidence from familial aggregation studies to suggest that positive family history of speech, language, and/or literacy difficulties is a risk factor for SSD (Campbell et al., 2003; Felsenfeld et al., 1995; Fox et al., 2002; Lewis et al., 1989; Shriberg & Kwiatkowski, 1994). For example, Shriberg and Kwiatkowski (1994) studied 62 children with SSD who were 2 to 6 years of age. They found that 39% of the children had one family member "with the same speech problem" (p. 1113) and an additional 17% had more than one family member with the same speech problem. That is, a total of 56% had one or more family members with SSD. Campbell et al. (2003) studied 639 three-year-olds and indicated that the odds ratio of having a positive family history was 1.67; that is, children with a positive family history were 1.67 times more likely to be identified as having SSD than those who did not have members of their family who had had speech, language, or stuttering difficulties. Lewis et al. (2007) tested the speech of 147 parents of children with SSD. The more first-degree family members who had a history of SSD or language impairment, the greater the risk of SSD. They found that the odds of having SSD increased by 1.99 times if the child had another family member with SSD, and the odds for language impairment increased by 4.12 times with another family member with language impairment. The 36 parents in the Lewis et al. (2007) study with histories of attending speech therapy produced more speech errors than parents who did not attend speech therapy as children on tasks involving multisyllabic words, nonsense words, tongue twisters, spelling, reading, and receptive language. Parents who had language impairment performed more poorly than those with SSD alone. The link between family history and SSD may be interpreted as a genetic and/ or an environmental influence, necessitating additional research to differentiate these aspects.

> **COMMENT:** *Family history interview*
>
> Lewis and Freebairn (1993) created a family history interview questionnaire for con-sidering familial aggregation of SSD. The questions enable SLPs to document whether each family member (over three generations) had difficulties with speech, language, reading, spelling, learning, or stuttering. A pedigree (chart) is drawn to illustrate the family history. Chapter 7 provides more information about eliciting background infor-mation during children's speech assessments.

Parent factors: Maternal and paternal education level

There is some evidence to suggest that low maternal (mothers') education is a risk factor for SSD (Campbell et al., 2003; Fox et al., 2002; To et al., 2013b; Yliherva et al., 2001). For exam-ple, Campbell et al. (2003) indicated that the odds ratio of low maternal education was 2.58; that is, in their study of 639 three-year-old children, those whose mothers had not completed high school education were 2.58 times more likely to be identified as having SSD than those whose mothers had completed high school.

There is less (and conflicting) evidence to suggest that low paternal (fathers') edu-cation is a risk factor for SSD. For example, Tomblin et al. (1991) found, in their study of 662 children in the United States, that paternal education level was a risk factor for "poor communication" status (that included measures of speech and language), whereas mater-nal education was not. In contrast, To et al. (2013b) found, in their study of 937 children in Hong Kong, that while maternal education level was a risk factor for SSD, paternal educa-tion level was not. Differently again, Weindrich et al. (2000) found that both maternal and paternal education were risk factors for speech and language impairment in their study of 320 children in Germany.

Family factors: Socioeconomic status

Socioeconomic status (SES) has been measured in different ways, including yearly income, occupational prestige, education levels, and some measures are combinations of these factors. There is evidence to indicate that SES does not impact children's acquisition of speech sounds (e.g., Dodd, Holm, et al., 2003; Smit et al., 1990); however, other stud-ies have shown that children from low SES backgrounds do not perform as well as those from higher ones (Templin, 1957; To et al., 2013b). SES has been found to have an effect on the acquisition of phonological awareness, and pre-literacy skills (e.g., Burt, Holm & Dodd, 1999; Lonigan, Burgess, Anthony, & Barker, 1998), and this effect is moderated by the age of the child, with those in high SES groups benefitting as they get older (McDowell, Lonigan, & Goldstein, 2007).

APPLICATION: *Case history questionnaire*

When SLPs assess children with suspected SSD, they often discuss background information relevant to the child using a case history questionnaire. Consider the risk and protective factors outlined in this chapter. What questions would you ask parents based on the information you have just read? Remember, having a risk factor is not predictive of having SSD. Look at Luke's case history in Chapter 16. What additional information is given in Chapter 16? What additional information would you like to know about Luke? Regardless of whether children have SSD of known or unknown causes, the SLP's role is to assess their strengths and areas of difficulty, create an intervention plan, and provide intervention that will ultimately result in their achieving their best ability to produce intelligible and acceptable speech to enable participation in society.

■ ▬ ■ ▬ ■ ▬ ■ ▬ ■ ▬ ■ ▬ ■ ▬ ■ ▬ ■ ▬ ■ ▬ ■ ▬ ■ ▬ ■ ▬ ■ ▬ ■ ▬ ■ ▬ ■ ▬ ■

✓ **APPLICATION:** *Questions and comments from health and education professionals*

Early childhood educators, school teachers, doctors, and nurses draw on our knowledge as experts in the area of speech development and impairment. Respond to the following questions and comments from health and education professionals about children who have SSD.

1. "When is the best time to refer a child for a speech assessment?"
2. "I think some children watch too much TV and spend less time talking with their parents. That's why we have so many children here with speech problems. What do you think?"
3. "I find that many of the children in my class with reading problems have a history of speech problems. Is there a link?"
4. "What factors increase a child's risk of having a speech problem?"
5. "What is the impact of SSD on a family?"

Family size and birth order

The number of siblings in the home has not been found to be associated with speech acquisition in some studies (To et al., 2013b); however, Yliherva et al. (2001) found that having more than four children in the household increased risk of speech, language, and learning difficulties. There is evidence that birth order may have an effect on identification of speech and language impairment. According to Tomblin et al. (1991), children who hold later birth positions in the family are more likely to have a poor communication status between 2½ and 5 years of age. Similarly, Harrison and McLeod (2010) found that 4- to 5-year-old children were more likely to be identified by their parents as having expressive speech and language difficulties if they had an older sibling, but there was no indication of a risk or protective factor if they had a younger sibling. To provide additional insight, they found that children were protected for receptive language difficulties if they had an older sibling. Harrison and McLeod (2010) hypothesized that children with older siblings may have fewer opportunities to practice their speech since older siblings may be speaking for the younger child, but more opportunities to hear speech.

EVIDENCE-BASED PRACTICE

The subtitle of this book is *An Evidence-Based Approach to Assessment and Intervention*. This book teaches SLPs about how to make evidence-based decisions to work with children and their families. It is a book that is focused on how to undertake an assessment, analysis, and intervention supported by a comprehensive understanding of the underlying research. Because of the importance of EBP, we devote an entire chapter (Chapter 15) to this topic later in this book. However, we have infused this book with EBP, so have provided this quick summary in Chapter 1 to support your learning.

 Evidence-based practice (EBP) is a term that is used frequently in most SLPs' workplaces and is an important decision-making framework for guiding SLPs' interactions with children with SSD (e.g., Baker & McLeod, 2011a, b; Tyler, 2006, 2008; Williams, McLeod, & McCauley, 2010). Descriptions of EBP typically include the integration of three elements: **research evidence**, **clinical expertise**, and **client values and preferences** (Sackett, Straus, Richardson, Rosenberg, & Haynes, 2000) (see Figure 1-4). Dollaghan (2007) described a modified framework of EBP, known as E³BP, for use within speech-language pathology (see Figure 1-5). Dollaghan (2007) defined her concept of E³BP as "the conscientious, explicit, and judicious integration of 1) best available external evidence from systematic research, 2) best available evidence internal to clinical practice, and 3) best available evidence concerning the preferences of a fully informed patient" (p. 2). If you apply E³BP to children with SSD, these three sources of evidence include:

1. **External evidence** = published literature on the different assessment tools, diagnostic criteria, and intervention approaches for children with SSD.
2. **Internal clinical evidence** = assessment and intervention data from an individual clinician's practice with children with SSD and their families.
3. **Internal patient/client evidence** = information about the factors, values, and informed preferences of the children and families with whom clinicians work.

FIGURE 1-4 **The three elements of evidence-based practice (EBP)**

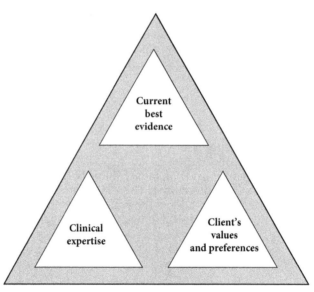

Source: Adapted from Sackett et al. (2000).

FIGURE 1-5 **The three elements of E³BP**

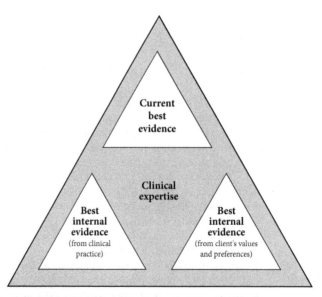

Source: Adapted from Dollaghan (2007).

Clinical expertise integrates all three sources of evidence in the provision of optimal clinical care (Dollaghan, 2007). E³BP encompasses clinical decisions regarding best practice in assessment and diagnosis and intervention (Dollaghan, 2007).

◼ Steps involved in clinical decision-making

There are a number of steps for using evidence-based practice when working with children with SSD (adapted from Gillam and Gillam, 2006). First, think of a clinical question you want to answer. Typically such a question relates to children with SSD to determine which intervention will result in the best outcome. For example, "Will intervention X be better than intervention Y for increasing the perception, production, and phonological awareness skills of a 4-year-old child with a moderate SSD of unknown origin?" Next, find and evaluate evidence from three sources: research (external) evidence that pertains to the question, internal evidence from your clinical practice, and evidence from children and their families regarding specific issues, values, and preferences. Finally, integrate these three sources of evidence, apply this to your clinical practice, and evaluate the outcome. Throughout this book, you will be provided with an integration of external research evi-

COMMENT: *Principles of evidence-based practice are woven throughout this book*

This book contains research undertaken by many different researchers in many different countries. Sometimes the evidence provides inconclusive guidance for practice. When this occurs, we have chosen to present a range of divergent evidence. Instead of telling you what to do, we provide you with the evidence to make up your own mind. As often as possible we provide information about the study (e.g., the number and age of participants, the language spoken, study design). We also provide the full reference at the end of the book so that you can look it up (online or via your library) and read the entire study yourself. We especially encourage you to read the entire studies when evidence provides inconclusive guidance for practice. We hope that this approach to presenting the evidence equips you to undertake evidence-based practice in your work with children with SSD.

APPLICATION: *Responding to a referral letter*

Consider the following referral letter from a pediatrician and write a short summary of what you think you might do for assessment and intervention of this child.

> *Dear SLP, Tom is difficult to understand. He was late to talk, and his father had speech therapy as a child. Tom has frequent ear infections. Tom is frustrated that others don't understand him. His behavior at preschool is problematic. His parents are anxious to send him to school next year. Please assess.*

Write answers to the following:

- ◼ What do you think you will do?
- ◼ What do you need to find out?

Compare and discuss your answers with a peer. Keep your summary and reconsider your recommendations, so that you can reexamine them after you have read this book to see how much you have learned and how your intuitive clinical practice has changed.

dence to apply to children and their families. You will also be given ideas for how to collect internal evidence from your own clinical practice, as well as from the children and families you work with. In Chapter 15 we provide you with a framework for applying evidence-based practice in your own clinical context.

Chapter summary

In this foundation chapter you learned about children with SSD, including the high prevalence of childhood SSD and the high proportion of children with SSD on SLPs' caseloads. You learned that risk factors associated with SSD include being male, having ongoing hearing problems, having a family history of speech and language impairment, and having a reactive temperament. Children with SSD can either normalize or continue to have difficulties with complex speech tasks (e.g., mul-

tisyllabic words, tongue twisters) and literacy into adolescence and adulthood. You learned that the lifelong effects of SSD can manifest in social, educational, and occupational contexts. Parents and siblings are also affected by childhood SSD. Finally, you had a brief introduction to the three aspects of evidence-based practice, so that you can use these insights in subsequent chapters.

Suggested reading

One prominent person who has conducted research into SSD for many years is Lawrence (Larry) Shriberg. In 2010 a book was written by his past students and colleagues to celebrate his career (Paul & Flipsen, 2010). This book commences with a historical summary of the field written by Shriberg (2010a).

■ Shriberg, L. D. (2010a). Childhood speech sound disorders: From postbehaviourism to the postgenomic era. In R. Paul & P. Flipsen Jr. (Eds.), *Speech sound disorders in children: In honour of Lawrence D. Shriberg* (pp. 1–33). San Diego, CA: Plural Publishing.

Other suggested reading includes:

Prevalence and natural history

■ Law, J., Boyle, J., Harris, F., Harkness, A., & Nye, C. (2000). Prevalence and natural history of primary speech and language delay: Findings from a systematic review of the literature. *International Journal of Language and Communication Disorders, 35*(2), 165–188.

Risk and protective factors

■ Harrison, L. J., & McLeod, S. (2010). Risk and protective factors associated with speech and language impairment in a nationally representative sample of 4- to 5-year-old children. *Journal of Speech, Language, and Hearing Research, 53*(2), 508–529.

Associated factors

■ McCormack, J., McLeod, S., McAllister, L., & Harrison, L. J. (2009). A systematic review of the association between childhood speech impairment and participation across the lifespan. *International Journal of Speech-Language Pathology, 11*(2), 155–170.

Impact

■ McLeod, S., Daniel, G., & Barr, J. (2013). "When he's around his brothers . . . he's not so quiet": The private and public worlds of school-aged children with speech sound disorder. *Journal of Communication Disorders, 46*(1), 70–83.

Application of knowledge from Chapter 1

You have read about Luke's case in Chapter 16. Luke represents a common clinical example of a child with SSD. Now read through the background information for Susie (7;4 years), Jarrod (7;0 years), Michael (4;2 years), and Lian (14;2 years) in Chapter 16. Compare and contrast each child's case history and assessment data.

1.   What are the similarities and differences between the children's case histories?

2.   Observe the children's speech samples and note down any similarities and differences in the types of errors present in their speech.

3.   List any terms that are unfamiliar to you. We encourage you to revisit your list as you read this book. Keep it as a working document—defining terms and adding others as you come across new concepts and ideas about SSD in children.

2

Classification, Causes, and Co-occurrence

1. Explain the difference between phonological impairment, inconsistent speech disorder, articulation impairment, childhood apraxia of speech (CAS), and childhood dysarthria.

2. Compare classification systems for children with SSD.

3. Identify known origins of SSD.

4. Describe the co-occurrence of SSD with difficulties with language, literacy, voice, and stuttering.

KEY WORDS

Speech sound disorders (SSD): phonology (phonological impairment, inconsistent speech disorder), motor speech (articulation impairment, childhood apraxia of speech [CAS], childhood dysarthria)

Classification systems: Speech Disorders Classification System, Differential Diagnosis System, Psycholinguistic Framework, International Classification of Functioning, Disability and Health – Children and Youth Version (ICF-CY)

SSD of known origin: genetic causes, craniofacial anomalies, hearing loss, cognitive/intellectual impairment, motor impairment (e.g., cerebral palsy), autism spectrum disorders

Co-occurrence with SSD: language impairment, literacy difficulties, stuttering, oromotor difficulties, voice difficulties

OVERVIEW

This chapter describes ways that SSD have been studied and classified. You will learn that there is no agreed-upon classification system, and that each system serves a different purpose for understanding the nature of the problem and how SSD can be treated. You will also learn about known causes of SSD, including genetic causes, craniofacial anomalies, hearing loss, cognitive/intellectual impairment, motor impairment (including cerebral palsy), and autism spectrum disorders. You will learn about the co-occurrence of SSD with other types of communication disorders including language impairment, literacy difficulties, stuttering, and voice disorder in addition to oromotor difficulties.

TYPES OF SSD IN CHILDREN

In the definition of SSD adopted in this book (Chapter 1), SSD can stem from difficulties with the **perception**, **articulation/motor production**, and/or **phonological organization** and **representation[1] of speech**. A major focus of this book is to provide SLPs with guidance for clinical practice when working with children's speech, particularly during assessment, analysis, goal setting, and intervention. Consequently, after considering the literature on assessment and intervention for children with SSD, we have structured this book around five types of SSD grouped into two broad categories: phonology and motor speech (articulation) difficulties. The five different types of SSD are:

1. **Phonological impairment:** a cognitive-linguistic difficulty with learning the phonological system of a language. Phonological impairment is characterized by pattern-based speech errors.
2. **Inconsistent speech disorder:** a phonological assembly difficulty (i.e., difficulty selecting and sequencing phonemes for words) without accompanying oromotor difficulties (Dodd, 2013, 2014). Inconsistent speech disorder is characterized by inconsistent productions of the same lexical item (word).
3. **Articulation impairment:** a motor speech difficulty involving the physical production (i.e., articulation) of specific speech sounds. It is characterized by speech sounds errors typically only involving the distortion of sibilants and/or rhotics (typically /s, z, ɹ, ɝ/). (This definition is narrower than some historical uses of the term.)
4. **Childhood apraxia of speech (CAS):** a motor speech disorder involving difficulty planning and programming movement sequences, resulting in errors in speech sound production and prosody (ASHA, 2007b).
5. **Childhood dysarthria:** a motor speech disorder involving difficulty with the sensorimotor control processes involved in the production of speech, typically motor programming and execution (van der Merwe, 2009).

Figure 2-1 shows the interrelationship of these different categories, and Table 2-1 demonstrates the differences in production of the word *seven* that would be made by a child in each of these groups. As you read more of this book, you will notice that these categories provide you with guidance for working with children's speech in clinical practice. We have chosen to use this framework within the book because there are interventions that specifically target each type of SSD. For example, contrastive phonological interventions are predominantly used with children with phonological impairment (Baker, 2010), core vocabulary therapy is suited to children with inconsistent speech disorder (Dodd, 2014), while concurrent treatment guided by principles of motor learning is suitable for children with articulation impairment (Skelton, 2004a).

---

[1]Representation of speech can occur at a number of levels of abstraction: acoustic, phonetic, phonological, and motor (Munson, Edwards, & Beckman, 2005a; see Chapter 5).

FIGURE 2-1   Conceptualization of childhood SSD used in this book

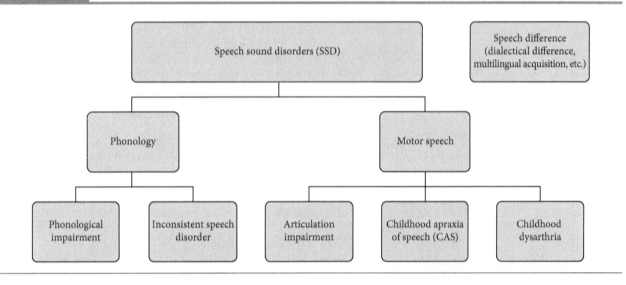

TABLE 2-1   Examples of speech sound errors for the production of *seven* /sɛvən/

	Nature of error	Possible examples
Phonological impairment	Cognitive-linguistic difficulty characterized by pattern-based errors.	[dɛbən]
Inconsistent speech disorder	Impaired phonological planning, resulting in inconsistent productions of the same word.	[tɛbən], [sɛbən], [dɛbən], etc.
Articulation impairment	Difficulty with the production (particularly phonetic placement) of specific speech sounds.	[θɛvən] OR [ɬɛvən]
Childhood apraxia of speech (CAS)	Impairment in planning and programming movement sequences impacting speech segments and prosody.	[dɛ.bɜn], [tɛbɜn]
Childhood dysarthria	Weakness, slowness, or incoordination of speech movements impacting speech systems including respiration, phonation, resonance, and articulation.	[sɛ::b̥ən]

Children's speech may fit neatly into one of these categories, or may be classified in a combination of ways. One reason for this is that throughout childhood, children are learning all aspects of perception, production, and representation. Consequently, while some children may have a primary difficulty with motor planning (e.g., CAS), their perceptual and phonological skills are still maturing, so it is possible that they may have some difficulties with these areas too. Figure 2-1 includes one more box that is not attached to the SSD framework. This box, labeled **speech difference**, is included to depict children whose speech may not be deemed acceptable or intelligible by people within their environment, but not because they have SSD. Although speech difference is not a focus of this book, speech differences as a result of speaking different dialects will be discussed briefly in Chapter 4. Our classification of SSD into these five types was driven by methods for assessment, analysis, and intervention reported in the literature. We now explain each type.

■ Speech sound disorders: Phonology

Phonology is about sounds (*phono*) and knowledge (*ology*). It refers to the speech sounds in languages and the rules for how those sounds combine to form words and how they are pronounced (Fromkin, Rodman, & Hyams, 2013). Phonology is one component of language, along with semantics (vocabulary), morphology (grammar), and syntax (sentence structure). Two types of SSD are considered phonological in nature: phonological impairment and inconsistent speech (phonological) disorder.

Phonological impairment

Children with phonological impairment have difficulty learning the phonological system of their language. They can have difficulty knowing which features, speech sounds, word shapes, and stress patterns are present in a language, how they are used, and how they mentally represent and organize that system. As Bowen (2009) states, "a phonological disorder is a *language* disorder that affects the phonemic organization level. The child has difficulty organizing his/her speech sounds into a system of sound contrasts" (p. 50).

During the early 20th century, all children with speech difficulties were thought to have problems with the physical production of speech (e.g., Blanton & Blanton, 1919). Around the 1970s and 1980s, phonological theories were applied to the study of children's speech, acknowledging that speech included a cognitive-linguistic component. This opened up the possibility that children with SSD had an underlying language component contributing to their unintelligibility. The application of phonological theories helped explain why some children with unintelligible speech could imitate particular speech sounds in isolation but not use them contrastively in words and/or in accordance with the phonotactic rules of a language.

One of the major changes to SLPs' practice of this time was that SLPs no longer considered that children had problems with the articulation of individual speech sounds, but had problems developing their phonological system. SLPs began to describe children's speech in terms of their error **patterns** or **phonological processes**. Children were described as having difficulty learning the rules of how sounds are used in the language(s) spoken, as well as learning how to perceive and produce speech sounds. As further research has been conducted into the nature of the problem, children's phonologically based error patterns have been considered symptomatic of underspecified phonological representations of words (e.g., Sutherland & Gillon, 2005). Chapter 5 describes the theoretical underpinnings of the shift in thinking from articulation to phonology and the abstract representation of speech.

In this book, phonological impairment has been used as an overarching term to include phonological delay and phonological disorder. A child with a **phonological delay** may exhibit systematic error patterns such as final consonant deletion (e.g., *seat* /sit/ → [si]) or cluster reduction (e.g., *blue* /blu/ → [bu]) that are typical in the speech of younger children but should have been resolved. A child with a **phonological disorder** may exhibit patterns such as initial consonant deletion (e.g., *feet* /fit/ → [it]) or glottal insertion (e.g., *feet* /fit/ → [ʔit]) that are not typical of the speech of younger children. In Chapter 6 we will discover that typical patterns in one language may not be typical patterns in others. For example, it is common for young children who speak

■ ■

 APPLICATION: *Luke (4;3 years), a child with a phonological impairment*

Luke is 4;3 and has a phonological impairment. Luke's case history and speech sample are found in Chapter 16. Look at Luke's speech sample in light of what you are beginning to learn about phonology. What patterns or rules do you notice in Luke's single-word sample of word-initial and word-final consonant clusters? We will keep coming back to the information about Luke in other chapters (e.g., Chapter 9 about analysis and Chapter 10 about goal setting) so that you can observe evidence-based speech-language pathology practice in action.

Read more about
Luke (4;3 years),
a boy with a phonological
impairment,
in Chapter 16 (Case 1).

Cantonese to realize some consonants as nasalized (e.g., producing /l/ as [n]) (To, Cheung, & McLeod, 2013a), whereas this would not be a common pattern in English (Shriberg & Kwiatkowski, 1980).

Inconsistent speech disorder

Inconsistent speech disorder is a type of SSD describing children who have "difficulty selecting and sequencing phonemes (i.e., in assembling a phonological template or plan for production of an utterance)" (Dodd, Holm, Crosbie, & McIntosh, 2010, p. 122). Dodd and colleagues state that a child has an inconsistent speech disorder if 40% or more of 25 words are produced variably during the three separate productions on an inconsistency assessment that mostly contains multisyllabic words (Dodd, Hua, Crosbie, Holm, & Ozanne, 2002). Approximately 10% of children with SSD are thought to have inconsistent speech disorder (Broomfield & Dodd, 2004b). The problem presents as lexical inconsistency—unpredictable pronunciations of the same word. These children often know how to articulate a range of speech sounds. Children with inconsistent speech disorder have difficulty with the assembly of phonemes that make up a word, in the absence of any oromotor signs of CAS (Dodd et al., 2010). For example, review Jarrod's speech sample (in Chapter 16 and the APPLICATION box below). Did you notice how his productions of the word *tongue* /tʌŋ/ differed, including [bʌns] [dʌn] [bʌʔm]. This occurred despite the fact that he could produce all the phonemes that made up the word. When Jarrod imitated the word, his intelligibility improved. This is an important characteristic of inconsistent speech disorder and highlights the type of intervention needed to address the problem. Children with inconsistent speech disorder need to learn how to phonologically plan words rather than simply imitate words.

Read more about Jarrod (7;0 years), a boy with inconsistent speech disorder, in Chapter 16 (Case 3).

■ Speech sound disorders: Motor speech

Motor speech difficulties refer to problems with the coordination and production of precise mouth movements, respiration, resonance, and/or phonation required for fluent and rapid speech. To put it another way, children with motor speech difficulties have trouble performing the articulatory gestures necessary for speech production. Motor speech difficulties may be simple or complex. A simple motor speech difficulty can be isolated to a problem with the articulation of specific speech sounds. Complex motor speech difficulties and the APPLICATION box, referred to as motor speech disorders (MSD), encompass problems with one or more of the sensorimotor control processes needed to produce speech including motor planning, motor programming, and execution that disrupt the respiratory, phonatory, resonatory, and/or articulatory systems used in speech production (Duffy, 2013; van der Merwe, 2009). Motor speech disorders may "result from a speech production deficit arising from impairment of the motor system . . . MSDs may be caused by disruption of high-level motor commands, neuromuscular processes, or both" (Maas et al., 2008, p. 278). In this book we consider a simple motor speech difficulty (articulation impairment) and two motor speech disorders (**CAS** and **childhood dysarthria**). Principles of motor learning guide intervention for these three types of SSD.

 APPLICATION: *Jarrod, a child with an inconsistent speech disorder*

We introduced you to Jarrod in Chapter 1. Jarrod's speech was 88% inconsistent (Dodd, Holm, Crosbie, & McIntosh, 2006) on the Diagnostic Evaluation of Articulation and Phonology (DEAP): Inconsistency assessment (Dodd et al., 2002). What do you notice about his productions of the following words?

- *witch* /wɪtʃ/ → [bwːːætʃ] [bwæ] [bweʔt]
- *tongue* /tʌŋ/ → [bʌns] [dʌn] [bʌʔm]
- *zebra* /zebɹʌ/ → [dʒeuwa] [jeiʊa] [jeʔdwʌ] (Dodd, Holm, et al., 2006)

> **COMMENT:** *Undifferentiated tongue movements*
>
> There is evidence from instrumental studies that some children with SSD are unable to perform precise tongue movements required for fluent and rapid speech. For example, some children move their whole tongue using undifferentiated lingual gestures (Gibbon, 1999), and in doing so, they demonstrate poor control of the tongue tip and poor lateral bracing and are unable to anchor the sides of their tongue along their teeth during speech (McAuliffe & Cornwell, 2008). Chapter 4 provides more information.

Articulation impairment

Articulation impairment is a type of motor speech difficulty typically reserved for speech errors limited to rhotics and/or sibilants. Common clinical manifestations of articulation impairment include distortions such as labialized /ɹ/, derhotacized /ɹ, ɝ, ɚ/, and lateralized or dentalized sibilants (typically /s, z/) (Shriberg, 1993). An articulation impairment is also apparent when children present with substitutions of the developmentally easier consonant [w] for the developmentally later consonant /ɹ/ in words like *ring*, *rock*, and *rabbit* and/or substitutions of interdental fricatives [θ, ð] for /s, z/ (in the absence of other speech difficulties).

We identify distortion and substitution errors involving sibilants and/or rhotics as an articulation impairment for three reasons. First, accurate perceptual distinction between distortion and substitution errors (particularly involving /ɹ/) can be challenging, as expert listeners have difficulty reliably classifying such errors as distortions versus substitutions (McAllister Byun & Hitchcock, 2012). Second, if a school-age child is identified as having an articulation error reminiscent of a younger child with typically developing speech (such as the substitution of [w] for /ɹ/) then the older child's difficulty might be identified as an articulation delay. If a child presents with an error that is not observed in typical speech acquisition (such as lateralized /s/) then the error might be identified as an articulation disorder. In this book we use the term *articulation impairment*, given the challenge of perceptually differentiating substitution from distortion errors involving rhotics and sibilants, and the subsequent potential for confusion about whether such errors constitute delayed versus disordered articulation. Third, distortion and/or substitution errors involving sibilants and/or rhotics (in the absence of other speech difficulties) are suited to similar intervention approaches influenced by principles of motor learning (e.g., Hitchcock & McAllister Byun, 2015; McAllister Byun & Hitchcock, 2012; Skelton, 2004b).

Within this book, we use a narrower definition of articulation than has been used in the past. Prior to the 1970s and 1980s, the predominant view was that all children with SSD had difficulties with **articulation** of speech sounds, and a major emphasis of speech-language pathology practice was on children's production of individual speech sounds (articulation). By restricting the definition of articulation impairment in this book to those children who have difficulties only with sibilants and rhotics, we are limiting the co-occurrence of articulation and phonology. Typically, children with articulation impairment do not have a concurrent difficulty with phonology. They have learned the phonological system and can make themselves understood. Children with articulation impairment have difficulty with the articulation (i.e., physical production) of sibilants and/or rhotics (Shriberg, 2010a; Shriberg, Flipsen, Karlsson, & McSweeny, 2001).

The underlying cause of articulation impairment limited to sibilants and/or rhotics is not well understood. It has been suggested that for some children, the problem lies in their perception of the speech sounds in error (Shuster, 1998) or difficulties with oromotor structure (e.g., dental occlusion, facial nerve palsy). Some children and adolescents may have prior history of other speech difficulties whereas others do not (e.g., Karlsson, Shriberg, Flipsen, & McSweeny, 2002; McAllister Byun & Hitchcock, 2012; McAllister Byun, Hitchcock, & Swartz, 2014; Shriberg, Flipsen, et al., 2001). Acoustic studies of the sibilant and rhotic speech errors produced by children and/or adolescents with and without

COMMENT: *Terminology for articulation errors*

Some researchers differentiate between developmental articulation errors in childhood and **residual articulation errors** that continue to occur beyond 9 years of age and into adulthood (Shriberg, Austin, Lewis, McSweeny, & Wilson, 1997b; Van Borsel, Van Rentergem, & Verhaeghe, 2007). Residual articulation errors include common clinical distortions, particularly with /s/ produced as a lateral [ɬ] or interdental lisp [θ] and /ɹ/ produced as [w] or a derhotacized consonant [ʊ], and "residual common distortions and imprecise speech (omissions and substitutions)" (Shriberg et al., 1997b, p. 725). Other terms include:

- misarticulations;
- residual articulation errors;
- common clinical manifestations;
- residual common distortions; and
- persistent speech errors.

MULTILINGUAL INSIGHTS: *When saying [ɬi] for see /si/ might not be an articulation impairment*

A child who says *see* /si/ as [ɬi] and speaks both English and Welsh may not be considered as having an articulation impairment, since lateral fricatives are part of the Welsh consonant inventory. A comprehensive analysis of the child's speech would be needed to determine why one consonant from one language is present in spoken words in another language.

■ ▬ ■ ▬ ■ ▬ ■ ▬ ■ ▬ ■ ▬ ■ ▬ ■ ▬ ■ ▬ ■ ▬ ■ ▬ ■ ▬ ■ ▬ ■ ▬ ■ ▬ ■ ▬ ■ ▬ ■

 APPLICATION: *Susie, a child with an articulation impairment*

Susie is a 7-year-old girl with a lateral lisp. Review Susie's production of /s, z/ in single-words in singleton and consonant cluster contexts, in initial, medial, and final-word positions in Chapter 16. What do you notice?

Read more about Susie (7;4 years), a girl with an articulation impairment (lateral lisp), in Chapter 16 (Case 2).

prior history of speech difficulties suggest that certain acoustic markers can differentiate individuals according to their speech error history (i.e., no history versus past history) (Karlsson et al., 2002; Shriberg, Flipsen, et al., 2001). Typically, children with articulation impairment are intelligible, but their speech errors may impact acceptability or clarity. Whether or not children and adolescents require different approaches to intervention for sibilants and/or rhotic errors based on prior history remains to be determined. Contemporary intervention approaches for articulation impairment are offered based on the presence of sibilant/rhotic errors, not speech error history (e.g., McAllister Byun & Hitchcock, 2012; McAllister Byun et al., 2014).

Childhood apraxia of speech (CAS)

CAS refers to a subgroup of children with SSD who have a motor speech disorder involving planning and programming movement sequences (ASHA, 2007b; Ozanne, 2013). CAS occurs in approximately one to two children per thousand (Shriberg, Aram, & Kwiatkowski,

1997). There have been a range of terms to describe the speech difficulties of this group of children (including *developmental dyspraxia*, *developmental verbal dyspraxia*, and *developmental apraxia of speech*); however, this century, CAS has become the standard term. The following definition was prepared by a committee of the American Speech-Language-Hearing Association (ASHA) and states:

> Childhood apraxia of speech (CAS) is a neurological childhood (pediatric) SSD in which the precision and consistency of movements underlying speech are impaired in the absence of neuromuscular deficits (e.g., abnormal reflexes, abnormal tone). Childhood apraxia of speech may occur as a result of known neurological impairment, in association with complex neurobehavioral disorders of known or unknown origin, or as an idiopathic neurogenic speech sound disorder. The core impairment in planning and/or programming spatiotemporal parameters of movement sequences results in errors in speech sound production and prosody. (ASHA, 2007b, pp. 3–4)

This definition means that children with CAS tend to have: "(a) inconsistent errors on consonants and vowels in repeated productions of syllables or words, (b) lengthened and disrupted coarticulatory transitions between sounds and syllables, and (c) inappropriate prosody, especially in the realization of lexical or phrasal stress" (ASHA, 2007b, p. 4). It has been noted that although children with CAS have an underlying motor speech disorder, this may impact their phonological and linguistic processing (Maassen, 2002).

Childhood dysarthria

Dysarthria is the term applied to a subgroup of children (and adults) with motor speech disorders and is used to describe a disorder in the ability to control and execute speech movements. Dysarthria is caused by a neurological impairment and can be described as flaccid, spastic, hyperkinetic, hypokinetic, ataxic, or mixed. In children, this could occur during or after birth (e.g., cerebral palsy), through traumatic brain injury, or a neurological condition (e.g., neurofibromatosis) (Pennington, Miller, & Robson, 2009). Children (and adults) with dysarthria have "weakness, slowness, or incoordination of the musculature used to produce speech" (Kent, 2000, p. 399). The speech of children with dysarthria has been described as follows:

> Children with dysarthria often have shallow, irregular breathing and speak on small, residual pockets of air. They have low pitched, harsh voices, nasalized speech and very poor articulation. Together, these difficulties make the children's speech difficult to understand. (Pennington, Miller, & Robson, 2009, p. 1)

Dysarthria is not as common as most other types of SSD. For example, cerebral palsy occurs in approximately 2 per 1,000 births (Anderson, Mjoen, & Vik, 2010), and approximately 35% of these children have a speech difficulty (Parks, Hill, Platt, & Donnelly, 2010).

 APPLICATION: Michael, a child with CAS

Michael (4;2 years) has CAS. Review the speech sample for Michael in Chapter 16. Notice how Michael produces the words *birthday cake* /bɝθde kek/ as [bɜf.de.kek], [bɜf.de.keʔ], and [bɜp.de.kek]. What similarities and differences do you notice between Jarrod's and Michael's productions of the words *birthday cake*?

Answer:

Like Jarrod, Michael's speech can be inconsistent. However, unlike Jarrod, Michael struggles with prosodic aspects of speech. The dots between the syllables in *birthday cake* reflect syllable segregation or short pauses between the syllables. Jarrod does not have this difficulty.

Read more about Michael (4;2 years), a boy with childhood apraxia of speech (CAS), and Jarrod (7;0 years), a boy with inconsistent speech disorder, in Chapter 16.

✓ APPLICATION: Lian, a bilingual child with childhood dysarthria

Lian is a 14-year-old who speaks both English and Cantonese and has childhood dysarthria due to cerebral palsy (specifically, right-sided spastic hemiplegia). Review Lian's speech sample in Chapter 16. What do you notice about Lian's production of the word *Jenny* /dʒɛni/ as [tsɛ̃ni̯]? The diacritic symbol above the vowel indicates that there was audible nasal air emission on the vowel (Chapter 4). What do you think this suggests about Lian's oral musculature and function for speech?

Read more about Lian (14;2 years), a girl with childhood dysarthria, in Chapter 16 (Case 5).

Differentiating between inconsistent speech disorder, CAS, and childhood dysarthria

Inconsistent speech disorder, CAS, and childhood dysarthria share some similarities such as substitution errors and error inconsistency. However, they are different types of problems requiring different approaches to intervention. For instance, Shriberg et al. (2006) used several diagnostic features to differentiate between apraxia of speech and spastic dysarthria. They indicated that generally speech characteristics were not specific for either disorder. Both groups of children had speech difficulties that ranged from mild to severe and included inconsistent errors and distortion errors. However, there were differences between prosody and voice characteristics. Children with CAS had the following characteristics:

- prosody: inappropriate phrasing, rate, sentential stress, lexical stress, and emphatic stress; and
- voice: appropriate loudness, pitch, laryngeal quality, and resonance.

Children with spastic dysarthria had the following characteristics:

- prosody: inappropriate rate, sentential stress, *but* appropriate phrasing, lexical stress, and emphatic stress; and
- voice: inappropriate loudness (too soft), pitch (too low), laryngeal quality (harsh), and resonance (hypernasal).

In contrast, children with inconsistent speech disorder typically do not have difficulty with prosody, voice, and fluency (Bowen, 2009; Dodd, 2013). Their difficulty stems from a problem with **phonological planning** rather than **motor planning**, **motor programming**, or **execution**. In addition, the speech intelligibility of children with inconsistent speech disorder is better in imitated than spontaneous contexts; children with CAS are better in spontaneous than imitated contexts (Dodd, 2014).

COMMENT: Why consider different classification systems?

Children are different from one another; that is, they are heterogeneous. Researchers have been working to understand and classify different groups of children for a range of reasons. As mentioned earlier in this chapter, in this book we use a symptomatology classification so that we can direct readers to appropriate intervention approaches. Other researchers have classified children based on the cause of SSD, while others have classified children using an explanatory framework. Each is valid, depending on the purpose of classifying children.

CLASSIFICATION SYSTEMS OF CHILDREN WITH SSD

Children with SSD are heterogeneous. The conceptualization of SSD used in this book (Figure 2-1) and described earlier has been driven by a need for understanding assessment and intervention research about clinical practice. However, there are a number of other ways to classify children with SSD. Waring and Knight (2013) provided an overview of broad and specific classification systems that are used to describe and differentiate subgroups of children with SSD. We will discuss four of these:

- Speech Disorders Classification System (Shriberg, 2010a): an etiological framework for children with SSD;
- Differential Diagnosis System (Dodd, 1995a, 2005, 2013): a descriptive-linguistic framework for children with SSD;
- Psycholinguistic Framework (Stackhouse & Wells, 1997): a processing-based framework for children with SSD; and
- International Classification of Functioning, Disability and Health (ICF-CY) (World Health Organization, 2007): a biopsychosocial framework for all children (including those with SSD).

The first three of classification systems are based on a **medical model** where impairment is located within the child and intervention focuses on "objective, separable and controllable parts of communication" (Duchan, 2001, p. 41). Some of these classification systems incorporate a **social model**, which considers the personal and environmental contexts that contribute to and impact a child's life (Byng, 2001). The final classification system, ICF-CY (WHO, 2007), is based on a **biopsychosocial model** (Engel, 1977), since it systematically considers biological, psychological, and social factors and their complex interactions.

■ Speech Disorders Classification System (Shriberg, 1980; 2010a)

The Speech Disorders Classification System (SDCS) provides an etiological framework for children with SSD. The SDCS initially was described by Shriberg in 1980, and over the years Shriberg has conducted systematic research to further refine this classification system (e.g., Shriberg & Kwiatkowski, 1982a, b; Shriberg, 1993; Shriberg, Austin, et al., 1997a, b; Shriberg, 2010a; Shriberg, Fourakis, et al., 2010a, b). Shriberg and colleagues give the following overarching rationale for the development of the SDCS: "the assumption is that next-generation personalized medicine for assessment, treatment, and eventual prevention of diseases and disorders will require international classification systems based on biological phenotypes" (Shriberg, Fourakis, et al., 2010a, p. 796). The SDCS can be used to support molecular genetics research into SSD by categorizing "antecedents" (Shriberg, 1993, p. 105) and "etiologic subtypes" (Shriberg, 2010a, p. 4) or causes of SSD, and Shriberg's ongoing publications document his work towards the identification of phenotypes and endophenotypes for SSD (e.g., Shriberg, Lohmeier, Strand, & Jakielski, 2012). The original SDCS outlined 10 categories to classify speech disorders in people from 2 years to adulthood (Shriberg, 1980).

In 2010 Shriberg and colleagues (Shriberg, Fourakis, et al., 2010a) described the SDCS as comprising a typology and etiology (see Figure 2-2). In the typological classification system there are children who have normal speech acquisition (NSA), and three types of speech disorders:

- Speech Delay (SD) (occurring between 3 and 9 years);
- Motor Speech Disorder (MSD) (occurring between 3 and 9 years); or
- Speech Errors (SE) (occurring between 6 and 9 years).

From 9 years of age, children in any of these groups may have normalized speech acquisition (NSA). Alternatively, children may have persistent speech disorders that are associated with their original typology:

- Persistent Speech Disorders – Speech Delay (PSD-SD);
- Persistent Speech Disorders – Motor Speech Disorder (PSD-MSD); or
- Persistent Speech Disorders – Speech Errors (PSD-SE).

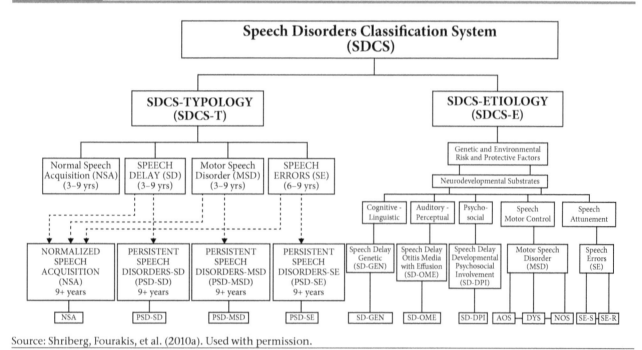

FIGURE 2-2 Speech Disorders Classification System

Source: Shriberg, Fourakis, et al. (2010a). Used with permission.

In the etiological classification system, the five etiologies (or causes) of SSD (Shriberg, Fourakis, et al., 2010a) are:

- Speech Delay – Genetic (SD-GEN): related to the cognitive/linguistic domain;
- Speech Delay – Otitis Media with Effusion (SD-OME): related to the auditory/perceptual domain;
- Speech Delay – Developmental Psychological Involvement (SD-DPI): related to the affective/temperamental domain;
- Motor Speech Disorder (MSD): related to the speech motor control domain and including Apraxia of Speech (AOS), Dysarthria (DYS), and Not Otherwise Specified (NOS); and
- Speech Errors (SE): related to speech attunement and including speech errors on sibilants (SE-S) and rhotics (SE-R).

These etiologies are described by Shriberg, Fourakis, et al. (2010a) as being overlapping, with origins in environmental and genetic domains.

Throughout the development of the SDCS, Shriberg and his colleagues created metrics and terminology that are now commonly used throughout the speech-language pathology profession, including:

- Percentage of Consonants Correct (PCC) (Shriberg & Kwiatkowski, 1982c; Shriberg, Austin, Lewis, McSweeny, & Wilson, 1997a);
- Articulation Competence Index (ACI) (Shriberg, 1993);
- Early-, middle-, and late-8 consonants (Shriberg, 1993); and
- Syllable Repetition Test (SRT) (Shriberg et al., 2009).

These and other assessment and analysis protocols have been described in the Madison Speech Assessment Protocol (MSAP) (Shriberg, Fourakis, et al., 2010a). You will learn more about early-, middle- and late-8 consonants in Chapter 6, assessments in Chapters 7 and 8, and how to calculate PCC and ACI in Chapter 9.

> **COMMENT:** *Incidence of subtypes of SSD based on Broomfield and Dodd (2004b)*
>
> Broomfield and Dodd (2004b) studied 1,100 children who were referred for speech-language pathology services in one region of the United Kingdom. There were 320 with SSD ("primary speech impairment") as their primary diagnosis. Of these 320 children:
>
> - 57.5% had phonological impairment;
> - 12.5% had articulation impairment;
> - 20.6% made consistent "nondevelopmental errors" (p. 135);
> - 9.4% made "inconsistent errors on the same lexical item" (p. 135); and
> - no children were diagnosed with CAS.

■ Differential Diagnosis System (Dodd, 1995a, 2005, 2013)

The Differential Diagnosis System (DDS) (Dodd, 1995a, 2005, 2013) provides a descriptive-linguistic framework for children with SSD. The DDS initially was developed to provide a surface-level classification of functional speech disorders with direct clinical application to decision-making regarding appropriate intervention techniques. The DDS comprises four subgroups:

- Articulation disorder: "an impaired ability to pronounce specific phonemes, usually /s/ or /r/" (Dodd, 2005, p. 9);
- Phonological delay: "all the error patterns . . . occur during normal development but are typical of younger children" (Dodd, 2005, p. 9);
- Consistent phonological disorder: "consistent use of some non-developmental error patterns" (Dodd, 2005, p. 9); and
- Inconsistent phonological disorder: "children's phonological systems show at least 40% variability (when asked to name the same 25 pictures on three separate occasions in one session)" (Dodd, 2005, p. 9).

In addition to the differences in the speech output of these groups of children, Crosbie, Holm, and Dodd (2009) found that children with consistent phonological disorder had greater difficulties with the executive functioning tasks of rule abstraction and cognitive flexibility than children with inconsistent phonological disorders.

Throughout the course of development of the Differential Diagnosis System, Dodd and colleagues developed assessments and intervention approaches to support the classification system that are commonly used throughout the speech-language pathology profession, including:

- Diagnostic Evaluation of Articulation and Phonology (DEAP, Dodd, Hua, et al., 2002, 2006); and
- Core vocabulary intervention for inconsistent speech disorder (Crosbie, Holm, & Dodd, 2005).

You will learn more about the DEAP in Chapter 8 and core vocabulary intervention in Chapter 13.

■ Psycholinguistic Framework (Stackhouse & Wells, 1997)

The Psycholinguistic Framework described by Stackhouse and Wells (1997) provides a processing-based framework to describe the speech and literacy skills of children with SSD. It was developed to explain rather than describe specific areas of difficulty for children with

SSD, and consequently to identify areas for intervention. The Psycholinguistic Framework draws on psycholinguistic explanations for children's speech perception and production that have been described for many years using box and arrow models (e.g., Smith, 1978; Menn, 1983; see Baker, Croot, McLeod, & Paul, 2001, for a review). The simplest version of the Psycholinguistic Framework is that a sound or word travels between a speaker and a listener along the following pathway: input → storage → output. In the case of speech, sound moves from the ear → brain → mouth, and in the case of writing (or sign language), words (or signs) move from the eye → brain → hand. Stackhouse and Wells (1997) developed this framework into the Speech Processing Model (see Figure 2-3), where an acoustic signal is heard as a sound (peripheral auditory processing), determined to be speech or not (speech/non-speech discrimination), and recognized as a word (phonological recognition). Stackhouse and Wells (1997) proposed a single underlying representation (called a lexical representation), represented by broad arrows and shaded boxes to indicate processes hypothesized to occur offline and including phonological and semantic representations. In order to produce speech, there is a pathway from motor programming, motor planning, and motor execution to speech input. Over the years, Stackhouse and Wells have created assessment and intervention resources to accompany the model (Pascoe, Wells, & Stackhouse, 2006; Stackhouse & Wells, 2001). The Psycholinguistic Framework is described in more depth in Chapter 5, and we illustrate how to address children's risk of literacy difficulties in Chapters 13 and 14.

FIGURE 2-3 **Speech processing model**

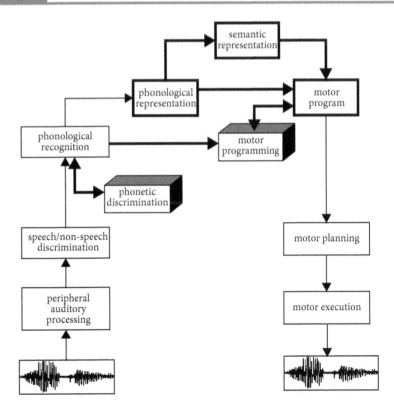

Source: From *Children's Speech and Literacy Difficulties: A Psycholinguistic Framework* (Figure 6.3 on page 166 and Appendix 4, p. 350) by J. Stackhouse and B. Wells, 1997. London, UK: Whurr. Copyright © 1997 John Wiley and Sons.

■ International Classification of Functioning, Disability and Health – Children and Youth Version (ICF-CY) (WHO, 2007)

The Children and Youth Version of the International Classification of Functioning, Disability and Health (ICF-CY) (World Health Organization, 2007) has been designed as a biopsychosocial framework for promoting and supporting health and wellness in children under 18 years (including those with SSD) so that they may participate fully in society. There are six interacting components of the ICF-CY (Figure 2-4):

- **Body Function:** "Physiological functions of body systems (including psychological functions)" (WHO, 2007, p. 9);
- **Body Structure:** "Anatomical parts of the body such as organs, limbs and their components" (WHO, 2007, p. 9);
- **Activity:** "The execution of a task or action by an individual" (WHO, 2007, p. 9);
- **Participation:** "Involvement in a life situation" (WHO, 2007, p. 9);
- **Environmental Factors:** "Make up the physical, social and attitudinal environment in which people live and conduct their lives" (WHO, 2007, p. 9). Environmental factors may be barriers or facilitators or both; and
- **Personal Factors:** Include "gender, race, age, other health conditions . . . habits, upbringing, coping styles, social background, education, . . . past and current experience . . . overall behavior pattern and character style . . ." (WHO, 2007, p. 15).

Each of these components are described by a set of codes that can be used for statistical and research purposes. The term SSD is not used within the ICF-CY (World Health Organization, 2007). Using the ICF nomenclature, the closest domain that encapsulates the notion of SSD would be an impairment of Voice and Speech Functions (b3), specifically Articulation function (b320). This in turn would have an impact on a child's Activities and Participation, particularly in the domain of Communication (d3).

The importance of the ICF-CY is that it presents a holistic framework for considering children in context. It focuses on capacity and performance and enables consideration of the impact of the environment and personal factors as either barriers or facilitators to functioning. As Tomblin and Christiansen (2010) argue, "the locus of the disorder in communication disorder will not be found in the characteristics or behavior of the individual but rather in the cultural context" (p. 40). The following core set of ICF-CY codes is suggested

FIGURE 2-4   **Interactions between the components of the International Classification of Functioning, Disability and Health – Children and Youth Version (ICF-CY)**

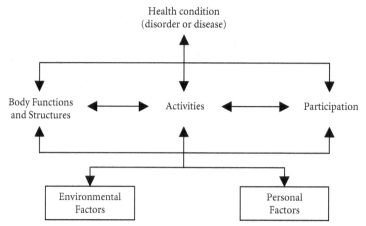

as a minimum for considering children with SSD (based on McLeod & McCormack, 2007). The most relevant codes are italicized:

- **Body Functions:** b117 Intellectual functions, b126 Temperament and personality functions, b230 Hearing functions, b1560 Auditory perception, b1670 Reception of language, b1671 Expression of language, b310 Voice functions, *b320 Articulation functions*, b330 Fluency and rhythm of speech functions;
- **Body Structures:** s1 Structure of nervous system, s240 Structure of external ear, s250 Structure of middle ear, s260 Structure of inner ear, s310 Structure of nose, *s320 Structure of mouth*, s330 Structure of pharynx, s340 Structure of larynx, s430 Structure of respiratory system;
- **Activities and Participation:** d1 Learning and applying knowledge (including d115 Listening, d140 Learning to read, d145 Learning to write), *d3 Communication* (including all domains), d6 Domestic life (including d660 Assisting others in communication), d7 Interpersonal interactions and relationships (including most domains), d810–820 Education, d9 Community, social and civic life;
- **Environmental Factors:** e1 Products and technology, e3 Support and relationships, e4 Attitudes, e5 Services, systems and policies; and
- **Personal Factors**

The ICF (World Health Organization, 2001) (the version for people 18+ years old) and the ICF-CY (World Health Organization, 2007) have been endorsed by many speech-language pathology professional associations throughout the world, including the American Speech-Language Hearing Association (ASHA), Speech-Language and Audiology Canada (previously known as Canadian Association of Speech-Language Pathologists and Audiologists, CASLPA), International Association of Logopedics and Phoniatrics (IALP), Royal College of Speech and Language Therapists (RCSLT), and Speech Pathology Australia (SPA). For example, ASHA endorsed the ICF in the Scope of Practice in Speech-Language Pathology (ASHA, 2007a), where they indicate, "The ICF framework is useful in describing the breadth of the role of the speech-language pathologist in the prevention, assessment, and habilitation/rehabilitation, enhancement, and scientific investigation of communication and swallowing." In addition, the ICF-CY specifically has been applied to children with SSD. For example, McLeod (2006b) considered a 7-year-old child, Jarrod, and classified each aspect of his case history and assessment using ICF-CY codes. A case study of Jarrod is found in Chapter 16. Neumann and Romonath (2012) applied the ICF-CY to children with cleft lip and palate. McLeod and Threats (2008) provided an extensive appendix where common assessments for children with SSD were classified using ICF-CY codes. We will consider the use of ICF-CY in assessments in Chapters 7 and 8. McLeod and Bleile (2004) provided recommendations for how to create goals for children with SSD that were focused on both the individual and society (community) in which they function, and we will consider goal setting using the ICF-CY in Chapter 10. McCormack, McLeod, McAllister, and Harrison (2009) conducted a review of the outcomes for children with SSD using the ICF-CY as the framework and identified that SSD in childhood may be associated with the following Activity Limitations and/or Participation Restrictions: d140 Learning to read, d166 Reading, d145 Learning to write, d170 Writing, d160 Focusing attention, d163 Thinking, d172 Calculating, d3 Communication, d4 Mobility, d5 Self-care, d7400 Relating to persons in authority, d7500 Informal relationships with friends, d7504 Informal relationships with peers, d7600 Parent-child relationships, d7602 Sibling relationships, d820 School education, and d845 Acquiring, keeping and terminating a job. This list demonstrates both the breadth of information that can be captured using the ICF-CY and the breadth of impact of SSD that was discussed in Chapter 1.

Read more about Jarrod (7;0 years), a boy with inconsistent speech disorder, in Chapter 16 (Case 3).

SSD of Known and Unknown Origins

The majority of children with SSD have what Shriberg and colleagues have termed "speech sound disorders of currently unknown origin" (Shriberg et al., 2005, p. 834). That is, at the moment there is no known cause for the majority of children's SSD. Known causes of SSD include genetic syndromes, craniofacial anomalies, hearing loss, cognitive/intellectual impairment, motor impairment, and there is some evidence that children with autism can have SSD. With the advance of genetic research it is proposed that additional causes or genetic pathways for SSD may be uncovered. For children with currently unknown origins, a number of risk and protective factors for SSD have been identified (see Chapter 1).

■ SSD of known origins

Some of the known origins of SSD may include:

- genetic causes, including genetic syndromes (e.g., cri du chat syndrome);
- craniofacial anomalies (e.g., cleft palate);
- cognitive/intellectual impairment (e.g., Down syndrome);
- hearing loss (e.g., sensorineural hearing loss);
- motor impairment (e.g., cerebral palsy); and
- autism spectrum disorders.

Children with known origins for SSD often receive services from health professionals such as doctors, psychologists, and audiologists from an early age. Thus, it is likely that the children will be referred earlier to speech-language pathology, and potentially receive an earlier identification of SSD. For this reason, if you are working with a child who has a known origin for his or her SSD, source journal articles and textbooks about the specific area. For example, there are many textbooks that specifically discuss children with cleft palate (e.g., *Cleft Palate and Craniofacial Anomalies* by Kummer, 2014; *Cleft Palate Speech* by Peterson-Falzone, Hardin-Jones, & Karnell, 2010).

Children with identified genetic causes

The human genome comprises DNA (deoxyribonucleic acid) consisting of 23 pairs of chromosomes and approximately 20,500 genes (National Human Genome Research Institute, 2012). While 99% of our genome is shared with other humans, differences lie in the remaining 1% (Ng et al., 2009). To identify genetic causes of diseases and disorders, researchers consider the association between the genotype (genetic makeup) and phenotype (observable behavior). For many years, SLPs have suspected genetic associations with SSD, especially considering the high number of males with SSD and familial aggregation of SSD is common. In 2001 a breakthrough in genetic research impacted the speech-language pathology profession. The *FOXP2* gene was announced as being associated with speech and language (Lai, Fisher, Hurst, Vargha-Khadem, & Monaco, 2001). This breakthrough was made across three generations of one family known as the KE family. Affected members of this family had difficulties with orofacial movements that were described as "developmental verbal dyspraxia" (Lai et al., 2001, p. 519), as well as difficulties with processing language and grammar. Later, Shriberg and colleagues speculated that affected members of the KE family "may have some form of dysarthria as well as some type of craniofacial dysmorphology" (Shriberg et al., 2006, p. 501). Subsequently, Shriberg et al. (2006) described the TB family as possibly having similar speech characteristics to the KE family. The mother and daughter of the TB family had "a breakpoint in a balanced 7;13 chromosomal translocation that disrupted the transcription gene, *FOXP2*" (Shriberg et al., 2006, p. 500) and were described as having "spastic dysarthria, an apraxia of speech, and residual developmental distortion errors" (p. 500) as well as difficulties with orofacial movements and speech motor control.

These breakthroughs have led to a greater understanding of the complex link between SSD and genetics. Morgan (2013) summarized genetics research and indicated that at least five chromosomes have been associated with speech difficulties:

- chromosome 1 (Miscimarra et al., 2007);
- chromosome 3 (Stein et al., 2004) and 3p14 (Horn et al., 2010; Pariani, Spencer, Graham, & Rimoin, 2009; Vernes et al., 2008);
- chromosome 6p (Smith, Pennington, Boada, & Shriberg, 2005);
- chromosome 7 (Lai et al., 2001); and
- chromosome 15q (Smith et al., 2005).

From current understanding, the gene *FOXP1* on chromosomal region 3p14 has the strongest association with SSD, but it should be noted that, in addition to SSD, *FOXP1* also is associated more broadly with autism spectrum disorders and cognitive impairment (Bacon & Rappold, 2012; Morgan, 2013).

Some genetic syndromes are associated with children having difficulty with speech sound production and include:

- Beckwith Wiedemann syndrome (Shipster, Oliver, & Morgan, 2006);
- Coffin-Siris syndrome (Swillen, Glorieux, Peeters, & Fryns, 1995);
- Cri du chat syndrome (Kristoffersen, 2008; Kristoffersen, Garmann, & Simonsen, 2014);
- Down syndrome (Kent & Vorperian, 2013; Sokol & Fey, 2013);
- Fragile X syndrome (Barnes et al., 2009);
- Galactosemia (Shriberg, Potter, & Strand, 2011);
- Joubert syndrome (Braddock, Farmer, Deidrick, Iverson, & Maria, 2006);
- Nager syndrome (Vallino, Peterson-Falzone, & Napoli, 2006);
- Nemaline myopathy (Bagnall, Al-Muhaizea, & Manzur, 2006);
- Rett syndrome (Woodyatt & Ozanne, 1992);
- Silver-Russell syndrome (Lai, Skuse, Stanhope, & Hindmarsh, 1994);
- Treacher Collins syndrome (Vallino, Peterson-Falzone, & Napoli, 2006); and
- Velocardiofacial syndrome (22q11.2 deletion syndrome) (Mills, Gosling, & Sell, 2006).

Many children with these syndromes have concomitant cognitive impairment and/or craniofacial anomalies.

The speech of children with cri du chat syndrome provides one example of the association between genetic syndromes and SSD. Kristoffersen (2008) reviewed publications about the speech and language of children with cri du chat syndrome and concluded that "substitutions, omissions, and distortions are frequent; consonant inventories are small; syllable shapes are restricted; and vowels are variable and overlap with each other acoustically" (p. 443). Consequently, SLPs play an important role in supporting children and their families with genetic syndromes that manifest with SSD.

Children with craniofacial anomalies

Orofacial clefting is one of the most common craniofacial conditions that can be associated with SSD. However, children also may have a cleft lip (unilateral or bilateral), a submucous cleft palate (either overt or occult), or anomalies extending to other parts of the face and jaw. Multidisciplinary team–based management, including surgical repair of structural anomalies, is available in many countries for very young children with craniofacial conditions. SLPs are members of craniofacial teams alongside surgeons, audiologists, orthodontists, psychologists, and other health professionals. With surgery and intervention, acceptable and intelligible speech is an achievable goal for most children with craniofacial anomalies (Van Demark, 1997). Children with cleft lip and palate have been identified as having:

- increased nasal resonance (hypernasality);
- abnormal nasal airflow during speech (including nasal emission and/or nasal turbulence);
- compensatory (active) and/or obligatory (passive) speech characteristics;
- voice disorder;
- reduced complexity of babbling;
- reduced consonant inventory size (especially high-pressure oral consonants);
- delayed onset in transitioning to first words; and
- slow early vocabulary acquisition
  (Chapman, Hardin-Jones, & Halter, 2003; Harding & Grunwell, 1998; Jones, Chapman, & Hardin-Jones, 2003; Scherer, Williams, & Proctor-Williams, 2008; Zajac, 2013).

Although young children with cleft lip and palate are reported to vocalize as frequently as children without clefts, their vocalizations are typically less complex (Scherer, Williams, & Proctor-Williams, 2008) and they are at increased risk for speech and language delay (Scherer, D'Antonio, & Kalbfleisch, 1999). There is some evidence to suggest that 1- to 2-year-old children with cleft lip and palate use nonverbal communicative behaviors (gestures) to a greater extent than typically developing children do to supplement their conversational attempts (Scherer, Boyce, & Martin, 2013). Therefore, consideration of gesture, complexity of babbling, first word transition, and consonant inventory size is relevant when considering whether young children with cleft lip and palate have SSD. Reduced intraoral pressure in children with craniofacial anomalies may result in abnormal nasal airflow and nasalization of voiced plosives and fricatives (Sweeney & Sell, 2008; Zajac, 2013). Compensatory (active) speech characteristics occur when specific articulatory gestures replace intended consonants (e.g., glottal stop substitution, atypically backed distortions) (Harding & Grunwell, 1998). Obligatory (passive) speech characteristics include audible nasal emission of high-pressure consonants (stops, fricatives, and affricates) (Harding & Grunwell, 1998).

Children with cognitive/intellectual impairment

Some children with communication impairment have associated cognitive/intellectual impairment. For example, in a large study that included 1,667 children with communication impairment in the United States, 4% were identified with an intellectual impairment (Pinborough-Zimmerman et al., 2007). In another large study that included 1,862 children with communication impairment in Australia, there was a highly significant association that students identified as having an intellectual impairment were also identified as having a communication impairment (McLeod & McKinnon, 2007).

There have been few studies that specifically have considered SSD in children with cognitive/intellectual impairment apart from those with identified genetic syndromes. One of the most described genetic syndromes co-occurring with cognitive/intellectual impairment is Down syndrome. Kent and Vorperian (2013) conducted a systematic review of voice, speech sounds, fluency, prosody, and intelligibility in individuals with Down syndrome. They concluded, "Children and adults with this syndrome face serious challenges in spoken communication, which may substantially interfere with their participation in social, educational, and vocational activities. The difficulties in communication are rooted in virtually all aspects of speech production . . ." (p. 189). Included in the systematic review was a summary of 45 studies that considered aspects of SSD (articulation, phonology, and resonance) and oromotor functioning in over 700 individuals with Down syndrome. They indicated that by 3 years of age delayed and disordered speech sounds were evident in children with Down syndrome, and variability in speech productions was evident on acoustic analysis. They also indicated that severity of SSD in children with Down syndrome was not highly correlated with measures of cognition or language, and may in part be related to anatomical differences (e.g., large tongue). Additionally, they suggested that there is some evidence that children with Down syndrome show differences in canonical babbling compared with typically developing peers. Sokol and Fey (2013) compared the speech of 26 two-year-old children with Down syndrome and 22 children who had similar cognitive and communication impairment but did not have Down syndrome (the majority with unknown etiology). They found that at 2 years of age the two groups of children had similar consonant inventory size, syllable shape complexity, and number of communication acts with canonical vocalizations. For example, stops and nasals were more prevalent than fricatives, affricates, and liquids. Whereas, 18 months later, the children with Down syndrome were not performing as well as the group who did not have Down syndrome. Reasons for this difference were hypothesized to include increased occurrence of otitis media, hypotonicity, and anatomical variations (cf. Cleland, Wood, Hardcastle, Wishart, & Timmins, 2010).

Children with hearing loss

The ability to hear includes sound detection, sound discrimination, localization of the sound source, lateralization of sound, and speech discrimination (World Health Organization, 2007, p. 65). A number of types of hearing loss have been described:

■ conductive hearing loss: reduced or distorted transmission of the sound through the external and middle ear (e.g., otitis media, atresia);
■ sensorineural hearing loss: reduced or distorted transmission of the sound in the inner ear (cochlea, cochlear hair cells, or auditory nerves);

■ mixed hearing loss: difficulty perceiving sound that has both a conductive and sensorineural component; and

■ retrocochlear and central auditory hearing loss: difficulty with interpreting sound occurs along the auditory pathway (e.g., auditory neuropathy, central auditory processing disorder) (Northern & Downs, 2002; Rance et al., 2007; Rappaport & Provencal, 2002).

Children with significant hearing loss (sometimes called children who are deaf and hard of hearing) may communicate with oral (i.e., speech), manual (e.g., sign), or mixed communication (oral and manual) modes. For example, in a population study of 406 three-year-old Australian children with hearing loss, the majority (75.3%) used oral communication only, regardless of whether they used a hearing aid or had a cochlear implant. Almost a quarter of children (23.9%) used mixed communication at home, and only 3 (0.7%) exclusively used manual communication (Crowe, McLeod, & Ching, 2012).

Children who have hearing loss can have difficulty perceiving and producing speech sounds, regulating prosody, and being intelligible. In addition, children with hearing loss may have delayed phonological awareness skills and have more difficulty on formal testing that assesses phonemes compared with formal testing that measures words, rhymes, and syllables (Webb & Lederberg, 2014). A cross-linguistic systematic review of 117 studies describing speech and language outcomes for children with hearing loss who spoke one or more of 20 languages revealed that better outcomes were associated with less severe hearing loss, earlier age of diagnosis of hearing loss, use of oral communication, earlier age of amplification, and type of amplification (cochlear implants or hearing aids) (Crowe & McLeod, 2014). Typically, speech intelligibility was better in children with cochlear implants than those using hearing aids (e.g., Van Lierde, Vinck, Baudonck, De Vel, & Dhooge, 2005). With early identification, early amplification, and early intervention, the prognosis for children with hearing loss continues to improve. For example, researchers who studied 12 preschool children with early identified severe to profound hearing loss indicated that their speech (including production of consonant clusters and morphophonemes), receptive language, and expressive language was within normal limits and "commensurate with expectations for typically-developing hearing peers" (Fulcher, Baker, Purcell, & Munro, 2014, p. 69).

Children with otitis media with effusion (OME)

There is continuing debate over the relationship between SSD and otitis media with effusion (OME, also called middle-ear infection or glue ear) (Roberts, Rosenfeld, & Zeisel, 2004). Campbell et al. (2003) did not support a link between speech delay at 3 years of age and an abnormal hearing test or an incidence of otitis media with effusion between 6 and 18 months. Shriberg, Friel-Patti, Flipsen, and Brown (2000) considered the speech outcomes of children aged 3, and stated that the risk of SSD for children with hearing levels greater than 20dB at 12–18 months was 33%. Similar results were obtained in a prospective study by Miccio, Gallagher, Grossman, Yont, and Vernon-Feagans (2001). Shriberg, Flipsen, et al. (2000) indicated that there was an increased risk of SSD for children of Native American background with otitis media with effusion. Roberts et al. (2004) conducted 11 meta-analyses regarding the association between OME and various aspects of speech and language. Overall, they found that hearing, but not OME, was a significant predictor in outcomes. One of the meta-analyses was based on three studies specifically relating to speech output (Paradise, Dollaghan, et al., 2000; Paradise, Feldman, et al., 2001; Shriberg, Friel-Patti, et al., 2000). The conclusion by Roberts et al. (2004) was that there was "no association between OME and speech development at 3 years old" (p. e242). However, they recommended hearing screening be conducted to ensure an optimal language and learning environment.

Children with motor impairment such as cerebral palsy

Children with impaired motor skills, such as those with cerebral palsy, early onset muscular dystrophy, and conditions such as Moebius syndrome (which affects the cranial nerves) can have dysarthric speech as a result of weakness, slowness, and lack of tone in their muscles for respiration and speech (Hodge, 2010). Cerebral palsy is the most common cause of severe motor impairment in young children, and up to 60% of children with cerebral palsy can have communication impairment (Bax, Tydeman, & Flodmark, 2006). Hustad, Gorton, and Lee (2010) developed four categories of communication profiles for children with cerebral palsy, with speech variables accounting for 93% of the variance. They were:

■ no evidence of speech-motor involvement (NSMI);
■ evidence of speech-motor involvement, typically developing language ability (SMI-LCT);
■ evidence of speech-motor involvement and language impairment (SMI-LCI); and
■ anarthria, unable to produce functional speech (ANAR).

Read more about
Lian (14;2 years),
a girl with childhood
dysarthria,
in Chapter 16 (Case 5).

Children in the SMI-LCT and SMI-LCI groups had slower speech rate, smaller vowel spaces, and lower intelligibility ratings than those in the NSMI group (Hustad et al., 2010). Additionally, for children in the SMI-LCT and SMI-LCI groups, intelligibility decreased (or fluctuated) as the length of the utterance increased (Hustad, Schueler, Schultz, & DuHadway, 2012). Throughout this book, additional information about childhood dysarthria will be presented, and this information will be relevant to many children with cerebral palsy, particularly those within the SMI-LCT and SMI-LCI groups.

Children with autism spectrum disorders

Most research regarding the communication of children with autism spectrum disorders (ASD) typically reports difficulties with social and language skills (Tomblin, 2011). Some researchers who have considered the speech of children with ASD have indicated that "articulation skills were spared" (Kjelgaard & Tager-Flusberg, 2001, p. 287) and that expressive and receptive prosody is similar to typically developing peers (Grossman, Bemis, Plesa Skwerer, & Tager-Flusberg, 2010). However, other researchers have found that children with ASD can have difficulty producing speech sounds (e.g., Cleland, Gibbon, Peppé, O'Hare, & Rutherford, 2010; Rapin, Dunn, Allen, Stevens, & Fein, 2009). For example, Cleland et al. (2010) considered the speech of 5- to 13-year-old children in the United Kingdom: 30 with high-functioning autism and 39 with Asperger syndrome. Overall, 41% of the children produced at least some speech errors (e.g., cluster reduction, gliding, final consonant deletion, and non-developmental distortions such as nasal emission) and 12% were identified with SSD. The same research team compared the prosodic abilities of 31 children with high-functioning autism and 72 typically developing children and found that the children with ASD had significantly poorer prosodic skills than the control group (McCann, Peppé, Gibbon, O'Hare, & Rutherford, 2007). Occasionally, children with SSD can be misdiagnosed as having ASD if the children are difficult to test and have a family history of ASD (e.g., Camarata, 2014).

Other known causes

There are other known causes for SSD that do not fit in the categories above. For example, in a study of 108 children with SSD (+/– language impairment), children with SSD and language impairment have been found to have increased risk for attention-deficit/hyperactivity disorder (McGrath et al., 2008). Additionally, children have been reported to have difficulty producing consonants after severe traumatic brain injury (TBI) (Campbell et al., 2013). In a longitudinal study of 56 children aged between 1 and 11 years who experienced TBI, gains in percentage of consonants correct was associated with the age of the child and severity of the injury. Younger children whose consonant inventory was still developing at the time of the injury were more likely to be affected (Campbell et al., 2013).

CO-OCCURRENCE OF SSD WITH OTHER TYPES OF COMMUNICATION IMPAIRMENT

Speech is only one aspect of communication (see Chapter 1). Children do not fit neatly into boxes, and many children with SSD have co-occurring difficulties with other aspects of communication. Next we will consider co-occurrence of speech, language, literacy, oromotor, and voice difficulties and stuttering. We have discussed co-occurrence of SSD with hearing difficulties previously in this chapter. However, it is important to note that the interaction can extend further than two ways. For example, Shriberg, Friel-Patti, et al. (2000) found that language skills had a significant mediating effect on the speech of children with hearing loss: a three-way interaction between speech, language, and hearing.

■ Co-occurrence of SSD and language impairment

The correlation between speech and language in the early years has been supported in many studies of young children's speech acquisition (Stoel-Gammon, 2011). In a study of 1,127 children who were 25 months old, children whose language was at the single-word stage had more phonological errors than children whose language was at the two- or four-word stage (Roulstone, Loader, Northstone, Beveridge, & the ALSPAC team, 2002). For example, when Roulstone et al. considered fricative production, children whose language was at the single-word stage had 61% errors; children at the two-word utterance stage had 48% errors; while children at the three- to four-word utterance stage only had 30% errors. Similarly, children with precocious language skills (advanced vocabulary) had phonological skills that were superior to their age-matched peers and similar to their language-matched peers (Smith, McGregor, & Demille, 2006).

Children with SSD can have concomitant difficulties with expressive and/or receptive language. Shriberg and Kwiatkowski (1994) studied 178 children with SSD and found that 50–70% had expressive language problems and 10–40% had expressive and receptive language problems. Aguilar-Mediavilla, Sanz-Torrent, and Serra-Raventos (2002) studied the phonology of two groups of children with specific language impairment (SLI) and language delay (LD) at age 3 and compared them with two control groups based on age and language level. They found that children with SLI and LD showed a delay in the acquisition of many aspects of phonology compared with their age-matched control group. However, children with SLI also displayed significant differences compared to their language-matched control group in the acquisition of early phonological structures such as vowels, nasals, stops, and consonant-vowel syllable structures. Deletion of unstressed syllables was more prevalent in the children with SLI than those in the language-matched control group. Macrae and Tyler (2014) studied 28 children aged 3;6 to 5;5 in two groups: 13 children with SSD only and 15 children with SSD plus language impairment (LI). The children with SSD+LI presented with more omissions and fewer distortions than the children with SSD only, whereas there was no significant difference in the substitutions or the use of typical or atypical error patterns.

■ Co-occurrence of SSD and literacy difficulties

Children with SSD are more likely to have difficulties with phonological awareness and literacy (reading and spelling) than their typically developing peers (Anthony et al., 2011; Bird, Bishop, & Freeman, 1995; Foy & Mann, 2012; Larrivee & Catts, 1999; Raitano et al., 2004). According to the **critical age hypothesis**, children who still have SSD at the beginning of literacy instruction (around 5 years old) are most at risk of having literacy difficulties (Bishop & Adams, 1990; Nathan, Stackhouse, Goulandris, & Snowling, 2004a). Researchers have demonstrated that underlying phonological processing skills (specifically, the quality and accessibility of phonological representations) may explain difficulties in phonological awareness and reading for children with SSD (Anthony et al., 2011).

Children are likely to have greater difficulties on phonological awareness tasks if they exhibit atypical or non-developmental speech errors (Leitão & Fletcher, 2004; Preston & Edwards, 2010; Rvachew, Chiang, & Evans, 2007), and children with CAS can have difficulties with phonological awareness, reading, and spelling (Gillon & Moriarty, 2007; McNeill, Gillon, & Dodd, 2009a). Children with SSD and concomitant language impairment are at greater risk of having difficulties with phonological awareness, reading, and writing than those who only have SSD (Lewis, Freebairn, & Taylor, 2002; Peterson, Pennington, Shriberg, & Boada, 2009; Preston & Edwards, 2010; Raitano et al., 2004; Sices et al., 2007). For example, Preston and Edwards (2010) studied 43 children with SSD and found that vocabulary and age predicted 33% of variance in the phonological awareness composite score, and an additional 6% of the variance was accounted for by the production of atypical errors.

■ Co-occurrence of SSD and oromotor difficulties

Previously in this chapter we considered the impact of orofacial anomalies (e.g., cleft palate) on children's speech. Known structural causes of SSD attest to the co-occurrence of SSD and oromotor difficulties. Children with motor speech disorders, including CAS and childhood dysarthria, can have difficulties with oromotor functioning. For example, children with CAS can have difficulty producing speech and non-speech oromotor movements on command (Ozanne, 2013). Children with childhood dysarthria can have difficulty with non-speech oromotor functions such as drinking, eating, and controling saliva (Hodge, 2010). Children with SSD of unknown origin also can have co-occurring difficulties with oromotor functioning. For example, McCabe, Rosenthal, and McLeod (1998) found that 32% of 50 children with SSD had "oral apraxia/problems with oral volitional movement" (p. 112). Children with speech and language impairment have greater difficulty with isolated and repeated oral movement tasks than typically developing children (Stark & Blackwell, 1997).

■ Co-occurrence of SSD and voice difficulties

There are few reports of the co-occurrence of SSD and voice difficulties. Warr-Leeper, McShea, and Leeper (1979) indicated that of 107 US children in grades 6 to 8, 6% demonstrated "inadequate articulation and voice," 37% demonstrated "inadequate articulation," and 48% demonstrated "inadequate voice" (p. 16). The main area of overlap between SSD and voice occurs when prosody is considered. As we will learn in Chapter 4, prosody includes stress, rhythm, intonation, and lexical and grammatical tones. Children may have increased difficulty with prosody-voice characteristics if they have phonological impairment (Shriberg, 1993), CAS (Odell & Shriberg, 2001), childhood dysarthria (Hodge, 2010), or hearing loss (Lenden & Flipsen, 2007).

■ Co-occurrence of SSD and stuttering

The co-occurrence of SSD and stuttering is described frequently, with up to 30–40% of children who stutter reported to have co-occurring SSD (Nippold, 2002). For example, in a study of 2,628 children who stuttered, SSD was the most frequently co-occurring disorder, with 33.5% being identified with "articulation disorders" and 12.7% with "phonology disorders" (Blood, Ridenour, Qualls, & Hammer, 2003, p. 427). Arndt and Healey (2001) surveyed 241 SLPs from 10 US states who described 467 children who stuttered on their caseloads. Of these, 205 children had verified concomitant disorders: 66 (32%) had verified phonological disorders, and 67 (33%) had verified phonological and language disorders. In addition, of the 109 children with suspected concomitant disorders, 13% had suspected phonological disorders.

The type of stuttering has been found to be different between children who do and do not have concomitant SSD. For example, preschool children who stuttered and had SSD produced more sound prolongations and fewer iterations per whole-word repetition than children who stuttered and did not have concomitant SSD (Wolk, Edwards, & Conture, 1993). Nippold (2004) indicated that children who stuttered and had a concomitant disorder such as SSD were more likely to be provided with intervention. While many SLPs treat stuttering and speech separately (Unicomb, Hewat, Spencer, & Harrison, 2013), some interventions to simultaneously treat stuttering and speech have been found to be feasible and effective (Conture, Louko, & Edwards, 1993), and children's phonological development does not predict the length of time required for stuttering intervention (Rousseau, Packman, Onslow, Harrison, & Jones, 2007).

The reason for the association between SSD and stuttering has been considered in a number of studies throughout the world. Phonetic and phonotactic complexity of words has been found to have an impact on the occurrence and type of stuttering, particularly for those over 6 years of age (Howell, Au-Yeung, Yaruss, & Eldridge, 2006). Increased stuttering was found to be associated with the phonetic complexity of words (based on place of articulation, manner of articulation, word length, word shape, and consonant length) in a study of children and adults (aged 6 to 18+ years) who stuttered and spoke Jordanian Arabic (Al-Tamimi, Khamaiseh, & Howell, 2013). Increased stuttering was found in phonetically complex German content words, but not German function words (Dworzynski & Howell, 2004). In a study that compared English-speaking preschoolers who stuttered with those who did not stutter, researchers found that place of articulation contributed to the disruption of fluency (Chang, Ohde, & Conture, 2002). In another study of English-speaking preschool children who stuttered, there was no increase in the overall susceptibility of words to stuttering based on phonotactic probability (e.g., word length, familiarity); however, phonotactic probability had an impact on the type of disfluency (Anderson & Byrd, 2008). Howell et al. (2006) indicated that factors that were most likely to lead to stuttering in English were, in order: "consonant by manner, consonant by place, word length, and contiguous consonant clusters" (p. 703). You will learn about manner and place in Chapter 4. Contiguous consonant clusters are two consonants produced together that are in the same place of articulation (e.g., /sn, ld/).

Despite many studies demonstrating that children who stutter can have speech difficulties, the link between phonology and stuttering has been questioned in studies that have compared the speech skills of children who do and do not stutter. Clark, Conture, Walden, and Lambert (2013) compared 277 preschool children's scores on the Goldman-Fristoe Test of Articulation-2 (GFTA-2) (Goldman & Fristoe, 2000) and found that there was no significant difference between the scores of 128 children who stuttered and 149 children who did not stutter. Furthermore, Gregg and Yairi (2007) studied two groups of 29 preschool children separated according to whether they exhibited "minimal phonological deviations" or "moderate phonological deviations" (p. 97). There was no difference in the amount of stuttering between the two groups.

Chapter summary

In this chapter you learned that SSD is an umbrella term for phonological impairment, inconsistent speech disorder, articulation impairment, CAS, and childhood dysarthria. You also learned four ways to classify children with SSD: Speech Disorders Classification System (Shriberg, 1980, 2010a), Differential Diagnosis System (Dodd, 1995a, 2005, 2013), Psycholinguistic Framework (Stackhouse & Wells, 1997), and the International Classification of Functioning, Disability and Health – Children and Youth Version (ICF-CY) (WHO, 2007). You learned that most children with SSD have no known origin; however, some of the known origins include genetic causes, craniofacial anomalies, and hearing loss. Finally, you learned about the co-occurrence of SSD with language impairment, literacy difficulties, oromotor difficulties, voice difficulties, and stuttering.

Suggested reading

This following text contains information on SSD classification systems and insights into genetics research and concomitant conditions observed in children with SSD (e.g., language impairment, traumatic brain injury, autism, hearing impairment).

■ Paul, R., & Flipsen, P., Jr. (Eds.). (2010). *Speech sound disorders in children: In honor of Lawrence D. Shriberg.* San Diego, CA: Plural Publishing.

Application of knowledge from Chapter 2

1. Discuss the similarities and differences between the Speech Disorders Classification System (Shriberg, 2010a), the Differential Diagnosis System (Dodd, 1995a, 2005, 2013), the Psycholinguistic Framework (Stackhouse & Wells, 1997), and the International Classification of Functioning, Disability and Health (ICF-CY) (World Health Organization, 2007) for describing SSD in children.
   a. Which system do you think would be most helpful for families to understand the impact of SSD on children?
   b. Which system do you think would be most helpful for identifying causes of SSD?
2. Prepare a brochure for families about the five types of SSD described in this chapter. Assume you are preparing it for Luke, Susie, Jarrod, Michael, and Lian's families (i.e., the case study children in Chapter 16). As part of your brochure, include a description of each type of SSD, the underlying nature of the problem, and information about possible causes. Make sure you note that for many children with SSD, there is no known cause for the problem.

3

Articulatory Foundations of Speech

LEARNING OBJECTIVES

1. Describe the anatomical structures involved in the production of speech: tongue, lips, nose, teeth, hard palate, soft palate, mandible, pharynx, and larynx.

2. Draw a schematic sagittal section of the head showing articulators and places of articulation.

3. Predict possible impacts of structural problems with the hard and soft palate on children's speech production.

4. Describe the ear, the primary anatomical structure involved in the detection of speech.

5. Describe the neurological and respiratory systems that support speech production and perception.

6. Predict the impact of neurological impairments on children's articulation, phonation, resonance, and respiration.

KEY WORDS

Structures involved in speech production: tongue, lips, teeth, mandible (jaw), hard palate, soft palate (velum), nose, pharynx, larynx, respiratory system

Structure involved in speech perception: ear

Structures involved in speech perception and production: neurological system

OVERVIEW

In order to work with children with SSD it is helpful to have a clear understanding of how speech sounds are produced and perceived. This chapter introduces important anatomical structures for speech production and perception. The mechanisms of speech production and speech perception paradoxically are both simple and complex. A sound or word travels between a speaker and a listener, moving from the brain → mouth → ear → brain (see Figure 3-1). The steps that are involved are as follows: speech occurs when a person decides to communicate a message (e.g., the person wants to say the word *sun*). In order to do this, a person retrieves the word from his or her brain (and the series of sounds /s/ /ʌ/ /n/). The motor pathways are activated so that air is moved from the speaker's lungs via the larynx and the word is shaped (articulated) through the oral and nasal cavities using the tongue, lips, nose, teeth, hard palate, soft palate, mandible, and pharynx. This word travels through air as an acoustic signal and reaches the listener's outer ear. The signal travels through the middle ear to the inner ear and moves from the cochlea to the auditory nerves. The sound is interpreted as speech within the brain, and assuming the listener is familiar with the meaning of the word, the word is accessed and the meaning is shared. For the rest of this chapter we will consider the anatomical structures needed for speech production and perception. In chapter 4 this knowledge will be combined with knowledge of how to transcribe children's speech.

ANATOMICAL STRUCTURES FOR SPEECH PRODUCTION AND PERCEPTION

The main anatomical structures involved in speech production include the tongue, lips, nose, teeth, hard palate, soft palate, mandible, pharynx, larynx, and respiratory system. The primary anatomical structure involved in the detection and perception of speech is the ear, and its constituent components. Speech production and perception are supported by the neurological system. Each of these anatomical structures will be examined in turn. They will be discussed with respect to structural and functional integrity in typical adults and children, and, where relevant, will be applied to structural impairments that can impact children's speech sound production and perception. Refer to your textbooks and notes from your classes on anatomy and physiology of speech and hearing structures (e.g., Fuller, Pimentel, & Peregoy, 2012; Seikel, Drumright, & Seikel, 2014; Zemlin, 1998) in order to supplement the overview provided in the current text.

STRUCTURES INVOLVED IN SPEECH PRODUCTION

The mouth, or oral cavity, contains the majority of important structures involved in speech production that you will observe when you are working as an SLP with children with SSD. The oral cavity consists of the tongue, lips, teeth, hard palate, soft palate, mandible, and pharynx. Figure 3-2 presents photographs and Figure 3-3 presents a schematic drawing of the oral cavity.

FIGURE 3-1 **A schematic diagram of how the word *sun* is stored, retrieved, produced, and perceived**

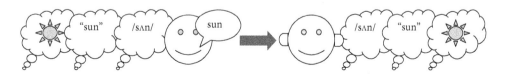

FIGURE 3-2   **Photographs of oral cavities**

(a) adult female and (b) adult male.

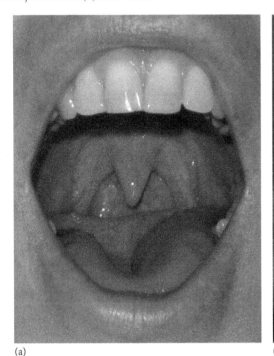 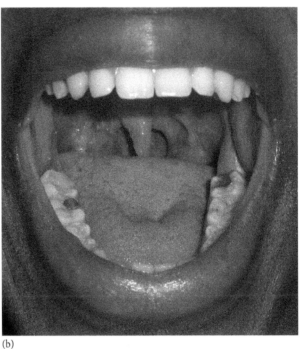

(a)   (b)

Source: Used by permission from Sharynne McLeod.

FIGURE 3-3   **Schematic of oral cavity and related structures**

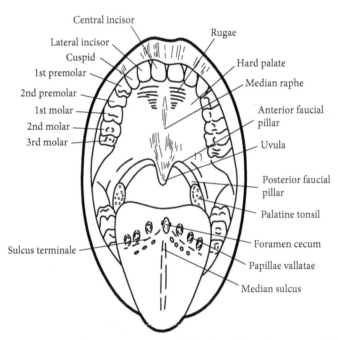

Source: Reprinted from Zemlin, W. R. (1998). *Speech and hearing science: Anatomy and physiology* (4th ed.). Boston, MA: Allyn and Bacon. Figure 4–30, p. 226.

▬ ▬

 APPLICATION: *Draw some mouths*

It is a useful skill for an SLP to be able to quickly draw an accurate representation of a person's mouth, such as in Figures 3-3 and 3-4. It is also important to have an understanding of the typical range of variability in adults' and children's mouths. Ask your family, friends, and fellow students to let you examine their oral cavity (with a flashlight), and draw what you see. Pay attention to the shape of the palate, the shape of the uvula, and whether or not they have palatal tonsils (these typically are not seen in adults, even if they have not had them surgically removed). Chapter 8 describes the assessment of children's oromusculature.

▇ Tongue

The tongue sits within the mouth and is made of eight muscles. Tongues lack a skeleton, so are classified as **muscular hydrostats**, similar to elephants' trunks and octopus' tentacles (Kier & Smith, 1985). The volume of a muscular hydrostat remains constant, regardless of whether it is elongated, shortened, bent, or twisted. Therefore, "any decrease in one dimension will cause a compensatory increase in at least one other dimension" (Kier & Smith, 1985, p. 307).

Function of the tongue

The main biological functions of the tongue relate to tasting, eating, swallowing, cleaning, and clearing food from the mouth. In addition, the tongue is the most important articulator in the production of speech. The tongue changes the shape of the oral cavity by restricting or stopping airflow, enabling the production of the majority of the world's consonants and vowels. Rapid and subtle movements of the tongue are possible because of the complex arrangement of the muscles and high innervation.

Structure of the tongue

The **dorsum** of the tongue can be divided into two anatomical parts. The **body** consists of the front two-thirds that sits horizontally in the mouth at rest and primarily consists of mucous-covered muscles and taste buds. The **root** consists of the back third of the tongue that anchors to the mandible, the walls of the pharynx, and the hyoid bone. The body of the tongue can be divided into four regions based on the contact with the palate during speech: **tip, blade, front, back** (Zemlin, 1998) (see Figure 3-4). During eating, the tip is used for licking and the entire tongue supports chewing and moving the bolus of food into the esophagus. During speech, the tip or blade touches the teeth to produce dental consonants /θ, ð/. The tip of the tongue is also used to touch the alveolar ridge to produce /t, d, n, l/; however, later we will see that the sides of the tongue are also used to anchor the tongue during the production of speech. The front of the tongue is used to produce postalveolar consonants /ʃ, ʒ/ and velar consonants /k, g/, and the back of the tongue is used to produce pharyngeal consonants /ħ, ʕ/ (these occur in languages such as Arabic).

There are eight muscles of tongue that change the shape of the tongue. The four **intrinsic muscles** are not attached to bone: genioglossus, styloglossus, palatoglossus, and the hyoglossus. The four **extrinsic muscles** are anchored to bone: superior longitudinal, inferior longitudinal, verticalis, and transversus (Zemlin, 1998). Hardcastle (1976) outlined seven articulatory parameters that account for the tongue positions during speech (see Figure 3-5 and Table 3-1). If you have the opportunity to visit an anatomy laboratory or to study a working model of the human tongue, use Table 3-1 to consider the effect different muscles have on the movement of the tongue.

| **FIGURE 3-4** | **A schematic sagittal section of the head showing articulators and places of articulation** |

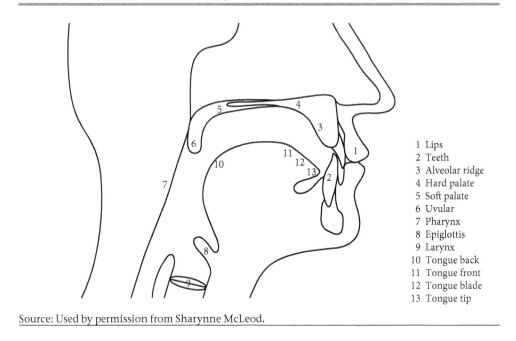

1 Lips
2 Teeth
3 Alveolar ridge
4 Hard palate
5 Soft palate
6 Uvular
7 Pharynx
8 Epiglottis
9 Larynx
10 Tongue back
11 Tongue front
12 Tongue blade
13 Tongue tip

Source: Used by permission from Sharynne McLeod.

| **FIGURE 3-5** | **Children's and adults' shapes, ranges of excursion, and movements of the tongue for people with typical speech** |

Note the variation in the tongue tip elevation across speakers; particularly consider the 10-year-old child and second adult male (both could elevate to the alveolar ridge but could not elevate the tongue tip towards the nose).

Child (female aged 2;7)				
Child (female aged 3;6)				
Child (female aged 4;6)				

(Continued)

FIGURE 3-5 (*Continued*)

Child (female aged 6;11)	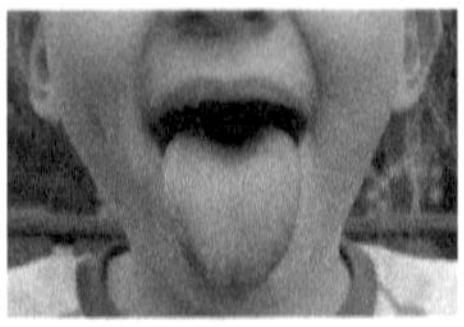	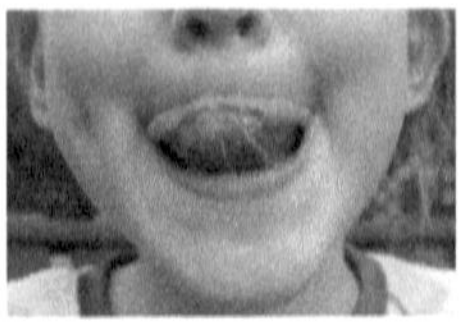	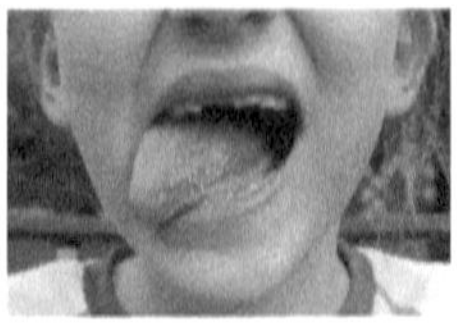	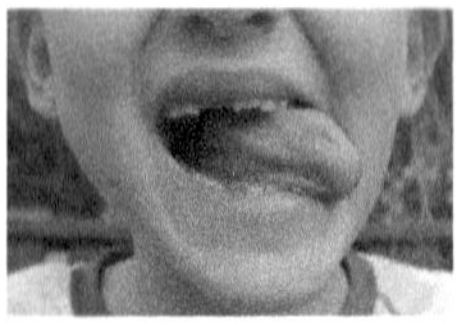
Child (male aged 10;4)	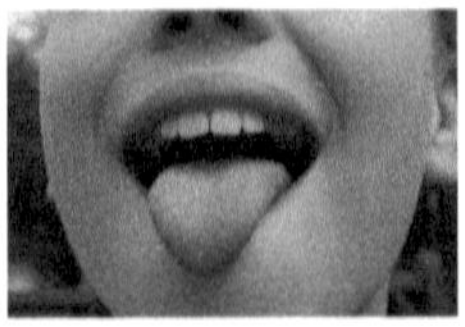	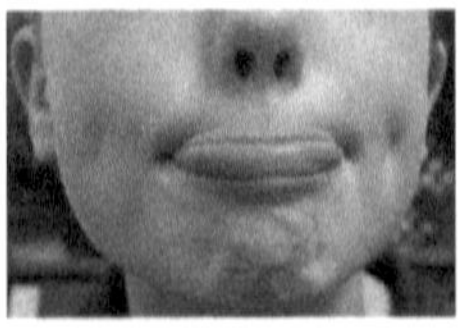	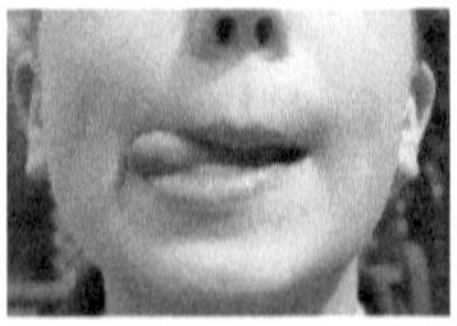	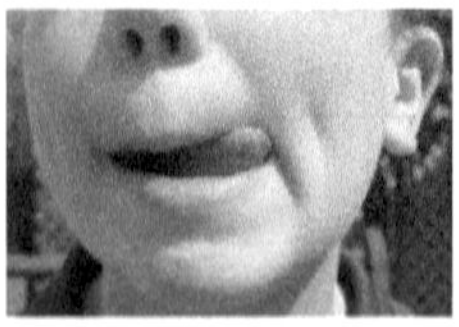
Adolescent (female aged 15;1)	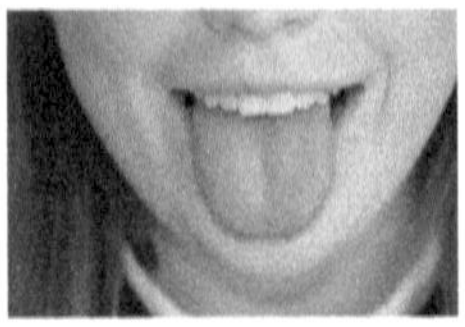	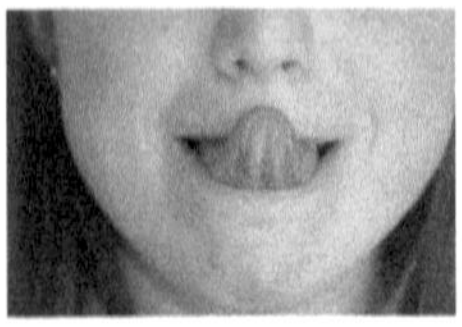	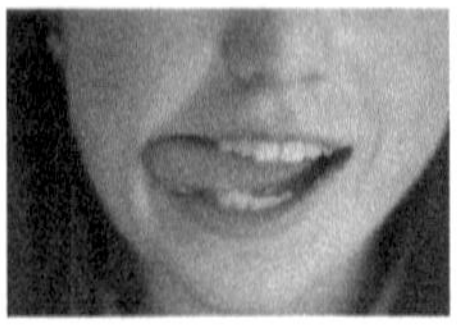	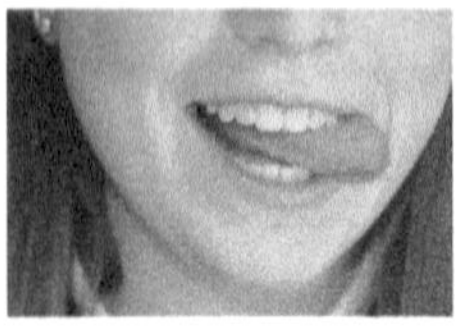
Adolescent (male aged 17;9)	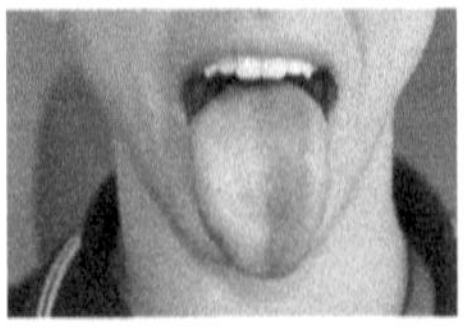	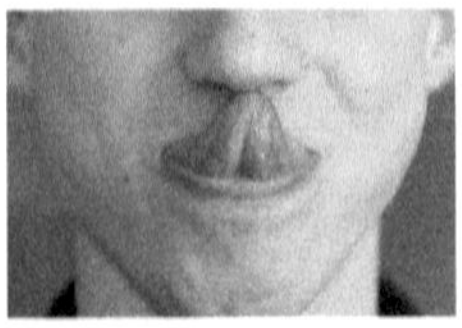	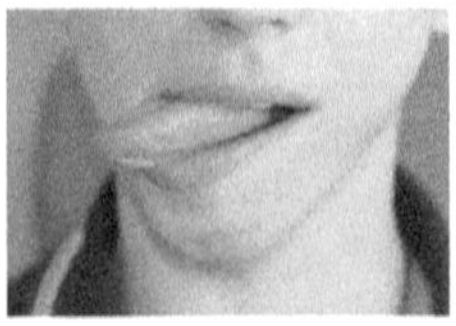	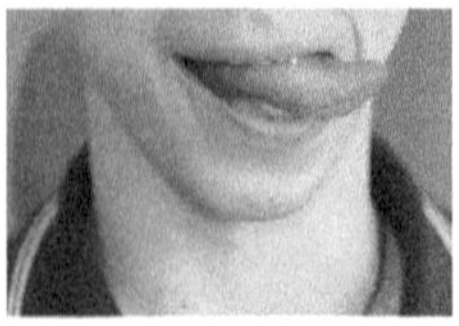
Adult (male)	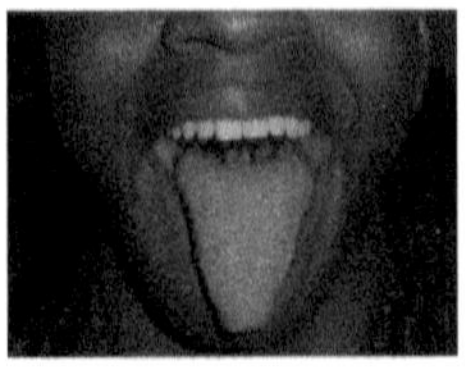	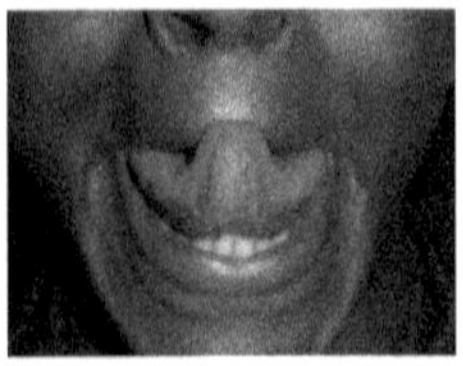	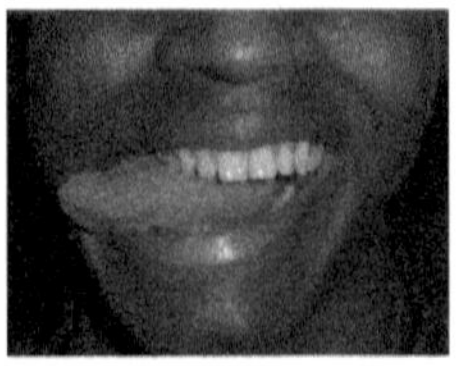	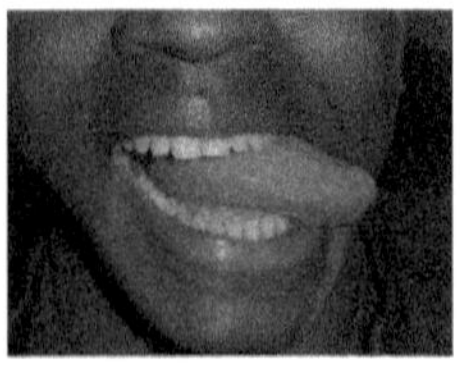
Adult (male)	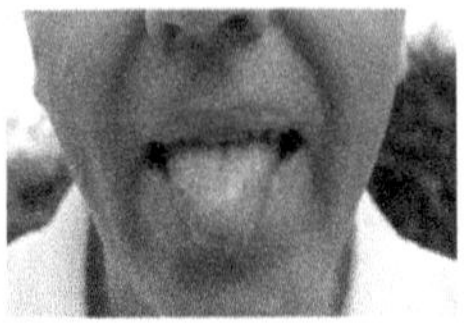	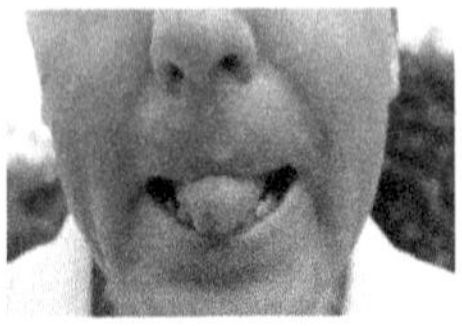	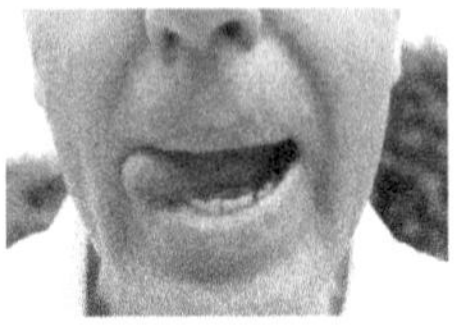	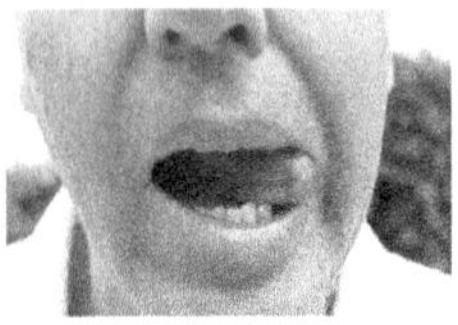
Adult (female)	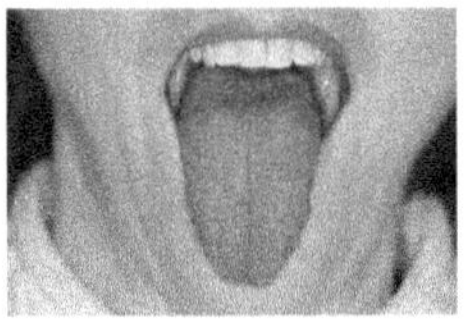	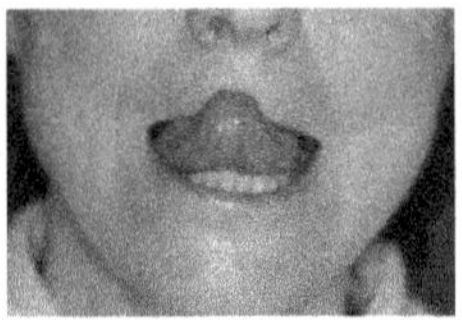	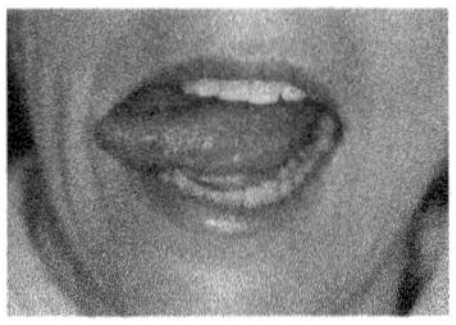	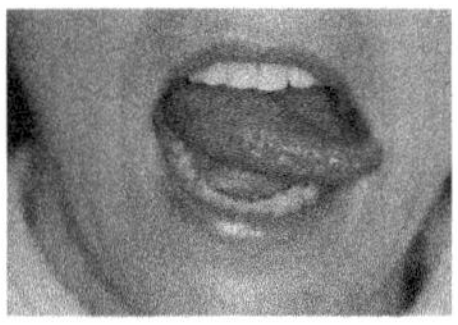
Adult (female)	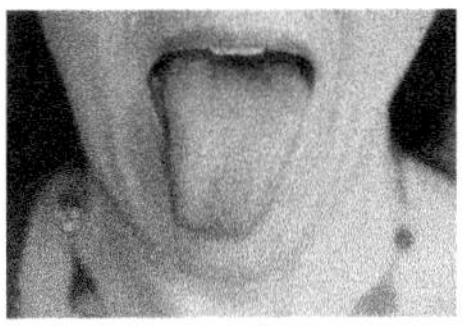	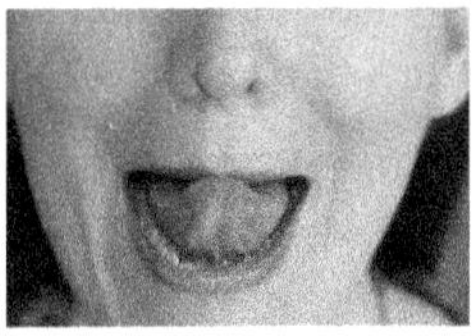	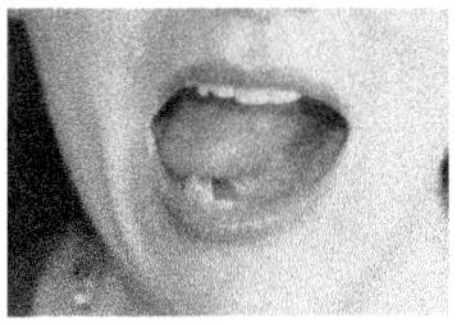	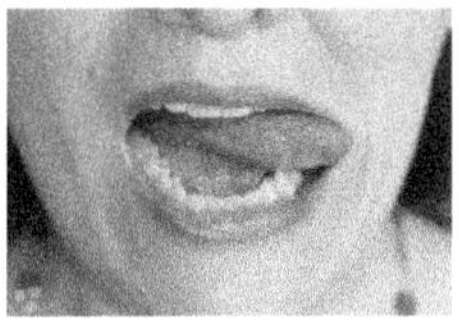

Source: Used by permission from Sharynne McLeod and Elise Baker.

TABLE 3-1 The seven articulatory parameters and associated muscles that account for tongue positions during speech

Movement	Speech sounds	Part of the tongue	Muscle(s)
Horizontal forward-back	Vowel: /a/	Body	Genioglossus
Vertical upward-downward	Central vowels Palatal consonants	Body	Styloglossus, palatoglossus, inferior longitudinal
Horizontal forward-backward	Consonants: retroflex	Tip-blade	Transversus, posterior genohyoid
Vertical upward-downward	Vowel: /i/ Consonants: /t, n, s/	Tip-blade	Superior longitudinal
Transverse convex-concave	Consonant: /t/	Body	Styloglossus, palatoglossus, transversus
Transverse cross-sectional central grooving	Consonant: /s/	Tip-blade	Transversus, verticalis
Spread or tapered surface	Vowels: /i, e/ Consonants: /t, s, l/	Dorsum	Transversus, hyoglossus

Source: Adapted from Hardcastle (1976).

FIGURE 3-6 Examples of the underside of adolescents' and adults' tongues showing the lingual frenulums

These photographs show the typical range of movement, and are not examples of tongue-tie. (a) adolescent female, (b) adult male, (c) and (d) adult females.

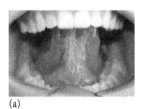 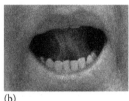 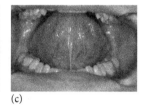 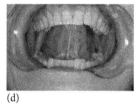

   (a)   (b)   (c)   (d)

Sources: Used by permission from Sharynne McLeod and Elise Baker.

Structural impairments of the tongue

The **lingual frenulum** (or lingual frenum) is the membrane that extends from the underside of the tongue to the floor of the mouth (see Figure 3-6). A short tight lingual frenulum can result in a **tongue-tie** or **ankyloglossia**. The prevalence of tongue-tie in newborns is typically reported in the United States to be between 3.2% (Ballard, Auer, & Khoury, 2002) and 4.2% (Ricke, Baker, Madlon-Kay, & DeFor, 2005), with a higher prevalence of 10.7% reported for infants in the United Kingdom (Hogan, Westcott, & Griffiths, 2005) and 16.4% in schoolchildren in India (Bai & Vaz, 2014). Almost half of these Indian schoolchildren were reported to have a mild tongue-tie, with range of movement being between 12 and 16 mm. Between 25 and 60% of infants with tongue-tie may have difficulties with breast-feeding (Segal, Stephenson, Dawes, & Feldman, 2007). Breast-feeding difficulties that may be associated with tongue-tie include difficulty latching onto the nipple, inability to feed continuously, and maternal nipple pain (Ballard, Auer, & Khoury, 2002; Buryk, Bloom, & Shope, 2011; Emond et al., 2014; Hogan, Westcott, Griffiths, 2005; Ricke et al., 2005). Fewer difficulties have been reported with bottle-feeding for infants with tongue-tie (Catlin, 1971).

While members of the public often believe that "tongue-tie" is the reason for children's SSD, the majority of children with SSD do not have a tongue-tie (i.e., short tight lingual frenulum). If a child with SSD does have a tongue-tie, then the SLP should consider children's ability to pronounce the alveolar consonants /t, d, n, l, s, z/, lick their lips, and clear food from their gums (Fernando, 2000; Wright, 1995).

■ ■

✅ **APPLICATION:** *Comparing a surgeon's view of tongue-tie with a systematic review*

Wright, a pediatric surgeon, reviewed his surgical records over 18 years. He reported that 158 frenulotomies were conducted after seeing 287 children with "simple tongue-tie" and two children with "true ankyloglossia" (Wright, 1995, p. 276). Wright concluded: " . . . there is no place for division of tongue-tie without anaesthesia in the newborn. Speech difficulties related to tongue-tie are over-rated and mechanical problems are underestimated. The indications for frenulotomy include articulation difficulties confirmed by a speech pathologist, mechanical limitations such as inability to lick the lips, to perform internal oral toilet or play a wind instrument" (p. 276). The systematic review titled "The Effect of Tongue-Tie Division on Breastfeeding and Speech Articulation" by Webb, Hao, and Hong (2013) was published almost 20 years after Wright's summary of his practice. Some of the major findings of the review are outlined in this chapter. What similarities and differences do you note? How would you advise a parent about the impact of tongue-tie?

Management of tongue-tie is controversial, with differing opinions between otolaryngologists, pediatricians, lactation consultants, and SLPs regarding the impact and treatment options (Messner & Lalakea, 2000). In some cases, a **frenulectomy** (also called fraenectomy, frenectomy, frenulotomy, or frenotomy) may be indicated and should be performed by a surgeon (Heller, Gabbay, O'Hara, Heller, & Bradley, 2005; Wright, 1995) (see "Comparing a Surgeon's View of Tongue-Tie With a Systematic Review"). A systematic review of the effect of frenulectomy on breast-feeding and speech was conducted by Webb, Hao, and Hong (2013). Of the 20 studies reviewed, only 5 were randomized controlled trials (sometimes comparing different surgical approaches), and the remainder presented observational reports. Webb et al. found that after frenulectomy there was some evidence of improvements in breast-feeding, but "no definitive improvements in speech function were reported" (Webb et al., 2013, p. 635). Since this time, a few additional studies have been published. Emond et al. (2014) conducted a randomized controlled trial of infants in the United Kingdom who received either early frenulectomy or standard care (i.e., no frenulectomy). They found by "8 weeks, there were no differences between groups in the breastfeeding measures or in the infant weight" (p. F189). Another study documented the outcomes after a frenectomy of 13 people with a short lingual frenulum who spoke Brazilian Portuguese. The participants had improved tongue mobility and number of alveolar consonant productions, but did not have an improvement in the production of the tap consonant (Camargo, Marchesan, Oliveira, Svicero, Pereira, & Madureira, 2013).

Macroglossia (large tongue) can be associated with speech difficulties and is found in people with acromegaly or gigantism and Beckwith-Wiedemann syndrome (Van Borsel, Van Snick, & Leroy, 1999). Additionally, macroglossia is associated with people with Down syndrome (Desai, 1997); however, some suggest people with Down syndrome do not have true macroglossia, but a large tongue in relation to a small oral cavity (Guimaraes, Donnelly, Shott, Amin, & Kalra, 2008).

A **bifid tongue** (a tongue with two points) is a feature of oro-facial-digital syndrome, Mohr's syndrome, and may be associated with Klippel-Feil syndrome (Whelan, Feldman, & Dost, 1975; Widgerow, 1990). A bifid tongue can also be a complication of tongue piercing (Fleming & Flood, 2005) or a result of a cosmetic tongue split (Bressman, 2006). With a bifid tongue, speech is intelligible, although the sibilants /s, z/ may be distorted (Bressman, 2006).

A **glossectomy** occurs when the tongue is surgically removed (typically as a result of cancer). Speakers who have undergone a glossectomy can be intelligible by using compensatory gestures to produce consonants and vowels (Bressman, Thind, Uy, Bollig, Gilbert, & Irish, 2005; Greven, Meijer, & Tiwari, 1994; Kaipa, Robb, O'Beirne, & Allison, 2012). However, vowels are typically more clearly articulated than consonants (Kaipa et al., 2012).

■ Lips

Lips form the entrance to the mouth and primarily consist of the circular orbicularis oris muscle.

Function of the lips

The lips are more important than many of us realize. They provide key facial cues regarding emotions (e.g., upturned corners = smiling = happy). They enable us to kiss and to hold our breath to swim underwater. Lips keep saliva inside our mouths. They also guide food into our mouths and away from our gums while eating. For babies, they enable a strong attachment during breast-feeding and bottle-feeding. They provide an airtight seal when sucking through a straw or when playing the clarinet or saxophone. They vibrate air when playing the French horn or trombone. Lips direct air when blowing out birthday candles or producing the bilabial fricatives /ɸ, β/ (e.g., /ɸ/ is the first consonant in the Japanese pronunciation of *futon*). They form a barrier to enable air to build up and then be released to produce consonants /p, b/. They can be rounded to produce consonants such as /w/ and vowels such as /u, ʊ, ɔ/ or spread to produce vowels such as /i, ɪ/. During the production of /m/, the lips restrict air from escaping through the mouth (so it can escape through the nose). They also enable the production of a bilabial trill /ʙ/, a sound that many babies produce, that is also a consonant in New Guinean languages such as Kele and Titan (Ladefoged, 2005).

Structure of the lips

The upper and lower lips are made up of muscles, glandular tissues, and fat, and are covered with skin (externally) and mucous membrane (internally). The most important muscle of the lips is the circular **orbicularis oris muscle** that enables the lips to move (pucker, smile, and compress). The orbicularis oris also provides insertion points for eight to nine facial muscles, including the transverse muscles (buccinator and risorius), angular muscles (levator labii superioris, levator labii superioris alaeque nasi, zygomaticus minor, zygomaticus major, and depressor labii inferioris muscles), labial or vertical muscles (mentalis, depressor anguli oris, and levator anguli oris muscles), and the parallel muscles (incisivus labii superioris and incisivus labii inferioris muscles). The **philtrum** is the vertical groove that extends from the upper lip to the nasal septum.

Structural impairments of the lips

Some children are born with a cleft of the upper lip (**cleft lip**). Cleft lips may be unilateral or bilateral and may be associated with a cleft palate (discussed later in this chapter). Cleft lips may be incomplete or complete: a complete cleft of the lip extends into the base of the nose (Peterson-Falzone, Hardin-Jones, & Karnell, 2010). In many Western countries, children with cleft lip undergo surgery within the first six months of life. Some children who have had a cleft lip may have difficulty producing consonants such as /p/ and /b/ that require a buildup of air behind the lips.

■ Teeth

Teeth are hard structures that are attached to the mandible and maxilla.

Function of the teeth

The primary function of the teeth is for biting and chewing during eating, and they are important determinants of the appearance of the face. However, they also have a number of roles during speech. The upper teeth form the boundary of the upper palate, much like a fence around a sporting field. Chapter 4 includes electropalatographic images of tongue/palate contact during speech, and the classic horseshoe shape of contact for /t, d, n, s, z/ occurs because the tongue is anchored along the margins of the palate beside (and sometimes touching) the teeth. The teeth are important for the production of the dental consonants /θ, ð/, where the tongue touches the teeth. The teeth are also important for the production of the labiodental consonants, where the lips touch the teeth. The English labiodental consonants are /f, v/, and labiodental consonants found in other languages around the world are /ɱ, v, ʋ/.

Structure of the teeth

There are four types of teeth. **Incisors** have a sharp cutting edge. **Canine** teeth (also called cuspids or eye teeth) are tusk-like and are for ripping or tearing. **Premolars** (also called bicuspids) are for cutting and tearing. **Molars** are the largest teeth and are for crushing and grinding. Teeth consist of a crown, neck, and root that anchors into the maxilla or mandible and gums. Teeth are made of dentin, dental pulp, enamel, and cementum.

FIGURE 3-7   Children's and adults' teeth

(a) First teeth of a child aged 8 months, (b) primary dentition of a child aged 3;6 years, (c) mixed dentition of a child aged 7;1 showing decayed deciduous teeth and healthy permanent teeth, (d) mixed dentition of a child aged 7;4 years (note the front incisor ready to fall out!), (e) mixed dentition of the same child aged 7;4 years (a few hours later), (f) mixed dentition of a child aged 6;11 years, (g) mixed dentition of a child aged 10;4 years, (h) permanent dentition of an adolescent aged 15;1 years, (i) permanent dentition of an adult male, and (j) permanent dentition of an adult male.

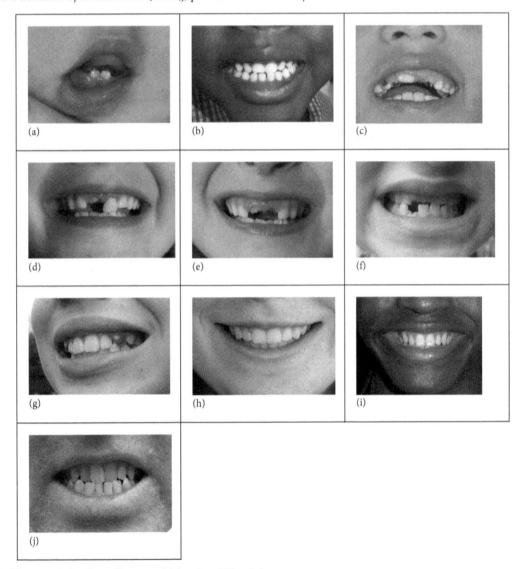

Sources: Used by permission from Sharynne McLeod and Elise Baker.

Children's primary teeth erupt during their first year of life and continue erupting over the next two years (see Figure 3-7 and Figure 3-8). When eruption ceases, children have 20 primary (deciduous) teeth: four incisors, two canines, and four molars on the maxilla and mandible. When children are 5 to 7 years old, they begin to lose their primary teeth, typically beginning with the incisors. Eventually the deciduous teeth are replaced by 32 permanent teeth: the permanent incisors, "canines," and premolars plus an additional 12 permanent molars (see Figure 3-3).

Structural impairments of the teeth

Structural impairments of the teeth primarily are the domain of dentists, orthodontists, and oro-maxillo-facial surgeons; however, SLPs should consider the presence/absence of

FIGURE 3-8 **Dentition displayed using an orthopantomogram (OPG) panoramic X-ray**

(a) the primary and permanent dentition of a child aged 5;5 (note the two rows of teeth on the upper and lower jaws),
(b) permanent dentition of an adolescent aged 16;3 years (note the wisdom teeth under the gums at the back of the maxilla).
A bite block is held between the front incisors to take the X-ray.

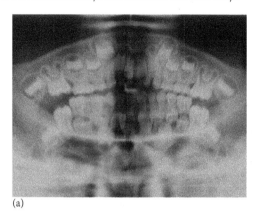
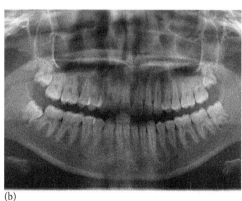

(a)   (b)

Source: Used by permission from Sharynne McLeod.

teeth, the condition of the teeth, and the occlusion (bite). One consideration during the speech-language pathology assessment of a 5- to 6-year-old is whether the central incisors are present, because this can impact the production of fricatives such as /s, z/ and possibly other consonants.

■ Mandible

The mandible is the movable lower jaw.

Function of the mandible

The mandible houses the lower teeth. Lowering and raising the mandible enables mastication (chewing). It also facilitates the production of many speech sounds by supporting the movement of the lower lip and tongue. The jaw never fully closes during speech; however, it can move very rapidly even in young children, such as in the production of /papapapa/ (Williams & Stackhouse, 2000). The movement of the jaw is important in the earliest phases of speech production. For example, **babbling** (e.g., *mamama* and *dadada*) is associated with "rhythmic mandibular oscillation" (Davis & MacNeilage, 1995, p. 1199). Vowel height is associated with opening and closing of the jaw. Look at yourself in the mirror as you contrast a high vowel /i/ "eee" with a low vowel /ɑ/ or /a/ "aah."

Structure of the mandible

The mandible is a single U-shaped bone that is connected to the temporal bone via the **temporomandibular joint**. The upper surface (alveolar arch) contains a socket for each tooth. The muscles associated with the mandible that are used for mastication are masseter, temporalis, internal pterygoid, external pterygoid, and the depressors of the mandible. The mandibular branch of the **trigeminal nerve** (cranial nerve V) "supplies the lower teeth and gums, the muscles of mastication, the skin of the ear and adjacent temporal regions, the lower facial region, and the mucous membrane of the anterior two-thirds of the tongue" (Zemlin, 1998, p. 371).

Structural impairments of the mandible

Occlusion refers to the skeletal and dental alignment of the teeth in the upper and lower jaws (McNamara, 1981) (see Figure 3-9). Edward H. Angle (1899, 1907) described four main types of occlusion, and these definitions are still used today: Class I occlusion, and Class I, Class II (division 1 and division 2), and Class III malocclusions. **Class I occlusion** refers

FIGURE 3-9   **Examples of Class I, II, and III occlusion and malocclusion**

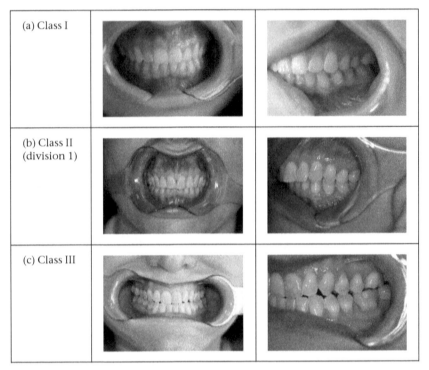

(a) Class I		
(b) Class II (division 1)		
(c) Class III		

Source: Used by permission from Sharynne McLeod.

to normal occlusion where the mesiobuccal cusp of the upper first molar is aligned over the buccal groove of lower first permanent molar. In Class I, incisors have positive overbite and overjet. The usual range for Class I is for the upper incisors to be 2–4 mm horizontally ahead of the lowers (overjet) and the vertical overlap of the upper incisors over the lower incisors to be 20–50% (overbite). **Class I malocclusion** covers occlusal features ranging from crowding, spaced and proclined incisors, overbite and overjet variations. **Class II malocclusion** occurs when the mesiobuccal cusp of the upper first permanent molar is positioned half a cusp in front of the buccal groove of the lower first permanent molar. People with Class II division 1 have a large or excessive overjet (horizontal protrusion greater than 5 mm) and often a deep overbite (greater than 50% overlap of the mandibular incisors) or long overjet (frequently called a deep bite). People with Class II division 2 have the maxillary (upper) central incisors that are lingually inclined, leading to a reduced overjet. **Class III malocclusion** refers to when the lower molars are half a cusp ahead of the corresponding upper molars, and the lower incisors are more prominent than and sometimes in front of the upper incisors. People with Class I, II, and III malocclusions can have an open bite or deep bite. People with Class II division 1 and division 2 can have the deepest overbites. In addition, people may have a cross bite where maxillary teeth are inside the mandibular teeth (on the same side) and this can be unilateral, bilateral, or anterior. An open bite occurs when there is a vertical space between the upper and lower front teeth.

   Orthodontists and **dentists** work to prevent and correct malocclusion. Children with malocclusions may have some difficulty producing speech sounds. For example, children with Class III malocclusion may invert the production of /f/ and /v/ so that the upper lip contacts the lower teeth. Children with Pierre Robin syndrome and Treacher Collins syndrome typically have micrognathia (unusually small mandible or lower jaw) that is often associated with dental malocclusions (Rotten, Levaillant, Martinez, Le Pointe, & Vicaut, 2002).

▇ Hard palate

The hard palate literally is the roof of the mouth, acting as a barrier between the oral and nasal cavities.

Function of the hard palate

The hard palate prevents air, saliva, and food from escaping through the nose. The hard palate also houses the upper teeth. Continuing the analogy of the roof, the palate is vaulted. The palatal height (vaulting) has direct impact on the individual vocal characteristics including the resonance and acoustics of the voice (Zemlin, 1998).

Structure of the hard palate

The maxilla (upper jaw) includes a body and the frontal, zygomatic, palatine, and alveolar processes (Fehrenbach & Herring, 2007). The **palatine and alveolar processes** form the hard palate. The hard palate primarily consists of bone that is covered by a mucous membrane. The bone is thicker at the front (alveolar arch) and sides of the palate, and thinner in the center. The wrinkled membranous covering across the slope of the alveolar arch is called the **rugae** (see Figure 3-10). The **midline raphe** is the slightly raised ridge that runs from the alveolar ridge along the midline of the palate, and its length varies across individuals.

Structural impairments of the hard palate

The most common structural impairment of the hard palate is **cleft palate**. There are a number of types: cleft palate only, unilateral cleft lip and palate, bilateral cleft lip and palate, and submucosal cleft palate, as well as cleft lip as discussed previously (Peterson-Falzone, Hardin-Jones, & Karnell, 2010). Children may have a cleft of the hard and/or soft palates. Children with cleft palate have difficulties with feeding and speech, and also can have problems with weight gain, hearing, and dentition. Murray (2002) described the differing frequency of clefts amongst racial groups, with a higher frequency (1:500) in Asian and American Indian populations, a moderate frequency in Caucasian populations, and a lower frequency (1:2,500) in African-derived populations. In many Western countries, multidisciplinary teams (that include SLPs) support babies' feeding and speech development, and many other aspects of the lives of children with cleft palate. Surgical repair of a cleft typically occurs within the first 18 months of life within Western countries.

A **submucosal cleft** (see Figure 3-11) is an anatomical abnormality along the midline of the posterior hard palate and musculature and can be associated with a bifid uvula. Smyth (2014) provides a clinical grading system for describing submucous clefts by considering the

- hard palate: normal, absent posterior nasal spine, palpable bony notch, or visible bony defect;
- soft palate: normal, midline groove, translucent midline (zona pellucida), or congenital fistula; and
- uvula: normal, groove, incomplete bifid, or complete bifid.

FIGURE 3-10 **An adult's hard palate showing the teeth, rugae, and midline raphe**

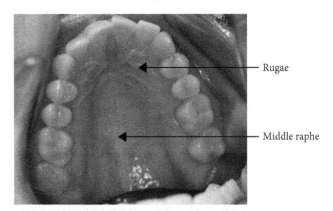

Rugae

Middle raphe

Source: Used by permission from Sharynne McLeod.

FIGURE 3-11 A submucosal cleft showing a complete bifid uvula, midline translucent area (zona pellucida), and palpable and visible bony defect, which is greater than the posterior third of the hard palate

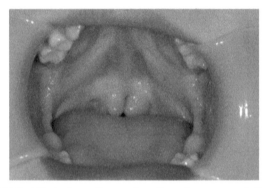

Source: Smyth, A. (2014). Clinical grading system for submucous cleft palate. *British Journal of Oral and Maxillofacial Surgery, 52*(3), 275–276. (Figure 1, p. 276). Reprinted with permission from Elsevier.

A submucosal cleft may be identified by shining a flashlight up a child's nose and looking into the child's mouth to see the light shining through the palate. Children with a submucous cleft may exhibit hypernasality, nasal emission, and problems with velopharyngeal closure (Sommerlad et al., 2004; Sullivan, Vasudavan, Marrinan, & Mulliken, 2010). However, there is a poor correlation between the severity of velopharyngeal insufficiency during speech and the anatomical presentation (Smyth, 2014).

Soft palate (Velum)

The soft palate consists of muscles and connective tissue that extends between the bones of the hard palate and the muscles of the pharynx.

Function of the soft palate

The soft palate can be lowered or raised. Breathing through the nose and mouth is facilitated when the soft palate is lowered. The resonance of the oral cavity is changed with the lowering and raising of the soft palate. When the soft palate is lowered, air can pass through the nose, enabling the production of the nasal consonants and nasalized vowels. In English the nasal consonants are /m, n, ŋ/ and there are no nasalized vowels (although languages such as French and Spanish have nasalized vowels). When the soft palate is raised, the soft palate touches the posterior palatal wall, preventing air from passing through the nose. This enables oral production of the majority of the world's consonants and vowels. It also prevents food from passing into the nasal cavity during eating. Another function of the muscles of the soft palate (particularly the tensor veli palatini) is to enable the Eustachian tube to open and equalize air pressure between the middle ear and the atmosphere.

Structure of the soft palate

The soft palate attaches to the bones of the hard palate and the muscles of the pharynx. It consists of connective tissue and muscles that comprise the **anterior** and **posterior faucial pillars**, and the **uvula** (see Figure 3-12). There are five muscles of the soft palate. The palatoglossus (anterior faucial pillar) inserts into the tongue and functions to depress the soft palate and elevate the tongue. The palatopharyngeus (posterior faucial pillar) moves the soft palate and posterior palatal wall. The levator veli palatini raises the soft palate to contact the posterior pharyngeal wall in order to prevent air from passing through

FIGURE 3-12   Soft palate showing the faucial pillars and uvula

(a) a child (aged 6;9 years) and (b) an adult. Note the tonsils are still present in the child.

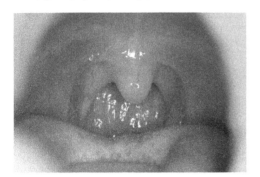

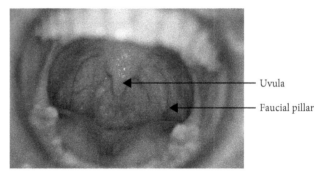

Uvula

Faucial pillar

Source: Used by permission from Sharynne McLeod.

the nose. The tensor veli palatini tenses and lowers the soft palate. The uvular muscle elevates the palate. The faucial or palatal tonsils reside between the anterior and posterior faucial pillars, and the lingual tonsils reside on the lower portion of the tongue dorsum.

Structural impairments of the soft palate

As mentioned earlier, children may have a **cleft** of the soft and/or hard palate and may experience associated difficulties with hypernasality, nasal emission, and velopharyngeal closure. A **bifid uvula** (see Figure 3-11) typically is not associated with speech difficulties; however, it is important for genetic documentation of craniofacial anomalies and may be associated with a submucosal cleft (Peterson-Falzone et al., 2010). Enlarged **palatine tonsils** (see Figure 3-13) rarely have an impact on speech production; however, if the tonsils are severely hypertrophied they may restrict velar movement and impact breathing.

■ Nose

The nose is the facial protrusion above the mouth.

Function of the nose

The nose has a number of functions. First, the nose is an avenue for the air that we breathe to be warmed, humidified, and filtered. Second, the nose is used for smelling and facilitating

FIGURE 3-13   Enlarged palatine tonsils of an adolescent aged 13;5 years

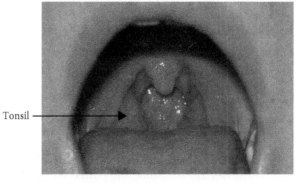

Tonsil

Source: Used by permission from Sharynne McLeod.

tasting. Third, the floor of the nose forms the roof of the palate, so it is the barrier between the two cavities, keeping food and saliva from coming through the nose. Fourth, it is a defining facial feature due to the variability of the shape and size of the nose. Finally, the nose acts as an extension to the oral cavity in the production of nasal consonants and vowels. In English there are only three nasal consonants, /m, n, ŋ/. However, there are seven nasal consonants listed in the International Phonetic Alphabet, and languages such as Vietnamese and Wiradjuri (an Australian Aboriginal language) use more nasal consonants than English. Nasalization of vowels is an important feature in languages such as French and Spanish.

Structure of the nose

The **bridge** of the nose is made of the nasal bone. The remainder of the external nose is made of septal, lateral, and alar **cartilage**. The **nasal septum** divides the nose vertically into two **nostrils** (nares). There are five muscles of the nose that contribute to facial expression, but have a limited role in speech: procerus, nasalis, depressor septi, and the anterior and posterior nasal dilators. The floor of the nasal cavity is made of the maxillae and palatine bones (recall that the palatine bone forms the hard palate). The **nasal cavity** contains the branches of the **olfactory nerve** and communicates with the paranasal sinuses.

Structural impairments of the nose

Deviation of the nasal septum may result in difficulty breathing. When air is blocked from passing through the nose (e.g., during a cold), speech sounds **hyponasal**, and nasalized consonants /m, n, ŋ/ sound more like the oral consonants [b, d, g]. In contrast, **hypernasal** speech occurs when the velum does not have adequate closure (or the person has a cleft palate) and allows too much air to pass through the nasal cavity during speech.

▓ Pharynx

The pharynx is the back of the throat. It connects and extends from the nasal cavity to esophagus.

Function of the pharynx

The main purpose of the pharynx is as a tube that "communicates with the tympanic, oral, laryngeal and nasal cavities, as well as the esophagus" (Zemlin, 1998, p. 227) conveying air, food, saliva, and mucous. The pharynx is the destination for the velum during velopharyngeal closure (i.e., to block the nasal cavity in order to produce oral consonants and vowels). However, in young children "velopharyngeal closure is actually *velum-adenoid closure*" (Peterson-Falzone et al., 2010, p. 252).

Structure of the pharynx

The pharynx is an oval-shaped tube of approximately 12 cm in length in adults. It is made of connective tissue and becomes more muscular as it joins with the **esophagus**. The **pharynx** is divided into three parts: the nasopharynx, oropharynx, and laryngopharynx. The **nasopharynx** extends from the nasal cavity (specifically, it begins at the "rostrum of the sphenoid bone and the pharyngeal protuberance of the occipital bone," Zemlin, 1998, p. 226) to the soft palate. The **Eustachian tube** extends from the middle ear to the nasopharynx. The **adenoid** pad (sometimes called the pharyngeal tonsils) sits within the nasopharynx behind the soft palate, so cannot be viewed on intraoral examination. The **oropharynx** extends from the soft palate down to the hyoid bone. The **laryngopharynx** extends from the hyoid bone until the pharynx joins with the esophagus.

Structural impairments of the pharynx

An enlarged adenoid pad may result in denasalized speech, and may impact sleep, appetite, and exercise tolerance. Surgical removal of the adenoid pad can impact velopharyngeal competence (Peterson-Falzone et al., 2010).

■ Larynx

The larynx, or vocal folds, is colloquially known as the "voice box" or "Adam's apple." It is the site of the production of voicing.

Function of the larynx

The primary function of the larynx (vocal folds) is to prevent food and fluids from entering the lungs. These are expelled by coughing or clearing the throat. The secondary function of the larynx is for vocalization. When the vocal folds vibrate they create voicing. The English voiced consonants are /b, d, g, m, n, ŋ, v, ð, z, ʒ, ɹ, j, l, w, ʤ/, and all vowels and diphthongs are voiced. The space between the vocal folds is called the **glottis**, and three consonants are produced at the glottis: /ʔ, h, ɦ/. The glottal stop /ʔ/ is produced in some dialects of English in the middle of words such as *bottle* and *button*. Vibration of the vocal folds enables us to produce different pitches (low, habitual, high, falsetto) and differing degrees of breathiness (whisper, breathy, harsh, hoarse) (see Figure 3-14).

Structure of the larynx

The larynx sits between the laryngopharynx and the **trachea** (windpipe). It is suspended from the **hyoid bone** by muscles and ligaments. The **vocal folds** are shelflike structures made of muscles and connective tissue that are lined with mucous membrane. There are three primary cartilages of the larynx: **thyroid cartilage**, **arytenoid cartilages**, and **cricoid cartilage**. The vocal folds are attached anteriorly to the thyroid cartilage and posteriorly to the arytenoid cartilages that move to open and close the vocal folds, or to allow them to approximate one another (e.g., during whispering). The cricoid cartilage

---

FIGURE 3-14   Schematics of various glottal configurations

Apex of arytenoid cartilage (A), vocal fold (VF), epiglottis (E), ventricular (false vocal) fold (V).

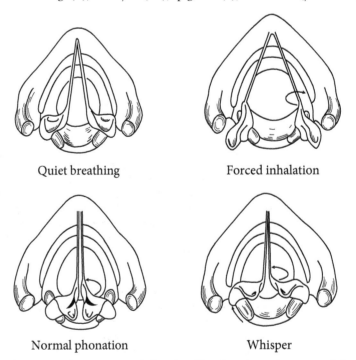

Quiet breathing   Forced inhalation

Normal phonation   Whisper

Source: Reprinted from Zemlin, W. R. (1998). *Speech and hearing science: Anatomy and physiology* (4th ed.). Boston, MA: Allyn and Bacon. Figure 3-31A and B, p. 120.

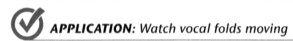

APPLICATION: *Watch vocal folds moving*

Type *vocal fold vibration movies* into your browser's search engine to see movies of different people's vocal folds vibrating. You should be able to view men and women speaking, singing, and whispering. Some movies show people with normal/typical vocal folds. If you add words such as *vocal nodules*, *polyps*, and *cancer*, you can see vibrating vocal folds of people with voice disorders.

forms the base of the larynx above the trachea. The extrinsic muscles of the larynx are sternothyroid muscles, thyrohyoid muscles, and the inferior pharyngeal constrictor. The intrinsic muscles (that are always found in pairs) are abductor muscles, adductor muscles, tensor muscles, and relaxer muscles. The **thyroarytenoid muscle** is the intrinsic muscle that constitutes the main mass of the vocal folds. The **vocalis muscle** vibrates during phonation (and is a portion of the thyroarytenoid muscle) (Zemlin, 1998).

Structural impairments of the larynx

The larynx can be affected by vocal abuse, allergies, neoplasms (e.g., polyps), and disease (e.g., laryngitis) that results in a change in voice quality. The most common impairment of the larynx in children is when **vocal nodules** appear on the vocal folds, typically as a result of vocal abuse (e.g., excessive shouting). Sometimes adults may have a **laryngectomy**, a surgical procedure to remove the larynx, typically as a result of laryngeal cancer. Voicing cannot occur with the removal of the larynx, so people can be taught to use **esophageal speech** (vibration of the sphincter of the esophagus).

■ The respiratory system

The respiratory system consists of the lungs, trachea, ribs, and thoracic muscles but also relies on the mouth and nose to convey air. It is the primary anatomical structure for supplying oxygen to the body. It is also important for producing speech.

Function of the respiratory system

The major function of the respiratory system is for life support: to provide oxygen to the body and to remove carbon dioxide from the body. However, a secondary function is to provide the controlled airstream for speech and singing. During speech, exhalation takes approximately ten times longer than inhalation (Garn-Nunn & Lynn, 2004). Most speech is produced during exhalation (**egressive** air); however, some rare consonants are produced during inhalation (**ingressive** air) (e.g., clicks and ingressive stops) and some people (e.g., Icelandic speakers) occasionally speak during inhalation. /h/ is produced if the egressive airstream passes through an open larynx, and there is no constriction within the oral cavity. Voicing occurs when air pressure is built up beneath the glottis (larynx) and then is released in a rhythmic opening and closing of the glottis and vocal folds. /ɑ/ is produced if the egressive airstream passes through the vibrating vocal folds and there is no constriction within the oral cavity.

Structure of the respiratory system

The respiratory system includes the **trachea** (windpipe), **lungs**, **thoracic cage** (ribs), and the muscles of respiration: the **intercostal muscles** and **diaphragm**. The trachea is a cartilaginous tube that branches into two bronchi as it enters the lungs. The bronchi branch into smaller bronchioles, terminating in alveolar ducts, and leading to alveolar sacs. The **alveoli** are contained within the alveolar sacs, and enable the exchange of oxygen and carbon dioxide. The diaphragm is dome-shaped and sits below the lungs and above the abdominal organs. The diaphragm and intercostal muscles enable the inhalation and exhalation of air. Many believe that while the heart is the most important muscle of the body, the diaphragm is the second most important (Zemlin, 1998).

Impairments of the respiratory system

There are a number of respiratory diseases, including influenza, asthma, pneumonia, cystic fibrosis, emphysema, mesothelioma, and lung cancer. These will affect breathing, but will also impact phonation and resonance during speech. Children with Pierre Robin syndrome can also have respiratory problems, with a majority requiring treatment of their airways (e.g., intubation) (Van den Elzen, Semmekrot, Bongers, Huygen, & Marres, 2001). In addition, children and adults with dysarthria can have difficulties with the muscles involved in respiration that can impact speech intelligibility and breath control (e.g., shallow breathing and coordination of breathing on phrases during connected speech).

STRUCTURES INVOLVED IN SPEECH DETECTION

The main structures involved in speech detection are the ear and the brain.

■ Ear

The ears, located at each side of the head, are the primary anatomical structures involved with hearing. They extend from the outer ear to the inner ear.

Function of the ear

The two primary functions of the ear are to facilitate hearing and provide the sensation of balance, spatial orientation, and movement.

Structure of the ear

The ear has three main sections (see Figure 3-15). The external ear consists of the **auricle** (pinna) (see Figure 3-16) that directs sound waves downwards through the **external auditory meatus** (ear canal). The middle ear is contained within the tympanic cavity and begins with the **tympanic membrane** (eardrum). The tympanic membrane is small, cone shaped, and compliant (stretches), facilitating response to sound. On examination with an **otoscope**, a healthy tympanic membrane is translucent and pearl gray in color. The **auditory ossicles** are the three tiny bones of the middle ear: the **malleus, incus**, and **stapes**. The malleus is attached to the tympanic membrane, the incus sits between the malleus and stapes, and the foot of the stapes sits in the **oval window**: the opening into the inner ear. The functions of the middle ear are: (1) to transduce sound waves from air pressure waves into mechanical movements that will create waves in the fluid of the inner ear, and (2) to protect the inner ear from excessive vibration (Zemlin, 1998). The **Eustachian tube** runs between the middle ear and the nasopharynx. It permits middle ear pressure to equalize and allows drainage of secretions from the middle ear. In adults, it is approximately 35 mm in length and runs downward and forward. However, in children it is almost half the length, wider, and more horizontal (Zemlin, 1998), and children have an increased risk of middle ear infections (otitis media).

The **inner ear** facilitates hearing and balance. It receives sound in three ways: air conduction across the middle ear, bone conduction through the skull, and mechanical vibration across the ossicles. The inner ear consists of the **cochlea, internal auditory meatus, vestibular labyrinth,** and the **semicircular canals**. The cochlea is a spiral-shaped canal about 35 mm long, linked to the tympanic cavity via the **oval** and **round windows**. The **organ of Corti** (spiral organ) is situated on the basilar membrane, within the scala media. The organ of Corti contains the sensory hair cells that enable hearing. Four rows of hair cells (one row of inner hair cells and three rows of outer hair cells) run the length of the organ of Corti. Waves in the fluid of the cochlea cause the hair cells to move.

FIGURE 3-15 A schematic representation of the anatomical divisions of the hearing mechanism and their functional roles

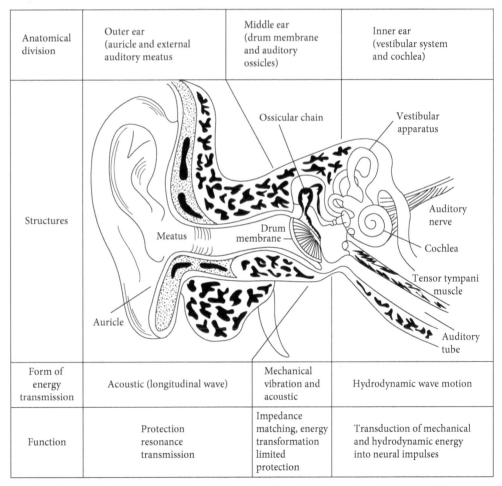

Anatomical division	Outer ear (auricle and external auditory meatus	Middle ear (drum membrane and auditory ossicles)	Inner ear (vestibular system and cochlea)
Structures			
Form of energy transmission	Acoustic (longitudinal wave)	Mechanical vibration and acoustic	Hydrodynamic wave motion
Function	Protection resonance transmission	Impedance matching, energy transformation limited protection	Transduction of mechanical and hydrodynamic energy into neural impulses

Source: Reprinted from Zemlin, W. R. (1998). *Speech and hearing science: Anatomy and physiology* (4th ed.). Boston, MA: Allyn and Bacon. Figure 4-129, p. 436.

The movement is transduced into an electrical signal that stimulates the auditory nerve (Palmer, 1993). The internal auditory meatus carries the facial and auditory nerves, nervus intermedius, and a branch of the basal artery. The **vestibular labyrinth** is composed of three semicircular canals and two otolith organs and is responsible for the sensation of balance, spatial orientation, and movement. The **semicircular canals** are three fluid-filled chambers oriented at right angles to each other on different planes, allowing for detection and discrimination of movements of the head in any direction. The otolith organs, the utricle and saccule, are located at the base of the semicircular canals and are responsible for the detection of movement and acceleration (Bhatnager & Andy, 1995).

Structural impairments of the ear

There are five types of hearing loss: conductive, sensorineural, mixed, retrocochlear, and central auditory. These five types of hearing loss are associated with difficulties with different anatomical structures. Problems with the structure or function of the outer or middle ear may lead to a **conductive hearing loss** (atresia, otitis media, and malformation of the bones of the middle ear). One of the most common causes of conductive hearing

FIGURE 3-16   The external ear

(a) child aged 3;6 years, (b) child aged 6;11 years, (c) adult male.

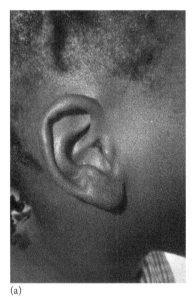 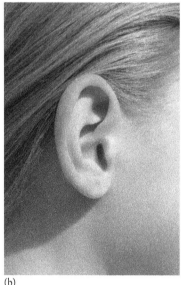 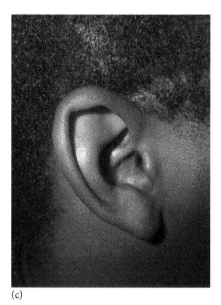

(a)   (b)   (c)

Sources: Used by permission from Sharynne McLeod and Elise Baker.

loss in children is otitis media with effusion (Robb & Williamson, 2011). **Otitis media with effusion (OME)**, a common childhood condition affecting up to 80% of children by 4 years (Williamson, 2007), occurs when there is fluid in the middle ear cavity without symptoms or signs of infection (Morris & Leach, 2009). The condition is also known as **glue ear**, because the fluid in the middle ear can be thick and glue-like, giving a sense of fullness in the ears. The fluid is usually the result of a buildup of negative pressure in the middle ear cavity because of Eustachian tube dysfunction (Cash & Glass, 2010). Hearing is reduced when the fluid inhibits the healthy vibration of the tympanic membrane or eardrum. OME is not to be confused with **acute otitis media (AOM),** a painful middle ear infection often accompanied by fever and general malaise (Toll & Nunez, 2012); however, OME can occur prior to or following AOM. It is also not to be confused with **chronic suppurative otitis media (CSOM)**, discharge in the ear canal and a perforated eardrum (often due to AOM) lasting greater than 2 to 6 weeks (Morris & Leach, 2009). If OME is persistent and does not spontaneously resolve after a period of active monitoring, an ear, nose, and throat specialist may surgically make a small hole in the eardrum (to drain out the fluid and equalize the pressure in the middle ear cavity) and insert eardrum ventilation tubes, also known as pressure equalizer tubes (PE tubes), grommets, or tympanostomy tubes (Robb & Williamson, 2011).

COMMENT: *Valsalva maneuver*

The **Valsalva maneuver** may be recommended when unequal ear pressure is experienced (e.g., when you have a cold, or when changing altitude in an airplane or car). The Valsalva maneuver is "the process of making a forceful attempt at expiration while holding the nostrils closed and keeping the mouth shut for the purpose of adjusting middle ear pressure" (Taylor, 1996, p. 8). This technique forces air up the Eustachian tube into the middle ear, enabling ear pressure to equalize and secretions to drain from the middle ear. This technique may be used in scuba diving to equalize pressure in the middle ear during descent (Taylor, 1996).

Problems with the structure or function of the inner ear are associated with **sensorineural hearing loss**. When people have a hearing loss with both conductive and sensorineural elements, they have a **mixed hearing loss**. Difficulty interpreting (rather than detecting sounds) occurs when there are problems with the structure or function of the auditory nerves and may be called **retrocochlear pathology** and **central auditory processing deficits** (Northern & Downs, 2002; Rance et al., 2007; Rappaport & Provencal, 2002). These difficulties include auditory neuropathy/dyssynchrony that is reported to occur in 7–10% of children with sensorineural hearing loss (Roush, 2011).

ADDITIONAL ANATOMICAL STRUCTURES THAT SUPPORT PERCEPTION AND PRODUCTION OF SPEECH

The neurological system is important in the perception, cognitive-linguistic processing, and production of speech.

■ The neurological system

The neurological system consists of the brain, brain stem, spinal cord, and nerves.

Function of the neurological system

One of the many functions of the brain and neurological system is to coordinate and enable the perception, storage, and production of speech. You will learn more about theories of perception, the abstract representation of speech, and the motor skills involved in speech production in chapter 5.

Structure of the neurological system

The neurological structures that support perception and production of speech are the brain and nervous system. The brain consists of four **cortical lobes** (frontal, temporal, parietal, and occipital), the midbrain, diencephalon, basal ganglia, cerebellum, brain stem, cranial nerves, gray and white matter, and corpus callosum. In a meta-analysis of 82 studies of word production and 26 studies of word perception, Indefrey and Levelt (2004) found that brain activation predominantly was **left lateralized** and that large parts of the brain were activated during speech production and perception (see Table 3-2). Regions that were NOT (or rarely) activated during word production were the superior and medial parietal lobe, right anterior and medial frontal lobe, anterior inferior temporal lobes bilaterally, bilateral posterior cingulate, bilateral hypothalamus, and the bilateral hippocampus (Indefrey & Levelt, 2004).

There are 12 cranial nerves (see Table 3-3). The major cranial nerve involved in hearing is the **acoustic nerve** (VIII). The major cranial nerve involved in the sensation and movement of the face is the **facial nerve** (VII). Movement of the tongue is controlled by the **trigeminal nerve** (V), **vagus nerve** (X), and the **hypoglossal nerve** (XII).

Impairments of the neurological system

Children who have impairments of the neurological system can have difficulties with motor execution and/or motor planning and programming. Children who have difficulty with **motor execution** include those who have cerebral palsy, muscular dystrophy, acquired brain injuries, and congenital conditions that affect the cranial nerves (e.g., Moebius syndrome). Many of these children have childhood **dysarthria**. The following quote by Hodge (2010) demonstrates the anatomical structures involved in dysarthria: " . . . impairments that interfere with signals sent from their brains to the muscle groups (diaphragm, rib cage, abdomen, vocal folds, pharynx, soft palate, tongue, lips, and jaw) that produce the rapid, precise, and coordinated movements of speech. These impairments result in weakness, slowness, and tone abnormalities in the affected muscles and reduce the accuracy and coordination of their actions" (p. 557).

TABLE 3-2	Areas of brain activation during word production and perception

Task	Areas of brain activation
Word generation and picture naming	11 left-hemispheric regions (posterior inferior frontal gyrus, ventral precentral gyrus, supplementary motor area [SMA], mid and posterior superior and middle temporal gyri, posterior temporal fusiform gyrus, anterior insula, thalamus, and medial cerebellum) four right-hemispheric regions (mid superior temporal gyrus, medial and lateral cerebellum, and right SMA)
Word generation (not picture naming)	Left anterior cingulate, right anterior insula, left lentiform nucleus, left dorsal precentral gyrus, left anterior and posterior (bilaterally) middle frontal gyri, and left posterior medial frontal gyrus
Picture naming (not word generation)	Six left and right occipital areas, left mid temporal fusiform gyrus, right posterior temporal fusiform gyrus, left mid and posterior sections of the inferior temporal gyrus, right posterior inferior frontal gyrus, and mid cingulate
Phonological coding	SMA, left anterior insula, and left posterior superior and middle temporal gyri (Wernicke's area)
Syllabification	Left posterior inferior frontal gyrus (Broca's area), left ventral precentral gyrus, bilateral mid superior temporal gyri, left posterior temporal fusiform gyrus, left thalamus, and right medial cerebellum
Phonetic encoding and articulation	12 regions of the central nervous motor systems (bilateral ventral motor and sensory regions, right dorsal motor region, right SMA, left and medial right cerebellum, bilateral thalami, right midbrain) plus five other regions (right posterior inferior frontal gyrus, left orbital gyrus, bilateral posterior lingual gyri, and right posterior medial temporal fusiform gyrus)

Source: Adapted from the meta-analysis by Indefrey and Levelt (2004).

TABLE 3-3	The twelve cranial nerves and their functions

No.	Nerve	Sensory/Motor	Function
I	Olfactory	Sensory	Smell
II	Optic	Sensory	Vision
III	Oculomotor	Motor	Muscles for visual convergence and accommodation
IV	Trochlear	Motor	Muscles for eye rotation (down and out)
V	Trigeminal	Sensory +	Sensation to the eye, nose, and face
		Motor	Muscles of mastication and the tongue
VI	Abducent	Motor	Lateral eye muscles
VII	Facial	Sensory +	Sensation to the tongue and soft palate
		Motor	Muscles of the face and stapedius
VIII	Acoustic	Sensory	Hearing and balance
IX	Glossopharyngeal	Sensory +	Sensation to the pharynx, soft palate, and tonsils
		Motor	Muscles of the pharynx and stylopharyngeus
X	Vagus	Sensory +	Sensation to the ear, pharynx, larynx, and viscera
		Motor	Muscles of the pharynx, larynx, tongue, and smooth muscles of the viscera
XI	Accessory	Motor	Muscles of the pharynx, larynx, soft palate, and neck
XII	Hypoglossal	Motor	Extrinsic and intrinsic muscles of the tongue, and strap muscles of the neck

Source: Adapted from Zemlin (1998).

Children who have **CAS** have difficulties with planning and programming sequences of motor movement, although it is not yet clear if all of these children have impairments of the neurological system. Shriberg (2010b) provided an extensive list of examples of children who have CAS as a secondary disorder to complex neurobehavioral disorders: "autism spectrum, chromosome translocations, Coffin-Siris syndrome, Down syndrome, Fragile-X syndrome, Joubert syndrome, galactosemia, Rett syndrome, Rolandic epilepsy, Russell-Silver syndrome, Velocardiofacial syndrome, and duplication of the Williams-Beuren locus" (p. 262). For example, children with galactosemia may have diffuse cerebellar damage and have been reported to have a high prevalence of coordination, strength, and speech disorders, including CAS and dysarthria (Potter, Nievergelt, & Shriberg, 2013; Shriberg, Potter, & Strand, 2011). We will discuss children with dysarthria and CAS in greater depth in other chapters in this book.

Chapter summary

In this chapter you have learned about the important anatomical structures that enable speech production and perception. You learned the structures that enable speech production include the tongue, lips, nose, teeth, hard palate, soft palate, mandible, pharynx, larynx, and the respiratory system. You learned the primary structure involved in the detection of speech is the ear, and speech production and perception are supported by the neurological system. In Chapter 4, you will add to this knowledge by learning how to transcribe children's speech. In Chapter 8 you will learn how to consider anatomical structures during an assessment of structure and function of the oromusculature.

Suggested reading

If you have not taken a class on speech science anatomy and physiology, we suggest that you consult a text designed for SLPs (e.g., Fuller, Pimentel, & Peregoy, 2012; Seikel, Drumright, & Seikel, 2014; Zemlin, 1998). If you would like to know more about the correspondence between anatomical structures and the articulation of individual consonants, you are encouraged to read chapter 4 and source McLeod and Singh (2009a).

- McLeod, S., & Singh, S. (2009a). *Speech sounds: A pictorial guide to typical and atypical speech*. San Diego, CA: Plural Publishing.

- Zemlin, W. R. (1998). *Speech and hearing science: Anatomy and physiology* (4th ed.). Boston, MA: Allyn and Bacon.

Application of knowledge from Chapter 3

Using the case-based information in Chapter 16, apply your knowledge about the anatomical structure and function foundations for speech by completing the following questions.

1. What type of dentition (deciduous or primary, mixed or adult) would you expect to see in the mouths of Luke (4;3 years), Susie (7;4 years), Jarrod (7;0 years), and Michael (4;2 years) (i.e., the case study children in chapter 16)? Review the case history information for each of these children in chapter 16. Was their dentition as you predicted?

2. Compare and contrast how oral musculature structure and function was assessed for Luke (4;3 years), Susie (7;4 years), Jarrod (7;0 years), Michael (4;2

years), and Lian (14;2 years) in Chapter 16. Why do you think Lian's assessment was more detailed than any of the other children?

3. Lian (14;2 years) has spastic dysarthria associated with congenital cerebral palsy (chapter 16). What motor-related difficulties might you observe in an assessment of Lian's respiration, phonation, articulation, and resonance? Compare your predictions with the assessment findings for Lian's case in Table 16-17.

4. Review Luke's assessment results in chapter 16 regarding "oral musculature structure and function." What structures and skills were assessed? Do you think Luke's (4;3 years) SSD is associated with a problem with his mouth?

4

Transcription of Speech

LEARNING OBJECTIVES

1 Explain the importance of phonetic transcription.

2 Transcribe speech using the International Phonetic Alphabet.

3 List the common diacritics used in the transcription of the speech of children with SSD.

4 Describe voice, place, and manner of characteristics of English consonants.

5 Describe phonotactic elements of language.

6 Compare and contrast sagittal and transverse images of English consonant production.

7 Indicate where the tongue touches the palate for a range of English consonants.

KEY WORDS

Transcription: systematic (phonemic, phonetic), impressionistic (simple/broad, detailed/narrow)

International Phonetic Alphabet: pulmonic consonants (voice, place, manner), non-pulmonic consonants, diacritics, vowels and diphthongs, suprasegmentals

Phonotactics: consonant clusters, syllable shapes, word positions

Understanding English consonants: sagittal and transverse diagrams

OVERVIEW

In this chapter you will gain an understanding of how to transcribe speech. You will be introduced to the study of phonetics, and then we will combine your knowledge of anatomy (from Chapter 3) and phonetics (from this chapter) and apply it to children with SSD of known and unknown origins. While the primary focus is on English, we also consider other languages, since SLPs also work with children who speak languages in addition to and other than English.

TRANSCRIPTION OF SPEECH

Transcription is the representation of speech using symbols "so as to furnish a record sufficient to render possible the accurate reconstruction of the utterance" (Wells, 2006, p. 386). In reality, speech is not neatly compartmentalized into words, consonants, or vowels. Speech is a continuum of sound. When speech is captured instrumentally, the transitions and fluidity of movement are obvious. The waveform depicted in Figure 4-1 shows the sound wave produced when counting *one, two, three, four, five, six, seven, eight, nine, ten*. You can see that there are 10 segments within the waveform: each corresponds to a different word because they were spoken with a short break between each word. The word *one* is darker and larger because it was at the beginning of the string, and emphasized, but also because all of the consonants /wʌn/ are **voiced** and the vowel and consonants are **sonorant** (you will learn about this later in the chapter). The number *six* is much smaller than the number *one*. The main peak in the number six is the vowel /i/. The smaller segments on either side of *six* correspond to the **voiceless** consonants /s/ and /ks/ (i.e., "x"). Number *seven* has two peaks, because there are two syllables (and two vowels) in the word *se-ven*. The number *nine* is also darker and larger (similar to number one) because it contains sonorant consonants.

The waveform depicted in Figure 4-2 shows the sound wave produced when saying, "This book is about children's speech." As you can see, the words are embedded in a continuous stream of sounds. The darker sections correspond to the vowels and voiced consonants. The sentence was spoken naturally, so that the boundaries between the words are not as distinct as in Figure 4-1. In order to understand, document, and analyze speech, we artificially segment the sound wave into consonants, vowels, and prosodic structures that in turn are combined into words, sentences, and conversations. In doing so, we make decisions about where the boundaries go. We need to be aware that we artificially segment speech during transcription. As Powell, Müller, and Ball (2003) stated: "Every transcription and coding system imposes categorizations on the data ... To put it simply, there is no such thing as 'raw' data ... forced decisions in transcribing and coding may hide important patterns and complexities in disordered language" (p. 425).

| **FIGURE 4-1** | **Waveform of the first author counting from one to ten** |

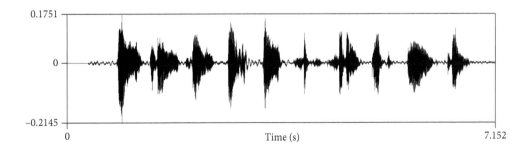

Source: Used by permission from Sharynne McLeod. Created using Praat (Boersma & Weenink, 2013).

FIGURE 4-2 Waveform of the first author saying, "This book is about children's speech."

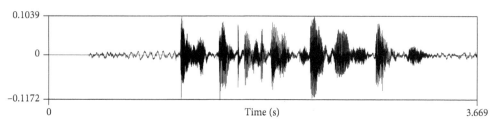

Source: Used by permission from Sharynne McLeod. Created using Praat (Boersma & Weenink, 2013).

COMMENT: *SLPs have a unique and valuable skill*

"Phonetic transcription ability is a skill unique to SLTs [SLPs] among the health care and education professions; no one else can provide this information about a child's speech. It is information that is essential to good practice and we need to use the skills inherent in our training in order to provide it" (UK and Ireland Specialists in Specific Speech Impairment Network [UK and Ireland SSSIN], 2013, p. 3).

If SLPs do not have good transcription skills, here are some potential problems identified by the UK and Ireland SSSIN (2013, p. 3):

■ Misdiagnosis and inappropriate management decisions;

■ Incorrect target choice;

■ Ineffective or inefficient therapy;

■ Not demonstrating progress objectively; and

■ Inadequate records.

A transcription decision-making tree is provided by the UK and Ireland SSSIN (2013) and reproduced in Appendix 4-1 to determine the amount and type of transcription that is necessary within different types of assessment.

Although speech is a continuum of sound, we have spent our lives segmenting the language(s) we speak into words, consonants, and vowels. Children learn to segment speech into words, consonants, and vowels in their first years of school. Have a look at the following words written by a 5-year-old child in his first year of school (Figure 4-3). What has he spelled? That's right, his letters I FEL LIK A SAD ALAGTA spell *I feel like a sad alligator*. At another time he wrote *good cat* as GUD KAT and *funny bird* as FUNI BRD. If we write these words using phonemic transcription, you will notice that they look closer to the child's writing than correct English spelling (orthography): /sæd æləgetɚ/, /gʊd kæt/, /fʌni bɝd/. Table 4-1 compares the three ways of writing these phrases, and adds up the number of consonants and vowels in each one (each diphthong in the last sentence was counted as one vowel). You will see that the number of the 5-year-old's letters closely corresponded to the number of phonemic symbols. So, in order to segment speech, it helps to think like a 5-year-old!

There are different terms to describe different types of auditory transcription. Different terminology is used for transcribing different groups of people, within research and practice, and within the fields of linguistics/phonetics, speech-language pathology, and foreign language teaching. Figure 4-4 has been developed to explain the different terminology.

| FIGURE 4-3 | "I feel like a sad alligator," written by a 5-year-old |

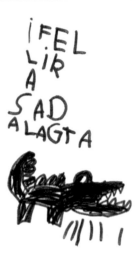

Source: Used by permission from Sharynne McLeod.

| TABLE 4-1 | A comparison between a 5-year-old's spelling, phonemic transcription, and an adult's spelling |

5-year-old's spelling	Phonemic transcription	Adult's spelling
I FEL LIK A SAD ALAGTA (17)	/aɪ fil laɪk ə sæd æləgetɚ / (18)	*I feel like a sad alligator* (22)
GUD KAT (6)	/gʊd kæt/ (6)	*good cat* (7)
FUNI BRD (7)	/fʌni bɝd/ (7)	*funny bird* (9)

Systematic transcriptions are used when "the transcriber knows in advance what all the possibilities are ..." (Abercrombie, 1967, p. 128). Systematic transcriptions primarily are used by linguists and phoneticians to transcribe typical, standard, or common realizations of speech. There are two types of systematic transcriptions: **phonemic** and **phonetic**. **Phonemic** transcription (sometimes called **phonological** transcription) documents phonemes or sounds that convey different meanings within a language. Phonemic transcription is written within virgules or slashes / /. For example, in English /p/ and /t/ are different phonemes and the two consonants create different words, as shown in the phonemic transcription of the words *pit* /pɪt/ and *tip* /tɪp/. Phonemic transcription is used within many dictionaries to provide the common pronunciation of words. **Phonetic** transcription (sometimes called **allophonic** transcription) documents differences within phones that do not change the meaning of a word but provide a more thorough description of the pronunciation. Phonetic transcription is written within square brackets [ ]. As mentioned earlier, /p/ and /t/ are different phonemes in English, and while the phonemic transcription of the word *pit* is /pɪt/, the phonetic transcription would be [pʰɪt˺], since in many English dialects the /p/ is aspirated [pʰ] at the beginning of a word (produced with a lot of air) and the /t/ is unreleased [t˺] at the end of a word (the air is not released).

Impressionistic transcriptions are used when "an almost infinite number of possibilities stretches before a transcriber" (Abercrombie, 1967, p. 128). When making an impressionistic transcription the transcriber may not know the pronunciation patterns of the person being recorded (e.g., when transcribing the speech of children with SSD). Impressionistic transcriptions primarily are used by SLPs to transcribe atypical speech and

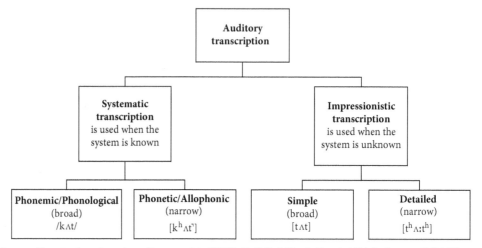

FIGURE 4-4 **Terminology for the transcription of speech**

The example for systematic transcription provides the standard pronunciation of the word cut.
*The example for impressionistic transcription provides the transcription of a child with an SSD
producing* [tʌt] *for* cut.

Source: Terminology based on Abercrombie (1967); Ball, Rahilly, & Tench (1996); Grunwell (1987).

by linguists who are working on poorly described languages, regional dialects, and social
dialects. Ball, Rahilly, and Tench (1996) describe the tension between speed and depth felt
by SLPs in clinical settings. As a result, they suggest that impressionistic transcriptions can
be classified as either **simple** (broad) or **detailed** (narrow). Simple transcription is less
time-consuming and may be all that is required, for example, if a child uses the voiceless
lateral fricative in the word *sun* /sʌn/ → [ɬʌn], as was the case for Susie (7;4 years) (see Chapter 16). Detailed impressionistic transcription is needed for children who are more complex—for example, a child who is displaying covert contrasts by voicing a consonant to
indicate knowledge of a consonant cluster, and lengthening a vowel to indicate knowledge
of the deleted final consonant (e.g., *stick* /stɪk/ → [ţɪː]). We will explain the diacritics used
in this example in more detail later in the book, so at the moment, just consider the different types of transcriptions that are available to you. Within this book we primarily use
phonemic transcription to indicate the target sound/word (e.g., *cat* /kæt/) and **simple
impressionistic transcription** to indicate a child's production of a sound/word (e.g.,
cat /kæt/ → *tat* [tæt]). All of the transcription symbols we have used in these examples are
found within the International Phonetic Alphabet transcription system.

Read more about Susie
(7;4 years), a girl with an
articulation impairment
(lateral lisp), in Chapter 16
(Case 2).

■ International Phonetic Alphabet (IPA)

The International Phonetic Alphabet (IPA) (see Figure 4-5) is an important tool to assist
SLPs with the transcription of speech sounds. The IPA chart contains symbols to transcribe
each speech sound produced by typically developing speakers across the world. The
IPA chart contains symbols for **consonants** (pulmonic and non-pulmonic), **vowels**,
suprasegmental features, **tones and accents**, as well as **diacritics** to distinguish
between different productions of consonants and vowels. The IPA chart is so important
that we have placed a full-sized copy on the inside front cover of this book (so you can find
it easily), a smaller-sized copy is provided in Figure 4-5 so that you can compare it with the
text describing consonants and vowels, and it can be downloaded from the International
Phonetic Association website.[1]

---

[1]https://www.internationalphoneticassociation.org/content/ipa-chart

FIGURE 4-5 **The International Phonetic Alphabet chart**

THE INTERNATIONAL PHONETIC ALPHABET (revised to 2015)

CONSONANTS (PULMONIC) © 2015 IPA

	Bilabial	Labiodental	Dental	Alveolar	Postalveolar	Retroflex	Palatal	Velar	Uvular	Pharyngeal	Glottal
Plosive	p b			t d		ʈ ɖ	c ɟ	k ɡ	q ɢ		ʔ
Nasal	m	ɱ		n		ɳ	ɲ	ŋ	N		
Trill	ʙ			r					R		
Tap or Flap		ⱱ		ɾ		ɽ					
Fricative	ɸ β	f v	θ ð	s z	ʃ ʒ	ʂ ʐ	ç ʝ	x ɣ	χ ʁ	ħ ʕ	h ɦ
Lateral fricative				ɬ ɮ							
Approximant		ʋ		ɹ		ɻ	j	ɰ			
Lateral approximant				l		ɭ	ʎ	ʟ			

Symbols to the right in a cell are voiced, to the left are voiceless. Shaded areas denote articulations judged impossible.

CONSONANTS (NON-PULMONIC)

Clicks	Voiced implosives	Ejectives
ʘ Bilabial	ɓ Bilabial	ʼ Examples:
ǀ Dental	ɗ Dental/alveolar	pʼ Bilabial
ǃ (Post)alveolar	ʄ Palatal	tʼ Dental/alveolar
ǂ Palatoalveolar	ɠ Velar	kʼ Velar
ǁ Alveolar lateral	ʛ Uvular	sʼ Alveolar fricative

OTHER SYMBOLS

ʍ Voiceless labial-velar fricative ɕ ʑ Alveolo-palatal fricatives

w Voiced labial-velar approximant ɺ Voiced alveolar lateral flap

ɥ Voiced labial-palatal approximant ɧ Simultaneous ʃ and x

ʜ Voiceless epiglottal fricative

ʢ Voiced epiglottal fricative

ʡ Epiglottal plosive

Affricates and double articulations can be represented by two symbols joined by a tie bar if necessary. t͡s k͡p

VOWELS

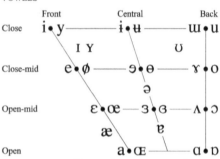

Where symbols appear in pairs, the one to the right represents a rounded vowel.

SUPRASEGMENTALS

	ˈ Primary stress	ˌfoʊnəˈtɪʃən
	ˌ Secondary stress	
	ː Long	eː
	ˑ Half-long	eˑ
	˘ Extra-short	ĕ
	ǀ Minor (foot) group	
	‖ Major (intonation) group	
	. Syllable break	ɹi.ækt
	‿ Linking (absence of a break)	

DIACRITICS Some diacritics may be placed above a symbol with a descender, e.g. ŋ̊

̥ Voiceless	n̥ d̥	̤ Breathy voiced	b̤ a̤	̪ Dental	t̪ d̪
̬ Voiced	s̬ t̬	̰ Creaky voiced	b̰ a̰	̺ Apical	t̺ d̺
ʰ Aspirated	tʰ dʰ	̼ Linguolabial	t̼ d̼	̻ Laminal	t̻ d̻
̹ More rounded	ɔ̹	ʷ Labialized	tʷ dʷ	̃ Nasalized	ẽ
̜ Less rounded	ɔ̜	ʲ Palatalized	tʲ dʲ	ⁿ Nasal release	dⁿ
̟ Advanced	u̟	ˠ Velarized	tˠ dˠ	ˡ Lateral release	dˡ
̠ Retracted	e̠	ˤ Pharyngealized	tˤ dˤ	̚ No audible release	d̚
̈ Centralized	ë	̴ Velarized or pharyngealized ɫ			
̽ Mid-centralized	e̽	̝ Raised	e̝ (ɹ̝ = voiced alveolar fricative)		
̩ Syllabic	n̩	̞ Lowered	e̞ (β̞ = voiced bilabial approximant)		
̯ Non-syllabic	e̯	̘ Advanced Tongue Root	e̘		
˞ Rhoticity	ɚ a˞	̙ Retracted Tongue Root	e̙		

TONES AND WORD ACCENTS

LEVEL		CONTOUR	
e̋ or ˥ Extra high		ě or ˩˥ Rising	
é ˦ High		ê ˥˩ Falling	
ē ˧ Mid		e᷄ ˦˥ High rising	
è ˨ Low		e᷅ ˩˨ Low rising	
ȅ ˩ Extra low		e᷈ ˧˦˧ Rising-falling	
ꜜ Downstep		↗ Global rise	
ꜛ Upstep		↘ Global fall	

Source: Copyright © 2015 International Phonetic Association. IPA Chart, https://www.internationalphoneticassociation.org/sites/default/files/IPA_Kiel_2015.pdf

COMMENT: *Hint for typing phonetic symbols*

If you want to type using phonemic and phonetic symbols, phonetic fonts are freely available from the SIL International.[1] Commonly used fonts are Doulos SIL[2] and Charis SIL.[3] Additionally, an IPA Palette is available for Macintosh computer users.[4]

[1] http://www.sil.org
[2] http://software.sil.org/doulos/
[3] http://software.sil.org/charis/
[4] http://www.blugs.com/IPA/index.html

COMMENT: *International Phonetic Association is more than 130 years old*

The International Phonetic Association first met in Paris in 1886. One of the major roles of the phoneticians who are members of the International Phonetic Association has been to document the world's speech sounds and provide a standard notation system to be used throughout the world. The most recent version of the chart was published in 2015. The International Phonetic Association has made the IPA chart freely available[1] so you are able to make copies for your own use (make sure you place a copy on your noticeboard). They also publish the *Journal of the International Phonetic Association*[2] and a handbook (International Phonetic Association, 1999) that contains a description of a range of languages.

[1] https://www.internationalphoneticassociation.org/content/ipa-chart
[2] http://journals.cambridge.org/action/displayJournal?jid=IPA

■ Pulmonic consonant chart

All spoken languages contain consonants, and most languages (including English) contain pulmonic consonants. A **pulmonic** consonant is produced on air expelled from the lungs. The IPA pulmonic consonant chart is organized according to the concepts of **voice**, **place**, and **manner** (see Figure 4-6).

> **Voice:** whether vocal fold vibration is present (voiced consonant) or absent (voiceless consonant).
>
> **Place:** where the articulators stop or slow the airstream.
>
> **Manner:** how the consonant is articulated.

On the IPA chart, paired voiceless and voiced consonants are found within the same box, with the voiceless consonants appearing on the left-hand side of the box. Some boxes contain only one consonant, so look to see if it is aligned with the left (voiceless) or right (voiced) side of the boxes. The columns of the pulmonic consonant chart represent the place of articulation. The left-hand columns begin with the lips (**bilabial** consonants) and move back into the mouth to end with the glottis (**glottal** consonants). The rows of the pulmonic consonant chart represent the manner of articulation. There are eight ways that pulmonic consonants can be articulated: **plosive, nasal, trill, tap/flap, fricative, lateral fricative, approximant,** and **lateral approximant**. The blank cells indicate that it is possible to produce these consonants, but they have not been found in any of the world's languages to date. The shaded cells indicate that these consonants are not possible to produce. The location of consonants on the pulmonic chart helps you determine the voice, place, and manner characteristics of individual consonants. For example, /t/ is the voiceless alveolar plosive and /ɸ/ is the voiceless bilabial fricative.

FIGURE 4-6 The pulmonic consonant chart from the International Phonetic Alphabet

CONSONANTS (PULMONIC) © 2005 IPA

	Bilabial	Labiodental	Dental	Alveolar	Postalveolar	Retroflex	Palatal	Velar	Uvular	Pharyngeal	Glottal
Plosive	p b			t d		ʈ ɖ	c ɟ	k ɡ	q ɢ		ʔ
Nasal	m	ɱ		n		ɳ	ɲ	ŋ	N		
Trill	ʙ			r					R		
Tap or Flap		ⱱ		ɾ		ɽ					
Fricative	ɸ β	f v	θ ð	s z	ʃ ʒ	ʂ ʐ	ç ʝ	x ɣ	χ ʁ	ħ ʕ	h ɦ
Lateral fricative				ɬ ɮ							
Approximant		ʋ		ɹ		ɻ	j	ɰ			
Lateral approximant				l		ɭ	ʎ	L			

Where symbols appear in pairs, the one to the right represents a voiced consonant. Shaded areas denote articulations judged impossible.

Source: IPA Chart, http://www.internationalphoneticassociation.org/content/ipa-chart, available under a Creative Commons Attribution-Sharealike 3.0 Unported License. Copyright © 2005 International Phonetic Association. Copyright © 2005 International Phonetic Association.

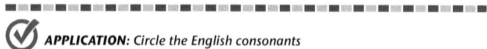

✓ APPLICATION: *Circle the English consonants*

Circle each of the 24 English consonants on the IPA chart (Figure 4-5). Most (21) of these will be found on the pulmonic consonant chart. Three of these consonants /w, ʧ, ʤ/ are found on the other symbols chart (discussed later in the chapter).

English pulmonic consonants

English has 24 pulmonic consonants: /p, b, t, d, k, g, m, n, ŋ, f, v, θ, ð, s, z, ʃ, ʒ, h, ɹ, j, l, w, ʧ, ʤ/. There are a few English consonant symbols that can be difficult for students to remember, mostly because they are depicted with non-English symbols:

- /ŋ/ is often written as "ng" and is found in the middle and end of the word *singing* /sɪŋɪŋ/. It is also found in the middle of the word *monkey* /mʌŋki/. It is not found at the beginning of words in English. However, /ŋ/ is found at the beginning of words in languages such as Cantonese and Vietnamese.
- /θ/ is the voiceless "th" consonant. It is found at the beginning of the word *think* /θɪŋk/, the middle of the word *toothache* /tuθeɪk/, and the end of the word *mouth* /maʊθ/.
- /ð/ is the voiced "th" consonant. It is one of the most often produced consonants in English because it is found at the beginning of the word *the* /ðə/. It is also found in the middle of the word *rhythm* /ɹɪðəm/ and the end of the word *bathe* /beɪð/.
- /ʃ/ is often written as "sh" and is found in the beginning of the word *shoe* /ʃu/, the middle of the word *nation* /neɪʃən/, and the end of the word *push* /pʊʃ/.
- /ʒ/ can be written as "zh" but is often spelled as "s" or "g." It is found at the beginning of the word *genre* /ʒɑnɹə/ (US), /ʒɒnɹə/ (UK), in the middle of words like *measure* /mɪʒɚ/ (US), /mɛʒə/ (UK), and the end of the word *mirage* /mɪɹɑʒ/ (US, UK), /məɹɑʒ/ (Australia).

COMMENT: */ɹ/ versus /r/*

The consonant /ɹ/ is often written as /r/ in English textbooks. In this book, we use /ɹ/ to indicate the alveolar approximant found in English, since in the IPA chart, the /r/ symbol is used for an alveolar trill that occurs in the Scottish English dialect as well as many other languages including Afrikaans, Arabic, Filipino, Finnish, French, German, Hungarian, Icelandic, Spanish, Thai, Vietnamese, Welsh, and many Australian Aboriginal languages. In fact, a trilled /r/ occurs in more languages than the voiced approximant /ɹ/. Ladefoged (2001b) states that it is permissible to use /r/ for the Standard English /ɹ/ when you are only referring to the Standard English /ɹ/. He wrote: "When you are not trying to make such precise distinctions, the IPA recommends that you use the simplest possible phonetic symbol, which in this case is r. Then at the end of the transcript, you should simply say r = upside-down-r" (p. 176).

- /ɹ/ is written as "r" and is found in the beginning of the word *run* /ɹʌn/, the middle of the word *hurry* /hʌɹi/, and the end of the word *car* /kɑɹ/ in US, Irish, and Scottish English (but not most other English dialects). Some textbooks use /r/ for /ɹ/ when referring to the English "r" (see "/ɹ/ versus /r/").
- /j/ is written as "y" and is found in the beginning of the word *you* /ju/ and the middle of the word *onion* /ʌnjən/. It is not found at the end of words in English.
- /ʧ/ is often written as "ch" and is found in the beginning of the word *chew* /ʧu/, the middle of the word *teacher* /tiʧɚ/ (US), /tiʧə/ (UK), and the end of the word *much* /mʌʧ/.
- /ʤ/ is often written as "j" or "g" and is found in the beginning and end of the word *judge* /ʤʌʤ/ and the middle of the word *unjust* /ʌnʤʌst/.

Features of pulmonic consonants: Voice, place, manner

Pulmonic consonants can be differentiated using the concepts of voice, place, and manner, and the subcategories under these concepts (see Table 4-2). For example, /m/ can be described as a voiced bilabial nasal and /f/ can be described as a voiceless labiodental fricative.

Voice

There are two degrees of voicing differentiated in English consonants: voiceless and voiced. Voiceless consonants, as the name suggests, are produced without vibration of the vocal cords. Voiced consonants are produced with vibration of the vocal cords to produce voicing. To determine the difference, place your hand on your throat, and say a consonant (but remember not to say it with a vowel, because all vowels are voiced). In English the nine voiceless consonants are: /p, t, k, θ, f, s, ʃ, h, ʧ/; all other consonants are voiced. Within the world's languages, many voiceless and voiced consonants are paired, sharing the same place and manner. Remember that paired voiceless and voiced consonants are

COMMENT: *Vowels in this book*

Some vowels (or the way that they have been transcribed) are fairly similar across many of the English dialects: /i, ɪ, u, ʊ, ɔ, ə, æ, ʌ/. Within this book we have tried to use words containing these vowels when we provide examples so that whether you are reading this book in Australia, Canada, Hong Kong, Ireland, New Zealand, Singapore, South Africa, the United Kingdom, or the United States, you will be able to make sense of most of our examples. However, when this is not possible we have provided the IPA transcription of the word using pronunciations based on General American English (US).

TABLE 4-2	Features of English pulmonic consonants as labeled in the International Phonetic Alphabet

Voice	Place	Manner
Voiceless	Bilabial	Plosive
Voiced	Labiodental	Nasal
	Labial-velar*	Fricative
	Dental	Affricate
	Alveolar	Approximant
	Postalveolar	Lateral approximant
	Palatal	Affricate*
	Velar	
	Glottal	

*The terms *Labial-velar* (describing the place of articulation for /w/) and *Affricate* (describing the manner of articulation for /ʧ, ʤ/) are found in the "Other symbols" section of the International Phonetic Alphabet.

found within the same box on the IPA chart, with the voiceless consonants appearing near the left-hand side of the box. In English, the eight pairs are: /p-b/, /t-d/, /k-g/, /θ-ð/, /f-v/, /s-z/, /ʃ-ʒ/, /ʧ-ʤ/ (/h/ is not paired in English). In some languages the amount of aspiration rather than degree of voicing distinguishes between plosives. For example, in Cantonese, plosive consonants are unaspirated or aspirated (e.g., /p/ versus. /pʰ/). In Korean, tenseness and aspiration are important: plain (fortis), aspirated, and tense (lenis) (e.g., /p/ versus. /pʰ/ versus. /p*/), as shown in the words /pul/ "fire," /pʰul/ "grass," and /p*ul/ "horn" (Kim & Pae, 2007, p. 473).

Place
In English there are nine places where the articulators stop or slow the airstream:

1. **Bilabial**: /p, b, m/ are produced with the lips together.
2. **Labial-velar**: /w/ is produced with the lips rounded, and the tongue on the velum.
3. **Labiodental**: /f, v/ are produced with the top teeth touching the bottom lip.
4. **Dental**: /θ, ð/ are produced with the tongue touching the front teeth.
5. **Alveolar**: /t, d, n, s, z, ɹ, l/ are produced at the alveolar ridge. All of these consonants, with the exception of /ɹ/, are produced with the tongue tip on the alveolar ridge behind the teeth. For most of these consonants, /t, d, n, s, z/, the tongue is also in horseshoe-shaped contact with the palate along the edges of the teeth.
6. **Postalveolar**: /ʃ, ʒ/ are produced with the tongue raised towards the palate, behind the alveolar ridge. The tongue is anchored along the sides of the teeth.
7. **Palatal**: /j/ is produced with the tongue raised towards the palate and the sides anchored along the lateral margins of the palate.
8. **Velar**: /k, g, ŋ/ are produced with the tongue touching the velum (approximately at the juncture between the hard and soft palate).
9. **Glottal**: /h/ is produced with the air passing through the glottis.

Manner
Consonants and vowels can be classified into two broad manner categories depending on the degree of constriction of the vocal tract: obstruents and sonorants (see Figure 4-7). **Obstruents** are characterized by either a complete or narrowed constriction of the vocal tract. Most English consonants are obstruents: /p, b, t, d, k, g, f, v, θ, ð, s, z, ʃ, ʒ, h, ʧ, ʤ/. **Sonorants** are produced with a relatively open vocal tract (either oral or nasal). All vowels, diphthongs, and vowel-like consonants (approximants and nasals) are sonorants. The sonorant English consonants are: /m, n, ŋ, w, j, ɹ, l/.

In English there are six manners of articulation identified in the IPA:

1. **Plosive**: /p, b, t, d, k, g/ use the articulators to stop the airflow, then typically release the air quickly. Some textbooks use the term **stop** instead of *plosive*.
2. **Nasal**: /m, n, ŋ/ are produced with a nasal airflow. All other English consonants are produced with the air passing through the mouth.

3. **Fricative**: /f, v, θ, ð, s, z, ʃ, ʒ, h/ are produced by constricting (but not stopping) the airflow. This constriction creates turbulence or friction. For fricatives that are made using the tongue, the passage or channel through which the air travels is called the **groove**.

4. **Approximant**: /w, j, ɹ/ are the most vowel-like of the consonants. The articulators approach one another, but not closely enough to create turbulence. Some English texts use the terms **glide** for /w, j/ and **liquid** for /ɹ, l/.

5. **Lateral approximant**: /l/ is produced with lateral airflow around the sides of the tongue.

6. **Affricate**: /ʧ, ʤ/ initially are produced by stopping the air and then are released as a fricative.

FIGURE 4-7   **A typology of the manner of articulation of English consonants and vowels**

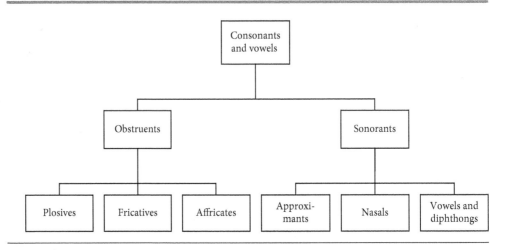

COMMENT: *Documenting children's progress using a visual analogue scale*

Sometimes when transcribing children's speech, it seems that children are producing a sound that is in between two consonants. Munson and colleagues have recommended using a visual analogue scale (VAS) for documenting gradual change in speech-sound learning (Juliena & Munson, 2012; Munson, Edwards, Schellinger, Beckman, & Meyer, 2010; Munson, Schellinger, & Urberg Carlson, 2012). A VAS is a 10 cm line with the endpoints marked as different consonants. Munson and colleagues have used the following endpoints: /s/–/ʃ/, /s/–/θ/, /t/–/k/, and /d/–/g/. They found high correlations with the acoustic measures of the consonants being scored and high levels of intra-rater reliability (Munson et al., 2012). SLPs can adapt this technique by drawing a 10 cm line on paper, inserting a mark along the line that best represents the distance from the two endpoints (e.g., the distance between [s] and [ʃ], or the distance between [s] and [ɬ] if the child is producing a lateral lisp), then using a ruler to measure the distance in millimeters. Changes in this distance over time can indicate gradual changes in speech-sound learning.

[s]   [ɬ]

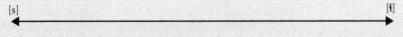

◼ Non-pulmonic consonant chart

The non-pulmonic consonant chart provides symbols for clicks, voiced implosives, and ejectives (see Figure 4-8). Clicks are "stop(s) produced with an ingressive velaric airstream" (Shriberg & Kent, 2003, p. 83). Implosives are "a combination of glottalic ingressive airflow, with a small amount of pulmonic egressive (just enough to create vocal fold vibration)" (Ball, Müller, Rutter, & Klopfenstein, 2009, p. 138). Ejectives are "a sound (usually a stop) produced by releasing a closure after holding the vocal folds together and moving them upward so as to compress the air in the vocal tract" (Ladefoged, 2005, p. 200). All ejectives are voiceless. People who have undergone a laryngectomy (typically after cancer of the larynx) are taught to use ejective forms of plosives, fricatives, and affricates to produce esophageal speech (Ashby, 2005). Non-pulmonic consonants do not occur in English, but occur in African languages including isiXhosa and isiZulu, Native American languages, and Sindhi, spoken by 50 million people in Pakistan (Ball, Müller, Klopfenstein, & Rutter, 2009; Maddieson, 2008b). Ejectives have been reported in the speech of children with hearing loss (e.g., Chin, 2002), and clicks have been reported in the speech of children with SSD (e.g., Bedore, Leonard, & Gandour, 1994) and cleft palate (Howard, 1993).

Pulmonic and non-pulmonic consonants in the world's languages

The world's languages range from having an inventory of six consonants (Rotokas spoken in Papua New Guinea) to 122 consonants (!Xóõ spoken in Botswana), with an average of 22.7 consonants per language (Maddieson, 2008a). This number includes pulmonic and non-pulmonic consonants. Consider the number and type of consonants that are used in a few of the world's languages on the next page. We have put them in order from the

---

FIGURE 4-8 The non-pulmonic consonant chart and other symbols chart from the International Phonetic Alphabet

CONSONANTS (NON-PULMONIC)

Clicks		Voiced implosives		Ejectives	
⊙	Bilabial	ɓ	Bilabial	'	Examples:
ǀ	Dental	ɗ	Dental/alveolar	pʼ	Bilabial
ǃ	(Post)alveolar	ʄ	Palatal	tʼ	Dental/alveolar
ǂ	Palatoalveolar	ɠ	Velar	kʼ	Velar
ǁ	Alveolar lateral	ʛ	Uvular	sʼ	Alveolar fricative

OTHER SYMBOLS

ʍ	Voiceless labial-velar fricative	ɕ ʑ	Alveolo-palatal fricatives
w	Voiced labial-velar approximant	ɺ	Voiced alveolar lateral flap
ɥ	Voiced labial-palatal approximant	ɧ	Simultaneous ∫ and X
ʜ	Voiceless epiglottal fricative		
ʢ	Voiced epiglottal fricative	Affricates and double articulations can be represented by two symbols joined by a tie bar if necessary.	k͡p t͡s
ʡ	Epiglottal plosive		

Source: IPA Chart, http://www.internationalphoneticassociation.org/content/ipa-chart, available under a Creative Commons Attribution-Sharealike 3.0 Unported License. Copyright © 2005 International Phonetic Association.

smallest to largest number of consonants. The consonants are listed in the same order as they appear on the IPA chart:

- Hawai'ian (8): /p, k, ʔ, m, n, h, l, w / (Pukui & Elbert, 1992)
- Finnish (13): /p, t̪, d, k, m, n, ŋ, r, s, h, ʋ, j, l/, with four additional consonants used by some speakers, /b, g, f, ʃ/ (Kunnari & Savinainen-Makkonen, 2007)
- Spanish (18): /p, b, t, d, k, g, m, n, ɲ, r, ɾ, f, s, x, j, l, w, ʧ/[2] (Goldstein, 2007)
- Cantonese (19): /p, pʰ, t, tʰ, k, kʰ, m, n, ŋ, f, s, h, j, l, w, ts, tsʰ, kʷ, kʷʰ/ (Zee, 1999)
- German (22): /p, b, t, d, k, g, ʔ, m, n, ŋ, f, v, s, z, ʃ, ʒ, ç, χ, ʁ, h, j, l/ (Kohler, 1999)
- French (20–24): /p, b, t, d, k, g, ʔ, m, n, ɲ, ŋ, r, ʀ, ɾ, f, v, s, z, ʃ, ʒ, ʁ, h, j, ɥ/ (Rose & Wauquier-Gravelines, 2007)
- English (24): /p, b, t, d, k, g, m, n, ŋ, f, v, θ, ð, s, z, ʃ, ʒ, h, ɹ, j, l, w, ʧ, ʤ/ (Smit, 2007)
- Jordanian Arabic (29): /b, t, t̪, d, d̪, k, q, ʔ, m, n, r, f, θ, ð, ð̪, s, s̪, z, ʃ, χ, ʁ, ħ, ʕ, h, j, l, w, ʧ, ʤ/, with six additional consonants used by some speakers, /g, ɢ, v, v, z̪, ʒ/ (Dyson & Amayreh, 2007)
- isiXhosa (41): Pulmonic /pʰ, b, tʰ, d, cʰ, ɟ, kʰ, g, m, n, ɲ, ŋ, r, f, v, s, z, ʃ, x, ɣ, ɦ, ɬ, ɮ, j, l̪, w, tsʰ, dz, ʧʰ, ʤ/ Non-pulmonic /ɓ, p', t', k', c', ts', ʧ', kx', ǀ, ǁ, !/ (Mowrer & Burger, 1991)

■ Other symbols chart

The other symbols chart (see Figure 4-8) contains symbols that do not neatly fit onto the pulmonic and non-pulmonic consonant charts, mostly because they are produced at two places of articulation. There are two entries on the other symbols chart that are important for the transcription of English. /w/ is listed here because it has two places of articulation: bilabial and velar. Affricates are listed on the other symbols chart, and although the examples /kp/ and /ts/ are not English affricates, this entry also includes the English affricates /ʧ/ and /ʤ/.

■■■ ■■ ■■ ■ ■■ ■ ■■ ■■ ■ ■ ■■ ■ ■ ■ ■ ■■ ■ ■ ■ ■ ■■ ■ ■■ ■ ■ ■■ ■ ■

 APPLICATION: *Comparing consonants across languages*

Appendix 4-2 contains a comparison of consonants across languages. Have a look at the consonants that are common and rare across languages. You may not recognize some of the consonants in the languages above and in the appendix. There are some excellent websites that enable you to hear how each consonant and vowel is produced by clicking on a symbol within the IPA chart. The following people have created websites:

- Eric Armstrong (York University, Canada)[1]
- John H. Esling (University of Victoria, Canada)[2]
- Peter Ladefoged (University of California, Los Angeles)[3]
- The University of Iowa[4]

A website created by researchers at six Scottish universities allows you to see and hear productions of the sounds of the IPA[5] (Lawson et al., 2015).

---

[1] http://www.yorku.ca/earmstro/ipa/index.html

[2] http://web.uvic.ca/ling/resources/ipa/charts/IPAlab/IPAlab.htm

[3] http://phonetics.ucla.edu/course/chapter1/chapter1.html

[4] http://www.uiowa.edu/~acadtech/phonetics/

[5] http://www.seeingspeech.arts.gla.ac.uk

---

[2]There is some disagreement about the phonemic status of /b, d, g/ and the spirants /β, ð, ɣ/. The list of consonants reflects those spoken in North and South America; there may be some differences with European Spanish.

▪▪ ▪ ░ ▪ ░ ▪ ░ ▪ ░ ▪ ░ ▪ ░ ▪ ░ ▪ ░ ▪ ░ ▪ ░ ▪ ░ ▪ ░ ▪ ░ ▪ ░ ▪ ░ ▪ ░ ▪ ░ ▪ ░ ▪▪

☑ APPLICATION: *Voice, place, and manner characteristics of English consonants*

Review the following words selected from Luke's (4;3 years) speech sample that is also found in Chapter 16.

sun [dʌn]	*zip* [dɪp]	*seat* [dit]	*feet* [bit]
van [bæn]	*meat* [mit]	*chip* [dɪp]	*bike* [baɪk]
light [laɪt]	*like* [laɪk]	*ship* [dɪp]	*that* [dæt]
fat [bæt]	*bite* [baɪt]	*thin* [dɪn]	*fun* [bʌn]

In this sample, Luke produces eight different consonants [p, b, t, d, k, m, n, l]:

1. Using the IPA chart, describe the voice, place, and manner characteristics of each of those speech sounds.
2. What do you notice about the voicing characteristic of the speech sounds he uses at the beginning of words—are they all voiced or voiceless?
3. What do you notice about his use of the velar consonant /k/?
4. What manners of articulation are not present in this sample of Luke's speech?

Answers:

1. [p] voiceless bilabial plosive, [b] voiced bilabial plosive, [t] voiceless alveolar plosive, [d] voiced alveolar plosive, [k] voiceless velar plosive, [m] voiced bilabial nasal, [n] voiced alveolar nasal, [l] voiced alveolar lateral approximant.
2. Speech sounds in word-initial position are all voiced.
3. [k] is only used in word-final position in words. When you review Luke's entire speech sample in Chapter 16, you will notice he uses velars in within word and word-final positions.
4. Across the 16 words, fricative, approximant, and affricate manners are not present. When you review Luke's entire sample in Chapter 16, the approximants [w, j] are present.

▪ Diacritics chart

Diacritics are "small letter-shaped symbols or other marks which can be added to a vowel or consonant symbol to modify or refine its meaning in various ways" (International Phonetic Association, 1999, p. 15). The IPA diacritics chart (see Figure 4-9) contains 31 symbols and marks. Ball, Müller, Klopfenstein, and Rutter (2010) divided the diacritics chart into six categories that are relevant for the clinical setting:

1. Voicing diacritics: voiceless, voiced,
2. Consonant release diacritics: aspirated, no audible release, nasal release, lateral release (the last two are used with the syllabic diacritic),
3. Consonant place diacritics: advanced, retracted, dental, apical, laminal,
4. Consonant manner diacritics: raised, lowered, syllabic,
5. Vowel diacritics: more rounded, less rounded, advanced, retracted, centralized, mid-centralized, advanced tongue root, retracted tongue root, rhoticity, non-syllabic,
6. Secondary articulation diacritics: labialized, palatalized, velarized, pharyngealized.

The remaining diacritics relate to voicing: breathy voiced, creaky voiced (for additional categorizations of diacritics see Ball, 2001).

The diacritics chart is useful for a number of reasons. First, if you plan to use narrow transcription, then you can use the symbols to describe the nuances of consonants and vowels. Second, you will find that some dialects and languages use diacritics to differentiate

FIGURE 4-9 **The diacritics chart from the International Phonetic Alphabet**

DIACRITICS   Diacritics may be placed above a symbol with a descender, e.g. ŋ̊

̥	Voiceless	n̥ d̥	̤	Breathy voiced	b̤ a̤	̪	Dental	t̪ d̪
̬	Voiced	s̬ t̬	̰	Creaky voiced	b̰ a̰	̺	Apical	t̺ d̺
ʰ	Aspirated	tʰ dʰ	̼	Linguolabial	t̼ d̼	̻	Laminal	t̻ d̻
̹	More rounded	ɔ̹	ʷ	Labialized	tʷ dʷ	̃	Nasalized	ẽ
̜	Less rounded	ɔ̜	ʲ	Palatalized	tʲ dʲ	ⁿ	Nasal release	dⁿ
̟	Advanced	u̟	ˠ	Velarized	tˠ dˠ	ˡ	Lateral release	dˡ
̠	Retracted	e̠	ˤ	Pharyngealized	tˤ dˤ	̚	No audible release	d̚
̈	Centralized	ë	~	Velarized or pharyngealized	ɫ			
̽	Mid-centralized	e̽	̝	Raised	e̝ (ɹ̝ = voiced alveolar fricative)			
̩	Syllabic	n̩	̞	Lowered	e̞ (β̞ = voiced bilabial approximant)			
̯	Non-syllabic	e̯	̘	Advanced Tongue Root	e̘			
˞	Rhoticity	ɚ a˞	̙	Retracted Tongue Root	e̙			

Source: IPA Chart, http://www.internationalphoneticassociation.org/content/ipa-chart, available under a Creative Commons Attribution-Sharealike 3.0 Unported License. Copyright © 2005 International Phonetic Association.

phonemes in their language. For example, US English uses the rhoticity diacritic /˞/ to indicate that vowels are rhotacized (or have an "r" like quality). US speakers use /ɝ/ and /ɚ/ whereas most other English dialects use /ɜ/ and /ə/ (e.g., *bird* /bɝd/ US versus /bɜd/ UK). Another example is that languages such as Cantonese have consonants that differ according to their aspiration (e.g., /p/ and /pʰ/). In Cantonese /pɔ/ and /pʰɔ/ are different words. /pɔ/ means *ball* 波 and /pʰɔ/ means *grandmother* 婆. The final reason why the diacritics chart is useful is because it is where you will be able to find symbols that represent the subtle differences between the child's production and the typical adult form. This is especially useful for transcribing the speech of young children who have not achieved adultlike pronunciation skills and children with SSD. For example, children may not pronounce a final nasal /n/ in the word *sun* /sʌn/, but may instead lengthen /ː/ and nasalize /˜/ the vowel, possibly to indicate that they know a nasal sound comes at the end so that *sun* /sʌn/ would be produced as [sʌ̃ː]. Some common diacritics that are used in the transcription of the speech of English-speaking children with SSD are voiceless [̥], voiced [̬], aspirated [ʰ], labialized [ʷ], dental [̪], nasalized [˜], and no audible release [̚]. If you are transcribing the speech of children with (unrepaired) cleft palate you are likely to use even more of these diacritics, non-pulmonic consonants, and other symbols (Fitzsimons, Jones, Barton, & North, 2012).

■ Vowel chart

Vowels are "sounds which occur at syllable centres, and … involve a less extreme narrowing of the vocal tract than consonants" (International Phonetic Association, 1999, p. 10). All languages contain vowels. The IPA vowel chart contains a representation of the vowels of the world's languages (see Figure 4-10). They are depicted as a **vowel quadrilateral** (Figure 4-10a). The shape of the vowel quadrilateral bears a general relationship to the tongue position during the production of the vowels [i], [a], [u], [o] (see Figure 4-10b). In the early 1900s, Daniel Jones defined a set of eight **cardinal vowels** (reference points) that were evenly spaced around the vowel quadrilateral. The International Phonetic

FIGURE 4-10 **Vowel chart from the International Phonetic Alphabet**

(a) The vowel chart from the International Phonetic Alphabet (b) Midsagittal section of the vocal tract with the outline of the tongue shape for each of the four extreme vowels superimposed

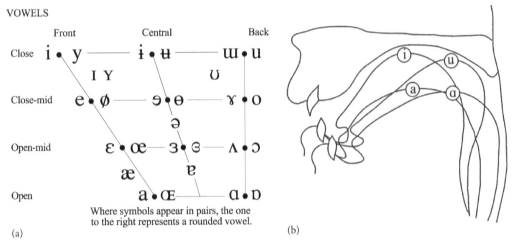

(a)

(b)

Source: (a) IPA Chart, http://www.internationalphoneticassociation.org/content/ipa-chart, available under a Creative Commons Attribution-Sharealike 3.0 Unported License. (b) 1999, Figure 3, p. 11. Copyright © 2005 International Phonetic Association.

Association (1999) describes the current conceptualization of cardinal vowels as: 1 [i], 2 [e], 3 [ɛ], 4 [a], 5 [ɑ], 6 [ɔ], 7 [o], 8 [u]. Notice that they are ordered anticlockwise around the perimeter of the vowel quadrilateral. Cardinal vowels were designed to be "arbitrary reference points" (Ladefoged, 1975, p. 195) and do not represent an exact match with English vowels (although some are close to French realizations of vowels).

The IPA vowel chart demonstrates four dimensions that impact the quality of the vowel sound:

1. Height: close, mid, open (vertical plane of the IPA vowel chart)—sometimes described as high, mid, low.
2. Advancement: front, central, back (horizontal plane of the IPA vowel chart).
3. Rounding (lip position): rounded, unrounded (pairs on the IPA vowel chart; left = unrounded, right = rounded).
4. Tenseness: tense, lax (tense vowels are indicated with a dot, lax vowels are not).

Other dimensions of vowels that are not depicted on the IPA vowel chart are:

5. Nasality: nasal, oral.
6. Vowel length: short, long.
7. Diphthongs: "a vowel sound forming a single syllable, but including a change from one vowel quality to another" (Ladefoged, 2005, p. 200).

Transcription of vowels is sometimes difficult. The exact location of the vowel can be unclear since vowels are not created by the articulators (e.g., tongue, lips) coming into contact with one another (although the approximate location is quite easily defined). The description of the vowel space was originally based on the relationship of the sound in question with the cardinal vowels. More recent descriptions of the vowel space have been based on formant frequencies (e.g., Cox, 2008).

Knowledge of the transcription of vowels is important in professional practice as an SLP. Many dialects of languages of the world differ in the use of vowels. Multilingual speakers frequently have different repertoires of vowels within the languages that they speak. There is increasing evidence for children with SSD exhibiting difficulties with vowels (e.g., Ball & Gibbon, 2012).

> **COMMENT:** *Everyone has an accent*
>
> "Everyone speaks with an accent. This accent tells his/her life story, where he/she has been, where he/she is from, where he/she learned his/her language, what cultures he/she has been exposed to. In sum, it is the way to tell the world who he/she is" (Cheng, 1999, p. 1).

English vowels and diphthongs

Each English dialect differs between the number and type of vowels and diphthongs spoken. There are some excellent volumes that describe the different English accents and go into depth about the usage of vowels in each dialect (e.g., Gimson & Cruttenden, 1994; Wells, 1982). However, there is no "neutral, all-purpose, international pronunciation of English" (Gimson & Cruttenden, 1994, p. 271). Indeed, there are differences in the vowels spoken by people across countries such as the United States (e.g., General American English, African-American English, Cajun English, Appalachian English) and the United Kingdom (e.g., General British, Cockney English, Northern Irish English, Scottish English). Other countries that use English as their primary language include both similar and different vowels and diphthongs from the United States and United Kingdom (e.g., Australia, Canada, New Zealand). Kachru (1985, 1997) proposed three circles of English and that the English spoken in each of these countries differs in the production of vowels, diphthongs, consonants, and prosody (e.g., stress versus syllable timing):

1. Inner circle varieties of English (native English-speaking countries): United Kingdom, United States, Canada (anglophone), Australia, and New Zealand.
2. Outer circle varieties of English (former British colonies): examples include Jamaica, Trinidad, Hong Kong, India, Singapore, South Africa, and Nigeria.
3. Expanding circle varieties of English (countries where English is used in business, science, technology, and education): examples include China, Japan, Korea, and Turkey.

General American English vowels and diphthongs

The following vowels and diphthongs have been used within the current book to describe the repertoire of General American English (GAE) vowels and diphthongs: /i, ɪ, e, ɛ, æ, ə, ɚ, ɝ, u, ʊ, o, ʌ, ɔ, ɑ, aɪ, aʊ, ɔɪ/ (see Table 4-3). In order to generate this list, we have used the conventions of the International Phonetic Alphabet and have relied on the work of Ladefoged (2001a, b, 2005), Shriberg and Kent (2003), Garn-Nunn and Lynn (2004), and Smit (2004). However, defining the list of vowels and diphthongs within GAE is not straightforward. Transcription differs according to the chosen text. As Shriberg and Kent (2003) indicate, "The choice of a diagraph symbol for the English diphthongs is not easy. An examination of this problem takes us into another part of the phonetic swamp" (p. 39).

TABLE 4-3 **The transcription conventions of General American English (GAE) vowels used in the current book**

Position	IPA transcription	Comments
Front vowels	/i, ɪ, e, ɛ, æ/	Most texts agree with the transcription of these vowels.
Central vowels	/ə, ɚ, ɝ/	The rhotic symbol / ˞ / that is used to transcribe /ɚ, ɝ/ is found on the IPA diacritics chart. Some authors (e.g., Wells, 1982) use /ᵊɪ/.
Back vowels	/u, ʊ, o, ʌ, ɔ, ɑ/	Shriberg and Kent (2003) and Smit (2004) describe /ʌ/ as a central vowel.
Diphthongs	/aɪ, aʊ, ɔɪ/	Shriberg and Kent (2003) describe [e] – [eɪ] and [o] – [oʊ] as allophones.

Most dialects of American English (e.g., African-American English, Appalachian English, Cajun English, Southern American English, New England English) typically have a similar vowel inventory as GAE, with context-specific variations.

Canadian English vowels and diphthongs

The following vowels and diphthongs are used in Canadian English: /i, ɪ, e, ɛ, æ, ə, ɚ, ɝ, ʉ, ʊ, o, ʌ, ɔ, ɑ, ʌɪ, ʌʊ, ɔɪ/ (Bernhardt & Deby, 2007). Canadian English vowels and diphthongs are similar to those in GAE, with four major exceptions: (1) the use of /ʉ/ instead of /u/, (2) the use of /ɔ/ only before /ɪ/, (3) the raising of the onset of the diphthongs /aɪ, aʊ/ to /ʌɪ, ʌʊ/, and (4) a disappearing distinction between /æ/ and /ɛ/ (Bernhardt & Deby, 2007; Brinton & Fee, 2001).

General British vowels and diphthongs

General British is the reference or standard accent within England (Cruttenden, 2014). General British was previously known as Received Pronunciation (RP), and it is important to note it is "not a different accent being described, but an evolved and evolving version of the same accent under a different name" (Cruttenden, 2014, p. 80). The following vowels and diphthongs are used in General British: /i, ɪ, ɛ, æ, a, ə, ɜ, u, ʊ, ʌ, ɔ, ɒ, aɪ, aʊ, ɔɪ, eɪ, oʊ, ɪə, ɛə, ʊə/ (Howard, 2007a). General British differs from GAE and Canadian English by the increased number of diphthongs and the fact that it is non-rhotic; that is, it does not use the r-colored vowels /ɚ, ɝ/ (see Table 4-4).

Australian English vowels and diphthongs

Australian English is non-rhotic, and is more closely related to General British than GAE (Cox, 2012; McLeod, 2007b). There are two transcription systems currently used to describe Australian English vowels and diphthongs. According to Harrington, Cox, and Evans (HCE) (1997), the following vowels and diphthongs are used in Australian English: /iː, ɪ, e, æ, ɐː, ə, ɜ, ʉː, ʊ, ɐ, oː, ɔ, ɑe, æɔ, ɔɪ, æɪ, əʉ, ɪə, eː, ʊə/. According to Mitchell (1946), the following vowels and diphthongs are used in Australian English: /i, ɪ, ɛ, æ, a, ə, ɜ, u, ʊ, ʌ, ɔ, ɒ, aɪ, aʊ, ɔɪ, eɪ, oʊ, ɪə, ɛə, ʊə/. Cox (2008) explains that the HCE system more closely relates to modern pronunciation of Australian English as verified by acoustic analysis.

New Zealand English vowels and diphthongs

Like General British, New Zealand English is non-rhotic. Bauer and Warren (2004) list the New Zealand English vowels and diphthongs as: /i, ɪ, ɛ, æ, ə, ɜ, u, ʊ, ʌ, ɔ, ɒ, ɑ, aɪ, aʊ, ɔɪ, eɪ, oʊ, ɪə, eə, ʊə/. Maclagan (2009) lists the New Zealand English vowels and diphthongs as: /i, ɪ, e, æ, a, ə, ɜ, ʊ, ʌ, ɔ, ɒ, ai, aʊ, ɔi, ei, oʊ, iə, eə, ʊə/. She states that the diphthongs /eə, ʊə/ are sometimes replaced by /iə, ɔ/ respectively. One of the characteristics of the New Zealand English accent is the closeness of the /ɪ/ and /ə/ vowels (e.g., production of the phrase *fish and chips* is often used to differentiate Australian and New Zealand English speakers), and the merger of the /iə/ and /eə/ diphthongs (Maclagan & Gillon, 2007).

Vowels in the world's languages

Languages and dialects differ regarding the number, type, and classification of vowels. The world's languages range from an inventory of two vowels (Yimas spoken in Papua New Guinea) to 13 or 14 vowels (German), with an average of just under six vowels per language (Maddieson, 2008c). When calculating these inventories, Maddieson (2008c) considered the vowel qualities of height, advancement, and lip position and did not include differences in vowel length, vowel nasalization, and diphthongs. Have a look at the number and type of vowels that are used in a few of the world's languages below. We have put them in order from the smallest to largest number of vowels and have extended the definition beyond that used by Maddieson:

- Spanish (5 vowels): /i, e, a, o, u/ (Maddieson, 2008c)
- Greek (5 vowels): /i, ɛ, ɐ, o, u/ (Jongman, Fourakis, & Sereno, 1989)

- Finnish (8 vowels + 18 diphthongs + 20 two-vowel combinations): /i, e, æ, y, ø, ɑ, o, u/ (Kunnari & Savinainen-Makkonen, 2007)
- Hawai'ian (5 vowels + 5 displaying lengthening contrasts + 8 diphthongs): /a, aː, e, eː, i, iː, o, oː, u, uː, ei, eu, oi, ou, ai, ae, ao, au/ (Pukui & Elbert, 1992)
- Cantonese (11 vowels + 11 diphthongs): /i, y, ɛ, œ, a, ɔ, u, ɐ, ɪ, θ, ʊ, ai, ei, ɐi, ui, ɔi, au, ɐu, iu, ou, θy, ɛu/ (Zee, 1999)
- German (13 vowels + 2 displaying lengthening contrasts + 3 diphthongs): /i, ɪ, e, ɛ, ɛː, y, ʏ, ø, a, aː, ə, u, ʊ, o, ɔ, aɪ, ɪc, aʊ/ (Kohler, 1999)
- General American English (14 vowels + 3 diphthongs): /i, ɪ, e, ɛ, æ, ə, ɚ, ɝ, u, ʊ, o, ʌ, ɔ, ɑ, aɪ, aʊ, ɪc/ (Smit, 2007) (Smit also lists 5 'r'-colored diphthongs)

TABLE 4-4   **A comparison between the pronunciation of General American English and General British vowels**

Location	General American English (GAE) (Smit, 2004)	General British (GB) (Wells, 1982)	Examples
High-front	i	i	*beat*
	ɪ	ɪ	*bit*
	e		*bait*
Mid-low-front	ɛ	ɛ	*bet*
	æ	æ	*bat*
High-back, rounded	u	u	*boot*
	ʊ	ʊ	*put*
Mid-back, rounded	o		*boat*
	ɔ	ɔ	*bought*
		ɒ	*pot*
Low-back	ɑ	ɑ	*bother*
		ɜ	*bird*
Central	ə	ə	*above*
	ʌ	ʌ	*but*
[r]-colored	ɝ		*bird*
	ɚ		*better*
	ɪɹ		*beer*
	ɛɹ		*bear*
	ʊɹ		*tour*
	ɔɹ		*bore*
	ɑɹ		*bar*
Diphthongs	aɪ	aɪ	*bite*
	aʊ	aʊ	*bout*
	ɪc	ɪc	*boy*
		eɪ	*bait*
		oʊ	*boat*
		ɪə	*beer*
		ɛə	*bear*
		ʊə	*tour*

> **COMMENT:** *Assessing changes in vowels across time*
>
> In 1952 Peterson and Barney assessed 11 American English vowels using a neutral /hVd/ context (*heed, hid, head, had, hard,* etc.) and determined the average formant frequencies (F1, F2, and F3) for each vowel for 28 women, 33 men, and 15 children. In 1995 Hillenbrand, Getty, Clark, and Wheeler replicated the study on 45 men, 48 women, and 46 children, showing some differences between the results of the two studies including the average formant frequencies (especially F1 and F2) and degree of overlap between the vowels that were adjacent in the vowel quadrilateral. The original data are available so you can listen to the men, women, and children's vowels.[1]
>
> [1] http://homepages.wmich.edu/~hillenbr/voweldata.html

◼ Suprasegmentals chart

The suprasegmentals chart (Figure 4-11) provides symbols to describe "properties of speech that tend to extend over more than one segment, and/or to vary independently of the segmental targets" (International Phonetic Association, 1999, p. 13). A term that is synonymous with suprasegmentals is **prosody** (Peppé, 2009). Suprasegmentals, or prosody, include stress, rhythm, intonation, and lexical and grammatical tones. Suprasegmentals can have a linguistic impact (i.e., they can directly affect the meaning of a word or phrase) or a paralinguistic impact (i.e., they add information) (Peppé, 2009).

Stress

Two levels of stress are differentiated on the IPA chart. The **primary** and **secondary stress** symbols provide cues for where the emphasis is placed within a word. The primary stress symbol is used to identify strong syllables in words that have the most emphasis. The primary stressed syllable is represented by the high vertical stroke mark on the IPA chart or the capital S. The secondary stress symbol is used to identify strong syllables in words that

FIGURE 4-11 The suprasegmentals chart and the tones and word accent chart from the International Phonetic Alphabet

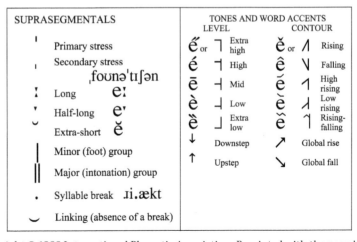

Source: Copyright © 1999 International Phonetic Association. Reprinted with the permission of Cambridge University Press.

have less emphasis than the primary stressed syllables, but greater emphasis than weak syllables in words. The secondary stressed syllable is represented by the the low vertical stroke mark on the IPA chart or the lowercase s. Weak syllables are not marked with a stress symbol, or are indicated using the lowercase w. Consider the word *helicopter* /ˈhɛliˌkɑptɚ/. It is made up of four syllables: the primary stressed syllable /ˈhɛ/, the secondary stressed syllable /ˌkɑp/, and two weak syllables /li/ and /tɚ/. The stress pattern can be summarized as Swsw.

English is said to have a left-dominant lexical stress pattern, as the most common stress pattern in English disyllabic words is **trochaic**. Trochees are stressed-unstressed, or strong-weak (Sw) (e.g., splinter /ˈsplɪntɚ/). A less common stress pattern in English is **iambic**. Iambs are unstressed-stressed or weak-strong (wS) (e.g., *attract* /əˈtɹækt/). McGregor and Johnson (1997) found that young English-speaking children were more likely to produce trochees in their early words. Disyllabic words with equal stress (e.g., *football*) are called **spondees**.

Some languages have variable stress (e.g., English, Dutch, Spanish); that is, syllables can vary in the placement of stress. In contrast, some languages have fixed stress; for example, they stress the first syllable (e.g., Icelandic, Finnish, Hungarian) or the last syllable in a word (e.g., Hebrew) (Peppé, 2012). Some languages reduce the vowel length in unstressed syllables (typically to a schwa /ə/) (e.g., English, Dutch, Hebrew, Icelandic, Norwegian, Swedish). Other languages do not reduce the vowel length in unstressed syllables (e.g., Finnish, French, Italian, Portuguese, Spanish, Turkish) (Peppé, 2012).

Stress in English can also be used to:

- differentiate **homographs**, or words that are spelled the same way but have different pronunciations and meanings (e.g., *SUBject* versus *subJECT*);
- differentiate compound words from phrases (e.g., *CHOCOLATE milk and cakes* versus *chocolate, MILK, and cakes*—note the placement of the commas); or
- mark contradictory or new information in a sentence (e.g., *I like the PURPLE shoes* versus *I like the purple SHOES*) (Velleman, 1998).

Rhythm

Languages can be described as stress-timed or syllable-timed. In stress-timed languages, each syllable varies in duration during connected speech. Stress-timed languages include English, Dutch, Hebrew, Icelandic, Norwegian, and Swedish. In syllable-timed languages, each syllable, whether in a monosyllabic word or a polysyllabic word, is of a similar duration in connected speech. Syllable-timed languages include Cantonese, Finnish, French, Italian, Portuguese, Spanish, and Turkish (Peppé, 2012).

Intonation

Intonation refers to the melody or pitch of speech. Intonation can change the meaning of words. Intonation can indicate whether a sentence is a question or a statement. Say these sentences:

She likes apples.
She likes apples?

Read more about Michael (4;2 years), a boy with childhood apraxia of speech (CAS), in Chapter 16 (Case 4).

COMMENT: *Transcribing syllable breaks*

Michael (4;2 years) has CAS. His speech has a characteristic feature of CAS—difficulty sequencing syllables (Chapter 16). If you listened to Michael's speech, you would have heard small breaks between his syllables—a difficulty known as syllable segregation. There is a symbol on the suprasegmentals chart (Figure 4-11) to capture this break between syllables—a small dot between the syllables. Review Michael's sample of polysyllabic words in Table 16-15. Read the transcription aloud and say it in the way that Michael did, with very brief pauses of syllable breaks between the syllables.

> **MULTICULTURAL INSIGHTS:** *Cantonese tones*
>
> The nine tones of Cantonese (see Figure 4-12) are distinguished by tone height, contour, and duration. Syllables with tone 1 to tone 6 end with a vowel, diphthong, or nasal, while syllables with tone 7 to tone 9 end with /p, t, k/. Traditionally, Cantonese tones are transcribed by marking the tone number on the right of the transcription. For example, "the syllable /ji/ can combine with the six level and contour tones to form different words: namely, 衣 *clothes* /ji₁/, 椅 *chair* /ji₂/, 意 *meaning* /ji₃/, 兒 *son* /ji₄/, 耳 *ear* /ji₅/ and 二 *two* /ji₆/" (To & Cheung, 2012, p. 166).

FIGURE 4-12 Nine Cantonese tones showing the tone number, tone height, and contour

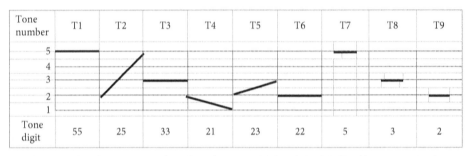

Source: Reprinted with permission from To, Cheung, & McLeod (2013a). Used by permission from American Speech-Language-Hearing Association (ASHA).

The first sentence has falling intonation to indicate it is a sentence. The second sentence has rising intonation, to indicate that it is a question. Questions are signaled by rising intonation in many languages (e.g., English, Spanish, Turkish); however, for Hungarian, questions are signaled by falling intonation (Peppé, 2012). The tones and word accents chart (Figure 4-11) includes symbols to indicate global rise and fall across words within phrases.

■ Tones and word accents chart

Tones are the pitch patterns associated with syllables or words. The tones and word accents chart (Figure 4-11) provides two alternative symbol sets for indicating tones. The symbols in the left column are used for tone languages that differentiate word meanings using fundamental frequency or pitch levels (e.g., Cantonese, Putonghua [Mandarin] , Thai, Vietnamese). For example, there are four tones in Putonghua (Mandarin) and nine tones in Cantonese (see Figure 4-12). The symbols in the right column are used for languages that can use differing pitch heights in each syllable (e.g., English, Spanish). The left and right columns of symbols are not meant to be comparable; they were produced in the two columns to save space on the chart (International Phonetic Association, 1999). Upstep is used in languages such as Hausa, and downstep is used in the Ghanaian language Akan (International Phonetic Association, 1999).

EXTENSIONS TO THE IPA

The Extensions to the IPA (extIPA) (Duckworth, Allen, Hardcastle, & Ball, 1990; ICPLA 2015) (Appendix 4-3) and the Voice Quality Symbols (VoQS) (Ball, Esling, & Dickson, 1995; 2015) (Appendix 4-4) were designed to transcribe the speech of people who do not have typical speech production. That is, they include additional symbols to describe sounds that are not found in the world's languages. The extIPA includes symbols and diacritics for the transcription of segments, as well as transcription of voice quality, rate, and intensity during connected speech. Additionally, the level of certainty of transcription is also included. An account of the origins of the extIPA is found in Duckworth, Allen, Hardcastle, and Ball (1990). Rutter, Klopfenstein, Ball, and Müller (2010) describe how to use the extIPA in clinical contexts where clients use "unattested sounds ... that have not been recorded in any natural language but have been noted as occurring in disordered speech of various types" (p. 118). The unattested sounds presented in the extIPA relate to consonant manner, consonant place, diacritics that can apply to consonants or vowels, connected speech, voicing, and other symbols relating to the certainty of transcription. For example, * can be used to indicate a "sound with no available symbol" (p. 119). The VoQS (Ball et al., 1995) (Appendix 4-4) includes symbols to describe the airstream, phonation, and supralaryngeal settings.

PHONOTACTICS

The IPA primarily describes individual segments and suprasegmental aspects of speech. Each language also has phonotactic constraints (rules) regarding aspects including:

■ the number of syllables that can occur within a word;
■ the number and type of consonants and vowels that can combine to form a syllable;
■ the number, type, and locations of consonants in consonant clusters;
■ the presence (or absence) of final consonants, diphthongs, and triphthongs;
■ the presence (or absence) of lexical tones;
■ harmony patterns whereby consonants and vowels become similar to one another; and
■ phrase- and sentence-level pronunciation effects (adapted from Velleman, 1998; see Chapter 5 for more information).

Understanding the phonotactic constraints for the primary language(s) spoken by children with SSD enables us to determine whether their difficulties lie at the segmental level (e.g., production of /s/), the syllable level (e.g., production of /s/ consonant clusters), or the word, phrase, or sentence level. Now let's consider the phonotactic constraints of English and some other languages. In Chapters 5 and 6 we will build on this understanding by applying it to theories of phonology and speech acquisition.

Most words in most languages contain consonants (C) and vowels (V) (e.g., *cat* /kæt/ = CVC). Some words only contain one vowel (e.g., *a* /ʌ/ = V) or one diphthong (e.g., *eye* /aɪ/ = V). Some words, in languages such as Cantonese, contain only one consonant and a tone, but no vowels (e.g., 五 *five* /ŋ₅/ = C). Words are made up of syllables. Typically, each syllable contains a vowel. In rare cases, syllables only contain a consonant, such as in Cantonese (see above), or in the final syllable of English words such as *apple* /æpl̩/ = VC,C or *button* /bʌtn̩/ = CVC,C (although some English speakers pronounce these words with two syllables by inserting a schwa: *apple* /æpəl/= VCVC or *button* /bʌtən/ = CVCVC). Some words are **monosyllabic** (e.g., *do* /du/ = CV), because they contain only one syllable and one vowel. Some are **disyllabic** because they contain two syllables (e.g., *doing* /duɪŋ/= CV,VC), or **polysyllabic** because they contain three or more syllables (e.g., *undoing* /ʌnduɪŋ/= VC,CV,VC).

■ Consonant clusters

Consonant clusters occur "when two or more consonants co-occur at the same position in syllable structure" (Grunwell, 1987, p. 14). In English, consonant clusters occur in the syllable-initial and syllable-final position. English two-element syllable-initial consonant clusters are: /pl, pj, pɹ, bl, bɹ, bj, tɹ, tw, tj, dɹ, dw, dj, kl, kɹ, kw, kj, gl, gɹ, gw, fl, fj, fɹ, vj, θɹ, sp, st, sk, sm, sn, sf, sl, sw, ʃɹ, mj, nj/ (e.g., *shrimp* /ʃɹɪmp/). English three-element syllable-initial consonant clusters are: /spl, spj, spɹ, stɹ, stj, skj, skɹ, skw/ (e.g., *splash*

/splæʃ/). Many dialects of American English do not include all of the /j/ clusters listed above (e.g., *tune* is pronounced as /tun/ not /tjun/ and *news* is pronounced /nuz/ not /njuz/). English syllable-final consonant clusters can range from two to four consonants in length. Common English syllable-final consonant clusters include /st, sk, ns, nd, nt, mp, ŋk, ntʃ, ndʒ/ (e.g., *lunch* /lʌntʃ/). Many other English syllable-final consonant clusters are **morphophonemic**. That is, they are created by adding a morpheme (e.g., plural, possessive, past tense, third person singular) to the end of the word. Examples of morphophonemic consonant clusters are /ts/ in *cats* and /mpt/ in *jumped*. In General American English, additional syllable-final consonant clusters include /ɹ/ clusters such as /ɹp, ɹb, ɹt, ɹd, ɹk, ɹg, ɹm, ɹn, ɹs, ɹʃ, ɹtʃ/ (e.g., *arch* /ɑɹtʃ/). In a study of 104 world languages, Locke (1983) calculated that the majority of the world's languages contain both word-initial and word-final consonant clusters, 39% have word-initial consonant clusters only, and 13% had word-final consonant clusters only:

- Word-initial and word-final consonant clusters (e.g., English, Dutch, French, German, Hungarian, Israeli Hebrew, Maltese, Norwegian, Welsh)
- Word-initial consonant clusters only (e.g., Greek, Japanese, Portuguese, Spanish, Thai)
- Word-final consonant clusters only (e.g., Turkish)
- No word-initial and word-final consonant clusters except in words borrowed from other languages (e.g., Filipino, Finnish, Korean, Putonghua, Vietnamese) (McLeod, 2007a)

Syllable shapes and word positions

In English, the shortest syllable is V (e.g., *a* /ʌ/) and longest syllable that can be produced is CCCVCCCC (e.g., *strengths* /stɹɛŋkθs/). Therefore, the English syllable shape is described as $C_{(0-3)}VC_{(0-4)}$ since there can be between zero and three initial consonants and between zero and four final consonants. The phonotactics of other languages differ. Let's compare a few:

- $C_{(0-3)}VC_{(0-4)}$ (e.g., English, Dutch)
- $C_{(0-3)}VC_{(0-3)}$ (e.g., French, German, Hungarian)
- $C_{(0-3)}VC_{(0-2)}$ (e.g., Maltese, Norwegian, Welsh)
- $C_{(0-3)}VC_{(0-1)}$ (e.g., Greek)
- $C_{(0-2)}VC_{(0-2)}$ (e.g., Israeli Hebrew, Spanish, Portuguese)
- $C_{(0-1)}VC_{(0-2)}$ (e.g., Turkish)
- $C_{(1-2)}V_{(1-2)}C_{(0-2)}$ (e.g., Jordanian and Lebanese Arabic)
- $C_{(0-1)}V_{(0-1)}C_{(0-1)}$ (e.g., Cantonese)
- $CVC_{(0-1)}$ (e.g., Filipino) (McLeod, 2007a)

In English, we often say that consonants occur in word-initial, within word (medial), and word-final positions. For example, the word *running* /ɹʌnɪŋ/ = CVCVC has word-initial /ɹ/, medial /n/, and final /ŋ/. However, many words contain more than one consonant within the word. As a result, it is better to consider both the syllable and word position simultaneously. A consonant within a **disyllabic** (two-syllable) English word can occur in one of four syllable positions: syllable-initial word-initial (SIWI), syllable-final within word (SFWW), syllable-initial within word (SIWW), and syllable-final word-final (SFWF) (see Figure 4-13). You can see in Figure 4-13 that there are now two within word positions. Consequently, in a word like *mustang*, /mʌstæŋ/ the /s/ is in the SFWW position and the /t/ is in the SIWW position. A word like *monster* presents another challenge since there are three consonants within the word: /nst/. Grunwell (1987) recommends that the SIWW position should be more complex than the SFWW, so the /nst/ would be separated into /n/ in the SFWW position and /st/ in the SIWW position. This rule does not apply for compound words, where the syllable boundaries reflect the word boundaries (e.g., *handbag* /hænd.bæg/ would have /nd/ in the SFWW position and /b/ in the SIWW position). The special issue of *Clinical Linguistics and Phonetics* (2002), volume 16(3),[3] provides more information about intervocalic consonants.

---

[3] http://www.tandfonline.com/toc/iclp20/16/3

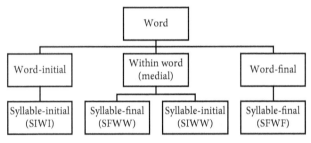

FIGURE 4-13   Conceptualization of word and syllable positions for English disyllabic words

Source: Copyright © 2005 International Phonetic Association.

COMMENT: *Cantonese syllables*

Cantonese syllables are described as $C_{(0-1)}V_{(0-1)}C_{(0-1)}$; that is, they may have the form CV, VC, CVC, V or syllabic consonant (C_{syll}). Most Cantonese words are disyllabic; however, words also can be monosyllabic, trisyllabic, and very occasionally polysyllabic. There are differing opinions as to whether Cantonese contains the consonant clusters /kw, k^hw/ (So & Dodd, 1994) or whether these should be classified as labial velars /k^w, k^{wh}/ (To, Cheung, & McLeod, 2013a; Zee, 1999).

UNDERSTANDING ENGLISH CONSONANTS USING KNOWLEDGE OF ANATOMY AND AUDITORY TRANSCRIPTION

The voice-place-manner descriptions of consonants provide a simple way of understanding where and how consonants are articulated. Think about the placement of your tongue when you say the [t] in *tea* /ti/. When producing /t/, your tongue tip makes contact with your alveolar ridge. Additionally, the sides of your tongue anchor against your upper molars. In this final section of the chapter, we provide a rich description of the articulation of each English consonant based on instrumental analysis (electropalatography and ultrasound) to combine and extend your knowledge of anatomy, transcription, and the voice-place-manner characteristics of each of the English consonants. For each English consonant, we provide:

1. Two images of the position of the articulators when adults produce the consonant, based on:
   (a) a sagittal diagram of the oral cavity
   (b) a transverse diagram of the hard palate
2. A description of how the consonant is articulated
3. An overview of common errors observed in children's speech for that consonant. In Chapter 12 we provide an overview of auditory and production cues (e.g., auditory stimulation, auditory discrimination, visual-phonetic cues, visual-prosodic cues, verbal-phonetic cues, motokinesthetic cues, orthographic cues, metaphonological cues, facilitating phonetic contexts and shaping) that can be used to help children learn how to produce and use each of the consonants in words.

Before we address each consonant, it is important to understand the two types of images, how they were obtained, what they depict, and how to interpret them.

■ Sagittal diagrams of English consonants

The sagittal diagrams depict the oral cavity along the sagittal plane (an imaginary plane that divides a person into right and left halves). In this chapter, each schematic sagittal image represents an ultrasound trace of the tongue during one production of a consonant produced by the first author of this book. To create the schematic sagittal diagrams, the first author recorded key words (within a carrier phrase) using simultaneous acoustic, ultrasound, and electropalatography (EPG). Figure 4-14 demonstrates the first author wearing a helmet to keep the ultrasound probe in place under the chin, an electropalatographic palate (a palate containing 68 electrodes to indicate tongue contact during connected speech—note the wires coming from her mouth), and a microphone for recording the acoustic signal. To create the schematic sagittal diagrams, word-initial consonants were identified by considering the acoustic signal, waveform, spectrograph, and EPG frames. Next, the exact midpoint of the consonant was calculated by looking at the string of EPG frames. Then, the corresponding ultrasound image for the midpoint of the consonant was identified and drawn onto a template of the oral cavity. For additional information on the creation of these images, see McLeod and Wrench (2008), and for a comprehensive description of the production of each consonant in English, see McLeod and Singh (2009a).

There are five questions to ask when considering each sagittal diagram:

1. Is the tongue touching a part of the mouth?
2. What is the shape of the tongue? Is it bunched at the back of the mouth, or elongated towards the front?
3. Are the lips touching each other (to indicate a bilabial consonant) or touching the teeth (to indicate a labiodental consonant)?
4. Does the velum (soft palate) extend to the pharynx (back of the throat) for an oral sound, or is there a gap to allow the air to pass through the nose for a nasal sound?
5. Does the diagrammatic representation of voicing at the larynx indicate a voiceless sound via the presence of a (−) or a voiced sound indicated via a (+)?

■ Transverse diagrams of English consonants

The transverse diagrams depict the hard palate along the **transverse** plane (an imaginary plane that divides a person horizontally). The transverse diagrams of the hard palate

---

FIGURE 4-14   **Instrumentation used to create schematic diagrams**

(a) A not very glamorous photo showing the first author wearing an electropalatograph (EPG) palate (see wires extending from the mouth and going into the multiplexer [white box]), and a helmet to anchor the ultrasound probe under her chin, while the acoustic signal is recorded via a microphone. (b) Equipment to record signals from the electropalatograph (EPG), ultrasound, and audio signal.

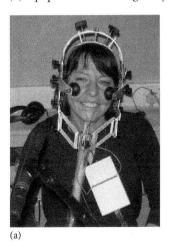 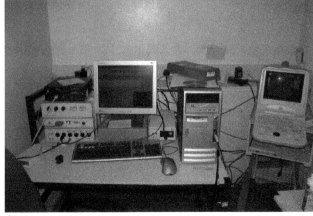

(a)   (b)

Source: Used by permission from Sharynne McLeod.

represent a flattened version of the hard palate using an electropalatographic (EPG) display. To create the transverse images, an average diagram was created for each consonant based on greater than 67% contact on a cumulative palate for at least 240 productions of each consonant by eight typical adults (30+ productions each). The creation of the averaged images is outlined in McLeod (2011), and all of the 240+ productions for each consonant are in McLeod and Singh (2009a).

Figure 4-15 shows the relationship between the transverse EPG diagram and the electrode placement in the palate that is worn during speech. The black squares represent the points where the tongue contacts the palate. Each EPG diagram represents contact during 10 milliseconds of speech. There are five questions to ask when considering each transverse diagram:

1. Is the tongue touching a part of the hard palate (i.e., are there any black squares)?
2. If so, is there minimal contact (e.g., /p/) or extensive contact (e.g., /ʧ/)?
3. What is the shape of the tongue/palate contact (e.g., horseshoe for /t, d, n/)?
4. Is the tongue predominantly touching the front of the palate (e.g., /l/), the back of the palate (e.g., /k, g, ŋ/), or is it distributed more equally across the palate?
5. Is there a central groove, and if so, is it narrow (e.g., /s, z/) or wide (e.g., /ʃ, ʒ/)?

A summary of the place and features of tongue/palate contact for English consonants is found in Table 4-5.

■ Bilabial plosives /p, b/

■ /p/ voiceless bilabial plosive
■ /b/ voiced bilabial plosive

Bilabial plosives are produced by stopping then releasing the airstream with the lips (see Figure 4-16). There is limited tongue contact with the palate, occurring only at the posterior lateral margins. The plosion (release of the air) occurs through the oral cavity, and the nasal cavity is closed by the velum.

The /p, b/ consonants are two of the earliest occurring consonants for typically developing English-speaking children, so most children with SSD of unknown origin do not have difficulty producing them. However, some children have difficulty with voicing; consequently they voice voiceless consonants, producing [b] for /p/ (e.g., *pin* /pɪn/ produced as [bɪn]). Few children have difficulty with the place of articulation for /p, b/, although some children who have micrognathia (unusually small jaw) or other craniofacial anomalies involving the mandible and maxilla may have difficulty making the lips meet. Some children (particularly those with a cleft palate) have difficulty with the manner of articulation for /p, b/. These children

FIGURE 4-15 **Electropalatographic (EPG) diagram and electrode placement**

An (a) EPG display of tongue contact (in black) during the production of [d], *and (b) an electropalatographic (EPG) palate on a dental cast showing the position of the 68 electrodes*

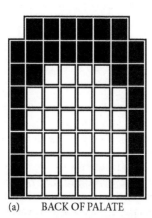
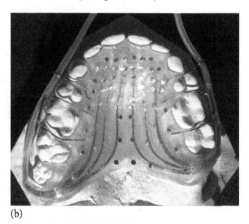

(a)   BACK OF PALATE   (b)

Source: (a) and (b) Sharynne McLeod. Used by permission from Sharynne McLeod.

TABLE 4-5   Place and features of tongue/palate contact for English consonants

Consonant	Alveolar contact	Palatal contact	Velar contact	Lateral contact	Midpalate contact	Groove present
/p/	no	no	sometimes	sometimes	no	no
/b/	no	no	yes	yes	no	no
/t/	yes	yes	yes	yes	no	no
/d/	yes	yes	yes	yes	no	no
/k/	no	no	yes	sometimes	no	no
/g/	no	no	yes	sometimes	no	no
/m/	sometimes	no	sometimes	yes	no	no
/n/	yes	yes	yes	yes	no	no
/ŋ/	no	no	yes	sometimes	no	no
/f/	no	no	no	no	no	no
/v/	no	no	yes	yes	no	no
/θ/	no	no	yes	yes	no	no
/ð/	no	yes	yes	yes	no	no
/s/	yes	yes	yes	yes	no	yes
/z/	yes	yes	yes	yes	no	yes
/ʃ/	no	yes	yes	yes	no	yes
/ʒ/	no	yes	yes	yes	no	yes
/h/	no	no	sometimes	sometimes	no	no
/tʃ/	yes	yes	yes	yes	no	partially
/dʒ/	yes	yes	yes	yes	no	partially
/w/	no	no	yes	yes	no	no
/l/	yes	no	no	no	no	no
/ɹ/	no	no	yes	yes	no	no
/j/	no	yes	yes	yes	no	no

Source: Adapted from McLeod (2011).

Key. Alveolar contact = contact across first 2–3 rows of the EPG palate. Palatal contact = contact across the middle 3 rows. Velar contact = contact across last 2–3 rows. Lateral contact = along the sides. Midpalate = contact in the middle of the palate. Groove present = no contact in the middle of the palate (only relevant for s, z [narrow groove], /ʃ/, /ʒ/ [wide groove]).

may have difficulty building up enough air pressure behind the lips and instead may produce bilabial fricatives such as [ɸ, ß] or release the consonant through the nose.

Alveolar plosives /t, d/

- /t/ voiceless alveolar plosive
- /d/ voiced alveolar plosive

Alveolar plosives are produced by stopping the airstream with the tongue (see Figure 4-17), then allowing the stopped airstream to escape. In order to stop the airstream, the tongue contacts the palate in a horseshoe shape along the teeth. The consonants are made orally and the nasal cavity is closed.

The consonants /t, d/ are mastered early by typically developing children, so most children with SSD of unknown origin do not have difficulty producing them. Indeed, some authors suggest that these are **default** consonants that children use for many other consonants (Bernhardt & Stemberger, 2000). Some children may voice the voiceless consonant /t/ and produce [d] instead. For example, a child may say *tin* /tɪn/ as [dɪn]. A second area of

COMMENT: *The need for combining sagittal and transverse diagrams of English consonants*

Most textbooks that describe consonant production provide a sagittal diagram for each consonant; however, few provide both sagittal and transverse diagrams that have been created during speech production. We believe it is important to include both diagrams to have an integrated knowledge of the articulatory placement for each consonant. Many SLPs have good knowledge of sagittal contact but poor knowledge of tongue/palate contact on the transverse plane, particularly along the lateral margins of the palate. McLeod (2011) asked 175 SLPs who worked with children with SSD to draw transverse diagrams of tongue/palate contact for 24 English consonants. Their mean accuracy score was only 38%! These SLPs did not show awareness of the horseshoe contact (lateral bracing) for alveolar consonants /t, d, n, s, z/, the groove for /s, z, ʃ, ʒ/, or posterior lateral contact for most other consonants. These SLPs were most accurate for consonants with no contact /p, f, h/, then velar consonants /k, g, ŋ/. The remaining consonants were rarely accurate (from most to least accurate: /l, t, ɹ, z, n, ʃ, s, ʒ, j, v, θ, d, m, b, w, ð, ʧ, ʤ/). This is of concern, since many of the consonants that are difficult for children with SSD are found in the least accurate list. Consequently, in this book we are making sure to show both a sagittal and transverse diagram of each English consonant. The sagittal diagram only represents a cross-sectional image along the midline, or sagittal plane. Therefore, it is possible for a schematic sagittal image to demonstrate no palatal contact at all, whereas the transverse image created via the EPG may demonstrate some contact along the edges of the palate (e.g., /p, b, m/).

 APPLICATION: *Where does your tongue touch your palate?*

Where do you think your tongue touches your palate during the production of consonants? Copy the blank palate below so that you have enough for 24 consonants. Next, color the squares where you think your tongue touches the palate for each of the English consonants: /p, b, t, d, k, g, m, n, ŋ, f, v, θ, ð, s, z, ʃ, ʒ, h, ɹ, j, l, w, ʧ, ʤ/. Once you have done this, have a look at the figures in rest of this chapter to see if you are correct.

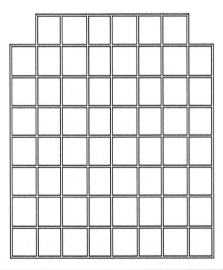

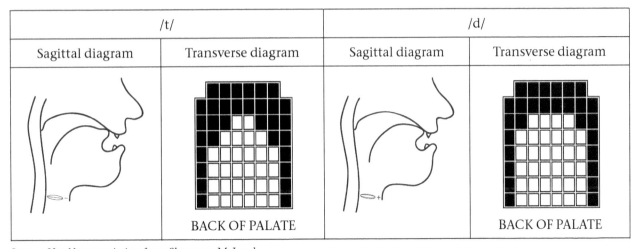

FIGURE 4-16 Bilabial plosives /p, b/

Sagittal (midline) diagram of placement of the articulators and transverse diagram of tongue/palate contact for /p/ and /b/

/p/		/b/	
Sagittal diagram	Transverse diagram	Sagittal diagram	Transverse diagram
	BACK OF PALATE		BACK OF PALATE

Source: Used by permission from Sharynne McLeod.

FIGURE 4-17 Alveolar plosives /t, d/

Sagittal (midline) diagram of placement of the articulators and transverse diagram of tongue/palate contact for /t/ and /d/

/t/		/d/	
Sagittal diagram	Transverse diagram	Sagittal diagram	Transverse diagram
	BACK OF PALATE		BACK OF PALATE

Source: Used by permission from Sharynne McLeod.

difficulty relates to the accuracy of tongue placement. Gibbon (1999) reviewed EPG literature and showed that 71% of 17 school-aged children with SSD were producing **undifferentiated lingual gestures** (whole palate contact, see Figure 4-18). One context where undifferentiated gestures occurred was when attempting to produce the consonants /t, d/. Gibbon (1999) indicated that undifferentiated gestures were produced by using the whole tongue body to cover the whole palate, and may sound as though the production is a substitution or distortion, or even may sound correct. Figure 4-18 provides an example of an undifferentiated gesture, and you will note that the transverse palatal contact diagram is completely black. Typically, the margins of the tongue produce a horseshoe contact pattern for /t/ and /d/ and the center of the palate should have no contact (Figure 4-17), so intervention will require clear guidance regarding the tongue contacting only the lateral margins of the palate. Finally, the manner of articulation of /t, d/ can be affected when children (e.g., with a cleft palate) have difficulty building up enough air pressure to produce these consonants, so they may produce a fricative instead of a plosive.

Electropalatographic (EPG) image of an undifferentiated gesture

Electropalatographic image of a child producing an undifferentiated gesture during the production of [d], *indicating that the tongue has made contact across the entire palate*

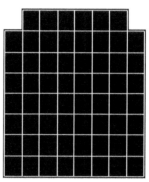

© Used by permission from Sharynne McLeod.

■ Velar plosives /k, g/

- ■ /k/ voiceless velar plosive
- ■ /g/ voiced velar plosive

Velar plosives are produced by stopping and then releasing the oral airstream with the back of the tongue, usually around the juncture between the hard and soft palate (see Figure 4-19). The transverse images in Figure 4-19 end at the juncture between the hard and soft palate. As a result, the images do not show that the tongue does have complete closure across the palate. If the image extended to the soft palate, complete closure would be demonstrated. There is some contact along the lateral margins of the palate. /k, g/ are oral consonants with no nasal air escape.

Many children with SSD of known or unknown origin have difficulty producing /k/ and /g/. When children have difficulty with voicing, they may produce [g] instead of /k/. The most common non-adult production involves a change of place of articulation when

Velar plosives /k, g/

Sagittal (midline) diagram of placement of the articulators and transverse diagram of tongue/palate contact for /k/ and /g/.
Some speakers would make complete contact across the palate.

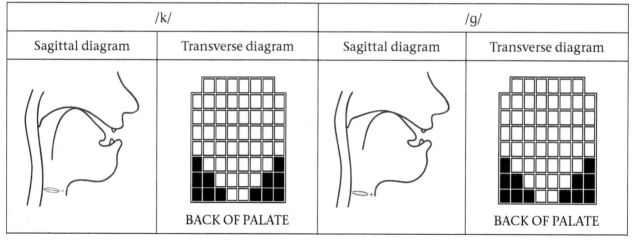

/k/		/g/	
Sagittal diagram	Transverse diagram	Sagittal diagram	Transverse diagram
	BACK OF PALATE		BACK OF PALATE

Source: Used by permission from Sharynne McLeod.

children produce [t] for /k/ and [d] for /g/. This is called **velar fronting** (see Chapter 5). Additionally, children may have difficulty with the manner of production of the plosives. For example, children with **velopharyngeal insufficiency** are unable to prevent the airstream from escaping through the nose. Consequently, the plosives /b, p/ may sound like [m], /t, d/ may sound like [n], and /k, g/ may sound like [ŋ].

Nasal consonants /m, n, ŋ /

- /m/ voiced bilabial nasal
- /n/ voiced alveolar nasal
- /ŋ/ voiced velar nasal

The bilabial nasal /m/ is produced by allowing the airstream to come through the nose, while stopping the airstream with the lips (see Figure 4-20). There is minimal tongue contact with the palate, occurring only at the lateral margins. The alveolar nasal /n/ is produced by allowing the airstream to escape through the nose while stopping the oral airstream with the tongue at the alveolar ridge (see Figure 4-20). In order to stop the airstream, the tongue is a similar shape to /t/ and /d/ because it contacts the palate in a horseshoe shape along the teeth. Similar to /n/, the velar nasal /ŋ/ is produced by allowing the airstream to escape through the nose while stopping the oral airstream with the tongue (see Figure 4-20). However, for /ŋ/, the tongue has similar oral contact to /k/ and /g/. The back of the tongue makes contact across the palate at the juncture between the hard and soft palate. Complete closure occurs across the back of the palate; however, this is not shown in Figure 4-20 since the transverse image does not extend to the soft palate. The manner of articulation for all three consonants is classified as nasal.

Few children with SSD of unknown origin have difficulty producing /m/ or /n/, and nasals are amongst the earliest phonemes to produce. Most children do not have difficulty with voicing of nasal consonants, since all English nasal consonants are voiced. Some children have difficulty with the tongue placement of /ŋ/. In fact, the most common non-adult production of /ŋ/ is [n], and this usually occurs when children also produce [t] for /k/ and [d] for /g/ (i.e., fronting). Finally, some children have difficulty with the manner of articulation of /m, n, ŋ/, and they produce an oral rather than a nasal consonant. For example, if a child has a cold or enlarged adenoids, and the passage of air is blocked to the nasal cavity, then the child may have **hyponasal speech**. Hyponasality can result in /m/ sounding more like [b], /n/ sounding more like [d], and /ŋ/ sounding more like [g]. So, *no*

FIGURE 4-20   Nasal consonants /m, n, ŋ /

Sagittal (midline) diagram of placement of the articulators and transverse diagram of tongue/palate contact for /m/, /n/, and /ŋ/

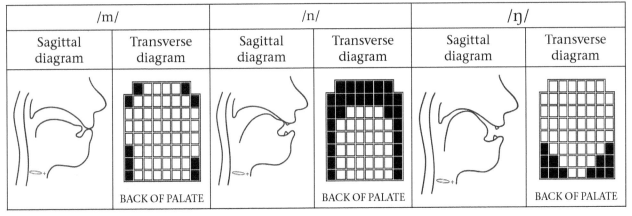

Source: Used by permission from Sharynne McLeod.

/noʊ/ will sound more like *dough* [doʊ]. If you compare the sagittal images of /b/ with /m/, /d/ with /n/, and /g/ with /ŋ/, you will notice that the main difference between the pairs relates to the positioning of the velum or soft palate against the pharyngeal wall. If it is against the pharyngeal wall, air cannot pass through the nose, so an oral consonant is produced: [b, d, g]. If it is away from the pharyngeal wall, then a nasal consonant is produced: [m, n, ŋ].

▪ Labiodental fricatives /f, v/

- ▪ /f/ voiceless labiodental fricative
- ▪ /v/ voiced labiodental fricative

The primary articulators involved in pronouncing /f, v/ are the teeth and lower lip. There is no tongue contact with the palate for /f/ and limited posterior lateral contact for /v/. The labiodental fricatives /f, v/ are produced by allowing the distributed airstream to escape through the slight opening between the upper teeth and lower lip (see Figure 4-21). /f, v/ are described as oral consonants since the nasal cavity is closed by the velum.

A common error pattern observed in children with SSD involves /f/ being produced as [p] and /v/ as [b] (e.g., *fan* /fæn/ as [pæn], and *van* /væn/ as [bæn]).

▪ Dental fricatives /θ, ð/

- ▪ /θ/ voiceless dental fricative
- ▪ /ð/ voiced dental fricative

The dental fricatives /θ, ð/ are produced by allowing the distributed airstream to escape through the opening (slit) between the tongue and the upper teeth (see Figure 4-22). Both /θ, ð/ are produced with limited contact of the tongue with the palate, with the only contact being along the posterior margins of the hard palate. The dental fricatives are oral consonants since no air escapes through the nose.

The dental fricatives /θ, ð/ are difficult for many children with SSD to pronounce correctly, and are often listed amongst the last consonants to be acquired. When children have difficulty with voicing they may produce [θ] instead of /ð/, although this is rare. Some

---

FIGURE 4-21   **Labiodental fricatives /f, v/**

Sagittal (midline) diagram of placement of the articulators and transverse diagram of tongue/palate contact for /f/ and /v/

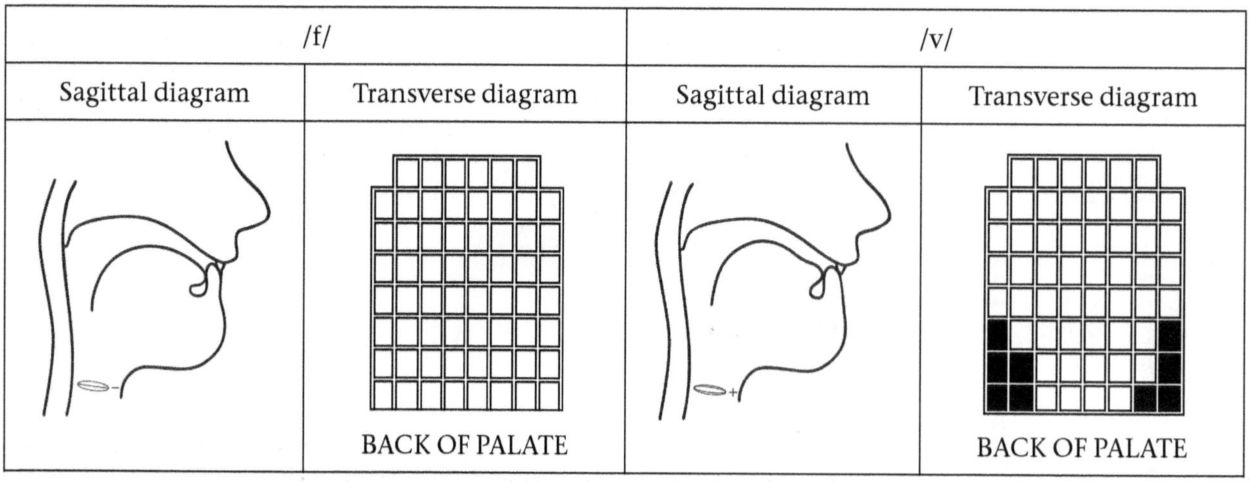

Source: Used by permission from Sharynne McLeod.

| FIGURE 4-22 | Dental fricatives /θ, ð/ |

Sagittal (midline) diagram of placement of the articulators and transverse diagram of tongue/palate contact for /θ/ and /ð/

/θ/		/ð/	
Sagittal diagram	Transverse diagram	Sagittal diagram	Transverse diagram
	BACK OF PALATE		BACK OF PALATE

Source: Used by permission from Sharynne McLeod.

> **COMMENT:** *Dental fricatives around the world*
>
> The dental fricatives /θ, ð/ occur frequently in Standard English, particularly in function words starting with /ð/ such as *the, this, that, there, then, though*. However, many dialects of English (e.g., Cockney English, Southern Irish English, and some researchers include General British) do not include /θ, ð/ in the consonant repertoire.
>
> The dental fricatives are amongst the most common consonants in Greek. In contrast, the consonants /θ, ð/ do not occur in many other languages, including Cantonese, Dutch, Filipino, French, German, Hungarian, Israeli Hebrew, Japanese, Korean, Maltese, Norwegian, Portuguese, Putonghua (Mandarin), Spanish, Thai, Turkish, and Vietnamese.

children change the place of articulation from the tongue tip touching the teeth, to the lower lip touching the teeth; consequently, they produce /θ, ð/ as [f, v], so, *thin* /θɪn/ will be produced as *fin* [fɪn]. This is called **fricative simplification** (see Chapter 5). Comparison of both the sagittal and transverse images for these consonants will assist you in determining the articulators involved in producing each sound, and the changes in tongue positioning. Some children who have difficulty producing /θ, ð/ change the manner of articulation, producing as a plosive rather than a fricative, so *thin* /θɪn/ will be produced as *din* [tɪn]. This is called stopping (see Chapter 5).

■ Alveolar fricatives /s, z/

- ▦ /s/ voiceless alveolar fricative
- ▦ /z/ voiced alveolar fricative

The alveolar fricatives /s, z/ are produced by directing the airstream through a narrow groove made by the tongue on the alveolar ridge (see the transverse diagram in Figure 4-23). In order to create the narrow groove, the tongue is anchored along the margins of the hard palate, creating horseshoe-shaped contact that is similar to the contact for /t, d, n/.

FIGURE 4-23   Alveolar fricatives /s, z/

Sagittal (midline) diagram of placement of the articulators and transverse diagram of tongue/palate contact for /s/ and /z/

/s/		/z/	
Sagittal diagram	Transverse diagram	Sagittal diagram	Transverse diagram
	BACK OF PALATE		BACK OF PALATE

Source: Used by permission from Sharynne McLeod.

The smaller the groove, the more **sibilant** (hissing) the sound. Thus, the most useful diagram for considering the production of /s/ and /z/ is the transverse diagram. The sagittal image may be misleading, since it depicts midline tongue contact with the alveolar ridge and does not indicate that a groove is formed. The groove may be directly in the midline (as suggested by the transverse images that were created by averaging 470 productions of /s/ and 310 productions of /z/ across eight speakers in Figure 4-23), or it may be slightly to the left or right of the midline (see all of the original images of /s/ and /z/ in McLeod & Singh, 2009a). The consonants /s, z/ are oral consonants, since the air is blocked from escaping through the nose by the velum.

Although /s/ (and to a lesser extent /z/) is common within the world's languages, these fricative consonants are difficult for children to produce. There are three major terms that explain most non-adultlike productions of /s/ and /z/ by children (and some adults): **interdental or dental lisp**, **lateral lisp**, and **stopping** (see Figure 4-24).

An **interdental lisp** occurs when /s/ and /z/ are produced as [θ] and [ð] respectively. While the manner and voicing remain the same for both consonants, the place of articulation changes. The tongue is placed further forward in the mouth for [θ] and [ð] (touching the teeth) compared with /s/ and /z/ where the tongue is on the alveolar ridge.

FIGURE 4-24   **Four productions of /s/**

Comparison between stylized transverse images of four productions of /s/: typical, interdental, lateral, and stopped

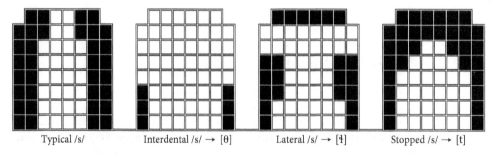

Typical /s/	Interdental /s/ → [θ]	Lateral /s/ → [ɬ]	Stopped /s/ → [t]

Source: Used by permission from Sharynne McLeod.

> **COMMENT:** *Production of /s/ and /z/ by preschoolers with SSD*
>
> In a study of 143 children with SSD who were 4 to 5 years old, 57.5% produced /s/ correctly and 45.5% produced /z/ correctly (McLeod, Harrison, McAllister, & McCormack, 2013). Of these 143 children, 39.9% produced interdental lisps on /s/ and /z/, 13.3% produced lateral lisps on /s/ and /z/, and 28.7% produced stopping on a range of fricatives including /s, z/ produced as [t, d], a pattern described in Chapter 5. Some children produced /s/ and /z/ in more than one of the ways indicated. None of these children had lost their front incisors.

The groove is very wide for the production of /θ/ and /ð/, and narrow for /s/ and /z/ (see Figure 4-24). This is the main anatomical difference between a sibilant and non-sibilant consonant. At times, children (and adults) may produce a consonant that is between an /s/ and [θ]. When this occurs a diacritic is used to indicate **dentalization**. The diacritic is easy to remember since it looks like a tooth underneath the consonant: [s̪, z̪]. Dentalized productions of /s/ have been labeled as "distortions" (Karlsson, Shriberg, Flipsen, & McSweeny, 2002, p. 403). Interdentalization and dentalization also may occur for other consonants, including /t, d, ʧ, ʤ/. While children do not have their front teeth and they await the growth of their adult dentition, their production of /s/ and /z/ may be dentalized.

A **lateral lisp** occurs when /s/ and /z/ are produced as [ɬ] and [ɮ] respectively. Lateral fricatives are produced by the air escaping over the sides of the tongue, and not through the central groove as in /s/ and /z/ (see Figure 4-24). This pattern was described by Hickey (1992) as being produced by a 10-year-old girl with a lateral lisp. Shriberg and Kent (2003, p. 223) describe lateral lisps as sounding "wet" or "slurpy." McLeod and Singh (2009a, pp. 175–176) considered previously published transverse images of tongue/palate contact during the production of lateralized /s/ and /z/ in English-speaking adults. There was a wide range of productions; however, the main differences between the lateral productions and /s/ and /z/ were the lack of a central groove, and greater palatal contact. An example of

APPLICATION: *Lateral fricatives*

Can you find the symbols /ɬ/ and /ɮ/ on your IPA chart? They are immediately under /s/ and /z/. Lateral fricatives occur in languages such as Welsh, African languages such as isiZulu and isiXhosa, and Native American languages such as Navajo but are not a part of the consonant repertoire for typical English speakers (Ball, 2012). Lateral productions of /s/ and /z/ are considered to be atypical in English. In contrast, in languages such as Greek, production of [ɬ] instead of /s/ is common in typically developing children (Mennen & Okalidou, 2007).

APPLICATION: *How do you make /s/?*

Susie (aged 7;4) said: "I can't make my 's' sound right. What do I do with my tongue so that is doesn't sound slushy when I say *super*?"

How would you answer Susie? As part of your answer, include a verbal explanation about how [s] is articulated and a visual explanation using a blank EPG palate. Revisit your answer once you have read Chapter 12.

Read more about Susie (7;4 years), a girl with an articulation impairment (lateral lisp), in Chapter 16 (Case 2).

a lateral production of /s/ is provided in Figure 4-24. Notice that the air cannot escape past the front teeth, since the alveolar ridge is blocked. Instead, there is an opening on either side of the alveolar ridge for the air to escape. Lateral productions of /s/ and /z/ are often resistant to traditional speech-language pathology intervention (Gibbon & Hardcastle, 1987). Consequently, if an English-speaking child exhibits a lateral lisp it may be appropriate to commence intervention earlier than for other productions of /s/, before motor patterns are ingrained.

Stopping of fricatives is another common phonological pattern observed in young children when children use plosives /t, d/ for fricatives. For example, /s/ produced as [t] (see Figure 4-24) and /z/ is produced as [d]. The sagittal images look exactly the same for /s, z, t, d/; however, the transverse images actually show the difference between tongue placements (see Figure 4-24). When [t] is used for /s/, the tongue makes contact around the palatal margins (like a horseshoe), and there is no groove for the air to escape. As you will learn in Chapter 5, the use of plosives for fricatives is often considered a phonological (rather than articulation) difficulty.

■ Postalveolar fricatives /ʃ, ʒ/

- ■ /ʃ/ voiceless postalveolar fricative
- ■ /ʒ/ voiced postalveolar fricative

The postalveolar fricatives /ʃ, ʒ/ are produced by directing the airstream through a wide groove made by the tongue anchored along the margins of the hard palate (see Figure 4-25). The groove is wider than that for the production of /s/ and /z/; however, /ʃ, ʒ/ are still classed as sibilants due to the large amount of acoustic energy. The consonants /ʃ, ʒ/ are oral consonants, since the air is blocked from escaping through the nose by the velum.

The two most common non-adult productions of /ʃ, ʒ/ involve change in manner with the fricatives /ʃ, ʒ/ being replaced by plosives [t, d], and a change in place with postalveolar fricatives /ʃ, ʒ/ being replaced by alveolar fricatives [s, z]. The consonants /ʃ, ʒ/ can also be lateralized (see /s, z/ earlier).

FIGURE 4-25 **Postalveolar fricatives /ʃ, ʒ/**

Sagittal (midline) diagram of placement of the articulators and transverse diagram of tongue/palate contact for /ʃ/ and /ʒ/.

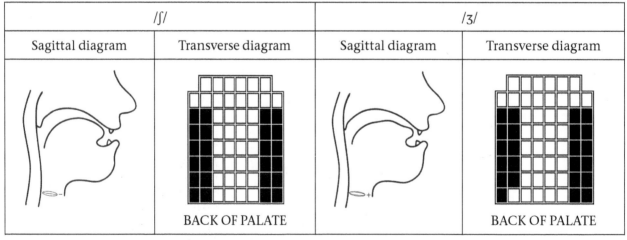

/ʃ/		/ʒ/	
Sagittal diagram	Transverse diagram	Sagittal diagram	Transverse diagram

Source: Used by permission from Sharynne McLeod.

▪ Glottal fricative /h/

- ▪ /h/ voiceless glottal fricative

The /h/ consonant is described as a glottal fricative because the turbulence in the airstream occurs just above the vocal folds. However, Ladefoged (2005, p. 118) suggests that this is not a good description of /h/ and proposes that it is "usually just a voiceless version of the adjacent sounds." He suggests that in a word like *hit* /hɪt/, the /h/ is a voiceless version of /ɪ/. You will learn in Chapter 5 that /h/ is considered a semivowel in phonological theories. There is limited (if any) contact of the tongue against the palate during the production of /h/ (Figure 4-26).

Few English-speaking children have difficulty producing /h/, since it requires little articulatory effort, and it is regarded as one of the "early-8" consonants (Shriberg, 1993, p. 119). If a child has a cleft palate, then **nasal emission** may occur during the production of /h/, where the airstream flows through the nose instead of solely through the mouth. The consonant /h/ does not occur in languages such as German, Greek, Hungarian, Spanish, or Portuguese, so children who speak these languages may have some difficulty pronouncing English words that contain /h/.

▪ Alveolar approximant /ɹ/

- ▪ /ɹ/ voiced alveolar approximant

The articulation of /ɹ/ is discussed widely. As Ladefoged (2005) states, "The sound **r** is more difficult to describe, partly because different speakers make it in different ways" (p. 54). Shriberg and Kent (2003) describe two classes of /ɹ/: **retroflex** and **bunched**. Figure 4-27 shows a slightly retroflexed /ɹ/ where the tongue tip is up and the tongue body is in the mid-central position. A bunched /ɹ/ is where the tongue tip is turned down and the blade is elevated. Cox (2012) described /ɹ/ as "an apical postalveolar sound" (p. 33). As with /h/, /ɹ/ is influenced by the surrounding consonants and vowels.

The consonant /ɹ/ is difficult for many children to acquire and is found amongst the "late-8" consonants (Shriberg, 1993, p. 119). It is unclear whether it is difficult to acquire because of its perceptual characteristics, articulatory demands, or both (Shriberg & Kent, 2013). A common difficulty with the production of /ɹ/ involves a change in the manner and place of articulation involving both the tongue placement and lip rounding with /ɹ/ → [w].

FIGURE 4-26 **Glottal fricative /h/**

Sagittal (midline) diagram of placement of the articulators and transverse diagram of tongue/palate contact for /h/

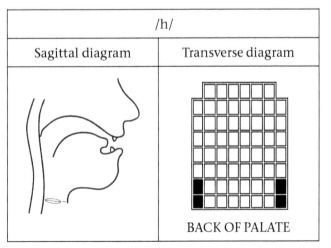

Source: Used by permission from Sharynne McLeod.

COMMENT: *Rhotic and non-rhotic dialects of English*

One of the defining features of English dialects is whether or not the dialect is rhotic or non-rhotic. Rhotic dialects pronounce /ɹ/ in syllable-initial, syllable-final, word-initial, and word-final positions, and have r-colored vowels (e.g., /ɝ, ɚ/). Rhotic English dialects include General American English, Scottish English, and Irish English. In contrast, non-rhotic dialects only use /ɹ/ in syllable-initial and word-initial position and do not have r-colored vowels (e.g., /ɜ, ə/). Non-rhotic English dialects include Bostonian English (US), General British (UK), Australian English, New Zealand English, and South African English. A famous sentence spoken in Boston (US) to distinguish between rhotic and non-rhotic English dialects is "Park the car in Harvard Yard." Those who use a rhotic pronunciation may pronounce the sentence as /pɑɹk ðə kɑɹɪn hɑɹvɝd jɑɹd/. In contrast, those who use a non-rhotic pronunciation may pronounce the sentence as /pɑk ðə kɑɹɪn hɑvəd jɑd/. Notice that the word *car* ends with an /ɹ/ in both sentences. This is because the word after *car* starts with a vowel. Non-rhotic dialects use linking-r in contexts when words that are spelled with a final "r" are followed by a word commencing with a vowel.

COMMENT: *The relative importance of /ɹ/ in different English dialects*

In England, /ɹ/ is frequently produced as the labiodental approximant [ʋ] or as the labiovelar approximant [w]. Foulkes and Docherty (2000) indicated that use of [ʋ] for /ɹ/ in England is reflective of social stratification, although this may no longer be true since many politicians, actors, and other public figures use these forms of /ɹ/ within the media. Consequently, many SLPs (called *speech and language therapists* in the UK) do not place a high priority on "correcting" children's pronunciation of /ɹ/. In contrast, /ɹ/ is a frequently targeted consonant by SLPs in the United States.

FIGURE 4-27 **Alveolar approximant /ɹ/ and palatal approximant /j/**

Sagittal (midline) diagram of placement of the articulators and transverse diagram of tongue/palate contact for /ɹ/ and /j/

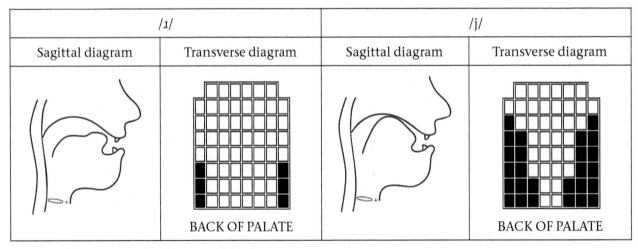

Source: Used by permission from Sharynne McLeod.

▨ Palatal approximant /j/

- ▪ /j/ voiced palatal approximant

The palatal approximant is produced with the tongue anchored along the lateral margins of the palate (see Figure 4-27). The tongue position for /j/ resembles /i/, but with greater constriction (Shriberg & Kent, 2013). /j/ is called a semivowel and in English it is always followed by a vowel, and /j/ is an oral consonant.

Few children have difficulty producing /j/. The most common word containing /j/ that children mispronounce is *yellow → lellow*, possibly due to the assimilation with the /l/ within the word. Some children produce /j/ → [l] or [w] in other contexts, demonstrating a change in place of articulation from palatal to alveolar or labiovelar.

▨ Alveolar lateral approximant /l/

- ▪ /l/ voiced lateral approximant

/l/ is the only lateral consonant found in English (there are a total of four lateral approximants that are used throughout the world's languages). There are two types of /l/ in English: clear [l] and dark [ɫ] (Recasens, 2004). Clear [l] is produced with the tongue tip on the alveolar ridge (see Figure 4-28), and dark [ɫ] is produced with the tongue tip on the alveolar ridge as well as contact along the lateral margins of the palate. In English, clear [l] is more likely to occur in word-initial positions (e.g., *leak* /lik/), and dark [ɫ] in word-final position (e.g., *feel* /fiɫ/), although prosodic word boundaries can also have an impact on which /l/ is produced (Oxley, Buckingham, Roussel, & Daniloff, 2006). /l/ is an oral consonant, because the velum is closed.

/l/ is a one of the later developing consonants in English. The most common error observed in children's speech involves a change in manner and placement of articulation with the liquid /l/ becoming [w] or [j], called **gliding** (see Chapter 5).

▨ Labiovelar approximant /w/

- ▪ /w/ voiced labiovelar approximant

/w/ is special since it has a double place of articulation. It is called a labiovelar consonant because the lips are rounded, so it is a labial consonant, and the back of the tongue is

---

FIGURE 4-28 **Alveolar lateral approximant /l/ and labiovelar approximant /w/**

Sagittal (midline) diagram of placement of the articulators and transverse diagram of tongue/palate contact for /l/ and /w/

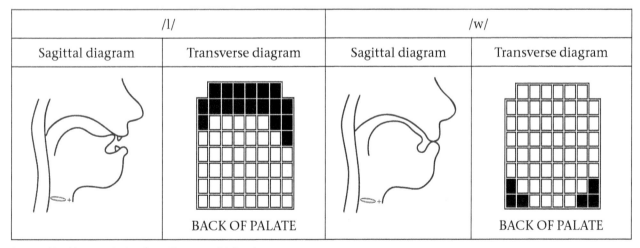

/l/		/w/	
Sagittal diagram	Transverse diagram	Sagittal diagram	Transverse diagram
	BACK OF PALATE		BACK OF PALATE

Source: Used by permission from Sharynne McLeod.

■■ ■■ ■ ■ ■■ ■ ■■ ■

 APPLICATION: *Chocolate* /ʧaklət/ *as* [tsɑ.kələʔ] *and teacher* /tiʧɚ/ *as* [ti.ʃɚ]

Lian (14;2 years) has spastic dysarthria associated with cerebral palsy. She is also multilingual—she speaks English and Cantonese. Affricates are one area of difficulty for Lian. She says *chocolate* /ʧaklət/ as [tsɑ.kələʔ] and *teacher* /tiʧɚ/ as [ti.ʃɚ]. Describe the voice place and manner of /ʧ/ and the two consonants that Lian substitutes for /ʧ/.

Read more about Lian (14;2 years), a girl with childhood dysarthria, in Chapter 16 (Case 5).

Answer: /ʧ/ is the voiceless postalveolar affricate; Lian substitutes the voiceless alveolar affricate /ts/ and the voiceless postalveolar fricative /ʃ/ for /ʧ/. You can more read more about Lian's difficulty with affricates in Chapter 16.

raised, so it is a velar consonant. The velum is closed and the airstream is directed out of the oral cavity (see Figure 4-28).

/w/ is an early developing consonant in English, and children rarely have difficulty with the production of this consonant.

■ Affricates /ʧ, ʤ/

- ■ /ʧ/ voiceless postalveolar affricate
- ■ /ʤ/ voiced postalveolar affricate

The affricates are produced with the body of the tongue bunching and touching the roof of the mouth, just behind the alveolar ridge. Notice in Figure 4-29 how much of the tongue (including the side) contacts the palate during the articulation of these two speech sounds. As the phonetic symbols suggest, the articulation is a combination of a short sharp production of something like /t/ followed by the frication of /ʃ/ for /ʧ/ and /d/ followed by the frication of /ʒ/ for /ʤ/.

Affricates can be difficult for children to master. Children may produce affricates /ʧ, ʤ/ as either a plosive (e.g., *chew* /ʧu/ changing to [tu], and *jump* /ʤʌmp/ changing to [dʌmp]) or a different fricative (e.g., *chew* /ʧu/ changing to [ʃu] or [su]). As you will learn in Chapter 5, other patterns involving affricates are possible.

FIGURE 4-29 **Affricates /ʧ, ʤ/**

Sagittal (midline) diagram of placement of the articulators and transverse diagram of tongue/palate contact for /ʧ/ and /ʤ/

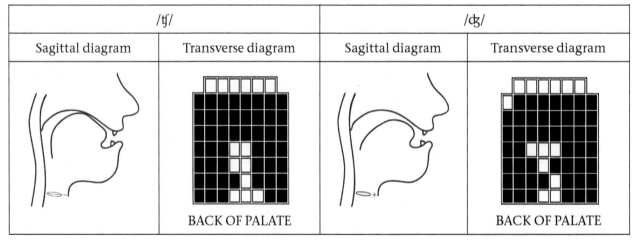

/ʧ/		/ʤ/	
Sagittal diagram	Transverse diagram	Sagittal diagram	Transverse diagram
	BACK OF PALATE		BACK OF PALATE

Source: Used by permission from Sharynne McLeod.

■ ■

 APPLICATION: *Do you really need to transcribe children's speech?*

Read more about
Luke (4;3 years),
a boy with a phonological
impairment,
in Chapter 16 (Case 1).

Imagine you are conducting an initial speech assessment with Luke (aged 4;3). Explain why it is important to phonetically transcribe Luke's speech sample (rather than simply marking Luke's productions of speech sounds in words as correct or incorrect).

Chapter summary

In this chapter you learned about the International Phonetic Alphabet, and how to use it to transcribe speech. The voice, place, and manner of consonants were described using diagrams of tongue/palate contact for English consonants. You were introduced to variations in the production of consonants by children with SSD of known and unknown origins. In Chapter 5, we add to this knowledge by considering the theories that have been developed to explain speech production and perception.

Suggested reading

Articulation of individual consonants

■ McLeod, S., & Singh, S. (2009a). *Speech sounds: A pictorial guide to typical and atypical speech*. San Diego, CA: Plural Publishing.

Transcription

■ Bauman-Waengler, J. (2009). *Introduction to phonetics and phonology: From concepts to transcription*. Boston, MA: Pearson.

■ Shriberg, L. D., & Kent, R. D. (2013). *Clinical phonetics* (4th ed.). Boston, MA: Pearson.

Application of knowledge from Chapter 4

Using the transcribed speech samples for Luke (4;3 years), Susie (7;4 years), Jarrod (7;0 years), Michael (4;2 years), and Lian (14;2 years) in Chapter 16, apply your knowledge about the transcription of speech by completing the following questions.

1. Compare and contrast the transcribed speech samples for Jarrod and Michael (in Tables 16-11 and 16-14 respectively), for the words *birthday*, *tongue*, and *witch*. What syllable-stress difficulty does Michael appear to have that Jarrod doesn't have?

2. Compare and contrast the transcribed speech samples for Michael (Table 16-14) and Lian (Table 16-18). Using your knowledge about the difference between CAS and childhood dysarthria, what do the speech samples tell you about their respective prosodic and voice characteristics?

3. Review the transcribed monosyllabic words for Luke in Table 16-6. What voice, place, and manners of articulation did Luke use in word-initial and word-final position?

4. Review the single-word sample of word-initial and word-final consonant clusters for Luke in Table 16-6.

Describe Luke's ability to produce consonant clusters with respect to (a) syllable position in words, and (b) the voice-place-manner characteristics of the consonants that make up the consonant clusters he can produce.

5. Review Susie's speech sample in Table 16-8. Using copies of the blank EPG palate in this chapter, color the squares where you think Susie's tongue touched the palate when she attempted to produce the /s/ in *rice* /ɹaɪs/ but realizes it as [ɹaɪɬ]. On another blank template, color in the squares where Susie's tongue should touch the palate when producing [s]. Compare your answer with the palates in Figure 4-24.

6. If you were to view Susie's articulation of [ɬ] using a coronal view of her tongue from an ultrasound image, what important tongue shape might be missing?

7. If you have access to an ultrasound machine, observe a coronal view of your own production of [s] and [ɬ]. What can you do with the lateral margins of your tongue, to make the [ɬ] sound slushy?

Appendix 4–1. Transcription decision-making tree

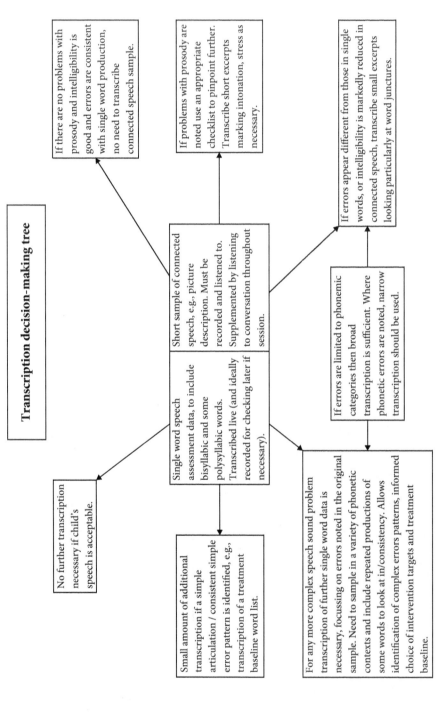

Transcription decision-making tree

No further transcription necessary if child's speech is acceptable.

If there are no problems with prosody and intelligibility is good and errors are consistent with single word production, no need to transcribe connected speech sample.

If problems with prosody are noted use an appropriate checklist to pinpoint further. Transcribe short excerpts marking intonation, stress as necessary.

If errors appear different from those in single words, or intelligibility is markedly reduced in connected speech, transcribe small excerpts looking particularly at word junctures.

Single word speech assessment data, to include bisyllabic and some polysyllabic words. Transcribed live (and ideally recorded for checking later if necessary).

Short sample of connected speech, e.g, picture description. Must be recorded and listened to. Supplemented by listening to conversation throughout session.

Small amount of additional transcription if a simple articulation / consistent simple error pattern is identified, e.g., transcription of a treatment baseline word list.

For any more complex speech sound problem transcription of further single word data is necessary, focussing on errors noted in the original sample. Need to sample in a variety of phonetic contexts and include repeated productions of some words to look at in/consistency. Allows identification of complex errors patterns, informed choice of intervention targets and treatment baseline.

If errors are limited to phonemic categories then broad transcription is sufficient. Where phonetic errors are noted, narrow transcription should be used.

Source: From UK and Ireland Specialists in Specific Speech Impairment Network [UK and Ireland SSSIN], 2013, p.3. Used by permission of Dr. Yvonne Wren.

Appendix 4-2. Inventory of consonants for 25 languages and dialects

Language/ Consonant — Plosives	Afrikaans	Arabic: Jordanian	Arabic: Lebanese	Cantonese	Dutch	Filipino	English	Finnish	French	German	Greek	Hungarian	Hebrew: Israeli	Icelandic	Japanese	Korean	Maltese	Norwegian	Portuguese	Putonghua	Spanish	Thai	Turkish	Vietnamese	Welsh
p	p		(p)	p pʰ	p	p	p	p	p	p	p (ᵐp)	p	p	p pʰ	p	p p* pʰ	p	p	p	p pʰ	p	pʰ ʔp	p	p	p
b	b	b	b		b	b	b	(b)	b	b	b (ᵐb)	b	b		b		b	b	b		b	b	b	b	b
t	t	t t̪	t tˤ	t tʰ	t	t	t t̪	t̪	t	t	t	t	t	t tʰ	t	t t* tʰ	t	t	t	t tʰ	t	tʰ ʔt	t	t̪ t	t̪
d	d	d dˤ	d dˤ		d	d	d d̪	d	d	d	d	d	d		d		d	d	d		d	d	d	d	d̪
ʈ																		ʈ							
ɖ																		ɖ							
c					(c)						(c)		(c)	(c) (cʰ)									c	c	
ɟ											(ɟ)		(ɟ)										ɟ		
k	k	k	(k)	k kʰ	k	k	k	k	k	k	k	k	k	k kʰ	k	k k* kʰ	k	k	k	k kʰ	k	kʰ ʔk	k	k	k
g	g	(g)	g		(g)	g	g	(g)	g	g	g (ᵑg)	g	g		g		g	g	g		g		g		g

(Continued)

Appendix 4-2. Inventory of consonants for 25 languages and dialects

(Continued)

Language/Consonant	Afrikaans	Arabic: Jordanian	Arabic: Lebanese	Cantonese	Dutch	Filipino	English	Finnish	French	German	Greek	Hungarian	Hebrew: Israeli	Icelandic	Japanese	Korean	Maltese	Norwegian	Portuguese	Putonghua	Spanish	Thai	Turkish	Vietnamese	Welsh
b		b	(b)																						
G		(G)																							
ʔ		ʔ	ʔ			(ʔ)	ʔ		ʔ	ʔ		ʔ		(ʔ)			ʔ					ʔ		ʔ	
Nasals																									
m	m	m	m	m	m	m	m	m	m	m	m	m	m	m	m	m	m	m	m	m	m	m	m	m
m̥											(m̥)		(m̥)	(m̥)											
n	n	n	n	n	n	n	n	n	n	n	n	n	n	n	n	n	n	n	n	n	n	n	n	n
n̥													(n̥)	(n̥)				ɳ							
ɲ					(ɲ)				ɲ		(ɲ)		ɲ	ɲ (ɲ̊)	(ɲ)				ɲ		ɲ			ɲ	
ŋ	ŋ			ŋ	ŋ	ŋ	ŋ	ŋ	ŋ	ŋ	(ŋ)			ŋ (ŋ̊)	ŋ	ŋ		ŋ		ŋ		ŋ		ŋ	ŋ
N						N									N										
Trills																									
ʙ																									
r		r	r					r		r				r r̥							r	r			r r̥ʰ
R									R																
Tap/flaps																									
ⱱ																									
ɾ	ɾ		ɾ		ɾ	(ɾ)	ɾ	ɾ	ɾ	ɾ	ɾ	ɾ	ɾ		ɾ	(ɾ)	ɾ	ɾ	ɾ		ɾ	ɾ	ɾ	ɾ	
ɽ																		ɽ						ɽ	
Fricatives																									
ɸ															ɸ										

Appendix 4-2. Inventory of consonants for 25 languages and dialects

Language/ Consonant	Afrikaans	Arabic: Jordanian	Arabic: Lebanese	Cantonese	Dutch	English	Filipino	Finnish	French	German	Greek	Hungarian	Hebrew: Israeli	Icelandic	Japanese	Korean	Maltese	Norwegian	Portuguese	Putonghua	Spanish	Thai	Turkish	Vietnamese	Welsh
β																									
f	f	f	f	f	f		f	(f)	f	f	f	f	f	f			f	f	f	f	f	f	f	f	f
v	v	(v)	(v)		v		v		v	v	v	v	v	v			v		v				v	v	v
θ		θ	(θ)				θ				θ			θ											θ
ð		ð	(ð)				ð				ð			(ð)											ð
ð̣		ð̣																							
s	s	s	s	s	s	s	s	s	s	s	s	s	s	s	s	s	s	s	s	s	s	s	s	s	s
sˤ		sˤ	sˤ													s*									
z	z	z	zˤ		z		z		z	z	z	z	z		z		z		z				z	z	z
ʃ	ʃ	ʃ	ʃ		ʃ	ʃ	ʃ	ʃ	ʃ	ʃ		ʃ	ʃ				ʃ		ʃ				ʃ	ʃ	ʃ
ʒ		(ʒ)	ʒ		(ʒ)		ʒ		ʒ			ʒ	ʒ						ʒ				ʒ	ʒ	
ʂ																		ʂ		ʂ					
zˤ																								zˤ	
ç										ç	(ç)		(ç)	ç	(ç)			ç							
ʝ											(ʝ)		(ʝ)	ʝ											
x		χ	x							x	x	x	(x)	(x)						x	x			x	x
ɣ			ɣ								ɣ		(ɣ)	ɣ										ɣ	
χ			(χ)		χ																				
ʁ		ʁ	(ʁ)						ʁ	ʁ		ʁ													
ħ		ħ	ħ																						
ʕ		ʕ	ʕ																						
h		h	h	h	h	h	h	h	h	h	h	h		h	h	h	h	h				h	h	h	h
ɦ	ɦ												(ɦ)												

(Continued)

Appendix 4-2. Inventory of consonants for 25 languages and dialects

Language/Consonant	Afrikaans	Arabic: Jordanian	Arabic: Lebanese	Cantonese	Dutch	Filipino	English	Finnish	French	German	Greek	Hungarian	Hebrew; Israeli	Icelandic	Japanese	Korean	Maltese	Norwegian	Portuguese	Putonghua	Spanish	Thai	Turkish	Vietnamese	Welsh
Lateral fricatives																									
ɬ																									ɬ
ɮ																									
Approximants																									
ʋ					ʋ			ʋ										ʋ						ʋ	
ɹ						ɹ											ɹ			ɹ				ɹ	
ɻ																									
j		j	j	j	j	j	j	j	j	j		j	j		j		j	j			j	j	j	j	j
ɥ																									
Lateral approximants																									
l		l	lˤ	l	l	l	l	l	l	l	l	l	l	l		l	l	l	l	l	l	l	l		l
ɭ														l̥											
ʎ											(ʎ)								ʎ						
ʟ																		ʟ					ɫ		
Other symbols																									
ʍ																									
w	w	w	w	w		w	w								w		w				w	w		w	w
ɥ									ɥ																
ʜ																									
ɕ															(ɕ)					ɕ					
ʑ															(ʑ)										
ɾ																									
ŋ																									

(Continued)

Appendix 4-2. Inventory of consonants for 25 languages and dialects

Language/Consonant	Afrikaans	Arabic: Jordanian	Arabic: Lebanese	Cantonese	Dutch	Filipino	English	Finnish	French	German	Greek	Hungarian	Hebrew: Israeli	Icelandic	Japanese	Korean	Maltese	Norwegian	Portuguese	Putonghua	Spanish	Thai	Turkish	Vietnamese	Welsh
Affricates																									
pf										pf															
ts				ts tsʰ						ts	ts	ts	ts		(ts)		ts			ts tsʰ					
ɸ											ɸ		ɸ*												
tʂ																				tʂ tʂʰ					
tɕ																tɕ tɕ* tɕʰ				tɕ tɕʰ		tɕ tɕʰ			
tʃ		tʃ				tʃ	tʃ					tʃ	tʃ				tʃ				tʃ		tʃ	tʃ	tʃ
dʒ		dʒ				dʒ	dʒ					dʒ	dʒ				dʒ						dʒ	dʒ	dʒ
cç													cç												
ɟʝ													ɟʝ												
cɕ															(cɕ)										
ɟʑ															(ɟʑ)										
Other				kʷ kʷʰ			dʲ						(x)					ʈɖ							

Source: Compiled using: McLeod, S. (Ed.). (2007a). *The international guide to speech acquisition*. Clifton Park, NY: Thomson Delmar Learning. Copyright © Sharynne McLeod, 2015.

Appendix 4-3. Extensions to the International Phonetic Alphabet

extIPA SYMBOLS FOR DISORDERED SPEECH
(Revised to 2015)

CONSONANTS (other than on the IPA Chart)

	bilabial	labio-dental	labio-alveolar	dento-labial	bidental	linguo-labial	inter-dental	alveolar	retroflex	palatal	velar	velo-pharyng.	(upper) pharyng.
Plosive		p̪ b̪	p̺ b̺	p̼ b̼		t̼ d̼	t̪ d̪						Q ʕ
Nasal		m̺̊ m̺	m̼̊ m̼			n̼̊ n̼	n̪̊ n̪						
Trill						r̼	r̪					ʜ̃ŋ ʜ̃ŋ	
Fricative median		f̪ v̪	f̺ v̺	h̪ h̪		θ̼ ð̼	θ̪ ð̪					fŋ fŋ	
Fricative lateral						ɬ̼ ɮ̼	ɬ̪ ɮ̪		ꞎ ꞎ	ʎ̝̊ ʎ̝	ʟ̝̊ ʟ̝		
Fricative lat. + med.								ls lz					
Fricative nasal	m̥̃ m̃	m̥̃ m̃						ñ̥ ñ	ñ̥ ɳ̃	ɲ̥̃ ɲ̃	ŋ̥̃ ŋ̃		
Approxt. lateral						l̼	l̪̃						
Percussive	ʬ				ʭ								

DIACRITICS

◌͖	labial spreading	s͖	◌̃	denasal	m̃ ñ	◌͐	main gesture offset right	s͐
◌͈	strong articulation	f͈	◌̰̃	fricative nasal escape	ṽ	◌͑	main gesture offset left	s͑
◌͉	weak articulation	v͉	◌̰̃	velopharyngeal friction	s̰̃ ʒ̰̃	◌̫	whistled articulation	s̫
\	reiteration	p\p\p	↓	ingressive airflow	p↓	◌͜◌	sliding articulation	θ͜s

CONNECTED SPEECH, UNCERTAINTY, ETC.

(.) (..) (...)	short, medium, long pause
f, ff	loud(er) speech: [{f laʊd f}]
p, pp	quiet(er) speech: [{p kwaɪ ət p}]
allegro	fast speech: [{allegro fast allegro}]
lento	slow speech: [{lento sloʊ lento}]
crescendo, rallentando, etc. may also be used	
Ⓞ, Ⓒ, Ⓥ	indeterminate sound, consonant, vowel
Ⓕ, Ⓟ, etc.	indeterminate fricative, probably [p], etc.
( )	silent articulation, e.g., (ʃ), (m)
(( ))	extraneous noise, e.g., ((2 sylls))

VOICING

◌̬	pre-voicing	̬z
◌̬	post-voicing	z̬
◌̬	partial devoicing	z̬ ʒ̬
◌̬	initial partial devoicing	z̬ ʒ̬
◌̬	final partial devoicing	z̬ ʒ̬
◌̥	partial voicing	s̥
◌̥	initial partial voicing	s̥
◌̥	final partial voicing	s̥
◌˭	unaspirated	p˭
ʰ◌	pre-aspiration	ʰp

OTHER SOUNDS

ɹ̺	apical-r
ɹ̈	bunched-r (molar-r)
s̺ z̺	laminal fricatives (incl. lowered tongue tip)
kꞎ etc.	[k] with lateral fricated release, etc.
tˡˢ dˡʑ	[t, d] with lateral and median release
tθ̞	[t] with interdental aspiration, etc.

t̼θ̼	linguolabial affricates, etc.
ʞ ʞ̥ ʞ̃	velodorsal oral and nasal stops
�	sublaminal lower alveolar percussive
ǃ̬	alveolar click with sublaminal percussive release
↺r̼	Buccal interdental trill (raspberry)
*	sound with no available symbol

© ICPLA 2015

Source: International Clinical Phonetics and Linguistics Association (ICPLA), 2015. Used with permission.

Appendix 4-4. Voice quality symbols

VoQS: Voice Quality Symbols

Airstream Types

⊕	buccal airstream	↓	pulmonic ingressive speech
Œ	œsophageal speech	Ю	tracheo-œsophageal speech

Phonation types

V	modal voice	F	falsetto
W	whisper	C	creak
V̬	whispery voice (murmur)	V̰	creaky voice
V̤	breathy voice	C̣	whispery creak
V̜	slack / lax voice	V!	harsh voice
V!!	ventricular phonation	V̬!!	diplophonia
V̤!!	whispery ventricular phonation	Vᴧᴧ	aryepiglottic phonation
V̬̈	pressed phonation / tight voice	Ẅ	tight whisper
ʌʌʌ	spasmodic dysphonia	И	electrolarynx phonation

Supralaryngeal Settings

L̝	raised larynx	L̞	lowered larynx
Vᵒᵉ	labialized voice (open rounded)	Vʷ	labialized voice (close rounded)
V̈↔	spread-lip voice	Vᶹ	labio-dentalized voice
V̺	linguo-apicalized voice	V̻	linguo-laminalized voice
V^	retroflex voice	V̪	dentalized voice
V̳	alveolarized voice	V̳ʲ	palatoalveolarized voice
Vʲ	palatalized voice	Vˠ	velarized voice
Vᴚ	uvularized voice	Vˤ	pharyngealized voice
V̝ˤ	laryngo-pharyngealized voice	Vᴴ	faucalized voice
Ṽ	nasalized voice	Ṽ̃	denasalized voice

J̞	open jaw voice	J̝	close jaw voice
J̪<	right offset jaw voice	J̪>	left offset jaw voice
J̟	protruded jaw voice	Θ	protruded tongue voice

USE OF LABELED BRACES & NUMERALS TO MARK STRETCHES OF SPEECH
AND DEGREES AND COMBINATIONS OF VOICE QUALITY:

[ˈðɪs ɪz ˈnɔɹməl ˈvɔɪs {3V! ˈðɪs ɪz ˈveɹi ˈhɑɹʃ ˈvɔɪs 3V} ˈðɪs ɪz ˈnɔɹməl ˈvɔɪs wʌns ˈmɔɹ {L̝ 1V! ˈðɪs ɪz ˈlɛs ˈhɑɹʃ ˈvɔɪs wɪð ˈloʊɚd ˈlæɹɪŋks 1V!L̝}]

© 2015 Martin J. Ball, John H. Esling, B. Craig Dickson

Source: VoQS, M. J. Ball, J. Esling, C. Dickson, 2015.

5

Theoretical Foundations of Children's Speech

LEARNING OBJECTIVES

1 Explain that spoken communication involves the perception, storage, and production of speech.

2 State the difference between phonetics and phonology.

3 Explain theoretical concepts and descriptive terms in phonology including phones, phonemes, allophones, minimal pairs, features, naturalness and markedness, implicational relationships, phonotactics, phonological rules, and phonological processes.

4 Briefly describe conventional and contemporary theories that have been applied to the study of SSD in children.

5 Identify common phonological processes evident in children's speech.

6 Explain what is involved in the perception of speech.

7 Describe the concepts of phonological planning, motor planning, motor programming, and motor execution.

KEY WORDS

Theoretical concepts in phonology: phones, phonemes, allophones, minimal pairs, features, naturalness, markedness, implicational relationships, sonority, phonotactics

Phonological theories: generative phonology, natural phonology, nonlinear phonology, optimality theory

Phonological processes: syllable structure processes (e.g., weak syllable deletion, reduplication, final consonant deletion, cluster reduction), substitution processes (e.g., fronting, stopping, gliding), assimilation processes

Speech perception: categorical perception, lack of invariance, speaker normalization

Speech production: motor planning, motor programming, motor execution, models of speech production: Nijmegen model, DIVA and GODIVA models, schema theory of motor learning, psycholinguistic speech processing model

OVERVIEW

Theory guides practice. Theory provides a way of thinking about and understanding phenomena. In this chapter you will learn concepts and theories about the perception of speech, the organization and abstract representation of speech, and the production of speech. You will learn that these three broad areas (perception, representation, and production) mirror a psycholinguistic framework for studying and understanding SSD in children (Stackhouse & Wells, 1997). While it would seem logical to start this chapter with the perception of speech, literature on speech perception assumes that you are familiar with ideas about the organization of spoken language in the mind. It assumes that you know about phonology. Therefore, we begin this chapter with the topic of phonology. We also dedicate much of this chapter to phonology because many children who have SSD have phonological difficulties. Additionally, many assessment, analysis, and intervention approaches used by SLPs are underscored by concepts in phonology. You need to be familiar with phonological concepts to understand elementary clinical methods and procedures. Following our overview of phonology, we consider ideas and theories about the perception of speech. Finally, we address the amazing phenomena of speech production—how words represented and stored in our mind can be transformed into spoken, intelligible words, through carefully timed sequences of motor movements.

For those of you who view the theoretical chapter of a textbook as less relevant or uninspiring, a word of caution. You might be tempted to skim over or even skip this chapter and go straight to the practical chapters on methods and procedures for working with children with SSD. However, methods and procedures are grounded in theory. An understanding of theory will help you understand why certain methods and procedures are used in practice. An understanding of theory will also help you be a critically thinking evidence-based clinician. So, read on and learn about theory with a clear mind ready to think, reflect, and ponder!

PHONOLOGY—WHAT IS IT?

There are over 7,000 known languages in the world (Gussenhoven & Jacobs, 2011; Lewis, Simons, & Fennig, 2014). However, as you learned in Chapters 3 and 4, there is a limit to the articulatory possibilities of the human vocal tract, and as such there is a limit to the consonants, vowels, tones, stress patterns, and syllable shapes that an individual can produce. So, what underlies the diversity across all these languages? The answer lies in the concept of phonology. Phonology, as its name implies, is about sounds (phono) and knowledge (ology). For example, if you speak English, you would know that /ki/ and /ti/ are two different words (*key* and *tea*) that begin with two different speech sounds, and that [tʰi] and [ti] are the same word (*tea*), despite the fact that they start with two similar yet different speech sounds. You also know that [ʃnɛ.kə] is not an English word. You are aware of this because you know (subconsciously) that English does not begin words with these two sounds [ʃn]. If you speak German, you would know this is *Schnecke*, the German word for "snail." You would also know that it is perfectly acceptable to begin a word with [ʃn] in German. This is what phonology is about—the sound system of languages, and the *rules* for how those

> **COMMENT:** *Are all theories helpful?*
>
> Theories can be helpful, but they are not infallible (Lof, 2011). Additionally, not all theoretically motivated methods are the most successful or most desired choice when working with children with SSD. As an evidence-based clinician you need to be selective about the theoretical influences on your practice. Look out for logical and rational theories that have been tested.

sounds can combine and are pronounced in languages (Fromkin et al., 2012). To put what you learned in Chapter 4 into context, phonetics is about the articulation or physical production of speech sounds, while phonology is about how those speech sounds are used and function in languages (Ball, Müller, & Rutter, 2010).

How much do you already know about the phonology of the language(s) you speak? Which sounds belong to your language(s)? What are all the rules for how those speech sounds are allowed to combine? Believe it or not, you know the answers to these questions, albeit subconsciously. What is more amazing is that most typically developing 5-year-old children know this too! The problem for many children with SSD is that they may not have a complete knowledge. To help these children, you need to develop a conscious awareness of your own phonological knowledge. What follows is an overview of theoretical concepts assumed in discussions of various phonological theories. Once you understand these basic concepts, you will be able to appreciate the similarities and differences across a range of classic and contemporary phonological theories.

■ Theoretical concepts: Phones, phonemes, allophones, and minimal pairs

The words *key* and *tea* are each made up of two speech sounds [kʰ] + [i] and [tʰ] +[i]. Each speech sound is called a **phone** when considered separately from the language in which it is used. However, in the context of a language, a speech sound that serves to contrast meaning between words is called a **phoneme**. To use /k/ and /t/ as an example, if /k/ replaced /t/ in the word *tea*, we would end up with the new word *key*. In this way, /t/ and /k/ are phonemes because the substitution of one for another alters the meaning of the word. When word pairs differ by a single phoneme, and the difference is enough to signal a change in meaning, they are called **minimal pairs** (Barlow & Gierut, 2002). Using this definition, *key* and *tea* are minimal pairs, as are *meat* and *seat*. When the distinguishing phonemes differ minimally, they are referred to as **minimally opposing minimal pairs**. For example, using your understanding about articulation from Chapter 4, the phonemes /k/ and /t/ differ minimally because they are both voiceless plosives, differing only by the place of articulation, whereas /m/ and /s/ are maximally opposing because they differ by voice, place, and manner of articulation. As you will learn later in this chapter, phonemes can be further described according to their distinctive features, and can be in minimal or maximal opposition with respect to the number of shared features. If word pairs differ simply by the presence or absence of a phoneme, as in *scar* and *car*, they are considered **near minimal pairs**. Remember this information about minimal pairs—you will need it to understand goal setting (Chapter 10) and phonological intervention approaches (Chapter 13).

What about subtle variations in the articulation of speech sounds, such as [k], [k⁼], and [kʰ]? Although they are the same phoneme in English, /k/, they are articulated in slightly different ways. Think for a moment about the differences in the production of /k/ in the words *key*, *ski*, and *back*. In *key*, the /k/ is aspirated [kʰ] (i.e., if you put the palm of your hand near your mouth, you will feel a little puff of air on your palm as you say /ki/), whereas the /k/ in *ski* is unaspirated [k⁼] (i.e., you will not feel any puff of air against the palm of your hand), while the /k/ in *back* can be unreleased [bæk ˺] at the end of a word

COMMENT: *What do phonemes have to do with SSD?*

Some children with SSD can be very difficult to understand. A common reason for this is that many of their words are **homonyms**—they sound the same. For instance, a child who does not use /k, s, ʃ, ɹ/ might pronounce the following words, *key* /ki/, *see* /si/, *ski* /ski/, *she* /ʃi/, and *tree* /tɹi/, all as *tea* [ti]. If you listen carefully to their speech, you will notice that many of the phonemes belonging to the language they are learning are missing—they have a small **phonemic repertoire**. You will learn more about how to analyze children's phonological systems in Chapter 9.

(i.e., no puff of air and no release of sound). Each of these subtle phonetic realizations of a phoneme is called an **allophone**. This means that a phoneme is an abstract, theoretical concept. Phonemes are stored in your mind. You do not actually articulate phonemes; rather, you produce allophones of phonemes. Remember from Chapter 4 that phonemes are written within virgules or slashes / /, and allophones are written within square brackets [ ].

Before you get too confused, let's integrate and illustrate these three fundamental terms—**phones**, **phonemes**, and **allophones**. If the substitution of one phone for another does not alter the meaning of the word, the phones would be considered allophones of a phoneme. If the substitution of one phone for another does alter word meaning, the phones would be phonemes. For example, if a child said [kʰi] and [ki], we would assume that they are saying the same word in English using subtly different versions or

APPLICATION: *Phones, phonemes, and allophones*

Explain the difference between phones, phonemes, and allophones, using the English words *cook* and *took*, pronounced as [kʰʊkˈ] and [tʰʊkˈ] and [kʰʊkʰ].

APPLICATION: *Phones, phonemes, and minimal pairs in Luke's (4;3 years) speech sample*

Review the following speech sample collected during the initial speech-language pathology assessment with Luke.

sun /sʌn/ [dʌn]	*zip* /zɪp/ [dɪp]	*seat* /sit/ [dit]	*feet* /fit/ [bit]
fan /fæn/ [bæn]	*meat* /mit/ [mit]	*chip* /ʧɪp/ [dɪp]	*bike* /baɪk/ [baɪk]
light /laɪt/ [laɪt]	*like* /laɪk/ [laɪk]	*ship* /ʃɪp/ [dɪp]	*that* /ðæt/ [dæt]
fat /fæt/ [bæt]	*bite* /baɪt/ [baɪt]	*thin* /θɪn/ [dɪn]	*fun* /fʌn/ [bʌn]

1. List all the phones (speech sounds) that Luke uses in word-initial position and word-final position. (There are no phones in medial position, because the sample only shows monosyllables. As discussed in Chapter 8, you would collect a much larger sample than this to get a broader understanding of Luke's speech production skills.)
2. Identify all the minimal pairs in Luke's speech sample.

    Hint: Look for Luke's productions of words that only differ by one phoneme, such as *fat* and *that*, and *ban* and *bat*.

3. What consonant phonemes (speech sounds used to contrast meanings between words) are present in Luke's speech sample, in word-initial and word-final position?

Answers:

1. Phones: initial [b, d, m, l] and final [p, t, k, n]
2. Luke's minimal pairs include:

sun /sʌn/ [dʌn]	*that* /ðæt/ [dæt]	*seat* /sit/ [dit]	*fan* /fæn/ [bæn]	*bike* /baɪk/ [baɪk]
fun /fʌn/ [bʌn]	*fat* /fæt/ [bæt]	*meat* /mit/ [mit]	*fat* /fæt/ [bæt]	*bite* /baɪt/ [baɪt]
feet /fit/ [bit],	*light* /laɪt/ [laɪt],	*zip* /dɪp/ [dɪp]	*seat* /sit/ [dit],	*like* /laɪk/ [laɪk]
meat /mit/ [mit]	*like* /laɪk/ [laɪk]	*thin* /θɪn/ [dɪn]	*feet* /fit/ [bit]	*bike* /baɪk/ [baɪk]

3. Phonemes: initial / b, d, m, l/ and final /p, t, k, n/

Read more about
Luke (4;3 years),
a boy with a phonological
impairment,
in Chapter 16 (Case 1).

allophones of the phoneme /k/. However, if the child said /ki/ and /ti/ to mean two different words, we know then that /k/ and /t/ are phonemes. It is important to emphasize that phonemes and allophones are language specific, so what is a phoneme in one language may be an allophone in another and vice versa. The Cantonese, Korean, and Thai phonological systems are helpful examples here, because these languages use aspiration in a contrastive way. For example, in Thai, the words *shoulder* and *forest* and the word for the action *to split* something are [baa], [paa], and [pʰaa] respectively (Davenport & Hannahs, 2010). To an English listener, [paa] and [pʰaa] would sound like the same word, making [p] and [pʰ] allophones. However, for a Thai speaker, [paa] and [pʰaa] have different meanings, thus making /p/ and /pʰ/ phonemes, and not allophones.

■ Theoretical concepts: Features

So far in this book, we have talked about speech sounds according to three broad articulatory characteristics or features—voice, place, and manner of articulation. For example, [t] is a voiceless alveolar plosive. We can also use these three terms to group speech sounds according to shared features. For example, [p, t, k] are all voiceless plosives. Using a binary coding system, where [+] means that the feature is present, and [−] means absent, we can also contrast phones. For example, [t] is [+] alveolar and [−] all other places of articulation, while [m] is [+] bilabial and [−] all other places.

[t]	[m]
− bilabial	+ bilabial
− labiodental	− labiodental
− dental	− dental
+ alveolar	− alveolar
− postalveolar	− postalveolar
− palatal	− palatal
− velar	− velar

What about if we wanted to describe the similarities and differences between phones such as [s] and [j]? The broad voice-place-manner system is not very helpful. Although we could say that they have nothing in common (because one is voiceless and the other is voiced, one is fricative and the other an approximant, and one is alveolar and the other is palatal), we have no way of classifying their similarity (continuous oral airflow), nor do we have any way of understanding their relationship in the phonological system (Bernhardt & Stemberger, 2000). For a phonological classification system or taxonomy to work, it needs to describe all the phonemes in a phonological system. Phonologists have attempted to do this by developing feature systems that capture more detailed articulatory and acoustic characteristics of speech sounds.

Across classic and contemporary phonology texts you will find that most authors refer to the pioneering feature system of Chomsky and Halle (1968) from their classic work *The Sound Pattern of English* (SPE). Their work was based on ideas proposed by Russian linguists Nikolai Trubetzkoy (1939) and Roman Jakobson (1941). In the SPE system, features are **binary**—either present [+] or absent [−]. The features are referred to as **distinctive features**, because the presence or absence of a feature distinguishes one phoneme from another phoneme. The presence of a distinctive feature across a group of phonemes also creates a **natural class** or group of phonemes. The broad voice-place-manner categories you learned about in Chapter 4 are types of natural classes. In other words, phonemes are each a unique set or bundle of distinctive features (Grunwell, 1987), and natural classes of phonemes share a particular distinctive feature.

Since the work of Chomsky and Halle (1968), phonologists have modified the names and range of features used to describe and classify speech sounds as a result of studying the phonological systems of different languages, children's acquisition of those features, and how features relate to one another in a phonological system (e.g., feature geometry theory: Sagey, 1986; underspecification theory: Archangeli, 1988). You will learn more about the relationships among features later in this chapter. What follows is a description of features used to describe English consonants and vowels. It is based on contemporary feature descriptions by Ball, Müller, and Rutter (2010), Bernhardt and Stemberger (2000), Davenport and Hannahs (2010), and Gussenhoven and Jacobs (2011). Like most phonologists, their work bears witness to the pioneering work of Chomsky and Halle (1968). The features are divided into four categories: major class features, followed by laryngeal, manner, and place features.

Major class features

There are three major class features: [± consonantal], [± sonorant], and [± approximant] (Ball, Müller, & Rutter, 2010; Gussenhoven & Jacobs, 2011).

1. **Consonantal** [± cons]: Distinguishes true consonants [+ cons] (plosives, affricates, fricatives, nasals, the lateral, and [ɹ]) from vowels and glides [w, j]. True consonants block, redirect, or narrow the airflow through the vocal tract. Glides are [– cons] because they are more like vowels, with the airflow being relatively unimpeded. The glottal sounds [h, ʔ] are also [– cons] because the constriction occurs at the larynx rather than in the oral or pharyngeal cavity. The consonantal status of [ɹ] is disputed—some authors suggest that it is [+ cons] (e.g., Gussenhoven & Jacobs, 2011) and others suggest it is [-cons] (e.g., Bernhardt & Stemberger, 2000). In this book [ɹ] is described as [+ cons].

2. **Sonorant** [± son]: Distinguishes sounds that allow airflow to be relatively unimpeded through the oral or nasal cavity [+ son] from sounds that either block or constrict the airflow [– son]. Vowels, nasals, glides, and liquids are all **sonorants**. Sonorants are usually voiced. Liquids are both [+ son] and [+ cons] because they redirect (rather than impede) the airflow. Plosives, fricatives, and affricates impede the airflow through the vocal tract, and are known as **obstruents**. Obstruents can be voiced or voiceless. The classification of [h] as a sonorant is controversial. Some authors classify [h] as [+ son], as the supraglottal pressure for [h] is low (Bernhardt & Stemberger, 2000), whereas other authors classify [h] as [– son], because the stricture for [h] is in the larynx rather than in the vocal tract (Gussenhoven & Jacobs, 2011). In this book [h] is described as [– son].

3. **Approximant** [± approx]: Distinguishes sounds that have a constriction in the vocal tract while still allowing frictionless escape of air (Gussenhoven & Jacobs, 2011). Vowels and non-nasal sonorants are considered [+ approx], and include [w, j, ɹ, l].

In summary, the three major class features create four classes of segments in English:

vowels (all) and glides [w, j]	– consonantal	+ sonorant	+ approximant
liquids [l, ɹ]	+ consonantal	+ sonorant	+ approximant
nasal [m, n, ŋ]	+ consonantal	+ sonorant	– approximant
obstruents [p, b, t, d, k, g, ʔ, f, v, θ, ð, s, z, ʃ, ʒ, h, ʧ, ʤ]	+ consonantal	– sonorant	– approximant

Note: [h] is not included in the table, because it is [– cons], [– son], and [– approx] because the stricture for [h] is in the larynx rather than in the vocal tract (Gussenhoven & Jacobs, 2011). In addition, some authors use the feature [± syllabic] rather than [± approximant] to separate vowels from all other consonants; however, because the term *syllabic* is used in a different way in nonlinear phonological theories, the term *approximant* is used to describe major class features (Ball, Müller, & Rutter, 2010).

Laryngeal features

There are three laryngeal features: [± voice], [± spread glottis], and [± constricted glottis].

1. **Voice [± voice]:** Distinguishes speech sounds involving vibration of the vocal folds (vowels and voiced consonants), from those produced with the vocal folds at rest. This means that all voiceless consonants are [– voice].

2. **Spread glottis [± s.g.]:** Distinguishes sounds in which the vocal folds are spread wide and accompanied by frication or turbulent airflow at the glottis (including [h] and the aspirated plosives [pʰ, tʰ, kʰ]) from sounds that do not.

   3. **Constricted glottis [± c.g.]:** Distinguishes sounds in which the vocal folds are pulled tight and drawn together (such as the glottal plosive [ʔ]) from those that do not. This feature is also used to describe a range of non-pulmonic sounds present in other languages, and occasionally, disordered speech. Bernhardt and Stemberger (2000) noted that the three plosives in English, [p, t, k], can be either [+] or [–] constricted glottis, depending on the phonetic context of the word in which they are produced.

Manner features

There are four manner features: [± continuant], [± nasal], [± lateral], and [± strident].

   1. **Continuant [± cont]:** Distinguishes speech sounds in which air moves uninterrupted or freely through the oral cavity, including vowels, glides, liquids, and fricatives, from those that block the airflow (plosives, affricates, and nasals). Nasals are [– cont] due to the block in the oral cavity and because of the way that they pattern similar to plosives [– cont]), even though they are characterized by continuous nasal airflow (Bernhardt & Stemberger, 2000).
   2. **Nasal [± nasal]:** Distinguishes speech sounds produced with the velum lowered, allowing nasal cavity airflow, from oral-only sounds. Note that air can also still flow out the mouth if [+ nasal] is specified. In English, [+ nasal] includes [m, n, ŋ]. In some languages, such as French, the feature is used to distinguish between vowels, as [+] or [–] nasal.
   3. **Lateral [± lat]:** Distinguishes speech sounds in which one or both sides of the tongue are lowered (while the tongue tip is in contact with the alveolar ridge), allowing air to flow over the sides of the tongue, from those that do not. The only lateral consonant in English is [l]. There are lateral consonants in other languages, such as the palatal lateral approximant [ʎ] in Italian and the voiceless lateral fricative [ɬ] in Welsh (Ball, 2012),
   4. **Strident [± strid]:** Distinguishes speech sounds that force air quickly through a small constriction creating a noisy or hissing airflow, including [f, v, s, z, ʃ, ʒ, tʃ, dʒ], from sounds that do not, including nasals, plosives, glides, liquids, and the dentals [θ, ð].

Place features

The major class features, manner features, and laryngeal features are binary. That is, consonants or vowels could have the feature present [+] or absent [–]. However, more recent descriptions of place features have introduced the concept of a **univalent feature**. A univalent feature simply serves as a superordinate term or umbrella feature (e.g., LABIAL) for a group of binary features (e.g., ± round) associated with the univalent feature (Gussenhoven & Jacobs, 2011). Univalent features are written in small capital letters to distinguish them from binary features. The idea of a univalent feature was introduced with the theory of feature geometry (described later in the chapter) to more concisely describe features of speech sounds and to account for how the features relate to one another in a phonological system. The univalent place features include LABIAL, CORONAL, and DORSAL (Bernhardt & Stemberger, 2000). Gussenhoven and Jacobs (2011) also include the feature RADICAL (or PHARYNGEAL). This feature refers to speech sounds produced with the root of the tongue, such as the voiceless pharyngeal fricative /ħ/ in varieties of Arabic (Gussenhoven & Jacobs, 2011). In this section we focus on features associated with English, based on the work of Bernhardt and Stemberger (2000) and Gussenhoven and Jacobs (2011). What follows is a description of the univalent features, LABIAL, CORONAL, and DORSAL, and their respective subordinate binary features.

   1. **LABIAL:** Speech sounds produced with one or both lips. This includes bilabials [p, b] and labiodentals [f, v], the approximants [w, ɹ] in English, and rounded vowels. LABIAL can be further specified as [+ round]. If a sound is not labial, then the feature [+ round] is irrelevant. Note that some authors do not consider [ɹ] to be [+ round].
      (a) **Round** [+ round]. The [+ round] feature includes [w, ɹ] and the rounded vowels [u, ʊ, ɒ, ɔ] in English. This means that the labial sounds [p, b, f, v] are all [– round]. Note that Bernhardt and Stemberger (2000) also include the feature [+ labiodental] as a sub-feature of LABIAL, which refers to a lip sound made with only one lip, including [f, v].

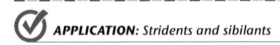

✓ APPLICATION: Stridents and sibilants

Strident and sibilant are similar but not synonymous terms. Strident is a distinctive feature in Chomsky and Halle's (1968) system that reflects an **acoustic** feature of speech sounds with noisy airflow. Stridents include [f, v, s, z, ʃ, ʒ, ʧ, ʤ]. By contrast, sibilant is a feature of Ladefoged's (1971) distinctive feature system, and refers to coronal (tongue tip or blade) fricatives. Sibilants include [s, z, ʃ, ʒ, ʧ, ʤ]. The key difference is that [f] and [v] are strident but not sibilant. The fricatives [θ] and [ð] are neither strident nor sibilant. Clinically, it is common to see 3- and 4-year-old children with phonological impairment who have difficulty contrasting fricatives from plosives. Occasionally, you will see children, like Mark (4;7 years), who use some but not all fricatives. In such cases, it can be helpful to use distinctive features to understand the nature of the child's difficulty. Review Mark's speech sample below. List the fricatives that he can produce in one column, and the fricatives he struggles to use contrastively in another column. Knowing that dental fricatives are neither sibilant nor strident, note down Mark's realization for dentals in a separate column and decide whether Mark has a difficulty with [+ sibilant] and/or [+ strident].

Word-initial fricatives and affricates in English	/h/	/f/	/v/	/s/	/z/	/ʃ/	/ʧ/	/ʤ/	/θ/	/ð/
Mark's production	heat /hit/ [hit]	feet /fit/ [fit]	vet /vɛt/ [vɛt]	see /si/ [ti]	zoo /zu/ [du]	shoe /ʃu/ [tu]	chew /ʧu/ [tu]	jeep /ʤip/ [dip]	thumb /θʌm/ [fʌm]	that /ðæt/ [væt]

Which distinctive feature best describes Mark's particular difficulty with fricatives and affricates?

Answer: As shown below, Mark has difficulty with sibilants, given that he can produce stridency in /f, v/.

Fricatives Mark produces and uses contrastively	Fricatives Mark does not produce	Mark's realization of dental fricatives
/h, f, v/	/s, z, ʃ, ʧ, ʤ/	/θ/→ [f]; /ð/ → [v]

2. **CORONAL:** Speech sounds produced with the tongue tip or blade, including alveolars, interdentals, postalveolars (also known as palatoalveolars), palatals, retroflexes, and front vowels (Bernhardt & Stemberger, 2000). CORONAL sounds are further specified using the binary features of anterior, distributed, and grooved.

   (a) **Anterior** [± ant]: Distinguishes coronal sounds produced in front of the postalveolar region in the oral cavity from those produced further back in the oral cavity. This means that alveolar and dental sounds are [+ ant]. The remaining coronal sounds (postalveolars, retroflex, palatal, and front vowels) are marked [– ant] for this feature. If a sound is not coronal, then the [± ant] feature is irrelevant, because it only relates to coronal sounds.

   (b) **Distributed** [± distr]: Distinguishes coronal sounds produced with a wide area of contact between the tip or blade of the tongue and the roof of the mouth or the teeth (laminal consonants) from those produced with a more narrow or specific point of contact (apical consonants) (Bernhardt & Stemberger, 2000; Gussenhoven & Jacobs, 2011). Interdentals, postalveolars, and palatals are [+ distr], and alveolars and retroflexes are [– distr].

   (c) **Grooved** [± grooved]: Distinguishes sounds produced with a narrow midline groove in the tongue [s, z, ʃ, ʒ, ʧ, ʤ] from those produced with a flatter tongue [θ, ð, j] or block in the airflow [t, d].

3. DORSAL: Sounds produced with bunching of the back of the tongue. This includes palatals, velars, vowels, glides, and the velarized dark [ɫ] in English. Uvular and pharyngeal sounds present in other languages are also DORSAL. Sounds can be further specified in terms tongue body features—where in the mouth the tongue bunching occurs (Gussenhoven & Jacobs, 2011). The subordinate features of DORSAL include:

   (a) **Tongue-body feature—High [± high]:** Distinguishes sounds in which the tongue body is raised above the neutral position (as in [ə]), including the vowels [i, ɪ, u, ʊ, ɛ] and consonants /k, g, ŋ, w, j/, from other DORSAL sounds.

   (b) **Tongue-body feature—Low [± low]:** Distinguishes sounds in which the bunched tongue body is lower than the neutral position, including the vowels [æ, ɔ, ɒ, ɑ, a]. Gussenhoven and Jacobs (2011) also specify [h, ʔ] as [+ low].

   (c) **Tongue-body feature—Back [± back]:** Distinguishes speech sounds in which the tongue is retracted back, including vowels [u, ʊ, ɑ, ɒ, ɔ, ʌ, ə, a] and [k, g, ŋ], from all other DORSAL sounds.

   (d) **Tense [± tense]:** Distinguishes longs vowels such as [i, e, a, o, u, ɔ] (considered [+ tense]) from short vowels such as [ɪ, ɛ, ɒ, ʌ, ə, ʊ] (considered [– tense]). The term Advanced Tongue Root ([+ ATR]) has been used interchangeably with the feature [+ tense], because both features capture the rising of the tongue body (Davenport & Hannahs, 2010). Vowels that are [– tense] have also been described as lax vowels.

Using the features, we now have a way of describing the similarity in continuous airflow between [s] and [j]. As shown in Table 5-1, they are both CORONAL and [+ continuant]. Table 5-2 provides a matrix of the features of all the English consonants.

TABLE 5-1   A matrix of the features of English consonants comparing [s] and [j]

	[s]	[j]
Major class features	+ [cons]	– [cons]
	– [son]	+ [son]
	– [approx]	+ [approx]
Laryngeal features	– [voice]	+ [voice]
	– [s.g.]	– [s.g.]
	– [c.g.]	– [c.g.]
Manner features	+ [cont]	+ [cont]
	– [nasal]	– [nasal]
	– [lat]	– [lat]
	+ [strid]	– [strid]
Place features	CORONAL	CORONAL
	+ [ant]	– [ant]
	– [distr]	+ [distr]
	+ [grooved]	– [grooved]
		DORSAL
		+ [high]
		– [low]
		– [back]

TABLE 5-2 Features for English consonants

	p	b	t	d	k	g	ʔ	tʃ	dʒ	f	v	θ	ð	s	z	ʃ	ʒ	h	m	n	ŋ	ɹ	l	w	j
MAJOR CLASS FEATURES																									
Consonantal [±cons]	+	+	+	+	+	+	+	+	+	+	+	+	+	+	+	+	+	−	+	+	+	+	+	−	−
Sonorant [±son]	−	−	−	−	−	−	−	−	−	−	−	−	−	−	−	−	−	−	+	+	+	+	+	+	+
Approximant [±approx]	−	−	−	−	−	−	−	−	−	−	−	−	−	−	−	−	−	−	−	−	−	+	+	+	+
LARYNGEAL FEATURES																									
Voice [±voice]	−	+	−	+	−	+	−	−	+	−	+	−	+	−	+	−	+	−	+	+	+	+	+	+	+
Spread glottis [±s.g.]	+/−	−	+/−	−	+/−	−	−	−	−	−	−	−	−	−	−	−	−	+	−	−	−	−	−	−	−
Constricted glottis [±c.g.]	+/−	−	+/−	−	+/−	−	+	−	−	−	−	−	−	−	−	−	−	−	−	−	−	−	−	−	−
MANNER FEATURES																									
Continuant [±cont]	−	−	−	−	−	−	−	−/+	−/+	+	+	+	+	+	+	+	+	+	−	−	−	+	+	+	+
Nasal [±nasal]	−	−	−	−	−	−	−	−	−	−	−	−	−	−	−	−	−	−	+	+	+	−	−	−	−
Lateral [±lat]	−	−	−	−	−	−	−	−	−	−	−	−	−	−	−	−	−	−	−	−	−	−	+	−	−
Strident [±strid]	−	−	−	−	−	−	−	+	+	+	+	−	−	+	+	+	+	−	−	−	−	−	−	−	−
PLACE FEATURES																									
LABIAL	✓	✓								✓	✓								✓					✓	
Round [±round]	−	−								−	−								−					+	−
Labiodentals [±labiodental]	−	−								+	+														
CORONAL			✓	✓				✓	✓			✓	✓	✓	✓	✓	✓			✓		✓	✓		✓
Anterior [±ant]			+	+				−	−			+	+	+	+	−	−			+		+	+		−
Distributed [±distr]			−	−				+	+			+	+	−	−	+	+			−		−	−		+
Grooved [±groove]			−	−				+	+			−	−	+	+	+	+			−		−	−		
DORSAL					✓	✓															✓			✓	✓
High [±high]					+	+															+			+	+
Low [±low]					−	−															−			−	−
Back [±back]					+	+															+			+	−
	Plosives							Affricates		Fricatives									Nasals			Liquids		Glides	
	Obstruents																		Sonorants						

Sources: Adapted from Bernhardt and Stemberger (2000); Davenport and Hannahs (2010); Gussenhoven and Jacobs (2011).

Note. ✓ = univalent feature applies to consonant. +/− means that the feature may be present in specific contexts (e.g., [+ spread glottis] on word-initial [pʰ] as in the word *pea /piː/*). The affricates are considered both −/+ (i.e., [− continuant] [+ continuant]) (Bernhardt & Stemberger, 2000). The classification of some consonants is controversial. For instance, Bernhardt and Stemberger (2000) specify [h, ʔ] as [+ son], and the place features for [j] including both CORONAL and DORSAL, whereas Gussenhoven and Jacobs (2011) specify [h] as [− son] and the place features for [j] as CORONAL only.

MULTILINGUAL INSIGHTS: *Non-pulmonic distinctive features across the world's languages*

Distinctive features are usually discussed across phonetics and phonology texts with the English language in mind. This limits to the focus to pulmonic consonants. Non-pulmonic features evident in other languages (and sometimes in disordered speech or speakers learning English) are usually not included. Two non-pulmonic features proposed by Chomsky and Halle (1968) relevant to other languages include:

■ Suction: Present in clicks such as the postalveolar click [!] in Xhosa and implosives such as the bilabial implosive [ɓ] in Sindhi) (Ladefoged, 2001a)

■ Pressure: Present in ejectives such as the velar ejective [k'] in Xhosa (Ball, 2012)

Clinically, you will come across children with SSD who use non-English speech sounds in addition to children with SSD who are learning languages other than or in addition to English (Ball, Müller, Klopfenstein, & Rutter, 2010). In such cases it is helpful to be familiar with the range of possible articulations and to be able to identify the distinctive features that characterize those phones, so that you can complete a more comprehensive phonological analysis.

APPLICATION: *Distinctive features in Luke's (4;3 years) speech sample*

Earlier in this chapter you thought about Luke's speech in terms of phones, phonemes, and minimal pairs. Reconsider the same speech sample thinking about the types of distinctive features that are present and absent in his production of consonants. Compare the distinctive features in word-initial and word-final position.

sun /sʌn/ [dʌn]	*zip* /zɪp/ [dɪp]	*seat* /sit/ [dit]	*feet* /fit/ [bit]
fan /fæn/ [bæn]	*meat* /mit/ [mit]	*chip* /tʃɪp/ [dɪp]	*bike* /baɪk/ [baɪk]
light /laɪt/ [laɪt]	*like* /laɪk/ [laɪk]	*ship* /ʃɪp/ [dɪp]	*that* /ðæt/ [dæt]
fat /fæt/ [bæt]	*bite* /baɪt/ [baɪt]	*thin* /θɪn/ [dɪn]	*fun* /fʌn/ [bʌn]

1. Using the distinctive feature matrix in Table 5-2, list major class, laryngeal, manner, and place features (specifying binary features as ±) in word-initial and word-final position consonants.
2. Given Luke's productions for the words *sun*, *feet*, and *ship*, what manner feature does Luke not use in word-initial position?
3. Consider Luke's use of [± sonorant] and [± voice] in word-final position. What do you notice?

Answers:

1. Major class features: *Initial* [+ cons], [± son], [± approx]: *Final* [+ cons], [± son], [− approx]
   Laryngeal features: *Initial* [+ voice]: *Final* [± voice]
   Manner features: *Initial* [± cont], [± nasal], [± lat] [− strid]: *Final* [− cont] [± nasal] [− lat] [− strid]
   Place features: *Initial* [LABIAL] [− round], [− labiodental], CORONAL [+ ant] [− distr] [− groove]: *Final* [LABIAL] [− round], [− labiodental], CORONAL [+ ant] [− distr] [− groove], DORSAL [+ high] [+ back] [− low].
2. [+ strident]
3. Sonorants are voiced (i.e., [+ son], [+ voice]) and obstruents always voiceless (i.e., [− son] [− voice]).

Read more about Luke (4;3 years), a boy with a phonological impairment, in Chapter 16 (Case 1).

■ Theoretical concepts: Naturalness, markedness, and implicational relationships

Listen to typically developing English-speaking 18-month-old toddlers and you will notice that they do not pronounce all speech sounds accurately. Although they might attempt words such as *run* and *look*, they will not pronounce all the speech sounds in the words accurately. What you will notice, however, is that the toddlers have similar errors, so that *run* is [wʌn] and *look* is [wʊk]. If you look at Appendix 4-2 in Chapter 4 and consider the consonants in five different languages, you will notice that most of the languages you choose have a range of sounds in common. (There may also be some sounds unique to one or more of the languages.) If you compare the sounds common to languages with the sounds accurately produced by the toddlers, you will find some similarities. Early developing sounds are common across the world's languages (Locke, 1983). Furthermore, if you were to compare the distinctive features of those sounds, you would find that groups of the sounds share a particular distinctive feature (e.g., [+ nasal]). When Trubetzkoy (1939) introduced the idea of distinctive features, he in fact proposed that some features were more natural while others were marked. **Natural features** are considered easier to articulate, more common within and/or across languages, and are likely to be acquired earlier by children (Johnson & Reimers, 2010). **Marked features** are quite the opposite. Marked features are thought to be phonetically more complex, less common across languages, and later developing. The concept of naturalness and markedness applies not only to features and segments but other aspects of phonology such as syllable shapes, stress patterns, and phonological rules or processes. For example:

- CV is considered to be the most natural syllable shape;
- obstruents are considered more natural than sonorants (this is because all languages have several obstruents, but many only have one liquid or nasal);
- of the obstruents, plosives are considered more natural than fricatives;
- voiceless obstruents are also considered more natural than voiced obstruents; and
- voiced sonorants are considered more natural than voiceless sonorants (Edwards & Shriberg, 1983).

Trubetzkoy's (1939) idea of naturalness and markedness was applied in the study of linguistic universals and implicational relationships (Jakobson, 1941). Linguistic universals reflect what is common across the world's languages. A **linguistic universal** may be **absolute** in nature if the phonological property is shared by all languages, or a **tendency** if it used by most but not all languages (O'Grady, Archibald, Aronoff, & Rees-Miller, 2005). The vowel [a] is considered an absolute universal, because it is used by all languages (Hyman, 1975). Plosives are another example of an absolute universal, because all languages have plosives. The fact that most but not all languages have at least one nasal makes it a linguistic universal tendency.

Jakobson (1941) studied linguistic universals across languages, trends in children's phonological acquisition, and common errors in adults with aphasia. Based on his observations, he described the interesting phenomenon of **implicational relationships**—the existence of a marked trait in a language implying the existence of the unmarked counterpart. Implicational relationships are unidirectional. If a language has a marked phonological property X it will have Y, but it will not have X if it does not have Y (Gierut, 2007). An analogy can be helpful at this point. A cake can have icing, but you cannot have icing without a cake. If you eat icing, it would assume that you also ate cake, but if you ate cake, you could not assume that you ate icing. For example, plosives and fricatives are related by implication because the existence of fricatives in a language implies the existence of plosives. Consider the list of implicational relationships in Table 5-3. They have been identified from studies of the world's languages, children's phonological acquisition, and children's responses to phonological intervention.

■ Theoretical concepts: Phonotactics

Phonotactics refers to the language-specific constraints about how speech sounds combine to form words in a phonological system. There are three types of constraints: inventory,

TABLE 5-3	Common implicational relationships observed in acquisition and intervention

- Consonants imply vowels (e.g., Robb, Bleile, & Yee, 1999)
- Fricatives imply plosives (e.g., Elbert, Dinnsen, & Powell, 1984)
- Voiced obstruents imply voiceless obstruents (e.g., McReynolds & Jetzke, 1986)
- Liquids imply nasals (e.g., Gierut, Simmerman, & Neumann, 1994)
- Velars imply coronals (e.g., Stoel-Gammon, 1996)
- Affricates imply fricatives (e.g., Schmidt & Meyers, 1995)
- Clusters imply singletons (e.g., Gierut & O'Connor, 2002)
- True clusters with small sonority differences imply true clusters with large sonority differences (e.g., Gierut, 1999)

Sources: Adapted from Gierut (2001, 2007); Gierut and Hulse (2010).

positional, and sequential constraints (Elbert & Gierut, 1986). **Inventory constraints** limit which phonemes are permitted in a language. For instance, the postalveolar click [ǃ] is permitted in Xhosa but not English. **Positional constraints** (also referred to as distributional constraints) limit where phonemes are permitted in words. For instance, in English the phonemes /ŋ/ and /ʒ/ are not permitted in syllable-initial position, whereas /h/ is not permitted in syllable-final position. Finally, **sequential constraints** (also known as combinational constraints) limit how phonemes combine to form syllables and words with respect to both the number of phonemes permitted in a syllable and how they combine to form the syllable. You learned about some of these restrictions in Chapter 4. For instance, a syllable can begin with up to three consonants, as long as the first consonant is /s/, the second is either /p, t, k/ and the third consonant is either /l, w, ɹ, j/ as in *strong* /stɹɪ/, *splash* /spl/, and *square* /skw/.

■ Theoretical concepts: Sonority

Sonority refers to the amount of sound present in a speech segment (Roca & Johnson, 1999). As a concept, sonority dates back to the mid-19th century (e.g., Whitney, 1865). Clinically it has only been examined since the late 20th century (e.g., Bernhardt, 1994; Gierut, 1999; Wyllie-Smith, McLeod, & Ball, 2006). So how is the amount of sound in a speech sound helpful when working with children with SSD? Firstly, speech sounds can be ordered by way of a numerical **sonority hierarchy**, with more sonorous sounds being lower in the hierarchy (e.g., vowels) and the less sonorous sounds higher in the hierarchy (e.g., voiceless plosives). An example of one such hierarchy by Steriade (1990) is shown in Figure 5-1.

■■■

 APPLICATION: *Phonotactic constraints in Luke's (4;3 years) speech*

Review Luke's speech sample in Table 16-4. This table shows Luke's attempt at producing words with word-initial and word-final consonant clusters. Describe Luke's sequence constraint in word-initial and word-final positions, with respect to consonant clusters.

Answer: Luke does not allow more than one consonant in syllable-initial position (i.e., no initial consonant clusters). However, Luke does allow two consonants in syllable-final word-final position, but only if they are a nasal followed by a homorganic (same place) voiceless plosive (e.g., [mp, nt, ŋk]).

Read more about
Luke (4;3 years),
a boy with a phonological
impairment,
in Chapter 16 (Case 1).

FIGURE 5-1 The sonority hierarchy

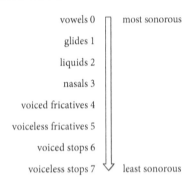

vowels 0 — most sonorous
glides 1
liquids 2
nasals 3
voiced fricatives 4
voiceless fricatives 5
voiced stops 6
voiceless stops 7 — least sonorous

Source: Adapted from Steriade (1990).

FIGURE 5-2 Sequence of speech sounds abiding by (*clump* /klʌmp/)
and violating ([lkʌpm]) the sonority sequencing principle

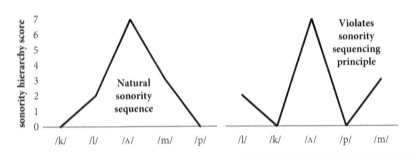

When we talk, we actually prefer to sequence the sounds in a syllable so that there is a natural rise and fall in sonority (Davenport & Hannahs, 2010). Consider the word *clump* /klʌmp/, in Figure 5-2. The word begins with a least sonorous segment, rises at the peak to the vowel, and falls to a least sonorous segment. Now try saying the word *clump* with the clusters in reverse /lkʌpm/—it will seem unnatural and difficult to pronounce.

This tendency to rise and fall is known as the **sonority sequencing principle** (SSP). There is also a tendency to start syllables with a large rise and end with a small fall, or as Gussenhoven and Jacobs (2011, p. 165) say, "start with a bang and end with a whimper." Gierut (1999) applied the concept of sonority and the SSP in an intervention study with six children who had a phonological impairment. She wanted to find out which types of clusters were more marked (e.g., /tɹ/ or /fl/). Using Steriade's (1990) sonority hierarchy, she classified clusters according to their **sonority difference** score. You calculate this difference by subtracting the sonority hierarchy score for the second sound from the first sound. For example, given that /t/ has a score of 7 and /w/ has a score of 1, /tw/ has a sonority difference score of 7 – 1 = 6. Similarly, /fl/ has a score of 3 because /f/ 5 – /l/ 2 = 3. Gierut (1999) suggested that consonant clusters with smaller sonority difference scores (e.g., /fl/) were more marked.

Gierut (1999) reported that intervention prioritizing more marked clusters (i.e., consonant clusters with smaller sonority difference scores) was associated with more widespread change in the children's phonological systems. Her results also confirmed suggestions that the onset clusters /sp, st, sk/ are adjuncts rather than true clusters, because they do not abide by the natural rise and fall in sonority, and may (for some children) need to be avoided as an initial intervention target when trying to help children learn principles about (rather than violations of) the phonological system. Other authors (e.g.,

■ ■■ ■■ ■■■ ■■ ■ ■■■ ■■■ ■■ ■ ■■■ ■ ■ ■■ ■ ■■ ■ ■■ ■ ■■ ■ ■ ■ ■

 APPLICATION: *Sonority difference scores and consonant clusters*

Using Steriade's (1990) numerical sonority hierarchy, calculate the sonority difference score for the following initial consonant clusters /kw, pl, kɹ, bɹ, gl, fl, sn, sp, st, sk/. What do you notice about /sp, st, sk/?

Answer: The sonority difference scores include

/kw/ 6   /pl/ 5   /kɹ/ 5   /bɹ/ 4   /gl/ 4   /fl/ 3   /sn/ 2   /sp/ -2   /st/ -2   /sk/ -2

/sp, st, sk/ all have a sonority difference score of -2. They are adjuncts rather than true consonant clusters.

Wyllie-Smith et al., 2006) have questioned the value of sonority for understanding the full range of consonant cluster difficulties in children's speech. You will learn more about the potential role of sonority in the complexity approach to selecting intervention targets for children who have SSD in Chapters 10 (on goals) and 13 (on intervention).

PHONOLOGICAL THEORIES

There are many different theories about how phonological systems are organized and operate. In this section you will read about classic and contemporary theories that offer different perspectives and insights into the nature of SSD in children. You will learn how these theories offer direction for assessing and analyzing children's speech, prioritizing phonological intervention goals, and evaluating intervention. To help you appreciate the historical context of the theories, refer to the timeline in Figure 5-3. The timeline shows you when key phonological concepts and theories emerged, in addition to the prominent authors and works associated with a concept or theory.

CLASSIC THEORIES OF PHONOLOGY

Why do toddlers produce words like *look* as [wʊk] and *key* as [ti]? Why is it that children of similar ages, who are learning the same language, show similar errors in their speech? In this section, we provide an overview of two classic derivational phonological theories: generative phonology and natural phonology. We review these theories because they offer interesting suggestions for why children make systematic errors like saying *look* as [wʊk], and because they continue to influence assessment and intervention practice in the field of childhood SSD. Later in this chapter, we address contemporary theories and ideas, including constraint-based nonlinear phonology, optimality theory, and representation-based accounts about how we encode and store speech. These theories offer alternate suggestions for why toddlers says *look* as [wʊk].

■ Generative phonology, underlying and surface representations, and rules

Generative phonology draws on a number of different phonological concepts, including phonemes, allophones, features, naturalness, markedness, and implicational relationships. Chomsky and Halle (1968) addressed the realization of phonemes as allophones in their theory of **generative phonology**. They proposed that we have two **levels of representations** of words. The most abstract is the **underlying phonological representation** where phonemes are stored. According to their theory, phonemes are

FIGURE 5-3 Timeline showing publication of key phonological concepts and theories, and clinical applications of those theories

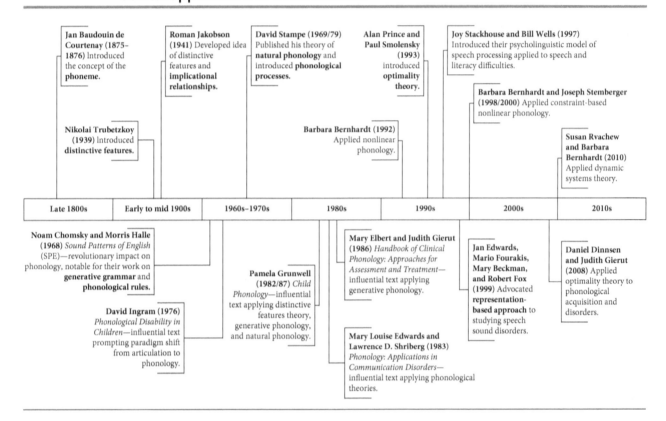

translated into allophones (i.e., phonetic realizations of phonemes) according to the rules or grammar of the phonology to create a **surface phonetic representation**. The rules help to describe the conditions under which phonemes are to be articulated in particular contexts. For example, in English, the words *key* /ki/, *ski* /ski/, and *book* /bʊk/ share the same phoneme /k/, yet the phonetic production of the /k/ in each word differs according to the linguistic rule for the context, with word-initial /k/ being aspirated [kʰ], the /k/ in clusters being unaspirated [k˭], and the /k/ in book being unreleased [k˺]. When allophones of a phoneme do not occur in the same environment in a word (e.g., [kʰ] occurs in syllable-initial word-initial position whereas [k˭] occurs in clusters after [s]), they are said to be in **complementary distribution** (Grunwell, 1987). However, when two allophones can occur in the same environment to produce subtly different pronunciations of the same word (e.g., [bʊk˺] and [bʊkʰ] they are said to be in **free variation**.

In generative phonology, rules are used to describe the conditions under which certain types of allophonic variations occur. It is important to emphasize that the rules describe rather than prescribe the changes between the underlying and surface forms of a phonological representation (Ball, Müller, & Rutter, 2010). Using the following notation, rules describe how a phoneme (i.e., / /) becomes (i.e., →) an allophone (i.e., [ ]) of that phoneme in the context of (i.e., /) a particular phonetic environment (i.e., _____):

$$/ / \rightarrow [ ] / \underline{\hspace{2cm}}$$

For example

(i) /p/ → [pʰ] / #___V
(ii) /p/ → [p˺] / V___#

The rule in (i) means that the phoneme /p/ becomes the allophone [pʰ] in the context of (noted by the slash /) a particular phonetic environment, such as word-initial

APPLICATION: *Complementary distribution of allophones*

David (4;5 years) has a severe phonological impairment of suspected genetic origin. Review the words below and list the speech sounds in his phonetic inventory in word-initial and word-final position. What do you observe about his production of /b, p/ and /t, d/?

seat /sit/ → [dit]	*patch* /pætʃ/ → [bæt]
ship /ʃɪp/ → [dɪp]	*stick* /stɪk/ → [dɪt]
cat /kæt/ → [dæt]	*cash* /kɹæʃ/ → [dæt]
toad /toʊd/ → [doʊt]	*cab* /kæb/ → [dæp]
dip /dɪp/ → [dɪp]	*trash* /tɹæʃ/ → [dæt]
beep /bip/ → [bip]	*pop* /pɑp/ → [bɑp]
bag /bæg/ → [bæt]	*bus* /bʌs/ → [bʌt]
chip /ʃɪp/ → [dɪp]	*sad* /sæd/ → [dæt]

Answer: In this example, David uses voiced sounds [b, d] in word-initial position and voiceless sounds [p, t] in word-final position. For David, [p] and [b] could be described as allophones in complementary distribution. A similar observation could be made about [t] and [d].

---

position and followed by a vowel (V). In the example above, the hash symbol # is used to signal a word boundary. The rule in (ii) means that the phoneme /p/ becomes the allophone [p˺] whenever it occurs in a word-final position and is preceded by a vowel (e.g., *up*). These rules apply to adult spoken English.

What about children's non-adult productions of words, like saying *look* as [wʊk]? According to Grunwell (1987), generative phonology provided a useful theoretical framework for describing and summarizing the systematic changes that take place between children's underlying phonological representations (that may or may not be adultlike) and their surface phonetic representations. The changes may involve distinctive features (e.g., [+ continuant] → [– continuant]) or the deletion, addition, or rearrangement of the order of sounds in words (Ball, Müller, & Rutter, 2010). For example, using distinctive features, we could express Luke's realization of /f/ as [b], in the word *feet*, as:

Read more about
Luke (4;3 years),
a boy with a phonological
impairment,
in Chapter 16 (Case 1).

$$
\begin{matrix}
[f] \\
+ \text{continuant} \\
+ \text{strident} \\
- \text{voice}
\end{matrix}
\rightarrow
\begin{matrix}
[b] \\
- \text{continuant} \\
- \text{strident} \\
+ \text{voice}
\end{matrix}
\Big/
[\# \_\_VC\,]
$$

Since the 1980s, generative phonology has been applied to the assessment, analysis, target selection, and treatment of children with phonological impairment (e.g., Gierut, 1989, 1990, 1991, 1992). One of the enduring ideas from applications of generative phonology to children with phonological impairment has been the concept of assessing the extent of children's **productive phonological knowledge**. Productive phonological knowledge refers to a speaker's competence and performance (i.e., tacit and explicit knowledge) of the sound system of the ambient language (Gierut, Elbert, & Dinnsen, 1987). Drawing on work by Gierut et al. (1987), although the individual speech sounds [s], [i], and [t] have no meaning, together they make the word *seat* /sit/. This sequence of sounds could actually be used to mean anything. There is nothing predictable about how [sit] has been associated with a piece of furniture, in the same way that there is nothing predictable about how you would decide on a meaning for the nonword [dut]. If we were to tell you that [dut] is a type of fruit, you would however be able to predict that as a noun, the plural of [dut] involves adding [s], [z] or [əz] depending on the final sound in the word; one [dut], two [duts]. Knowledge of the lexical representation of morphemes in addition to the

CHILDREN'S INSIGHTS: *I can't say* key *because my teeth are too little*

James (4;4 years) had a moderate-severe phonological impairment. He also had a very creative theory about speech and language acquisition and why children pronounce words differently from adults. During a phonological intervention session with James, he explained to Elise why he could not say velar sounds in words just yet. According to James, we store the words we know in our teeth. When we are born, we do not talk because we do not have teeth. When we are little, we have little teeth and so do not know many grown-up words. When we grow up, we have big strong teeth and so have room to store many big words and all the sounds for all the words. When we get old and lose our teeth, we lose the words we once knew. James reasoned that he was having difficulty saying some words, including words with velars, simply because his teeth were too little.

application of phonological rules reflects a child's **phonological competence** or tacit knowledge. The phonetic and phonemic inventories in conjunction with distributional properties about speech sounds reflect a child's **phonological performance** or explicit knowledge. A variety of informal assessment tools exist to examine a child's productive phonological knowledge, such as Gierut's (1985) Phonological Knowledge Protocol (PKP) (available in the appendix of Gierut et al., 1987) and Williams' (2003) Systemic Phonological Protocol (SPP).

Generative phonological descriptions of children's speech have been used to describe and sort children's knowledge of the ambient phonological system into one of six types, ranging from **most knowledge** (#1 = adultlike production in all contexts) through to **least knowledge** (#6 = inventory constraint). Intervention research has suggested that least knowledge targets (i.e., speech sounds typically not in a child's phonetic inventory and more marked in the ambient phonology) may facilitate more widespread change or implicationally related phonological generalization (e.g., Gierut, 1992). You will learn more about the clinical application of generative phonology in Chapter 9 on the analysis of children's speech and in Chapter 10 on goal setting.

■ Natural phonology and phonological processes

Natural phonology, proposed by David Stampe (1969, 1979), uses the idea of rules from generative phonology and the concepts of naturalness, markedness, and features to explain why young children often pronounce words in similar less mature ways, like saying *look* as [wʊk]. David Stampe proposed that phonology is governed by a collection of natural phonological processes or easier (less marked) ways of producing speech, and that acquisition involves suppression of these natural innate ways to make way for marked and unmarked contrasts. Stampe (1979) defined a **phonological process** as a "mental operation that applies in speech to substitute for a class of sounds or sound sequences presenting a common difficulty to the speech capacity of the individual, an alternative class identical but lacking the difficult property" (p. 1) and that a phonological process merges "a potential opposition into that member of the opposition which least tries the restrictions of the human speech capacity" (p. vii). In other words, phonological processes convert a difficult aspect of phonology into something that is phonologically similar but less difficult or challenging to produce. Stampe (1979) viewed phonological processes as psychologically real—actively changing underlying representations (that are difficult for a particular speaker to produce) into manageable surface representations. Unlike phonological rules, which need to be learned, Stampe (1979) suggested that processes were innate (and therefore need to be unlearned).

Although the existence or reality of phonological processes has not been proven (and indeed has been questioned), the concept has been adopted widely by SLPs simply as a way of *describing* the systematic error patterns in children's speech.

> **COMMENT:** *Phonological processes, phonological patterns, phonological deviations, and phonological deficit patterns. What's the difference?*
>
> The term **phonological process** was introduced by David Stampe (1969). His definition of the term was integral to his theory of natural phonology. The term was adopted by SLPs in response to David Ingram's (1976) book *Phonological Disability in Children*. Over the years, the term has been modified as different researchers have moved away from the theoretical assumptions originally associated with Stampe's (1969) work, particularly the idea that acquisition is a complex negative progression of undoing knowledge (e.g., un-delete final consonants, and un-front velars). This idea is considered counterintuitive to the idea that acquisition should be an additive process from little knowledge to more complex knowledge (Bernhardt & Stoel-Gammon, 1994). As researchers have moved away from the underlying concept, they have introduced different terms such as *phonological patterns, phonological deficiencies, phonological targets* (e.g., Hodson, 2007), and/or used the term with a different theoretical assumption (e.g., Bernhardt & Stemberger, 2000). If you ask a practicing SLP what the term *phonological process* or *phonological pattern* means, you would be told that they are terms for describing phonological error patterns in children's speech. For instance, the term *final consonant deletion* is used to describe the pattern of omitting final consonants from words. As a beginning clinician, you could assume that phonological processes and phonological patterns are synonymous unless an author writing about the terms specifies otherwise. If you are looking for *the* definitive or exhaustive list of universally accepted phonological processes—there is not one. What we have done in this book is synthesize various authors' work on phonological processes to generate a comprehensive list of terms in keeping with notable classic works in the field and more recent research (e.g., Cohen & Anderson, 2011; Dodd, 2013; Edwards & Shriberg, 1983; Grunwell, 1987; Ingram, 1976; Shriberg & Kwiatkowski, 1980; Stoel-Gammon & Dunn, 1985; Weiner, 1979).

What follows is an overview of phonological processes evident in children's speech based on terminology by Edwards and Shriberg (1983), Grunwell (1982, 1987, 1997), Ingram (1976), Stoel-Gammon and Dunn (1985), and Weiner (1979). The processes are divided into three categories: (1) syllable structure processes, (2) substitution processes, and (3) assimilatory processes, in keeping with Grunwell (1987). Within each category, we list common and then less common processes in typically developing English-speaking children's speech, followed by atypical or non-developmental processes (based on Cohen & Anderson, 2011; Dodd, 2013; Dodd & Iacono, 1989; Dyson & Paden, 1983; Haelsig & Madison, 1986; James, 2001a; Leonard & McGregor, 1991; McLeod, van Doorn, & Reed, 2001a, b; Roberts, Burchinal, & Footo, 1990; Watson & Scukanec, 1997b). In Chapter 6, you will learn more about when common phonological processes in English-speaking children disappear. In Chapters 7, 8, and 9, you will apply your knowledge of these phonological processes to the assessment and analysis of children's speech.

Syllable structure processes

Syllable structure processes describe changes to the syllable structure. Changes can involve (1) the repetition, deletion, or reduction of an entire syllable, (2) the deletion or reduction of consonants in a syllable, or (3) a change to the order of the sounds within a syllable.

Common structural processes in typically developing English-speaking children

1. **Weak syllable deletion (post-tonic and pre-tonic):** Omission of an unstressed syllable in a disyllabic or polysyllabic word. The most vulnerable weak syllables are pre-tonic syllables, because they occur before stressed syllables in words (Grunwell, 1985). Omission of a pre-tonic weak syllable is referred to as pre-tonic weak syllable

deletion (e.g., *potato* /pəteɪtoʊ/ → /teɪtoʊ/) (Grunwell, 1997). If the child omits weak syllables that occur after stressed syllables, the error pattern would be described as post-tonic weak syllable deletion (e.g., *telephone* [tɛləfoʊn] → [tɛfoʊn]).

2. **Reduplication (complete and partial):** Repetition of (usually the first) syllable in a disyllabic or polysyllabic word. When the entire first syllable is repeated, the pattern is referred to as complete reduplication (e.g., *messy* /mɛsi/ → [mɛmɛ]). If a child duplicates part of the syllable (usually the consonant) while retaining an element of the original syllable (usually the vowel) it is referred to as partial reduplication (e.g., messy /mɛsi/ → [mɛmi]) (Grunwell, 1997).

3. **Final consonant deletion:** Deletion of a consonant in syllable-final, word-final position (e.g., /sɪt/ → [sɪ]). Some children might omit all final consonants, while others might only omit one or more classes of consonants, such as nasals, plosives, fricatives, affricates, or clusters. Using the following limited speech sample from Kevin (3;7 years), you could describe his pattern of omitting word-final /f, v, s, z, ʃ, tʃ, dʒ/ as final consonant deletion of fricatives, affricates, and clusters.

off /ɑf/ → [ɑ]	*mash* /mæ/ → [mæ]
have /hæv/ → [hæ]	*watch* /wɑ/ → [wɑ]
miss /mɪs/ → [mɪ]	*badge* /bæ/ → [bæ]
buzz /bʌz/ → [bʌ]	*bus* /bʌs/ → [bʌ]
come /kʌm/ → [kʌm]	*can* /kæn/ → [kæn]
bag /bæg/ → [bæg]	*cat* /kæt/ → [kæt]

4. **Cluster reduction:** Deletion of (usually the marked) consonant in a cluster. Clusters may be reduced in word-initial position from three to two, three to one, or two to one consonants (e.g., *splash* /splæʃ/ → [plæʃ]; *please* /pliz/ → [piz]). If a child says please as [pwiz], this is a systemic rather than a structural phonological process, referred to as **cluster simplification**. Consonant clusters may also be reduced within words (e.g., *toothbrush* /tuθ.bɹʌʃ/ → [tuθ.bʌʃ]) and word-final position (e.g., *wrist* /ɹɪst/ → [ɹɪt]).

Example patterns of word-initial consonant cluster reduction:*

/s/ clusters	/ɹ/ clusters	/l/ clusters	/w/ clusters	/j/ clusters	3-element clusters
/sm/ → [m]	/pɹ/ → [p]	/pl/ → [p]	/tw/ → [t]	/tj/ → [t]	/stɹ/ → [st] or
/sn/ → [n]	/fɹ/ → [f]	/fl/ → [f]	/gw/ → [g]	/kj/ → [k]	[tr] but not [sɹ]
/sp/ → [p]	/tɹ/ → [t]	/kl/ → [l]		/mj/ → [m]	/spl/ → [pl]
/st/ → [t]	/gɹ/ → [g]			/nj/ → [n]	OR [sp] (but not [sl])
/sk/ → [k]					

*Adapted from Smit (1993b), Powell (1995), and McLeod, van Doorn, & Reed (2001b).

Less common structural processes in typically developing English-speaking children

1. **Coalescence:** Features associated with two adjacent consonants (typically in a cluster) combining into a new consonant. Using the /sp/ cluster as an example, coalescence occurs when a child combines the [+ continuant] feature of /s/ with the [LABIAL] place feature of /p/, resulting in [f]—which is [LABIAL] and [+ continuant] (e.g., *spoon* /spun/ → [fun]). Although typical, coalescence is not common in English-speaking children (McLeod et al., 2001a).

2. **Epenthesis:** Insertion of a segment (typically schwa) in the middle of a word (usually between two consonants that make up a consonant cluster) (e.g., *please* /pliz/ → [pəliz]). This process is typical but uncommon in English-speaking children (McLeod et al., 2001a; Smit, 1993b).

3. **Metathesis:** Reversal or swapping of the position of two consonants in a word. The consonants can be adjacent (e.g., *spaghetti* /spəgɛti/ → [psəgɛti]) or nonadjacent (e.g., *animal* /ænəməl/ → [æmənəl]). Like epenthesis, metathesis is uncommon yet typical in English-speaking children (James, 2001a; McLeod et al., 2001a).

4. **Migration:** The migration or movement of a sound from one position in a word to another (e.g., *ski* /ski/ → [kis]).

5. **Diminutization:** The addition of the vowel /i/ or /ɪ/ at the end of a word (e.g., *dog* /dɑg/ → [dɑgi]; *bird* /bɝd/ → [bɝdi]). This process is associated with "baby talk" and may occur during the first 50-word stage of language acquisition (Gordon-Brannan & Weiss, 2007).

Substitution (systemic) processes

Substitution processes describe the changes to consonants or vowels in words. Typically, a later developing, more marked articulatory feature of a phoneme is replaced with an easier feature. While it might appear that children substitute or replace one sound for another, the change usually involves a feature of a phoneme rather than an entire phoneme. This is an important concept to grasp, because it has implications for how you think about goals and your principles of intervention. Like the rules used to describe changes in children's speech using generative phonology, phonological processes capture the pattern or rule affecting a group of sounds (that often share a particular feature) rather than the substitution of a list of individual sounds. In addition, substitution processes can be evident across all word positions (initial, medial, and final) and syllable structure contexts (singleton and consonant cluster), or they might be constrained to a particular context. In Chapter 9, you will learn more about how to analyze patterns unique to individual children's speech. As you review the substitution processes in this chapter, identify which characteristics (voice, place, manner) have changed, which have remained constant, and the context in which the process applies (word-initial, within words, or word-final; singletons or consonant clusters).

Common substitution processes in typically developing English-speaking children

1. **Fronting:** Substitution of a consonant further back in the mouth with a consonant articulated further towards the front of the mouth. There are two main types of fronting: velar and palatal fronting.

   (a) **Velar fronting:** Substitution of a velar consonant with an alveolar, such as /k/ → [t]; /g/ → [d]; /ŋ/ → [n]. Notice how the voice and manner characteristic of the original consonant remains the same (e.g., *key* /ki/ → [ti]; *ski* /ski/ → [sti]; *bag* /bæg/ → [bæd]; *bang* /bæŋ/ → [bæn]). Like most substitution processes, velar fronting might be present across all places of articulation (e.g., *cake* /kek/→[tet] [US], /keɪk/→[teɪt] [UK]) or present in one or two word positions (e.g., *cake* /kek/→[tek] [US], /keɪk/→[teɪk] [UK]).

   (b) **Palatal fronting (depalatalization):** Substitution of a postalveolar consonant with an alveolar, such as /ʃ/ → [s]; /ʒ/ → [z]; /tʃ/ → [ts]; /dʒ/ → [dz]. Again, notice how the voice and manner characteristic of the original consonant remains the same (e.g., *shoe* /ʃu/ → [su]; *occasion* /əkeʒən/ → [əkezən]; *chip* /tʃɪp/ → [tsɪp]; jump /dʒʌmp/ → [dzʌmp]).

2. **Stopping of fricatives:** Substitution of a fricative consonant with a homorganic plosive. This means that the plosive is characterized by the same or nearest equivalent place of articulation, such as /f/ → [p]; /v/ → [b]; /θ/ → [p] OR [t]; /ð/ → [b] or [d]; /s/ → [t]; /z/ → [d]; /ʃ/ → [t]; /ʒ/ → [d] (e.g., *feet* /fit/→ [pit]; *van* /væn/ → [bæn]; *see* /si/ → [ti]; *zoo* /zu/ → [du]; *shoe* /ʃu/ → [tu]; *occasion* /əkeʒən/ → [əkedən]). A process similar to stopping of fricatives is **stridency deletion**, as described by Hodson and Paden (1991). Hodson uses stridency deletion to capture the substitution of a strident phoneme with a non-strident phoneme, which includes the substitution of strident fricatives with plosives (e.g., /s/ → [t]).

3. **Stopping of affricates:** Substitution of an affricate consonant for a plosive consonant having a similar place of articulation, such as /tʃ/ → [t] and /dʒ/ → [d] (e.g., *chew* / tʃu/→ [tu]; *jam* /dʒæm/ → [dæm]). Stopping of affricates is not to be confused with deaffrication or depalatalization.

4. **Deaffrication:** Substitution of an affricate consonant with a fricative such as /tʃ/→ [ʃ] and /dʒ/→ [ʒ] (e.g., *chew* /tʃu/ → [ʃu]; *jam* /dʒæm/ → [ʒæm]). This process is not to be confused with stopping of affricates or depalatalization.

5. **Gliding of liquids:** Substitution of a liquid /l, ɹ / with a glide /w, j/ such as /l/→ [w] or [j], and /ɹ/→ [w] or [j]. Gliding of liquids can occur in singleton and/or con-

sonant cluster contexts (e.g., *look* /lʊk/→[wʊk]; *lamb* /læm/ → [jæm]; *run* /ɹʌn/→ [wʌn]; *please* /pliz/→[pwiz]; *tree* /tɹi/→[twi]).

6. **Context sensitive voicing (CSV):** This process describes the loss of voice/voice-less contrasts within syllable-initial and syllable-final contexts (Grunwell, 1997): /p/ → [b], /t/ → [d], /k/ → [g], /f/ → [v], /s/→ [z], /ʃ/→ [ʒ], /ʧ/→ [ʤ]. There are two types: prevocalic and postvocalic voicing.

   (a) **Prevocalic voicing:** Whereby voiceless consonants are replaced by the voiced counterpart in syllable-initial position in words such as *pea* /pi/ → [bi]; *tea* /ti/ → [di]; *key* /ki/ → [gi].

   (b) **Postvocalic devoicing:** Substitution of a voiced consonant with the voice-less counterpart in syllable-final position in words such as *bib* /bɪb/ → [bɪp]; *lid* /lɪd/ → [lɪt]; *bag* /bæg/ → [bæk]; *love* /lʌv/ → [lʌf]; *buzz* / bʌz / → [bʌs]; *badge* /bæʤ/ → [bæʧ].

7. **Consonant cluster simplification:** Substitution of one or more consonants with an easier consonant. Consonant cluster simplification differs from consonant cluster reduction because it does not involve the deletion of a consonant. Instead, it typically involves the substitution of a more marked, later developing consonant within a cluster, with an earlier developing, less marked consonant in a cluster such as: /bl/ → [bw]; /dɹ/ → [dw]; /fl/ → [pl] or [pw]; /sk/→ [st]; /kɹ/→ [kw] or [tw]; /ʃɹ/→ [sw] or [tw]. Typically, the change is the result of another simplification process such as fronting, gliding of liquids, stopping of fricatives, and/or context sensitive voicing.

8. **Fricative simplification:** Substitution of an interdental consonant with a labial con-sonant, such as /θ/ → [f] and /ð/ → [v] (e.g., *thumb* /θʌm/ → [fʌm]; *that* /ðæt/ → [væt]).

Less common substitution processes produced by typically developing English-speaking children

1. **Alveolarization (apicalization):** Substitution of a labiodental or interdental consonant with an alveolar consonant such as /f/ → [s], /v/ → [z], /θ/ → [s], and /ð/ → [z] (e.g., *feet* /fit/ → [sit]; *van* /væn/ → [zæn]; *thumb* /θʌm/ → [sʌm]; *that* /ðæt/ → [zæt]).

2. **Vocalization:** Substitution of a syllabic consonant such as /l/ with a vowel, such as /l/ → [ʊ] (Grunwell, 1982) (e.g., *bottle* /bɑtl/→[bɑtʊ]; *apple* /æpl/→[æpʊ]). Edwards and Shriberg (1983) suggested that vocalization can also be evident in syl-labic nasals; however, Grunwell (1982) suggests that such instances may be better described as final consonant deletion.

3. **Labialization:** Substitution of a non-labial consonant with a labial (bilabial or labiodental) consonant, such as /ʧ/ → [f] (e.g., *chip* /ʧɪp/ → [fɪp]) and /s/ → [f] (e.g., *sun* /sʌn/ → [fʌn]). Edwards and Shriberg (1983) include the substitution of /θ/ → [f] and /ð/ → [v] as labialization. Given that this latter pattern of substitution is com-mon in typically developing English-speaking children's speech, we prefer the term *fricative simplification* exclusively for /θ/ → [f] and /ð/ → [v] substitutions.

4. **Stopping of liquids:** Substitution of a liquid consonant with a plosive consonant such as /l/ → [d] and /ɹ/ → [d] (e.g., *run* /ɹʌn/ → [dʌn]; *lamb* /læm/ → [dæm]).

Assimilation processes (consonant harmony)

Assimilation processes are where one sound becomes more like another sound in the same word. Three dimensions are used to describe assimilation (Edwards & Shriberg, 1983). First, it may be complete (total) or partial. **Complete assimilation** is equivalent to a sound being copied and then pasted from one position in a word, replacing another sound (e.g., *sip* /sɪp/ → [pɪp]). **Partial assimilation** occurs when a feature of a sound rather than an entire sound, such as labial place of articulation, is copied or assimilated onto another sound (e.g., *sip* /sɪp/ → [fɪp]). Second, assimilation may be contiguous or noncontiguous. According to Edwards and Shriberg (1983), **contiguous assimilation** is when the influ-ence is between two adjacent sounds (e.g., *swing* /swɪŋ/ → [fwɪŋ]), whereas **noncontigu-ous assimilation** is when there is at least another sound (consonant or vowel) between the two sounds involved in the assimilation (e.g., *sip* /sɪp/ → [pɪp]) (Lowe, 1994). Third, the direction of an assimilation may be progressive or regressive. **Progressive assimilation** is when a sound earlier in a word affects a sound later in a word (e.g., *pig* /pɪg/ → [pɪp]), whereas **regressive assimilation** is when a sound later in a word affects a sound earlier in a word (e.g., *pig* /pɪg/ → [gɪg]). So, in summary, assimilation patterns can be described according to the completeness, adjacency, and direction. Assimilation can be further categorized with respect to voice, place, or manner of articulation. Specific patterns of assimilation are described in the text that follows.

Common assimilation patterns produced by typically developing English-speaking children
Relative to the common segmental and substitution processes, assimilation is not widely used by typically developing English-speaking children (Grunwell, 1987). If it is used, regressive assimilation is thought to be more common than progressive (Edwards & Shriberg, 1983). With respect to voice, place, and manner, the following assimilation patterns are thought to be more common:

1. Velar assimilation (e.g., *pack* /pæk/ → [kæk])
2. Labial assimilation (e.g., *pig* /pɪg/ → [pɪp])
3. Assimilation of voice (equivalent to context sensitive voicing) (Grunwell, 1987)

Less common assimilation patterns produced by typically developing English-speaking children

1. Alveolar assimilation (e.g., *pad* /pæd/ → [dæd])
2. Palatal assimilation (e.g., *fish* /fɪʃ/ → [ʃɪʃ])
3. Nasal assimilation (e.g., *lamb* /læm/ → [næm])
4. Liquid assimilation (e.g., *yellow* /jɛlo/ → [lɛlo]) (this specific example commonly occurs in young children's speech)

■ ▪ ■ ▪ ■ ▪ ■ ▪ ■ ▪ ■ ▪ ■ ▪ ■ ▪ ■ ▪ ■ ▪ ■ ▪ ■ ▪ ■ ▪ ■ ▪ ■ ▪ ■ ▪ ■ ▪ ■ ▪ ■ ▪ ■

 APPLICATION: *Assimilation*

Assimilation patterns can be difficult to work out when you first look at a child's speech sample. We suggest that you start by determining which sound is influencing another sound in the word. Describe the voice, place, and manner characteristics of the influencing sound to identify the type of assimilation (e.g., velar assimilation). Next, consider the position of the sound in the word to determine whether the influence is regressive (sound later in a word influencing an earlier sound) or progressive (sound earlier in a word influencing a later sound). Note whether the influencing and influenced sounds are contiguous (adjacent) or noncontiguous (separated by one or more sounds). Finally, consider whether the assimilation is complete (two or more sounds are identical in the child's production of the word) or partial (the influencing sound is not repeated entirely, only a feature of the sound). Apply your understanding of assimilation by completing the following table.

Target word	Child's realization	Complete or partial	Contiguous or noncontiguous	Progressive or regressive	Type of assimilation
pig /pɪg/	[pɪp]	complete	noncontiguous	progressive	labial
lamb /læm/	[næm]				
duck /dʌk/	[gʌk]	partial		regressive	
swing /swɪŋ/	[fwɪŋ]		contiguous		labial
van /væn/	[næn]	complete		regressive	
web /wɛb/	[bɛb]		noncontiguous		labial
sheep /ʃip/	[pip]	complete			
fish /fɪʃ/	[ʃɪʃ]		noncontiguous		palatal
yellow /jɛlo/	[lɛlo]				
sip /sɪp/	[fɪp]				

Rare or atypical processes produced by English-speaking children

The question of how many atypical phonological processes exist is a little like asking how many different colors are there in the world. Across the literature on atypical phonological processes in English-speaking children's speech, many have been described (e.g., backing, initial consonant deletion, glottal insertion, nasal intrusion, tetism, nasal substitution, neutralization, gliding of intervocalic consonants, velarization) (Dodd, 2005; Edwards & Shriberg, 1983; Preston & Edwards, 2010). Additionally, children can create unusual realizations of common phonological processes. For example, Leonard and McGregor (1991) reported an unusual form of migration where word-initial stridents migrated to word-final position (e.g., *zoo* /zu/ → [uz]; *soup* /sup/ → [ups]). The issue is further compounded by the fact that what is uncommon and atypical in English may in fact be quite common and typical in another language! What follows is a description of the atypical processes for English reported across a number of authors (e.g., Dodd, 2005; Dodd & Iacano, 1989; Edwards & Shriberg, 1983; Grunwell, 1987). Once you are familiar with these processes, review Table 5-4 and you will then appreciate how atypical processes in one language (such as backing in English) are typical in other languages.

TABLE 5-4	Phonological processes evident in typically developing children's speech across languages
	Phonological process	**Example languages**
Syllable structure processes	Weak syllable deletion	Jordanian Arabic, Dutch, English, Finnish, French, German, Israeli Hebrew, Japanese, Maltese, Norwegian, Portuguese, Spanish, Turkish, Welsh
	Reduplication	Dutch, English, Greek, Korean, Turkish, Welsh
	Final consonant deletion	Jordanian Arabic, Cantonese, Dutch, English, German, Greek, Israeli Hebrew, Korean, Maltese, Portuguese, Putonghua, Spanish, Thai, Turkish, Welsh
	Cluster reduction	Dutch, English, French, Greek, Israeli Hebrew, Maltese, Spanish, Thai, Turkish, Welsh
	Initial consonant deletion	Finnish, Maltese, Spanish, Thai
Substitution processes	Fronting	Jordanian Arabic, Lebanese Arabic, Cantonese, English, German, Greek, Israeli Hebrew, Japanese, Korean, Maltese, Norwegian, Portuguese, Putonghua, Thai, Turkish, Welsh
	Stopping	Lebanese Arabic, Cantonese, Dutch, English, German, Greek, Israeli Hebrew, Japanese, Korean, Maltese, Norwegian, Portuguese, Putonghua, Thai, Turkish, Welsh
	Gliding of liquids	Lebanese Arabic, Cantonese, Dutch, English, French, Korean, Maltese, Portuguese, Putonghua, Turkish, Welsh
	Context sensitive voicing: Devoicing	Jordanian Arabic, Lebanese Arabic, Dutch, German, Hungarian, Israeli Hebrew, Maltese, Norwegian
	Context sensitive voicing: Voicing	English, German, Norwegian, Turkish, Welsh
	Backing	Lebanese Arabic, Cantonese, Greek, Japanese, Norwegian, Putonghua, Thai, Vietnamese
Assimilation/ Consonant harmony	Assimilation	Cantonese, Dutch, English, French, Greek, Maltese, Norwegian, Portuguese, Putonghua, Turkish, Welsh

Source: Adapted from McLeod (2007a, 2010).

Note: There are other processes evidenced in other languages not mentioned in this table.

1. **Initial consonant deletion:** Deletion of the initial consonant in syllable-initial word-initial position (e.g., *song* [sɒŋ] → [ɒŋ]; *feet* [fit] → [it]). This process is uncommon and atypical in English, but common and typical in some other languages (McLeod, 2010; see Table 5-4).

2. **Backing:** Substitution of a consonant further forward in the mouth with a consonant articulated further back in the mouth. Two types have been reported in the literature.

    (a) **Backing of velars**, characterized by /t/ → [k]; /d/ → [g]; /n/ → [ŋ]. This process is the opposite of velar fronting (e.g., *two* /tu/ → [ku]; *step* /stɛp/ → [skɛp]; *bat* /bæt/ → [bæk]; *bun* /bʌn/ → [bʌŋ]). The term *velarization* has also been used to describe the use of velars for a range of speech sounds produced further forward in the mouth (Edwards & Shriberg, 1983).

    (b) **Backing of fricatives**, characterized by /s/ → [ʃ]; /z/ → [ʒ]) is the opposite of palatal fronting (e.g., *Sue* /su/ → [ʃu]; *zoo* /zu/ → [ʒu]) and was reported by Dodd and Iacano (1989).

       While backing is listed here as uncommon and atypical in English-speaking children, it is common and typical in children who are learning to speak other languages such as Lebanese Arabic, Greek, Japanese, Norwegian, Putonghua (Mandarin), Thai, and Vietnamese (McLeod, 2010; see Table 5-4).

3. **Gliding of fricatives:** Substitution of fricatives with a glide. If this process is present, sibilants tend to be replaced by [j], and other fricatives replaced by [w] (e.g., *see* /si/ → [ji]; *feet* /fit/ → [wit]) (Grunwell, 1997).

4. **Denasalization:** Substitution of a nasal consonant with a homorganic plosive, such as /m/ → [b], /n/ → [d] and /ŋ/ → [g]. Some of the words in your own speech are denasalized (hyponasal) when you have a cold with blocked nose (e.g., *me* /mi/ → [bi]; *knee* /ni/ → [di]; *sing* /sɪŋ/ → [sɪg]).

5. **Affrication:** Substitution of fricatives with affricates (e.g., *shoe* /ʃu/ → [tʃu]; *zip* /zɪp/ → [dʒɪp]).

6. **Systematic sound preference:** Substitution of one speech sound for a range of other speech sounds, such as using [f] for all fricatives and affricates (e.g., *shoe* /ʃu/ → [fu]; *zip* /zɪp/ → [fɪp]) or [d] for all consonants in word-initial position in words (e.g., *shoe* /ʃu/ → [du]; *zip* /zɪp/ → [dɪp]; *run* /rʌn/ → [dʌn]; *spoon* /spun/ → [dun]; *me* /mi/ → [di]).

7. **Glottal insertion:** Substitution of a consonant with a glottal stop such as /t/ → [ʔ] in *hat* /hæt/ → [hæʔ], *happy* /hæpi/ → [ʔæʔi] and *catching* /kætʃɪŋ/ → [kæʔɪŋ]. Glottal insertion, while not a feature of typically developing speech, can occur in children with SSD and is considered to be the most common compensatory articulation used by children with a cleft palate (Peterson-Falzone, Hardin-Jones, & Karnell, 2010).

Multiple phonological processes

The task of identifying and describing phonological processes in children's speech can seem a little difficult at first. This is because a range of processes can be evident in a child's speech. You need to carefully examine the range of words spoken by a child and figure out which processes best describe the child's production of an intended adult word. An example is helpful for illustrating this point. Consider the following words spoken by Molly (4;2 years), who has a severe phonological impairment:

skip /skɪp/ → [tɪp]	*key* /ki/ → [ti]
ship /ʃɪp/ → [tɪp]	*leaf* /lif/ → [wip]
miss /mɪs/ → [mɪt]	*tree* /tɹi/ → [ti]
buzz /bʌz/ → [bʌt]	*bus* /bʌs/ → [bʌt]
please /pliz/ → [pit]	*peach* /pitʃ/ → [pit]
flat /flæt/ → [pæt]	*cat* /kæt/ → [tæt]

When you first begin the task of describing a child's speech patterns using phonological processes, consider one word at a time. Make a hypothesis about the processes that could describe the child's production of that word. For instance, what processes could

> **COMMENT:** *Why various theories?*
>
> Why are classic and contemporary theories included in this book? The simple answer is that theories and ideas are often ahead of practice. You need to understand classic theoretical accounts of children's speech, such as generative phonology and natural phonology, to understand the foundations of assessment and intervention practices currently used by SLPs working with children with SSD. You also need to understand more contemporary theories, to appreciate some of the less widely used yet promising or upcoming approaches to assessment and intervention. Knowledge of both classic and contemporary theoretical accounts will help you be discerning as you engage in evidence-based practice.

describe Molly's production of *cat* /kæt/ → [tæt]? Given that the same sound is present at the beginning and end of the word, it could be **complete noncontiguous regressive alveolar assimilation**. However, it could also simply be **velar fronting**, with /k/ → [t]. The answer to which process best describes the pattern is hidden in the rest of Molly's speech sample. You need to look for other instances of alveolar assimilation and velar fronting. If alveolar assimilation is evident, then alveolar assimilation should be present in other CVC words ending in /t/. Consider Molly's production of *flat* /flæt/ → [pæt]. Alveolar assimilation is not present. If it was, *flat* /flæt/ would have been produced as [tæt]. To confirm that velar fronting best describes one of the patterns in Molly's speech, you need to find other unequivocal instances of this process. Consider Molly's production of *skip* /skɪp/ → [tɪp] and *key* /ki/ → [ti]. The voiceless velar plosive /k/ in each context is produced as the voiceless alveolar plosive /t/, confirming that *cat* /kæt/ → [tæt] is an instance of velar fronting. Now while this sequence of reasoning from *cat* → *flat* → *key* and *skip* may seem slow, you will find that with practice you become quicker at identifying multiple processes in children's speech.

CONTEMPORARY THEORIES OF PHONOLOGY

In this section we provide a brief overview of two contemporary theories of phonology: constraint-based nonlinear phonology based on Bernhardt and Stemberger (2000) and optimality theory based on Prince and Smolensky (1993) and Dinnsen and Gierut (2008). Although these theories still use some of the enduring concepts in phonology such as the phoneme and distinctive features, they provide alternate accounts of children's phonological systems. As you learn more about phonological theories, you will realize that there are many more contemporary phonological theories in the literature (e.g., articulatory phonology: Browman & Goldstein, 1992; cognitive phonology: Bybee, 2001). As Bernhardt and Stoel-Gammon (1994) point out, not all phonological theories have direct clinical application to children with SSD, and even when they do, it can take many years for useful applications to be developed and used by clinicians in everyday practice. We have focused on these two theories primarily because there is some literature on the application of these theories to children with SSD.

■ Nonlinear phonology (based on Bernhardt & Stemberger, 2000)

Nonlinear phonology, as described by Bernhardt and Stemberger (2000), is based on a collection of phonological theories that together address a broad range of elements in a phonological system, from phrases through to the individual features that comprise speech sounds. Nonlinear phonological theories focus on "the hierarchical nature of the relationships among phonological units" (Bernhardt & Stoel-Gammon, 1994, p. 123). This is in contrast to linear theories of phonology, such as generative and natural phonology, where sounds are analyzed as a linear sequence of segments and sets of rules are used to account for changes in children's speech. Consider the phrase *blue canoe*. From a linear point of view, this phrase comprises a sequence of seven segments /blu kənu/. Nonlinear theories acknowledge that the phonological system is broader and more complex than just speech sounds—comprising an organized hierarchy of phrases, words, feet, syllables, onsets and rimes, timing units (mora), segments, and features (see Figure 5-4). Each phonological element in the hierarchy can be evaluated as an independent element and with respect to its interaction with other elements in the hierarchy. Elements are organized on separate

FIGURE 5-4   **Nonlinear phonological hierarchy**

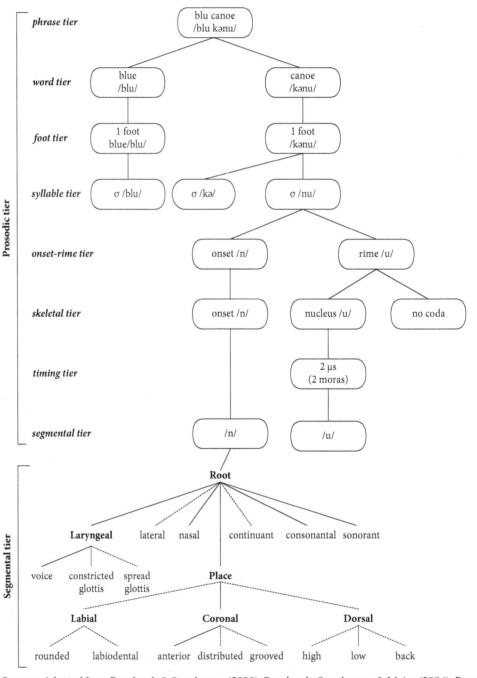

Sources: Adapted from Bernhardt & Stemberger (2000); Bernhardt, Stemberger, & Major (2006); Bernhardt, Bopp, Daudlin, Edwards, & Wastie (2010).

levels of representation called **tiers**, with tiers higher up in the hierarchy dominating lower tiers (Bernhardt, Bopp, Daudlin, Edwards, & Wastie, 2010). The two main tiers in nonlinear phonology are the **prosodic tier** and the **segmental tier** (see Figure 5-4). What follows is an overview of each of these two tiers, and the tiers comprising them.

The prosodic tier

The prosodic tier comprises all the phonological elements beyond the segment, such as phrases, words, feet, syllables, onsets and rimes, and timing units or mora. The concepts of phrases and words would be familiar to you. Some of the other elements may not. A **foot** is a phonological element consisting of one stressed syllable and any associated unstressed or weak syllables (Davenport & Hannahs, 2010). For example, the word *canoe* /kənu/ has two syllables but one foot, because there is only one stressed syllable, /nu/. The word *kangaroo* /kæŋgəɹu/ has three syllables and two feet, because there are two stressed **syllables**, /kæŋ/ and /ɹu/, with primary stress on the final syllable. The Greek letter *sigma* σ is the conventional symbol for syllable (Davenport & Hannahs, 2010). We have used the convention of putting the syllable with primary stress directly below the foot node, and the unstressed syllables and syllables with secondary stress being linked with a slanted line (Bernhardt & Stemberger, 2000).

Syllables in the prosodic tier are represented in the **onset-rime tier**. Onsets are consonants to the left of a vowel. Rimes contain a nucleus (typically a vowel) and possibly a coda. Codas typically comprise one or more consonants to the right of the nucleus in the same syllable. In the word *canoe* /kənu/, each syllable contains an onset and a rime, each comprising one vowel. Syllables also comprise a timing unit or **mora**, represented by the Greek letter *mu* μ. Syllables with one μ are considered *light*, whereas syllables with two μ are considered *heavy* (Bernhardt & Stemberger, 2000). Syllables with one μ typically comprise one short vowel, whereas syllables with two μ (or bimoraic syllables) may contain a long vowel, a diphthong, or a vowel plus a coda (Davenport & Hannahs, 2010). Syllable onsets are not counted in the weight of a syllable. In the phrase *blue canoe*, the first word contains two μ (because the syllable contains the long vowel /u/), the second syllable contains one μ (because the syllable contains the short vowel /ə/), and the final syllable contains two μ (because it contains the long vowel /u/). According to Bernhardt et al. (2010), the inclusion of a timing tier helps to account for phenomena observed in children with SSD such as compensatory lengthening of vowels when final consonants have been omitted, in order to maintain syllable timing (e.g., foot /fʊt/ → [fʊː]).

The segmental tier

The segmental tier comprises the features that characterize consonants and vowels. As Figure 5-4 shows, the segmental tier looks like a system of tree roots. This structural grouping of features in a segment is referred to as **feature geometry** (Bernhardt & Stemberger, 2000). Many of these features (e.g., [+ consonantal], [+ sonorant]) were described earlier in this chapter. In nonlinear phonology, these features are considered to be autonomous, combining in different ways to express different segments. The lines that link elements in the segmental tier are known as **association lines**, and make explicit the elements to be expressed at one point in time (Bernhardt & Stemberger, 2000). For instance, if the features [+ consonantal], [+ sonorant], [+ nasal], [+ voice], and LABIAL are specified, the resulting segment would be /m/. There are three main organizing features or nodes in the segmental tier: root node, laryngeal node, and place node. Manner features are typically linked to the root node and specify whether a segment is going to be a vowel or consonant, and, for consonants, the manner of the consonant. The laryngeal node specifies the presence or absence of voicing, in addition to the state of the glottis as [+ constricted] (as in the glottal stop /ʔ/) or [+ spread] (as in /h/, aspirated stops, and voiceless fricatives in English) (Bernhardt & Stemberger, 2000). The place node specifies the place of articulation of both consonants and vowels. Recall from the section on distinctive features, earlier in the chapter, that there are three univalent place features—LABIAL, CORONAL, and DORSAL—and that they each have respective subordinate features.

Central concepts in nonlinear phonology

In nonlinear phonology, like earlier classic phonological theories, the concept of markedness is important. Specifically, unmarked elements are designated as **default** elements in the system, while marked elements are considered **non-default**. On the prosodic tier, default elements include noncomplex onsets, nuclei, rimes, and feet, whereas the features [– voice], [CORONAL, + anterior] and [– continuant] (i.e., voiceless, coronal, and plosive) are considered the defaults on the segmental tier (Bernhardt et al., 2010). Additionally, only unpredictable non-default features are thought to be included in the underlying representation, with default features provided by the phonological processing system (Baker & Bernhardt, 2004). For example /t/ is considered the most underspecified consonant, because it is characterized by the three default features of voice, place, and manner—voiceless coronal stop. As Bernhardt and Stoel-Gammon (1994) point out, children with SSD often use this default [t] in words (e.g., *keep* /kip/, *sheep* /ʃip/, *seep* /sip/, and *cheap* /tʃip/ → [tip]). Using this example, the idea of a default offers a more concise description and explanation of the child's non-adult productions of *keep, sheep, seep,* and *cheap* than multiple phonological processes such as stopping of fricatives and affricates, and velar fronting. The idea also offers an insight into what children are doing over the course of speech development—learning the non-default elements of the phonological system, such as dorsal and continuant.

Constraints and **repair processes** are another component of nonlinear phonology. Using a fundamental concept in optimality theory (described in the next section), constraints are the limitations on what can be done, while repairs involve either the addition or deletion of a phonological element (e.g., feature, node, timing unit, syllable) or an association line. As Bernhardt and Stemberger (2000) indicate, this creates four possible processes:

1. Spreading: addition of an association line to an existing element
2. Delinking: deletion of an association line from an existing element
3. Insertion: addition of a new element and association line
4. Deletion: deletion of an element and its association line

Constraints and repairs can also be evident in specific interactions between the prosodic and segmental tiers (Bernhardt & Stemberger, 2000). For example, a preschool-aged child with an SSD might only use [DORSAL] in coda position in words. A toddler might only use the feature [LABIAL] in CVCV words. In Chapter 10 we apply this theoretical concept to goal setting for Billy (2;10 years), a toddler with a limited phonetic and syllable structure inventory.

In summary, nonlinear phonology offers insight into a range of skills beyond classic theories of phonology. We have provided you with a brief introduction—a detailed description is beyond the scope of this text. If you would like a more in-depth review of nonlinear theory, suggested readings include Bernhardt and Stemberger (1998, 2000), Bernhardt et al. (2010), and case studies of children with phonological impairment (e.g., Baker & Bernhardt, 2004; Bernhardt, 1992). You could also view online clinical tutorials on nonlinear phonology.[1]

■ Optimality theory (based on Dinnsen & Gierut, 2008)

Optimality theory was proposed by Prince and Smolensky (1993). Like generative phonology, this theory assumes two levels of representation: input (akin to an underlying representation) and output (akin to a surface representation) (Barlow & Gierut, 1999). However, this theory differs from classic phonological theories in that rules are not used to derive a surface representation from an underlying representation. Rather, a system of constraints influences a child's output representation.

Three basic mechanisms comprise the grammar in optimality theory: the **Generator (GEN)**, **Constraints (CON)**, and an **Evaluator (EVAL)** (Gierut & Morrisette, 2005). Using an input, the GEN generates or supplies a range of possible candidate outputs. For example, for an underlying form such as /pæt/, GEN may supply candidates such as [pæt], [pæ], [æt], [bæt], [pʰæt]. The outputs are universal, and therefore possible in any language. CON offers a library of universal constraints that limit and influence the range of possible outputs (Gierut & Morrisette, 2005). EVAL then selects which option best fits or is the most optimal for a specific language.

The difference between phonological systems across languages is the order in which the constraints are ranked. For instance, in English consonant clusters are allowed in

---

[1]http://phonodevelopment.sites.olt.ubc.ca

word-initial position in words. However, in Turkish, word-initial consonant clusters are not allowed. Consider the English word *please* /pliz/. An adult speaker competent in English would presumably have no difficulty matching the output of this word with the input. However, a Turkish speaker would need to find a solution to producing the word within the confines of a constraint in Turkish—words should not start with consonant clusters. This solution can involve inserting a vowel between the two consonants that comprise the word-initial consonant cluster (e.g., [pəliz]).

So what are constraints? In optimality theory there are two types of constraints: **markedness constraints** and **faithfulness constraints**. It can be helpful to think of them like constraints belonging to antagonistic or opposing teams. Markedness constraints want the output to be as simple as possible— having less rather than more marked phonological properties. By contrast, faithfulness constraints want the output to be as faithful or authentic to the input as possible. Just like the names of the players on a team, there are names for all the different constraints belonging to each type. There is also a universal convention about how those names are written—small capital letters. Some of the names for faithfulness and markedness constraints based on Barlow and Gierut (1999) and Gussenhoven and Jacobs (2011) include:

Example faithfulness constraints

MAX-IO	All segments in an input (I) should correspond maximally (MAX) with the output (O) (i.e., all segments should be present)
DEP-IO	All segments in an output (O) should be dependent (DEP) or correspond to segments in an input (I) (i.e., no insertion or addition of segments)
IDENT-MANNER	Preserve manner features from input segments
IDENT-PLACE	Preserve place features from input segments

Example markedness constraints

NOCODA	Syllables should not have a coda
NOCORCLUST	No coronal clusters such as /nd/ or /nt/
*COMPLEX	No consonant clusters (The * symbol means "no")
*DORSAL	No dorsal segments

There are also conventions about how to represent or depict inputs, the operations of the GEN, EVAL, and CON, and the eventual output using a **tableau**. In the example shown in Figure 5-5, we have used Davenport and Hannahs' (2010) convention. Specifically, the input (phonemic transcription of the target word) is entered into the top left corner cell of the tableau. Candidates supplied by GEN are listed in the first column below the input. Constraints are ranked in order on the top row next to the input, with the highest

FIGURE 5-5 Conventional tableau used in optimality theory

Showing the input (/sænd/), candidate outputs (/sænd/ and /sæn/), constraints (NOCORCLUST; MAX-IO), violations (* = violation, *! = fatal violation), and optimal output (☞= the winning candidate)

Input: /sænd/	NOCORCLUST	MAX-IO
sænd	*!	
☞ sæn		*

Source: Adapted from Davenport & Hannahs (2010).

ranked option first, followed by lower ranked constraints to the right along the row. An asterisk (*) is used to indicate a **violation** of the candidate for a particular constraint. An asterisk plus an exclamation mark (*!) represents a fatal violation—the candidate is no longer an option because it has violated the highest ranking constraint compared with other candidates. The shaded box indicates that the constraint for the candidate has not been considered, because a prior constraint has been fatally violated. The pointing finger (☞) shows you which is the optimal or winning candidate selected by EVAL for output.

Of the many recent phonological theories, optimality theory is considered to be the most successful because many phonologists now use the framework (Davenport & Hannahs, 2010). While a number of researchers have written articles and books on the application of theory to phonological acquisition and disorders in children (e.g., Barlow & Gierut, 1999; Bernhardt & Stemberger, 1998, 2000; Dinnsen & Gierut, 2008; Gierut & Morrisette, 2005), the theory is yet to be widely adopted by SLPs in everyday clinical practice. Further research and practical empirically supported assessment, analysis, and intervention resources are needed for optimality theory to become embedded into everyday clinical practice. Remember, Stampe's (1969/1979) idea of the phonological process did not enter into mainstream clinical practice until the 1980s. If you would like to learn more about optimality theory, Barlow and Gierut (1999) provide a helpful tutorial paper. Bernhardt and Stemberger (1998) and Dinnsen and Gierut (2008) provide more in-depth overviews with developmental and clinical relevance.

▪ Representation-based accounts of SSD in children

There are different views about the nature of children's underlying representations of words (Munson, Edwards, & Beckman, 2011). Phonology theories (e.g., generative phonology, optimality theory) focus on the abstract representation of spoken language. Some of the classic phonology theories such as generative phonology assume that children have adultlike underlying phonological representations of words, and that their pronunciation is due to the application of phonological rules that accommodate a developing speech production system (e.g., Smith, 1973). This idea forms the basis of the single-lexicon model of speech acquisition. Another position is that children have two lexicons—a perceptually based input lexicon and production-based representation—and that children's immature productions result from the application of reduction rules on phonological representations in the output lexicon (Menn & Matthei, 1992). See Baker, Croot, McLeod, and Paul (2001) for further discussion of these early models.

Since the late 20th century, research on SSD in children has explored the nature of children's underlying representations in broader theoretical contexts—considering how representations are first established from the perception of speech and how abstract representations are transformed into physically uttered words (e.g., Edwards, Fourakis, Beckman, & Fox, 1999; Edwards, Munson, & Beckman, 2011; Munson, Baylis, Krause, & Yim, 2010; Munson, Edwards, & Beckman, 2005b, 2011; Rvachew, 1994; Rvachew & Grawburg, 2006; Rvachew & Jamieson, 1989; Shriberg, Lohmeier, Strand, & Jakielski, 2012; Tourville & Guenther, 2011). Essentially, the focus has extended to include the mind, ear, and mouth. This research has given rise to representation-based accounts of speech acquisition and SSD in children (Edwards et al., 1999; Rvachew & Brosseau-Lapré, 2012). The main idea behind such accounts is that children's underlying representations are much more complex than an abstract bundle of phonological features transformed by rules. This does not mean that you dismiss what you learned earlier in this chapter about phonemes, allophones, features, processes, rules, and constraints; it means that you build on and extend what you have learned.

According to Munson et al. (2011), underlying representations comprise multiple levels from multiple sensory domains such as the auditory characteristics of words and sounds spoken and heard by the listener, the visual characteristics of the speech they have seen others produce, in addition to the tactile, kinesthetic, and somatosensory characteristics of the sounds that the speaker has produced. These multilayered representations are presumably learned via a **production-perception loop** (Edwards et al., 2011). It is thought that children who have SSD struggle to create detailed acoustic-perceptual and articulatory representations for words and that their non-adultlike productions are the consequence of less robust perceptual representations (Munson et al., 2010).

At this point, it is helpful to clarify the terms **phonological knowledge**, **phonological processing**, and **representation**, because they differ depending on the literature you read. Earlier in this chapter you learned about Gierut, Elbert, and Dinnsen's (1987) conceptualization of productive phonological knowledge. Their concept is based on a linguistic perspective. Within representation-based accounts of SSD, phonological knowledge has a broader meaning. Edwards et al. (1999) consider it to be multilayered, including several different types of complex representations and the mappings or relationships among them. **Phonological processing** refers to the way you mentally handle phonological information relevant to a particular language in order to read, write, and speak that language (Wagner & Torgesen, 1987). Three types of phonological processing skills include:

1. **Phonological awareness:** The ability to detect and manipulate the sounds in an oral language (Anthony et al., 2011). For example, segmenting and blending phonemes in words, such as blending /k/, /æ/, and /t/ together to make *cat* /kæt/.
2. **Phonological working memory:** The ability to temporarily store phonological information in memory so it can be processed (Wagner et al., 1997). For example, repeating spoken nonwords comprising multiple syllables.
3. **Phonological naming (aka rapid naming):** The ability to rapidly retrieve stored phonological information from long-term or permanent memory (Wagner et al., 1997). For example, quickly recalling names for pictured items such as numbers, letters, colors, and objects.

The term *phonological processing* is not to be confused with *phonological processes*. Literature on phonological processing is usually about abilities that are important for speaking, reading, and writing, while literature on phonological processes is about patterns in children's speech. As for representations—there are many ways that this term is used in the literature. Broadly speaking, a **representation** is an abstract mental store of information about a word. The term **lexical representation** can be used as an umbrella term for all the different types of information or representations that a person can have for a word. In this way, a lexical representation can include a **semantic representation** (i.e., word meaning), an **orthographic representation** (i.e., written word), a **phonological representation** (i.e., phonological information about a spoken word or its word form), **acoustic-phonetic or perceptual representation** (i.e., acoustic information about what a word sounds like), and an **articulatory-phonetic representation** (i.e., information about the physical production of the speech sounds comprising a word). In the literature focused on speech perception and production, the focus is typically on acoustic (i.e., perceptual), phonological, and/or articulatory representations (e.g., Munson, Baylis, et al., 2010; Rvachew & Brosseau-Lapré, 2012). To better understand representation-based accounts of children's speech, and the implications of the research on this approach for clinical practice, you need to understand what is involved in the perception and production of speech.

SPEECH PERCEPTION

How many words do you recognize? How did those words become part of your mentally stored knowledge? How is it that you can comprehend the same word spoken by different people in quiet or noisy conditions? The short answer is that you have developed good speech perception skills. You learned to transform or convert speech input into abstract phonological representations of that input (Samuel, 2011). You appreciate how amazing this skill is when you overhear a conversation between speakers talking in a language that is foreign to you. You know that they are talking, but you struggle to make much sense of what they are talking about, because you do not know the points at which one word ends and another word begins. Unlike this text, where there are white spaces between words, your ear simply hears a continuous acoustic speech signal that does not differentiate words, syllables, and phonemes (Nittrouer, 2002). In this section you will learn about ideas and theories of speech perception. It is important that you understand what is involved in the perception of speech, because poor speech perception can underlie unintelligible speech production.

■ How do we perceive speech?

When we listen to people talk, our brains sift, sort, and organize multiple sources of information. These sources include acoustic, visual, motor, contextual, and social input (Kim, Stephens, & Pitt, 2012; Kuhl, 2009; Samuel, 2011). Some of the earliest researchers on speech perception found that we make sense of acoustic input by sorting what we hear into abstract categories. For instance, if you were to listen to notes played on a piano in a sequential order from low to high, you would simply hear an incremental increase in pitch. However, if you were to listen to the syllable /ba/ followed by a series of syllables in which the acoustic parameter of voicing gradually changed, there would come a point that you would decide that the phoneme /b/ was no longer present in the syllable but had changed to /p/. This abrupt change in the perception of one phoneme to another was coined **categorical perception** (Liberman, Cooper, Shankweiler, & Studdert-Kennedy, 1967). If you look at a spectrogram and waveform of these two syllables, you might then think that your perception and subsequent segmentation of a continuous waveform into categories of speech sounds is the result of tuning into a specific acoustic cue unique to a specific speech sound. However, our perception of speech is not that simple.

Despite much study in search of definitive acoustic cues, there are no specific acoustic properties uniquely associated with each speech sound (Nittrouer, 2002). This is because the acoustic information associated with a given speech sound in a word overlaps, in time blurring the boundaries between sounds, syllables, and words (Kluender & Kiefte, 2006). We coarticulate, transferring phonetic features between adjoining sounds and making them more alike, such as vowels becoming nasalized when followed by nasal consonants (Fromkin et al., 2012). Acoustic information also varies greatly within and across speakers (e.g., men versus women versus children), speaking contexts (e.g., slow versus rapid speech rate; formal versus casual conversation), and phonetic contexts (e.g., Creel & Jimenez, 2012; Kim et al., 2012). This **lack of invariance** (Liberman et al., 1967)—that is, absence of clear, consistent acoustic cues corresponding to a speech sound within and across speakers, speaking contexts, and phonetic contexts—poses a challenge. What do we do with the acoustic signal?

It would seem that early in infancy, babies can hear differences between a wide range of speech sounds from their own and other languages (Kuhl, 2009). As they are exposed to spoken language, they engage in **statistical learning** and discover patterns in what they hear (Romberg & Saffran, 2010). They discover patterns for speech sounds and patterns for word boundaries. They learn how to encode acoustic-phonetic information and figure out what to pay attention to in an acoustic signal and what to ignore (Nittrouer, 2002). As young infants, they are not understanding or comprehending the meanings of the words they hear, but they are learning to make some sense of the acoustic signal. With experience, their "perception both shapes and is shaped by the acquisition of language-specific phonological categories" (Munson et al., 2011, p. 293). As infants listen to their native language, their ability to discriminate speech sounds in non-native language diminishes, while their ability to discriminate speech sounds in their language into phonemic categories improves (Kuhl, 2009). For example, through listening to language, children learn the acoustic characteristics of /s/ and develop a robust encoding of these characteristics that allows them to differentiate it from similar-sounding phonemes such as /θ, ð, ʃ/ (Edwards et al., 2011). Over the course of development, an infant's initial fragile perceptual or acoustic-phonetic representations become more detailed and robust.

As adults, our store of acoustic-phonetic representations is sufficiently detailed so that we can recognize words even in challenging acoustic contexts. For instance, we do not notice or perceive that any sounds are missing from a word when part of the acoustic signal associated with a speech sound has been deleted and replaced with white noise or a cough (Warren, 1970). It seems that we restore the intended signal using our established representations—a phenomena known as the **phoneme restoration effect** (Warren, 1970). Ganong (1980) discovered a similar phenomenon (**the Ganong effect**)—when we hear a word in which a segment within the word is ambiguous or acoustically unclear, we tend to fix up or adjust our perception of the ambiguous segment towards a word that we already know and have heard before. We use our prior knowledge of what the word sounds like to recognize the word (Calabrese, 2012). To cope with the great deal of acoustic variance among speakers, Johnson (2005) suggests that we actively work at **speaker**

normalization. Using his exemplar-based model of speech perception, we use stored category-based instances of people's speech and use these instances as a frame of reference to understand speech. The more experience we have listening to different speakers, the richer our store. For instance, Bradlow and Bent (2008) discovered that when American English-speaking adults were trained to listen and write down the sentences spoken by Chinese speakers with strong Chinese accents, the listeners who were trained with examples from a variety of speakers performed better over time compared with listeners who were trained with only one speaker. Similarly, when Japanese listeners were trained to hear the difference between /l/ and /ɹ/ in English words (a contrast that is not in Japanese), the listeners who heard productions from multiple speakers learned to understand the contrast with new words and new people, while listeners who were trained with one speaker only learned to hear the contrast in new words spoken by that same person they were trained to listen to, not new people (Lively, Logan, & Pisoni, 1993).

■ The theoretical relevance of speech perception for children with SSD

According to Shiller, Rvachew, and Brosseau-Lapré (2010), many children who have SSD have difficulty with the perception of speech. The problem is not with their ears—they can detect sound. Rather, they can have difficulty perceiving or making sense of what they hear. A study by Edwards et al. (1999) helps illustrate the problem. Edwards et al. (1999) examined the speech perception skills of six children who had SSD and six typically developing same-age peers. All the children had normal hearing, based on pure tone hearing screening. Edwards et al. (1999) reported that although all the children could point to pictures of words such as *cake* and *bird* spoken in live voice in a quiet room (i.e., they could perceive or recognize the spoken word given a complete acoustic signal in good listening conditions), the children who had an SSD had more difficulty perceiving the words when the acoustic signal had been altered—either when a portion of the acoustic signal at the end of the word had been removed or a portion of the vowel in the middle of a word had been removed and replaced with noise. These findings are important, because they suggest that children with SSD can have difficulty creating detailed, robust perceptual representations of speech (Munson et al., 2011), and that for some children at least, you will need to carefully assess (Chapter 8) and help improve (Chapter 13) their speech perception skills.

Clearly, listening to speech is important in the perception of speech. However, researchers have discovered that seeing speech and producing speech also helps us perceive speech. For instance, McGurk and MacDonald (1976) discovered that if you listen to the syllable [ba] but see the mouth produce the syllable [ga], then you perceive [da]! This phenomenon is known as the **McGurk effect**. Infants show this effect from around 4 to 5 months of age (Burnham & Dodd, 2004), with just over half of typically developing children showing the effect between 6 and 12 years (Nath, Fava, & Beauchamp, 2011). Most

COMMENT: *Indexical cues and speech perception*

When you listen to someone talk, your brain extracts all sorts of information from the acoustic signal. Not only do you process the signal to recognize the words being spoken, but you also process indexical cues or information in the signal about the person who is speaking. For instance, you can recognize your friend's speech over the phone because you have stored information about his or her speech (Calabrese, 2012). When you listen to someone you have never heard before, it is possible to extract information and ideas from the acoustic signal about the talker's sex, age, height, weight, perceived honesty, perceived femininity, social class, region of origin, and sexual orientation (Creel & Tumlin, 2011). Research on socioindexical learning and how children who have SSD learn to perceive and produce indexical cues is an emerging area of research (Munson et al., 2011).

children with SSD perform no differently to children with typically developing speech; however, some children with SSD may have difficulty integrating the speech they hear with the speech they see (Dodd & McIntosh, 2008).

Speech production also influences (and is influenced by) speech perception. The idea that production influences perception started with Liberman and colleagues, as part of their **motor theory of speech perception** (Liberman, Cooper, Harris, & MacNeilage, 1962). They suggested that because there are no clear and consistent acoustic cues for perceiving speech, we perceive speech based on intended motor gestures of the vocal tract (Liberman et al., 1962; Liberman et al., 1967). Although some of the tenets of their theory have attracted criticism (see Galantucci, Fowler, & Turvey, 2006, and Samuel, 2011, for helpful reviews), their idea about there being a connection between perception and production has not been dismissed. In fact, their idea of the perception-production connection was spurred on with the discovery of mirror neurons—special neurons that fire when you either do an action or when you watch (or listen) to someone else do the same action (Rizzolatti & Craighero, 2004). This means that just by listening to someone talk, your motor neurons activate! This connection is not present at birth but develops in early infancy. Specifically, Imada, Zhang, Cheour, Taulu, Ahonen, and Kuhl (2006) found that when newborn babies listened to speech, only auditory areas of the brain activated. However, by 3 months, auditory and motor areas show activation when listening to speech. Kuhl (2009) suggests that between birth and 3 months, infants are busy making connections between perception and production. This linkage coincides with the emergence of vowel-like sounds, and suggests that the ability to produce speech is preceded by the ability to perceive speech (Munson et al., 2011). This has helpful implications for intervention. Researchers have discovered that when children with SSD receive speech perception training, their ability to articulate specific speech sounds (i.e., speech sound stimulability) can improve (e.g., Rvachew, 1994). In the final section of this chapter, we explore theories and models about how the speech sounds we hear and words we know are produced by carefully planned sequences of muscle movements.

SPEECH PRODUCTION

The physical production of speech is an amazing human ability. On average, we articulate about 12–14 speech sounds per second (Werker & Tees, 1992). In Chapter 3 you learned about body structures needed to articulate speech. In the final section of this chapter, we consider concepts and models about how an abstract phonological representation can be transformed into a carefully timed sequenced of muscle movements. The concepts of phonological planning, motor planning, motor programming, and motor execution are described. Like the fields of phonology and speech perception, there are many different theories and models about the production of speech. We provide a brief overview of a few select theories that have been considered in clinical literature on children with SSD.

■ Phonological planning, motor planning, motor programming, and motor execution

When you say the word *cat* /kæt/, you are thought to retrieve your phonological representation for that word from memory and compile a phonological plan. This abstract information needs to be transformed into a motor plan. The plan then needs to be programmed and executed. These ideas are central to a range of models of speech sensorimotor control and production (e.g., Bohland, Bullock, & Guenther, 2009; Caruso & Strand, 1999; Levelt, Roelofs & Meyer, 1999; Stackhouse & Wells, 1997; Terband, Maassen, Guenther, & Brumberg, 2014; van der Merwe, 2009). These ideas also come up in discussions about the nature of the speech difficulties experienced by children who have inconsistent speech (phonological) disorder, CAS, and childhood dysarthria. What follows is an overview of four key ideas or concepts (phonological planning, motor planning, motor programming, and motor execution) that attempt to capture the processes involved in transforming the words in our head into intelligible speech.

Phonological planning is about selecting and sequencing the right combination of phonemes for words in keeping with the phonotactic constraints of the language (van de Merwe, 2009). Phonological planning is what children with inconsistent speech disorder are thought to find challenging. Without a model or phonological plan to imitate, children with inconsistent speech disorder produce variable productions of the same word. Table 16-11 illustrates Jarrod's (7;0 years) difficulty with phonological planning in his repeated productions of the words *witch*, *tongue*, and *birthday cake*. Each attempt was different. In Chapter 13 you will find out how you can help children like Jarrod learn how to phonologically plan words.

Read more about Jarrod (7;0 years), a boy with inconsistent speech disorder, in Chapter 16 (Case 3).

Unlike phonological planning, motor planning, motor programming, and motor execution all involve motor abilities. The first of the three motor concepts is **motor planning**. As the name implies, motor planning is about forming a strategy of action to say a word or utterance by outlining motor goals, with the plan being "articulator-specific not muscle-specific" (van der Merwe, 2009, p. 9). Motor plans have also been described as gestural scores (e.g., Browman & Goldstein, 1986) that provide instructions about what and when specific articulators are to be used. This can be likened to an orchestral musical score that specifies what and when specific notes are to be played in concert with other instruments to produce a song. In speech, this can be seen as multiple articulators needing to work together to produce a word. For instance, in the word /kæt/, the gestural score or motor plan might begin with mouth opening and the back of the tongue elevating to touch the velum to articulate [k], finishing with the tongue tip elevating towards the alveolar ridge to articulate the [t]. That is the plan.

Motor programming is responsible for specifying the parameters or scaling variables of muscle movement to realize the plan. Essentially, programming specifies what muscles you need to move, when, and how, with respect to spatiotemporal and force

COMMENT: *Knowing what is meant by motor planning and motor programming*

We have described motor planning, motor programming, and motor execution as different processes involved in the production of speech. You create a plan for what your articulators need to do to produce a sequence of speech sounds, you transform that plan into a program of specific muscle movements, then execute or perform the movement (van der Merwe, 2009). As you read literature on speech motor control, motor learning, and CAS, you will notice that the terms *motor planning* and *motor programming* are sometimes referred to as motor planning/programming (e.g., Murray, McCabe, & Ballard, 2015; Shriberg et al., 2012). This is because in reality it is difficult to separate planning from programming problems. You may also read different authors' work and notice that the terms *motor planning* and *motor programming* do not always mean the same thing. For instance, Stackhouse and Wells (1997) use the terms *motor program*, *motor programming*, and *motor planning* in their speech processing model. However, they identify motor programs as stored gestural targets that specify the sequence of articulators involved in saying specific words, motor programming as the process of creating new motor programs, and motor planning as the process of putting together gestural targets for words in the right order in real time to create connected speech that accounts for coarticulatory effects and speaking conditions (e.g., asking a question, whispering) (Stackhouse & Wells, 1997). Did you notice how motor programming and motor planning are presented in the reverse order and have different meanings in the Stackhouse and Wells (1997) model when compared with descriptions of motor planning and motor programming in literature on speech sensorimotor control (e.g., van der Merwe, 2009)? This example highlights the importance of carefully reading and understanding the terms *motor planning* and *motor programming*, as intended by different authors.

parameters including muscle tone, speed, direction, and range of movement to achieve the intended plan suited to your speaking context (van de Merwe, 2009).

Motor execution involves the physical production of the programmed movements. Children who have CAS are thought to primarily have difficulty with the motor planning and programming of speech, although recent evidence suggests that they can have difficulties with speech perception (encoding), memory processes involved in storing and retrieving abstract representations, and motor planning/programming (Shriberg et al., 2012). By contrast, children who have dysarthria are thought to have difficulty with motor programming and/or motor execution. The specific type of difficulty depends on the type of dysarthria.

■ Theories and models of speech production

Like the fields of phonology and speech perception, there are many different theories and models about the production of speech. Some of these theories are variations on box-and-arrow models (e.g., input → storage → output) while others are based on complex models of neural computation, both trying to capture specific skills and processes involved in the production of speech (e.g., **Nijmegen model** by Levelt, Roelofs, & Meyer, 1999; **speech processing model** by Stackhouse & Wells, 1997; **directions into velocities of articulators (DIVA)** model by Tourville & Guenther, 2011; **gradient order DIVA (GODIVA)** by Bohland, Bullock, & Guenther, 2009). Theories (e.g., **schema theory**, Schmidt, 1975) and principles of motor learning (e.g., Maas et al., 2008; Schmidt & Bjork, 1992) have also been used to inform our understanding about how children with unintelligible speech can learn to become intelligible.

Nijmegen model and the importance of syllables

The Nijmegen model (Levelt et al., 1999) is credited as being one of the first theories that attempted to describe how we transform our abstract phonological representations into spoken words. A key feature of the Nijmegen model is that we learn motor programs for frequently occurring syllables and store those syllables in a mental syllabary (Levelt et al., 1999). We then use these syllables to construct a plan for a word (Levelt et al., 1999). The idea that our motor plans are based on syllables (rather than isolated phonemes) has implications for how we think about the speech production difficulty facing children who have CAS. It also has implications for intervention—suggesting that we help children learn how to build and sequence syllables (as opposed to building words from a series of isolated phonemes). This idea is further discussed in Chapter 14.

DIVA and GODIVA models of speech acquisition and production

The DIVA and GODIVA models are complementary neurocomputational models that are designed to capture what goes on in specific regions of the brain when we produce speech. The DIVA model (the first of the two models to be developed) was designed to focus on the motor control processes involved in the articulation of speech (Tourville & Guenther, 2011), while the GODIVA model interfaces or links with the DIVA model, considering how our abstract phonological representation can be transformed into a motor plan then produced (Bohland et al., 2009). Both models are based on the work of Guenther and colleagues (e.g., Bohland, Bullock, & Guenther, 2009; Guenther, 1995; Tourville & Guenther, 2011). Before going any further, it is helpful to explain some of the concepts in the name of the models—Directions Into Velocities of Articulators. When you talk, your articulators move in specific **directions** (e.g., to produce [p], you close and then open your lips). **Velocity** captures both the speed of movement of the articulators, and the direction of that movement. Thus, the DIVA model attempts to describe the physical movement (speed and direction) of the articulators as speech is produced. One of the unique features of the DIVA model is that it accounts for the phenomenon of **motor equivalence**—the idea that various movements of the articulators can produce the same acoustic result (Tourville & Guenther, 2011). It does so by considering how what we hear and feel when we talk guides our production of speech (see Figure 5-6). Another feature of the DIVA model is the role of feedback and feedforward systems in the control and execution of a speech motor movement. You appreciate the role of these two systems when you try

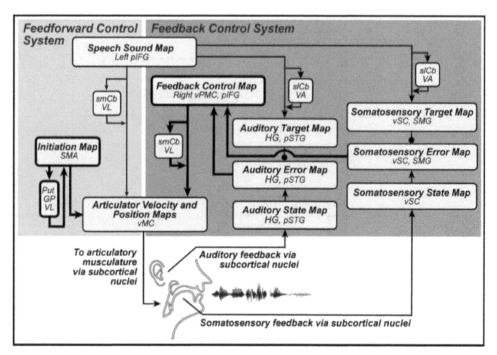

FIGURE 5-6 The DIVA model of speech acquisition and production

Abbreviations: GP globus pallidus; HG Heschl's gyrus; pIFg posterior inferior frontal gyrus; pSTG posterior superior temporal gyrus; Put putamen; slCB superior lateral cerebellum; smCb superior medial thalamus; SMA supplementary motor area; SMG supramarginal gyrus; VA ventral anterior nucleus of the thalamus; VL ventral lateral nucleus of the thalamus; vMC ventral motor cortex; vPMC ventral premotor cortex; vSC ventral somatosensory cortex.

Source: From The DIVA model: A neural theory of speech acquisition and production (Figure 1, p. 955) by J. A. Tourville and F. H. Guenther (2011). In *Language and Cognitive Processes 26*(7): 952–981, London, UK: Psychology Press. Copyright by Psychology Press. Used with permission.

to talk with a dental plate or similar device in your mouth. As you talk, your speech production system adjusts to match the intended acoustic target with what is actually being produced. A detailed description of both models is beyond the scope of this chapter. The models are also still being tested and refined (Bohland et al., 2009). If you would like to learn more, suggested readings include Guenther (1995), Bohland et al. (2009), and Tourville and Guenther (2011).

Schema theory of motor learning

The schema theory of motor control and learning was developed by Schmidt (1975). Although it was proposed to account for motor control and learning in general, concepts and principles have been applied to speech (Maas et al., 2008; Schmidt & Bjork, 1992). Briefly, Schmidt (1975) described a theory to account for the idea that motor movements are learned, stored in memory, and retrieved, as well as modified or created as needed. Motor learning is thought to occur when children figure out relationships between actions and outcomes—they learn what particular speech production movements sound like and/or feel like. They then create rules about those relationships. Schemas are sets of rules that guide decisions about how motor movements will be achieved under particular conditions (Schmidt & Lee, 2005). In Chapter 11, we provide a richer discussion about the principles of motor learning and how these principles guide intervention procedures. We also elaborate on aspects of Schmidt's schema theory relevant to intervention principles for children with SSD. Suggested readings on motor schema theory include Schmidt and Lee (2005) and Maas et al. (2008).

FIGURE 5-7 Speech processing model

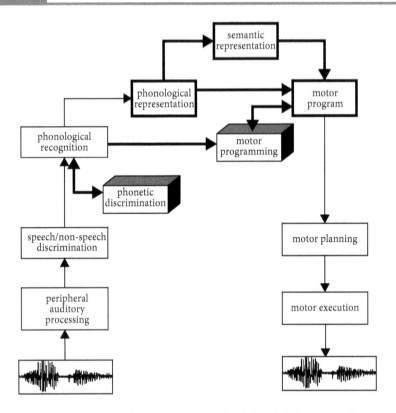

Source: From *Children's Speech and Literacy Difficulties: A Psycholinguistic Framework* (Figure 6.3 on page 166 and Appendix 4, p. 350) by J. Stackhouse and B. Wells, 1997. London, UK: Whurr. Copyright © 1997 John Wiley and Sons.

Psycholinguistic speech processing model

Stackhouse and Wells (1997) proposed a psycholinguistic box-and-arrow model of speech processing, depicted in Figure 5-7 and previously explained in Chapter 2. They designed their model to capture the full range of processes involved in the perception (input), storage, and production of speech (output). Their model assumes many of the concepts you have learned in this chapter. It also has been applied to speech and literacy skills for children with SSD. So, read the following summary of their model to see how much you have learned!

When a child hears a sound, the sound is input through the **peripheral auditory system** (i.e., ear). Having heard a sound, the first task facing the child is to determine whether what was heard was speech or something else (i.e., **speech/non-speech discrimination**). If the child recognizes the sound as speech, then the **phonological recognition** module is used to determine whether the speech belongs to a familiar phonological system (i.e., the spoken language the child knows) or another system. If the speech matches the child's phonological system (e.g., the word includes phonemes and sound sequences permissible in the language), then the word will be further processed. If the word is familiar, then an abstract underlying **phonological representation** will be activated, the meaning accessed, and the word recognized.

To produce a word, the child accesses and retrieves the underlying representation for the word. As shown in the model, three boxes are used to represent the main components that constitute a child's lexical representation relevant to speech: **phonological representation**, **semantic representation**, and abstract **motor program**. Stackhouse and

APPLICATION: *Identifying phones, processes, tiers, and markedness constraints in Luke's speech sample*

Luke (Case 1, Chapter 16) has a phonological impairment. Review the speech sample for Luke in Chapter 16, and apply what you have learned in this chapter by completing the following tasks.

1. List all the phones in syllable-initial and syllable-final position in Luke's speech sample.
2. Identify the phonological processes evident in the first 50 words of Luke's speech sample.
3. Using Bernhardt and Stemberger's (2000) clinical application of nonlinear phonology, decide whether Luke has difficulty primarily with the segmental tier or the prosodic tier.
4. Identify and describe three markedness constraints evident in Luke's speech sample. You might like to complete these tasks and then compare your answers with a peer.

Read more about
Luke (4;3 years),
a boy with a phonological
impairment,
in Chapter 16 (Case 1).

Wells (1997) acknowledge that abstract representations also include other elements such as grammatical and orthographic (written) representations. Having retrieved the word, it is transformed into a sequence of motor movements (through what they describe as motor planning), which are then executed. The arrows on the model indicate the direction of the processes involved in the perception, storage, and production of speech. For further information about this model, see Stackhouse and Wells (1997).

Chapter summary

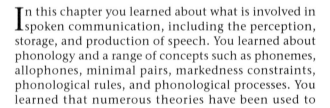

In this chapter you learned about what is involved in spoken communication, including the perception, storage, and production of speech. You learned about phonology and a range of concepts such as phonemes, allophones, minimal pairs, markedness constraints, phonological rules, and phonological processes. You learned that numerous theories have been used to describe how we perceive speech, how our phonological system is organized, and how we physically organize our speech muscles to produce an acoustic signal that matches how a word should sound. Having read this chapter, you have the basic theoretical foundations needed to understand the chapters on typical speech acquisition, assessment, analysis, and intervention.

Suggested reading

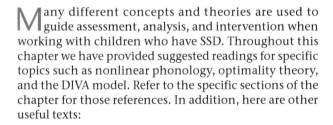

Many different concepts and theories are used to guide assessment, analysis, and intervention when working with children who have SSD. Throughout this chapter we have provided suggested readings for specific topics such as nonlinear phonology, optimality theory, and the DIVA model. Refer to the specific sections of the chapter for those references. In addition, here are other useful texts:

Phonology

- Davenport, M., & Hannahs, S. J. (2010). *Introducing phonetics and phonology* (3rd ed.). London, UK: Hodder Education.

- Gussenhoven, C., & Jacobs, H. (2011). *Understanding phonology* (3rd ed.). London, UK: Hodder Education.

Language (including syntax, semantics, morphology, phonetics, and phonology)

- Fromkin, V., Rodman, R., & Hyams, N. (2013). *An introduction to language* (10th ed.). Boston, MA: Wadsworth.

- McLeod, S., & McCormack, J. (Eds.). (2015). *Introduction to speech, language and literacy*. Melbourne, Australia: Oxford University Press.

Speech motor control

■ Maassen, B., & van Lieshout, P. (Eds.). (2010). *Speech motor control: New developments in basic and applied research*. New York, NY: Oxford University Press.

Speech perception

■ Moore, B. C. J., Tyler, L. K., & Marslen-Wilson, W. D. (Eds.). (2009). *The perception of speech: From sound to meaning*. New York, NY: Oxford University Press.

Application of knowledge from Chapter 5

Using the case-based data for Luke (4;3 years), Susie (7;4 years), Jarrod (7;0 years), Michael (4;2 years), and Lian (14;2 years) from Chapter 16, apply your knowledge about the theoretical foundations of speech by completing the following questions.

1. Provide a theoretically motivated explanation for why:
   a. Luke says *bike* /baɪk/ as [baɪk] but *cat* /kæt/ as [dæt].
   b. Susie says *sun* /sʌn/ as [ɬʌn] and *zip* /zɪp/ as [ʤɪp].
   c. Jarrod says *birthday cake* /bɜθdeɪ keɪk/ as [bɜθdeɪkʰeɪʔk] and [bɜfdeːpʰeɪʔt] and [bɜθdæɪˌtʰʌʔt].
   d. Michael says *caterpillars* /kætɚpɪlɚz/ as [kæʔ.pɪʔ.wəs].
   e. Lian says *chocolate* /tʃɑklət/ as [tsɑ.kələ̩ʔ].

Note: There will be no single perfect answer to this question. Use your knowledge of concepts, theories, and models to generate a feasible answer. Compare and contrast your answer with a peer.

2. Which of the five cases do you think might have a difficulty with speech perception? Why?

3. Prepare a lay description of phones, phonemes, and phonological processes for Luke's parents.

4. Using your knowledge of phonological concepts and theories, explain to Luke's parents why Luke pronounces *bike* /baɪk/ as [baɪk] but *cat* /kæt/ as [dæt].

5. Phonetically transcribe your own name and apply the phonological processes evident in Luke's speech. How would Luke most likely pronounce your name?

6

Children's Speech Acquisition

KEY WORDS

Factors: age, sex, socioeconomic status, language ability, elicitation, phonetic complexity, functional load, input frequency, phonotactic probability, neighborhood density

Theorists: Piaget, Vygotsky, Bronfenbrenner

Methodological issues: diary studies, cross-sectional studies, longitudinal studies, comparative studies

Typical speech acquisition: oral mechanism, perception, intelligibility, phonetic inventory, syllable and word shape inventory, mastery of consonants and vowels, percentage of consonants/consonant clusters/ vowels correct, common mismatches, phonological processes, syllable structure, prosody, metalinguistic and phonological awareness skills

Speech acquisition: monolingual, multilingual, English, Cantonese, Dutch, Spanish, etc.

LEARNING OBJECTIVES

1 Describe the difference between typical speech and acceptable speech.

2 Identify factors that influence speech acquisition.

3 Outline key child development theories that have influenced SLPs' understanding of children's speech acquisition.

4 Summarize aspects used by SLPs to consider children's speech acquisition.

5 Explain the overall sequence of development of English-speaking children's speech.

6 Outline similarities and differences between speech acquisition for children across different languages.

OVERVIEW

Speech acquisition begins in the womb. Before children are born, they learn to differentiate their mothers' voice from other voices and their mothers' native language(s) from other languages (Kisilevsky et al., 2009). From birth, the contours of babies' cries are similar to the prosody of their native language (Cross, 2009; Mampe, Friederici, Christophe, & Wermke, 2009). In the weeks and months following birth, there is a rapid growth in children's abilities to perceive, store, organize, and produce speech. As their oromusculature and structure (e.g., lips, teeth, tongue, palate) grow and change, coos and squeals make way for babbling, which in turn paves the way for spoken words—unique, meaningful, melodic sequences of consonants and vowels. As children's cognition develops, their perception and organization of categories of speech sounds becomes more sophisticated. By the time children are 5 years old they have learned to produce most consonants and vowels and their speech is intelligible to unfamiliar listeners (Flipsen, 2006b; McLeod, Crowe, & Shahaeian, 2015). During the school years, children continue to put the finishing touches on their ability to perceive speech (e.g., hear the difference between *it swings!* versus *it's wings*) (de Marco & Harrell, 1995), produce more complex consonant sequences (e.g., *statistical*), and refine their production of stress and timing in increasingly complex polysyllabic words and sentences (e.g., *My science project is about the process of photosynthesis*).

What do children do while they are learning to speak intelligibly? They make predictable and acceptable errors. Some of these errors will be familiar to you (e.g., *rabbit* /ɹæbət/ as [wæbət] and *spaghetti* /spəgɛti/ as [gɛti]). Over time, speech errors disappear and pave the way for mature adultlike speech. In principle, the idea is simple—[gɛti] becomes *spaghetti* /spəgɛti/. The reality is more complex. This is because different pronunciations of the same word are acceptable across and within young children of the same age. For example, at age 2;0 years it would be acceptable for three different English-speaking children (or indeed the same child) to pronounce *spaghetti* /spəgɛti/ in three different ways (e.g., [gɛti], [dɛti] and [pədɛti]). In addition, children's productions of the same word can (and need to) change over time as they become more intelligible. For instance, between 2;0 and 4;0 years is it possible for spaghetti /spəgɛti/ to change from [dɛti] to [gɛti] to [pəgɛti] to [pəsgɛti] to [spəgɛti].

This chapter is about children's speech acquisition—their journey from unintelligible to intelligible speech. Reading this chapter provides a rich understanding about how

■■

 APPLICATION: *Different types of caterpillars*

Review the following pronunciations of the word *caterpillar* by three different toddlers learning General American English (GAE).

	Luke (2;1 years)	Ryan (2;1 years)	Emily (2;1 years)
caterpillar /kætɚpɪlɚ/	[dæbɪwɚ]	[hæhɪjɚ]	[kæpɪwɚ]

Questions:

1. What phonological processes are evident in Luke's, Ryan's, and Emily's different pronunciations of *caterpillar*?
2. Do you think any of their pronunciations of caterpillar are atypical at 2;1 years?

Answers:

1. Luke: velar fronting, context sensitive voicing, weak syllable deletion, and gliding of liquids. Ryan: systematic sound preference for /h/, weak syllable deletion, and gliding of liquids Emily: weak syllable deletion and gliding of liquids.
2. Luke's and Emily's pronunciations are all acceptable at 2;1 years. Ryan's production is atypical, given his preference for /h/.

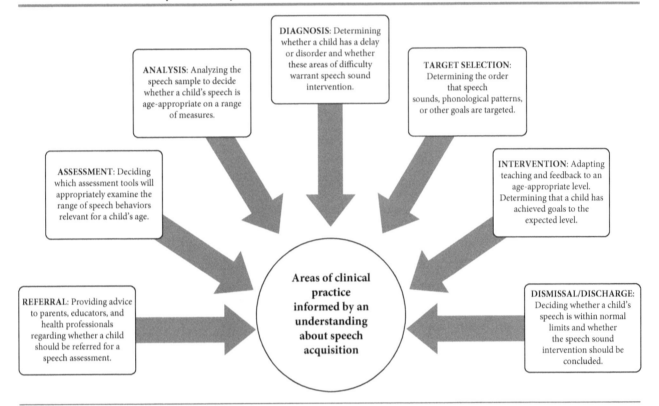

FIGURE 6-1 Areas of clinical practice informed by an understanding about speech acquisition

speech acquisition informs clinical decisions in seven different areas of clinical practice (see Figure 6-1). The most obvious decision is diagnosis—working out whether a child has typical or atypical speech. As we illustrate in this chapter, such decisions should be evidence-based—guided by research, information from children, their parents, teachers, and communities, and your own experience.

This chapter is divided into three parts. In Part 1 we provide an overview of issues that are important to consider when thinking about children's speech acquisition. In Part 2 we provide a summary of studies of typical speech acquisition for English-speaking children. Part 3 provides a brief overview of speech acquisition for children who speak languages other than English.

PART 1: IMPORTANT ISSUES WHEN CONSIDERING CHILDREN'S SPEECH ACQUISITION

The first part of this chapter outlines issues that underpin research and clinical practice regarding children's speech acquisition. Four aspects are considered. First, the importance of differentiating between statistically typical speech acquisition versus acceptable speech acquisition. Next, multiple factors influencing typical speech acquisition are outlined: age, sex, socioeconomic status, language ability, elicitation factors, phonetic complexity, functional load, input frequency, phonotactic probability, and neighborhood density. Third, an overview is presented of the work of three important theorists: Piaget, Vygotsky, and Bronfenbrenner. Finally, methodological issues in studying speech acquisition are described, drawing on research undertaken using diary studies, cross-sectional studies, longitudinal studies, and comparative studies.

TYPICAL VERSUS ACCEPTABLE SPEECH ACQUISITION

During clinical practice, SLPs take on the role of gatekeepers, deciding who is developing typically, who has an SSD, and consequently who requires intervention, what intervention should target, and when intervention should cease. As a result, it is important to consider what typical speech sounds like and to examine your own assumptions about what you think is acceptable, and what researchers report is acceptable. Within the child development literature there are two common uses of the word **typical** (or *normal*). The first is used to mean "statistical similarity or frequency" and the second to mean "desirability or acceptability" (Thomas, 2000, p. 101).

When SLPs apply the first definition of the word *typical* (i.e., "statistical similarity or frequency"), they consider sources such as:

■ research documenting children's competency at certain ages;
■ cutoff scores from normative tests that indicate typical acquisition; and
■ research and textbooks that document typical adult productions.

Research documenting children's speech acquisition at certain ages is summarized later in this chapter (e.g., English-speaking children can produce /p/ correctly by 3 years of age). By using typical speech acquisition data, SLPs compare the speech of the child they are assessing with the statistical data of children who are a similar age and sex, or children and adults who speak the same language and dialect.

The second definition of the word *typical* is "desirability or acceptability" (Thomas, 2000, p. 101). This definition includes both objective and subjective processes to determine desirable or acceptable pronunciations for each child. This second definition has received less focus within the speech acquisition literature. Thomas (2000) provides three criteria to consider desirable or acceptable behavior: (1) needs and developmental tasks that are especially prominent at different age levels, (2) typical abilities of children at successive ages and the accompanying rights and responsibilities that society holds for those age stages, and (3) attitudes (and stereotypes) held within society. He concludes by stating that ". . . normative information provides a useful starting point . . . that then needs to be verified and refined by information about the particular child whose development we are seeking to evaluate" (Thomas, 2000, p. 107). Thus, a complete understanding of speech acquisition includes far more than knowing the typical abilities of children at successive ages and should consider the life skills required by each unique individual in their context to determine acceptability at different stages. Listening to adults' pronunciations within the communities children live in is also important for determining desirability and acceptability. For example, historically, accurate production of the English consonant cluster /stɹ-/, as in the word *street*, was transcribed as [stɹ-]; however, [ʃtɹ-] is becoming an acceptable production for many English speakers in the United States (Rutter, 2011). In another example, the accepted production of 11 Cantonese consonants, tones, and consonant-vowel sequences has changed over the past century (To, Cheung, & McLeod, 2013a). One phonetic variant that is now an acceptable production is that word-initial /n/ is produced as [l] by over 90% of a sample of 1,838 adults and children in Hong Kong (e.g., 男 *boy* /nam/ → [lam]) (To, McLeod, & Cheung, 2015). Dialect is another example—different dialects have different acceptable pronunciations of speech sounds in words. For instance, in General American English *sleeve* is acceptable as /sliv/, in Spanish-influenced English it is acceptable as /esli/ or /eslif/, while in African-American English it is acceptable as /slif/.

To summarize, Thomas (2000) suggests that there are two ways of understanding typical speech acquisition: (1) knowledge of statistical similarity and (2) understanding of acceptability, attitudes, and desirability within the child's context. The majority of this chapter summarizes research on typical speech acquisition and describes ages of attainment over a wide range of measures based on the first definition. The summaries and tables will be useful as a resource in your clinical practice. However, you are also encouraged to interpret these data within the child's context (the second definition) to determine acceptable acquisition by thinking as an anthropologist within the community that you are working. Remember, your pronunciation is not the only standard you use to guide your clinical decisions. Understand and appreciate acceptable linguistic diversity around you.

APPLICATION: *Where do you draw the line?*

In order to highlight the difficulty you may have deciding who is developing typically and who is not, consider the box below.

1. Can you determine exactly when the box changes from black to white? Select a point in the box where it first changes from black to white and compare your cut-point with a peer. Did you both select the same point?

Answer: Probably not. On the left, it is clear that the box is black, on the right it is clear that the box is white, but the point at which it becomes white is indeterminate. There is a range of variation in the middle.

2. Imagine if you listened to a hundred 4-year-old children pronounce the same list of 50 words. How would you determine the point of differential between typical speech and SSD?

Answer: At either end of the group, it would be easy to determine that one child has an SSD (e.g., if the child is 4 years old and is unintelligible and cannot produce any consonants and only a few vowels) and another child does not have an SSD (e.g., if the child is 4 years old and is able to produce all consonants and consonant combinations accurately in complex contexts such as polysyllabic words and tongue twisters). However, among the remaining 98 children, there would be a range of abilities. You would need to use your professional judgment to decide which children are showing signs of typical speech acquisition and which children are not. What is professional judgment? It is based on your understandings of typical speech acquisition, the social acceptability of differing speech patterns, and conversely your understandings of impairment. As mentioned in Chapter 4, different English-speaking countries currently have different attitudes about acceptable pronunciations of /ɹ/. In the United Kingdom, clinicians place less emphasis on intervention on /ɹ/ since many public figures in the United Kingdom produce [w] and derhotacized versions of /ɹ/ within the media. In the United States and Australia, production of /ɹ/ is considered to be typical for adults. This example demonstrates that societal attitudes about the production of /ɹ/ may impact clinicians' decisions regarding what are *typical* (or socially acceptable and desirable) productions. Similar considerations should be made for speakers of different languages and dialects. There may be differences between the identification of "typical" and "impaired" production between different dialects of languages (e.g., African-American English compared with General American English; Aboriginal English compared with standard Australian English), resulting in differing priorities and speech intervention goals (Bleile & Wallach, 1992; Toohill, McLeod, & McCormack, 2012).

3. In a small group, discuss the issues involved in understanding the concept of typical, acceptable, and atypical speech, as it relates to your language and dialect.

Factors influencing typical speech acquisition

There are a range of factors that influence children's speech acquisition. In this section we consider (1) between child factors such as age and sex, (2) within child factors, (3) elicitation factors, and (4) phonetic, phonological, and lexical factors.

Between child factors

Speech production varies, both between and within children. Some factors that have been reported to influence the accuracy of children's speech acquisition **between** children include age, sex, socioeconomic status, maternal education, and language ability. You may

> **COMMENT:** *The validity of the typical-atypical divide*
>
> Since clinicians work within multidisciplinary contexts, it is also necessary to note that other fields have differing views of identifying children as typically developing or "normal" and conversely the validity of using the terms "disorder," "disability," or "impairment" (Deeley, 2002; Green & Kostogriz, 2002; Hedlund, 2000; Peters, 2000). For example, McDermott (1993, p. 272), in his thought-provoking chapter titled "The Acquisition by a Child of a Learning Disability," has argued that "there is no such thing as LD [Learning Disability], only a social practice of displaying, noticing, documenting, remediating and explaining it." Further, Coleman (1997, p. 217) states that "all human differences [including age, sex, speech] are potentially stigmatizable," with stigmas reflecting value judgments of a dominant group. Speech-language pathology literature has rarely questioned the validity of the typical-atypical divide.

recall that in Chapter 2 we outlined risk and protective factors for identifying SSD in children. The information below is related, but different, since it relies on information from studies of typical speech acquisition, rather than on studies of children with speech and language difficulties (including SSD).

- **Age:** As children grow older, their speech becomes more adultlike. The tables later in this chapter provide extensive evidence of this fact.
- **Sex:** The evidence is inconclusive regarding the impact of sex on children's speech acquisition. Some studies indicate that there is no difference between boys' and girls' acquisition of speech (e.g., McIntosh & Dodd, 2008); however, if a difference is significant, then typically girls are found to acquire speech earlier than boys (e.g., Dodd, Holm, Hua, & Crosbie, 2003; Gillon & Schwarz, 2001; Kenney & Prather, 1986; Poole, 1934; Smit et al., 1990).
- **Socioeconomic status:** Again, the evidence is inconclusive regarding the impact of socioeconomic status on children's speech acquisition. Some studies show no difference in speech acquisition across groups of children with different SES backgrounds (Dodd, Holm, et al., 2003; Smit et al., 1990); however, other studies have shown that children from higher SES backgrounds acquire speech earlier (e.g., Templin, 1957; To, Cheung, & McLeod, 2013b) and have better phonological awareness skills (e.g., Burt, Holm, & Dodd, 1999; Gillon & Schwarz, 2001; Lonigan, Burgess, Anthony, & Barker, 1998).
- **Maternal education:** Higher maternal education has been linked with more advanced speech and language skills across many studies (for a summary, see Harrison & McLeod, 2010). However, few studies of speech sound acquisition have considered this factor. Dollaghan et al. (1999) studied 240 three-year-old children and found no effect of maternal education on percentage of consonants correct in spontaneous speech samples. In contrast, To et al. (2013b) studied 937 two- to six-year-old Cantonese-speaking children and found that higher maternal education (but not paternal education) was significantly associated with better speech skills on a single-word task, but accounted for a small amount of variance in scores.
- **Language ability:** Children's speech and language skills are interlinked (Crystal, 1987a). Generally, children who have typical language skills also have typical speech skills. For example, Roulstone et al. (2002) studied 1,127 two-year-old children and found that the more advanced the children's language level, the fewer the number of phonological errors they produced. Despite this evidence, it is important to remember that some children have difficulties with speech and not language, and vice versa.
- **Between child factors that have not been associated with speech acquisition:** To date, factors that have not been associated with speech sound acquisition include paternal education, number of siblings, and having a foreign domestic helper (To et al., 2013b).

Elicitation factors

Methods used to elicit and study children's speech acquisition can influence our understanding about acquisition. Factors include whether the words were single words versus connected speech, spontaneous versus imitated productions, and whether they were elicited once or on a number of occasions. These issues will be covered more fully in Chapters 7 and 8 when we discuss how to assess children's speech.

Within child factors

Factors that influence children's speech production **within** children include pragmatic factors and personal factors.

- **Pragmatic factors:** Children might avoid saying specific words or sounds because others have found their speech difficult to understand. They may also avoid certain words because they know they are difficult to say. We have observed these phenomena in typically developing and clinically referred children. Adelaide (4;2 years) said, "I'm not saying it again," after being teased by her older brother for saying the word *ridiculous* /ɹədɪkjələs/ as [ɹədɪkləjəs]. Mark (4;7 years) refused to say words starting with initial consonant clusters during a single-word picture naming test, because he told the clinician he couldn't say those words. Conversely, children may repeat and improve their production of specific words when misunderstood (Gallagher, 1977; Gozzard, Baker, & McCabe, 2008).
- **Personal factors:** Young children's performance on a task may be influenced by the time of day they take a test and whether they are hungry, tired, bored, anxious, or disinterested in the task.

Phonetic, phonological, and lexical factors

As children learn to talk, there is a complex interplay between phonetic, phonological, and lexical factors. For instance, the sounds in babies' babble are often the sounds in children's first words (Stoel-Gammon, 2011). Children are more likely to learn the words *mommy*, *baby*, and *bed* (because they contain babbled sounds [m, b, d]) rather than *octopus*, *strawberry*, and *volcano*. Research on the interaction between children's developing phonetic, phonological, and lexical systems is both fascinating and puzzling. Figure 6-2 illustrates the range of phonetic, phonological, and lexical factors thought to influence children's speech acquisition. In this section we provide a brief overview about each factor and key findings. You will notice that the findings for some factors are clear and consistent; for others the research is inconclusive, inconsistent, or lacking.

- **Word frequency:** Words occur in languages at different rates—dichotomized as either high or low frequency. For instance, *have* and *their* are high frequency in English; *llama* and *fairy* are low frequency. High-frequency words have been reported as more accurate during speech acquisition (Tyler & Edwards, 1993) and better for facilitating progress in intervention (Gierut & Morrisette, 2012a). Others have

 APPLICATION: *"I didn't understand, what did you say?"*

Many factors influence a child's journey from unintelligible to intelligible speech. The experience of being misunderstood is an interesting one to think about. For example, "I didn't understand. Can you say that again?" We know that unintelligible words can become more intelligible (or less intelligible) when children respond to requests for clarification (Gozzard et al., 2008). We also know that children with SSD experience significantly more episodes of breakdown in communication relative to their typically developing peers (Gardner, 1989). How might the experience of being misunderstood influence speech acquisition? (Think about both positive and negative influences.) For example, children may be shy or withdrawn, or they may try harder to change their production.

FIGURE 6-2
Phonetic, phonological, and lexical factors thought to influence speech acquisition

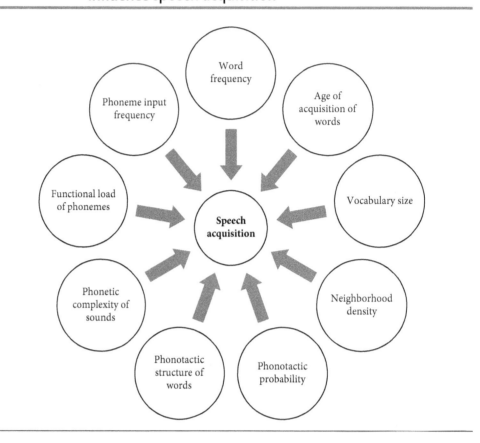

observed highly frequent words as the last to change when a new phonemic contrast is being learned by a child (Velten, 1943). More research is needed to understand the role of word frequency on speech acquisition.

■ **Age of acquisition of words:** Children learn words at different times. Some words are acquired early (e.g., *book*, *dog*) while others are acquired later (e.g., *skunk*, *microscope*). The role of the age of acquisition on speech accuracy is inconclusive. Tyler and Edwards (1993) reported that voicing was first learned in words that were early acquired (and also high in frequency). By contrast, Macken and Barton (1980) noted that voicing was first learned in later acquired words. Clinically, Gierut and Morrisette (2012a) reported that intervention using later acquired words induced greater phonological generalization compared with earlier acquired words. You will learn more about the importance of word selection in maximizing change in children's speech in Chapter 10.

■ **Vocabulary size:** Children vary in the number of words they know and use. Bidirectional relationships have been reported between vocabulary size (receptive and/or expressive measures) and speech accuracy. For instance, Oller et al. (1999) reported that infants with delayed onset of canonical babbling at 10 months had smaller expressive vocabularies at 18, 24, and 30 months relative to a control group. Smith et al. (2006) reported that lexically precocious 2-year-olds had better phonological abilities with respect to final consonants, compared to age-matched peers. Sosa and Stoel-Gammon (2012) found that 2-year-olds with larger expressive vocabularies had less intra-word variability, but not necessarily better accuracy. It seems that early speech production abilities drive word learning. As children learn more words, their speech improves. More words may mean more detailed underlying phonological representations (Mestala & Walley, 1998).

- **Neighborhood density:** Neighborhood density is "the number of words that differ from a given word by one phoneme and is thought to influence activation of lexical representations" (Storkel, Maekawa, & Hoover, 2010, p. 934). For example, using the Speech and Hearing Lab Neighborhood Database (Sommers, n.d.), the word *cat* is in a dense neighborhood (35 neighbors) that includes *bat, fat, mat, rat, cap, can, caught,* and *cast*; *family* is in a sparse neighborhood with no neighbors. Children can recall more words from dense neighborhoods, but recognize more words from sparse neighborhoods (Storkel et al., 2010). Sosa and Stoel-Gammon (2012) found that for 2-year-olds, words from dense neighborhoods were more accurate and less variable in their production than those from sparse neighborhoods. Clinically, the findings have been less clear. For children with phonological impairment, Gierut and Morrisette (2012a) reported that better intervention progress was associated with high-frequency words from dense neighborhoods, while Morrisette and Gierut (2002) reported an advantage for words from sparse neighborhoods.
- **Phonotactic probability:** Phonotactic probability is "the likelihood of occurrence of a given sound or pair of sounds in a language and is thought to influence activation of phonological representation" (Storkel, Maekawa, & Hoover, 2010, p. 934). For example, according to Edwards and Beckman (2008b), the consonant-vowel sequence /kæ/ (as in *cat*) begins 257 different words whereas the consonant-vowel sequence /kʌ/ (as in *cup*) only begins 48 words listed in the Hoosier Mental Lexicon. Edwards and Beckman (2008a) reported that common sound sequences (e.g., high-frequency consonant-vowel sequences) were more quickly learned and are more accurate than less common sound sequences during the course of typical speech acquisition. In contrast, Sosa and Stoel-Gammon (2012) found that phonotactic probability was not associated with measures of speech accuracy.
- **Phonotactic structure of words:** The length and syllabic complexity of a word influences children's accuracy of speech production. The longer the word length, the more likely children will have difficulty producing all of the consonants correctly. Children's productions of consonants and vowels are more accurate in monosyllabic words than in words of more than one syllable (James, van Doorn, McLeod, & Esterman, 2008). This finding has been documented for a range of languages. For example,

---

 APPLICATION: *Lexical characteristics of words—how do they compare?*

1. Using the table below, describe the words *ball, blanket, lamb, people,* and *their* with respect to word frequency and neighborhood density. Words with a frequency count greater than 100 are considered to be high frequency; words with more than 10 neighborhoods are considered to be high density (Storkel & Morrisette, 2002).
2. Compare the word frequency and neighborhood density characteristics with age of acquisition—what do you notice?
3. Explain why speech acquisition cannot be explained easily by an individual lexical characteristic.

Word	Age of acquisition, based on % of 2-year-olds producing the word[1]	Word frequency[2]	Neighborhood density[2]
ball	91.6%	110	24
blanket	75.7%	30	0
lamb	40.2%	7	27
people	31.8%	847	5
their	2.8%	5,394	17

[1]From Dale and Fenson (1996);

[2]From the Speech and Hearing Lab Neighborhood Database (Sommers, n.d.).

Brosseau-Lapré and Rvachew (2014) found that for French-speaking children with developmental phonological disorders, consonants were more likely to be present in one- and two-syllable words, and omitted in three- and four-syllable words. Similarly, consonants within **complex syllables** containing word-initial or word-final consonant clusters were more likely to be produced incorrectly than consonants within simpler syllables (McLeod, van Doorn, & Reed, 2001a, b; Smit et al., 1990).

■ **Phonetic/articulatory complexity:** This factor describes how difficult a consonant is to produce from an articulatory perspective. For example, /h/ is one of the least complex consonants because the lips are open, the tongue sits low within the mouth, and the larynx allows the air to pass through unobstructed. In comparison, the trilled /r/ found in languages such as Spanish and Icelandic is phonetically complex. Kent (1992) proposed the following four-level scale of articulatory complexity for English consonants, with respect to the degree of motor control required to articulate each sound: Level 1: [p, m, n, w, h]; Level 2: [b, d, k, g, f, j]; Level 3: [t, ɹ, l]; and Level 4: [s, z, ʃ, ʒ, tʃ, dʒ, v, θ, ð]. In English, early emerging consonants tend to be lower in articulatory complexity (Stokes & Surendran, 2005).

■ **Functional load of phonemes:** This factor describes how often a phoneme contrasts with other phonemes within a language. Think of it like "the amount of 'work' that the phoneme does in distinguishing words in communication" (Wedel, Kaplan, & Jackson, 2013, p. 179). Word-initial English consonants that have a high functional load include /w, m, b, ɹ, h, s, k, n, t/, because many English words contain these consonants (Baayen, Piepenbrock, & Gulikers, 1995). A consonant in English with a low functional load is /ð/, because it appears in a small number of words; whereas in Greek /ð/ appears in many different words (Ingram, 2012). In a comparison of the three factors (functional load, articulatory complexity, and phoneme input frequency), functional load was the best predictor of the age of emergence of consonants in English—sounds emerging first had a high functional load (Stokes & Surendran, 2005).

■ **Phoneme input frequency:** This factor describes how often a phoneme occurs in a language. For example, in English the few words that contain /ð/ are used frequently (e.g., *the, this, that, then, there*), so /ð/ has a high input frequency. In general, more frequently heard phonemes are learned earlier; however this trend is not universal or absolute. This is because the influence of one factor can be offset by the influence of another factor. The phoneme /ð/ is a good example—although it has a high input frequency, it is later acquired in English, presumably because of its articulatory complexity and lower functional load.

Information regarding language-specific factors that influence children's speech acquisition leads us to acknowledge that it is not appropriate to apply normative data from children who speak English to children who speak another language (e.g., Spanish, Romanian, Turkish). If children speak more than one language (i.e., they are multilingual), then the combination of languages and dialects spoken, the ages each are acquired, and the contexts in which they are heard and spoken have a complex influence on children's speech acquisition. To this end, Davis (2007) stated, "As SLPs increasingly assess and treat children from varying linguistic backgrounds, knowledge of typical acquisition must expand beyond descriptions of developmental milestones based predominantly on studies of English" (p. 51). Hambly et al. (2013) conducted a systematic review into the influence of bilingualism on speech acquisition and reported limited evidence to suggest that bilingual children acquire speech at a different rate to their monolingual peers. Instead, there

 APPLICATION: *What's the difference between* ball *and* their?

The words *ball* and *their* are both high density and high frequency (as you determined in the previous application exercise). However, *ball* is acquired earlier by most typically developing toddlers at 24 months, while *their* is not. In light of what we know about phonetic complexity and functional load in English, why might more toddlers have acquired *ball* than *their*?

COMMENT: *The influence of phonetic, phonological, and lexical factors varies across languages*

There has been cross-linguistic evidence that input frequency, functional load, and articulatory complexity influence children's speech acquisition across a range of languages (Ingram, 2012). For example, Stokes and Surendran (2005) studied children's acquisition of American English, Cantonese, and Dutch and provided evidence that variance in acquisition was accounted for by input frequency for Cantonese and Dutch, whereas variance in acquisition of American English was accounted for by functional load and articulatory complexity. Edwards and Beckman (2008b) suggested that consonants that are not articulatorily complex are more likely to have a high input frequency and functional load within languages. Later, Beckman and Edwards (2010) demonstrated that input frequency accounted for children's production accuracy for different phonemes when learning Cantonese, Greek, Japanese, and English, although the strength of the relationship differed across languages.

was evidence for transfer between phonology from the first language (L1) to the second language (L2) as well as from L2 to L1. If you are considering the speech of a child who is bilingual, or speaks a dialect that is different from the dialect and language used to create the normative data for a speech assessment you are using, then it is important to consider the second definition of *typical* as outlined above. That is, "desirability or acceptability" (Thomas, 2000, p. 101) for the child's family and community. We will consider children's acquisition of languages other than English in more detail later in this chapter.

THEORIES OF CHILD DEVELOPMENT THAT HAVE INFLUENCED OUR UNDERSTANDING OF SPEECH ACQUISITION

There are three major theorists in the field of child development who have influenced our understanding of children's speech acquisition: Jean Piaget, Lev Vygotsky, and Urie Bronfenbrenner. Each theorist's perspective will be outlined briefly.

■ Jean Piaget

When clinicians describe the stages children progress through and facilitate children's active construction of learning during the acquisition of speech, they are drawing on understandings from the work of Piaget. Jean Piaget (1896–1980), a Swiss psychologist, described children's cognitive development and believed that children are constructive and active thinkers. Piaget believed that children use **schemas**, or organizational frameworks, to organize their experiences and construct their world. He suggested that development resulted in continual **organization** of information and that children incorporated knowledge into their schemas via **assimilation**, or adjusted their environment via **accommodation** (Piaget, 1952). He proposed four stages of development:

■ **Sensorimotor stage (0–2 years):** During this stage infants construct their understanding of the world as they coordinate sensory information (e.g., hearing, tasting) with motoric actions (e.g., touching), hence the label *sensorimotor*. **Object permanence**, or knowing that an object still exists even when it is not seen, is an important milestone during this stage.

■ **Preoperational stage (2–7 years):** During this stage children describe their understanding of the world with words and images. They begin in the **symbolic function** substage (2–4 years), where they use language to represent objects that are not present, and have an **egocentric** (or self-centered) worldview. The **intuitive thought** substage (4–7 years) follows, where they use primitive reasoning that often focuses on one attribute to the exclusion of others (or **centration**). During this stage children are likely to ask many questions about the world. Children in this stage also do not understand **conservation**; that is, that an object may change in appearance, but stays the same. In Piaget's most famous conservation experiment, he showed that children in the preoperational stage did not understand that the same amount of water poured into glasses of different sizes was still the same amount of water.

■ **Concrete operational stage (7–11 years):** During this stage children are able to classify objects using several characteristics. They can use logical reasoning within concrete (but not abstract) situations. Children in the concrete operational stage understand **seriation** (e.g., ordering objects along a continuum from smallest to largest) and **transitivity** (e.g., using logic to determine relationships between objects).

■ **Formal operational stage (11 years–adulthood):** During this stage adolescents and adults think about the world in logical, abstract, and idealistic ways. They use **hypothetical-deductive reasoning** to create hypothetical solutions to problems to test theories.

Piaget's contributions include his insights into how to observe children and how cognitive growth occurs in stages. However, over the years there has been criticism of Piaget's theories; particularly that he did not focus on the impact of training, culture, and education and that he suggested that skills within a stage should emerge at the same time (Santrock, 2004). Neo-Piagetians have revised Piaget's theories and provide more emphasis on attention, memory, and strategies (Case, 2000). Clinicians' understanding that children progress through stages of speech acquisition that build on one another (as provided later in this chapter) draw on Piaget's theory of child development.

■ Lev Vygotsky

When clinicians describe children's acquisition of speech by learning through interaction with others, they are drawing on understandings from the work of Vygotsky. Lev Vygotsky (1896–1934) was a Russian psychologist who, like Piaget, advocated a constructivist approach to learning. However, unlike Piaget, Vygotsky did not describe stages of development and did not advocate the idea of children's egocentricity. He believed in the **social construction** of understanding; that is, that knowledge is gained by interacting with others in cooperative activities. He also believed that language is an important tool for constructing knowledge, planning, solving problems, and monitoring behavior. One of his most famous ideas (and one that frequently is used by SLPs) is the **zone of proximal development** (Vygotsky, 1978). Many tasks are too difficult for children to master alone, but can be learned through the guidance of others (older children or adults including parents, teachers, and SLPs). The zone of proximal development extends from the level that the child can attain without assistance to the level that the child can attain with assistance from others. **Scaffolding** refers to the assistance provided to children. Skills can be learned by scaffolding or changing the level and type of support to fit the child's current performance. Social construction of learning occurs through dialogue. Vygotsky's major contribution is the importance of collaboration and the understanding that knowledge is mutually constructed and learned. Clinicians' use of dynamic assessment approaches (see Chapter 7) and scaffolding learning during intervention (see Chapters 10–14) draw on Vygotsky's social-constructivist approach.

■ Urie Bronfenbrenner

When clinicians describe the importance of context or environment during the acquisition of speech, they are drawing on understandings from the work of Bronfenbrenner. Urie Bronfenbrenner (1917–2005) was a Russian American psychologist. He developed the ecological systems theory of development (Bronfenbrenner, 1979) to describe the relationship between the social and psychological aspects of children's development and the contexts and influences on their development. Bronfenbrenner stated:

[the ecological] . . . understanding of *human development* demands more than the direct observation of behavior on the part of one or two persons in the same place; it requires examination of multiperson systems of interaction not limited to a single setting and must take into account aspects of the environment beyond the immediate situation containing the subject. (Bronfenbrenner, 1979, p. 21)

He described an ecology of five interdependent systems that influenced development (Bronfenbrenner, 1994):

- **Microsystem:** represents those who have regular and close contact with the child (e.g., family, friends, professionals such as teachers and SLPs).
- **Mesosystem:** represents the links or interactions between important people within the child's microsystems (e.g., discussions between parents, teachers, and SLPs).
- **Exosystem:** represents settings that do not include the child as an active participant, but have an impact on the child (e.g., health and education departments).
- **Macrosystem:** represents how cultural ideologies and societal factors impact on the child (e.g., culture, race, and socioeconomic status).
- **Chronosystem:** represents change and/or consistency over time within the child and the child's environment (e.g., the influence of technology over time).

Typically these five systems are drawn as a series of concentric circles or nested spheres with the child in the middle. However, such an image was described but never drawn by Bronfenbrenner. As a result, there are a multitude of representations available.

Within the microsystem, Bronfenbrenner (1979) described three types of dyadic relationships that aid skill development and have been used by clinicians to support children's speech acquisition:

- **Observational dyads:** where the child observes another person.
- **Joint activity dyads:** where the child simultaneously completes a task with someone else.
- **Primary dyads:** where the relationship and influence between the child and another person continue to exist even when they are apart.

Bronfenbrenner's ecological systems theory has gained wide acceptance within health and education fields. However, some consider that it does not provide enough emphasis on biological and cognitive factors, nor does it provide information on stages of development (Santrock, 2004). Clinicians' application of Bronfenbrenner's ecological theory occurs when predictors of SSD are considered (e.g., maternal education), children's contexts are considered within comprehensive assessments (e.g., home language), facilitators and barriers that impact intervention are considered (e.g., support provided by their preschool teacher), and context is varied when promoting generalization beyond the clinic (e.g., practicing speech tasks with school friends) (McLeod, Daniel, & Barr, 2013).

METHODOLOGICAL ISSUES IN STUDYING SPEECH ACQUISITION

Research about children's typical speech sound acquisition is a primary source of data used by clinicians to decide whether a child is acquiring speech typically. It is useful to understand how speech acquisition data are elicited in order to interpret our subsequent discussion of these data. Some studies of speech acquisition are based on small samples of children (sometimes only one or two) taken over a long period of time, whereas other studies are based on large groups of children who are seen once. Therefore, the data that are gained from these studies need to be interpreted differently. Appendix 6-1 lists the English speech acquisition studies described in this chapter, and pertinent details about the number of participants, the research technique (diary, cross-sectional, longitudinal, comparative), sampling method, and country where the data were collected. There are four major techniques that have been used for determining how children acquire speech: diary studies, large-scale cross-sectional group studies, longitudinal studies, and comparative studies.

■ Diary studies

Diary studies are exactly as the name suggests: researchers keep a detailed diary of a child's speech acquisition. Sometimes diaries are supplemented with audio recordings (this technology was not available for the earlier diary studies). Many diary studies have been conducted by linguists or psychologists who have studied their own children:

- Velten's (1943) daughter's (Joan) growth of speech and language patterns
- Leopold's (1947) daughter's (Hildegarde) bilingual speech acquisition
- Smith's (1973) son's (Amahl) phonological acquisition
- Menn's (1971) son's (Daniel) early sound sequence constraints
- Waterson's (1971) son's (P) prosodic development
- Elbers' son's words and babbling within the first word period (Elbers & Ton, 1985)
- Stemberger's (1988) eldest daughter's between-word processes
- Stemberger's (1989) daughters' nonsystemic errors within and across phrases
- French's (1989) son's acquisition of word forms within the first 50 word stage
- Lleó's (1990) daughter's use of reduplication and homonymy

One of the critiques of diary studies is that children of linguists may not be typical, either as a result of genetic endowment or the environment in which they have grown up. Despite this criticism, diary studies have enabled detailed analyses of speech acquisition over time within the same child. Such detailed analyses have provided evidence for theory generation, but have not been used widely by clinicians as a guide to typical speech acquisition.

■ Cross-sectional studies

Large-scale cross-sectional studies emerged as the primary method for examining speech acquisition between the 1950s and 1970s in association with the major theoretical paradigm of the time, behaviorism. Within large-scale cross-sectional studies, developmental norms are generated by using the same testing protocols for groups of children of the same age, sex, socioeconomic status, and intelligence. Typically, within speech acquisition studies, children are shown pictures and then produce single words containing different consonants and vowels. The accuracy of their production is scored and their errors are analyzed. Large-scale cross-sectional studies (also called **normative studies**) are still considered to be the most important source of information for comparing a child's speech acquisition to what is expected for a child of a similar age, sex, and context. Examples of large-scale cross-sectional studies of English children's speech include:

- Templin (1957), who examined the acquisition of consonants by 480 three- to eight-year-old children from the United States.
- Smit, Hand, Freilinger, Bernthal, and Bird (1990), who studied 997 three- to nine-year-old children from the United States to examine the acquisition of consonants and consonant clusters. Later, Smit (1993a, b) categorized these children's non-adult productions of consonants and consonant clusters by age and frequency of occurrence.
- Dodd, Holm, Hua, and Crosbie (2003), who studied 684 three- to six-year-old children from the United Kingdom to examine the acquisition of consonants and vowels and the use of phonological processes.
- Roulstone, Loader, Northstone, Beveridge, and the ALSPAC team (2002), who studied 1,127 two-year-old children from the United Kingdom to examine the acquisition of consonants and vowels, the use of phonological processes, and interrelationship between speech and language.
- Kilminster and Laird (1978), who studied 1,756 three- to nine-year-old children from Australia to examine their age of acquisition of consonants.

In addition, there are many large-scale cross-sectional studies of children who speak languages other than English. For example:

- **Cantonese:** To, Cheung, and McLeod (2013a), who studied 1,726 two- to eleven-year-old Cantonese-speaking children from Hong Kong to examine their age of acquisition of consonants, vowels, and tones.

- **French:** MacLeod, Sutton, Trudeau, and Thordardottir (2011), who studied 156 two- to four-year-old French-speaking children in Canada to examine their inventory and age of acquisition of consonants.
- **Hungarian:** Nagy (1980), who studied 7,602 three- to eight-year-old children in Hungary to examine their age of acquisition of consonants.
- **Japanese:** Nakanishi, Owada, and Fujita (1972), who studied 1,689 four- to six-year-old children in Japan to examine their age of acquisition of consonants.
- **Spanish:** Linares (1981), who studied 148 five- to eight-year-old children in Mexico and the United States to examine their age of acquisition of consonants.

A critique of large-scale cross-sectional studies is that by providing information about the means, standard deviations, and average age of acquisition, the range of individual variation is obscured. Furthermore, in order to provide similar data on a large number of children, the data collection methods are rarely naturalistic; for example, they rely on single-word speech samples and rarely include connected speech sampling. Consequently many longitudinal studies of children's speech acquisition use connected speech sampling and provide information on individual variability.

Longitudinal studies

Longitudinal studies document speech acquisition of a group of children over time. The number of children and the length of time vary, but typically studies of speech acquisition include 10–20 children who are studied for 1–2 years. Examples of longitudinal studies of children's speech acquisition include:

- Watson and colleagues' longitudinal study of the acquisition of consonants and vowels by 12 children between 24 and 36 months (Watson & Scukanec, 1997a, b; Watson & Terrell, 2012);
- Robb and Bleile's (1994) longitudinal study of the growth of consonants inventories by seven children aged 8 to 25 months; and
- McLeod, van Doorn, and Reed's (2001b) longitudinal study of 16 two-year-old children's acquisition of consonant clusters.

An advantage of longitudinal studies is that any changes in the area of interest are attributable within the child, rather than because a different child has been selected at an older age group. Longitudinal sampling enables examination of individual variability and provides connected data that can be used to document developmental trends. For example, Lleó and Prinz (1996) used longitudinal data to report that word shapes were acquired by German- and Spanish-speaking children in the following developmental sequence: CV → CVC → CVCC → CCVCC (where C = consonant and V = vowel).

Comparative studies

Comparative studies have been used to test hypotheses and theories of children's speech acquisition. Comparisons have been made between:

- typically developing children and children with SSD. For example, Storkel, Maekawa, and Hoover (2010) considered the effect of phonotactic probability and neighborhood density on comprehension and production of vocabulary for 20 children with SSD and 34 typically developing age-matched peers;
- typically developing children and adults. For example, Giannakopoulou, Uther, and Ylinen (2013) compared the ability of 40 children aged 7 to 8 years (20 Greek-speaking and 20 English-speaking) and 40 adults aged 20 to 30 years (20 Greek-speaking and 20 English-speaking) on speech perception tasks that varied in vowel duration cues; and
- cross-linguistic studies of typically developing children. For example, Beckman and Edwards (2010) compared database transcriptions of toddlers learning Cantonese, English, Greek, or Japanese to determine the interaction between consonant accuracy and input frequency within the lexicon for each language. In another study, Yavaş, Ben-David, Gerrits, Kristoffersen, and Simonsen (2008) used sonority theory to explain children's acquisition of consonant clusters containing /s/ in English, Hebrew, Dutch, and Norwegian.

COMMENT: *What makes a good normative (large-scale cross-sectional) sample?*

McCauley and Swisher (1984a) provide 10 psychometric criteria for reviewing norm-referenced tests designed to assess the speech and language of young children. The first two criteria relate to normative sampling. Criterion 1 relates to the description of the normative sample. McCauley and Swisher (1984a) indicate that there should be a clear description of the geographic residence and socioeconomic status of the children included in the sample. When you look at normative studies and tests, consider how well the geographic residence and socioeconomic status of the children match the children in your clinic. Also included under criterion 1 is that there should be a description of the "'normalcy' of subjects in the sample, including the number of individuals excluded because they exhibited nonnormal language or nonnormal general development" (McCauley & Swisher, 1984a, p. 38). There has been a lot of discussion about whether normative samples should or should not include children who have speech and language (and other) difficulties. Indeed, Peña, Spaulding, and Plante (2006) wrote a paper titled "The Composition of Normative Groups and Diagnostic Decision Making: Shooting Ourselves in the Foot" and analyzed simulated and test manual data. They indicated that by including children with language impairment within the normative sampling, the group mean was lowered, the standard deviations were increased, and the ability to classify children accurately (typical versus impaired) was decreased. When you look at normative studies and tests, consider whether the normative sample included children with SSD and other difficulties.

Criterion 2 relates to the size of the normative sample used in standardizing tests. McCauley and Swisher (1984a) indicate that the lower limit for adequate sampling is to have subgroups of 100 or more children. That means, if data are provided on boys and girls in 6 monthly age groups from the age of 3;0 to 5;11, then there should be at least 1,200 children within the sample (and 100+ children in each subgroup). When you look at normative studies and tests, consider the size of the sample and number of children within the subgroups to see if an adequate number of children have been sampled. Few English studies of speech acquisition meet this criterion. Examples where the sample size is adequate, with subgroups of 100 or more children, are found in the following speech sound assessments reviewed in McLeod and Verdon (2014):

- Contextual Probes of Articulation Competence: Spanish (Goldstein & Iglesias, 2006) (*n* = 1,127), which assesses production of Spanish

- Hong Kong Cantonese Articulation Test (Cheung, Ng, & To, 2006) (*n* = 1,838), which assesses production of Cantonese

- Türkçe Sesletim-Sesbilgisi Testi [Turkish Articulation and Phonology Test] (Topbaş, 2005) (*n* = 735), which assesses production of Turkish

Within comparative studies, experiments can be undertaken to appreciate relationships between groups or concepts. Comparative studies enhance our understanding of the nuances of children's speech acquisition, providing insights and pathways for supporting the speech of children whose speech is not developing typically.

■ Summary of Part 1

The first part of this chapter outlined four important issues for considering children's speech acquisition: (1) the importance of differentiating between statistically typical speech acquisition versus acceptable speech acquisition, (2) factors influencing typical speech acquisition, (3) theories of child development, and (4) methodological issues in research on children's speech acquisition. It is now time to apply this foundational knowledge to considering data on children's speech acquisition.

PART 2: TYPICAL SPEECH ACQUISITION FOR ENGLISH-SPEAKING CHILDREN

The second part of this chapter provides a summary of studies of typical speech acquisition for English-speaking children. It is organized according to three age groups (0–2 years, 3–5 years, 6+ years) to reflect children's typical developmental sequence and to enable you to have the information at your fingertips when considering whether a child's speech is developing in a typical manner. Within each age group the following aspects are considered:

- Oral mechanism
- Perception
- Intelligibility
- Phonetic inventory
- Syllable and word shape inventory
- Mastery of consonants and vowels
- Percentage of consonants, consonant clusters, and vowels correct
- Common mismatches
- Phonological processes
- Syllable structure
- Prosody
- Metalinguistic and phonological awareness skills

When considering the information, it should be noted that rates of development vary among typically developing children. Where possible, data from more than one study are presented under each heading at each age to allow for comparison and to encourage consideration of diversity and individuality. Key features of the studies of English-speaking children's speech acquisition that have been used in the chapter are summarized in Appendix 6-1. When considering which data are relevant for the children in your clinical context, look at Appendix 6-1 to determine the sample size, the country the data were collected in, and whether single-word or connected speech sampling techniques were used.

SPEECH ACQUISITION FOR ENGLISH-SPEAKING INFANTS AND TODDLERS FROM BIRTH TO 2 YEARS

The birth of a child is an exciting event in most families. During the first two years of life children undergo significant change. They almost double their height, and quadruple their weight (Waterlow et al., 1977). Their reflexive movements become more purposeful. They are creative and entertaining as they increase their independence. They learn to crawl, then walk, then run. Their visual and aural perception becomes refined as they explore their world.

Children are born vocalizing; however, it takes some time for them to acquire intelligible speech. Early communicative acts include gaze, gesture, and vocalization (Wetherby & Prizant, 1993). During their first year of life, children produce their first words, and these tend to be ones they have frequently heard from their parents (Hart, 1991). Between the ages of 1 and 2, most children produce single words. During this time, children's early lexical attempts are supplemented by gestures such as pointing. There is evidence that their word-gesture combinations predict the onset of two-word combinations, acting as a stepping-stone to increasingly complex language (McGregor, 2008; Özçalışkan, & Goldin-Meadow, 2005). High-frequency words have been found to be less variable in production (Sosa & Stoel-Gammon, 2012) than low-frequency words. There is a wide range of variability in young children's speech. This variability is reduced when children shift to a rule-based strategy of phonological learning around 2 years of age (Scherer, Williams, Stoel-Gammon, & Kaiser, 2012).

■ Oral mechanism

At birth, the purpose of the oromusculature is threefold: for nutrition (sucking), breathing, and for gaining attention via crying. Compared with adults, infants' oral spaces are smaller. Their lower jaws are smaller and retracted. Sucking pads in the cheeks provide stability during sucking. Their tongues are large compared to size of oral cavity and therefore have more restricted movement. Their tongues move with their jaws. Newborns breathe and swallow at the same time, so they breathe through their nose. Their epiglottis and soft palates are in approximation as a protective mechanism. The larynx is higher in newborns than in adults and the Eustachian tube lies in a horizontal position, compared with the more vertical position in adults. During the first year of life, teeth emerge (Kent & Tilkens, 2007).

Within the first three years of life, children's oral spaces enlarge as their lower jaws and other bony structures grow. Their oromusculature develops to enable sophisticated movements for speech, eating, and swallowing. They have increased muscle tone, and tongue movement becomes more skilled. Their tongue movement becomes dissociated from jaw movement, a feature that enables increased skill in eating and speech. One- to 2-year-olds' jaw movement is similar to adults'; however, upper and lower lip movement is variable and takes longer to mature (Green, Moore, & Reilly, 2002). There is separation of the epiglottis and soft palate, and their larynx is lowered. In a longitudinal study of 98 children's oromotor development from 2 to 24 months for eating, Carruth and Skinner (2002) showed increased efficiency in the children's jaw stability (open and close mouth), lateral tongue movements (move food in mouth), and lip closure (keep food in mouth).

Diadochokinesis (DDK) and maximum phonation time

While there are no data on diadochokinesis (DDK) for 1-year-old children, we know that typically developing 2-year-old children can produce between three and four syllables per second on a DDK task and can sustain the vowel /a/ for 5–6 seconds (Robbins & Klee, 1987) (see Table 6-1).

■ Perception

Babies only a few days old have shown that they can perceive differences in phonemes. In fact, within the first year of life, children have shown that they can perceive differences in **manner** between plosives versus glides, plosives versus nasals, fricatives versus affricates, the approximants [ɹ] versus [l], and oral versus nasal vowels. Additionally, young children have shown that they can perceive differences in **place** of articulation for stops, glides, fricatives, and vowels (for a review, see Rvachew & Brosseau-Lapré, 2012). The vowels [i], [u], [a] are particularly salient for infants (Polka & Bohn, 2011) (look at the vowel quadrilateral in Chapter 4 and you will see that these are located at the corners). A number of studies have shown that young children can differentiate between phonemes that are not contrastive in the language that they typically hear. For example, Ruben (1997) states: "By at least 2 days of age, the neonate has an ability to discriminate language specific acoustic

TABLE 6-1	Diadochokinesis (DDK) and maximum phonation time for 2-year-old children
Task	**2;6–2;11 years**
/pʌ/	3.7/sec
/tʌ/	3.7/sec
/kʌ/	3.7/sec
patticake	1.3/sec
Maximum phonation time for /a/	5.6 seconds

Source: Adapted from Robbins & Klee (1987).

> **COMMENT:** *Methods for testing young children's speech perception*
>
> Very young children (some only a few days old) have been able to indicate whether or not they can perceive differences in speech thanks to the innovations of creative researchers.
>
> - **High amplitude sucking technique** is where babies suck on a teat and are presented with a sound (e.g., /pa/). Once they become used to hearing the sound (as determined by their regular rhythmical sucking), another sound is presented (e.g., /ba/). The babies' sucking pattern typically changes on presentation of the new stimuli, indicating that they perceive a difference in the sounds (e.g., Eimas, Siqueland, Jusczyk, & Vigorito, 1971).
>
> - **Visually reinforced head-turn procedure** is a behavioral technique where babies learn to turn their head to look at a new stimuli when they hear a new sound (e.g., Polka, Rvachew, & Mattock, 2007)
>
> - **Event-related potentials (ERPs)** involve a non-invasive neurophysiological device that determines sensory and cognitive processing by recording patterns of electrical activity in the brain through the skull (e.g., Cheour, Korpilahti, Martynova, & Lang, 2001; Dehaene-Lambertz & Gliga, 2004).
>
> - **Functional magnetic resonance imaging (fMRI)** is another non-invasive neurophysiological device that measures neural activity by recording changes in blood flow in the brain (e.g., Dehaene-Lambertz, Dehaene, & Hertz-Pannier, 2002).

distinctions. The 12 month old human has developed the capacity to categorize only those phonemes which are in its native language" (p. 203), and the better the speech perception as an infant, the larger the vocabulary as a toddler (Tsao, Liu, & Kuhl, 2004). Jusczyk (1999) indicated that 2-year-old children's speed and accuracy identifying words in speech is similar to adults'; however, it takes until at least 12 years of age for children's perception to be adultlike (de Marco & Harrell, 1995).

◼ Crying, vocalization, and babbling

In the first 12 months of life, children cry. McGlaughlin and Grayson (2003) undertook a cross-sectional study of 297 children between 1 and 12 months to determine the mean amount of crying per 24 hours. They found that from 1 to 3 months of age, children cried, on average, for 90 minutes per 24 hours, mostly in the evening. From 4 to 6 months, children cried for 64.7 minutes, mostly in the afternoon. From 7 to 9 months, they cried for an average of 60.5 minutes, mostly in the afternoon/evening. By 10–12 months, children cried for an average of 86.4 minutes, mostly in the evening.

In addition to crying, children's vocalization skills develop over the first year of life. There are two classification systems that are frequently used to describe the progression of children's vocalization. First, Stark, Bernstein, and Demorest (1993) suggest that from 0 to 6 weeks children produce reflexive vocalizations; that is, they cry and fuss. Between 6 and 16 weeks children coo and laugh, producing vowel-like sounds. Between 16 and 30 weeks children produce syllable-like vocalizations that contain consonant-like and vowel-like sounds. Between 31 and 50 weeks they use reduplicated babbling—that is, a series of consonant and vowel-like elements (Mitchell, 1997).

The second classification system by Oller, Eilers, Neal, and Schwartz (1999) describes the first stage, between birth and 2 months, as including phonation, quasi-vowels, and glottal sounds. Between 2 and 3 months, children are in the primitive articulation stage and "goo." Between 4 and 5 months, children are in the expansion stage, where they produce full vowels, raspberries, and marginal babbling. After 6 months, children are in the canonical stage, where they produce well-formed canonical syllables and reduplicated sequences (e.g., [babababa]). According to Oller et al. (1999), ". . . late onset of canonical babbling may be a predictor of disorders ... [i.e.] smaller production vocabularies at 18, 24, and 36 months" (p. 223).

Children's babbling increases and becomes refined as children develop control of their jaw movements, using "rhythmic mandibular oscillation" (Davis & MacNeilage, 1995, p. 1199). Babbling may be reduplicated (e.g., /dada/) or variegated (e.g., /bada/) forms. As children practice different babbled forms and their babbling is acknowledged by others in their environment, they transition to intentional word use. Vihman and Croft (2007) proposed that children learn to use new words via phonological word templates. Children's first words appear around 1 year of age, and their lexicon rapidly increases. By their second birthday they have begun to put two words together.

■ Intelligibility

Unfamiliar listeners can have difficulty understanding the speech of very young children, particularly if the child is not known to them. Roulstone, Loader, Northstone, Beveridge, and the ALSPAC team (2002) studied 1,127 children and reported that by age 2;1 "children were mostly intelligible to their parents with 12.7% parents finding their child difficult to understand and only 2.1% of parents reporting that they could rarely understand their child" (p. 264).

■ Phonetic inventory

A phonetic inventory outlines the consonants, consonant clusters, and vowels children produce regardless of whether they matched the adult target.

Phonetic inventory of consonants

In the first year of life, children's phonetic inventories include the following consonant types: nasal, plosive, fricative, approximant, labial, and lingual (Grunwell, 1981). In a study of 1-year-old children, it was found that children's phonetic inventories contained an average of 4.4 consonants (median 4; range 0–16), with [b, d, m, n] being the most frequently reported (Ttofari Eecen, Reilly, & Eadie, 2007). Grunwell (1987) suggested that children between 1 and 2 years of age produce the following consonants in their inventory: [p, b, t, d, m, n, w], which expands to [p, b, t, d, (k), (g), m, n, (ŋ), h, w] between 2;0 and 2;6.

Robb and Bleile (1994) described the emergence of children's phonetic inventories within a longitudinal study of the connected speech produced by seven children from 8 months (0;8) to 25 months (2;1). Notice that square brackets are used to indicate that these are consonants that are used by the children but are not necessarily produced correctly as the intended target consonant.

- 0;8 = five consonants in initial position (typically [d, t, k, m, h]); three consonants in final position (typically [t, m, h])
- 0;9 = five consonants in initial position (typically [d, m, n, h, w]); two consonants in final position (typically [m, h])
- 0;10 = six consonants in initial position (typically [b, t, d, m, n, h]); four consonants in final position (typically [t, m, h, s])
- 0;11 = four consonants in initial position (typically [d, m, n, h]); two consonants in final position (typically [m, h])
- 1;0 = five consonants in initial position (typically [b, d, g, m, h]); two consonants in final position (typically [m, h])
- 1;3 = six consonants in initial position (typically [b, d, g, n, h, w]); two consonants in final position (typically [n, h])
- 1;6 = six consonants in initial position (typically [b, d, m, n, h, w]); three consonants in final position (typically [t, s, h])
- 2;0 = 10 consonants in initial position (typically [p, b, t, d, k, m, n, s, h, w]); four consonants in final position (typically [t, k, n, s])

- 2;1 = 15 consonants in initial position (typically [p, b, t, d, k, g, m, n, f, s, ʃ, h, w, j, ʤ]); 11 consonants in final position (typically [p, t, d, k, m, n, f, s, h, l, ɹ]) (Robb & Bleile, 1994)

After children's second birthdays, their phonetic inventory continues to increase. Stoel-Gammon (1987) indicated that 2-year-old children have 9–10 word-initial consonants and 5–6 word-final consonants in their phonetic inventory. Other studies have provided a list of consonants produced by typically developing 2-year-old English-speaking children:

- Word-initial [p, b, t, d, k, m, n, s, h, j, w] and word-final [p, t, k, m, n, s, z] (Watson & Scukanec, 1997b)
- Word-initial [p, b, t, d, k, g, m, n, f, s, h, ts, (ʧ), (ʃ), (ɹ), j, l, w] and word-final [p, t, d, k, (g), m, n, ŋ, f, (v), s, z, ʃ, (ts), ʧ, (ɹ), ʔ] (Dyson, 1988)

Phonetic inventory of consonant clusters

Consonant clusters can occur in word-initial, within word, or word-final position (see Chapter 4). Two-year-old children can produce consonant clusters (Stoel-Gammon, 1987); however, children take many years to master consonant cluster production (well into the school years) (McLeod & Arciuli, 2009). According to McLeod, van Doorn, and Reed (2001b), 2-year-olds predominantly produce word-initial consonant clusters containing /w/ (e.g., [bw, kw]) in their phonetic inventory. Remember, these are the consonant clusters that they can produce, not the targets (e.g., the targets may have been /bɹ, kl/). Common word-final clusters in the phonetic inventories of 2- to 3-year-olds contain nasals (e.g., [-nd, -nt, -ŋk]) (McLeod et al., 2001b). The following example shows the development of an inventory of word-initial and word-final consonant clusters for children within a longitudinal study:

- 2;6 = [pw, bw, -nd, -ts]
- 2;9 = [pw, bw, pl, -nd, -ts, -nt, -nz]
- 3;0 = [st, sp, pl, -nd, -ts, -nt, -nz, -st, -ɹŋk] (Watson & Scukanec, 1997b)

Phonetic inventory of vowels

According to Donegan (2002), "Low, non-rounded vowels are favored in the first year. Front-back vowel differences appear later than height differences" (p. 2). Selby, Robb, and Gilbert (2000) described the longitudinal acquisition of vowels by four children living in the United States as follows:

- 1;3 = [ɪ, ʊ, ʌ, ɑ]
- 1;6 = [i, u, ʊ, ʌ, ɔ, ɑ, æ]
- 1;9 = [i, ɪ, u, ɛ, o, ʌ, ɔ, ɑ]
- 2;0 = [i, ɪ, u, ɛ, e, o, ɔ, ɑ, æ]

As can be seen, for these four children, the number and diversity of vowels increased as they came closer to their second birthdays. In another study of six children living in the United States aged from 18 to 48 months, vowel space (remember our discussion of the vowel quadrilateral in Chapter 4) was established early in life and did not change significantly beyond 30 months, apart from the effects of regional dialectal variation in some children (McGowan, McGowan, Denny, & Nittrouer, 2014).

◼ Syllable and word shape inventory

Syllable shape refers to the structure of a syllable within a word. When describing syllables and words, the following convention is used: C = consonant and V = vowel. Two-year-olds have the following syllable and word shape inventory:

- CV, CVC, CVCV, CVCVC (Stoel-Gammon, 1987)
- CV, VC, CVC, two-syllable (Shriberg, 1993)
- CV, VC, CVC, CCVC, CVCC, CVCV, VCV, CC(C)VCC (Watson & Scukanec, 1997b)

■ Age of acquisition of consonants, consonant clusters, and vowels

Age of acquisition of consonants

Age of acquisition is frequently defined as the age at which a certain percentage (often 75% or 90%) of children have acquired a phoneme in initial, medial, and final position in single words. Only a handful of studies have considered the age of acquisition of English consonants by children under 3 years of age. As will be seen later in the chapter, the youngest children in most age-of-acquisition studies are 3-year-olds. Table 6-2 provides a summary of the age of acquisition of consonants by children who are 2 years old. Many of these studies indicate that early consonants to be mastered are plosives and nasals, the fricative /h/, and the approximant /w/. The study by McIntosh and Dodd (2008) also suggests early acquisition of /s/. The documented age of acquisition of /s/ and /z/ is one of the most diverse for any English consonant; as you will see later, some studies suggest that it takes until a child is 9 years old to acquire /z/ (Chirlian & Sharpley, 1982).

Age of acquisition of consonant clusters

Two-year-old children begin to master the production of consonant clusters. McLeod et al. (2001b) indicated that 2-year-olds were more likely to correctly produce word-initial /l/ and /s/ and word-final nasal consonant clusters than other consonant clusters. They indicated that /ɹ/ consonant clusters were rarely produced correctly by 2-year-olds. There was a wide range of variability between young children's abilities to produce consonant clusters (McLeod & Hewett, 2008).

Age of acquisition of vowels

Otomo and Stoel-Gammon (1992) found that for children between the ages of 1;10 and 2;6 the order of acquisition was: /i, ɑ/, then /e, æ/, followed by /ɪ, ɛ/. Donegan (2002) indicated that there was considerable variability in the production of vowels, but that most vowels were acquired early.

■ Percentage of consonants, consonant clusters, and vowels correct

The percentage of consonants, consonant clusters, and vowels that are produced correctly is often used as an overview of children's competence. Percentage of consonants correct (PCC) is calculated by using the following formula, initially described by Shriberg and Kwiatkowski (1982c, p. 267) and expanded in Chapter 9.

$$PCC = \frac{\text{number of correct consonants}}{\text{number of correct plus incorrect consonants}} \times 100$$

Frequently, PCC is calculated using children's spontaneous speech; however, some researchers calculate PCC on a single-word speech assessment. A similar formula is used to calculate percentage of consonant clusters correct, percentage of vowels correct, and percentage of phonemes correct. Table 6-3 provides a summary of studies that have considered 1- to 2-year-old children's percentage of consonants, consonant clusters, and vowels that are produced correctly. It is important to note the wide variability in these young children's skills, as demonstrated by the wide range between the minimum and maximum scores in Table 6-3. On average, when 2 years old, children are producing approximately 70% of consonants correctly. Scherer, Williams, Stoel-Gammon, and Kaiser (2012) found that typically developing children aged 1;6–3;0 were more likely to produce nasals (97.9%), stops (96.0%), and fricatives (94.5%) correctly than liquids (84.3%), affricates (79.7%), and glides (78.1%). Non-rhotic vowels are more likely to be produced correctly than rhotic vowels (Pollock, 2002). Consonant clusters pose the greatest difficulty for children, with McLeod et al. (2001b) indicating that less than 30% are correct (see Table 6-3).

TABLE 6-2 Age of acquisition of English consonants for children aged 0 to 2 years
Gray cells indicate that the consonant was not acquired by 2;11

Study	Chirlian & Sharpley (1982)		McIntosh & Dodd (2008)	McIntosh & Dodd (2008)	Paynter & Petty (1974)	Prather et al. (1975)
Age range	2;0–9;0		2;1–2;11	2;1-2;11	2;0–2;6	2;0–4;0
Criterion	75%		75%	90%	90%	75%
No. of children in sample	1,357		62	62	90	147
Sex	F	M	F&M	F&M	F&M	F&M
Plosives						
p	2;6	3;0	2;5	2;5	2;6	2;0
b	3;6	3;0	2;5	2;5	2;6	2;8
t	2;6	3;6	2;5	2;5	2;6	2;8
d	2;6	2;6	2;5	2;5	**	2;4
k	2;6	3;0	2;5	2;5	**	2;4
g	2;0	3;0	2;5	2;5	**	3;0
Nasals						
m	2;0	2;0	2;5	2;5	2;6	2;0
n	2;0	2;0	2;5	2;5	**	2;0
ŋ	2;6	2;6	2;5	2;11	**	2;0
Fricatives						
f	3;0	3;6	2;5	**	**	2;4
v	5;0	9;0	—	—	**	>4;0
θ	7;6	8;0	**	**	**	>4;0
ð	7;6	7;6	—	—	**	4;0
s	3;6	4;0	2;5	2;5	**	3;0
z	9;0	**	2;5	**	**	>4;0
ʃ	3;6	3;6	**	**	**	3;8
ʒ	4;0	4;6	—	—	**	4;0
h	2;0	3;0	2;5	2;11	2;0	2;0
Approximants						
ɹ	5;0	5;0	**	**	**	3;4
j	3;0	3;6	2;5	2;11	**	2;4
l	4;0	3;6	2;5	**	**	3;4
w	2;6	3;0	2;5	2;5	2;0	2;8
Affricates						
tʃ	3;6	3;6	**	**	**	3;8
ʤ	4;0	3;6	**	**	**	>4;0

— not assessed; ** not acquired by the oldest age in the study. F = female, M = male.

TABLE 6-3	Percentage correct for English consonants, consonant clusters, and vowels for children aged 1 to 2 years

Blank cells indicate that the age range was not studied

Aspect	Study	Age				
		1;6	2;0	2;3	2;6	2;9
Consonants	McIntosh & Dodd (2008)		63.9% (range 13–93)		73.4% (range 49–95)	
	Pollock (2002)	53.2% (SD = 10.0)	70.4% (SD = 9.5)		80.9% (SD = 10.4)	
	Scherer, Williams, Stoel-Gammon, & Kaiser (2012)	86.5% (SD = 15.1)				
	Stoel-Gammon (1987)		70%			
	Watson & Scukanec (1997b)		69.2% (range 53–91)	69.9% (range 51–91)	75.1% (range 61–94)	82.1% (range 63–96)
Consonant clusters	McLeod, van Doorn & Reed (2001b)		29.5% (range 0.0–79.1)			
Vowels (non-rhotic)	McIntosh & Dodd (2008)		88.2% (range 19–100)		94.9% (range 83–100)	
	Pollock (2002); Pollock & Berni (2003)	82.2% (SD = 8.3; range = 69–96)	92.4% (SD = 5.5; range 78–100)		93.9% (SD = 6.4; range 78–100)	
Vowels (rhotic)	Pollock (2002)	23.5% (SD = 24.1; range = 0–70)	37.5% (SD = 30.7; range 0–87)		62.5% (SD = 30.0; range 0–100)	

A different way to consider the percentage of consonants correct is to calculate the percentage of error. Roulstone et al. (2002) calculated the mean *error* rates for children aged 2;7 as follows: velars = 31%, fricatives = 38%, liquids = 57%, and consonant clusters = 72%.

■ Common mismatches

Currently there is no information about common mismatches for English-speaking children aged between 0 and 1 years. Smit determined common mismatches for the production of consonants (Smit, 1993a) and consonant clusters (Smit, 1993b) by English-speaking children aged 2;0 to 9;0. Common mismatches that occurred at least 15% of the time by the youngest groups of children (ranging from 2;0 to 3;6) are listed below. Note that Ø indicates an omitted consonant.

■ Stops (word-initial position): /p/ → [b]; /k/ → [t]; /g/ → [d]
■ Stops (word-final position): /p/ → Ø; /b/ → [p], Ø; /t/ → Ø; /d/ → [t], Ø; /g/ → [k]
■ Nasals (word-final position): /ŋ/ → [n]
■ Fricatives (word-initial position): /v/ → [b]; /θ/ → [f]; /ð/ → [d]; /s/ → [s̺]; /z/ → [d]; /ʃ/ → [s]
■ Fricatives (word-final position): /v/ → [b]; /f/ → [s̺]; /θ/ → [f], [s]; /s/ → [s̺]; /z/ → [s], [ts]; /ʃ/ → [s]
■ Approximants (word-initial position): /j/ → Ø; /l/ → [w]; /ɹ/ → [w]
■ Approximants (word-final position): /l/ → vowel
■ Affricates (word-initial position): /tʃ/ → [t, d]; /dʒ/ → [d]
■ Affricates (word-final position): /tʃ/ → [ts] (Smit, 1993a)
■ /w/ clusters: /tw/ → [t]; /kw/ → [k]
■ /l/ clusters: /pl/ → [p, pw]; /bl/ → [b, bw]; /kl/ → [k, kw]; /gl/ → [g, gw]; /fl/ → [f, fw]; /sl/ → [s, sw]

- /ɹ/ clusters: /pɹ/ → [p, pw]; /bɹ/ → [b, bw]; /tɹ/ → [t, tw]; /dɹ/ → [d, dw]; /kɹ/ → [k, kw]; /gɹ/ → [g, gw]; /fɹ/ → [f, fw]; /θɹ/ → [f, θw]
- /s/ clusters (2 element): /sw/ → [w]; /sm/ → [m]; /sn/ → [n]; /sp/ → [p, b]; /st/ → [t, d]; /sk/ → [k]
- /s/ clusters (3 element): /skw/ → [k, t, kw, gw]; /spl/ → [p, b, pl, pw, spw]; /spɹ/ → [p, pw, pɹ, sp, spw]; /stɹ/ → [t, d, st, tw, sw]; /skɹ/ → [k, w, kw, gw, fw, skw] (Smit, 1993b)

◼ Phonological processes

Children use most if not all phonological processes during the first year (Grunwell, 1987). In Chapter 5 you were introduced to the different phonological processes, so you may like to take a moment to review the terminology. Between 1;6 and 2 years, the following phonological processes are present in English-speaking children's speech: final consonant deletion, cluster reduction, velar fronting, stopping, gliding, context sensitive voicing, and assimilation. Reduplication is declining in use. Table 6-4 documents the phonological processes that are used by 1- to 3-year-olds according to different authors.

◼ Syllable structure

When English-speaking children are 1 to 2 years old, they primarily produce monosyllabic utterances. For example, Dyson (1988) found that 2- to 3-year-olds mostly produce CVC syllable shapes and two-syllable words make up about 12% of words produced.

◼ Prosody

As mentioned in Chapters 3 and 4, mastery of prosody involves perception and production of stress, rhythm, and intonation. It also includes mastery of lexical and grammatical tones for tone languages such as Cantonese. Within the literature on speech

TABLE 6-4 **Phonological processes reported to be used by children from 1;0 to 2;11 across six studies (mean occurrence > 10%)**

Phonological process	1;6	2;0	2;6
SYLLABLE STRUCTURE PROCESSES			
Weak syllable deletion	G, PHP	G, J, MD, PHP	G, MD
Reduplication	G	(G)	
Final consonant deletion	G	G, J, MD, WS	G, MD
Cluster reduction	G, PHP	G, J, MD, PHP, WS	G, MD, PHP, RBF, WS
SUBSTITUTION (SYSTEMIC) PROCESSES			
Velar fronting	G, PHP	G, J, MD, PHP	(G), PHP, RBF
Palatal fronting (depalatalization)		J	
Stopping	G, PHP	G, J, MD, PHP, WS	G, MD, PHP, WS
(De)affrication		J, MD	
Gliding of liquids	G, PHP	G, J, MD, PHP, WS	G, MD, PHP, RBF, WS
Context sensitive voicing (CSV)	G	G, J, MD	(G), MD
Consonant cluster simplification			WS
Fricative simplification		J	
ASSIMILATION			
ASSIMILATION	G	G, J, MD	(G), MD

G = Grunwell (1987); J = James (2001a); MD = McIntosh & Dodd (2008); RBF = Roberts, Burchinal, & Footo (1990); PHP = Pressier, Hodson, & Paden (1988); WS = Watson & Scukanec (1997b).

acquisition, the majority of attention has been on the acquisition of stress, particularly lexical stress (i.e., stress within a word), with limited attention on the acquisition of rhythm and intonation.

Intonation

Intonation, also called pitch variation, refers to the "relative pitch-height of the beginnings and ends of syllables and differences of pitch-range" (Gibbon & Smyth, 2013, p. 428). Children produce varying intonation during their babbling, and use intonation to convey adult-like meanings in their early words and sentences (Cruttenden, 1982). Young children are able to control their intonation earlier than they can control syllable timing or stress (Snow, 1994).

Stress

Young children are able to perceive lexical stress differences. For example, children as young as 7 months have been found to be able to differentiate alternating stress patterns of English (Jusczyk, Houston, & Newsome, 1999). By 14 months, children can recognize novel words that contain differences in stress patterns according to syllable duration, intensity, and frequency (Curtin, 2010). Young children are also able to produce different stress patterns. Children aged 7 to 14 months are able to produce adultlike stress patterns during babbling by altering duration, intensity, and frequency (Davis, MacNeilage, Matyear, & Powell, 2000). Children's early words typically contain stressed syllables, and unstressed syllables may be deleted (Salidis & Johnson, 1997). Kehoe (2001) analyzed children's syllable deletion patterns and observed that non-final unstressed syllables (e.g., *balloon, banana*) are more likely to be deleted than stressed syllables (e.g., *balloon*) and word-final unstressed syllables (e.g., *banana*). Additionally, stress errors were less frequent in spontaneous than imitated productions (Kehoe, 1997).

■ Metalinguistic skills

One- to 2-year-old children learn to monitor and spontaneously repair their own utterances, adjust their speech to different listeners, and practice sounds, words, and sentences (Owens, 1996).

SPEECH ACQUISITION FOR ENGLISH-SPEAKING PRESCHOOLERS FROM 3 TO 5 YEARS

Between the ages of 3 and 5 years, children become more independent. They can run, jump, and climb. Their fine motor skills develop as they dress themselves and use cutlery, pencils, scissors, puzzles, and blocks. They have conversations using increasingly longer sentences. They constantly seem to ask questions such as "Why?" They learn grammatical structures such as plurals, past tense, and possessives. As summarized by James (1990), "Five-year-old children are producing long, complex sentences ... and maintaining a topic for several turns. In a few short years, children move much closer to the adult level of linguistic and communicative competence" (p. 74). Many children attend early years educational settings, so they may have more conversational partners. The ability for others to understand their expanding observations of the world increases in importance. Let's consider features of children's speech acquisition between 3 and 5 years of age.

■ Oral mechanism

Children's oral mechanism continues to grow and change throughout the preschool years and into adolescence (Walsh & Smith, 2002). Their 20 primary (deciduous) teeth typically are in place before they begin school: four incisors, two canines, and four molars on the maxilla and mandible. By 3 years of age, children's swallow is more adultlike. The refinement of tongue-tip, tongue-body, and jaw movements for speech continue to be refined throughout childhood and into late adolescence (Cheng, Murdoch, Goozée, & Scott, 2007).

Diadochokinesis (DDK) and maximum phonation time

Children's ability to produce rapid consonant-vowel sequences increases with age. Typically developing 3- to 5-year-old children can produce approximately four syllables per second on a diadochokinesis (DDK) task and can sustain the vowel /a/ for 5 to 9 seconds. Table 6-5 provides a summary of children's DDK rates and maximum phonation time according to Robbins and Klee (1987).

Intelligibility

Between 3 and 5 years of age, children's overall intelligibility increases, but this is moderated by the familiarity of the speaker and the complexity of the message. Gordon-Brannan (1993 cited in Gordon-Brannan, 1994) suggested that by 4;0 children are on average 93% (range = 73–100%) intelligible in conversational speech with unfamiliar listeners. Flipsen (2006b) reported that a transcriber can reliably understand an average of 95.68% (range = 88.89–100.00%) of words spoken by a 3-year-old, an average of 96.82% (88.42–100.00%) of words spoken by a 4-year-old, and an average of 98.05% (89.84–100.00%) of words spoken by a 5-year-old. By 5 years of age, children should be intelligible most of the time, even to unfamiliar people (McLeod, Crowe, & Shahaeian, 2015).

Phonetic inventory

A child's phonetic inventory consists of the consonants, consonant clusters, and vowels produced regardless of whether they match the adult target.

Phonetic inventory of consonants

Three- to 4-year-old children are reported to have the following consonants in their phonetic inventory:

- [p, b, t, d, k, g, m, n, ŋ, f, s, h, w, j, (l)] (2;6–3;6) (Grunwell, 1987)
- [p, b, t, d, k, g, m, ŋ, f, v, s, z, ʃ, h, ʧ, ʤ, (ɹ), j, l, w] (3;6–4;6) (Grunwell, 1987)

Word-initial consonants in phonetic inventory:

- [p, b, t, d, k, g, m, n, ð, f, s, h, ʧ, w, j, l, ɹ] (Watson & Scukanec, 1997b)
- [p, b, t, d, k, g, m, n, f, s, (ʃ), h, w, j, l, ɹ] (Dyson, 1988)

Word-final consonants in phonetic inventory:

- [p, t, d, k, m, n, s, z, l, ɹ] (Watson & Scukanec, 1997b)
- [p, t, d, k, (g), ʔ, m, n, ŋ, f, v, s, z, ʃ, ɹ, (ʧ)] (Dyson, 1988)

Four- to 5-year-old children are reported to have the following consonants in their phonetic inventory:

- [p, b, t, d, k, g, m, n, ŋ, h, θ, ð, f, v, s, z, ʃ, ʒ, h, ʧ, ʤ, ɹ, j, l, w] (Grunwell, 1987)

| TABLE 6-5 | Diadochokinesis (DDK) and maximum phonation time for children aged 3 to 5 years |

Task	3;0–3;5	3;6–3;11	4;0–4;5	4;6–4;11	5;0–5;5	5;6–5;11
/pʌ/	4.7/sec	4.8/sec	4.9/sec	4.6/sec	4.8/sec	5.1/sec
/tʌ/	4.6/sec	4.8/sec	4.8/sec	4.5/sec	4.8/sec	5.2/sec
/kʌ/	3.8/sec	4.8/sec	4.6/sec	4.3/sec	4.6/sec	4.9/sec
patticake	1.4/sec	1.8/sec	1.6/sec	1.3/sec	1.6/sec	1.7/sec
Maximum phonation time for /a/	5.5 sec	7.8 sec	8.0 sec	9.2 sec	8.1 sec	9.4 sec

/sec = per second.

Source: Adapted from Robbins & Klee (1987).

Phonetic inventory of consonant clusters

By 3 years, children can produce a range of word-initial clusters, and these typically contain /l/, /w/, or /s/. They can also produce word-final clusters such as [-nd, -nt, -ŋk]) (McLeod et al., 2001b). In a longitudinal study of 12 children, Watson and Scukanec (1997b) found that the 3-year-olds' word-initial and word-final consonant cluster inventory was: [st, sp, pl, -nd, -ts, -nt, -nz, -st, -ɪŋk]. Grunwell (1987) described 3- to 4-year-olds' consonant cluster inventory as containing obstruent + approximant and /s/ clusters (that may be "immature").

Phonetic inventory of vowels

Selby, Robb, and Gilbert (2000) studied four 3-year-old children from the United States and summarized the vowels in their inventory as: [i, ɪ, ɛ, e, u, ʊ, o, ʌ, ɔ, ɝ, ɑ, æ]. Robb and Gillon (2007) described the inventories of 20 three-year-old children in United States as [i, e, u, o, ɒ, ɪ, ɛ, æ, ə, ʌ, ɔ, ʊ, ɝ, ɚ] and New Zealand as [i, e, u, o, ɒ, ɪ, ɛ, æ, ə, ʌ, ɔ, ʊ] based on connected speech samples. If you recall from Chapter 4, the vowels produced by adults in these two countries are slightly different; consequently, both groups of children were able to produce vowels within their ambient dialect.

■ Syllable and word shape inventory

Between 3 and 5 years old, children's syllable and word shape inventory expands. Flipsen (2006a) indicated that the average number of syllables per word increased from 1.26 at 3;0 to 1.27 at 4;0 and 1.29 at 5;0. Shriberg (1993) found that 3- to 4-year-olds could produce words of the following syllable shapes: CV, VC, CVC, Cn_ or _Cn, two-syllable (where Cn indicates a consonant cluster). He indicated that 4- to 5-year-olds could produce words of the following syllable shapes: CV, VC, CVC, Cn_, _Cn, Cn_Cn, two-syllable, three-syllable.

■ Age of acquisition of consonants, consonant clusters, and vowels

Between 3 and 5 years is the time that children acquire (i.e., accurately produce) the majority of consonants, consonant clusters, and vowels.

Age of acquisition of consonants

One of the most commonly studied features of preschool children's speech is the age of acquisition of consonants, and the majority of English consonants are acquired between the ages of 3 and 5 years. According to Porter and Hodson (2001), "3-year-olds had acquired all major phoneme classes, except liquids ... sibilant lisps were still common until the age of 7 years" (p. 165). Table 6-6 provides a summary of age of acquisition of English consonants by children aged 2;0 to 9;0 from eight studies that were conducted in the United States, United Kingdom, and Australia. From this table, it is evident that plosives /p, b, t, d, k, g/ and nasals /m, n, ŋ/ are acquired early, with most studies showing that they are acquired before children are 4 years old. In contrast, while the fricatives /f/ and /h/ are acquired by 4 years old, the other fricatives take longer to acquire according to most studies. In fact, the voiceless interdental fricative /θ/ was acquired by 5 years in only three of the studies of English speech acquisition in Table 6-6. Thus, English consonants that are acquired after 5 years according to the majority of studies in Table 6-6 are /θ, ð/. Four additional consonants are acquired after 5 years according to at least two studies: /v, z, ɹ, l/.

Age of acquisition of consonant clusters

Three- to 5-year-old children can produce two-element word-initial /w/, /l/, and /ɹ/ consonant clusters correctly (e.g., /tw/ in *twin*, /pl/ in *plant*, /kɹ/ in *crash*). They can also produce some two-element word-initial /s/ consonant clusters (e.g., /sp/ in *spoon* and /st/ in *star*). Most three-element word-initial /s/ consonant clusters are not acquired by 6 years (see Table 6-7).

TABLE 6-6 Age of acquisition of English consonants for children aged 2 to 9 years

Gray cells indicate that the consonant was acquired after 5;11

Study	Arlt & Goodban (1976)	Chirlian & Sharpley (1982)		Dodd, Holm, et al. (2003)	Kilminster & Laird (1978)	Prather et al. (1975)	Smit et al. (1990)		Templin (1957)
Age range	3;0–6;0	2;0–9;0		3;0–6;11	3;0–9;0	2;0–4;0	3;0–9;0		3;0–8;0
Criterion	75%	75%		90%	75%	75%	75%		75%
No. of children in sample	240	1,357		684	1756	147	997		480
Sex	F&M	F	M	F&M	F&M	F&M	F	M	F&M
Plosives									
p	3;0	2;6	3;0	3;0	3;0	2;0	<3;0	<3;0	3;0
b	3;0	3;6	3;0	3;0	3;0	2;8	<3;0	<3;0	4;0
t	3;0	2;6	3;6	3;0	3;0	2;8	<3;0	<3;0	6;0
d	3;0	2;6	2;6	3;0	3;0	2;4	<3;0	<3;0	4;0
k	3;0	2;6	3;0	3;0	3;0	2;4	<3;0	<3;0	4;0
g	3;0	2;0	3;0	3;0	3;0	3;0	<3;0	<3;0	4;0
Nasals									
m	3;0	2;0	2;0	3;0	3;0	2;0	<3;0	<3;0	3;0
n	3;0	2;0	2;0	3;0	3;0	2;0	<3;0	<3;0	3;0
ŋ	3;0	2;6	2;6	3;0	3;0	2;0	5;6	6;0	3;0
Fricatives									
f	3;0	3;0	3;6	3;0	3;6	2;4	<3;0	3;6	3;0
v	3;6	5;0	9;0	3;0	6;0	>4;0	4;0	4;6	6;0
θ	5;0	7;6	8;0	*	8;6	>4;0	5;6	6;0	7;0
ð	5;0	7;6	7;6	*	8;0	4;0	4;0	5;6	6;0
s	4;0	3;6	4;0	3;0	4;6	3;0	3;0	5;0	4;6
z	4;0	9;0	**	3;0	4;6	>4;0	5;0	6;0	7;0
ʃ	4;6	3;6	3;6	5;0	4;0	3;8	4;0	5;0	4;6
ʒ	4;0	4;0	4;6	4;0	4;6	4;0	—	—	7;0
h	3;0	2;0	3;0	3;0	3;0	2;0	<3;0	<3;0	3;0
Approximants									
ɹ	5;0	5;0	5;0	6;0	5;0	3;4	6;0	5;6	4;0
j	—	3;0	3;6	3;0	3;0	2;4	3;6	3;6	3;6
l	4;0	4;0	3;6	3;0	4;0	3;4	4;6	6;0	6;0
w	3;0	2;6	3;0	3;0	3;0	2;8	<3;0	<3;0	3;0
Affricates									
tʃ	4;0	3;6	3;6	3;0	4;0	3;8	4;0	5;0	4;6
dʒ	4;0	4;0	3;6	4;0	4;6	>4;0	4;6	4;0	7;0

— = not assessed; * = not achieved by 6;11; ** = not achieved by 9;0. F = female, M = male.

TABLE 6-7	Age of acquisition of word-initial English consonant clusters for children aged 3 to 12 years

Gray cells indicate that the consonant was acquired by or after 5;11

Study	McLeod & Arciuli (2009)	Smit et al. (1990)		Templin (1957)
Age range	5;0–12;11	3;0–9;0		3;0–8;0
Criterion	90%	75%		75%
No. of children in sample	74	997		480
Sex	F&M	F	M	F&M
/w/ clusters				
tw	—	3;6	3;6	4;0
kw	—	3;6	3;6	4;0
/l/ clusters				
pl	—	4;0	5;6	4;0
bl	—	4;0	5;0	4;0
kl	—	4;0	5;6	4;0
gl	—	4;6	4;6	4;0
fl	—	4;6	5;6	5;0
/ɹ/ clusters				
pɹ	9;0–10;0	6;0	5;6	4;0
bɹ	5;0–6;0	6;0	6;0	4;0
tɹ	5;0–6;0	6;0	5;6	4;0
dɹ	5;0–6;0	6;0	5;0	4;0
kɹ	5;0–6;0	4;6	5;6	4;0
gɹ	5;0–6;0	6;0	5;6	4;6
fɹ	7;0–8;0	6;0	5;6	4;6
θɹ	9;0–10;0	7;0	7;0	6;0
2-element /s/ clusters				
sp	5;0–6;0	4;6	5;0	4;0
st	5;0–6;0	4;6	5;0	4;0
sk	5;0–6;0	4;6	6;0	4;0
sm	5;0–6;0	5;6	7;0	4;0
sn	5;0–6;0	6;0	5;0	4;0
sl	5;0–6;0	6;0	7;0	4;0
sw	5;0–6;0	4;6	6;0	6;0
3-element /s/ clusters				
spl	7;0–8;0	6;0	7;0	6;0
spɹ	9;0–10;0	8;0	8;0	5;0
stɹ	5;0–6;0	8;0	8;0	5;0
skw	5;0–6;0	4;6	7;0	6;0
skɹ	5;0–6;0	8;0	8;0	6;0

— = not assessed, F = female, M = male.

> ### COMMENT: *Early-8, middle-8, and late-8 consonants*
>
> Many SLPs use the terms *early-8*, *middle-8*, and *late-8* to describe consonant mastery. This terminology is not based on the acquisition of speech by typically developing children. Here is how the concept developed. The consonant mastery of a group of 64 three- to six-year-old children with SSD was studied by Shriberg, Kwiatkowski, and Gruber (1992). Later, Shriberg (1993) used these data to divide the 24 English consonants into three groups of eight sounds based on the average number of consonants correct during spontaneous conversational speech.
>
> Early-8 (averaging over 75% correct): /m, b, j, n, w, d, p, h/
> Middle-8 (averaging 25%–75% correct): /t, ŋ, k, g, f, v, ʧ, ʤ/
> Late-8 (averaging less than 25% correct): /ʃ, θ, s, z, ð, l, ɹ, ʒ/

Age of acquisition of vowels

According to Donegan (2002), ". . . most studies suggest that vowel production is reasonably accurate by age 3, although some studies call this into question" (p. 2). Paradigmatic production (i.e., production of individual vowels in words such as *moon* /mun/) is generally mastered by 3 years. However, syntagmatic production (production of vowels in contexts such as polysyllabic words) takes up to at least 6 years (James, van Doorn & McLeod, 2001).

◼ Percentage of consonants, consonant clusters, and vowels correct

Data for the percentage of consonants correct across studies of English-speaking children are presented in Table 6-8. Young children typically produce more vowels correctly than consonants and consonant clusters. Non-rhotic vowels (e.g., /i, a/) are more likely to be correct at a younger age than rhotic vowels (e.g., /ɝ/). Most studies indicate that by 5 years of age children can produce over 90% of vowels, consonants, and consonant clusters correctly.

◼ Common mismatches

Smit determined common mismatches for the production of consonants (Smit, 1993a) and consonant clusters (Smit, 1993b) by children aged 2;0 to 9;0. Common mismatches that occurred at least 15% of the time by children aged between 2 and 3 years old were listed in the previous section outlining speech acquisition for 1- to 3-year-olds. Common mismatches that occurred at least 15% of the time by children aged between 4 and 5 years old were rare, mostly related to the production of consonant clusters, and are listed below:

- ◼ Stops (word-final position): /t/ → Ø
- ◼ Fricatives (word-initial position): /θ/ → [f]; /s/ → [s̺]
- ◼ Fricatives (word-final position): /θ/ → [f]; /s/ → [s̺]
- ◼ Approximants (word-initial position): /ɹ/ → [w]
- ◼ Approximants (word-final position): /l/ → vowel (Smit, 1993a)
- ◼ /l/ consonant clusters: /pl/ → [pw], /bl/ → [bw], /kl/ → [kw], /gl/ → [gw], /fl/ → [fw], /sl/ → [s̺]
- ◼ /ɹ/ consonant clusters: /pɹ/ → [pw]; /bɹ/ → [bw]; /tɹ/ → [tw]; /dɹ/ → [dw]; /kɹ/ → [kw]; /gɹ/ → [gw]; /fɹ/ → [fw]; /θɹ/ → [fɹ]
- ◼ /s/ consonant clusters (2 element): /sn/ → [s̺n], /st/ → [s̺t]
- ◼ /s/ consonant clusters (3 element): /skw/ → [s̺kw]; /spl/ → [s̺pl, spw]; /spɹ/ → [s̺pɹ, spw]; /stɹ/ → [s̺tɹ, stw]; /skɹ/ → [s̺kɹ, skw] (Smit, 1993b)

TABLE 6-8	Percentage correct for English consonants, consonant clusters, and vowels for children aged 3;0 to 5;11 years

Blank cells indicate that the age range was not studied

Aspect	Study	Age					
		3;0	3;6	4;0	4;6	5;0	5;6
Consonants	Dodd et al. (2003)	82.1%		90.4%			
	James, van Doorn & McLeod (2002)	76.8% (SD = 10.8; range = 51–97) (MSW)		84.0% (SD = 7.6; range = 65–97) (MSW)		89.5% (SD = 7.3; range = 68–98) (MSW)	
	James, van Doorn & McLeod (2002)	76.4% (SD = 7.0; range = 63–85) (PSW)		82.5% (SD = 5.6; range = 66–93) (PSW)		88.4% (SD = 6.1; range = 71–95) (PSW)	
	Waring, Fisher, & Aitken (2001)		85.2%	88.5%		93.4%	
	Watson & Scukanec (1997b)	86.2% (range 73–99)					
	Pollock (2002)	91.5 (SD = 4.9)	92.6% (SD = 4.1)	92.9% (SD = 5.1)	94.2% (SD = 4.0)	93.3% (SD = 4.1)	95.9% (SD = 3.9)
	Ballard, Wilson, Campbell, Purdy, & Yee (2011)					92.4%	92.7%
Consonant clusters	McLeod & Arciuli (2009)					92.4%	
	Waring, Fisher, Aitken (2001)		86.4%	88.1%		94.9%	
Vowels (non-rhotic)	Dodd, Holm, et al. (2003)	97.4%		98.9%			
	James, van Doorn, & McLeod (2001)	94.9% (SD = 3.9, range = 88–95) (MSW)		95.2% (SD = 1.8, range = 92–99) (MSW)		94.9% (SD = 1.5, range = 91–97) (MSW)	
	James, van Doorn, & McLeod (2001)	88.3% (SD = 3.2, range = 80–92) (PSW)		92.0% (SD = 2.5, range = 86–97) (PSW)		94.3% (SD = 2.5, range = 88–100) (PSW)	
	Pollock, 2002; Pollock & Berni (2003)	97.3% (range = 89–100)	97.2% (range = 91–100)	98% (range = 91–100)	99% (range = 94–100)		
	Ballard, Wilson, Campbell, Purdy, & Yee (2011)					98.0%	98.3%
Vowels (rhotic)	Pollock (2002)	79.2% (range = 4–100)	76.5% (range = 4–100)	90.1% (range = 37–100)	86.8% (0–100)		

MSW = monosyllabic words; PSW = polysyllabic words.

It is interesting to note that common mismatches for consonant clusters preserved the number of elements (i.e., 2 element clusters contained two consonants, 3 element clusters contained three consonants), whereas in children younger than 3;0 the most common realizations were the deletion of consonants within the consonant cluster.

▪ Phonological processes

As children's speech matures, there are fewer phonological processes occurring. The following phonological processes are still occurring in the speech of 3- to 5-year-old children:

weak syllable deletion, final consonant deletion, cluster reduction, fronting, stopping, deaffrication, and gliding. Reduplication and context sensitive voicing rarely occurred within this age group (see Table 6-9).

■ Prosody

Children's speaking rate was determined by Robb and Gillon (2007). They found that in the United States, 3-year-old children produced an average of 208 syllables per minute and 8.17 phones/sec; whereas in New Zealand, 3-year-old children spoke more slowly. They produced an average of 182 syllables per minute and 7.15 phones/sec.

Children's ability to produce and differentiate stressed and unstressed syllables continues to develop during the preschool years. Kehoe (2001) stated: ". . . after 2 years of age, deletion of stressed syllables is relatively infrequent, and after 3 years of age, deletion of unstressed syllables is less frequent" (p. 291). By 3 years of age, children typically have mastered trochaic stress patterns (i.e., strong-weak stress patterns, such as in the word _garden_ or _butterfly_). However, it takes until approximately 7 years for children to master words with non-final weak syllables in words, such as _ambulance, behind, caterpillar, computer, potato,_ and _vegetables_ (Ballard, Djaja, Arciuli, James, & van Doorn, 2012; James, van Doorn, McLeod, & Esterman, 2008).

TABLE 6-9 Phonological processes reported to be used by children from 3;0 to 7;11 (mean occurrence > 10%)

PHONOLOGICAL PROCESS	3;0	3;6	4;0	4;6	5;0	5;6	6;0	6;6	7;0
SYLLABLE STRUCTURE PROCESSES									
Weak syllable deletion	D, G, HM, J	D, (G) HM, J	HM, J	HM, J	HM, J	J	J	J	J
Reduplication									
Final consonant deletion	(G), HM, J	HM, J	J	HM, J	J	J	J	J	J
Cluster reduction	D, G, HM, J, RBF	D, (G), HM, J, RBF	HM, J, RBF	HM, J	J	J	J	J	J
SUBSTITUTION (SYSTEMIC) PROCESSES									
Fronting	D, (G), HM, J	D, J	J	J	J				
Stopping	D, G, HM, J, WS	G, HM, J	G, J	G, J	(G) J	J	J	J	J
Deaffrication	D, J	D, J	D, J	D, J			J	J	J
Gliding of liquids	D, (G), HM, J, RBF	D, (G), HM, J	D, (G) HM, J	D, (G), HM, J	D, (G) J	D, J	J	J	J
Context sensitive voicing (CSV)									
Consonant cluster simplification	WS								
Fricative simplification	J	J	J	J	J	J	J	J	J
ASSIMILATION									
Assimilation	HM, J	HM, J	HM, J						

D = Dodd, Holm, et al. (2003); G = Grunwell (1987); HM = Haelsig & Madison (1986); J = James (2001a); RBF = Roberts, Burchinal, & Footo (1990); WS = Watson & Scukanec (1997b) (only tested 2;0–3;0). James (2001a) was based on small sample sizes in each age group (typically < 10 children) and relied on production in polysyllabic as well as monosyllabic words.

Acoustic analysis of children's acquisition of lexical stress confirms that consistency in the length of segment durations (particularly unstressed syllables) continues to be refined during the preschool years and until at least 7 years (Allen & Hawkins, 1980; Kim & Stoel-Gammon, 2010).

■ Phonological awareness

Phonological awareness skills are precursors to literacy and involve syllable-level awareness, onset-rime (rhyme) awareness, and phonemic awareness (Rvachew & Grawburg, 2006). Three-year-old children can demonstrate awareness of rhyming words (MacLean, Bryant, & Bradley, 1987).

Carroll, Snowling, Stevenson, and Hulme (2003) studied 62 children aged 3;2 to 4;5 prior to formal school entry and then twice more within the year, as many entered formal schooling. They compared the children's skills in syllable, rime, and phoneme awareness and letter knowledge over time. They found that children's syllable and rime awareness preceded and predicted children's phoneme awareness skills and were associated with their articulation of speech sounds. Anthony, Lonigan, Driscoll, Phillips, and Burgess (2003) studied 947 children aged 2 to 5 years and similarly found that children's skills in manipulating syllables preceded their ability to manipulate smaller units such as individual phonemes. They demonstrated that after children could identify individual phonemes, then they learn skills to:

- Blend onset + rime /s/ + /it/ = /sit/
- Blend individual phonemes /s/ + /i/ + /t/ = /sit/
- Segment words into phonemes /sit/ = /s/ + /i/ + /t/
- Delete phonemes /sit/ /s/ = /it/

The acquisition of skills in the perception and production of speech, as well as phonological awareness skills, lays the foundation for children's ability to read and write.

Speech Acquisition for English-Speaking School-Aged Children from 6 Years

There are still a few speech skills that remain to be learned from 6 years old. Most relate to fine motor movements to produce consonants such as /θ/, consonant clusters, and appropriate stress within polysyllabic words. By 6 years of age, most English-speaking children have begun formal schooling, and have begun to learn to read and write. This places additional demands on children's phonological knowledge as they move from an oral to literate expression of their phonological knowledge. Indeed, the **critical age hypothesis** proposed by Bishop and Adams (1990) suggests: "children who have speech difficulties that persist to the point at which they need to use phonological skills for learning to read are at high risk for reading problems" (Nathan, Stackhouse, Goulandris, & Snowling, 2004a, p. 378). Difficulties with speech and literacy are covered in other chapters; however, it is important to keep in mind the interrelationship between speech and literacy when considering typical speech acquisition for children aged 6 years and older.

■ Oral mechanism

Between the ages of 5 and 7, children start to lose their primary teeth, beginning with their incisors (recall the photographs in Chapter 3). As the years progress, their 32 permanent (adult) teeth emerge. By 6 years of age, a child's skull reaches adult size. The lower face grows from the ages of 7 to 10 years, and the tongue and lips grow between ages 9 and 13. The mandible, tongue, and lips continue to grow until 16 years for girls and 18 years for boys (Bauman-Waengler, 2014). Throughout childhood and into late adolescence, refinement of tongue-tip, tongue-body, and jaw movements for speech continues (Cheng, Murdoch, Goozée, & Scott, 2007).

CHILDREN'S INSIGHTS: *What is it like to lose your two front teeth?* *(by Adelaide, 6;9 years)*

Elise: "Tell me what it is like to have your two top front teeth missing." (See Figure 6-3.)

Adelaide: "It feels very weird when I say /f/ because my lip just goes into the big tooth gap and when I say /s/ more air comes out of my mouth than before. It's hard to make my 'es' sharp. My tongue just goes through the big hole because my teeth use to stop my tongue from getting out. It's weird also when I bite something because nothing happens at my front teeth because they are missing. When I drink water though, I don't have to really open my mouth because the water just goes through the gap."

Elise: "What are you looking forward to when you get your grown-up front teeth?"

Adelaide: "I'm looking forward to getting big teeth so I can bite again, smile properly, open my drink bottle with my teeth, and so I can say my 'es' sharply."

FIGURE 6-3 **Adelaide's mixed dentition two months later at 6;11 years as her "grown-up front teeth" began to grow** *(You also saw Adelaide's teeth in Chapter 3.)*

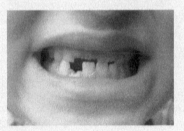

Source: Used by permission from Elise Baker.

Diadochokinesis (DDK) and maximum phonation time

Typically developing 6-year-old children can produce five syllables per second on a diadochokinesis (DDK) task and can sustain the vowel /a/ for 10 to 11 seconds (see Table 6-10, adapted from Robbins & Klee, 1987).

TABLE 6-10 **Diadochokinesis (DDK) and maximum phonation time for children aged 6 to 7 years**

Task	6;0–6;5	6;6–6;11
/pʌ/	5.4/sec	5.5/sec
/tʌ/	5.3/sec	5.4/sec
/kʌ/	4.9/sec	4.9/sec
patticake	1.6/sec	1.6/sec
Maximum phonation time for /a/	11.0 sec	11.5 sec

/sec = per second.

Source: Adapted from Robbins & Klee (1987).

■ Intelligibility

Six-year-olds are intelligible (Gordon-Brannan, 1994). Specifically, according to Flipsen (2006b), transcribers can reliably understand 98.43% (91.67–100.00%) of words spoken by 6-year-olds, 99.51% (97.36–100.00%) of words spoken by 7-year-olds, and 99.01% (97.07–100.00%) of words spoken by 8-year-olds. Note the very small range in the older children, indicating that there is limited variability between children.

■ Phonetic inventory

English-speaking children who are 6 years and older typically have all English consonants [p, b, t, d, k, g, m, n, ŋ, f, v, θ, ð, w, s, z, ʃ, ʒ, h, ʧ, ʤ ɹ, j, l, w] and vowels within their inventory (Grunwell, 1987). In addition, they will have most consonant clusters within their inventory.

■ Syllable and word shape inventory

English-speaking children who are 6 years old are able to produce all English syllable shapes (Shriberg, 1993). Flipsen (2006a) indicated that the average number of syllables per word increased from 1.30 at 6;0 to 1.32 at 7;0 and 1.33 at 8;0.

■ Age of acquisition of consonants, consonant clusters, and vowels

By the time children reach 6 years old there are few consonants, consonant clusters, or vowels left to master. Earlier in this chapter, Table 6-6 documented when English consonants were acquired by children aged 2;0 to 9;0 years, with shaded cells indicating that the consonant was acquired after 5;11 years. According to this table, the fricatives /v, θ, ð, z/ and the approximant /ɹ/ are among the latest consonants to be acquired by typically developing English-speaking children. Six-year-old children can produce most two-element word-initial consonant clusters correctly (see Table 6-7); however, during the school years children are still mastering some two-element word-initial /ɹ/ and /s/ consonant clusters (e.g., /θɹ/ in *three*) and most three-element word-initial /s/ consonant clusters (e.g., /spl/ in *splash*) (see Table 6-7). While many vowels are mastered at a young age, there are still aspects of vowel production that extend into the school years. Paradigmatic production (i.e., production of individual vowels) is generally mastered by 3 years. However, syntagmatic production (i.e., production of vowels in context such as polysyllabic words) takes up to at least 6 years of age (James et al., 2001). Even older children are challenged by the timing of vowels, particularly schwa /ə/ within polysyllabic words such as *hippopotamus*.

COMMENT: Hippopotamus *is so hard to say*

Deb James titled her Ph.D. thesis *Hippopotamus Is So Hard to Say: Children's Acquisition of Polysyllabic Words* (James, 2006). Within her thesis she described how the acquisition of polysyllabic words lasted until at least 7;11 years. She described the "complex interaction between segmental and prosodic features" (p. 268). The most difficult words for children to produce correctly were *ambulance, animals, caterpillar, elephant, escalators, hippopotamus,* and *spaghetti.* She described the features of these words that made them difficult as: "non-final weak syllables, within-word consonant sequences that often required an anterior-posterior movement, velar and liquid sounds, and segments that shared manner or place features" (p. 240).

■ Percentage of consonants, consonant clusters, and vowels correct

By 6 years of age, the percentage of consonants, consonant clusters, and vowels that are produced correctly is above 90% (see Table 6-11). The only exception is that rhotic vowels are still difficult to produce, and, as can be seen by the range in Table 6-11, Pollock (2002) has indicated that some children who are 6 and above are still unable to produced rhotic vowels correctly.

TABLE 6-11 **Percentage correct for English consonants, consonant clusters, and vowels for children aged 5;6 to 12 years**
Blank cells indicate that the age range was not studied

Aspect	Study	Age								
		5;6	6;0	6;6	7;0	8;0	9;0	10;0	11;0	12;0
Consonants	Dodd, Holm, et al. (2003)		95.9%							
	James, van Doorn, & McLeod (2002)		93.7% (SD = 4.0; range = 81–100) (MSW)		93.9% (SD = 4.7; range = 79–99) (MSW)					
	James, van Doorn, & McLeod (2002)		90.8% (SD = 3.7; range = 79–99) (PSW)		91.0% (SD = 4.1; range = 75–97) (PSW)					
	Pollock (2002)		97.2%	93.1%						
	Waring, Fisher, Aitken (2001)		95.1%		98.4%					
Consonant clusters	Waring, Fisher, Aitken (2001)		96.6%		98.3%					
	McLeod & Arciuli (2009)		92.4%		89.7%			96.5%		98.8%
Vowels (non-rhotic)	Dodd, Holm, et al. (2003)		99.2%							
	James, van Doorn, & McLeod (2001)		95.4% (SD = 1.7, range = 91–97) (MSW)		95.1% (SD = 1.4, range = 88–97) (MSW)					
	James, van Doorn, & McLeod (2001)		94.9% (SD = 2.0, range = 87–99) (PSW)		95.4% (SD = 1.8, range = 89–100) (PSW)					
	Pollock, 2002; Pollock & Berni (2003)		98.5% (SD = 1.3; range = 94–100)	99.2% (SD= -; range = n/a)						
Vowels (rhotic)	Pollock (2002)		77.2% (SD = 42.2; range = 2–100)							

MSW = monosyllabic words; PSW = polysyllabic words.

■ Prosody

Mastery of the complexity of adult intonation patterns extends into the school years, with children over the age of 10 years still developing these skills (Cruttenden, 1982).

■ Phonological awareness and literacy

Children's entry into formal schooling typically heralds the acquisition of literacy skills (reading and writing). However, as discussed earlier in this chapter, children have been developing phonological awareness skills including syllable-level awareness, onset-rime (rhyme) awareness, and phonemic awareness. Phoneme identification often emerges around the time of transition to formal schooling (Paulson et al., 2003). You will learn more about the importance of including phonological awareness and letter knowledge activities as a component of intervention for young children with SSD in Chapters 13 and 14.

PART 3: TYPICAL SPEECH ACQUISITION FOR ALL CHILDREN

Many SLPs work in settings where they see children who speak many different languages. The remainder of this chapter has been designed to support clinicians to understand general trends in acquisition across languages. Studies based on monolingual and multilingual children who speak a range of languages provide us with insights into typical speech acquisition for all children, regardless of the languages spoken. Some of these studies have examined more than one language at once and have made comparisons between speech acquisition for children who speak different languages (e.g., German-Turkish, Maltese-English, Spanish-English), whereas most studies have considered speech acquisition for a group of children who speak one language (e.g., Cantonese, Norwegian, Spanish). The summary of cross-linguistic trends in children's speech acquisition below is based on McLeod (2010, 2012b) and relies on information from over 250 studies of typical speech acquisition described within McLeod (2007a). Additional information is available in Goldstein and McLeod (2012) and Hua and Dodd (2006).

There is a famous quote from Jakobson (1941/1968) that subsequently has not been proven:

> Whether it is a question of French or Scandinavian children, of English or Slavic, or Indian or German, or of Estonian, Dutch or Japanese children, every description based on careful observation repeatedly confirms the striking fact that the relative chronological order of phonological acquisitions remains everywhere and at all times the same ... the speed of this succession is, in contrast, exceedingly variable and individual and two "newly added phenomena" which directly succeed each other in one child can in another child be separated by many months, and even by years. (Jakobson, 1941/1968, p. 46)

Since Jakobson's famous quote, we have been able to study children's speech acquisition with greater breadth and depth. We have found that there are both similarities and differences between the acquisition of speech by children learning different languages. In a systematic review of 66 studies describing 23 bilingual populations, Hambly, Wren, McLeod, and Roulstone (2013) indicated that the research revealed a complex picture of rate of acquisition of phonemes, with some studies showing:

■ no difference in rate of acquisition;
■ slower acquisition; or
■ accelerated acquisition compared with monolingual English peers.

They found that typically bilingual children showed a different pattern of development to monolingual peers and that most studies provided evidence of transfer between languages, but the amount of transfer varied.

■ Intelligibility

Children's intelligibility primarily has been studied for speakers of English, Finnish, and Portuguese. Overall, 2-year-olds are intelligible at least 50% of the time (more often with

> ### MULTICULTURAL INSIGHTS: *Children's acquisition of Spanish*
>
> The typical age of acquisition of Spanish consonants has been examined in the following studies:
>
> - De la Fuenta (1985) studied 55 monolingual Dominican Spanish-speaking children aged 23–77 months in the Dominican Republic.
> - Fabiano-Smith and Goldstein (2010a, b) studied 24 children aged 36–48 months in the United States: eight monolingual Spanish-speaking children, eight bilingual Spanish-English-speaking children, and eight monolingual English-speaking children.
> - Jimenez (1987) studied 120 mono- and multilingual Mexican Spanish-speaking children aged 36–67 months in the United States.
> - Linares (1981) studied 97 monolingual Mexican Spanish-speaking children aged 36–83 months in Mexico and an additional 14 multilingual Mexican Spanish-speaking children in the United States.
>
> Fabiano-Smith and Goldstein (2010b) compared the three groups of children described above. They found that the children exhibited a similar pattern of early-, middle-, and late-8 acquisition for English consonants when compared with Shriberg (1993). For Spanish, they found the following pattern:
>
> - Early 6: /ŋ, t, m, n, k, x/
> - Middle 6: /s, f, p, ʧ, β, ɣ/
> - Late 4: /l, ð, r, ɾ/

their parents), whereas 4- and 5-year-olds' speech is intelligible most of the time, even to strangers. For example, Luotonen (1998) studied 1,618 Finnish-speaking children's intelligibility and found that only 6.9% of 3-year-old boys and 1.9% of 3-year-old girls' speech was not intelligible.

◼ Phonetic inventory

Young children's phonetic inventories (i.e., consonants and vowels produced regardless of the adult target) have been studied in many languages including Arabic, Cantonese, English, Finnish, and Maltese. Vowels, nasals, and plosives appear to be the earliest sounds to be produced by children. Children produce more sounds and greater articulatory variation as they grow older. For example, consonants within the phonetic inventories of at least five of 13 Jordanian Arabic 1- to 2-year-olds were plosives [b, d, t, ʔ], fricatives [ʃ, ʕ, ħ, h], nasals [m, n], a lateral [l], and approximants [w, j] (Amayreh & Dyson, 2000). Phonetic inventories of 21 Maltese children aged 2;0 contained nasals [m, n], plosives [p, b, t, d, k, ʔ], a fricative [h], and approximants [w, l, j] (Grech, 1998).

◼ Syllable and word shape inventory

There are very few languages for which studies have been made of children's acquisition of syllable and word shape inventories. CV has been found to be a universal syllable shape (Locke, 1983) and is the earliest syllable structure to emerge in many languages. The next syllable shapes to emerge are CVC (e.g., English, Israeli Hebrew, Maltese, Spanish), V (e.g., Korean), and VC (e.g., Israeli Hebrew, Spanish). For example, Goldstein and Cintrón (2001) examined the syllable inventories of three monolingual Puerto Rican Spanish-speaking children aged 1;10, 2;4, and 2;5. The majority of syllables produced by the children were CV (67%), followed by V (22%), CVC (7%), VC (4%), and CCVC (1%). The majority of words contained two syllables (67%), and the remaining words were one-syllable (25%), three-syllable (6%), four-syllable (2%), and five-syllable (1%) words.

■ Mastery of consonants and vowels

Children's age of acquisition of consonants has been studied in many different languages. For example, MacLeod, Sutton, Trudeau, and Thordardottir (2011) examined the acquisition of consonants by 156 French-speaking children aged 20 to 53 months in Québec, Canada. They found three stages of consonant acquisition: (1) /t, m, n, z/ were acquired before 36 months; (2) /p, b, d, k, g, ɲ, f, v, ʁ, l, w, ɥ/ were acquired between 36 and 53 months; and (3) /s, ʒ, ʃ, j/ were acquired after 53 months.

Within the international speech acquisition literature, there is wide diversity of reported ages (> 2;6 years) of the acquisition of consonants, even for languages sharing similar consonants. In contrast, children's acquisition of vowels has been studied in very few languages, mostly English and Cantonese; however, from the limited data available, it appears that vowels are acquired earlier than consonants. For example, a large cross-sectional study of the acquisition of Cantonese was undertaken in Hong Kong. To, Cheung, and McLeod (2013a) studied the age of acquisition of consonants, vowels, and tones in 1,726 children aged 2;4 to 12;4 years (see Table 6-12). The majority of consonants were acquired by 4;6, whereas most vowels, diphthongs, and tones were acquired by 2;6.

■ Percentage of consonants, consonant clusters, and vowels correct

Many languages have documented the percentage of consonants correct, including English, Finnish, French, German, Hungarian, Putonghua, and Welsh. Overall, it appears that 2-year-olds produce consonants correctly at least 70% of the time, whereas 5-year-olds produce consonants correctly at least 90% of the time. For example, Fox and Dodd (1999) studied 178 German-speaking children to determine the percentage of consonants incorrect (PCI) (notice, that this is the reverse of the percentage of consonants correct). They found a progression, similar to that found across the world:

TABLE 6-12   Age of acquisition of Cantonese consonants, vowels, diphthongs, and tones

Age	Word-initial consonants (males)	Word-initial consonants (females)	Word-final consonants (males + females)	Vowels (males + females)	Diphthongs (males + females)	Tones (males + females)
2;6	p-	p-, ŋ-/Ø-		i, a, u, ɔ, ɛ, ɪ	ɔi, ai, ɐi, ɵy, ou, au	All 9 tones
3;0	j-, m-	j-, w-, m-	-k	y	ui, ei, iu, ɛu	
3;6	pʰ-, f-, h-, w-, ŋ-/Ø-	pʰ-, t-, f-, h-	-t	ʊ, ɐ		
4;0	t-, l-	k-, kʰ-, kʷ-, kʷʰ-, l-		œ	ɐu	
4;6	tʰ-, kʷ-, ts-	tʰ-, ts-, tsʰ-	-p, -m, -n, -ŋ	ɵ		
5;0	k-, kʰ-, kʷʰ-		-k			
5;6						
6;0	tsʰ-, s-	s-				

Note: The word-final consonants /-n, -ŋ, -t/ were not acquired by the oldest children; however, this may be due to acceptable variants in the production of Cantonese.

Source: Adapted from To, Cheung, & McLeod (2013a).

1;6–1;11 PCI = 26.05% (SD = 11.1)

2;6–2;11 PCI = 12.59% (SD = 8.1)

3;6–3;11 PCI = 5.75% (SD = 4.1)

4;6–4;11 PCI = 3.80% (SD = 4.0)

5;6–5;11 PCI = 1.92% (SD = 2.3)

(Note: Additional data were available for the intervening ages, but were not reproduced here.)

■ Common mismatches

Common mismatches have been considered within a few languages, including English, Greek, Japanese, Hungarian, and Dutch. Although there are some similarities, common mismatches do differ between languages. For example, common mismatches for /s/ include: [t] (e.g., English, Dutch, Finnish, Hungarian, and Portuguese), dentalized [s̪] (e.g., English), [ɮ] (e.g., Greek), palatalized fricative (e.g., Japanese), and [ʃ] (e.g., Israeli Hebrew).

■ Phonological processes

Phonological processes have been described as occurring in many languages (McLeod, 2007a, 2010). Processes that are considered to be atypical in some languages (e.g., backing in English) are considered to be typical in others (e.g., backing in Cantonese). Common systemic simplifications include:

- Fronting (e.g., Jordanian Arabic, Lebanese Arabic, Cantonese, English, German, Greek, Israeli Hebrew, Japanese, Korean, Maltese, Norwegian, Portuguese, Putonghua, Thai, Turkish, Welsh)
- Backing (e.g., Lebanese Arabic, Cantonese, Greek, Japanese, Norwegian, Putonghua, Thai, Vietnamese)
- Stopping (e.g., Lebanese Arabic, Cantonese, Dutch, English, German, Greek, Israeli Hebrew, Japanese, Korean, Maltese, Norwegian, Portuguese, Putonghua, Thai, Turkish, Welsh)
- Gliding/liquid deviation (e.g., Lebanese Arabic, Dutch, English, French, Korean, Maltese, Portuguese, Putonghua, Turkish, Welsh)
- Devoicing (e.g., Jordanian Arabic, Lebanese Arabic, Dutch, German, Hungarian, Israeli Hebrew, Maltese, Norwegian)
- Voicing (e.g., English, German, Norwegian, Turkish, Welsh)

Common structural simplifications include:

- Assimilation/consonant harmony (e.g., Cantonese, Dutch, English, French, Greek, Maltese, Norwegian, Portuguese, Putonghua, Turkish, Welsh)
- Cluster reduction (e.g., Dutch, English, French, Greek, Israeli Hebrew, Maltese, Spanish, Thai, Turkish, Welsh)
- Initial consonant deletion (e.g., Finnish, Maltese, Spanish, Thai)
- Final consonant deletion (e.g., Jordanian Arabic, Cantonese, Dutch, English, German, Greek, Israeli Hebrew, Korean, Maltese, Portuguese, Putonghua, Spanish, Thai, Turkish, Welsh)
- Reduplication (e.g., Dutch, English, Greek, Korean, Turkish, Welsh)
- (Weak) syllable deletion (e.g., Jordanian Arabic, Dutch, English, Finnish, French, German, Israeli Hebrew, Japanese, Maltese, Norwegian, Portuguese, Spanish, Turkish, Welsh)

■ Prosody

Acquisition of prosody involves acquisition of intonation, stress, and tones. The acquisition of intonation has been studied in only a few languages. There is evidence that language-specific intonation patterns begin between 1 and 2 years of age (e.g., English and

Hungarian) and is not fully acquired until at least 5 years. Perception continues to develop until 10 and 11 years (Wells, Peppé, & Goulandris, 2004). Acquisition of stress appears to be language-dependent. Children acquire stress very early in some languages, particularly those with predictable stress patterns. For example, Israeli Hebrew has stress on the word-final syllable, and there were only 12 errors in the production stress patterns in Ben-David's (2001) comprehensive longitudinal analysis of 10 children's acquisition of speech and language. In contrast, children acquire stress later in languages with variable stress placement (e.g., Dutch and English). Finally, tones have been reported to be acquired by 2-year-olds in studies of Cantonese (To et al., 2013a) and Putonghua (Mandarin) (Hua, 2002).

Chapter summary

In this chapter you learned there are two ways to consider typical speech acquisition: (1) "statistical similarity or frequency" and (2) "desirability or acceptability" (Thomas, 2000, p. 101). You also learned about factors influencing typical speech acquisition, theories of child development, and methodological issues in research on children's speech acquisition. The final half of this chapter provided a summary of studies of typical speech acquisition for English-speaking children organized according to three age groups (0–2 years, 3–5 years, 6+ years). You are encouraged to consider both the information about typical speech acquisition summarized within this chapter but also to consider each child within his or her milieu and listen as anthropologists to the speech of those within their local communities. The significance of considering each child as a unique individual cannot be overemphasized when making decisions about typical speech acquisition.

Recommended reading

The following books provide extensive information about children's speech acquisition in English and many other languages:

- Hua, Z., & Dodd, B. (Eds.) (2006). *Phonological development and disorders in children: A multilingual perspective*. Clevedon, UK: Multilingual Matters.

- McLeod, S. (Ed.). (2007a). *The international guide to speech acquisition*. Clifton Park, NY: Thomson Delmar Learning.

Application of knowledge from Chapter 6

Apply your knowledge about typical speech acquisition by completing the following tasks.

1. Luke (4;3 years) and Michael (4;2 years) are both preschool-age children profiled in Chapter 16. What errors would you expect to see in Luke and Michael's speech, if they had typically developing speech?
2. Prepare a brochure for parents about typical speech acquisition including (1) what to expect of children from birth to age 6 years, (2) examples of typical speech production errors, and (3) warning signs for children of different ages.

3. Review the speech samples for Luke (4;3 years), Susie (7;4 years), Jarrod (7;0 years), Michael (4;2 years), and Lian (14;2 years) from Chapter 16. Do you notice any typical errors? Do you notice any atypical errors? (Remember to consider the languages that the children are learning, and the types of errors that are typical of those languages.)
4. Read more about Luke (4;3 years, Case 1), Susie (7;4 years, Case 2), Jarrod (7;0 years, Case 3), Michael (4;2 years, Case 4), and Lian (14;2 years, Case 5) in Chapter 16.

Appendix 6-1. Summary of studies of English-speaking children's speech acquisition

Authors	Year	Country	No. of children	Age of children	Sample type	Data collection method
Anthony, Bogle, Ingram, & McIsaac	1971	UK	510	3;0–6;0	SW	Cross-sectional
Arlt & Goodban	1976	USA	240	3;0–6;0	SW	Cross-sectional
Ballard Wilson, Campbell, Purdy, & Yee	2011	New Zealand	106	5;0–5;11	SW	Cross-sectional
Ballard, Djaja, Arciuli, James, & van Doorn	2012	Australia	73 (+24 adults)	3;0–7;10	SW	Cross-sectional
Chirlian & Sharpley	1982	Australia	1,357	2;6–9;0	SW	Cross-sectional
Dodd	1995b	UK & Australia	5	1;8–3;0	CS	Longitudinal
Dodd, Holm, Hua, & Crosbie	2003	UK	684	3;0–6;11	SW	Cross-sectional
Donegan	2002	UK & USA	—	—	—	Compilation
Dyson	1988	USA	20	2;0–3;3	CS	Cross-sectional & longitudinal
Flipsen	2006a, b	USA	320	3;1–8;10	CS	Cross-sectional
Grunwell	1987	UK	—	—	—	Compilation
Haelsig & Madison	1986	USA	50	2;10–5;2	SW	Cross-sectional
James	2001a	Australia	50	2;0–7;11	SW	Cross-sectional
James	2001b	Australia	99	2;0–7;11	SW	Cross-sectional
James, McCormack, & Butcher	1999	Australia	240	5;0–7;11	SW	Cross-sectional
James, van Doorn, & McLeod	2001, 2002	Australia	354	3;0–7;11	SW	Cross-sectional
Kehoe	1997	USA	18	1;10–2;10	SW	Cross-sectional
Kehoe	2001	USA	—	1;6–2;10	—	Compilation
Kilminster & Laird	1978	Australia	1,756	3;0–9;0	SW	Cross-sectional
Lowe, Knutson, & Monson	1985	USA	1,048	2;7–4;6	SW	Cross-sectional
McGlaughlin & Grayson	2003	UK	297	0;1–1;0	Crying	Cross-sectional
McIntosh & Dodd	2008	Australia	62	2;1–2;11	SW	Cross-sectional & longitudinal
McLeod & Arciuli	2009	Australia	74	5–12 years	SW	Cross-sectional
McLeod, Crowe, & Shahaeian	2015	Australia	803	4;0–5;5	Parent report	Cross-sectional
McLeod, van Doorn, & Reed	2001a	Australia	—	—	—	Compilation

(Continued)

Appendix 6-1. (*Continued*)

Authors	Year	Country	No. of children	Age of children	Sample type	Data collection method
McLeod, van Doorn, & Reed	2001b	Australia	16	2;0–3;4	CS	Longitudinal
McLeod, van Doorn, & Reed	2002	Australia	16	2;0–3;4	CS	Longitudinal
Oller, Eilers, Neal, & Schwartz	1999	USA	3,400	0;10–1;0	CS; Parent report	Cross-sectional & longitudinal
Otomo & Stoel-Gammon	1992	USA	6	1;10–2;6	SW	Longitudinal
Paynter & Petty	1974	USA	90	2;0–2;6	SW	Cross-sectional
Pollock	2002	USA	162	1;6–6;10	SW & CS	Cross-sectional
Pollock & Berni	2003	USA	165	1;6–6;10	SW & CS	Cross-sectional
Porter & Hodson	2001	USA	520	2;6–8;0	SW	Cross-sectional
Prather, Hedrick, & Kern	1975	USA	147	2;0–4;0	SW	Cross-sectional
Preisser, Hodson, & Paden	1988	USA	60	1;6–2;5	SW	Cross-sectional
Robb & Bleile	1994	USA	7	0;8–2;1	CS	Longitudinal
Robb & Gillon	2007	New Zealand & USA	20	3;1–3;5 (NZ) 2;11–3;5 (US)	CS	Cross-sectional
Robbins & Klee	1987	USA	90	2;6–6;11	SW	Cross-sectional
Roberts, Burchinal, & Footo	1990	USA	145	2;6–8;0	SW	Cross-sectional & longitudinal
Roulstone, Loader, Northstone, Beveridge, & ALSPAC team	2002	UK	1,127	2;1	SW; Parent report	Single age group
Scherer, Williams, Stoel-Gammon, & Kaiser	2012	USA	42 (+26 with cleft lip and palate)	1;6–3;0	CS	Cross-Sectional
Selby, Robb, & Gilbert	2000	USA	4	1;3–3;0	CS	Longitudinal
Shriberg	1993	USA	—	—	—	Compilation
Smit	1993a, b	USA	997	3;0–9;0	SW	Cross-sectional
Smit, Hand, Freilinger, Bernthal, & Bird	1990	USA	997	3;0–9;0	SW	Cross-sectional
Snow	1994	USA	9	1;0–1;8	CS	Longitudinal
Stoel-Gammon	1985	USA	34	1;3–2;0	CS	Longitudinal
Stoel-Gammon	1987	USA	33	2;0	CS	Cross-sectional
Stokes & Surendran	2005	USA	40	2;1	CS	Single age group

(*Continued*)

Appendix 6-1. (*Continued*)

Authors	Year	Country	No. of children	Age of children	Sample type	Data collection method
Templin	1957	USA	480	3;0–8;0	SW	Cross-sectional
Ttofari Eecen, Reilly, & Eadie	2007	Australia	1,734	1;0	Parent report	Single age group
Waring, Fisher, & Aitken	2001	Australia	299	3;5–7;11	SW	Cross-sectional
Watson & Scukanec	1997a, b	USA	12	2;0–3;0	CS	Longitudinal
Wells, Peppé, & Goulandris	2004	UK	120	5;6–13;0	SW and CS	Cross-sectional

SW = single word, CS = connected speech

7

Assessment Preparation, Purpose, and Types

LEARNING OBJECTIVES

1 Outline the typical structure and components of a speech assessment session.

2 Discuss issues to consider when preparing an assessment: the SLPs' competence and knowledge, child- and family-friendly factors, and context of the assessment.

3 Describe multidisciplinary, interdisciplinary, transdisciplinary ways to work with other professionals during assessment.

4 Outline the scope of background information required to undertake an assessment.

5 Explain the individualized, comprehensive, and strategic nature of assessment.

6 Discuss the difference between assessment for the purposes of description, diagnosis, intervention planning, and outcome measurement.

7 Compare and contrast different types of assessments: standardized versus informal, norm-referenced versus criterion-referenced, screening versus diagnostic, static versus dynamic assessments, and response to intervention.

KEY WORDS

Preparation: SLPs' competence and knowledge, child- and family-friendly assessments, context

Work with professionals: multidisciplinary, interdisciplinary, transdisciplinary

Background information: referral, developmental, medical, and family history, language use and proficiency

Purposes: description, diagnosis, intervention planning, outcome measurement

Types: standardized, informal, norm-referenced, criterion-referenced, screening, diagnostic, static, and dynamic assessments, and response to intervention

OVERVIEW

An assessment involves consideration of children's areas of strength, difficulty, and communicative capacity. Assessments typically are conducted as the first and last contact with children and their families. As an SLP, your key roles during an assessment are to describe children's speech, determine whether children's speech is typical or not (i.e., as a diagnostician), decide whether intervention is warranted (i.e., as a gatekeeper to services), plan intervention goals, and document the outcome of intervention using evidence-based decision-making. The outcome of the time you spend during assessment can have a significant impact on a child's life. As Hobbs (1975) wrote,

> Classification can profoundly affect what happens to a child. It can open doors to services and experiences the child needs to grow in competence, to become a person sure of his [or her] worth, and appreciative of the worth of others, to live with zest and to know joy. (p. 3)

TYPICAL ASSESSMENTS FOR CHILDREN WITH SUSPECTED SSD

To orient you to these two chapters on assessment (Chapters 7 and 8) we begin by describing what SLPs typically do during an assessment for a child with suspected SSD. Let's begin by considering studies from across the world where SLPs have been surveyed to describe their typical assessment practices for children with suspected SSD: Skahan, Watson, and Lof (2007), who surveyed 333 SLPs in the United States; Joffe and Pring (2008), who surveyed 98 SLPs in the United Kingdom; McLeod and Baker (2014), who surveyed 231 SLPs in Australia; Priester, Post, and Goorhuis-Brouwer (2009), who surveyed 85 SLPs in the Netherlands; and Oliveira, Lousada, and Jesus (2015), who surveyed 88 SLPs in Portugal.

- **Pre-assessment tasks** typically include reviewing the case history, reviewing educational and medical reports from other professionals, completing paperwork, conducting parent and teacher interviews, and preparing the assessment tasks. Pre-assessment tasks typically took up to 40 minutes.
- **Face-to-face assessments** typically include single-word speech sampling, connected speech sampling, and consideration of stimulability and intelligibility. The surveyed SLPs also assessed oromotor skills, hearing (often supported by an audiologist), phonemic awareness skills, perception/discrimination, and determined phonetic context effects. Some SLPs also conducted parent interviews during the face-to-face assessment phase (in addition to, or instead of during the pre-assessment phase). Classroom observation was a frequent component of assessments in the United States. Face-to-face assessments were reported to take up to 60 minutes (or more).
- **Post-assessment tasks** typically include scoring tests, analyzing results, and writing reports. These post-assessment tasks typically took up to 60 minutes.

Overall, SLPs in the United States and Australia reported that an entire initial assessment would take from 2 to 2½ hours.

PREPARATION

Preparation to undertake assessments requires consideration of many factors. The first is to consider the knowledge, skills, and cultural competence you bring to the assessment as the SLP. Other factors include consideration of child- and family-friendly assessment practices, the environment in which you will conduct the assessment, and other professionals you will work with in order to assess children with suspected SSD.

■ ■

 APPLICATION: *What would you include within a 90-minute assessment session?*

In 2002 the *American Journal of Speech-Language Pathology* published a clinical forum where a number of experts discussed what they would do within a 90-minute assessment session for "Bobby," a 4-year-old with phonological impairment (Williams, 2002).

- Bleile (2002) said that his assessment would begin by gathering background information (communication, birth/medical, social, and educational history). He would then assess receptive language skills and listen to the child's conversational speech (recording at least 50 utterances) to consider intelligibility, expressive language, voice, and fluency. An assessment of articulation and phonology would be undertaken to determine major speech errors and areas of abilities (e.g., imitation). After completing an oral structure examination and hearing assessment, the results of the assessment would be conveyed to the parents.

- Miccio (2002) indicated that she would include an interview (prior to the face-to-face assessment), articulation test, receptive language test, audiological (hearing) screening, oral structure and function screening, probe list, play, book reading, conversational speech, stimulability, and discussion of prognosis and recommendations.

- Tyler and Tolbert (2002) indicated that their assessment would include a parent case history questionnaire (prior to the face-to-face assessment), single-word phonology assessment, a stimulability task, oral structure and function examination, and screening of receptive and expressive language skills. A 50-utterance spontaneous language sample would be elicited to further consider language skills as well as intelligibility, pragmatics, voice, and fluency, followed by an audiometric (hearing) screening, and recommendation session with the parents. Data analysis and report writing would be completed after the assessment.

Make a list of the similarities and differences between these lists. What do you think you would include in an assessment of a 4-year-old with suspected SSD? Since the publication of the clinical forum, additional areas have been highlighted as important when assessing children's speech (e.g., perception, phonological processing, phonological awareness). After reading Chapters 7 and 8, revise your list of what you would include in an assessment.

■ The most important assessment tool: The SLP

The SLP is ultimately responsible for developing a relationship with children and their families, planning for and undertaking appropriate, individualized, and thorough assessments, and determining the outcome of the assessment through appropriate interpretation of the data collected from multiple sources. This is not an easy task. Each assessment plan needs to be individualized for each child. This requires professional expertise and application of the three domains of evidence-based practice: external evidence, internal clinical evidence, and internal patient/client evidence. Assessment tools form only one part of the assessment process. Professional judgment is required to select and administer assessment tools and analyze the results. Results of assessments need to be complemented with information from children, families, teachers, other professionals, knowledge of the children's community, and a critical appraisal of relevant research literature.

Foundational knowledge and skills

Throughout your studies as an SLP you will have developed foundational knowledge and skills that support your professional competence during an assessment. You are aware of prevalence, risk and protective factors, and outcomes for children with SSD (Chapter 1). Your knowledge includes an understanding of features and types of SSD, and co-occurrence with other areas of difficulty (see Chapter 2). You have developed knowledge about anatomical structures and functioning relevant to speech perception and production (see Chapter 3), the theoretical foundations of phonology and motor speech (see Chapter 5), and typical speech and language acquisition (see Chapter 6). The integration of this knowledge strengthens your decision-making.

A fundamental and specific skill that every SLP needs to draw on during an assessment of children's speech is the ability to transcribe and describe children's speech (Chapter 4). This skill is akin to a carpenter's ability to hammer a nail—if this basic skill is applied correctly, a solid structure is built. Repeated practice and refinement of transcription skills increases your ability to perceive subtle difference in speech production and the accuracy of your observations, interpretation, and decision-making.

Professional knowledge and skills

Your professional knowledge and skills include your own communicative competence, interpersonal skills, and ethical practice. Before assessing the communicative competence of children, it is important to consider your own communicative competence. Consider the skills you possess to process, interpret, and respond appropriately to verbal and non-verbal information from others. Interpersonal skills refer to your ability to relate to other people. You use your interpersonal skills during an assessment when you develop rapport with children and their families and gather information via direct, reflective, and responsive questioning. For example, good interpersonal skills are required in order to respectfully "obtain [a] client's perception and description of the communication condition, . . . [its] importance and relation to other life factors, . . . [their] goals and life circumstances" (Speech Pathology Association of Australia, 2011, p. 11). Collaboration with children, their families, and other professionals to make decisions requires good interpersonal skills. Additional expertise is required when offering counseling and support to families as they face the outcome of assessment and planning for their future.

SLPs also need to engage in ethical practice throughout the assessment process, to a similar extent as they would during all of their work with children and their families, colleagues, employers, and the general public. Ethics is "a process of deliberation about how best to act in the presence of others' lives" (Seedhouse, 1998, p. 47). Ethical practice involves respecting autonomy, avoiding harm (nonmaleficence), relieving or preventing harm (beneficence), and fair distribution of benefits and risks (justice) (Beauchamp & Childress, 2012). Speech-language pathology associations worldwide have ethical practice guidelines (e.g., American Speech-Language-Hearing Association, 2010), and you should be familiar with the code of practice that is relevant to your jurisdiction (see Chapter 15).

You should also have professional knowledge of key documents, legislation, and guidelines that are relevant to your professional association, country, state, and local community. In some locations different assessment tools (and cutoff scores) are recommended to enable children to access services or receive insurance benefits. Access to services has been described as a "postcode [zip code] lottery" (Bercow, 2008), where people living in different locations (countries, states, and even streets) receive different services. While it is important to adhere to recommended guidelines, critique of current services and advocacy for better services are also roles of a professional.

Cultural competence

SLPs need to have insight into their own practice, beliefs, and culture. It is important for SLPs to be aware of potential biases and assumptions that they bring to assessments and interactions. This is often referred to as cultural competence. Cultural competence "acknowledges and incorporates—at all levels—the importance of culture, assessment of cross-cultural relations, vigilance toward the dynamics that result from cultural differences, expansion of cultural knowledge, and adaptation of services to meet culturally unique needs" (Betancourt, Green, Carrillo & Ananeh-Firempong, 2003, p. 294). Cultural competence requires an understanding that children and families are different from one another, with priorities and goals that may be different from your own. Cultural competence is not just required when interacting with children and families from culturally and linguistically diverse backgrounds; it involves consideration of gender, race, sexual orientation, and level of ability. Acknowledge that throughout your career you will need to continually seek new knowledge and reflect on your practices as new cross-cultural challenges are presented. Consideration of cultural competence is important because it is our duty as

■■ ■■

 APPLICATION: *Consider who you are*

- Who am I? What words do I use to describe myself to others? (*male, student, young, professional, mother, white, Hispanic, Jewish, athletic, organized, empathetic, middle-class, artistic,* etc.)
- What is my cultural heritage? What are my current cultural beliefs and practices?
- What are my attitudes towards people of different gender, race, language background, sexual orientation, or level of ability to my own?
- Why do I have these beliefs/attitudes?
- What biases do I bring to assessment and intervention?

Moxley (2003) provides a questionnaire to assess your "multicultural IQ," and the American Speech-Language-Hearing Association (2010b) provides a Cultural Competency Checklist.[1]

---

[1]http://www.asha.org/uploadedFiles/Cultural-Competence-Checklist-Personal-Reflection.pdf

professionals and our clients' right to receive culturally appropriate services (International Expert Panel on Multilingual Children's Speech, 2012).

Cultural competence and professional judgment are particularly important when working with children from non-dominant backgrounds. Many of the standardized speech assessment tools available for SLPs have been developed in WEIRD societies. WEIRD is an acronym that stands for Western, Educated, Industrialized, Rich, and Democratic (Henrich, Heine, & Norenzayan, 2010). Therefore, many standardized speech assessment tools and procedures have been normed on WEIRD populations: middle-class children in English-dominant countries such as the United States, United Kingdom, Canada, Australia, and New Zealand. Henrich et al. (2010) suggested that "members of WEIRD societies, including young children, are among the least representative populations one could find for generalizing about humans" (p. 61). Normed assessments are only able to be used in a standardized manner with children who were represented within the norming population (see Chapter 6). Therefore, the SLP is required to seek additional information, and use additional techniques, requiring cultural competence, professional judgment, and insight.

There are three key elements to building cultural competence:

- **Self-awareness, self-reflection, and cultural humility (Verdon, 2015):** When thinking about your own culture, consider your beliefs, perspectives, communication styles, skills, and biases. Be aware that others see the world differently from the way you do (see "Consider Who You Are").
- **Knowledge of culture and language:** Knowledge of cultures includes consideration of family and gender roles, religion, beliefs, cultural practices, and nonverbal communication style. Cross-cultural assessments require time for building trust and relationships, getting to know the children and families, and for discussing what is important to them to ensure that goals are client-oriented. A thorough case history is essential, and guidelines are provided later in this chapter. To reflect on your own knowledge of cultures, you may wish to complete the American Speech-Language-Hearing Association (2010b) Cultural Competence Checklist.[1] Knowledge of language involves accessing basic information about speech (e.g., consonants, vowels, tones) and language (e.g., morphology, syntax) as well as common errors that are relevant to the language and dialect of the child. Chapters 4 and 6 provided some information, and additional information is available from McLeod (2010) and the Multilingual Children's Speech website.[2]
- **Adaptation of services:** What can you do to adapt your services to appropriately address cultural and linguistic diversity? Assessment (and intervention) must be

---

[1]http://www.asha.org/uploadedFiles/Cultural-Competence-Checklist-Personal-Reflection.pdf
[2]http://www.csu.edu.au/research/multilingual-speech

adaptable and tailored to the individual needs of clients based on their language, culture, interests, beliefs, and goals. Selection of culturally appropriate and sensitive tools is a key to accurate assessment and diagnosis (cf. McLeod & Verdon, 2014). Technology can be used to reach across cultural, linguistic, and geographical barriers (e.g., Skype). Be flexible. Every client requires a unique approach; one size does not fit all.

■ Child-friendly assessments

Within many workplaces and jurisdictions, the assessment process is prescribed, and a range of assessment tools are recommended to determine whether children meet cutoff scores for access to intervention and services. However, foregrounding the uniqueness of individual children and their families is also important to determine the best outcome of an assessment. When creating child-friendly assessment plans, acknowledge "that children are competent, capable, and creative and have individual characteristics, interests, and circumstances" (International Expert Panel on Multilingual Children's Speech, 2012, p. 1). Remember that in Chapter 1 we considered Article 12 from the United Nations Convention on the Rights of the Child: "Parties shall assure to the child who is capable of forming his or her own views the right to **express those views freely in all matters affecting the child**, the views of the child being given due weight in accordance with the age and maturity of the child" (UNICEF, 1989, p. 4) (emphasis added). In Chapter 8 we will consider child-friendly assessment tools that ask children about their own lives (e.g., McLeod, 2004), and "Talking to the SLP" shows children's insights into talking with their SLP. Prior to the assessment, it may also be appropriate to gain a child's **assent** to participate (Hurley & Underwood, 2002; Merrick, 2011). Here is an example of what you could say, and have printed for the child to "sign":

> Hi, my name is [NAME]. Today we are going to do some fun activities together, like looking at pictures, listening, and talking. It will take a little while to do all the activities, but you can say "stop" if you don't want to talk or if you need a rest at any time—that's OK. I'd like to video and tape record what we say, so that I can listen to it later and don't forget anything you tell me. Your mom/dad said this is OK. Does all this sound OK to you? If this is OK, please write your name or draw a smiley face here. If this is not OK, let me know.

CHILDREN'S INSIGHTS: *Talking to the SLP*

Building rapport between children and their SLP is an important (but sometimes overlooked) consideration regarding whether a full appraisal of the child's abilities can be gained during an assessment session. SLPs should be aware that children have a lot to communicate (as well as a right to communicate) about matters that are important to them. Drawings were created by 143 four- to five-year-old children from the Sound Effects Study during their speech-language pathology assessments (McLeod, Harrison, McAllister, & McCormack, 2013). The children with SSD were asked to draw themselves talking to someone. Seven of these children chose to draw themselves talking to the SLP (see Figure 7-1). In most of the drawings the SLP and the child were close to one another, and in many instances were smiling or talking. Often, the SLP was larger than the child (showing an understanding of sense of self). The focal points in the drawings highlight individual differences in the drawings. Victoria drew herself and the SLP with open mouths, possibly to indicate talking. Otto demonstrated "talking" by writing letters above the people. Maddison drew an eye between herself and the SLP, possibly indicating that the SLP had been watching her during the assessment. Owen, who had the most severe SSD (PCC = 20.2), did not draw another person but indicated that he was speaking to the SLP. Tessa and Krystal's drawings were full of color and vitality. Young children can provide insights into their lives and worlds through their drawings (Holliday, Harrison, & McLeod, 2009). Child-friendly techniques for listening to children will be explored in more depth in Chapter 8.

(Continued)

FIGURE 7-1 **Children's drawings of talking with their SLP.**

PCC = percentage of consonants correct

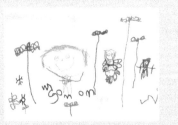

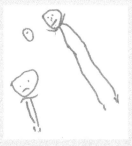

Tessa (4;3, PCC = 36.7) on the left talking "about nothing in particular" with the SLP (middle) and her mother (right) in the "garden." The SLP was drawn wearing a "necklace" that matched the one worn by the SLP during the assessment.
How I feel about my talking: ☺

Otto (4;10, PCC = 69.0) on the right talking with the SLP about "going to the park." The letters above the figures' heads were "talking."
How I feel about my talking: ☹ "Not very good . . . Sometimes I talk right and sometimes I don't."

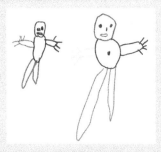

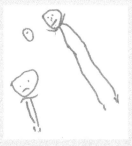

Victoria (4;10, PCC = 59.7) on the left talking to the speech-language patholo-gist (interviewer) "at kinder."
How I feel about my talking: ☺

Maddison (5;0, PCC = 47.2) on the left talking with the SLP about "people." The object between the two figures is "an eye."
How I feel about my talking: ☺

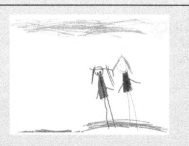

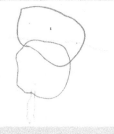

Krystal (4;10, PCC = 75.9) on the left talking with the SLP at the "park" about "the stuff what we did."
How I feel about my talking: ☺

Owen (4;6, PCC = 20.2) drew only him-self, but stated that in the drawing he was talking to the SLP about "nothing." When asked who he liked talking to, he said, "no one."
How I feel about my talking: ?

■ Family-centered and family-friendly assessments

When undertaking family- centered and family-friendly assessments, SLPs need to "recognize, value, and promote genuine, reciprocal and respectful partnerships between children, families, communities, SLPs, interpreters, educators, and all who support the acquisition of communicative competence" (International Expert Panel on Multilingual Children's Speech, 2012, p. 1). In a survey of 277 SLPs' assessment practices for children with SSD, it was found that while the majority (84%) of parents were always or usually present during assessment sessions for children with SSD, fewer SLPs asked parents if they agreed with their child's diagnosis (68%) or involved parents in goal setting (67%) (Watts Pappas, McLeod, McAllister, & McKinnon, 2008). In order to create family-friendly assessment practices, the following phrases can be used to facilitate collaboration with families:

- "We value what you know about your child."
- "We want to gather information from you and others important to your child."
- "We know that you know your child best so we need your help."
- "We will try to figure out together what's best for your child." (Crais, 2009, pp. 119–120)

Using an ecological approach to assessment, Crais (2009) also recommended that SLPs collaborate with the family to determine who is important in the child's life and who should be involved in providing information and decision-making during the assessment. Families can be involved in pre-assessment planning to determine location, time, participants, and structure of the assessment, as well as to provide background information about the child (we discuss case history information in the following pages). Families can be asked whether they want to observe, take notes, and interpret the child's behaviors during the assessment process. Families can be asked to attend an additional session to discuss the assessment results and set goals for intervention with the SLP and other relevant professionals. They can review a draft of the report before it is finalized and sent to the school and others (Crais, 2009). By conducting child- and family-friendly assessments, valid descriptions and diagnoses will be made, and goal setting is more likely to be appropriate for the child and family. Chapter 11 outlines the difference between family-centered and family-friendly practice.

■ Assessment contexts

The environment in which you conduct an assessment may influence the outcome of the assessment. Assessments may be conducted within a clinical context, school, home, or community center. Think about what context will enable you to best assess children's **performance** (on the day) and **capacity** (the best they can do). You may need to assess children in more than one context. Child- and family-friendly assessment environments provide practical support for attending the session, for example, easy appointment booking systems, available parking, friendly reception staff, information about what to bring and what will be expected in a range of languages, play equipment, and space for other children and family members. The assessment room should be welcoming, with furniture and equipment that is suitable for children and adults. The room should have good lighting and not be noisy. The signal-to-noise ratio within the room should enable high-quality audio and video recording so that recorded speech samples can be replayed, analyzed, and compared with future recordings to consider whether changes have taken place and intervention has been successful. Vogel and Morgan (2009) indicated that the choice of hardware, software, and microphone significantly impacts the quality of the recording and suggested that "highest quality recording would be made using a stand-alone hard disk recorder, an independent mixer to attenuate the incoming signal, and insulated wiring combined with a high quality microphone in an anechoic chamber or sound treated room" (p. 431). In clinical contexts, adjustments may need to be made; however, high-quality recording equipment with a microphone that is located close to the child's mouth is important.

If you are conducting an assessment within a home, school, or community context, ensure that you spend time observing the child interacting with others in a typical way. This will enable you to have a sense of the child's daily communicative capacity. Spend time talking to significant people within the child's life (parents, grandparents, siblings, friends, teachers). If you are conducting standardized assessments with the child, try to find a quiet space where the child will not be distracted so that you can determine his or her best performance on the tests.

■ Collaboration with other professionals

When assessing children, it is likely that you may work in a team with other professionals. These professionals may have referred the children to you, or you may refer children to them for additional assessments. Professionals who may be involved in the assessment of children with possible SSD include:

- **Audiologists:** hearing and speech perception
- **Psychologists:** behavior and cognition
- **Doctors** such as pediatricians, ear, nose, and throat specialists, oral surgeons, psychiatrists: causal factors (e.g., cleft palate, cerebral palsy), health, and well-being
- **Teachers:** academic skills (including reading, spelling, numeracy), socialization, approach to learning
- **Physical (physio) therapists:** gross and fine motor skills, strength, functioning
- **Occupational therapists:** daily functioning
- **Social workers:** family functioning
- **Optometrists:** vision

Interprofessional practice is a fundamental skill for SLPs working effectively in medical or educational settings (Goldberg, 2015). There are three different terms that describe how professionals work together when conducting assessments and intervention with children and their families: multidisciplinary, interdisciplinary, and transdisciplinary (Dyer, 2003). Within **multidisciplinary** teams, professionals typically work independently within their own discipline-specific parameters. Multidisciplinary assessments occur when professionals from different disciplines work in parallel to assess the child independently, and then communicate their unique discipline-specific findings and recommendations to other professionals within the team (Dyer, 2003; Hoeman, 1996). Within multidisciplinary teams, professionals may be invited to undertake an assessment by a case manager, or gatekeeper (Garner, 1995). Within **interdisciplinary** teams, professionals work **inter**dependently. That is, they maintain their discipline-specific identities, but they have a coordinated organizational structure to identify children's areas of need, and they share responsibility for children's outcomes across the team (Crow & Pounder, 2000; Dyer, 2003). Within **transdisciplinary** teams, a group of professionals jointly provide an integrated service to the family. Professionals within transdisciplinary teams share aims, information, tasks, and responsibilities. While transdisciplinary team members are the authoritative resource about their discipline, all team members have to expand their traditional roles (Briggs, 1997; Watson, Townsley, & Abbott, 2002). Choice of working in multidisciplinary, interdisciplinary, or transdisciplinary teams should be made in the child and families' best interests, rather than based on workforce shortages (Speech Pathology Association of Australia, 2009a).

Referral and Background Information

An assessment typically begins with a referral. Information gathered during the referral process (whether it is via a phone call, email, report, or conversation) helps you generate a hypothesis about children's areas of strength and difficulty. For example, a phone call from a preschool teacher indicating that a child is difficult to understand and has trouble saying a range of consonants might prompt you to suspect that the child has a phonological impairment (cf. Luke, Chapter 16). A phone call from a parent of a school-age child who describes difficulty pronouncing /s/ might prompt you to suspect articulation impairment limited to /s/ and /z/ (cf. Susie, Chapter 16)—perhaps a lateral or interdental lisp. A referral from a pediatrician for a child diagnosed with cerebral palsy might prompt you to suspect dysarthria (cf. Lian, Chapter 16). A more formal referral or report can be received from a

Read more about
Luke (4;3 years, Case 1),
Susie (7;4 years, Case 2),
and Lian (14;2 years,
Case 5) in Chapter 16.

pediatrician, teacher, audiologist, psychologist, or other health professional requesting that an assessment be conducted to assist with diagnosis. Once you receive the referral, you need to collect information (based on direct assessment, parent and teacher interview/ questionnaire, and other sources). The first task typically involves collecting case history information.

■ Case history information

Taking time to gather and understand background information about children and their families is essential for considering the child in context, making informed diagnoses, and planning appropriate intervention. Many speech-language pathology clinics, health centers, and schools use case history questionnaires to collect information about children even before a face-to-face assessment begins. Some SLPs ask parents to complete questionnaires, while others interview parents (and teachers, with parental permission) over the telephone, or during a separate face-to-face interview.

SLPs typically request a range of background information within a case history, including potential causes for SSD as well as identified risk and protective factors (as discussed in Chapter 1). Topics frequently covered within a case history questionnaire include:

- **Demographic information:** Name, date of birth, age, sex, address, telephone, email address (see the MULTICULTURAL INSIGHTS box).
- **Areas of concern:** Reason for referral. Other areas of concern.
- **Communication history:** Babbling, first words, combined two words, current communication abilities, areas of concern, previous assessment and intervention from SLP. Family history of speech, language, communication and academic difficulties.
- **Cultural and language history:** Countries the family has lived in. Languages spoken at home and school (and competency in each language) (see below).
- **Hearing history:** Number of ear infections and how they were treated, hearing tests, diagnosis of hearing loss, hearing aids, cochlear implant.
- **Birth history:** Pregnancy, significant birth events, gestation age at birth (prematurity).
- **Developmental history:** Milestones (sitting, walking), significant events during childhood.
- **Health and medical history:** General health and well-being, diagnosis of any health conditions (e.g., cleft lip and palate, cerebral palsy, Down syndrome), hospitalizations, medications.
- **Feeding and eating:** Difficulties with breast-feeding, bottle-feeding, swallowing, food preferences and allergies.
- **The child and his or her environment:** Interests, strengths, and concerns, family members, friends, school, activities (e.g., sports, music, religious, community).
- **Family preferences:** family preferences for assessment and intervention (including service delivery), parent/caregiver roles.

Read more about Luke (4;3 years, Case 1), Susie (7;4 years, Case 2), Jarrod (7;0 years, Case 3), Michael (4;2 years, Case 4), and Lian (14;2 years, Case 5) in Chapter 16.

Examples of information collected during a case history are found in Chapter 16 for Luke, Susie, Jarrod, Michael, and Lian.

■ Documenting family history of speech, language, and communication difficulties

Lewis and Freebairn (1993) created a clinical tool for considering the family history (and potential familial basis) for speech, language, and communication difficulties. They recommended conducting a 15-minute family history interview with the child's parent(s) where each member of the family for three generations (i.e., mother, father, siblings, aunts, uncles, cousins, grandparents) is considered to document whether or not they have had:

- Speech and language disorder
- Reading and spelling difficulties
- Learning disability
- Stuttering
- Hearing loss

A genetic pedigree is drawn using squares for males, circles for females. Lines are drawn to connect family members, and the focus child is identified by an arrow. Dark shading is used to indicate when a family member has an identified area of difficulty. Lewis and Freebairn (1993) did not provide guidelines for interpreting family history information and differentiating between environmental or genetic (familial) causes of SSD. However, this information can be used to consider whether there may be some familial involvement, whether other family members (e.g., siblings) should be assessed, and which family members may be helpful collaborators during the assessment and intervention. On rare occasions, the outcome of family history interviews (plus your direct assessment) may lead you to request that the family doctor or pediatrician undertake further assessment to consider a genetic cause or syndrome that is associated with the child's SSD.

■ Documenting children's language use and proficiency

Approximately half of the world speaks more than one language (Grosjean, 1982), and the majority of the world's children will acquire two or more languages (Tucker, 1998). Therefore, you are likely to assess multilingual children. Additional background information regarding language use and proficiency is required for multilingual children, particularly those who live in multilingual families and multilingual communities. First, determine which language(s) and dialects are spoken by the child, and those who live with the child (e.g., parents, siblings, grandparents, cousins). To assist with the docu-

MULTICULTURAL INSIGHTS: *Take care when documenting a child's name, date of birth, and age*

During your first contact with children and their families, take time to ensure that you have their names, date of birth, and age correct. Check the correct spelling and pronunciation of their names. Transcribe their name phonetically on the file so that each time you see them, you pronounce their name correctly. If they have non-Western heritage, check carefully which name is their surname versus first name. Many Asian countries typically write their names with the surname first. For example, people in Vietnam write surname + middle name(s) + first name. So, the Vietnamese name *Phạm Thị Bền* would be pronounced as /fam⁶ tʰi⁶ ben²/ and would be written in a Western way as *Ben Phạm*, with the first name = *Bền* and the surname = *Phạm*. In Vietnam *Thị* = female (a dot should be above and under the letter i) and *Văn* = male (*Van* is also a first name). The Chinese name *To Kit Sum* would be pronounced as /toʊ kɪt sʌm/ and would be written in a Western way as *Kit Sum To*, with the first name = *Kit Sum* and the surname = *To*. Some people write their names by using the Western ordering and adding a Western name. In fact, you have read the research of *Carol Kit Sum To* from the University of Hong Kong in Chapters 1 and 6 (e.g., To, Cheung, & McLeod, 2013a, b). Some families will use their traditional names and some will adapt to the Western traditions—so check with each child and family.

Documenting children's dates of birth is also important to get right. Check whether families provide the child's date of birth and age using a Western calendar or another calendar. For example, in China and Vietnam, traditional families use the lunar calendar and count the child's age from the time of conception to the beginning of the Lunar New Year instead of the time of birth. If they are using the lunar calendar, then the age that they report will be approximately 1 to 2 years more than if they were using the Western calendar.

mentation of less common languages, consult *Ethnologue*[3] (Lewis, Simons, & Fennig, 2016) for a list of over 7,000 world languages, alternate spellings, and countries where these languages are typically spoken. Next, for each language spoken by the child and family, document:

- **Length of time spoken. Simultaneous** language learners learn languages during the first years of life; **sequential** language learners learn additional languages once their first language(s) are established, often upon the commencement of schooling (Paradis, Genesee, & Crago, 2011).
- **Proficiency** in listening, speaking, reading, and writing (if appropriate). For example, Goldstein and Bunta (2012) used a 5-point scale to determine language proficiency, where 4 = native-like proficiency with few grammatical errors and 0 = cannot speak the indicated language.
- **Frequency of use.** Parents could estimate the percentage of time that each language is spoken each day within a typical week. For example, Sunday (at home) = 90% Spanish, 10% English; Monday (at school) = 30% Spanish, 70% English. Goldstein, Bunta, Lange, Rodriguez, and Burrows (2010) asked parents to outline their child's weekly schedule. Percentage of language use was calculated by "multiplying the number of hours of output of that language by 100 and then dividing that number by the total number of hours of activities reported per week" (p. 240).
- **Contexts** where the language is used. For example, home, school, weekend activities (e.g., Greek school), community events, and religious ceremonies. The context also includes countries the child has lived in and, if known, where they intend to live in the near future. Some families may practice **circular migration** (Hugo, 2010), where families regularly travel to their home country to maintain links with their family, community, culture, and language.
- **Exposure** to reading and other literacy activities in a language(s) (Gutiérrez-Clellen & Kreiter, 2003).
- **Attitudes** of the child, parents, siblings, and community towards the different languages spoken and how many languages a child should speak. Some families may choose to use one or multiple languages. Some languages may be perceived as having higher status than others (Jordaan, 2008; Stow & Dodd, 2003).

Some parent-report questionnaires that have been designed to consider speech and language competency of multilingual children include:

- Alberta Language and Development Questionnaire (ALDeQ) (Paradis, Emmerzael, & Duncan, 2010) quantifies children's early milestones, language use, preferences, and family history via a psychometrically validated measure. This free questionnaire was normed on 139 typically developing children and 29 children with language impairment. It takes into account the impact of war, refugee status, and other events that may have impacted children's development.
- Bilingual English-Spanish Assessment (BESA) (Peña, Gutiérrez-Clellen, Iglesias, Goldstein, & Bedore, 2014) contains two parent and teacher surveys. The Bilingual Input Output Survey (BIOS) can be used to determine whether the child should be assessed in Spanish, English, or both. The Inventory to Assess Language Knowledge (ITALK) can be used to consider parents' and teachers' perceptions of the children's speech and language competence.

Questionnaires can be used to consider the language competency of adults as well:

- Language Experience and Proficiency Questionnaire (LEAP-Q) (Marian, Blumenfeld, & Kaushanskaya, 2007)
- History of Bilingualism Questionnaire (Paradis, 1987)
- Bilingual Dominance Scale for Spanish-English bilingual adults (Dunn & Fox Tree, 2009)
- Language Background Questionnaire (Rickard Liow & Poon, 1998)
- A self-report language dominance questionnaire for Mandarin-English bilinguals (Lim, Liow, Lincoln, Chan, & Onslow, 2008)

---

[3]https://www.ethnologue.com

COMMENT: *Comparing academic outcomes for monolingual and multilingual children*

A longitudinal population study ($n = 4,983$) was conducted to compare academic outcomes for four groups of children: (1) typically developing monolingual (English-only) children, (2) typically developing multilingual children, (3) monolingual children whose parents were concerned about their speech and language, and (4) multilingual children whose parents were concerned about their speech and language. The study commenced when the children were 4 to 5 years old and followed the children until they were 8 to 9 years old. Monolingual and multilingual children had similar literacy and numeracy outcomes. The main predictor of literacy and numeracy outcomes at school was parental concern about children's speech and language in early childhood. Typically developing children (regardless of whether they were monolingual or multilingual) had significantly higher literacy and numeracy outcomes than children with parental concern (McLeod, Harrison, Whiteford, & Walker, 2016).

■ Learning from those who know the child the best: Parents, grandparents, teachers, siblings, and friends

When you gather background information about children and their families, it is useful to talk with a range of people: parents, grandparents, teachers, siblings, and friends. Typically SLPs take a case history from the mother. If possible, also talk with the child's father. If children have contact with their grandparent(s), you may also wish to ask them about their areas of concern, as well as their perspectives about the child's interests and strengths. Ask children's parents about any other people who may provide useful background information, such as a sports coach or music teacher. The Speech Participation and Activity – Children (SPAA-C) (McLeod, 2004) contains a range of questions for important people in a child's life and is designed to consider children's ability to participate fully in society. Questions from the SPAA-C for parents include:

- "What is important to your child and your family?"
- "What would be a typical weekly timetable? Who are all the people your child would speak to within a normal week?"
- "Have you observed differences between different confidence levels and communication skills at: mealtimes, school, with friends, with his/her grandparents and other family members, during hobbies and extracurricular activities (e.g., swimming lessons)?"
- "Does s/he get invited to play at other children's homes/invited to birthday parties?" (McLeod, 2004, p. 80)

Questions from the SPAA-C for others include:

- "Tell me about (this child)."
- "How well does this child get his/her message across?"
- "What helps you understand what s/he says?"
- "What do you do when you don't understand him/her?" (McLeod, 2004, p. 81)

Children's preschool or school teachers can provide valuable information about children's communicative competence in the classroom and playground, as well as the impact of their speech and language difficulties on their socialization, academic skills (including reading, spelling, mathematics), and their approach to learning. Perusing school reports, writing samples, curriculum materials, and adaptations will enhance your understanding of children in the educational context. The following teacher-report scales have been used within large-scale research (e.g., McLeod & Harrison, 2009) to indicate areas of strength and difficulty:

- Academic Rating Scale: Language and Literacy Scale (National Center for Education Statistics, 2002) has nine items (e.g., conveys ideas when speaking, reads fluently) to rate children's performance in oral and written language according to a 5-point scale (not yet = 1, beginning = 2, in progress = 3, intermediate = 4, and proficient = 5).

- Academic Rating Scale: Mathematical Thinking Scale (National Center for Education Statistics, 2002) has nine items (e.g., creates and extends patterns, recognizes shape properties and relationships) to rate children's ability on the same 5-point scale.
- Approach to Learning Scale (ALS) (Gresham & Elliott, 1990) has six items (e.g., works independently, persists in completing tasks) that were taken from the Social Skills Rating System (Gresham & Elliott, 1990), and children's performance is rated on a 4-point scale (never = 1 to very often = 4).

Children's siblings and friends may be important informants when gathering background information about participation, socialization, strengths, and difficulties (remember the CHILDREN'S INSIGHTS box in Chapter 1). Siblings play important roles in the lives of children with SSD, especially if they attend the same school. Siblings can take on (or are enlisted to) the roles of interpreter, protector, and additional parent, being described as the "cavalry on the hill" (Barr, McLeod, & Daniel, 2008, p. 21). The SPAA-C (McLeod, 2004) contains questions for friends and siblings that have been developed to maintain positivity within the discussion. Questions from the SPAA-C include:

- "Tell me about your sister/brother/friend."
- "What do you like about your sister/brother/friend?"
- "What do you like doing together?"
- "Is there anything your sister/brother/friend has trouble with?"
- "What do you do when you don't understand your sister/brother/friend?" (McLeod, 2004, p. 80)

Gaining background information about children from their parents, grandparents, teachers, siblings, and friends equips you to understand children in context. In turn, this promotes a person-centered approach to assessment, diagnosis, goal setting, and intervention.

PURPOSES OF ASSESSMENT

Not all children should be assessed in the same way. An assessment should be individualized and strategic. You should plan an assessment that is appropriate for each child's age, context, and referred areas of strength and difficulty. An assessment should be planned yet flexible, screening all areas of communication then exploring in greater depth the nature of the area(s) of difficulty that are unique to an individual. An assessment also should be iterative: gather information, reflect on this information, and then gather more information based on what you learn about children's areas of strength and difficulty. The final phase of an assessment involves analysis of the information gathered (see Chapter 9) and possibly collection of additional information until you confirm or revise your hypotheses. There are four major purposes of assessment:

- **Description:** Assessments can be used to describe children's areas of strength and difficulty, and how children function in the context of their daily lives.
- **Diagnosis:** Assessments can be used to formulate a differential diagnosis. Does the child have an SSD? Does the child require intervention?
- **Intervention planning:** Assessments can be used to determine whether a child would benefit from intervention and, if so, what should be targeted.
- **Outcome measurement:** Once a child is receiving intervention, assessments can be used to monitor progress and determine outcomes.

As described above, assessments can be undertaken for four main purposes: description, diagnosis, intervention planning, and outcome measurement. At times the first three purposes can be merged into the same assessment. Be clear about the purpose(s). This will influence the choice of assessment tools (e.g., to use standardized assessments during a diagnostic assessment) and the time allocated for undertaking an assessment. We will now consider factors relating to assessing for the purpose of description, diagnosis, and outcome measurement. Descriptions of specific tools and areas of assessment are provided in Chapter 8. Intervention planning and goal setting are considered in Chapter 10.

COMMENT: *The purposes of speech assessment*

Why should you assess speech? There are a number of answers to this question, depending on whether you are thinking about an individual or society.
Questions to ask when assessing the speech of individual children.

- Is their speech is developing typically? Do they have an SSD?
- What are their areas of strength and difficulty along the speech chain (perception, storage, production)?
- Which factors may be causing or contributing to their SSD?
- Do they require intervention?
- Are they eligible to receive speech-language pathology services?
- Which type of intervention will be most suitable?
- Which factors are facilitators and/or barriers to speech production and to increasing their communicative competence?
- What is the outcome of intervention? Has their speech improved as a result of intervention?
- Are they ready to be discharged from intervention? Are there other areas that require intervention (e.g., literacy)?

Questions to ask when assessing the speech of a group of children:

- What are typical ages of acquisition for speech sounds across children?
- Which aspects of speech (e.g., consonants, vowels, prosody) are easy and difficult for children to produce?
- What are children's common non-adult productions of speech sounds?
- What are children's common error patterns?

Questions to ask when assessing the speech of a group of adolescents and adults:

- Is there a shift in pronunciation occurring in the younger population? Have adolescents changed in the pronunciation of consonants and vowels in certain words and contexts compared with the adult productions (e.g., /stɹ/ → [ʃtɹ] in words such as *street*, Rutter, 2011)?
- What consonants, vowels, and stress patterns of one language (e.g., Standard American English) are difficult for non-native speakers of the language (e.g., immigrants to the United States from Mexico, China, or Slovenia)?

■ Descriptive assessments

Descriptive assessments can be used to describe a child's speech function, hearing, oral structure and function, activities and participation, and to understand barriers and facilitators from the environment that contribute to children's ability to participate. Descriptive assessments should outline children's strengths and weaknesses, profiling personal and environmental factors that may be facilitators or barriers to promoting children's communicative competence. Most of the assessment tools outlined in Chapter 8 can be used within descriptive assessments, including those that assess speech segments (production and perception of consonants, vowels, consonant clusters, polysyllabic words), prosody, and intelligibility. Descriptive assessments are often used by researchers. For example, researchers undertaking a community (non-clinical) study of 143 preschool children documented the occurrence of interdental lisps (39.9% of children), dentalization of sibilants (17.5%), and lateral lisps (13.3%) (McLeod, Harrison, McAllister, & McCormack, 2013). Most SLPs do not have funding or time to undertake descriptive assessments; instead, their main mandate is to undertake diagnostic assessments and, if a child is diagnosed with SSD, then to undertake assessments for intervention planning and eventually outcome measurement.

■ Diagnostic assessments

Diagnostic assessments are used for comprehensively assessing children's speech to determine whether or not children have an SSD, whether or not they require intervention, and what intervention goals should be targeted. Most speech assessment tools are created for diagnostic assessments. A diagnostic assessment tool should have high sensitivity and specificity to identify whether a child has difficulty producing speech sounds when compared with other children of the same age. It also should be extensive enough to enable intervention planning. Many diagnostic assessments are formulated based on a theoretical premise. For example, the Diagnostic Evaluation of Articulation and Phonology (DEAP) (Dodd, Hua, et al., 2002, 2006) has been designed using the framework of the Differential Diagnosis System (Dodd, 2005), a descriptive-linguistic framework to differentiate subgroups of children with SSD (see Chapter 2). Subtests of the DEAP are designed to assess articulation disorder, phonological delay/disorder, and inconsistent speech disorder, as well as to screen oromotor skills. The DEAP has been normed on 650 children in the United States (Dodd, Hua, et al., 2006) and over 600 children in the United Kingdom (Dodd et al., 2002), check normed on 144 children in Australia, and standardized and normed in Ireland. It provides standard scores and percentile ranks for sounds in words, phonological process use, and single words versus connected speech agreement criterion. Additional diagnostic measurement tools are outlined in Chapter 8.

■ Intervention planning

When the purpose of assessment is intervention planning, there are two main questions: Will a child benefit from intervention? And if so, what should be targeted? To determine appropriate intervention targets, SLPs often probe specific areas that were difficult for children in order to understand the extent of difficulty and contexts in which the difficulties occur. The Secord Contextual Articulation Test (S-CAT, Secord & Shine, 1997) includes a range of probes that can be used to consider the context of different consonants, to enable planning of goals and target words for intervention. Noncommercial probes are also available. For example, if children have difficulty producing consonant clusters on a standardized single-word assessment such as the Goldman-Fristoe Test of Articulation – Second Edition (Goldman & Fristoe, 2000), then SLPs may not have enough information about their consonant cluster production in different contexts (e.g., this assessment does not sample word-final consonant clusters). Therefore, SLPs may consider using a non-standardized assessment to probe consonant cluster production in a range of contexts (e.g., McLeod, Hand, Rosenthal, & Hayes, 1994; Powell, 1995).

■ Outcome measurement

Outcome measurement is used to determine whether intervention is effective and whether intervention can cease. Lollar and Simeonsson (2005) state ". . . improvement in function is often the litmus text that society uses to evaluate effectiveness of programs and treatments" (p. 323). It is important that outcome measurements are able to differentiate change as a result of intervention rather than change as a result of other factors. If possible, a stable baseline over at least two time points should be obtained before intervention begins. A measure used to document change over time should be stable, reliable, and sensitive to provide an accurate indicator of functioning. Sources of instability that may occur as a result of biological variation (e.g., ageing) and technological error (e.g., equipment, analysis) should be minimized (Vogel & Maruff, 2014).

While most speech assessments primarily are created as diagnostic assessments, many can also be used as outcome measurements, to consider change over time and to document change as a result of intervention. To use a diagnostic assessment as an outcome measurement tool, a comparison is made between the standard scores, percentile ranks, or percentage of consonants correct over time. A limitation of using a diagnostic assessment to measure outcomes is that unless the child has achieved a level that is comparable with typically developing peers, it is not known whether or not a change in scores is significant. For example, Lousada et al. (2014) used two intelligibility measures (based on intelligibility in words and connected speech) and indicated that these measures were sensitive enough to demonstrate changes in a group of children who received phonological intervention, but not in a group of children who received articulation intervention.

Assessment tools that have specifically been designed to assess outcomes of intervention include:

■ American Speech-Language-Hearing Association National Outcome Measurement System (ASHA NOMS) (American Speech-Language-Hearing Association, 2003)
■ Focus on the Outcomes of Children Under Six (FOCUS) (Thomas-Stonell et al., 2012)
■ Therapy Outcome Measures (TOMs) (Enderby & John, 1997, 2015)

For example, the ASHA NOMS (American Speech-Language-Hearing Association, 2003) includes a series of 7-point functional communication measures that range from level 1 (least functional) to level 7 (most functional). It includes a scale for Articulation/Intelligibility, and a certified SLP enters the appropriate scores on admission to speech-language pathology services and at discharge, along with demographic information and intervention characteristics (e.g., frequency and intensity of intervention). Web-based data collection is now available to registered ASHA members. Comparative data from the ASHA NOMS is available in Mullen and Schooling (2010) and was discussed in Chapter 1. Both the TOMs and the FOCUS have been designed using the International Classification of Functioning, Disability and Health (World Health Organization, 2001).

TYPES OF ASSESSMENTS

There are five different types of assessments, and these types apply to most developmental assessments, including those designed for children with suspected SSD:

■ standardized versus informal assessments
■ norm-referenced versus criterion-referenced assessments
■ screening versus diagnostic assessments
■ static versus dynamic assessments
■ response to intervention

Careful consideration of the selection of assessment types is essential when working with children suspected of SSD. Some speech sampling tools have specifically been designed to be used in one of the ways mentioned earlier (e.g., as a standardized norm-referenced static diagnostic assessment tool), whereas others can be used in more than one way.

■ Standardized assessments

Standardized assessments play a key role in speech-language pathology practice, as they "serve as gateways to services" (Crais, 2011, p. 342) since they are used to differentially diagnose the presence or absence of SSD in children. The term **standardized assessment** means that there are consistent test materials, consistent procedures for test administration, and consistent scoring rules (American Educational Research Association, American Psychological Association, & National Council on Measurement in Education, 1999). Most commercially available speech assessments are standardized. Examples include:

- Goldman-Fristoe Test of Articulation-2 (Goldman & Fristoe, 2000)
- Bankson-Bernthal Test of Phonology (Bankson & Bernthal, 1990)
- Diagnostic Evaluation of Articulation and Phonology (Dodd, Hua, et al., 2002, 2006)

That is, they provide standardized elicitation procedures (e.g., colored pictures of stimulus words to sample the consonants and vowels of a language) and an examiners' manual that outlines how to administer and score the assessment. Standardized assessments are designed (and can be evaluated) by considering psychometric properties. These psychometric properties include aspects of test design such as validity (predictive, concurrent, construct, content) and reliability (internal consistency, test-retest reliability, inter- and intra-rater reliability) (Friberg, 2010; McCauley & Swisher, 1984a, b). **Predictive validity**, or identification accuracy, of standardized assessment tools is often considered the most important aspect of a standardized assessment (Friberg, 2010). Predictive validity is whether an assessment is able to differentiate between children who do and don't have difficulties. Related to predictive validity is the sensitivity and specificity of the measure. **Sensitivity** refers to the ability of the assessment to accurately identify children who have the specified area of difficulty, and **specificity** refers to the ability of the tool to accurately identify absence of difficulty in children who do not have difficulty (see "What Are Sensitivity and Specificity, and Why Do I Need to Know?"). If the psychometric properties of a standardized assessment tool are not rigorous, or if the tool is used with a population other than the intended population, then it may result in "inappropriate provision or denial of clinical services" (Friberg, 2010, p. 86). Standardized assessments can be norm-referenced or criterion-referenced, concepts that are described below.

■ Informal assessments

In contrast to standardized assessments, informal assessments typically do not have standardized processes for administration, analysis, or scoring. Informal assessments are not accompanied with normative data, although results may be compared with functional standards (AERA, APA, & NCME, 1985). Informal measures are often "self-made" by speech-language pathologists and researchers (Priester, Post, & Goorhuis-Brouwer, 2009, p. 1101), rather than commercial publishers, and usually are developed for an intended purpose and population. For example, informal assessments have been developed when speech assessments are not available for a particular dialect or language (e.g., Samoan:

COMMENT: *What are sensitivity and specificity, and why do I need to know?*

Sensitivity is the ability to identify the presence of SSD in children who have an SSD. **Specificity** is the ability to identify the absence of SSD in children who do not have SSD (i.e., are typically developing). If an assessment does not have an appropriate level of sensitivity, then children who have an SSD will not be identified as such and are unlikely to receive intervention. If an assessment does not have an appropriate level of specificity, then children who are developing typically will be identified as having an SSD and may be referred for unnecessary intervention; thus clinical resources are not used optimally. Sensitivity and specificity are measured between 0 and 1.0, indicating the level of precision of making an accurate diagnosis. Values closest to 1.0 indicate the most accurate diagnosis. Plante and Vance (1994) recommend that values over .80 are acceptable and over .90 are optimal. A caveat to the determination of sensitivity and specificity is that a tool needs to be measured against a "gold standard." Although sensitivity and specificity are important, keep in mind that all children are individuals, and difficulty producing speech sounds will have a different impact depending on the attitudes and norms of the community in which they live (see Chapter 6). Consequently, it is also important to consider environmental and personal factors when deciding on whether intervention is necessary.

Ballard & Farao, 2008), and many SLPs report that they use informal assessments with multilingual children (Skahan et al., 2007; Williams & McLeod, 2012). Surveys reveal that SLPs also create or use informal measures when evaluating the speech of monolingual children, even when standardized assessments are available (Limbrick, McCormack, & McLeod, 2013; McLeod & Baker, 2014; Oliveira et al., 2015; Priester et al., 2009). Reasons for this include the use of informal assessments as probes to supplement data obtained from standardized measures (e.g., to assess polysyllabic words, consonant clusters, morphopho-nemes), or due to the high cost of purchasing standardized norm-referenced assessments and score forms (Limbrick et al., 2013). Selecting informal assessments only for financial reasons may not be cost-effective in the long run, since standardized norm-referenced assessments are designed to have high predictive validity, and reduce the chance of misdiagnosis.

■ Norm-referenced assessments

Norm-referenced assessments are tools that "indicate the standing of an individual . . . within a population of individuals" (American Educational Research Association et al., 1999, p. 49). Norm-referenced assessments are usually standardized and compare performance against normative samples to determine whether a specific child's performance is typical or delayed (Sodoro, Allinder, & Rankin-Erickson, 2002). Most commercially available norm-referenced assessments include an examiner's manual that contains information about the demographics of the normative sample (e.g., age, sex, language, dialect, socioeconomic status, location) as well as the normative information about the age of acquisition of different consonants and vowels, and the percentage of consonants correct at different ages, which is typically presented in tables or appendices. You may recall that in Chapter 6 we also presented normative information for the age of acquisition, percentage of consonants correct, and other aspects of speech acquisition. Some of the information presented in Chapter 6 is normative data collected during the norming of standardized norm-referenced assessments (e.g., Dodd, Holm, et al., 2003, is based on the normative sampling for the United Kingdom/Australian version of the DEAP, Dodd, Hua, et al., 2002). It is recommended that a normative sample should have over 100 children in each of the groups that are assessed (100+ three-year-old children, 100+ four-year-old children, etc.) (McCauley & Swisher, 1984a, b).

■ Criterion-referenced assessments

Criterion-referenced assessments measure performance against the ability to produce a target skill, but "make no direct reference to the performance of other examinees" (American Educational Research Association et al., 1999, p. 50). Criterion-referenced assessments may be either standardized or informal. Examples of standardized criterion-referenced assessments include the Metaphon Resource Pack (Dean, Howell, Hill, & Waters, 1990) and Secord Contextual Articulation Test (S-CAT, Secord & Shine, 1997), which are suitable for probing production of different speech sounds or different phonological processes. Informal criterion-referenced assessments include assessments of consonant clusters (McLeod, et al., 1994; Powell, 1995), which have been developed since consonant clusters are not fully sampled in commercially available standardized assessments.

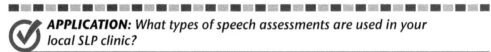

APPLICATION: *What types of speech assessments are used in your local SLP clinic?*

Look at the speech assessments in your SLP clinic. Which assessments are used the most often? What speech skills do they assess? Can you determine whether they are standardized assessments, informal assessments, norm-referenced assessments, criterion-referenced assessments, screening assessments, diagnostic assessments, outcome measures, static assessments, and/or dynamic assessments?

COMMENT: *Determining the quality of assessment measures*

When selecting an assessment to use, it is important to consider whether the purpose, intended population, target skill, and scope match your intended use of the tool. In addition, consider the psychometric properties of the tool: validity (predictive, concurrent, construct, content) and reliability (internal consistency, test-retest reliability, inter- and intra-rater reliability). Some review articles that critique speech assessment tools include:

- Psychometric properties of single-word speech tests (Flipsen & Ogiela, 2015)
- Consonants and vowel inventories (Eisenberg & Hitchcock, 2010)
- Speech and language assessments (McCauley & Swisher, 1984a)
- Screening assessments (Nelson, Nygren, Walker, & Panoscha, 2006; Sturner et al., 1994)
- Intelligibility assessments (Kent, Miolo, & Bloedel, 1994)
- Nonword assessments (Archibald & Gathercole, 2006)
- Oral and speech motor assessments (McCauley & Strand, 2008)
- Phonological error patterns (Kirk & Vigeland, 2014)
- Informal assessments (Limbrick, McCormack, & McLeod, 2013)
- Speech assessments in languages other than English (McLeod & Verdon, 2014)

One website that publishes reviews of assessments is the Buros Center for Testing.[1]

[1]https://marketplace.unl.edu/buros/

Screening assessments

A screening assessment "is intended to separate out the children who need further investigation of their speech and language skills from those with normally developing speech and language . . . Resources can then be concentrated on the children failing the screen" (Law et al., 1998, p. 38). Screening assessments can be undertaken by parent report, direct assessment, or observation (Law et al., 1998). When selecting a screening assessment, it is important to consider whether it has high sensitivity and specificity, whether it is valid, and whether it has normative information that is relevant for your speech community. There are two types of screening assessments: first-level (primary) and second-level (secondary) screening (Sturner et al., 1994).

Primary screening assessments are for mass-level population screening. Primary screening assessments are typically undertaken by non-SLPs, such as doctors, community nurses, teachers, and other health professionals (e.g., audiologists, psychologists). After primary screening, most children will be considered to be developing typically, requiring no further contact. Some will be considered to be at risk, and may be rescreened at a later date. Others will be referred to the appropriate professional (SLP, audiologist, psychologist) for further assessment. During primary screening assessments, screening of speech and language may be embedded within a protocol to screen children's broader development, including hearing, vision, and cognition. One example of a published primary screening assessment is the Parents' Evaluation of Developmental Status (PEDS) (Glascoe, 2000), a parent report measure consisting of 10 questions (two relating to speech and language) that has been used in large-scale prevalence studies of speech and language (e.g., McLeod & Harrison, 2009).

An example of a primary screening assessment available for teachers to screen children's speech is the Phoneme Factory Phonology Screener (Wren, Hughes, & Roulstone, 2006), a computerized assessment that enables teachers to score only one phoneme at a time, and generates a report to indicate whether additional assessment is required. Another example of a primary screening procedure, developed for doctors to screen the speech of children aged 4;6, was described by Rigby and Chesham (1981) and reported by Law et al. (1998) as having high sensitivity (> .8) and specificity (> .9). The procedure included four sections: (1) production of the following words: *"penny, teapo(t), knife, bu(s), cup, duck, chair, fish, wheel, lett(er), gun, (s)ock, watch, light*" (Rigby & Chesham, 1981, p. 449), (2) production of a "spontaneous, understandable 2-word sentence" (p. 449), (3) parental concern, and if the child failed any part of the screening test, and (4) a hearing test. The Triage 10 is a list of 10 words analyzed using a mean word complexity measure that can be used by SLPs to identify preschool children who would benefit from additional assessment (Anderson & Cohen, 2012).

Secondary screening assessments occur within a selected population and typically are undertaken by SLPs to determine which children may need a more comprehensive assessment. Secondary screening assessments are used when a "child referred for one type of speech-language problem (e.g., articulation) is checked further to determine if there are additional communication system deficits" (Sturner et al., 1994, p. 25). For example, when a child's main area of concern is production of speech sounds, SLPs may conduct a comprehensive assessment of speech and screening assessments of other aspects of communication due to the co-occurrence of SSD with these areas: expressive and receptive language, stuttering, voice, oral structure and function, swallowing/feeding, and hearing (Chapter 2 provides more information about co-occurrence). Some examples of published secondary screening assessments that consider speech and language skills include:

- Fluharty Preschool Speech and Language Screen Test: Second Edition (Fluharty-2) (Fluharty, 2001)
- Preschool Language Scales: Fifth Edition (PLS-5) (Zimmerman, Steiner, & Pond, 2012), available as either an English or Spanish edition

Children's hearing and oral structure and function also may be screened during secondary screening.

A secondary speech screening undertaken by an SLP is a brief (usually 5–10 minutes) rather than comprehensive assessment, and it may consider either common problematic sounds (e.g., /s, ɹ/) or phonemes within a language (e.g., consonants, vowels, and some consonant clusters). Examples include:

- Quick Screener (Bowen, 1996)
- Diagnostic Screen subtest of the Diagnostic Evaluation of Articulation and Phonology (DEAP) (Dodd, Hua, et al., 2002, 2006)
- The Articulation Survey (Aitken & Fisher, 1996)

Some SLPs may be surprised to learn that the Goldman-Fristoe Test of Articulation (Goldman & Fristoe, 2000) is also considered a screening assessment. In addition, there are some screening assessments that English-speaking SLPs can use for screening the speech of children in languages other than English. For example:

- Spanish Articulation Measures (Mattes, 1995)
- Bilingual Speech Sound Screen: Pakistani Heritage Languages (Stow & Pert, 2006)

If children pass a secondary screening assessment, then no further assessment is required at that time, and it is likely that they do not have SSD. If they do not pass a secondary screening assessment, then more detailed diagnostic assessment is required to determine what areas of difficulty they have, to verify whether or not they have an SSD, whether they need intervention, and what should be targeted in intervention.

Screening assessments may be useful diagnostically, but they may not provide enough information in order to determine appropriate intervention goals that align with a specified intervention approach. Currently, there are no universally accepted protocols for screening children's speech (Nelson, Nygren, Walker, & Panoscha, 2006). Sturner et al. (1994) suggested that many screening measures lack predictive validity data and instead rely on subjective judgments.

▪ Static assessments

Most traditional standardized norm-referenced speech assessments are static assessments. During a static assessment, children's **performance** at a particular time is assessed; however, their full **capacity** may not be assessed, since they are typically are asked for only one production of a word in one context. Children are not provided feedback on their speech production during a static assessment. Instead, SLPs will comment on children's attention to the task rather than their accuracy of production.

■ Dynamic assessments

In contrast to a static assessment, a dynamic assessment enables consideration of children's **capacity** to learn as well as their **performance** at a particular time (Hasson & Joffe, 2007). During a dynamic assessment, children's capacity is assessed as they are provided with cues to assist them to make the best possible production of a word or sound. Typically, children are asked for more than one production of a word and are provided feedback on their speech production. Dynamic assessment provides more details about children's skills and can be used to provide greater evidence of change over time. Dynamic assessment was inspired by the work of Vygotsky (1978), and his concept of the **zone of proximal development** (see Chapter 6). Initially, dynamic assessment was adopted for use with children when norm-referenced standardized assessments were inappropriate—for example, children with cognitive delays, children who were multilingual and/or were English language learners (Gutiérrez-Clellen & Peña, 2001; Peña, Iglesias, & Lidz, 2001). However, more recently, dynamic assessments have been included within assessment protocols and are an important aspect of considering children's response to intervention (RTI). Some dynamic assessments of speech include:

- Dynamic Assessment of Preschoolers' Proficiency in Learning English (DAPPLE) (Hasson, Camilleri, Jones, Smith, & Dodd, 2013)
- Dynamic Evaluation of Motor Speech Skill (DEMSS) (Strand, McCauley, Weigand, Stoeckel, & Baas, 2013)
- Glaspey Dynamic Assessment of Phonology (GDAP) (Glaspey & MacLeod, 2010; Glaspey & Stoel-Gammon, 2007)

Dynamic assessments of stimulability are useful for determining whether a child with SSD is able to say a sound after provision of cues and prompts and the level at which instruction needs to start. The GDAP (Glaspey & MacLeod, 2010; Glaspey & Stoel-Gammon, 2007) is a standardized dynamic assessment that assesses children's production of consonants and consonant clusters. Children's productions of each consonant or consonant cluster is rated on a 1–15 scale where 1 = best, indicating the lowest level of support is needed, and 15 = worst, indicating the highest level of support is needed. The assessment is able to document incremental changes over time. Figure 7-2 demonstrates the steps and scoring procedures for each consonant or consonant cluster.

FIGURE 7-2 | **Glaspey Dynamic Assessment of Phonology (GDAP)**

Hierarchy of cues and linguistic environments ranging from 1 to 15

Linguistic environments	Cues			
	Level 0: No assistance	Level 1: Instructions, verbal model	Level 2: Instructions, verbal model, prolongation, segmentation	Level 3: Instructions, verbal model, prolongation, segmentation, tactile cues
Not stimulable				15
A. Isolation			12	14
B. Word	10	11	8	13
C. 3-word sentence	6	7		9
D. 4-word sentence	4	5		
E. Target sentence	2	3		
F. Connected speech	1			

Source: Reprinted with permission from the Appendix (p. 299) of Glaspey, A. M., & MacLeod, A. A. N. (2010). A multi-dimensional approach to gradient change in phonological acquisition: A case study of disordered speech development. *Clinical Linguistics and Phonetics*, 24(4-5), 283–299. Used with permission.

Dynamic assessment has also been used to assess the speech of children with suspected CAS. The DEMSS (Strand et al., 2013) is a motor speech assessment that "systematically varies the length, vowel content, prosodic content, and phonetic complexity within sampled utterances" (p. 506). During administration of the nine subtests of the DEMSS, children's responses to cueing and facilitation in the production of syllables and utterances of increasing length and complexity (e.g., CV, VC, CVC, disyllables, multisyllables) are scored on the following areas: overall articulatory accuracy, vowels, prosody, and consistency. Administration time with children with SSD ranged from 7 to 25 minutes. Initial evidence for acceptable reliability and validity was determined in a study of 81 children with severe SSD or suspected CAS (Strand et al., 2013).

■ Response to intervention

Within education settings, particularly within the United States, response to intervention (RTI) is used to determine children's eligibility for special education services. Assessment of progress is an important component of the response to intervention model. The premise behind the response to intervention model is to help children succeed by embracing a school-wide prevention approach to support struggling learners before they fail. A three-tiered approach is advocated (Fuchs & Fuchs, 2007), although schools may opt for more tiers. **Tier one** includes universal screening for all children and the provision of short-term monitoring programs for children at risk within a general education setting. **Tier two** involves targeted small-group, school-based interventions that are validated and standardized and includes assessment to determine children's response to this intervention. **Tier three** involves multidisciplinary interventions (including from SLPs) with individualized intervention and regular assessment and monitoring of progress. For example, the DEAP (Dodd, Hua, et al., 2002, 2006) has been identified by the publishers as appropriate for assessments in tiers 1, 2, and 3 (Pearson, 2014). When surveyed, SLPs indicated that they valued the response to intervention model and the focus on progress monitoring, assessment, and prevention (Sanger, Mohling, & Stremlau, 2011); however, SLPs have also highlighted the importance of resourcing and collaboration between school administrators, educators, and SLPs for this model to succeed (Snow, Sanger, Childers, Pankonin, & Wright, 2013).

Chapter summary

This chapter provided you with an overview of the contents of assessments of children's speech. You learned that preparation for undertaking an assessment included consideration of the knowledge, beliefs, and skills of the SLP, consideration of child- and family-friendly assessment practices, consideration of the assessment context, and other professionals. You learned that collaboration with the children's parents and others who are important in their lives (e.g., grandparents, teachers, siblings) will provide important background information to understand children in context. Four purposes of assessment were discussed: description, diagnosis, intervention planning, and outcome measurement. You learned that descriptive assessments can be used to describe children's areas of strength and difficulty and how children function in the context of

their daily lives. Diagnostic assessments can be used to determine whether a child has SSD, and if so, which type. Assessments can be used to determine whether a child would benefit from intervention, and if so, what should be targeted. You learned that once a child is receiving intervention, outcome measures can be used to monitor progress and decide when intervention should conclude. You learned about the psychometric properties of assessments for diagnosis and differentiated between standardized, informal, norm-referenced, criterion-referenced, screening, diagnostic, outcome measures, response to intervention, static, and dynamic assessments. The next chapter will examine assessment tools that can be used during an assessment of children's speech and will provide guidance for developing assessment plans for children with different types of SSD.

Suggested reading

■ Flipsen, P., Jr., & Ogiela, D. A. (2015). Psychometric characteristics of single-word tests of children's speech sound production. *Language, Speech, and Hearing Services in Schools*, 46(2), 166–178.

■ Skahan, S. M., Watson, M., & Lof, G. L. (2007). Speech-language pathologists' assessment practices for children with suspected speech sound disorders: Results of a national survey. *American Journal of Speech-Language Pathology*, 16(3), 246–259.

Application of knowledge from Chapter 7

Consider each of the case study children in Chapter 16.

1. Which people would have been contacted by the SLPs in order to write the background descriptions of these children (e.g., parents, siblings, teachers)?
2. Would it be appropriate for any of the case study children to be assessed by other professionals? If so, who?
3. Consider your own professional knowledge, skills, and cultural competence. What would you need to prepare or learn in order to assess the children profiled in Chapter 16?
4. What speech assessments do you have available at your university, school, or clinic? Can you describe them according to the different types of assessments outlined in this chapter (e.g., standardized, informal, norm-referenced, criterion-referenced)? You will need to look at the examiner's manuals in order to answer this question.
5. Search for and administer a standardized or informal articulation assessment on a peer. If you do not have ready access to assessments at a university clinic, then search for readily available informal assessment tools on the Internet such as the Quick Screener by Caroline Bowen (1996). If you administer a standardized test, reflect on the time it took and the skill needed to administer the test in accordance with the instructions in the test manual. If you administer an informal assessment tool, reflect on type of information obtained, the administration and scoring procedures.

8

Assessment of Children's Speech

LEARNING OBJECTIVES

1 Select tools suitable for assessing intelligibility, speech production, oral structure and function, speech perception, hearing, phonological processing, literacy skills, psychosocial aspects, communicative participation in educational and social contexts, language, voice, and fluency.

2 Debate the advantages and disadvantages of single-word and connected speech sampling.

3 Use the International Classification of Functioning, Disability and Health – Children and Youth Version (ICF-CY) as a framework for planning speech assessments.

4 Generate assessment plans suitable for children with different types of SSD.

KEY WORDS

Intelligibility, acceptability, comprehensibility

Speech production elements: consonants, consonant clusters, vowels and diphthongs, polysyllables, prosody, and tones

Speech production methods: single word, connected speech, stimulability, inconsistency/variability

Body structures and functions that support speech: Oral structure and function, hearing, speech perception

Additional areas of communication: language, voice, and fluency

Phonological processing: phonological access, phonological memory, phonological awareness

Literacy: emergent literacy, early literacy, conventional literacy

Psychosocial aspects: temperament, communicative participation in educational and social contexts

International Classification of Functioning, Disability and Health: (World Health Organization, 2001, 2007)

Strategic assessments: phonological impairment, articulation impairment, inconsistent speech disorder, CAS, childhood dysarthria, hearing loss, and craniofacial anomalies

OVERVIEW

In this chapter we present an overview of assessment practices for children with suspected SSD for the four purposes outlined in the previous chapter: description, diagnosis, intervention planning, and outcome measurement. We describe aspects of speech, communication, and daily functioning that typically are assessed and methods and types of assessments that can be used within an individualized iterative approach. We describe the range of tests, tasks, and questions that can be used to assess children with suspected SSD. Inclusion of an assessment tool (commercially available or freely available) is not intended as an endorsement of a particular assessment or approach. In order to determine if particular assessment tools are suitable for your context, you are encouraged to read the manuals of assessment tools to consider their validity and reliability. Search the literature (especially journal articles) to reflect on how different assessment tools have been used, validated, and critiqued. Next we outline use of the International Classification of Functioning, Disability and Health – Children and Youth Version (ICF, ICF-CY) (WHO, 2001, 2007) as a framework for planning speech assessments. At the end of the chapter we provide information for planning individualized and strategic assessments for the different types of SSD described in Chapter 2. That is, we discuss appropriate assessment plans for describing and diagnosing different types of SSD: phonological impairment, articulation impairment, inconsistent speech disorder, CAS, and childhood dysarthria.

COMPONENTS OF CHILDREN'S SPEECH ASSESSMENTS

The following components may be included in a comprehensive assessment of children's speech:

1. Children's context and development (case history, as outlined in Chapter 7)
2. Intelligibility
3. Speech production
   (a) Elements: consonants, consonant clusters, vowels and diphthongs, polysyllables, prosody, and tones (if appropriate)
   (b) Methods: single word, connected speech, stimulability, inconsistency/ variability
4. Oral structure and function
5. Speech perception
6. Hearing
7. Phonological processing: phonological access, phonological memory, phonological awareness
8. Literacy skills
9. Psychosocial aspects
10. Participation in educational and social contexts
11. Language, voice, and fluency

Next we will describe the principles of assessment for each of these aspects and include examples of assessments that you may be able to use in your clinical practice. In most cases, there are a number of other assessments that could have been included, so talk with your colleagues about what assessment tools are suitable for your context and the children and families you work with.

ASSESSMENT OF INTELLIGIBILITY

Intelligibility is "the degree to which the listener understands what the speaker says when the target is uncertain" (Camarata, 2010, p. 382). Intelligibility has been described as ". . . the single most practical measurement of oral communication competence" (Gordon-Brannan, 1994). Intelligibility requires a two-way interaction between the speaker and listener, so it is beneficial to consider assessments of intelligibility that take into consideration both communicative partners. Intelligibility is frequently considered by SLPs when determining presence of an SSD, the need for intervention, and whether intervention has been successful (Baker, 2010a; Hustad, 2012; Mullen & Schooling, 2010; Williams, McLeod, & McCauley, 2010). Development of intelligibility assessments has been informed by research undertaken with children and adults with SSD (Flipsen, 2006b; Lagerberg, Åsberg, Hartelius, & Persson, 2014; McLeod, Harrison, & McCormack, 2012b), hearing loss (Ertmer, 2011), dysarthria, including children with cerebral palsy (Hustad, Schueler, Schultz, & DuHadway, 2012; Yorkston & Beukelman, 1978), and craniofacial anomalies (Johannisson, Lohmander, & Persson, 2014; Whitehill, 2002). There are three main ways that intelligibility can be assessed (cf. Kent, Miolo, & Bloedel, 1994): rating scales, single-word measures, and connected speech measures. Significant differences between these intelligibility measures have been found (Johannisson et al., 2014). Intelligibility has also been found to differ depending on whether the listener is a family member, a stranger, or an SLP (Baudonck, Buekers, Gillebert, & Lierde, 2009; Flipsen, 1995; Kwiatkowski & Shriberg, 1992). For example, Kwiatkowski and Shriberg (1992) found that caregivers accurately understood an average of 73% of words and 58% of the utterances in connected speech compared with the SLPs' reference gloss that was created by repeated listening of the sample and knowledge of the context. Intelligibility measurement is also affected by the listeners' task, whether it was multiple choice, or orthographic versus phonetic transcription of single words, sentences, or connected speech (Johannisson et al., 2014). The listener's task can be affected by the phonological, grammatical, and syllabic complexity, word position, and utterance length (Weston & Shriberg, 1992). Finally, the medium of transmission (e.g., live, audio, or video recording) can also impact intelligibility scores (Lagerberg et al., 2014; Whitehill, 2002). Therefore the measurement tool, listener type, listener task, and medium of transmission need to be considered carefully when assessing intelligibility. Miller (2013) calls for the use of diagnostic intelligibility testing in order to explain why someone is difficult to understand rather than just quantifying the overall level of intelligibility.

■ Rating scales that quantify perceptions of intelligibility

There are a number of different rating scales that can be used to quantify perceptions of intelligibility, including:

- Intelligibility in Context Scale (ICS) (McLeod, Harrison, & McCormack, 2012a)
- Meaningful Use of Speech Scale (MUSS) (Robbins & Osberger, 1990)
- Speech Intelligibility Rating Scale (Allen, Nikolopoulos, Dyar, & O'Donoghue, 2001)
- 5-point Intelligibility Rating Scale (Bleile, 1995)

For example, the Intelligibility in Context Scale (ICS) (McLeod, Harrison, & McCormack, 2012a) is a rating scale for parents to report their children's intelligibility in a range of contexts outside of the clinical setting (see Table 8-1 for the English version and Table 8-2 for the Spanish version). The 7-item scale was based on concepts from the International Classification of Functioning, Disability and Health – Children and Youth Version (ICF-CY) (WHO, 2007). The ICS is available for free in 60 languages[1] and has been validated for use with young children for a variety of languages including English (McLeod, Crowe, & Shahaeian, 2015; McLeod, Harrison, & McCormack, 2012b), traditional Chinese/Cantonese (Ng, To, & McLeod, 2014), Slovenian (Kogovšek & Ozbič, 2013), Croatian (Mildner, 2014), and Jamaican Creole (Washington, McDonald, McLeod, Crowe, Devonish, 2015). Miller (2013) indicated that the ICS offered a measure for considering functional success and stated that the ICS "permits one to gain inroads into what counts as a clinically, communicatively, as opposed to merely statistically significant change in intelligibility" (p. 608). While rating scales offer quick screening measures of intelligibility, disadvantages of relying on rating scales of intelligibility include the interdependence of the listener and speaker (therefore different listeners will make different judgments), and specific intervention targets are unable to be determined from the results (Miller, 2013).

---

[1]http://www.csu.edu.au/research/multilingual-speech/ics

TABLE 8-1 Intelligibility in Context Scale: English

The following questions are about how much of your child's speech is understood by different people. Please think about your child's speech over the past month when answering each question. Circle one number for each question.

	Always	Usually	Sometimes	Rarely	Never
1. Do you understand your child?	5	4	3	2	1
2. Do immediate members of your family understand your child?	5	4	3	2	1
3. Do extended members of your family understand your child?	5	4	3	2	1
4. Do your child's friends understand your child?	5	4	3	2	1
5. Do other acquaintances understand your child?	5	4	3	2	1
6. Do your child's teachers understand your child?	5	4	3	2	1
7. Do strangers understand your child?	5	4	3	2	1
TOTAL SCORE	/35				
AVERAGE TOTAL SCORE	**/5**				

Source: McLeod, Harrison, & McCormack (2012a). Reprinted with permission from the authors and available in 60+ languages from http://www.csu.edu.au/research/multilingual-speech/ics

TABLE 8-2 Escala de Inteligibilidad en Contexto: Español
[Intelligibility in Context Scale: Spanish]

Las siguientes preguntas son acerca de que tan bien entienden diferentes personas el habla de su hijo/a. Al responder a cada pregunta, por favor piense sobre el habla de su hijo/a durante el mes pasado. Para cada pregunta, dibuje un círculo alrededor de un número.

	Siempre	Usualmente	A veces	Raramente	Nunca
1. ¿Usted le entiende a su hijo/a?	5	4	3	2	1
2. ¿Su familia inmediata le entiende a su hijo/a?	5	4	3	2	1
3. ¿Su familia extendida le entiende a su hijo/a?	5	4	3	2	1
4. ¿Los/Las amigos/as de su hijo/a le entienden?	5	4	3	2	1
5. ¿Otros conocidos le entienden a su hijo/a?	5	4	3	2	1
6. ¿Los profesores le entienden a su hijo/a?	5	4	3	2	1
7. ¿Gente extraña le entienden a su hijo/a?	5	4	3	2	1
PUNTUACIÓN TOTAL	/35				
PROMEDIO DE PUNTUACIÓN TOTAL	**/5**				

Source: McLeod, Harrison, & McCormack (2012c), R. Prezas, R. Rojas, & B. A. Goldstein, Trans. Reprinted with permission from the authors and available in 60+ languages from http://www.csu.edu.au/research/multilingual-speech/ics

■ Single-word measures that quantify intelligible phonetic contrasts

There are many different single-word assessments that have been developed to assess children's intelligibility. In most of these assessments, children produce a set of single words and listeners determine which word was spoken via either transcription of the word or multiple-choice selection. Single-word intelligibility tests of English include:

- Children's Speech Intelligibility Measure (CSIM) (Wilcox & Morris, 1999)
- Computer Mediated Single-Word Intelligibility Test (Zajac, Plante, Lloyd, & Haley, 2011)

- Picture Speech Intelligibility Evaluation (Picture SPINE) (Monsen, Moog, & Geers, 1988)
- Preschool Speech Intelligibility Measure (PSIM) (Morris, Wilcox, & Schooling, 1995)
- Speech Intelligibility Probe for Children with Cleft Palate (SIP-CCLP) (Hodge & Gotzke, 2007)
- Test of Children's Speech Plus (TOCS+) (Hodge, Daniels, & Gotzke, 2009)
- Weiss Intelligibility Test (Weiss, 1982) (also includes spontaneous speech)

For example, the CSIM (Wilcox & Morris, 1999) has been developed to measure the intelligibility of 3- to 10-year-old children. Children produce single words either as a picture-naming task or by repeating words spoken by the examiner. Listeners are presented with a multiple-choice task to determine the words spoken. The TOCS+ (Hodge, Daniels, & Gotzke, 2009) relies on orthographic transcription of open-set word identification tasks. It has been validated on 15 adults, 48 three- to six-year-old children with typical speech, 48 children with SSD, and 22 children with dysarthria and cerebral palsy. The TOCS+ has been found to differentiate between children with SSD and typically developing children, as well as children with SSD with and without dysarthria (Hodge & Gotzke, 2014). The Computer Mediated Single-Word Intelligibility Test (Zajac et al., 2011) assesses children's intelligibility when producing 50 single words. It was found to be valid and reliable when tested on 22 four- to nine-year-old children with repaired cleft lip and palate and 16 typically developing children.

Researchers in Sweden have contributed to our understanding of intelligibility in children and adults with SSD, dysarthria, and cleft lip and palate. Single-word intelligibility tests of Swedish include:

- Swedish Intelligibility Test (SWINT) (Lillvik, Allemark, Karlström, & Hartelius, 1999) (68 single words and 10 nonsensical sentences)
- Swedish Test of Intelligibility for Children (STI-CH) (Lagerberg et al., 2015)

For example, the STI-CH (Lagerberg et al., 2015) relies on the repetition of single words after an examiner and listeners are required to provide an orthographic transcription. In a study of 10 children with SSD, 10 children who were typically developing, and 20 listeners, inter- and intra-judge reliability was found to be high, and there was a significant difference between the scores of children with SSD compared with typically developing children, and a high correlation with PCC and intelligibility in spontaneous speech (Lagerberg et al., 2015).

While single-word measures offer time-efficient and standardized tools for examining intelligibility, in order to keep the length of the assessment to a manageable level, single-word measures only cover sounds, combinations, and contexts that are likely to cause difficulties with intelligibility, but are unable to comprehensively sample children's speech (Miller, 2013).

■ Connected speech measures that quantify word and syllable identification

Eliciting and analyzing connected speech to judge intelligibility provides an assessment context with face validity. That is, judgments of intelligibility are made in naturalistic speech contexts more closely reflecting day-to-day interactions. Speake, Howard, and Vance (2011) found that intelligibility was affected by word juncture when comparing a 7-year-old's intelligibility across single-word naming, sentence repetition, and spontaneous conversation tasks, providing additional evidence for the importance of considering intelligibility using connected speech measures.

Connected speech measures of intelligibility primarily have relied on sentence repetition (Beginners' Intelligibility Test: Osberger, Robbins, Todd, & Riley, 1994), sentence reading (e.g., Lillvik, Allemark, Karlström, & Hartelius, 1999), or on conversational speech (Flipsen, 2006b; Lagerberg et al., 2014; Shriberg, Austin, Lewis, McSweeny, & Wilson, 1997a, b). Significant differences between intelligibility measures requiring reading versus spontaneous speech have been found, and Johannisson et al. (2014) concluded that measures involving reading were invalid for use with 10-year-olds due to the significant influence of their reading ability on intelligibility scores.

There have been a number of methods for quantifying intelligibility in children's conversational speech. The Intelligibility Index (Shriberg, Austin, Lewis, McSweeny, & Wilson, 1997a, b; Flipsen, 2006b) is a measure that quantifies the number of words understood by a listener. Flipsen (2006b) compared four versions for calculating the Intelligibility Index using speech samples from 320 typically developing children and 202 children with SSD (speech delay). He concluded that the original version of the Intelligibility Index, "in which a transcriber takes an utterance-by-utterance approach and groups the unintelligible syllables into words during transcription" (p. 308) differentiated the two groups of children and resulted in lower scores that may "better represent reality" (p. 310) and was more efficient than the other methods. An alternative to the Intelligibility Index for the assessment of children's spontaneous speech was proposed by Lagerberg et al. (2014). They recommended counting the percentage of syllables that were perceived as understood. They suggested that this method was quicker than transcribing words, and that it had high validity when correlated with PCC in single words for children with SSD and typically developing children.

While connected speech measures of intelligibility offer face validity, disadvantages include the inability to determine children's intended target words (particularly if they are very unintelligible) and therefore to determine whether or not the children have been understood, the possibility that children will select to use more intelligible words within their repertoire (and avoid difficult words), the time demands on listeners to transcribe connected speech, and the diminishing pool of available naive listeners over time (since people within your workplace will become accustomed to listening to unintelligible speech). Therefore, SLPs need to consider the advantages and disadvantages of each approach when determining the most appropriate measure of intelligibility.

■ Assessment of acceptability and comprehensibility

It is important to distinguish between **intelligibility** (whether a speaker's message is understood), **acceptability** (whether a speaker's message is different from what is accepted by the linguistic community) (Henningsson et al., 2008), and **comprehensibility** (whether a message can be conveyed) (Yorkston, Strand, & Kennedy, 1996). For example, if an adult pronounced the word *thinking* /θɪŋkɪŋ/ as [fɪnkən], it would be intelligible (people would know that the target word was *thinking*), but may not be considered to be an acceptable pronunciation for speakers that usually hear Standard American English. Acceptability is an important consideration for children who have dysarthria, CAS, craniofacial anomalies (e.g., cleft palate), cerebral palsy, or hearing loss. For example, children with craniofacial anomalies who produce extremely hypernasal speech containing nasal snorts may not be acceptable to some listeners. While there are numerous methods for assessing intelligibility (described earlier), assessment measures of acceptability have rarely been described in the literature. Henningsson et al. (2008) provide a 4-point rating scale of acceptability to be used when considering speech samples from children with cleft palate:

> 0 = Within normal limits: Speech is normal
>
> 1 = Mild: Speech deviates from normal to a mild degree
>
> 2 = Moderate: Speech deviates from normal to a moderate degree
>
> 3 = Severe: Speech deviates from normal to a severe degree (p. 5)

Comprehensibility is another construct that is particularly relevant for speakers with dysarthria (Yorkston et al., 1996) and speakers of English as a second or subsequent language (Munro & Derwing, 1995). Comprehensibility includes signal-independent information beyond the acoustic speech signal, such as environmental cues, gestures, and orthographic cues (e.g., the first letter of words). Assessment of comprehensibility has been studied less frequently than intelligibility but includes consideration of the communication partners as well as the speaker. For example, Yorkston et al. (1996) indicate that the following aspects of the communication partners be considered: "(a) their role in improving comprehensibility, (b) procedures for manipulating the environment, (c) techniques involved in maximizing hearing acuity, and (d) strategies to be adapted for dealing with communication breakdown" (p. 61).

ASSESSMENT OF SPEECH PRODUCTION: ELEMENTS

Assessment of children's speech production is the most common type of assessment undertaken for children with SSD (Joffe & Pring, 2008; McLeod, & Baker, 2014; Priester, Post, & Goorhuis-Brouwer, 2009; Skahan, Watson, & Lof, 2007). The assessment of speech production can include consideration of the following elements: consonants, consonant clusters, vowels and diphthongs, polysyllables, prosody, and tones (see Table 8-3). As discussed in Chapter 4, some languages do not include all of these elements. For monolingual English-speaking children, assessment of consonant clusters is necessary, but assessment of tones is not necessary. For monolingual Cantonese-speaking children, the reverse is true: assessment of consonant clusters is not necessary, but assessment of tones is important. Assessment of required elements can occur during single-word sampling (standardized or strategic), connected speech sampling, and during assessment of stimulability and consistency. These different methods of sampling will be discussed later in this chapter.

■ Consonants

Assessment of consonant production is the most common and fundamental aspect of any assessment of children's speech, regardless of the purpose. SLPs typically aim to provide opportunities for children to produce the entire consonant repertoire for the language(s) and dialect(s) spoken by children (see Chapter 4 for a list of consonants within different languages). Most English single-word assessments include words that commence with each of the following word-initial consonants: /p, b, t, d, k, g, m, n, f, v, θ, ð, s, z, ʃ, h, ɹ, j, l, w, tʃ, dʒ/. Most English assessments also contain words to assess each of the following word-final consonants: /p, b, t, d, k, g, m, n, ŋ, f, v, θ, ð, s, z, ʃ, l, tʃ, dʒ/, and words concluding with /ɹ/ (e.g., *car*) in assessments constructed for rhotic dialects (e.g., General American English). Some authors of single-word assessments also attempt to elicit consonants across three word positions (e.g., word-initial /p/ = *pig*, within word /p/ = *happy*, word-final /p/ = *cup*). However, many commercially available single-word assessments primarily consist of monosyllabic words, so do not include many opportunities for assessing within word consonants, and few consider the syllabic boundaries of within word consonants (i.e., syllable-final within word consonants versus syllable-initial within word consonants). The English consonant /ʒ/ typically is only sampled within words (e.g., *measure, television*). There is some research that provides evidence for the importance of sampling consonants across word positions. For example, Rvachew and Andrews (2002) examined consonant productions of 10 children with moderate to severe SSD in word-initial, within word, and word-final positions. They found that while 46% of productions were correct in all three word positions, 25% had different word-initial productions compared with within word and word-final productions. A further 13% had different within word productions compared with word-initial and word-final productions, and there was wide variability between participants for patterns of matches and mismatches based on the position in the word.

It is recommended that at least two examples of each consonant in each word position be elicited in order to account for variability in production. The surrounding consonants,

TABLE 8-3	Speech production elements and methods
Elements of assessment	**Methods of assessment**
■ Consonants (e.g., /p/)	■ Single-word elicitation
■ Consonant clusters (e.g., /sp, kl/)	■ Connected speech elicitation
■ Vowels and diphthongs (e.g., /i/)	■ Stimulability assessment
■ Polysyllables (e.g., *ambulance*)	■ Inconsistency/variability assessment
■ Prosody (e.g., intonation)	
■ Tones (only applicable for tone languages such as Cantonese)	

■■ ■■

✓ **APPLICATION:** *Word selection can influence accuracy of consonant production*

Consider a child who has emerging accuracy of production of the consonant /k/. Which of these words would you predict would be more likely to be produced correctly: *key, car, cow, kick, kit, clown, book, caterpillar, helicopter*? The phonotactic and coarticulatory contexts can provide some clues. Phonotactic constraints can have an effect:

- Consonants produced in monosyllables may be easier to produce than in polysyllabic words (e.g., /k/ in *cat* may be easier to produce than /k/ in *caterpillar* and *helicopter*)

- Consonants produced in singleton contexts may be easier to produce than in consonant cluster contexts (e.g., /k/ in *cow* may be easier to produce than /k/ in *clown*)

Coarticulation can have an effect:

- Velar consonants produced with back vowels may be easier than front vowels (e.g., /k/ in *car* may be easier to produce than /k/ in *key*)

- Velar consonants produced in the context of other velar consonants may be easier than those produced in a word with alveolar consonants (e.g., /k/ in *kick* may be easier to produce than /k/ in *kit*)

- Velar consonants produced in word-final position may be easier than those produced in word-initial positions (e.g., /k/ in *book* may be easier to produce than /k/ in *cob*) (Morrisette, Dinnsen, & Gierut, 2003)

Morphophonology (i.e., grammar + phonology) also can have an effect:

- Velar consonants produced in words that do not have additional grammatical morphemes may be easier than in words that contain a grammatical morpheme (e.g., /k/ in *box* [bɑks] may be easier to produce than /k/ in *licks* [lɪks] since it requires the addition of the third-person singular morpheme)

---

vowels, and syllable structure may influence the accuracy of children's production of consonants during an assessment (see "Word Selection Can Influence Accuracy of Consonant Production"). In Chapter 6 we discussed the influence of phonetic complexity, functional load, input frequency, phonotactic probability, and neighborhood density on the acquisition of consonants. These factors also play a role in the assessment of consonants.

Most commercially available standardized single-word assessments target children's production of consonants. For example:

- Bankson-Bernthal Test of Phonology (BBTOP) (Bankson & Bernthal, 1990)
- Diagnostic Evaluation of Articulation and Phonology: Articulation Assessment (DEAP) (Dodd, Hua, et al., 2002, 2006)
- Goldman-Fristoe Test of Articulation – Second Edition (GTFA-2) (Goldman & Fristoe, 2000)
- Hodson Assessment of Phonological Patterns – Third Edition (HAPP–3) (Hodson, 2004)
- Nuffield Centre Dyspraxia Programme (Williams & Stephens, 2004)
- Photo-Articulation Test – Third Edition (PAT–3) (Lippke, Dickey, Selmar, & Soder, 1997)
- Secord Contextual Articulation Test (S-CAT) (Secord & Shine, 1997)
- South Tyneside Assessment of Phonology (Armstrong & Ainley, 1988)

Some measures are designed to probe accuracy in multiple productions of one or two target consonants at a time. For example, the Secord Contextual Articulation Test (S-CAT) (Secord & Shine, 1997) enables SLPs to assess consonants and vowels in multiple contexts within words and stories.

> **MULTILINGUAL INSIGHTS:** *Locating assessments of consonants, vowels, and tones in english and other languages*
>
> There are two websites that provide a list of speech (articulation and phonology) assessments:
>
> ■ American Speech-Language-Hearing Association's Directory of Speech-Language Pathology Assessment Instruments includes information about speech assessments in English and other languages[1]
>
> ■ Multilingual Children's Speech website includes a list of children's speech assessments in over 30 languages[2]
>
> A review of 30 commercially available speech assessments in 19 languages was undertaken by McLeod and Verdon (2014). The languages were Cantonese, Danish, Finnish, German, Greek, Japanese, Korean, Maltese-English, Norwegian, Pakistani-heritage languages (Mirpuri, Punjabi, Urdu), Portuguese, Putonghua (Mandarin), Romanian, Slovenian, Spanish, Swedish, and Turkish. There were many similarities between these commercially available assessments and those available in English. Only two of the assessments that had English manuals provided information about the sensitivity and specificity of the assessment:
>
> ■ Bilingual English-Spanish Assessment (BESA) (Peña, Gutiérrez-Clellen, Iglesias, Goldstein, & Bedore, 2014)
>
> ■ Contextual Probes of Articulation Competence: Spanish (CPAC-S) (Goldstein & Iglesias, 2006)
>
> [1]http://www.asha.org/uploadedFiles/practice/multicultural/EvalToolsforDiversePops.pdf
> [2]http://www.csu.edu.au/research/multilingual-speech/speech-assessments

■ Consonant clusters

Consonant clusters occur "when two or more consonants co-occur at the same position in syllable structure" (Grunwell, 1987, p. 14; see Chapter 4). Consonant clusters are one of the most protracted elements of English to be mastered, since children begin to acquire consonant clusters when they are around 2 years old, whereas some consonant clusters are not mastered until well into the school years (e.g., Smit 1993b; see Chapter 6). Difficulty producing consonant clusters contributes to high levels of unintelligibility in children with SSD (Dodd & Iacano, 1989; Hodson & Paden, 1981), particularly as a result of cluster reduction. Consonant clusters are often targeted in intervention, since learning to produce consonants within consonant clusters may generalize to singleton contexts, thus increasing the efficiency of intervention.

While many commercially produced single-word assessments elicit a sample of consonant clusters, most do not comprehensively sample all consonant clusters within the language (Eisenberg & Hitchcock, 2010). For example, the Goldman-Fristoe Test of Articulation (Goldman & Fristoe, 2000) samples 11 word-initial consonant clusters and no word-final consonant clusters. Consequently, a number of assessments of consonant clusters have been developed and can be used when strategic single-word sampling is required:

- Clinical Procedure for Assessing Consonant Cluster Production (Powell, 1995)
- Single Word Test of Consonant Clusters (McLeod, Hand, Rosenthal, & Hayes, 1994)
- Story Retell to Elicit Consonant Clusters (McLeod et al., 1994)
- Consonant Cluster Homonym Task (McLeod, van Doorn, & Reed, 1998)
- Consonant Cluster Conversational Speech Task (McLeod, 1997; McLeod, van Doorn, & Reed, 2001b)

Powell (1995) developed a single-word screening assessment of General American English consonant clusters and validated the assessment on a hundred 4- to 5-year-old children. The 62-item word list includes 34 word-initial consonant clusters (e.g., *snow* /sn/, *shrub* /ʃɹ/, *music* /mj/) and 30 word-final consonant clusters (including /ɹ/ final consonant clusters such as in *card* /ɹd/, and consonant clusters created as a result of morphophonemes such as in *cans* /nz/). Powell (1995) included the 62-item word list in his appendix and a pattern analysis within the journal article.

Complementary single-word and connected speech consonant cluster assessments have been developed by McLeod and colleagues in order to assess the speech of children ranging from 2 years of age through school-age (McLeod, 1997; McLeod, Hand, Rosenthal, & Hayes, 1994; McLeod, van Doorn, & Reed, 2001b). For example, the appendix of McLeod et al. (1994) includes a 72-item single-word test that elicits two examples of 27 word-initial consonant clusters (e.g., *blue* /bl/, *stop* /st/, *splash* /spl/) and nine word-final consonant clusters (e.g., *fence* /ns/); morphophonemic consonant clusters were not included. The associated photographs and score sheet are freely available to be downloaded.[2] To supplement the single-word assessment, the appendix of McLeod et al. (1994) also contains two stories to elicit a range of consonant clusters within a structured connected speech context. McLeod et al. (1994) studied 40 children with SSD and found that the single-word context resulted in more instances of epenthesis (e.g., *blue* /blu/ produced as [bəlu]), and the connected speech context resulted in more instances of cluster reduction (e.g., *blue* /blu/ produced as [bu]) and final consonant deletion (*fence* /fens/ produced as [fe]); however, there was wide individual variability.

Vowels and diphthongs

As indicated in Chapter 6, most children acquire the ability to produce vowels and diphthongs in monosyllabic words at an early age, although mastery of the production of vowels in polysyllables continues into the school years. In contrast, some children with SSD have difficulty producing vowels even in monosyllabic words, resulting in a significant impact on intelligibility. Children who have vowel errors may have severe SSD, CAS, or dysarthria. They may also have (undetected) hearing loss, resulting in difficulties perceiving and thus producing vowel contrasts.

Although it is impossible to assess children's speech without eliciting vowels, many speech assessments specifically target consonants but do not focus on the production of vowels and diphthongs. Vowels and diphthongs are not specifically targeted because of the assumption that most children do not have difficulty producing vowels. The following single-word speech assessments specifically target vowels (and diphthongs):

- Arizona Articulation Proficiency Scale – Third Edition (AAPS–3) (Fudala, 2000)
- Diagnostic Evaluation of Articulation and Phonology: Articulation Assessment (DEAP) (Dodd, Hua, et al., 2002, 2006)
- Fisher-Logemann Test of Articulation (FLTA) (Fisher & Logemann, 1971)
- Hodson Assessment of Phonological Patterns – Third Edition (HAPP–3) (Hodson, 2004)
- Photo-Articulation Test – Third Edition (PAT–3) (Lippke, Dickey, Selmar, & Soder, 1997)
- Templin-Darley Tests of Articulation (TDTA) (Templin & Darley, 1969)

Typically each vowel or diphthong is targeted in one word, so the influence of coarticulatory context cannot be examined. Consequently, a comprehensive assessment of vowels and vowel inventories cannot be obtained when using a single-word speech assessment (Eisenberg & Hitchcock, 2010; Pollock, 1991).

Transcription of the whole word during a speech assessment, rather than just the targeted consonant, can enable SLPs to consider children's vowel production to a greater extent. However, if you are concerned about a child's production of vowels and diphthongs, you will need to conduct a strategic assessment using a specifically designed sampling tool that is relevant to the language(s) and dialect(s) of the child.

A strategic assessment of vowels should consider the phonetic context. Pollock and colleagues (Pollock, 1991; Pollock & Berni, 2003; Pollock & Keiser, 1990) recommend that

[2]http://athene.riv.csu.edu.au/~smcleod/Consonantclustertest.pdf

the consonant following the vowel has more impact on vowel quality than the consonant preceding the vowel. Therefore, when assessing vowels in different phonetic contexts, attempt to assess a vowel in an open syllable (e.g., *pea* /pi/) and then in the context of more than one word-final consonant (e.g., *peep* /pip/, *peek* /pik/, *peach* /pitʃ/). Postvocalic liquids such as /l/ can change the vowel quality (e.g., *peel* /pil/). Selection of the syllable length and stress within the word is also important when assessing vowels. You will recall that children have greater difficulty producing vowels correctly in polysyllabic words than monosyllabic words (James, van Doorn, McLeod, & Esterman, 2008). Additionally, children have greater difficulty producing vowels in unstressed syllables, particularly at the beginning of words. They may delete the unstressed syllable, or use the incorrect stress (and therefore the incorrect vowel). For example, they may say *computer* as COM-PUT-TER /ˈkom.ˈpju.ˈtɝ/ instead of com-PU-ter /kəmˈpjutɚ/. So, consider the impact of syllable length and stress patterns when assessing vowels.

Some examples of strategic vowel assessments follow:

■ Pollock (2002) created the Single Word Elicitation Task and Story Retelling Task for the Memphis Vowel Project (US) and the tasks found in her appendix (Pollock, 2002, pp. 104–107). These tasks assess vowels in open and closed monosyllables as well as in syllables with primary stress and non-primary stress in polysyllabic words. For example, the vowel /i/ is assessed in open monosyllables (*three, key*), closed monosyllables (*green, eat*), primary stress (*zebra, peanuts*), and non-primary stress (*cookies, Ernie, party*).

■ Speake, Stackhouse, and Pascoe (2012) created a strategic vowel assessment for use in their research in the United Kingdom that included four tasks: (1) 12 CV words commencing with an initial plosive, fricative, or nasal + vowel (e.g., *key, shoe, near*); (2) 12 VC words concluding with a final plosive, fricative, or nasal (e.g., *eat, ice, arm*); (3) 52 CVC words (e.g., /i/ in *sheep, teeth, team, wheel*); and (4) eight imitated sentences that included words with a range of vowels (e.g., "You *might* do the *ironing* with an *iron*." "Charlie left his *kite out* in the *rain*.")

■ Reid (2003) developed the Vowel House to support children's production and writing of Scottish English vowels. She used the following assessment tasks: an auditory discrimination task to differentiate between minimal pairs (e.g., *pin* versus *pen*), a lexical judgment task to determine when the target word was spoken from a list (e.g., Target = *tin*; List = *ten, tin, tan, tin*), a nonword listening task to determine when the vowel changed (e.g., *pix pix pix pix pex*), and spelling of real words and nonwords.

■ Peterson and Barney (1952) created the /hVd/ context task, where vowels are embedded within the neutral consonants /h/ and /d/ (*heed, hid, head, had, hard*, etc.). This task can be used to plot a child's vowel space. A child's vowel space can be described by

■ creating an inventory of vowels and plotting it on the International Phonetic Alphabet vowel quadrilateral (e.g., Stoel-Gammon and Herrington, 1990, found that corner vowels were more likely to be produced accurately before non-corner vowels)

■ plotting the F1 and F2 formants, measured at the midpoint of the vowel (e.g., Hillenbrand, Getty, Clark, & Wheeler, 1995) using acoustic analysis software (see Chapter 9).

One of the difficulties with assessing vowels is that people produce vowels differently according to the dialect of the language spoken. Therefore, designation of a correct production of a vowel or diphthong must be defined within the child's ambient language and dialect. Chapter 4 described vowels and diphthongs in greater depth and provided details for which dialects of English include rhotic vowels and diphthongs (General American English, Scottish English, Irish English) and which do not (General British English, Australian English, New Zealand English, South African English). Pollock (2002) recommends consideration of four categories of American English vowels: non-rhotic monophthongs, non-rhotic diphthongs, rhotic monophthongs, and rhotic diphthongs. Prior to assessment of vowels, it is important to determine the inventory of vowels that is appropriate for the language(s) and dialect of the children you assess.

■■ ■■

 APPLICATION: *Comma gets a cure*

Comma Gets a Cure[1] (Honorof, McCullough, & Somerville, 2000) is a standard reading passage that can be used to differentiate between speakers with different accents. It was created by incorporating Wells' (1982) key words, thus providing a good representation of English vowels and diphthongs. The first phrase from *Comma Gets a Cure* says, "Well here's a story for you." Listen to your friends' vowels in this sentence to hear differences in pronunciation. There are many examples on the Internet of people with different accents reading *Comma Gets a Cure*.

[1]http://www.dialectsarchive.com/comma-gets-a-cure

■ Polysyllables

Assessment of children's ability to produce polysyllabic words (words of 3+ syllables) can provide insights into children's speech, phonotactics, prosody (especially stress), language, literacy, and phonological processing skills (James, van Doorn, & McLeod, 2008; Larrivee & Catts, 1999; Lewis & Freebairn, 1992; Masso, McLeod, Baker, & McCormack, 2015). You will recall from Chapter 6 that during typical speech acquisition there is a shift around 5 years of age where the focus changes from paradigmatic aspects (production of vowels in isolation) to syntagmatic aspects (production of vowels in context) of speech production. Syntagmatic aspects of speech production can be measured during production of polysyllables. Polysyllables enable SLPs to consider children's ability to accurately use timing, stress, and the schwa vowel.

A criticism of many single-word speech assessments is that they rely on the assessment of monosyllabic and disyllabic words, but contain very few polysyllabic words (James, van Doorn, & McLeod, 2008). Children may be able to produce consonants and vowels in monosyllabic contexts but be unable to produce them in more complex words; thus, if polysyllabic words are not assessed then an SSD may be "concealed or underestimated" (James, van Doorn, & McLeod, 2008, p. 347). There are a number of informal assessments of polysyllabic words:

- 10 Clinically Useful Words (James, 2009)
- Single Word Polysyllable Test (Gozzard, Baker, & McCabe, 2004)
- Polysyllable Preschool Test (POP) (Baker, 2013)
- Toddler Polysyllable Test (T-POT) (Baker, 2010c)
- Assessment of Children's Articulation and Phonology: 199 word test including 17 polysyllables, 77 disyllables, and 105 monosyllables (James, 2001b)

For example, James (2006, 2009) identified 10 polysyllabic words that were clinically useful in revealing speech production difficulties in children. The words were *ambulance, hippopotamus, computer, spaghetti, vegetables, helicopter, animals, caravan, caterpillar,* and *butterfly*.

 CHILDREN'S INSIGHTS: *Long words are hard to say*

Production of polysyllabic words can be important for individual children who enjoy talking about dinosaurs, characters from animations and games, and other things that have long names (e.g., *tyrannosaurus rex, brontosaurus*). The sibling of a child with SSD said: "When he tries to say long words he can't say them properly" and "he first started off saying *speech therapist* like 'beach berry'. . . And then it turned into 'beach fairy'. And then, he still calls it 'beach fairy'. . ." (McLeod, Daniel, & Barr, 2013, p. 79). What does this make you think about the importance of assessing polysyllabic words in school-aged children?

■ Prosody

You will recall from Chapter 4 that prosody (or suprasegmentals) includes stress, rhythm, intonation, and lexical and grammatical tones. Prosody can either directly affect the meaning or it can add information to a word or phrase (Peppé, 2009). As mentioned in Chapter 6, children's ability to produce prosodic contours develops early in life. However, refinement of prosody can take well into the school years (Ballard, Djaja, Arciuli, James, & van Doorn, 2012; Cruttenden, 1982; James, van Doorn, McLeod, & Esterman, 2008). Difficulty with prosody has been documented in children and adults with SSD (Howard, 2007b), CAS (Odell & Shriberg, 2001), dysarthria (Bunton, Kent, Kent, & Rosenbek, 2000), developmental delay (Shriberg & Widder, 1990), Williams syndrome (Setter, Stojanovik, Van Ewijk, & Moreland, 2007), hearing loss (Lenden & Flipsen, 2007), Down syndrome (Zampini et al., 2015, in press), and autism spectrum disorders (McCann, Peppé, Gibbon, O'Hare, & Rutherford, 2007; Shriberg, Paul, McSweeny, Klin, Cohen, & Volkmar, 2001). Conversely, prosody has not been found to be a core area of difficulty for English-speaking children with specific language impairment (SLI) or dyslexia (Marshall, Harcourt-Brown, Ramus, & Van der Lely, 2009).

There are a number of different ways to assess prosody depending on whether or not it is perceived as an area of difficulty. Many SLPs begin by informally listening to children's prosody during connected speech testing. They may use a checklist to consider whether a child's stress, rhythm, and intonation are appropriate. SLPs may transcribe prosodic features when undertaking a phonetic/phonemic transcription using the International Phonetic Alphabet and extIPA (Rutter, Klopfenstein, Ball, & Müller, 2010). There are a few assessments that focus on prosody during speech production. For example:

- Prosody-Voice Screening Profile (Shriberg, Kwiatkowski, & Rasmussen, 1990)
- Prosody-Voice Profile (Shriberg, 1993)
- Prosody Profile (PROP) (Crystal, 1982)
- Profiling Elements of Prosody in Speech-Communication (PEPS-C) (Peppé & McCann, 2003a; Peppé, 2015)

The Prosody-Voice Profile (Shriberg, 1993) enables SLPs to profile a child's connected speech sample on three prosodic domains (phrasing, rate, and stress) and three voice domains (loudness, pitch, and quality of laryngeal and resonance features) that are further divided into 31 types of inappropriate prosody-voice codes (see Figure 8-1).

While the Prosody-Voice Profile (Shriberg, 1993) and PROP (Crystal, 1982) can be used to describe prosody during connected speech, the PEPS-C consists of 14 subtests designed to assess both the comprehension (input) and production (output) of prosody (Peppé & McCann, 2003a; Peppé, 2015). The prosodic function tasks include turn end, affect, lexical stress chunking/boundary, and contrastive stress, and the prosodic form tasks include an auditory discrimination and imitation task. For example, in a chunking task children have to differentiate between "chocolate cake and buns" and "chocolate, cake, and buns" (notice the commas). The computerized PEPS-C was designed for children aged 4 years and above and has been normed on 120 Southern British English-speaking children (Wells, Peppé, & Goulandris, 2004). It has been used with children with SSD as well as children with high-functioning autism/Asperger syndrome and is available in Dutch, English (Australian, North American, Southern British, Scottish, Irish), French, Norwegian, and Spanish (Martínez-Castilla & Peppé, 2008; Peppé, Coene, Hesling, Martínez-Castilla, & Moen, 2012). Details of PEPS-C tasks, instructions for administration, scoring procedures, and task items are outlined in the appendix of McCann, Peppé, Gibbon, O'Hare, and Rutherford (2007) and information about the 2015 revision is on the PEPS-C website.[3]

One aspect of prosody that has diagnostic significance is lexical stress (Ballard, Djaja, Arciuli, James, & van Doorn, 2012). Accuracy of lexical stress can be measured in familiar polysyllabic words commencing with strong-weak (e.g., *elephant*) and weak-strong (e.g., *computer*) stress patterns. Words commencing with weak-strong stress are more difficult, and this can be a diagnostic feature of the speech of children with CAS.

---

[3]http://www.peps-c.com

FIGURE 8-1 **Prosody-voice profile**

Prosody-Voice Codes
Prosody

Phrasing		Rate		Stress	
1 Appropriate	___	1 Appropriate	___	1 Appropriate	___
2 Sound/Syllable Repetition	___	9 Slow Articulation/Pause Time	___	2 Multisyllabic Word Stress	___
3 Word Repetition	___	10 Slow/Pause Time	___	14 Reduced/Equal Stress	___
4 Sound/Syllable and		11 Fast	___	15 Excessive/Equal/	
Word Repetition	___	12 Fast/Acceleration	___	Misplaced Stress	
5 More than One Word Repetition	___			16 Multiple Stress Features	___
6 One Word Revision	___				
7 More than One Word Revision	___				
8 Repetition and Revision	___				

Voice

Loudness		Pitch		Quality			
				Laryngeal Features		**Resonance Features**	
1 Appropriate	___	1 Appropriate	___	1 Appropriate	___	1 Appropriate	___
17 Soft	___	19 Low Pitch/Glottal Fry	___	23 Breathy	___	30 Nasal	___
18 Loud	___	20 Low Pitch	___	24 Rough	___	31 Denasal	___
		21 High Pitch/Falsetto	___	25 Strained	___	32 Nasopharyngeal	___
		22 High Pitch	___	26 Break/Shift/			
				Tremulous	___		
				27 Register Break	___		
				28 Diplophonia	___		
				29 Multiple Laryngeal			
				Features	___		

Source: Shriberg (1993). Used by permission from American Speech-Language-Hearing Association (ASHA).

■ Tones

A number of the world's languages use contrastive tones to differentiate meaning (e.g., Cantonese, Mandarin/Putonghua, and Vietnamese). Assessing perception and production of tones is not relevant for monolingual English speakers but is relevant for speakers of tonal languages, since meaning is lost if tones are perceived or produced incorrectly. Examples of assessments that include consideration of production of tones are:

- Cantonese Segmental Phonology Test (CSPT) (So, 1993)
- Hong Kong Cantonese Articulation Test (HKCAT) (Cheung, Ng, & To, 2006)
- Putonghua Segmental Phonology Test (PSPT) (So & Jing, 2000)

Tests that enable consideration of the perception of tones include:

- Cantonese Basic Speech Perception Test (Lee, 2006)
- Hong Kong Cantonese Tone Identification Test (Lee, 2010)

ASSESSMENT OF SPEECH PRODUCTION: METHODS

There are four main methods used to assess speech production: single-word testing, connected speech testing, stimulability testing, and inconsistency/variability testing. Each will be considered next.

▪ Single-word speech assessments

Single-word speech assessments are the most commonly used assessment format for children with suspected SSD (Joffe & Pring, 2008; McLeod, & Baker, 2014; Priester et al., 2009; Skahan et al., 2007) because the repertoire of consonants (and vowels) for a language can be sampled and analyzed in a time-efficient manner. Single-word speech assessments typically consist of a series of pictures (or objects) that are shown to a child to elicit single-word productions (e.g., *duck*). Originally single-word speech assessments were designed to assess the **articulation** of speech sounds, and many are still used today:

- Arizona Articulation Proficiency Scale – Third Edition (Arizona-3) (Fudala, 2000)
- Edinburgh Articulation Test (Anthony, Bogle, Ingram, & McIsaac, 1971)
- Fisher-Logemann Test of Articulation (FLTA) (Fisher & Logemann, 1971)
- Goldman Fristoe Test of Articulation – Second Edition (GFTA-2) (Goldman & Fristoe, 2000)
- New Zealand Articulation Test (Moyle, 2004)
- Photo Articulation Test (PAT) (Lippke et al., 1997)
- Structured Photographic Articulation Test II: Featuring Dudsberry (SPAT-D II) (Dawson & Tattersall, 2001)
- Templin-Darley Tests of Articulation (TDTA) (Templin & Darley, 1969)
- Weiss Comprehensive Articulation Test (WCAT) (Weiss, 1980)

Typically articulation assessments have been designed to sample each consonant (and some have also considered vowels and consonant clusters) in different word positions. Some single speech word assessments have been designed to assess children's **phonology**:

- Hodson Assessment of Phonological Patterns – Third Edition (HAPP-3) (Hodson, 2004)
- Bankson-Bernthal Test of Phonology (BBTOP) (Bankson & Bernthal, 1990)

For example, the Bankson-Bernthal Test of Phonology (BBTOP) (Bankson & Bernthal, 1990) is organized so different sets of words assess the occurrence of velar fronting, cluster reduction, and other phonological processes/patterns. Finally, some single-word speech assessments are designed to consider both articulation and phonology:

- Clinical Assessment of Articulation and Phonology (CAAP) (Secord, & Donohue, 2002)
- Computerized Articulation and Phonology Evaluation System (CAPES) (Masterson & Bernhardt, 2001)
- Diagnostic Evaluation of Articulation and Phonology (DEAP) (Dodd, Hua, et al., 2002, 2006)
- Smit-Hand Articulation and Phonology Evaluation (SHAPE) (Smit & Hand, 1997)

Surveys of SLPs have revealed that SLPs commonly used single-word speech assessments that were developed in the countries where they worked. For each country, the most commonly used assessments were:

- United States: Goldman-Fristoe Test of Articulation (Goldman & Fristoe, 2000) and the Photo Articulation Test (Lippke, Dickey, Selmar, & Soder, 1997), as reported in a survey of 333 SLPs (Skahan et al., 2007).
- United Kingdom: South Tyneside Assessment of Phonology (Armstrong & Ainley, 1988) and the Nuffield Centre Dyspraxia Programme (Williams & Stephens, 2004), as reported in a survey of 98 SLPs (Joffe & Pring, 2008).
- Australia: Articulation Survey (Aitken & Fisher, 1996) and the Diagnostic Evaluation of Articulation and Phonology (Dodd, Hua, et al., 2002), as reported in a survey of 231 SLPs (McLeod & Baker, 2014).
- The Netherlands: Logo-Art (Baarda, de Boer-Jongsma, & Haasjes-Jongsma, 2005) and Metaphon (Leydekker-Brinkman & Bast, 2002), as reported in a survey of 85 SLPs (Priester et al., 2009).
- Portugal: Teste de articulação verbal (TAV) (Guimarães & Grilo, 1996) and Teste fonético-fonologico–avaliação da linguagem pré-escolar (TFF-ALPE) (Mendes, Afonso, Lousada, & Andrade, 2013), as reported in a survey of 88 SLPs (Oliveira et al., 2015).

When authors create single-word speech assessments, they consider the conceptualization and operationalization of the measure (McLeod, 2012a). We will describe the operationalization later in this chapter when we discuss standardized testing. During the conceptualization phase, decisions are made regarding the content. Specifically, words within a single-word speech assessment frequently are selected to represent each of the consonants within the targeted language and dialect. For example, in the Goldman-Fristoe Test of Articulation (Goldman & Fristoe, 2000) there are opportunities to produce each English consonant in word-initial, within word, and word-final positions. A number of authors of single-word speech assessments also consider the representativeness of the sampled vowels, diphthongs, consonant clusters, stress, and phonotactic complexity (e.g., monosyllabic versus polysyllabic words). Despite the care taken by the authors when conceptualizing single-word speech assessments, Eisenberg and Hitchcock (2010) found that none of 11 commonly used single-word speech assessments provided sufficient opportunities for the production of word-initial consonants, word-final consonants, and vowels to make conclusions about a child's phonetic inventory. They suggested that in order to create a consonant inventory, the sample should elicit consonants in contexts with different:

- syllable stress (e.g., /k/ in *kitchen* = strong-weak versus *koala* weak-strong),
- number of syllables (e.g., /k/ in *cat* = one syllable versus *caterpillar* = four syllables),
- consonant cluster contexts (e.g., /k/ in *clown* = /kl/ versus *crown* = /kɹ/ versus *sky* = /sk/ versus *screw* = /skɹ/ versus *ask* = /sk/),
- morpheme contexts (e.g., /ks/ in *box* versus *locks*, the plural of *lock*),
- assimilation contexts (e.g., /k/ in *cat* = velar-alveolar versus *kick* = velar-velar), and
- vowel-consonant combinations (e.g., /k/ with *key* = front vowel versus *car* = back vowel versus *core* = rounded vowel).

To ensure that a comprehensive sample is elicited, at least two productions of a consonant should be elicited in each word position within different words containing different vowels and syllable shapes. Eisenberg and Hitchcock (2010) found that many published single-word speech assessments did not meet this guideline. Some authors recommend that a single-word sample should consist of at least 100 words and include a complete inventory of consonants across word positions and a variety of word shapes, lengths, and stress patterns (Bernhardt & Holdgrafer, 2001a, b; Eisenberg & Hitchcock, 2010).

Many SLPs use single-word speech assessments because they can efficiently sample children's productions of each consonant (and possibly other elements of speech) to provide an overview of sounds/processes across word positions. Additionally, many single-word speech assessments provide standard scores and percentile ranks, enabling comparison with the tested population and determination of eligibility for speech-language pathology services. However, there are limitations of single-word speech assessments that are eloquently described by Miccio (2002):

> I view all articulation tests as screening devices because of the limitations in the size of the sample and because of the way the sample is obtained. Standardized scores allow comparison to a normative sample, but they do not provide adequate information on the systematic nature of a child's phonology or how it is used in connected speech, a crucial aspect of any assessment. (p. 224)

Additional limitations of single-word speech assessments include that a limited range of words and word types are assessed (frequently monosyllabic and disyllabic nouns are favored). In some assessments, consonants are only elicited in one word per word position, so phonological information and the impact of stress and prosody cannot be determined. For example, elicitation of /ʤ/ in the word *giraffe* is likely to be produced differently than in the word *jump*. Furthermore, the test environment of picture naming is not naturalistic and may encourage children to overemphasize production.

There are a number of factors that have been considered regarding whether or not they influence children's speech production during single-word testing.

- **Imitated versus spontaneous production:** It is possible that inclusion of imitated productions may overestimate children's speech production skills. Differences between children's imitated and spontaneous production of words has been examined, with some studies indicating fewer errors occurring during imitated

> **COMMENT:** *Desirable characteristics of sampling tools*
>
> ■ Easily identifiable pictures or objects (by children)
> ■ Assesses all phonemes in a variety of contexts
> ■ Allows sufficient sampling for phonological analysis
> ■ Assesses single words, sentences, and spontaneous speech
> ■ Appropriate for various ages
> ■ Reflective of the cultures within the community
> ■ Attractive
> ■ Durable and portable
> ■ Computerized administration and scoring
> ■ Valid and reliable
> ■ High sensitivity and specificity
> ■ Large normative sample that reflects the community

productions of words (DuBois & Bernthal, 1978; Johnson & Somers, 1978; Kresheck & Socolofsky, 1972), some studies showing varying results (Goldstein, Fabiano, & Iglesias, 2004), and others showing no difference (Andrews & Fey, 1986; Powell, 1997). For example, Kresheck and Socolofsky (1972) compared imitated and spontaneous productions during a single-word testing. Forty of the 45 children achieved a higher overall score for the imitated condition. DuBois and Bernthal (1978) studied 18 children with SSD and documented significantly more errors on a continuous speech task compared with a modeled continuous speech task. Goldstein et al. (2004) studied 12 Spanish-speaking children with SSD producing single words and indicated identical production of consonants across the tasks 62% of the time, more adultlike production in spontaneous productions 25% of the time, and more adultlike productions for imitated productions 13% of the time. Leonard, Schwartz, Folger, and Wilcox (1978) found that young children avoided producing target words within a spontaneous speech task.

■ **Pictures versus written stimuli:** There were no significant differences in error rates during the production of consonant clusters elicited using pictures versus written words for 74 typically developing children aged 5 to 12 years. However, the younger children took more time and required significantly more prompting when reading the written words (McLeod & Arciuli, 2009).

■ **Color versus black and white stimuli:** There are some differences between using color in single-word naming versus connected speech elicitation. Typically developing 4-, 6-, and 8-year-old children named colored drawings significantly faster than black and white line drawings for words that were in their emerging lexicons. There was no significant difference for words that were established in their lexicons (Barrow, Holbert, & Rastatter, 2000). The color of images did not affect the content, length, or word variety used in narratives of typically developing 4-year-old children (Schneider, Rivard, & Debreuil, 2011).

■ Single-word testing for young children

The need for early identification of speech difficulties has led to the recent development of assessments for 2-year-old children, including:

■ Profiles of Early Expressive Phonological Skills (PEEPS) (Williams & Stoel-Gammon, in preparation)
■ Toddler Phonology Test (TPT) (McIntosh & Dodd, 2011)

> **COMMENT:** *Four-step process for eliciting single words*
>
> The following four-step protocol for eliciting single words may increase the likelihood of spontaneous versus imitated productions within a single-word speech assessment (McLeod, Hand, Rosenthal, & Hayes, 1994). For example, to elicit the word *bird*:
>
> 1. Ask, "What's this?"
> 2. Provide a clue (e.g., it has wings and flies).
> 3. Provide a binary choice with the target word produced first: "Is it a *bird* or a *house*?" The decoy word should not be similar to the target word in meaning or in phonetic structure.
> 4. Provide delayed imitation. "It's a *bird*. What is it?" It is important to add a phrase after the production of the target word so that the child is not repeating the last word heard. If possible, a short while after the word has been elicited using delayed imitation, the word should be elicited spontaneously by asking, "What's this again?"

Profiles of Early Expressive Phonological Skills (PEEPS) (Williams & Stoel-Gammon, in preparation) uses toy manipulatives (toys) to elicit 60 developmentally appropriate words that are based on lexical norms from the MacArthur-Bates Communicative Developmental Inventories, in basic and expanded word lists. The authors indicate that by using manipulatives and age-appropriate vocabulary, a high proportion of the words are able to be elicited spontaneously (Stoel-Gammon & Williams, 2013). The Toddler Phonology Test (TPT) (McIntosh & Dodd, 2011) was designed to assess children aged 2;0–2;11 and uses 37 picture stimuli to elicit single-word productions and includes normative data.

■ Connected speech assessments

The second method used to assess speech production is connected speech testing. Connected speech testing can be achieved in a number of different ways, including conversation during play (Andrews & Fey, 1986; Morrison & Shriberg, 1992), narrative retell (DuBois & Bernthal, 1978; Kenney, Prather, Mooney, & Jeruzal, 1984; McLeod et al., 1994), picture description (Healy & Madison, 1987), and sentence repetition (Bankson & Bernthal, 1982). In some instances, reading passages may also be used. For example, Patel et al. (2013) recommended that "The Caterpillar" passage could elicit a variety of segmental and prosodic variables and be used to diagnostically differentiate between apraxia of speech and dysarthria for 22 adults. Commercially available assessments that contain connected speech tasks include:

■ Diagnostic Evaluation of Articulation and Phonology (DEAP) (Dodd, Hua, et al., 2002, 2006)
■ Secord Contextual Articulation Test (S-CAT) (Secord & Shine, 1997)

The DEAP includes a short story retell component to compare words that were elicited within the single-word sampling subtests. The subtest of the S-CAT titled Storytelling Probes of Articulation Competence (SPAC) facilitates collection of connected speech samples that are focused on specific speech sounds.

Conversational speech samples are reported to be elicited by many SLPs around the world (McLeod & Baker, 2014; Priester, Post, & Goorhuis-Brouwer, 2009; Skahan, Watson, & Lof, 2007). For example, conversational speech sampling was reported to be used always (58%) or sometimes (25.7%) by 231 Australian SLPs (McLeod & Baker, 2014). Listening to connected speech provides a real-world (natural) view of children's intelligibility and ability to produce speech in context. Connected speech samples enable examination of prosody, intelligibility, and interactions between children's speech and other language abilities (Bernhardt & Holdgrafer, 2001a, b; Morrison & Shriberg, 1992). In addition, connected speech samples provide real-world data to analyze error patterns and monitor progress.

Eliciting an appropriate length of a conversational speech sample is important to ensure validity and reliability of the sample (Crary, 1983). Grunwell (1987) recommended that 100 different words is the minimum size of an adequate sample and 200–250 words is preferable. Similarly, Shriberg et al. (1997b) recommended eliciting a sample containing 100 different intelligible words and that a speech sample should contain "at least two tokens in two different words of any error or inventory item to be used in making a classification" (p. 735). Van Severen, Van Den Berg, Molemans, and Gillis (2012) considered the impact of the size of spontaneous speech samples when describing the consonant inventories of 30 Dutch-speaking 2-year-old children. They found a positive correlation between the size of children's reported consonant inventories and the number of words in the speech sample. The number of consonants in children's inventories differed within the same session and depended on which sample was selected. For example, one child's inventory varied from three to seven consonants within different samples selected within the same conversational speech session. The maximum sample size required to ensure a complete consonant inventory differed for each child. Next, Van Severen et al. (2012) determined that numbers of consonants (not amount of time or number of words) was the most appropriate unit for determining the best sample size. Finally, they determined that in order to compare consonant inventories between children and over time, speech samples containing at least 2,995 word-initial consonant tokens and 343 word-final consonant tokens should be drawn from randomly selected utterances within the same session. Dutch contains 21 word-initial consonants and 14 word-final consonants, so it is possible that a larger sample size would be required for English (since it contains a greater number of word-initial and word-final consonants).

> **COMMENT: *Assessment of connected speech processes***
>
> Connected speech testing can be helpful for assessing children's abilities to use **juncture**—that is, the way children join words together across syllable boundaries (Wells, 1994). Connected speech testing assesses children's use of the naturally occurring processes of elision, assimilation, and liaison, in addition to their connected speech ability across different types of contexts (neutral, facilitatory, and phonetically challenging) (Pascoe et al., 2006). As you read the example sentences below, say the sentences aloud using casual connected speech, so that you hear the processes.
>
> 1. Natural processes in connected speech
>   - **Elision** (omission of a speech sound in casual connected speech): *"the cat scratched me"* /ðə kæt skɹætʃt mi/ → [ðə kæ skɹætʃt mi] (omission of [t] in [kæt])
>   - **Assimilation** (one speech sound changing due to the influence of another speech sound): *"the brown cat"* /ðə braʊn kæt/ → [ðə braʊŋ kæt] (velar assimilation of /n/→ [ŋ])
>   - **Liaison** (phonological adjustment such as a glide being inserted between two words): *"they ate up"* /ðe et ʌp/ → [ðe jet ʌp] (insertion of /j/ between [e] and [e])
>
> 2. Neutral, facilitatory, and challenging phonetic connected speech contexts
>
>   - **Neutral context** (final consonant of one word is followed by word starting with a vowel) *"cat in"* /kæt ɪn/
>   - **Facilitating context** (the same consonant ends one word and begins the next) *"The cat too!"* /kæt tu/
>   - **Challenging context** (a word ending in a consonant is followed by a word starting with a different consonant) *"cat jumped"* /kæt dʒʌmpt/
>
> Stackhouse, Vance, Pascoe, and Wells (2007) provide a helpful compendium of sentence imitation tasks for examining children's use of these naturally occurring processes and different connected speech contexts.

COMMENT: *Technological transcriptions*

Connected speech sampling is often considered to be time-intensive, particularly for transcription and analysis of the sample (Tomasello & Stahl, 2004). Technological advances in recording and transcription may revive the practicality of this important sampling technique. For example, LENA technology can be used to record children's speech and language samples while they wear a vest containing a recording device. Xu, Richards, and Gilkerson (2014) reported that LENA recordings have been automatically transcribed and reliably differentiated between consonant and vowel production. Additionally, Thomas Campbell and colleagues at the University of Texas, Dallas, have been working on automated transcriptions of English single-word speech samples (UT Dallas, 2014). Subsequent advances in technology will impact SLPs' ability to transcribe and analyze connected speech samples in the future.

CHILDREN'S INSIGHTS: *Listen to my conversational speech, not just easy words*

James (aged 6 years) was assessed by an SLP whose mother reported that the SLP said, "He's really very mild . . . he is able to say every sound that is age-appropriate," and the SLP indicated that James did not need any intervention. The mother reported that the SLP showed James some pictures (possibly a single-word test predominantly comprised of monosyllables), but did not listen to his conversational speech. However, James' mother said: "We haven't got that [correct sounds] into everyday speech yet . . . He speaks either very quietly or very loudly and all his words run together, there are no spaces in between so it can be very hard to understand what he's saying" (McLeod, Daniel, & Barr, 2013, p. 74). James was involved in a research project and was asked to draw a picture of himself talking to someone. He described his picture as "talking to someone with listening ears" (see Figure 8-2). In the picture, James is on the left with a sad mouth, and his friend is on the right with large listening ears. James loved dinosaurs and computer games, so many of the words that were important to him were polysyllables, and would not be found within standardized single-word tests. What does this information about James make you think about when planning a speech assessment?

FIGURE 8-2 James drew himself talking to someone with listening ears

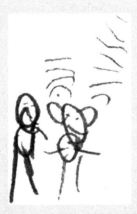

Source: From Using Children's Drawings to Listen to How Children Feel About Their Speech, S. McLeod, G. Daniel, & J. Barr, 2006, *Proceedings of the 2006 Speech Pathology Australia National Conference*, p. 41. Copyright 2006 by Speech Pathology Australia.

▪ Single-word versus connected speech assessments

Single-word and connected speech assessments may place different cognitive demands on the speaker. Table 8-4 provides a comparison of single-word and connected speech testing. Many studies have documented significant differences between single-word and connected speech testing, with some studies indicating that there are more errors occurring in connected speech (DuBois & Bernthal, 1978; Faircloth & Faircloth, 1970; Healy & Madison, 1987) and other studies indicating fewer errors in connected speech (Morrison & Shriberg, 1992). For example, Morrison and Shriberg (1992) documented differences between single-word and connected speech production for 61 children with SSD in the overall accuracy, occurrence of phonological processes, production of individual phonemes, types of errors and other aspects such as variations in manner and allophones. They indicated that established sounds were more likely to be correct in connected speech and emerging sounds were more likely to be correct in single-word testing. However, not all studies have documented a significant difference between the two sampling techniques, particularly when considering the occurrence of phonological processes (Andrews & Fey, 1986; Kenney, Prather, Mooney, & Jeruzal, 1984; McLeod, Hand, Rosenthal, & Hayes, 1994; Paden & Moss, 1985). For example, McLeod, Hand, Rosenthal, and Hayes (1994) considered the production of consonant clusters of 40 children with SSD under the two sampling conditions and indicated that while there was a large amount of variability, there was no significant difference overall; however, on the connected speech task, there were significantly more instances of cluster reduction and final consonant deletion and significantly fewer instances of epenthesis (e.g., *blue* /blu/ → [bəlu]).

▪ Assessment of stimulability

After eliciting children's speech using either single-word or connected speech sampling techniques, it is useful to list the sounds in error, and to determine whether or not children are stimulable for these sounds. Stimulability refers to a child's ability to "immediately modify a speech production error when presented with an auditory and visual model" (Miccio, 2009,

---

TABLE 8-4 **A comparison between single-word and connected speech elicitation**

	Single-word elicitation	Connected speech elicitation
Similarity with day-to-day speech	Less naturalistic	More naturalistic (inherent face validity)
Elicited phonetic and syllabic contexts	Controlled to elicit every consonant (and vowel) in the ambient language	More dependent on child, topic, stimuli. It is possible that some consonants, vowels, and word shapes may not be elicited
Elicited word types	Mostly nouns + a few verbs	All word types
Number of productions	Typically one production of each word	Scope for multiple productions of each word to determine variability in production and ability to change productions after requests for clarification
Standardization of procedures	Most have standardized elicitation and scoring protocols that can be reapplied to assess progress	Few have standardized elicitation and scoring protocols
Time	Faster to administer and analyze	More time-consuming to analyze
Knowledge of the target words	Known linguistic context	Unknown linguistic context, so the target of unintelligible words may be unknown
Selection and avoidance	Children are invited to produce a range of words	Children may avoid producing difficult words and may produce short utterances (single words)
Comparison with normative data	The majority of normative studies have used single-word sampling	Fewer normative studies have used connected speech word sampling
Scope of information	Sample is primarily used for considering speech sound production	Sample may be used to consider speech sound production, intelligibility, language, voice, fluency

p. 97). Stimulability provides insights into the difference between **capacity** (children's abilities under the most supportive circumstances) and **performance** (children's abilities in typical day-to-day situations) and is thought to reflect children's productive phonological knowledge (Dinnsen & Elbert, 1984). Stimulability can provide information about children's prognosis for change (Powell & Miccio, 1996), and children who are stimulable for sounds may not require direct intervention on these sounds (Powell, Elbert, & Dinnsen, 1991).

To assess stimulability, list the consonants that are absent from a child's inventory. Then, provide auditory and visual models, as well as instructions regarding the voicing, place, and manner of articulation (see Chapter 4). For example, if a child does not produce /k/ in single-word or connected speech testing, you may say, "Let's try to say the [k] sound. Remember to keep your tongue at the back of your mouth when you say it. [k, k, k]. Now you try." Miccio (2002) recommended that children be given 10 opportunities to produce a sound: in isolation, and in CV, VC, and VCV contexts with the vowels /i/, /u/, and /a/. Tyler and Tolbert (2002) recommended testing stimulability (1) in isolation first, then if correct in CV and VC syllables, (2) in word positions that are problematic, and (3) and in words and sentences for sounds that are produced inconsistently. In Chapter 7 we discussed the role of stimulability in dynamic assessment and profiled the Glaspey Dynamic Assessment of Phonology (GDAP) (Glaspey & MacLeod, 2010; Glaspey & Stoel-Gammon, 2007) as a standardized dynamic assessment.

■ Assessment of inconsistency and variability

Variability within children can occur in two different ways: (1) different realizations of a sound in *different* lexical items (e.g., /k/ is realized differently in *key* /ki/ → [ki] and *cat* /kæt/ → [tæt]) and (2) different realizations for different productions of the *same* lexical item (e.g., *sleep* /slip/ → [swip], [lip], [fliː]) (McLeod & Hewett, 2008). As discussed earlier in this chapter, the first type of variability can be influenced by the context of the word (e.g., whether the surrounding consonants share the same place and manner of articulation). The second type of variability can be influenced by the sampling condition (e.g., single word versus connected speech or imitated versus spontaneous production) or whether the production has changed because the child is responding to a request for clarification (Gozzard, Baker, & McCabe, 2008; Masso, McCabe, & Baker, 2014). However, if the assessment task remains the same and the child's productions of the words are different each time, it is important to differentiate between normal variability (i.e., productions that differ according to typical acquisition patterns) and inconsistency. "Inconsistency is speech characterized by a high proportion of differing repeated productions with multiple error types, both segmental (phoneme) and structural errors (consonant–vowel sequence within a syllable)" (Holm, Crosbie, & Dodd, 2007, p. 467) and is suggestive of speech processing difficulties. Variability has been described using the Error Consistency Index (Tyler, Lewis, & Welch, 2003). Dodd, Hua, et al. (2002, 2006) created a specific subtest of the DEAP called the Inconsistency Assessment that consists of 25 words of one to four syllables that sample most English consonants and vowels (e.g., *elephant*). During the Inconsistency Assessment, children are required to name the 25 words within the same session on three different occasions that are separated by an unrelated activity. Each word triplet is coded as: consistently correct, consistently incorrect, variable (with at least one word correct), variable (with no words correct). Holm et al. (2007) tested 409 typically developing British children aged 3;0 to 6;11 and found that the majority of the words were coded as consistently correct (e.g., 76.5% of the 3;0- to 3;5-year-olds' responses) and found that age and sex had an effect on consistency of productions. An inconsistency percentage score is created by determining the number of words that were produced variably, dividing by 25, and multiplying by 100. Inconsistent speech disorder is defined as 40% variable production on the Inconsistency Assessment (Dodd, Hua, et al., 2002, 2006; Holm, Crosbie & Dodd, 2013).

ASSESSMENT OF ORAL STRUCTURE AND FUNCTION

It is important that children's oral structure and function are examined during an assessment to identify possible underlying causes of SSD. Impaired body structures (for example, a cleft lip or palate) may impact children's ability to perceive or produce speech sounds, and therefore it is essential that identification occurs as early as possible to reduce possible long-term impacts upon children's speech. Assessment of oromotor function is particularly important for differential diagnosis of CAS and childhood dysarthria (McCauley & Strand, 2008).

An oral structure and function assessment will consider the anatomical structures used in speech: lips, tongue, teeth, mandible (jaw), hard palate, soft palate (velum), nose, pharynx, and larynx (see Chapter 3). Oral function assessments can consider oromotor function in three ways: nonverbal, during speech, and during feeding. An oral structure and function assessment may be conducted by systematically assessing structures of the face and oral cavity, and the function of relevant cranial nerves. For example, in the Oral and Speech Motor Control Protocol, Robbins and Klee (1987) recommend that assessment of the lips (cranial nerve VII) should include consideration of the structure of the lips at rest (symmetry and the relationship between open and closed lips), oral function (rounding, protrusion, retraction, pucker/smile, bite lower lip, puff cheeks, open/close lips), and speech function of the lips (rounding /oʊ/, protrusion /u/, retraction /i/, alternate /u/ and /i/, bite lower lip /f/, open-close lips /mʌ/). They recommend that assessment of the tongue (cranial nerve XII) should include consideration of the tongue at rest (symmetry, carriage, fasciculations, furrowing, atrophy, hypertrophy), oral function (protrusion, elevation to the alveolar ridge, anterior-posterior sweep, interdental protrusion), and speech function of the tongue (elevation to the alveolar ridge for /n, t, l/, lateral edges of tongue to teeth for /s, ʃ/, interdental /θ/, and posterior tongue to palate /k, g/). They provided similar tasks for assessing the mandible (cranial nerve V), tongue (cranial nerve XII), velopharynx (cranial nerve X), and larynx-respiration (cranial nerve X), as well as the maxilla, teeth, coordinated speech movements, prosody, and voice.

Oral-diadochokinesis (DDK) tasks are often used to examine oromotor function (Wertzner, Alves, & de Oliveira Ramos, 2008; Williams, & Stackhouse, 2000). DDK tasks require rapid repetition of syllables, typically at different places of articulation: /pʌpʌpʌ/, /tʌtʌtʌ/, /kʌkʌkʌ/, and /pʌtʌkʌ/. Real words, such as *buttercup* or *patty-cake*, are sometimes substituted for the nonsense word /pʌtʌkʌ/. Icht and Ben-David (2015) found that Hebrew-speaking preschool-aged children produced the real Hebrew word *bodeket* significantly faster than the nonword *pataka* and recommended that both real and nonsense words be included in assessment of DDK.

Maximum performance tasks can also be used to examine oromotor function and include prolongation of vowels (e.g., /a/) and consonants (e.g., /s/, /f/), and repetition of syllables (e.g., /mama/) including the syllables described in the DDK tasks above (Rvachew, Hodge, & Ohberg 2005; Thoonen, Maassen, Gabreels, & Schreuder, 1999). Maximum performance tasks are useful in differential diagnosis of motor speech disorders, as they provide information on "articulatory coordination, breath control, speaking rate, speech fluency, articulatory accuracy and temporal variability" (Thoonen, Maassen, Wit, Gabreels, & Schreuder, 1996, p. 312). Children with CAS are more likely to have slower trisyllabic repetition rates (e.g., /pʌtʌkʌ/) and short fricative durations (e.g., /f/ and /s/), whereas children with dysarthria are more likely to have shorter phonation durations (e.g., /a/) and slow monosyllabic repetition rates (e.g., /pʌpʌpʌ/) (Thoonen et al., 1996, 1999).

Some standardized assessments of oral structure and/or function include:

- Apraxia Profile (AP) Preschool and School-Age Versions (Hickman, 1997)
- Kaufman Speech Praxis Test for Children (KSPT) (Kaufman, 1995)
- Oral and Speech Motor Control Protocol (Robbins & Klee, 1987)
- Oral Speech Mechanism Screening Examination – Third Edition (OSMSE–3) (St. Louis & Ruscello, 2000)
- Screening Test for Developmental Apraxia of Speech – Second Edition (STDAS–2) (Blakeley, 2001)
- Verbal Dyspraxia Profile (VDP) (Jelm, 2001)
- Verbal Motor Production Assessment for Children (VMPAC) (Hayden & Square, 1999).

Currently there is no gold standard oral structure and function assessment tool even though assessment of oral structure is important for identifying underlying causes of SSD and assessment of oromotor function is important for differential diagnosis of CAS and childhood dysarthria (McCauley & Strand, 2008). McCauley and Strand (2008) considered the psychometric properties of six standardized assessments focused mostly on oromotor function and found that the tests varied considerably in task requirements (e.g., spontaneous versus imitated productions), complexity, and judgment required by the examiner. They indicated that few provided adequate reliability and validity measures. VMPAC (Hayden & Square, 1999) was the only test that met their definition for adequate norms and adequate content validity and included some information about reliability and construct validity. The five other tests provided some information about these psychometric properties but did not meet their operational definition for adequacy.

ASSESSMENT OF SPEECH PERCEPTION

Assessment of children's speech perception can only provide clues into their underlying knowledge of speech and language (Dinnsen, Barlow, & Morrisette, 1997). As Locke (1980a) stated,

> The processes of perception are inescapably private. There is, consequently, no way that perception can be tested. At best, one can put the child on a task in which his responses to his perceptions can be witnessed and infer from the entire pattern of activity the child's perceptions. (p. 433)

Locke (1980a) suggested that a clinically useful assessment of speech perception should include repeated opportunities to make a comparison between children's perception of target speech sounds with the sounds that they replace, as well as perceptually similar sounds. He also stated that children's required response should be within their capacity. Across the literature on speech perception assessment for children with SSD, tasks vary according to whether they involve the following factors:

- Live voice versus recorded voice
- Single versus multiple speakers
- Adult versus child speaker
- Female versus male speaker
- Own versus others' speech
- Phones versus phonemes versus syllables versus nonwords versus real words versus sentences
- Pictures versus no pictures
- Speech sounds produced incorrectly by the child versus a wide repertoire of speech sounds

There is no agreed upon standard about the best combination of factors or type of test for assessing the speech perception skills of children with SSD because "it is quite possible for a child to take two tests of auditory discrimination and pass one and fail the other!" (Stackhouse & Wells, 1997, p. 38). For this reason, we provide an overview of a selection of tasks described in the literature, classifying them into one of two types: auditory discrimination tasks and auditory lexical discrimination tasks (Stackhouse & Wells, 1997).

■ Auditory discrimination tasks

Auditory discrimination tasks require children to discriminate between phones or phonemes in isolation, syllables, or words (real or nonwords). For example, Bridgeman and Snowling (1988) developed and tested a 60-item real and nonword **auditory discrimination same/different task** for children with CAS. Their task required children to determine whether two words sounded the same or different (e.g., *lost* versus *lots*). They discovered that although the children with CAS were able to discriminate real words equally well as children with typically developing speech, the children with CAS had more difficulty with nonword discrimination. Another type of auditory discrimination task is the **ABX task** (Locke, 1980b). In this task a listener hears three syllables. The first two syllables are different, while the third syllable is identical to either the first or second syllable. This means that a listener could hear ABA or ABB. The listener's task is "to indicate whether the final or comparison syllable (X) is more like A or more like B" (Locke, 1980b, p. 457). One other type of task involves auditory discrimination of **legal versus illegal nonwords**. As part of this task, children listen to nonwords comprising phonotactically legal (e.g., [plik]) or illegal (e.g., [pnik]) syllable sequences and judge whether they are possible or not possible in the language they are learning (Stackhouse, Vance, Pascoe, & Wells, 2007). Standardized tests of auditory discrimination include:

- Wepman Auditory Discrimination Test-2 (Wepman & Reynolds, 1987)
- Word discrimination subtest of the Test of Auditory Processing Skills (Martin & Brownell, 2005)
- Word discrimination subtest of the Test of Language Development-Primary (TOLD-P) (Newcomer & Hammill, 1988; 2008)

■ Auditory lexical discrimination tasks

Auditory lexical discrimination tasks are designed to not only assess children's abilities to detect differences between words but their ability to compare what they hear with their own stored representations of words (Stackhouse & Wells, 1997). Lexical discrimination tasks can be undertaken either with or without the use of pictures. A common example of a lexical discrimination task involves **contrastive minimal pairs** where children are asked to point to a picture of one of the word pairs (Barton, 1980; Howell & Dean, 1994). The word pairs typically contain the target word and the child's error production of that word. For example, if a child was gliding /ɹ/ to [w], the task would involve the child listening and pointing to a picture of a *ring* or *wing*, in accordance with the speaker's production. In Chapter 13 you will learn more about how this type of task has been included in some interventions for children with phonological impairment. Constable, Stackhouse, and Wells (1997) created another type of lexical discrimination task containing four different productions of 10 polysyllabic words, including one correct production, two mispronunciations of the target word, and one perceptually similar word (e.g., *caterpillar* /kætɚpɪlɚ/ versus [kætɚtɪlɚ] versus [kæpɚtɪlɚ] versus *calculator*). They were interested in assessing a child's ability to detect mispronunciations of target words. Sutherland and Gillon (2005, p. 303) developed and tested a **phonological representation accuracy judgment** task and found that children with SSD "were more likely to make incorrect judgments of the accuracy of spoken words as compared to children with typical speech development."

The Speech Assessment and Interactive Learning System (SAILS) (Rvachew, 2009) is another type of speech perception assessment tool suitable for children with SSD. SAILS requires children to make lexical and phonetic perceptual judgments about the accuracy of a particular word, through a computer-based activity. As part of this task, children have to decide whether a word they hear matches a target word (i.e., lexical judgment) and whether the pronunciation is an accurate rendition of the word or whether it is distorted in some way (i.e., phonetic judgement). Multiple speaker stimuli are included (i.e., adults and children, including children with SSD), because children need to learn how to perceive the same word spoken by males and females, adults and children. As discussed in Chapter 5, children need to accommodate speaker variance (Johnson, 1997) and develop categorical perception in keeping with the phonological system they are learning. It is important to ensure that the speech stimuli in perception assessment tasks match the language and dialect spoken by the child. For example, SAILS (Rvachew, 2009) was developed for children learning US and Canadian English (additional dialects are under development). Additional information about creating individualized speech perception tasks can be found in Locke (1980b) and Stackhouse et al. (2007).

In addition to the speech perception assessments for children with SSD, a number of standardized speech perception assessments have been developed for use with children with hearing loss:

- Infant-Toddler Meaningful Auditory Integration Scale (IT-MAIS) (Zimmerman, Osberger, & McConkey Robbins, 2000)
- Meaningful Auditory Integration Scale (MAIS) (Robbins, Renshaw, & Berry, 1991)
- PLOTT Test and PLOTT Sentence Test (Plant & Moore, 1993; Plant & Westcott, 1983)

For example, the PLOTT Test (Plant & Westcott, 1983) contains nine subtests to assess children's ability to detect a range of phonemes as well as to discriminate between phonemes based on place, manner, and voice features.

ASSESSMENT OF HEARING

As discussed in Chapter 2, there is a significant association between children's hearing and their ability to perceive and produce speech (Keilmann, Kluesener, Freude, & Schramm, 2011). Children with suspected SSD should undergo routine audiological testing including tympanometry (to assess middle ear function) and audiometry (to assess perception of sounds of different loudness [dB] and pitches [Hz]). Audiometric testing is typically undertaken by an audiologist; however, in some countries screening audiometry may be conducted by trained SLPs, doctors, or nurses. If a child fails a hearing screening, then a full audiological examination is required. Comprehensive audiological assessment can be used to determine whether children have a hearing loss, the type of hearing loss (i.e., conductive, sensorineural, mixed, retrocochlear, or central auditory), and the potential impact of any loss on children's speech production difficulties. Intervention for hearing loss is prescribed by audiologists and medical specialists, and may include antibiotics and/or the insertion of PE tubes (grommets) in cases of otitis media, hearing aids, or cochlear implants.

ASSESSMENT OF PHONOLOGICAL PROCESSING

Phonological processing is important for the acquisition of speech, language, and literacy. As discussed in Chapter 4, phonological processing involves three components: phonological access, phonological memory, and phonological awareness (Anthony et al., 2003). Assessments that have been designed to comprehensively assess phonological processing include:

- Comprehensive Test of Phonological Processing – Second Edition (CTOPP-2) (Wagner, Torgesen, Rashotte, & Pearson, 2013)
- Preschool Comprehensive Test of Phonological and Print Processing (PCTPPP) (Lonigan, Wagner, Torgesen, & Rashotte, 2002)

For example, the CTOPP-2 is designed to assess phonological processing within the age range of 4;0 to 24;11 years and has been standardized on 1,900 individuals from six states of the United States. It includes 12 subtests: (1) elision, (2) blending words, (3) sound matching, (4) phoneme isolation, (5) blending nonwords, (6) segmenting nonwords, (7) memory for digits, (8) nonword repetition, (9) rapid digit naming, (10) rapid letter naming, (11) rapid color naming, and (12) rapid object naming. It provides the following composite scores: (1) phonological awareness composite score, (2) phonological memory composite score, (3) rapid symbolic naming composite score, and (4) rapid non-symbolic naming composite score. The individual components of phonological processing will be discussed next.

■ Phonological access

Phonological access typically is assessed using rapid automatic naming tasks where children name colors, letters, shapes, or illustrations of objects (Anthony, Williams, Aghara, Dunkelberger, & Novak, 2010). Children's rapid automatic naming skill is measured by counting either the number of words produced correctly or the number of words produced within a time limit. It is important that the targeted words are in children's receptive vocabularies; otherwise the rapidity of naming will be affected (Anthony et al., 2010). Rapid automatic naming tasks are found as subtests within assessments of broader speech, language, and phonological skills including:

- Clinical Evaluation of Language Fundamentals - Fifth Edition (CELF-5) (Semel, Wiig, & Secord, 2013)
- Preschool Comprehensive Test of Phonological and Print Processing (Lonigan et al., 2002)

For example, the Rapid Object Naming subset from the Preschool Comprehensive Test of Phonological and Print Processing (Lonigan et al., 2002) requires children to name common words of one syllable such as *car*, *ball*, and *tree*. The Rapid Size Naming Task (Lonigan et al., 2002) requires children to state the size of the object (e.g., *big* or *little*) when shown shapes of different sizes, for example, a big circle or a little square.

■ Phonological working memory: Nonword repetition tasks

Phonological working memory typically is assessed using nonword repetition tasks (and occasionally using real word repetition tasks). Nonword repetition tasks require children to repeat unfamiliar words and are used during screening and diagnostic assessments. Nonword repetition tasks manipulate different linguistic variables including phonetic content, word-likeness, and morphology. Ability on nonword repetition tasks has been linked to phonological memory, speech processing skills, vocabulary knowledge, understanding of spoken language, and reading achievement. Some examples of English nonword repetition tests include:

- Children's Test of Nonword Repetition (CN-REP) (Gathercole & Baddeley, 1996)
- Nonword Repetition Test (NRT) (Dollaghan & Campbell, 1998)
- Syllable Repetition Task (SRT) (Shriberg, Lohmeier, Campbell, Dollaghan, Green, & Moore, 2009)
- Test of Early Nonword Repetition (TENR) (Stokes & Klee, 2009)

Some of these nonword repetition tasks include phonetically complex words that have low word-likeness (e.g., /ɛmplifɔvənt/ from the CN-REP test). Children with specific language impairment (SLI) have more difficulties than typically developing children in the production of phonetically complex words (e.g., longer polysyllabic words and words containing consonant clusters) (Archibald & Gathercole, 2006). In contrast, the SRT only uses phonemes that are within the repertoires of most children: /b, d, m, n, ɑ/ (e.g., /bɑmɑ/, /nɑdɑmɑbɑ/) (Shriberg et al., 2009), thereby reducing the chance that children's results on the nonword repetition task will be influenced by their ability to produce the required consonants and vowels.

The majority of research studies that have used nonword repetition tasks focus on children with specific language impairments (see Coady and Evans, 2008, for a review). However, nonword repetition tasks have also been used with populations with SSD (Shriberg, Lohmeier, et al., 2009), apraxia (Van der Merwe, 2007), autism (Bishop et al., 2004), hearing loss (Briscoe, Bishop, & Norbury, 2001; Burkholder-Juhasz, Levi, Dillon, & Pisoni, 2007), stuttering (Hakim & Ratner, 2004; Sasisekaran & Byrd, 2013), Williams syndrome (Robinson, Mervis, & Robinson, 2003), and traumatic brain injury (Falconer, Geffen, Olsen, & McFarland, 2006).

Additionally, some researchers have advocated for the use of nonword repetition tests as a valid and reliable measure for assessing multilingual children's speech. For example, Windsor, Kohnert, Lobitz, and Pham (2010) assessed children using both a Spanish and English nonword repetition task and found a correlation between their scores for both languages, and children with language impairment achieved lower scores than typically developing children. However, when using nonword repetition tasks cross-linguistically, it is important to consider whether the requirements of the nonword repetition task matches the phonological and phonotactic features of the spoken language. Nonword repetition tasks have been developed for and used with speakers of many languages, including Arabic (Saiegh-Haddad, 2007), Dutch (de Bree, Rispens, & Gerrits, 2007), Finnish (Service, Maury, & Luotoniemi, 2007), Italian (Dispaldro, Leonard, & Deevy, 2013), Portuguese (Santos & Bueno, 2003), Putonghua (Mandarin) (Zhichao & Jing, 2006), Spanish (Ebert, Kalanek, Cordero, & Kohnert, 2008), and Turkish (Topbaş, Kaçar-Kütükçü, & Kopkalli-Yavuz, 2014).

■ Phonological awareness

Phonological awareness skills are the third component of phonological processing (Anthony, Lonigan, Driscoll, Phillips, & Burgess, 2003) and are a predictor of later reading and writing success (Kame'enui e al., 1997; Torgesen, Wagner, & Rashotte, 1994). Phonological awareness is the "explicit awareness of the sound structure of spoken words" (Gillon, 2005, p. 308). That is, phonological awareness tasks rely on auditory rather than print-based tasks. Phonological awareness tasks include rhyming, segmenting words and sentences, and phonemic awareness. Phonemic awareness "refers to the ability to isolate and manipulate the sounds used in spoken language" (McDonagh, 2015, p. 360) and includes:

- Sound isolation: What is the first sound in *moon*? /m/ What is the last sound in *moon*? /n/ What is the middle sound in *moon*? /u/.
- Phoneme identity: What sound is the same in: *sun, sand, sea*? /s/.
- Phoneme categorization: Which word doesn't belong? *moon, mat, fish. Fish.*
- Oral blending: Can you tell me what word these sounds make when you put them together? /f/ /i/ /t/. *Feet.*
- Oral segmentation: Tell me the sounds in the word *cup.* /k/ /ʌ/ /p/.
- Phoneme deletion: What word is *stop* without the /s/? *Top.*
- Phoneme addition: What word do you get if you add /b/ to *red*? *Bread.*
- Phoneme substitution: The word is *mat.* Now change the /m/ to /k/. What is the new word? *Cat.* (McDonagh, 2015)

Phonological (and phonemic) awareness tasks have been used to assess children with SSD, reading difficulties (Elbro, Borstrøm, & Petersen, 1998), and hearing loss (Webb & Lederberg, 2014). Standardized tools designed to assess phonological awareness include:

- Phonological Awareness Test (Robertson & Salter, 1997)
- Pre-Reading Inventory of Phonological Awareness (PIPA) (Dodd, Crosbie, McIntosh, Teitzel, & Ozanne, 2003)
- Preschool and Primary Inventory of Phonological Awareness (PIPA) (Dodd, Crosbie, McIntosh, Teitzel, & Ozanne, 2000)
- Preschool Comprehensive Test of Phonological and Print Processing (Lonigan et al., 2002)
- Sutherland Phonological Awareness Test – Revised (SPAT-R) (Neilson, 2003)
- Test of Auditory Analysis (TAAS) (Rosner, 1999).
- Test of Phonological Awareness – Second Edition: Plus (TOPA-2+) (Torgesen & Bryant, 2004)
- Test of Phonological Awareness Skills (TOPAS) (Newcomer & Barenbaum, 2003)

For example, the PIPA (Dodd et al., 2000, 2003) is designed for children aged 3;6–6;11 and includes six subtests: syllable segmentation, alliteration identification, rhyme identification, phoneme isolation, phoneme segmentation, and letter knowledge. The US version (Dodd et al., 2003) was standardized on 450 children in the United States. The Phonological Awareness Test (Robertson & Salter, 1997) was standardized and validated on 1,582 children and includes seven subtests: (1) rhyming discrimination and production, (2) deletion for compound words, syllables, and phonemes, (3) substitution (with and without manipulatives), (4) blending syllables and phonemes, (5) graphemes, (6) decoding, and (7) invented spelling. It was found to have good psychometric properties when used with 108 children who used cochlear implants and hearing aids (Webb & Lederberg, 2014). While most assessments of phonological awareness are static assessments, Kantor, Wagner, Torgesen, and Rashotte (2011) describe two dynamic phonological awareness assessments involving scaffolding and modifying items in response to errors (dynamic-supported assessment), and direct instruction on phonological awareness tasks (dynamic-instruction assessment).

ASSESSMENT OF EMERGENT LITERACY, EARLY LITERACY, AND CONVENTIONAL LITERACY SKILLS

Emergent literacy skills are often assessed in young children with suspected SSD due to the established links between speech, language, reading, and writing (e.g., Raitano et al., 2004; see Chapter 2). Emergent literacy skills (e.g., word and print awareness, letter knowledge, phonological awareness, oral language, name writing) are the foundation skills on which conventional literacy or reading is built (Justice, 2006). Reading requires skills in five areas: phonological awareness, alphabetic principle (phonics), vocabulary, comprehension, and accuracy and fluency with decoding connected text (National Reading Panel, 2000).

Collaboration between SLPs and teachers is important to assess and support literacy acquisition for children with SSD. There are a wide range of assessments that are used by SLPs and teachers to consider children's different stages of literacy acquisition (emergent literacy, early literacy, and conventional literacy), including:

- Dynamic Indicators of Basic Early Literacy Skills Next (DIBELS Next) (Good & Kaminski, 2011)
- Early Literacy Test (Gillham, 2000)
- Informal assessment of children's knowledge of letter name and sounds (e.g., Dodd & Carr, 2003)
- Neale Analysis of Reading Ability – Third Edition (Neale, 1999)
- Phonics and Early Reading Assessment (McCarty & Ruttle, 2012)
- Pre-Literacy Skills Screening (Crumrine & Lonegan, 1999)
- Pre-literacy rating scale of the Clinical Evaluation of Language Fundamentals: Preschool-2 (CELF-P2) (Wiig, Secord, & Semel, 2004)
- Preschool Word and Print Awareness Assessment (PWPA) (Justice & Ezell, 2001)
- Queensland University Inventory of Literacy (QUIL) (Dodd, Oerlemans, MacCormack, & Holm, 1996)
- Test of Word Reading Efficiency – Second Edition (TOWRE-2) (Torgesen, Wagner & Rashotte, 2012)
- Tests of Reading Comprehension – Third Edition (TORCH-3) (Australian Council for Educational Research, 2013)
- Woodcock-Johnson III Diagnostic Reading Battery (WJ III DRB) (Woodcock, Mather, & Schrank, 2004)

For example, the DIBELS Next (Good & Kaminski, 2011) is designed to detect reading risk in children from kindergarten to grade 6. The subtests include letter naming fluency, first sound fluency, phoneme segmentation, nonsense word fluency, oral reading fluency, retell, and daze.

ASSESSMENT OF PSYCHOSOCIAL ASPECTS

Psychosocial aspects including children's temperament have been associated with SSD (see Chapter 2). For example, Shriberg and Kwiatkowski (1994) list multiple psychosocial inputs (e.g., parental expectation, language stimulation) and behaviors (e.g., sensitivity to others, compliance) within the Causal-Correlates Descriptor Ratings for Speech-Delayed Children (Shriberg & Kwiatkowski, 1994). Collaboration between SLPs and psychologists can be helpful in the assessment of psychosocial aspects. There are some short assessments that can be completed by SLPs, parents, or teachers to consider the impact of psychosocial aspects on children's functioning:

- Strengths and Difficulties Questionnaire (SDQ) (Goodman, 1997)
- Short Temperament Scale for Children (STSC) (Sanson, Prior, Garino, Oberklaid, & Sewell, 1987)
- School-Age Temperament Inventory (SATI) (McClowry, 1995)

For example, the Strengths and Difficulties Questionnaire (Goodman, 1997) is available in over 80 languages and has been normed in 10 different countries (e.g., on 10,367 children in the United States). It can be completed by parents or teachers of children aged 4 to 16 years and consists of 25 items (e.g., often seems worried). The items are divided between five scales: emotional symptoms, conduct problems, hyperactivity/inattention, peer relationship problems, and prosocial behavior. Free translations of the SDQ, scoring protocols, and norms are available from youthinmind (2012).[4] The STSC (Sanson et al., 1987) consists of 12 items (e.g., "This child is shy when first meeting new children") and provides ratings for three subscales: sociability, persistence, and reactivity. Items are scored on a scale from (1) *almost never* to (6) *almost always* and are combined to generate a mean score for each

---

[4]http://www.sdqinfo.org/

subscale. The STSC (Sanson et al., 1987) has been used to compare risk and protective factors for 4,983 preschool children who were and were not identified with speech and language difficulties. It was found that having a reactive temperament was a consistent risk factor, and having a more persistent and more sociable temperament were consistent protective factors (Harrison & McLeod, 2010). Subscales from the SDQ (Goodman, 1997) and SATI (McClowry, 1995) have been used to compare outcomes at school age for 4,329 children who were and were not identified with speech and language difficulties in preschool. It was found that children who were identified with speech and language difficulties had higher emotional symptoms, lower persistence, and more difficulty managing stress and demands than their typically developing peers (McCormack, Harrison, McLeod, & McAllister, 2011).

ASSESSMENT OF CHILDREN'S COMMUNICATIVE PARTICIPATION

The Focus on the Outcomes of Children Under Six (FOCUS) (Thomas-Stonell et al., 2012) was listed as an outcome measure in Chapter 7 and was developed to consider children's communicative participation, a construct inspired by the International Classification of Functioning, Disability and Health – Children and Youth Version (ICF-CY) (WHO, 2007). The items on the FOCUS were developed by considering responses from 165 families and SLPs regarding observed change in communicative participation after speech and language intervention. Research has been undertaken to establish the validity and reliability of the FOCUS for use with children with speech and language disorders (Thomas-Stonell, Oddson, Robertson, & Rosenbaum, 2013; Washington et al., 2013). Using the FOCUS, a 16-point change in scores between initial assessment and after intervention is considered to be significant. Examples of questions on the FOCUS include "My child can talk to other children about what s/he is doing. . . My child is included in play activities by other children. My child is willing to talk to others" (Thomas-Stonell, Oddson, Robertson, & Rosenbaum, 2010, p. 53). The FOCUS (Thomas-Stonell et al., 2012) is available for free[5] and has been translated into Chinese, Danish, French, German, Hebrew, and Spanish.

■ Assessment of children's views of their speech within educational and social contexts

Children's current and future well-being and outcomes, both in educational and social contexts, can be affected by SSD in childhood (Felsenfeld, Broen, & McGue, 1994; Lewis, Freebairn, & Taylor, 2000a, b; see Chapter 1). In Chapter 1 we cited Article 12 from the United Nations Convention on the Rights of the Child (UNICEF, 1989), which indicates the importance of considering children's views about matters that impact their lives. There are a number of tools designed to help one listen to children's views about their speech and the impact upon their participation in educational and social contexts. These include:

- Communication Attitude Test (CAT) (Brutten & Dunham, 1989)
- Communication Attitude Test for Preschool and Kindergarten Children Who Stutter (KiddyCAT) (Vanryckeghem & Brutten, 2006)
- Index for Inclusion (Booth & Ainscow, 2002)
- Speech Participation and Activity Assessment of Children (SPAA-C) (McLeod, 2004)

For example, one component of the SPAA-C (McLeod, 2004) includes a questionnaire containing 10 items where children describe how they feel about talking in different contexts (see Figure 8-3). Children are invited to respond using a pictorial Likert scale (☺ ☺ ☹ O?) and to elaborate responses if they select "another feeling." The SPAA-C also can be used to gain perspectives of significant others who communicate with the child on a regular basis, including their parents, friends, and teachers (examples of questions are provided in Chapter 7). The KiddyCAT consists of 12 questions for children that can be answered

---

[5]http://research.hollandbloorview.ca/outcomemeasures/focus

FIGURE 8-3 A 6-year-old child's responses to the Speech Participation and Activity Assessment of Children (SPAA-C)

For questions 4 and 6, he indicated he felt "nerves" (nervous).

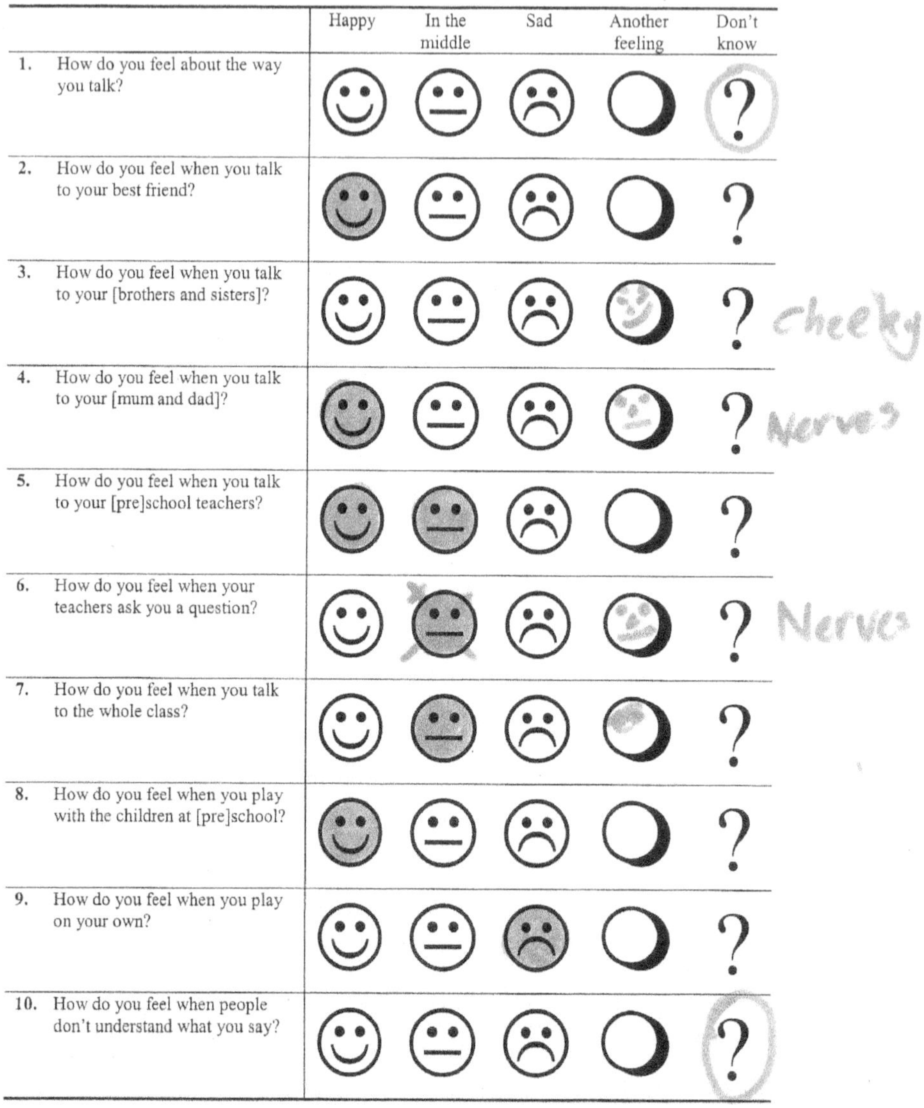

Source: McLeod (2004). Used by permission of Sharynne McLeod.

with yes or no (e.g., "Do people like how you talk?"). While the KiddyCAT and CAT were originally designed for children who stutter, they have been used with typically developing children (Johannisson et al., 2009; Vanryckeghem, Brutten, & Hernandez, 2005), children with SSD (McLeod, McCormack, McAllister, Harrison, & Holliday, 2011), and children with cleft lip and palate (Havstam, Sandberg, & Lohmander, 2011).

Another method for listening to children with SSD is to invite them to draw a picture of themselves talking to someone (Holliday, Harrison, & McLeod, 2009). You will have noticed that we have included children's drawings throughout this book. Each drawing was collected using the Sound Effects Study protocol, where a child is handed a blank piece of paper and 10 marker pens. They are asked to "draw yourself talking to someone." Once their drawing is completed, clarification questions include: "Who is in the drawing? How do you know this person (i.e., friend, brother, etc.)? Do you usually like talking to this person? Where are you? What are you/they doing? What are you saying/talking about?" Preschool and school-aged children with SSD have been able to provide insights into the frustration of being misunderstood in public contexts, and that they typically enjoy speaking with their families, via the SPAA-C, KiddyCAT, and drawings of themselves talking (e.g., McCormack, McLeod, McAllister, & Harrison, 2010; McLeod, Daniel, & Barr, 2013).

In addition, there have been a number of methods for considering children's quality of life. For example, Markham, van Laar, Gibbard, and Dean (2009) conducted focus group interviews with young people with speech, language, and communication needs who indicated the following themes were important when considering quality of life: achievement, emotions, independence, individual needs, relationships, relaxation, school, and support. There have been a few quality of life questionnaires developed for children and their parents. These include:

- Cerebral Palsy Quality of Life Questionnaire for Children (CP QOL-Child) (University of Melbourne, 2013)
- Cerebral Palsy Quality of Life Questionnaire for Adolescents (CP QOL-Teen) (Davis, Davern, et al., 2013)
- The KIDSCREEN Questionnaires – Quality of life questionnaires for children and adolescents (The KIDSCREEN Group Europe, 2006)
- TNO-AZL Preschool Children Quality of Life (TAPQOL) (Fekkes et al., 2000)

For example, the CP QOL-Child and CP QOL-Teen have been developed to consider quality of life in children with cerebral palsy (who may also have dysarthria). The CP QOL-Child measures the following constructs: social well-being and acceptance, feelings about functioning, participation and physical health, emotional well-being and self-esteem, access to services, pain and impact of disability, and family health. The scales have been validated (Chen et al., 2013; Davis, Mackinnon, et al., 2013), are being translated into a range of languages (e.g., Farsi, Greek, Hebrew, Korean, Spanish, Tamil), and are freely available.[6]

LANGUAGE, VOICE, AND FLUENCY ASSESSMENTS

Entire books have been written about the assessment of children's language, voice, and fluency, so these areas will be addressed briefly here. As indicated in Chapter 2, there may be co-occurrence of SSD with difficulties with language, voice, and stuttering, so it is important to screen each of these areas to determine if more in-depth assessment is required. It is recommended that a language sample be elicited to provide a naturalistic evaluation of children's language skills as well as an opportunity to determine whether the child's voice and fluency are within normal limits. Consider the loudness, pitch, and quality of the child's voice, and whether the child stuttered. Language assessments should consider children's expressive and receptive abilities and should cover semantics (vocabulary), morphology (grammar), syntax (sentence structure), discourse, and pragmatics. If children have had difficulty naming words during a single-word speech assessment, you may choose to assess their vocabulary knowledge on a specific test of expressive or receptive vocabulary. Pay particular attention to children's morphology due to the interrelationship between production of speech sounds and marking of tense and agreement. For example, children who have final consonant deletion or cluster reduction in word-final position will not produce finite morphemes such as regular past tense (winked /wɪŋkt/ → [wɪŋ] or [wɪ]), plural (e.g., beans /binz/ → [bin] or [bi]), and third-person singular morphemes (e.g., eats /its/ → [it] or [i]), so an assessment of morphology will be beneficial. In Chapter 13 you will learn about morphosyntax intervention (Tyler & Haskill, 2010). A few of the many language assessments that may be suitable include:

- Clinical Evaluation of Language Fundamentals – Fourth Edition, Screening Test (CELF-4 Screener) (Semel, Wiig, & Secord, 2004)
- Clinical Evaluation of Language Fundamentals – Fifth Edition (CELF-5) (Semel, Wiig, & Secord, 2013)

---

[6]http://cpqol.org.au/

- Expressive Vocabulary Test – Second Edition (EVT-2) (Williams, 2007)
- Peabody Picture Vocabulary Test – Fourth Edition (PPVT-4) (Dunn & Dunn, 2007)
- Rice/Wexler Test of Early Grammatical Impairment (RWTEGI) (Rice & Wexler, 2001)
- Structured Photographic Expressive Language Test – Preschool 2 (SPELT-P2) (Dawson et al., 2005)
- Test of Integrated Language and Literacy Skills (TILLS) (Nelson, Plante, Helm-Estabrooks, & Hotz, 2015)

Using the ICF-CY Framework to Scaffold Assessment Planning

The International Classification of Functioning, Disability and Health – Children and Youth Version (ICF-CY) (World Health Organization, 2007) was introduced in Chapter 2 as a classification system that can be used to consider children with SSD. Consequently, we will use the ICF-CY as the framework for holistic, individualized, comprehensive, and strategic assessments for children with suspected SSD. The ICF-CY considers a health condition (in our case, SSD) using five components: Body functions, Body structures, Activities and participation, Environmental factors, and Personal factors. Each component is listed below indicating first the area of primary focus (the most relevant and salient ICF-CY codes), then additional aspects to consider during an assessment. The letter/number combination relates to the alphanumeric coding within the ICF-CY.

- Body Functions
    - Primary focus: b320 Articulation functions (note this category also includes phonology), b1560 Auditory perception
    - Additional aspects: b230 Hearing functions, b144 Memory functions, b1670 Reception of language, b1671 Expression of language, b310 Voice functions, b330 Fluency and rhythm of speech functions, b117 Intellectual functions, b126 Temperament and personality functions
- Body Structures
    - Primary focus: s320 Structure of mouth
    - Additional aspects: s1 Structure of nervous system, s240 Structure of external ear, s250 Structure of middle ear, s260 Structure of inner ear, s310 Structure of nose, s330 Structure of pharynx, s340 Structure of larynx, s430 Structure of respiratory system
- Activities and Participation
    - Primary focus: d3 Communication (includes all domains)
    - Additional aspects: d1 Learning and applying knowledge (including d115 Listening, d140 Learning to read, d145 Learning to write), d6 Domestic life (including d660 assisting others in communication), d7 Interpersonal interactions and relationships (include most domains), d810–820 Education, d9 Community, social and civic life
- Environmental Factors
    - Primary focus: e3 Support and relationships
    - Additional aspects: e1 Products and technology, e4 Attitudes, e5 Services, systems and policies
- Personal Factors

Within the ICF-CY each component can be described in a positive or negative way. The dichotomies are:

- Function – Impairment
- Activities – Activity limitation
- Participation – Participation restriction
- Environmental facilitator – Environmental barrier

Here is an example of how to use ICF-CY terminology. You can say:

Sam has **impaired** articulation functioning that **limits** his communication **activities** and **restricts participation** at school. While **barriers** include the attitudes of some peers in the playground, **facilitators** supporting Sam's communication include his siblings, parents, teachers, and the SLP.

Each category within the ICF-CY can be coded using a qualifier: 0 = no problem, 1 = mild problem, 2 = moderate problem, 3 = severe problem, 4 = complete problem. Therefore, a child with a severe SSD would be coded as b320.3, with b = Body functions, 320 = the numerical code for Articulation functions, and .3 = severe problem. A comprehensive assessment plan based on the ICF-CY framework is provided in Appendix 8-1 and an example of a completed assessment plan for Luke is provided in Appendix 8-2. Use these appendices to consider where each of the components of a typical speech assessment (outlined next) fit into the ICF-CY framework. For example, assessment of consonant production is a Body Function and would be coded as b320 Articulation functions. Remember, this term is included in the ICF-CY to be used by people of different professions, in different countries, to describe people of different ages and abilities. SLPs need to consider the nuances of this term, including distinctions between articulation and phonology.

STRATEGIC ASSESSMENTS SUITED TO CHILDREN WITH DIFFERENT TYPES OF SSD

In Chapter 2 we described five types of SSD: phonological impairment, articulation impairment, inconsistent speech disorder, CAS, and childhood dysarthria. It is appropriate to plan to undertake different assessments depending on which type of SSD is suspected. Table 8-5 gives different referral scenarios that provide some clues towards which type of assessment should be planned. Once you meet the child and learn more information from the parents, you may change your hypothesis to a different type of SSD. Assessment is an iterative process. You gather information, consider it, and then gather further information. The final diagnosis will be made once the assessment and analysis is complete; however, it is useful to have a working hypothesis so that you ensure you assess the most relevant areas.

In the next sections we illustrate how different elements of assessment combine to form individualized, comprehensive strategic assessment. You will be provided with suggested areas of assessment for each of the different types of SSD. Do not think of these examples as prescriptive but suggestive. Remember—every child is an individual. What, when, and how you assess depends on the individual's needs. However, it is useful to undertake the following measures for every child with suspected SSD:

- **Case history:** outline important factors in a child's life.
- **Intelligibility rating:** describe the amount of speech that is understood.
- **Single-word and connected speech assessments:** document the consonants and vowels that are produced correctly and in error. Make sure you sample different

TABLE 8-5	Examples of referral scenarios for different types of SSD	
	Nature of error	**Possible referral scenarios**
Phonological impairment	Cognitive-linguistic difficulty	"Some people find my child difficult to understand. He is having difficulty putting the ends on words and saying sounds like 'c,' 'k,' 'g'" (i.e., patterns of errors)
Articulation impairment	Inadequate articulatory control	"My child is having difficulty saying the sounds 's' and 'r.' He has a lisp."
Inconsistent speech disorder	Impaired phonological planning, resulting in inconsistent productions	"My child is hard to understand. Every time he says the same word he pronounces it differently."
Childhood apraxia of speech (CAS)	Impaired motor planning and programming of movement sequences	"My child is very difficult to understand. He has difficulty moving his tongue within his mouth."
Dysarthria	Weakness, slowness, or incoordination of speech musculature	"My child's speech sounds slurry. Some sounds are hard to say, and people find it hard to understand him."

word positions, and compare singletons versus consonant clusters, monosyllables versus polysyllables, and single word versus connected speech.

- ■ **Stimulability assessment:** determine whether the child is able to produce the sounds in error with cues.
- ■ **Oral structure and function:** consider underlying causal factors.
- ■ **Hearing and speech perception:** determine whether the child can detect and perceive sounds in error.
- ■ **Contextual testing:** consider the child's response to requests for clarification (RQCL).
- ■ **Assessment of children's communicative participation** and their own views of their speech within educational and social contexts.
- ■ Screening of **language, voice, and fluency.**

In Chapter 9 you will learn how to analyze children's speech in order to determine whether they require intervention, and if so, what that type of intervention they need. So, in order to analyze children's speech, you need to have elicited enough information to make the right decisions. The areas in the analysis of speech production in Chapter 9 include:

- ■ **Severity**
- ■ **Intelligibility**
- ■ **Independent analysis:** phonetic inventory (singleton consonants, consonant clusters, vowels), syllable shape inventory, word length inventory, syllable stress inventory
- ■ **Relational analysis:** percentage of consonants correct, percentage of vowels correct, phonological processes/patterns, systemic analysis

If there are sampling constraints, you will not be able to describe each of these components. For example, if you select a speech assessment that primarily elicits words that have a CVC word shape (e.g., *pig, soap, moon, duck, house*), then you will not be able to comment on children's ability to produce a variety of consonant clusters, syllable shapes, word length, and stress patterns.

■ Assessments for children with suspected phonological impairment

If a preschool or school-aged child who is referred to an SLP is described as being difficult to understand, having trouble saying sounds (e.g., "My child can't say the letters c, k, g"), putting sounds on the ends of words, or other patterns of errors, then you may hypothesize that the child has a phonological impairment. In order to confirm your tentative diagnosis, it would be useful to plan to undertake the following assessments:

- ■ Comprehensive single-word speech sample from a standardized phonology test.
- ■ Connected speech assessment: targeting specific areas of difficulty (e.g., consonant clusters, fricatives, affricates, liquids).
- ■ Informal probes of patterns of errors (e.g., fronting, stopping, cluster reduction). This may include assessment of the production of relevant minimal pairs (e.g., *spot-pot*).
- ■ Speech perception ability (e.g., percent correctly identified target sounds given an array of correct, incorrect, and other sounds).

If during the assessment it is clear that more than sibilant and rhotic consonants are affected, the child's errors seem consistent, and prosody is relatively unaffected, then it is likely that the child has a phonological impairment. The most appropriate speech sample analysis to confirm this diagnosis may include:

- ■ Independent phonological analysis: inventory of phones (consonants, vowels), syllable and word shapes, and stress patterns.
- ■ Relational phonological analyses: measure of speech accuracy (e.g., PCC); inventory of phonemes; systemic analysis to identify collapses of contrast (Williams, 2003), and/or generic phonological process analysis.

You will learn more about these analyses in Chapter 9.

Assessments for children with suspected inconsistent speech disorder

If a child referred to an SLP is described as being difficult to understand, and produces words differently each time, you may hypothesize that the child has inconsistent speech disorder. In order to confirm your tentative diagnosis, it would be useful to plan to undertake the following assessments in addition to the ones listed for every child with suspected SSD:

- Inconsistency assessment: sample 25 words on three occasions from the Diagnostic Evaluation of Articulation and Phonology: Variability assessment (Dodd, Hua et al., 2002; 2006).
- Assessment of the same words in imitated and spontaneous speech contexts.
- Stimulability testing of any consonants not present.

If the child's speech errors are inconsistent, imitated speech is better than spontaneous speech, and the child's prosody and fluency are relatively unaffected, you may tentatively diagnose inconsistent speech disorder (a problem with phonological planning). The most appropriate speech sample analysis may include:

- Independent phonological analysis: inventory of phones (consonants, vowels), syllable and word shapes, and stress patterns.
- Relational phonological analysis: Calculate percent inconsistency to determine whether the child's repeated productions of single words show ≥ 40% variability (Dodd, Holm, et al., 2006).

Assessments for children with suspected articulation impairment

If a child referred to an SLP is described as having a lisp, or having difficulty producing one or two speech sounds only (typically /s, z, ɹ/), you may hypothesize that the child has an articulation impairment involving sibilants and/or rhotics where phonemic contrasts are preserved. In order to confirm your tentative diagnosis, it would be useful to plan to undertake the following assessments:

- Single-word standardized articulation assessment: determine exactly which consonants (and vowels) are in error, and any phonotactic constraints (e.g., whether the errors occur in all word positions, only in consonant clusters, only in polysyllabic words).
- Informal probes of consonants in error (e.g., /s, z, ɹ/): sample 10–20 words containing the consonants in error to determine the consistency of production and any phonotactic constraints that were not tested or were not apparent during single-word testing.
- Connected speech assessment: to consider the impact on intelligibility and acceptability.
- Ultrasound imaging of tongue body if /ɹ, ɚ, ɝ/ distortion detected (optional).

The most appropriate speech sample analysis may be a SODA (substitution, omission, distortion, addition) analysis (Van Riper, 1939). An acoustic analysis of /s, z, ɹ/ may also be suitable. You will learn more about these analyses in Chapter 9.

Assessments for children with suspected CAS

If a child referred to an SLP is described as being very difficult to understand, having difficulty pronouncing many consonants and vowels, problems saying long words, and unusual sounding speech, you may hypothesize that the child has CAS. In order to confirm your tentative diagnosis, it would be useful to plan to undertake the following assessments:

- Comprehensive single-word sample from standardized phonology assessment.
- Informal assessment of words of increasing length (e.g., *but, butter, butterfly*).
- Assessment of polysyllables (real and nonwords) reflecting varying stress patterns (e.g., SS, Sw, wS, Sws, Sww, Swsw, wSwsw).
- Assessment of the same words in imitated and spontaneous speech contexts.

■ Connected speech assessment: pay particular attention to intelligibility, juncture, and prosody (look for inappropriate phrasing, rate, sentential stress, lexical stress, and emphatic stress in addition to syllable segregation).
■ Stimulability testing: determine whether the child is able to produce the sounds in error with cues.
■ Oral structure and function: particularly elicit maximum performance tasks (look for slower trisyllabic repetition rates on /pʌtʌkʌ/ and short fricative durations on /f/ and /s/).
■ Assessment of children's views of their speech within educational and social contexts, quality of life, friendships, and differences between communication at home and school.

Some assessments that are specifically designed for children with CAS include:

■ Apraxia Profile (Hickman, 1997)
■ Kaufman Speech Praxis Test (Kaufman, 1995)
■ Screening Test for Developmental Apraxia of Speech – Second Edition (STDAS–2) (Blakeley, 2001)
■ Verbal Dyspraxia Profile (Jelm, 2001)
■ Verbal Motor Production Assessment for Children (Hayden & Square, 1999)
■ The Nuffield Centre Dyspraxia Programme (NDP-3) (Williams & Stephens, 2004)

If these assessments show that the child has difficulty producing consonants and vowels, difficulty with phonotactics (e.g., syllable shape and length), and inappropriate prosody (e.g., lexical stress), it is possible that the child has CAS, a motor speech disorder involving planning and programming. The most appropriate speech sample analysis may include:

■ Independent phonological analysis: inventory of phones (consonants, vowels), syllable and word shapes, and stress patterns.
■ Relational phonological analysis such as measure of speech accuracy (e.g., PCC); naturalness rating and/or measures of accuracy of suprasegmentals/prosody; phonological process analysis; acoustic analysis followed by calculation of pairwise variability index of lexical stress (Ballard et al., 2010).

■ Assessments for children with suspected childhood dysarthria

If a child referred to an SLP is described as being difficult to understand, with slurred speech and difficulty producing sounds, you may hypothesize that the child has childhood dysarthria. Dysarthria is a motor speech disorder involving motor execution. You will recall that there are different forms of dysarthria (flaccid, spastic, dyskinesia, ataxic, or mixed), and children are likely to have respiratory, phonatory, resonance, articulation, and prosodic difficulties in addition to increased or decreased muscle tone, uncoordinated mouth movements, and/or imprecise or weak articulation (particularly for plosives, fricatives, and affricates). Depending on the child's age, severity, and possible cause of dysarthria, it would be useful to plan to undertake the following assessments:

■ Comprehensive single-word sample from a standardized phonology test.
■ Informal probe of specific speech sounds in error (particularly plosives, fricatives, and affricates) across word positions, compare singletons versus consonant clusters, monosyllables versus polysyllables and single word versus connected speech.
■ Intelligibility test (single word): especially if the child's speech is highly unintelligible and severely affected.
■ Connected speech assessment and/or reading passage, such as "The Caterpillar" (Patel et al., 2013): take note of respiration, phonation, prosody (e.g., inappropriate rate, sentential stress, but appropriate phrasing, lexical stress, and emphatic stress), voice (e.g., inappropriate loudness—too soft, low pitch, harsh laryngeal quality, and hypernasal resonance), intelligibility, and acceptability.
■ Stimulability testing: determine whether the child is able to produce the sounds in error with cues.

- Oral structure and function: particularly elicit maximum performance tasks (look for shorter phonation rate on prolonged /a/ and slow monosyllabic repetition rates on /pʌpʌpʌ/).
- Assessment of the child's views of his or her speech within educational and social contexts, including the child's perspectives on his or her quality of life.

Some assessments that are specifically designed for children with dysarthria include:

- Communication Function Classification System (Hidecker, et al., 2011)
- Quick Assessment for Dysarthria (Tanner & Culbertson, 1999)

A speech sample analysis may include:

- Independent phonological analysis: inventory of phones (consonants, vowels), syllable and word shapes, and stress patterns.
- Relational phonological analysis: include a measure of speech accuracy (e.g., PCC), naturalness rating or measure of accuracy of suprasegmentals/prosody, and measurement of speech intelligibility (e.g., percentage of words understood by familiar and unfamiliar listeners).

You will learn more about these analyses in Chapter 9. If a diagnosis of either CAS or dysarthria is unclear, consider Shriberg's (2010a) classification of motor speech disorder-not otherwise specified (MSD-NOS)

■ Assessment of SSD for child with craniofacial anomalies

Children who have had craniofacial anomalies, such as cleft lip and palate, will be in contact with an SLP soon after birth to assist with feeding, hearing, speech, and language acquisition. Children who have a history of cleft lip and palate will benefit from assessments using the measures listed above for every child with suspected SSD (speech production, stimulability, etc.). In addition, five universal parameters have been recommended by the Universal Speech Parameters Group to be reported for all children with cleft lip and palate: "(1) hypernasality, (2) hyponasality, (3) audible nasal air emission and/or nasal turbulence, (4) consonant production errors, (5) voice disorder" (Henningsson et al., 2008, p. 1), as well as "global parameters of speech understandability and speech acceptability" (p. 4). The following factors may contribute to differences in the speech of children with cleft lip and palate compared with typically developing children:

- Palate may be absent or healing after surgery (reduces ability to produce alveolar, postalveolar, and palatal consonants)
- Reduced ability to produced intraoral pressure (reduces ability to produce stops)
- Reduced practice in using stops and alveolar and palatal consonants (reduces intelligibility, and increases compensatory articulations)
- Poor Eustachian tube functioning (reduces hearing) (Scherer & Chapman, 2014)

Some recommendations for assessing the speech of children who have a history of cleft lip and palate include:

- Assess consonants and vowels, paying particular attention to high-pressure consonants (e.g., plosives) and high vowels that are more susceptible to hypernasality. Assess consonants in isolation, words, and sentences. Compare children's total consonant inventories (that may include glottal stops and compensatory articulations such nasal fricatives) with consonants that are in the ambient language.
- Assess short sentences that are loaded with several consonants of the same type to consider hypernasality (e.g., /p/) and hyponasality (e.g., /m/).
- Assess oral structure and function, including velopharyngeal function (Hirschberg & Van Demark, 1997).

Instrumentation can be used to enhance assessments of children with craniofacial anomalies. Assess nasal resonance and nasal escape using a nasometer, or nasopharyngoscopy, and velopharyngeal competence using videofluoroscopy. It is important to note that nasal resonance and the use of glottal stops may be related to either velopharyngeal insufficiency or phonological learning. Therefore, a short period of intervention to reduce nasalization and the use of glottal stops is indicated before undergoing assessment of velopharyngeal insufficiency. Tongue placement can be assessed using ultrasound or electropalatography (EPG). Some articulation and phonology tests are not sensitive enough to provide comprehensive data for children who have a history of cleft lip and palate (Van Demark, 1997). Therefore it is useful to administer an assessment that is specifically designed for these children and is heavily weighted with plosives, fricatives, and affricates. Examples include:

- Iowa Pressure Articulation Test (IPAT) (Templin & Darley, 1969)
- Great Ormond Street Speech Assessment (GOS.SP.ASS) (Sell, Harding, & Grunwell, 1999)
- SVANTE—Svensktartikulations-och Nasalittets Test [Swedish Articulation and Nasality Test] (Lohmander et al., 2005). This assessment is in Swedish.

In addition, the Profiles of Early Expressive Phonological Skills (PEEPS) (Williams & Stoel-Gammon, in preparation) has been used to assess the speech of 2- to 3-year-old children with cleft lip and palate (Scherer, Williams, Stoel-Gammon, & Kaiser, 2012).

■ Assessment of SSD for child with hearing loss

Children with hearing loss typically are identified at a young age, after newborn infant hearing screening. They will have had contact with audiologists and may have had contact with SLPs soon after birth. Children who have a hearing loss will benefit from speech assessments using the measures listed above for every child with suspected SSD (speech production, stimulability, etc.). However, there are additional factors to consider. When children with hearing loss attend a speech-language pathology assessment, ask to see their most recent audiogram and consider their aided and unaided thresholds (if they are wearing hearing aids). It is important to discuss with the family whether the child uses speech, manual communication (e.g., American Sign Language), or mixed communication (Crowe, McLeod, McKinnon, & Ching, 2014). If the child uses speech or mixed communication, consider how the child's hearing thresholds affect the audibility of speech sounds. For example, nasals /m, n/ are usually easier to hear than voiceless fricatives /f, s/. Assessments that may be useful in assessing sound detection and discrimination are:

- The Ling Sounds (Ling, 1976, 1989) /a/, /i/, /u/, /s/, /ʃ/, /m/ can be used to determine which frequencies (250–8000 Hz) the child is able to perceive and discriminate. This is a good, quick check prior to an assessment to ensure the child's hearing aids and/or cochlear implant is working.
- The PLOTT Test (Plant & Westcott, 1983) contains nine subtests to assess children's ability to detect a range of phonemes as well as to discriminate between phonemes based on place, manner, and voice features.

Assessments that may be useful in assessing speech perception for children with hearing loss are:

- Functional Auditory Performance Indicators (FAPI) assesses seven categories of auditory development: sound awareness, sound is meaningful, auditory feedback, localizing sound source, auditory discrimination, short-term memory, and linguistic auditory processing (Stredler-Brown & Johnson, 2003).
- The Meaningful Auditory Integration Scale (MAIS) (Robbins, Renshaw, & Berry, 1991) and the Infant-Toddler Meaningful Auditory Integration Scale (IT-MAIS) (Zimmerman, Osberger, & McConkey Robbins, 2000) are scales developed for professionals to administer to the parents of children with hearing loss and describe children's use of amplification/cochlear implant and behaviors regarding environmental sounds and speech.
- Parents' Evaluation of Aural/Oral Performance of Children (PEACH) (Ching & Hill, 2007) and Teachers' Evaluation of Aural/Oral Performance of Children (TEACH) (Ching, Hill, & Dillon, 2008) are parent/teacher diaries containing examples of the listening behavior of children in everyday life in different contexts. Parent and teacher forms are available in a number of languages.[7]

---

[7]http://outcomes.nal.gov.au/peach.html

> **COMMENT:** *The role of analysis in assessment*
>
> In clinical practice, analysis is integral to the process of assessment and diagnosis. Although it can occur once you complete an assessment, analysis can also occur partway through an assessment. For instance, you might collect a speech sample from a child, analyze it, and then decide that you need to conduct further assessment. In this chapter we present an overview of the assessment process. Chapter 9 provides you with the knowledge and skills needed to analyze speech samples gathered during an assessment.

Speech production assessments may include:

- The Meaningful Use of Speech Scale (MUSS) (Robbins & Osberger, 1990) is a scale administered to the parents of children with hearing loss. Parents are asked to answer questions describing the way their child verbalizes and uses speech in everyday life.
- Picture Speech Intelligibility Evaluation (Picture SPINE) (Monsen, Moog, & Geers, 1988) is a speech assessment that is specifically designed for children aged 5 to 15 years with hearing loss.

DIFFERENTIAL DIAGNOSIS AND PROGNOSTIC STATEMENTS

The final step of any assessment process confirms your hypothesis about a child's SSD. You reach a point of differential diagnosis. You consider all the information you have gathered and generate a description about the nature of a child's SSD. This description forms your diagnostic statement, and includes the type and severity of SSD. The findings from your assessment help to generate intervention goals. Goals are addressed in Chapter 10. Of course, a comprehensive assessment is not complete without the analysis of the speech samples you gather during an assessment. The findings from your analysis not only help you understand the nature of a child's SSD, but offer direction about speech goals. The knowledge and skills needed to analyze speech are addressed in the next chapter. At this point, you may also include a prognostic statement to estimate the course or outcome of a problem based on a collection of conditions and child and family characteristics. A well-written prognostic statement contains a goal statement, a judgment of success, and prognostic variables that justify the judgment. An example of a prognostic statement is:

> Even though David's phonological impairment was diagnosed as severe, his prognosis for improved speech intelligibility with effective intervention was judged to be good, based on the following variables: his cooperative behavior, good attention and task persistence during the assessment, his stimulability for some errored sounds, the absence of any structural problems, and the high level of support from his parents.

Chapter summary

In this chapter you learned about a variety of tools to assess the following areas during children's speech assessments: intelligibility, speech production, oromotor structures and functioning, speech perception, hearing, phonological processing, literacy skills, psychosocial aspects, communicative participation in educational and social contexts, language, voice, and fluency. Next we considered the International Classification of Functioning, Disability and Health – Children and Youth Version (ICF, ICF-CY) (WHO 2001, 2007) as a framework for planning speech assessments. Finally, this chapter provided directions for generating strategic assessment plans based on hypothesized diagnostic categories of SSD types. Despite the range of resources given in this chapter, the most important focus in assessment is on creating an individualized assessment that is appropriate for individual children and their families.

Suggested reading

■ Shriberg, L. D. (1993). Four new speech and prosody-voice measures for genetics research and other studies in developmental phonological disorders. *Journal of Speech and Hearing Research, 36,* 105–140.

■ De Lamo White, C., & Jin, L. (2011). Evaluation of speech and language assessment approaches with bilingual children. *International Journal of Language and Communication Disorders, 46*(6), 613–627.

Application of knowledge from Chapter 8

Using the assessment plan from Appendix 8-1, and the example plan for Luke in Appendix 8-2, create an assessment plan for Michael, Susie, Jarrod, and Lian (see Chapter 16 for details about these children).

Appendix 8-1. Assessment plan

Name: _____ Date of birth: _____ Age: _____

Reason for referral: _____ Language(s) spoken: _____

		Areas to be assessed	Assessment tools	Priority areas
Function and disability	Body functions	b320 Articulation functions (includes phonology)		
		b1560 Auditory perception		
		b230 Hearing functions		
		b144 Memory functions (includes phonological processing)		
		b1670 Reception of language		
		b1671 Expression of language		
		b310 Voice functions		
		b330 Fluency and rhythm of speech functions		
		b117 Intellectual functions		
		b126 Temperament and personality functions		
	Body structures	s320 Structure of mouth		
		s1 Structure of nervous system, s240–260 Structure of ear, s310 Structure of nose, s330 Structure of pharynx, s340 Structure of larynx, s430 Structure of respiratory system		
	Activities and participation	d3 Communication		
		d1 Learning and applying knowledge (including d115 Listening, d140 Learning to read, d145 Learning to write)		
		d6 Domestic life (including d660 Assisting others in communication)		
		d7 Interpersonal interactions and relationships		
		d810–820 Education		
		d9 Community, social and civic life		
Contextual factors	Environmental	e3 Support and relationships		
		e4 Attitudes		
		e1 Products and technology		
		e5 Services, systems and policies		
	Personal			

SESSION PLAN

The assessment plan can be freely copied with acknowledgment of the source being McLeod & Baker (2017)

Appendix 8-2. Assessment plan for Luke

Name: *Luke*   Date of birth: _____   Age: *4;3* _____

Reason for referral: _____   Language(s) spoken: *English* _____

		Areas to be assessed	Assessment tools	Priority areas
Function and disability	**Body functions**	b320 Articulation functions (includes phonology)	■ Single words (SW): Diagnostic Evaluation of Articulation and Phonology (DEAP) Phonology (Dodd, Hua, et al., 2002, 2006) ■ Single words: Production of polysyllables ■ Connected speech (CS): conversation with playdough and simple book ■ Contextual testing during connected speech ■ Stimulability testing informal ■ Intelligibility rating informal	High
		b1560 Auditory perception	■ Phonological processing ■ Phonological working memory via nonword repetition task (nonword repetition test)	Medium
		b230 Hearing functions	■ Hearing Test: audiologist ■ Tympanometry: audiologist	High
		b144 Memory functions (includes phonological processing)	■ Comprehensive Test of Phonological Processing – Second Edition (CTOPP-2; Wagner, Torgesen, Rashotte, & Pearson, 2013)	Medium
		b1670 Reception of language	■ Peabody Picture Vocabulary Test – Fourth Edition (PPVT-4) (Dunn & Dunn, 2007)	Medium
		b1671 Expression of language	■ Basic subtests of Clinical Evaluation of Language Fundamentals: Preschool-2 (CELF-P2) (Wiig, Secord, & Semel, 2004) to assess receptive and expressive language ■ Use of finite morphemes (via CS sample)	Medium
		b310 Voice functions	■ Informal observation during connected speech	Low
		b330 Fluency and rhythm of speech functions	■ Informal observation during connected speech	Low
		b117 Intellectual functions	■ Primary Test of Nonverbal Intelligence (PTONI) (Ehrler & McGhee, 2008)	Low
		b126 Temperament and personality functions	■ Strengths and Difficulties Questionnaire (SDQ) (Goodman, 1997)	Low
	Body structures	s320 Structure of mouth	■ Oral and speech motor control protocol (Robbins & Klee, 1987)	High
		s1 Structure of nervous system, s240–260 Structure of ear, s310 Structure of nose, s330 Structure of pharynx, s340 Structure of larynx, s430 Structure of respiratory system	■ Informal observation and referral to doctor if necessary	Low
	Activities and participation	d3 Communication	■ Speech Participation and Activity Assessment of Children (SPAA-C) (McLeod, 2004) interview with: Luke and Family ■ Luke's drawing	High

Appendix 8-2. (*Continued*)

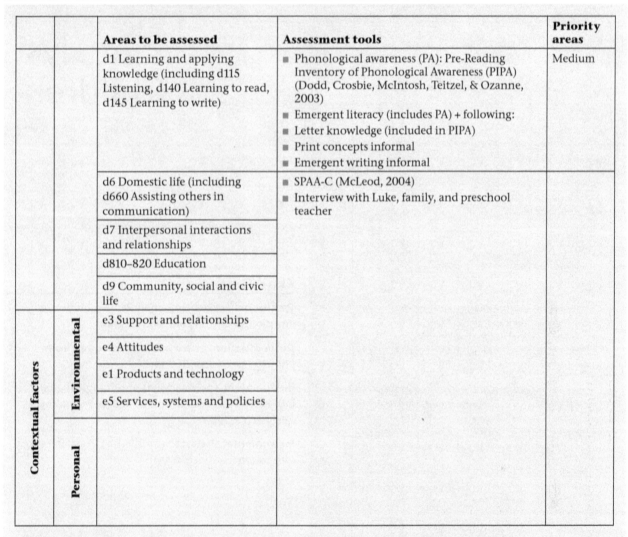

		Areas to be assessed	Assessment tools	Priority areas
		d1 Learning and applying knowledge (including d115 Listening, d140 Learning to read, d145 Learning to write)	■ Phonological awareness (PA): Pre-Reading Inventory of Phonological Awareness (PIPA) (Dodd, Crosbie, McIntosh, Teitzel, & Ozanne, 2003) ■ Emergent literacy (includes PA) + following: ■ Letter knowledge (included in PIPA) ■ Print concepts informal ■ Emergent writing informal	Medium
		d6 Domestic life (including d660 Assisting others in communication)	■ SPAA-C (McLeod, 2004) ■ Interview with Luke, family, and preschool teacher	
		d7 Interpersonal interactions and relationships		
		d810–820 Education		
		d9 Community, social and civic life		
Contextual factors	Environmental	e3 Support and relationships		
		e4 Attitudes		
		e1 Products and technology		
		e5 Services, systems and policies		
	Personal			

SESSION PLAN

Assessment session(s) plan: This plan very full—pending the outcome of any of the assessments, additional speech, language, or emergent literacy testing may need to be conducted in a subsequent session.

SESSION 1: Interview with parents (10 minutes) while Luke does a drawing of himself and his family—and invite Luke to write his name on his drawing; DEAP Phonology (10 minutes); oral structure and function (10 minutes); PPVT (10 minutes); and Basic Receptive and Expressive subtests of CELF-Preschool (20 minutes) (Intelligibility ratings to be done between sessions by parents/grandparent and teacher; referral to audiology given for hearing tests) = 60 minutes

SESSION 2: Conversational speech sample (includes contextual testing, voice, fluency observations) (10 minutes); print concepts evaluation with book (5 minutes); children's nonword repetition test (5 minutes); production of polysyllables (5 minutes); PIPA (15 minutes); Stimulability testing (5–10 minutes); interview with Luke using SPAA-C (5 minutes); and Luke to complete a drawing of himself talking while clinician talks with parent about general results (10 minutes) = 60 minutes *(This plan assumes that Luke will be compliant and get on with the various tasks—assessment with children sometimes does not go to plan, and the information that you will gather will still provide a valuable insight into a child's individual profile of strengths and areas of difficulty.)*

9

Analysis of Children's Speech

LEARNING OBJECTIVES

1 Distinguish between phonetic and phonemic errors.

2 Complete an articulation analysis of a speech sample, using the substitution, omission, distortion, addition (SODA) framework.

3 Analyze and describe sibilant errors in a speech sample.

4 Complete phonological process analysis on a given speech sample.

5 Complete an independent and relational phonological analysis, using the Children's Independent and Relational Phonological Analysis (CHIRPA) template, on a speech sample for a child with SSD.

6 Understand the benefits of undertaking a simple acoustic analysis of a digitally recorded speech sample to identify vowel formants and fricative noise on a spectrogram, and calculate measures such as voice onset time and vowel and syllable duration.

7 Visually inspect and describe a child's tongue placement, using an electropalatographic image of lingual consonants.

KEY WORDS

Traditional articulation analysis: substitution, omission, distortion, addition (SODA)

Differentiation: phonemic (phonological) from phonetic (articulation) errors

Independent and relational phonological analyses: Children's Independent and Relational Phonological Analysis (CHIRPA)

Instrumental analyses: acoustic, electropalatography, ultrasound

OVERVIEW

In this chapter, you will learn how to analyze children's speech. You will learn about traditional articulation analysis, phonological analysis, and instrumental analysis. Analysis is essential for identifying specific speech production abilities to be targeted in intervention. It is an important step between determining that there is a problem (i.e., assessment) and generating a plan to solve the problem (i.e., goal setting). Analysis is also a prerequisite for doing something about the problem (i.e., intervention).

The steps involved in analysis are similar to the steps involved in the completion of a jigsaw puzzle. The speech samples collected during an assessment are like the puzzle pieces. Through analysis you figure out what a child already knows about the sound system (i.e., the portions of the puzzle the child has already completed), what the child is yet to learn (i.e., the puzzle pieces that have not been put in place yet), and what a child may have learned incorrectly (i.e., the puzzle pieces that are in the wrong spots or belonging to other puzzles). Once you have identified all the pieces to be worked on, you are in a better position to determine a child's goals of intervention (i.e., the order in which the missing or incorrect puzzle pieces will be worked on) and suitable intervention approaches for working on the goals. Intelligible speech that can be used to participate in society is the desired end product or completed puzzle.

If you enjoy puzzles, you will enjoy this chapter. If puzzles are not one of your favorite pursuits, be patient. You might be tempted to think that time spent analyzing children's speech is like time wasted sorting all the pieces of an incomplete jigsaw puzzle without actually putting any puzzle pieces in place. It might seem appealing to begin intervention on an obvious, noticeable error or missing puzzle piece. However, if you start intervention without analysis, you risk meandering through the pieces of children's phonological systems from one session to the next, wasting the very thing you planned to use wisely in the first place—time. As Bernhardt and Holdgrafer (2001a) point out, inaccurate or incomplete analysis can result in intervention continuing for much longer than it needs to. At some point you will need to sit down and analyze a child's speech to determine the most effective and efficient way to help the child complete the puzzle and become intelligible. So, find a quiet place to read, and get ready to learn methods for articulation, phonological, and instrumental analysis.

TRADITIONAL ARTICULATION ANALYSIS: SUBSTITUTION, OMISSION, DISTORTION, ADDITION (SODA)

As you learned in Chapter 8, the speech sample that you end up analyzing for an individual child is influenced by your initial thoughts about the nature of the child's SSD. If a child presents with only one or two speech sounds in error, and phonemic contrasts are preserved, then you will have collected a single-word sample, a portion of connected speech, and probes of the specific speech sound(s) in error. Taking into consideration other findings from your assessment (e.g., hearing, speech perception, oromotor structure and function), you may have tentatively diagnosed the SSD as an articulation impairment. In such cases, the most simple and common approach to analysis is traditional articulation analysis, colloquially known among SLPs as SODA (Van Riper, 1939): sorting errors in the speech sample into **substitution, omission, distortion,** and **addition**.

- **Substitution:** one speech sound has been replaced by another speech sound (e.g., *see* /si/ → [ti])
- **Omission:** a speech sound has been omitted from the expected position in the word (e.g., *see* /si/ → [i])
- **Distortion:** the articulation of a speech sound is altered such that a listener perceives the target **phoneme** as unclear (i.e., the phonemic contrast is preserved) (e.g., *see* /si/ → [ɬi])
- **Addition:** a speech sound has been added to the word (e.g., *see* /si/ → [sis])

The **SODA taxonomy** was introduced by Charles van Riper in 1939. Prior to the 1970s, this framework was the standard method for analyzing children's speech. Many decades on, other frameworks are available for organizing and making sense of complicated error patterns in children's speech. This does not mean that SODA analysis is old-fashioned or out-of-date. The SODA framework still has a place in the analysis and differential diagnosis of SSD in children (e.g., Shriberg, 2010a), particularly for speech errors involving rhotics /ɹ, ɝ, ɚ/ and sibilants /s, z/. What follows is a description of common speech errors using the SODA taxonomy.

- **Lateral lisp:** distortion of /s, z/ with a lateral fricative across word-initial, within word, and word-final positions including singleton and consonant cluster contexts (e.g., *see* /si/ → [ɬi]; *zip* /zɪp/ → [ɮɪp]; *skip* /skɪp/ → [ɬkɪp]; *missing* /mɪsɪŋ/ → [mɪɬɪŋ]; *bus* /bʌs/ → [bʌɬ]; *buzz* /bʌz/ → [bʌɮ]). While the lateral lisp typically affects /s, z/, phonetically similar sounds including /ʃ, ʒ, ʧ, ʤ/ can also be distorted (Shine, 2007).
- **Interdental lisp:** substitution of [ð, θ] for /s, z/ across word-initial, within word, and word-final positions in singleton and consonant cluster contexts (e.g., *see* /si/ → [θi]; *zip* /zɪp/ → [ðɪp]; *skip* /skɪp/ → [θkɪp]; *missing* /mɪsɪŋ/ → [mɪθɪŋ]; *bus* /bʌs/ → [bʌθ]; *buzz* /bʌz/ → [bʌð]). Shine (2007) points out that acoustic analysis of the phone used by children perceived as having an interdental substitution (i.e., /s/ → [θ]) can show stridency. Correctly produced interdentals do not have stridency. Therefore, if in doubt about the nature of a child's lisp, consider the child's error as a distortion, and use the dentalized diacritic [s̪] rather than substitution.
- **Misarticulations involving consonantal /ɹ/ and vocalic /ɝ, ɚ/:** Errors involving /ɹ, ɝ, ɚ/ are typically divided into either:
  - **substitutions:** consonantal /ɹ/ in word-initial and within word position substituted with [w] (e.g., *read* /ɹid/ → [wid]; *carrot* /kæɹət/ → [kæwət]) or in syllable-final /ɹ/ position (sometimes described as a rhotic diphthong, as in *hear* /hɪɚ/) substituted with a derhotacized schwa or a back rounded vowel (Bernhardt & Stemberger, 1998) such as *hear* /hɪɚ/ → [hɪə].
  - **distortions** of /ɹ, ɝ, ɚ/: distorted /ɹ, ɝ, ɚ/ productions occur when a child's attempts at /ɹ, ɝ, ɚ/ are not clearly and easily identified as /ɹ, ɝ, ɚ/ but are not readily confused with [w]. The child's production may be produced as a labiodental approximant [ʋ] or be along the continuum that sounds like /ɹ, ɝ, ɚ/ but is not quite right.

COMMENT: */s/ was slushy in* see *but not as slushy in* soup: *How do I analyze distorted consonants?*

Accurate and reliable description of distorted consonants can be challenging. This is because a child's production of a particular consonant might sound closer or further away from an acceptable production. We suggest that analysis of distorted production can be done in one of three ways:

1. Categorize consonant productions as either correct or incorrect/distorted no matter how distorted or almost accurate a child's production (McAllister Byun & Hitchcock, 2012).
2. Use a simple visual analogue scale (VAS) (e.g., Juliena & Munson, 2012) (as described in Chapter 4) and note where along a continuum a child's production is—more or less accurate. For example, is a distorted /ɹ/ more like [ɹ] or [w]? Is a distorted /s/ more like [s] or [ɬ]?
3. Complete an instrumental analysis (e.g., acoustic analysis) to visualize the productions and objectively describe perceived distortions (see the section on acoustic analysis later in the chapter for further information).

■ When and how do I use traditional SODA analysis?

Traditional SODA analysis is primarily suited to children who have one or two speech errors involving sibilants (usually /s, z/), consonantal /ɹ/, and vocalic /ɚ, ɝ/; however, it could be used with children who present with multiple speech sound errors. Researchers (e.g., Shriberg, 2010a) also use SODA analysis as part of a wider repertoire of analysis methods to inform research on the characteristics of children with SSD.

To undertake a SODA analysis you use the speech samples gathered during an initial assessment to calculate the percent occurrence of a particular error (typically, distortion) across word-initial, within word, and word-final positions, in singleton and consonant cluster contexts. You could also calculate the percent occurrence in single-word and conversational speech contexts. This latter calculation is particularly important if you notice that a child produces a speech sound clearly in single words but struggles to do the same during conversational speech.

How do you work out the percent occurrence of a particular substitution, omission, distortion, or addition? You count number of instances of a particular error (e.g., distorted [s]) over the number of opportunities to produce the specific speech sound (e.g., /s/). The findings from your analysis then guide your clinical decisions about the specific speech sound(s), word positions, and contexts (single words and/or connected speech) requiring intervention.

■ ▨ ■ ▨ ■ ▨ ■ ▨ ■ ▨ ■ ▨ ■ ▨ ■ ▨ ■ ▨ ■ ▨ ■ ▨ ■ ▨ ■ ▨ ■ ▨ ■ ▨ ■ ▨ ■ ▨ ■

 APPLICATION: *SODA analysis*

Review the speech sample in Table 16-8, collected from Susie during an initial speech-language pathology assessment. The speech sample contains 24 words and was designed to strategically probe Susie's production of /s, z/ in word-initial, within word, and word-final positions in singleton and consonant cluster contexts. The sample was gathered following the identification of lateralized /s, z/ during the administration of a standardized articulation test.

1. Analyze the errors on /s, z/ using the SODA taxonomy, tallying correct and distorted productions according to word-initial, within word, and word-final positions, in singleton and consonant cluster contexts.
2. Calculate the percentage of distortion errors on /s, z/ in Susie's speech sample.
3. Based on your analysis, describe the nature of Susie's articulation impairment.

Answers:

1. Sorted and analyzed table of responses:

	Word-initial	Within word	Word-final
/s/	3/3 distortions /s/ → [ɬ]	2/2 distortions /s/ → [ɬ]	2/2 distortions /s/ → [ɬ]
/z/	3/3 distortions /z/ → [ɮ]	3/3 distortions /z/ → [ɮ]	2/2 distortions /z/ → [ɮ]
Consonant cluster context	2/2 distortions /sk/ → [ɬk, ɬt]	2/2 distortions /st/ → [ɬt]	5/5 distortions /ndz/ → [ndɮ, ɬt]

2. 100% (15/15) lateralization of /s, z/ in singleton contexts, in word-initial, within word, and word-final positions, and 100% (9/9) lateralization of /s/ in cluster contexts.
3. Susie has an articulation impairment characterized by lateralization of /s, z/, in singleton and consonant cluster contexts, in mono-, di-, and polysyllabic words, across word-initial, within word, and word-final positions.

Read more about Susie (7;4 years), a girl with an articulation impairment (lateral lisp), in Chapter 16 (Case 2).

DIFFERENTIATING PHONEMIC (PHONOLOGICAL) FROM PHONETIC (ARTICULATION) ERRORS

As described in Chapter 2, there are different types of SSDs. The most common is a phonological impairment. Children who have a **phonological impairment** can be difficult to understand because many of their words sound the same. The phonemic contrast between words is lost. Children with an articulation impairment (usually limited to sibilants or rhotics) have a different problem—although speech sounds may be distorted, word meaning is usually preserved. The problem is phonetic. Consider the following two cases depicted in Figure 9-1.

In Figure 9-1, Susie says *sea* /si/ as [ɬi]. Sally says *sea* /si/ as [ti]. For the word *tea* /ti/, Susie says *tea* /ti/ as [ti] while Sally says *tea* /ti/ as [ti]. If you had to decide whether Susie said *sea* or *tea*, you could. This is because Susie has preserved or maintained the phonemic contrasts in her speech. You know what she tried to say despite the fact that her production of /s/ in the word *sea* /si/ was unclear or distorted. By contrast, if you had to decide whether Sally said *sea* or *tea*, you would struggle. If Sally's errors were consistent, you would consistently choose *tea* /ti/, even if she intended to say *sea*. The result would be a misunderstanding, because Sally had not preserved the phonemic contrasts between the two words. This is because both /s/ and /t/ are realized as [t]. Susie's difficulty is phonetic, because phonemic contrasts are preserved. Sally's difficulty is phonemic, because the phonemic contrast is lost. Revisit Chapter 2 for further discussion about the differential diagnosis of SSD in children and Chapter 5 for further discussion about the difference between phones, phonemes, and allophones.

INDEPENDENT AND RELATIONAL PHONOLOGICAL ANALYSES

The independent and relational phonological analysis framework was developed by Stoel-Gammon and Dunn (1985). This analysis framework offers insight into what children can produce regardless of the errors in their speech (independent analysis), and what

FIGURE 9-1 **The difference between phonetic and phonemic speech errors: Breakdown in communication**

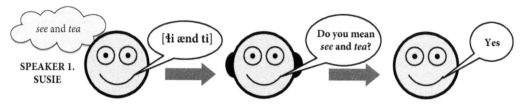

Phonetic difficulty
Phonemic contrast is preserved and communication is successful.

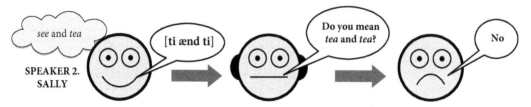

Phonemic difficulty
Phonemic contrast is lost, resulting breakdown in communication.

> **COMMENT:** *The value of hindsight in understanding the nature of children's speech errors—phonetic difficulty underlining an apparent phonemic error*
>
> Masterson and Daniels (1991) describe a case study of a child (3;8 years) who presented with errors on /ɹ/ and sibilants. His receptive and expressive language skills were above average. He had recurrent middle ear infections during his first 18 months, with pressure equalization tubes inserted at 1;7 years. His hearing tested as normal at 1;9 years. He had a habitual open-mouth posture with his tongue resting on his lower incisors or in an interdental position. He was also observed to use a dentalized swallow. Masterson and Daniels used traditional SODA analysis to describe the child's errors: 100% dentalized distortion of all sibilants, and substitution of [w] for pre-vocalic /ɹ/ and vocalization of post-vocalic /ɹ/. The authors noted that given that there was a loss of phonemic contrast between the sibilants, and between /w/ and /ɹ/, the authors initially trialed a contrastive phonological approach to intervention. The child's production of /ɹ/ improved with this approach. Although the child's production of sibilants improved, consistent improvement in sibilants did not happen until the child engaged in drill practice involving nonsense syllables and words (Masterson & Daniels, 1991)—that is, until they treated the sibilant errors as phonetic (rather than phonemic) errors. This case study helps to illustrate the challenge of differentiating phonetic from phonemic errors, and the fact that some children can have both phonetic and phonemic errors (Ruscello, 2008). This case also highlights how SODA analysis can be a helpful framework for sorting and describing the errors in children's speech, but that it is not infallible—different methods of analysis (e.g., acoustic analysis, electropalatography) and/or children's responses to intervention can also help you understand the phonetic and phonemic nature of children's speech sound errors.

children can produce correctly (relational analysis). Consider the following sample of speech, [bæt]. Not knowing the intended word or the language(s) spoken by the child, it is apparent that the child can produce the sounds [b] [æ] [t], can sequence the voiced bilabial plosive and the voiceless alveolar plosive in the monosyllable shape CVC, and can produce a word length of one syllable. You can make these observations independent of the target phonological system. The production [bæt] was produced by Luke (4;3 years) (see Chapter 16). If you have read previous chapters, you would know that Luke is monolingual and is learning to speak General American English. The target word was *splash*. Knowing this information, you can undertake a relational analysis, and it becomes apparent that Luke produced the word incorrectly. Using your knowledge of SODA analysis, he substituted [b] for /spl/ and [t] for /ʃ/. Using your knowledge of phonological processes, it is likely that cluster reduction and context sensitive voicing are present in syllable-initial word-initial position, and stopping of fricatives in word-final position. Luke produced 0/4 consonants correctly (/s/, /p/, /l/, and /ʃ/ were incorrect) and 1/1 vowels correctly. His production of the syllable shape (CCCVC) was incorrect. We arrive at these observations by comparing

Read more about Luke (4;3 years), a boy with a phonological impairment, in Chapter 16 (Case 1).

Luke's production of *splash* [bæt] with the intended production /splæʃ/. Together, the findings from an independent and relational analysis provide helpful insight into children's speech production skills. The findings complement one another, providing a rich understanding about what a child knows and does not know, phonologically. So what exactly does an independent and relational analysis involve?

In Stoel-Gammon and Dunn's (1985) original description of the independent and relational analysis framework, an independent analysis comprised three components: a phonetic inventory, syllable inventory, and word shape inventory. A relational analysis primarily consisted of phonological processes analysis (Stoel-Gammon & Dunn, 1985). Since the introduction of the independent and relational analysis framework, different authors have included different components or types of analyses within the framework, often motivated by different phonological theories. Table 9-1 lists components of independent and relational analyses described throughout the literature.

TABLE 9-1	Components of independent and relational phonological analysis	
Independent analysis	**Relational analysis**

Independent analysis	Relational analysis
■ inventory of singleton phones (consonants and vowels) ■ inventory of voice, place, and manner classes ■ inventory of minimal pair words, minimal pair syllables, and near-minimal pairs (Stoel-Gammon & Dunn, 1985; Velleman, 1998, 2003) ■ positional constraints (e.g., /k, g/ only evident in word-initial position) (e.g., Bernhardt & Stemberger, 2000; Elbert & Gierut, 1986) ■ sequence constraints between adjacent consonants and vowels (e.g., labials only with mid central vowels) (Bernhardt & Stemberger, 2000) (similar to consonant-vowel dependency analysis [Velleman, 1998]) ■ sequence constraints between consonants separated by a vowel (e.g., consonants in CVCV limited to same place of articulation) (Bernhardt & Stemberger, 2000) ■ inventory of consonant clusters according to constituent cluster elements and word position (McLeod et al., 2001a) ■ sequence constraints between elements comprising a cluster (e.g., /pw, bw, ɸw/ clusters constrained to a sequence of the place of articulation) (Bernhardt & Stemberger, 2000) ■ syllable shape, word shape, and stress pattern inventory (e.g., Long, 2008) ■ proportion of whole-word variation (PWV) (Ingram, 2002), similar to percent variability (Dodd, Hua, et al., 2006). ■ observation about other prosodic characteristics: pitch, loudness, syllable duration, rate, and intonation (Davis, 2005)	■ inventory of singleton consonants and vowels correct and incorrect ■ inventory of consonant voice, place, and manner classes correct and incorrect ■ percentage of consonants, vowels, consonant clusters, syllable shapes, word lengths, stress patterns correct (e.g., Shriberg & Kwiatkowski, 1982a; Velleman, 1998) ■ phonological mean length of utterance (pMLU); proportion of whole-word proximity (PWP); proportion of whole-word correctness (PWC) (Ingram, 2002; Ingram & Ingram, 2001) and whole-word accuracy (WWA) (Schmitt, Howard, & Schmitt, 1983) ■ inventory of consonant clusters according to constituent cluster elements and word positions correct and incorrect ■ place-voice-manner (PVM) analysis (Elbert & Gierut, 1986; Williams, 2003) (similar to phoneme and cluster realization analysis [Grunwell, 1985] and target error analysis [Long, 2008]), involves description of each target phoneme as correct, or as substitution, omission, or distortion across word-initial, within word, and word-final positions (e.g., /s/ → [t] 8/10, [d] 1/10, and ø (omission) 1/10, in word-initial position) according to voice, place, and manner characteristics (e.g., all velars produced as alveolars; all fricatives and affricates produced as homorganic stop) ■ target error analysis of syllable shapes, word lengths, and stress patterns (e.g., weak strong [wS] → strong strong [SS] 5/5) (Long, 2008) ■ phonological process analysis (e.g., Grunwell, 1982; Shriberg & Kwiatkowski, 1980; Weiner, 1979) ■ distinctive feature analysis (e.g., Grunwell, 1982; McReynolds & Huston, 1971) ■ contrastive analysis of singleton consonants, consonant clusters, and syllable shapes (a component of Phonological Assessment of Children's Speech, PACS: Grunwell, 1985), similar to analysis of phonemic contrasts (e.g., Elbert & Gierut, 1986; Stoel-Gammon & Dunn, 1985) ■ identification of collapses of contrast (Williams, 2003) based on contrastive analysis of singleton consonants and consonant clusters ■ analysis of productive phonological knowledge (PPK) (Elbert & Gierut, 1986) to determine the child's knowledge along a continuum of six different types from most versus least. PPK can be used to derive a measure of the percent correct underlying representations (PCUR) (e.g., Williams, 2000a)

As Table 9-1 shows, there are many different ways in which children's speech samples can be analyzed. Where do you start? Which ones do you choose? Over the years, different authors have compiled and described their own combination of components in Table 9-1 for conducting an independent and relational analysis. Some comprise a series of paper-based templates to be completed by hand. For example:

■ Phonological Assessment of Children's Speech (PACS) (Grunwell, 1985)
■ Systemic Phonological Analysis of Child Speech (SPACS) (Williams, 2003)
■ Phonetic and Phonological Systems Analysis (PPSA) (Bates & Watson, 2012)
■ Nonlinear Scan Analysis (Bernhardt & Stemberger, 2000)
■ Procedures for the Phonological Analysis of Children's Language (PPACL) (Ingram, 1981)

■■ ■■

 APPLICATION: *Computerized phonological analysis*

There are a number of computer-based approaches for conducting phonological analysis. Here is one that you can try.

1. Visit Steven Long's Computerized Profiling website.[1]
2. Find out what the PROPH+ module is and the types of independent and relational analyses it can generate.
3. Download PROPH+ and analyze a speech sample that you have gathered (or one of the speech samples supplied in Chapter 16).

[1]http://www.computerizedprofiling.org/

Given the potential for phonological analysis to be time-consuming (Long, 2001), some authors have developed helpful computer-based systems for analyzing children's speech. For example:

- Computerized Profiling, including Profile in Phonology (PROPH+) (Long, 2008)[1]
- Computerized Assessment of Articulation and Phonology (CAPES) (Masterson & Bernhardt, 2001)
- Computer Aided Speech and Language Assessment (CASALA) (Blamey, 1997)
- Hodson Computerized Analysis of Phonological Patterns (HCAPP) (Hodson, 2003)
- Phon (Rose et al., 2006; Rose & MacWhinney, 2014)[2].

CHILDREN'S INDEPENDENT AND RELATIONAL PHONOLOGICAL ANALYSIS (CHIRPA)

Phonological analysis needs to be comprehensive. It also needs to be efficient or relatively quick to complete. In this chapter we provide a practical step-by-step guide for conducting a straightforward independent and relational phonological analysis—the Children's Independent and Relational Phonological Analysis (CHIRPA) (Baker, 2016). It comprises a total of 18 boxes to be filled in or checked: six boxes comprise the independent analysis, nine comprise the relational analysis, and three boxes are used to summarize additional observations and ratings about a child's speech (e.g., intonation, speech rate, consistency) and to indicate whether additional speech samples are needed to analyze a specific speech skill. The independent analyses of the CHIRPA include:

- phonetic inventory for singleton consonants, consonant clusters, and vowels; and
- syllable shape, word length, and stress pattern inventories.

The relational analyses of the CHIRPA include:

- inventory of consonants correct (based on Shriberg, 1993);
- inventory of vowels, syllable shapes, word lengths, and stress patterns correct;
- singleton consonant and consonant cluster error analysis;
- phonological process analysis (based on Edwards & Shriberg, 1983; Grunwell, 1982, 1987, 1997; Ingram, 1976; Stoel-Gammon & Dunn, 1985; Weiner, 1979); and
- analysis of the loss of phonemic contrast (based on Grunwell, 1985; Williams, 2003).

A complete copy of the CHIRPA is available in Appendix 9-1. Take a look at it now, and then return to this section of the chapter to learn how to complete each of the boxes. What follows is a case-based explanation of how you can complete each box, based on single-word and connected speech samples collected from Luke during his initial assessment. Refer to Chapter 16 for further information and examples of Luke's speech. It would

[1]http://www.computerizedprofiling.org/
[2]https://www.phon.ca

Read more about
Luke (4;3 years),
a boy with a phonological
impairment,
in Chapter 16 (Case 1).

help if you had pencil and paper (or equivalent) to use as you read, to complete some of the exercises. A worked example of the CHIRPA for Luke is available in Appendix 9-2. This worked example was based on the complete list of words from the Diagnostic Evaluation of Articulation and Phonology: Phonology Assessment (Dodd, Hua, et al., 2006), strategic single-word samples of consonant clusters and polysyllables, and two 10-minute conversational speech samples.

■ Independent phonological analysis

(1) Phonetic inventory: Singleton consonants

A basic and often first step in phonological analysis involves compiling a list of phones or speech sounds produced by a child. (As shown in Figure 9-2, the first box of the CHIRPA lists the range of singleton consonants relevant to English.) To do this, you simply highlight the phones produced by a child more than once, regardless of accuracy. Luke's production of *splash* /splæʃ/ as [bæt], and *fat* /fæt/ as [bæt], mean that the speech sounds [b] and [t] can be highlighted—they are both present in his phonetic inventory. As shown in Figure 9-2, Luke (4;3 years) produced 12 phones. The classes of nasals, plosives, and glides are circled, because all nasals, glides, and plosives are present. Luke also produced [l] (but not [ɹ]), so his limited presence of liquids is shown in parentheses. Luke produced no fricatives or affricates, so they are not highlighted or given parentheses. Positional constraints are present if a child uses a particular speech sound but only in specific word positions. For instance, in Luke's case "Yes" is shaded ■, because Luke only produced velars in within word and word-final positions, and /j/ in word-initial position. The voiceless plosive [p] is also limited to word-final position only, and there is a tendency for Luke to primarily use [+ voice] in word-initial position. There is a space in the box to note such comments. Finally, depending on the child's age and your observations, you would indicate whether your observations constitute a problem. Given Luke's age (4;3 years), his limited phonetic inventory compared with other children his age (see Chapter 6), and his positional constraints, phonetic inventory (Box 1) is a problem area.

(2) Phonetic inventory: Consonant clusters

Box 2 (Figure 9-3) of the CHIRPA lists the range of consonant clusters relevant to General American English. Like the phonetic inventory of singleton consonants, you need to highlight any consonant clusters produced by a child more than once. Parentheses are used to mark consonant clusters occurring once only. Notice how the consonant clusters

---

FIGURE 9-2 **(1) Phonetic inventory: Singleton consonants for Luke (4;3 years)**

(a) CHIRPA template

(1) Phonetic inventory: singleton consonants
- Highlight consonants produced more than once
- Parentheses ( ) around consonants produced once
- Circle if most consonants in a sound class are present and use ( ) if only one or few sounds in a sound class are present

[p b t d k g m n ŋ f v θ ð s z ʃ ʒ h tʃ dʒ ɹ j l w]
Sound classes present
nasals plosives glides liquids fricatives affricates
Positional constraints ☐ yes ☐ no
Comments

Problem area ☐ yes ☐ no

(b) CHIRPA based on Luke's speech sample

(1) Phonetic inventory: singleton consonants
- Highlight consonants produced more than once
- Parentheses ( ) around consonants produced once
- Circle if most consonants in a sound class are present and use ( ) if only one or few sounds in a sound class are present

[p b t d k g m n ŋ f v θ ð s z ʃ ʒ h tʃ dʒ ɹ j l w]
Sound classes present
(nasals) (plosives) (glides) (liquids) fricatives affricates
Positional constraints ■ yes ☐ no
Comments
- *Velar [k, g] limited to medial and final position*
- *[j] limited to word-initial position*
- *[p] limited to word-final position*
- *Tendency for [+ voice] in word-initial position only*

Problem area ■ yes ☐ no

Source: Used by permission from Elise Baker.

are grouped by word-initial and word-final positions, and further grouped into categories according to a common consonant (e.g., /l/ clusters). As discussed in Chapter 4, there are many different consonant clusters in word-final position, primarily due to the addition of suffixes to mark morphemes (e.g., plural: *cats* /kæts/; past tense: *jumped* /dʒʌmpt/). Rather than listing all the possible word-final clusters, use the space in each cluster category to list the consonant clusters produced by the child. They are highlighted in Figure 9-3 to draw your attention to the fact that they were added to the template based on what was evident in Luke's comprehensive speech sample. Space is also provided for you to note any additional consonant clusters produced by a child. As discussed in Chapter 4, some dialects of English have more word-initial clusters than others (e.g., /nj/ in *new*). Also, some children produce non-adult consonant clusters as a result of errors on the consonants that comprise the cluster. For example, a child who says *flip* /flɪp/ → [fwɪp] and *sleep* /slip/ → [fwip] has the cluster [fw] in his or her independent inventory. In such cases, you write down the additional non-adult consonant clusters produced by a child. Notice Luke's limited production of consonant clusters—no word-initial consonant clusters and only a few word-final consonant clusters. Of his word-final clusters, the combinations were limited to nasal + plosive and lateral + plosive. There is space in the box to describe such limitations or sequence constraints. In the event that one or more consonant clusters were not sampled, indicate these with an asterisk (*) as shown in Figure 9-3. In Luke's case the infrequently occurring consonant clusters /fj, vj, sf/ were not sampled during his initial assessment. Given the absence of all word-initial consonant clusters (including early developing clusters) and singleton fricatives, it was considered unlikely that he would have these more complex clusters. As with the other boxes comprising the CHIRPA, you also indicate whether a child's consonant cluster inventory is a problem for his or her age. For Luke, his general absence of consonant clusters was a problem.

(3) Phonetic inventory: Vowels

Phonetic inventory of vowels is captured in Box 3 (Figure 9-4) on the CHIRPA template. In keeping with Boxes 1 and 2 addressing phonetic inventory, completion of Box 3 involves reviewing a child's speech sample and identifying instances of each of the vowels and diphthongs listed in Box 3. In Luke's case, all monophthongs and diphthongs not requiring

---

FIGURE 9-3 **(2) Phonetic inventory: Consonant clusters for Luke (4;3 years)**

(a) CHIRPA template

(2) Phonetic inventory: consonant clusters
- Highlight consonant clusters produced more than once
- Parentheses ( ) around consonant clusters produced once

Initial	Final
[tw kw sw]	[s] + consonant e.g.,
[pj bj kj mj fj vj]	consonant + [s] or [z] e.g.,
[pl bl kl gl fl sl]	[l] + consonant e.g.,
[pɹ bɹ tɹ dɹ kɹ gɹ fɹ θɹ ʃɹ]	[ɹ] + consonant e.g.,
[sp st sk sm sn sl sw sf]	nasal + consonant e.g.,
[spɹ stɹ skɹ spl skw]	e.g.,

Additional consonant clusters
Sequence constraints ☐ yes ☐ no
Comments

Problem area ☐ yes ☐ no

(b) CHIRPA based on Luke's speech sample

(2) Phonetic inventory: consonant clusters
- Highlight consonant clusters produced more than once
- Parentheses ( ) around consonant clusters produced once

Initial	Final
[tw kw sw]	[s] + consonant e.g.,
[pj bj kj mj fj*vj*]	consonant + [s] or [z] e.g.,
[pl bl kl gl fl sl]	[l] + consonant e.g., ([lt])
[pɹ bɹ tɹ dɹ kɹ gɹ fɹ θɹ ʃɹ]	[ɹ] + consonant e.g.,
[sp st sk sm sn sl sw sf*]	nasal + consonant e.g., [nt, ŋk, mp]
[spɹ stɹ skɹ spl skw]	

Additional consonant clusters
Sequence constraints ■ yes ☐ no
Comments
- *Limited to nasal + plosive and lateral+ plosive word-final clusters*
- *No word-initial consonant clusters*
- ** = not sampled during assessment*
Problem area ■ yes ☐ no

Source: Used by permission from Elise Baker.

FIGURE 9-4 | **(3) Phonetic inventory: Vowels for Luke (4;3 years)**

(a) CHIRPA template

(3) Phonetic inventory: vowels
- Highlight vowels produced more than once
- Parentheses ( ) around vowels produced once

Monophthongs [i ɪ e ɛ æ u ʊ o ɔ ɑ ə ʌ ɝ ɚ]

Diphthongs [ɔɪ ʊə ɪə ɛə ɪɔ ɪʊ aɪ aʊ ɔɪ]

Comments

Problem area ☐ yes ☐ no

(b) CHIRPA based on Luke's speech sample

(3) Phonetic inventory: vowels
- Highlight vowels produced more than once
- Parentheses ( ) around vowels produced once

Monophthongs [i ɪ e ɛ æ u ʊ o ɔ ɑ ə ʌ ɝ ɚ]

Diphthongs [ɪɔ ɛɪ ʊɔ ɔɪ aɪ aɪ aʊ ɔɪ] Also [ɛə]

Comments
- *No rhotic vowels*

Problem area ■ yes ☐ no

Source: Used by permission from Elise Baker.

COMMENT: *Sequence constraints and consonant clusters*

Using the constraint-based nonlinear phonological analysis framework developed by Bernhardt and Stemberger (2000), Baker and Bernhardt (2004) described one boy's system for realizing consonant clusters. During an assessment James (4;4 years) only produced the word-initial consonant clusters [pw, fw]. What do these clusters have in common? They are both labial-labial sequences. James' consonant clusters were constrained to segments that shared the same place of articulation—labial. Other discoveries were made about James' phonological system using a constraint-based nonlinear analysis. See Baker and Bernhardt (2004) for further insights.

COMMENT: *Can I use the CHIRPA to analyze speech samples for children who speak another dialect of English and/or speak another language?*

The CHIRPA template in Appendix 9-1 was designed for use with children learning General American English. CHIRPA templates for a selection of other English dialects are available from the second author.

rhotic vowels were present. As seen in Luke's production of *square* /skwɛɪ/ → [dɛə], the non-rhotic diphthong [ɛə] was added to his list of diphthongs produced. Overall, his inventory of vowels was indicated as a problem area only because rhotic vowels were not present.

(4) Syllable shape inventory

A child's syllable shape inventory is summarized in Box 4 (Figure 9-5). Recall that a syllable can occur in word-initial, within word, or word-final position. Luke produced the word *animals* /ænɪməlz/ → [ænɪməlt] with three syllables. The first syllable ([æ]) is a vowel, and therefore simply has the shape V. The second syllable ([nɪ]) has the shape CV. The third syllable ([məlt]) has the shape CVCC. Syllable shapes occurring more than once are highlighted in Box 4. Notice how some of the syllable shapes listed have parentheses. The use of parentheses denotes a core syllable shape that has a range of possible combinations (cf. Bernhardt & Stemberger, 2000). For instance, the core shape of [C+]VCC may have zero, one, two, or three consonants to the left of the vowel (e.g., VCC, CVCC, CCVCC, CCCVCC).

| FIGURE 9-5 | **(4) Syllable shape inventory for Luke (4;3 years)** |

(a) CHIRPA template

(4) Syllable shape inventory
- Highlight syllable shapes produced more than once
- Parentheses ( ) around syllable shapes produced once
- [C+] = 0 or more consonants

V   CV   VC   CVC   CCV[C+]   [C+]VCC
CCCV[C+]   [C+]VCCC
Others
Comments

Problem area ☐ yes ☐ no

(b) CHIRPA based on Luke's speech sample

(4) Syllable shape inventory
- Highlight syllable shapes produced more than once
- Parentheses ( ) around syllable shapes produced once
- [C+] = 0 or more consonants

V   CV   VC   CVC   CCV[C+]   [C+]VCC
CCCV[C+]   [C+]VCCC
Others
Comments
- *Mostly CV and CVC syllables*
- *[C+]VCC included CVCC and VCC syllable shapes*
- *No evidence of CCV[C+], CCCV[C+], or [C+]VCCC*

Problem area ■ yes ☐ no

Source: Used by permission from Elise Baker.

In the comments section you can include your general observations about a child's syllable structure inventory and note the range of consonant clusters used by a child for those shapes containing parentheses, particularly when the range is limited. This was the case for Luke. Although [C+]VCC is highlighted, we noted that this shape was limited to VCC and CVCC. Overall, syllable shape was indicated to be a problem area primarily because Luke's inventory did not include CCV[C+], CCCV[C+], and [C+]VCCC.

(5) Word length inventory

The range of word lengths produced by English speakers is documented in Box 5 (Figure 9-6) of the CHIRPA. As you review a speech sample, it can be helpful to highlight words of different lengths (particularly words comprising three, four, and five syllables) using different colored pens or pencils and write down their corresponding syllable shape. This way when you come to complete Box 5, you can find the longer words produced by a child more easily. In Luke's case he produced words comprising one through to five syllables. Notice that 5+ syllables is in parentheses. This is because the only five-plus syllable word said by Luke was *hippopotamus* /hɪpəpɑtəməs/ → [ɪpəbɑtəmət]. The syllable shapes produced by Luke for each word length are also listed. An opportunity is also provided for you to note whether any sequence constraints were evident in a child's speech sample. Drawing on the work of Bernhardt and Stemberger (2000), it can be helpful to notice whether there are interactions between speech sounds and syllable shapes. For example, if a child only ever produced two-syllable words whereby the consonants in the words had the same place of articulation (e.g., *nanny* /næni/ → [næni]; *daddy* /dædi/ → [dædi]; *bunny* /bʌni/ → [bʌbi]; *dinner* /dɪnɚ/ → [dɪnə]), this constraint could be described in the comments section. In Luke's case, he had no sequences involving postalveolar place of articulation; however, this was thought to be due to his phonetic inventory constraint. Given that Luke produced a range of word lengths, each with a range of syllable shapes (apart from syllable-initial consonant clusters), word length was not considered to be a problem area for Luke.

(6) Syllable stress inventory

A child's syllable stress inventory is the sixth and final independent analysis box (Figure 9-7) on the CHIRPA. As you review a child's speech sample, take note of the different types of syllable stress patterns produced by the child. Weak syllables can be found by identifying the rhotic /ɚ/ and non-rhotic schwa /ə/ in rhotic dialects of English (e.g., General American English, Scottish English, and Irish English). Similarly, schwa /ə/ occurs in weak syllables in non-rhotic dialects of English (e.g., Bostonian English [US], General British English [UK], Australian English, New Zealand English, and South African English). Like the other boxes, highlight the stress patterns occurring more than once, and mark those stress patterns produced once only with parentheses. Be on the lookout for words that begin with a weak syllable. Of the stress patterns listed in Box 6, those with weak onsets (e.g., wS, wSw) are more challenging and are less likely to be included in an inventory if a child has difficulty with stress. When we reviewed Luke's speech sample, he produced a range of syllable stress patterns, including two- and three-syllable words with weak onsets (see Figure 9-7). His syllable stress inventory was therefore not considered to be a problem area.

FIGURE 9-6 (5) Word length inventory for Luke (4;3 years)

(a) CHIRPA template

(5) Word length inventory
- Highlight word lengths produced more than once
- Parentheses ( ) around word lengths produced once
- List common and most complex syllable shape for each word length such as monosyllables CV and CVCC; disyllables CVCV and CVC,CV; 3-syllables CVCVCV and CVCVCVC

Monosyllables e.g.,

Disyllables e.g.,

3-syllables e.g.,

4-syllables e.g.,

5+ syllables e.g.,

Sequence constraints ☐ yes ☐ no
Comments

Problem area ☐ yes ☐ no

(b) CHIRPA based on Luke's speech sample

(5) Word length inventory
- Highlight word lengths produced more than once
- Parentheses ( ) around word lengths produced once
- List common and most complex syllable shape for each word length such as monosyllables CV and CVCC; disyllables CVCV and CVC,CV; 3-syllables CVCVCV and CVCVCVC

Monosyllables e.g., V; CV; VC; CVC; CVCC

Disyllables e.g., CVCV; CVCVC; CVCVCC; CVC,CV; CVC,CVC ; VCVCC

3-syllables e.g., CVCVCV; CVCVCVC ; CVC,CVCV ; VCVCVCC; CVVCVC

4-syllables e.g., VCVCVCV; CVCVCVCV

(5+ syllables) e.g., VCVCVCVCVC

Sequence constraints ■ yes ☐ no
Comments
- Sequence constraint due to small phonetic inventory as no sequences involving postalveolar place of articulation
- Overall, word length does not appear to be a problem

Problem area ☐ yes ■ no

Source: Used by permission from Elise Baker.

FIGURE 9-7 (6) Syllable stress inventory for Luke (4;3 years)

(a) CHIRPA template

(6) Syllable stress inventory
- Highlight syllable stress patterns produced more than once
- Parentheses ( ) around stress patterns produced once

SS e.g., *rainbow*	**Swsw** e.g., *watermelon*
Sw e.g., *carrot*	**Other polysyllabic words**
wS e.g., *giraffe*	e.g., *hippopotamus*
Sww e.g., *elephant*	
Sws e.g., *dinosaur*	
wSw / wSs e.g., *potato*	
Comments	

Problem area ☐ yes ☐ no

(b) CHIRPA based on Luke's speech sample

(6) Syllable stress inventory
- Highlight syllable stress patterns produced more than once
- Parentheses ( ) around stress patterns produced once

SS e.g., *rainbow*	**Swsw** e.g., *watermelon*
Sw e.g., *carrot*	**Other polysyllabic words**
wS e.g., *giraffe*	e.g., *(Swsww) hippopotamus*
Sww e.g., *elephant*	
Sws e.g., *dinosaur*	
wSw / wSs e.g., *potato*	
Comments	
• No obvious difficulties with stress	

Problem area ☐ yes ■ no

Source: Used by permission from Elise Baker.

> **COMMENT:** *Phonotactics in CAS*
>
> If you are analyzing a speech sample from a child who you suspect may have CAS, pay particular attention to the child's phonotactics—that is, syllable and word shapes. Limited repertories of syllable and word shapes are considered particularly indicative of CAS (Velleman, 2003). For instance, a child may be limited to CV and CVCV syllables only. Children who have CAS may also limit or have constraints on the types of speech sounds used in particular syllable and word shapes. For instance, the velar consonant /g/ may only ever occur with the back vowel /u/, such as the word *giggle* /ɡɪɡəl/ being pronounced as [gugu] (Velleman, 2003). Velleman (2003) provides a helpful overview of the phonotactic difficulties commonly observed in children with CAS. She also includes templates to guide more in-depth phonotactic analysis. Remember that children with CAS also have difficulties with prosody—this issue is addressed in Box 16 of the CHIRPA.

■ Relational phonological analysis

Relational analysis considers a child's performance relative to the adult target. That is, we compare the child's productions (e.g., [bæt]) with target words (e.g., *splash*) to determine whether there is an error and describe the error.

(7) Consonants correct

Boxes 7 through 15 comprise the relational analyses of the CHIRPA. One of the most common analyses involves the identification of correct consonants. As shown in Figure 9-8, English consonants can be divided into early-, middle-, and late-8 consonants (Shriberg, 1993).

There are two methods for completing Box 7 (Figure 9-8): quantitative calculation and qualitative observation. You could adopt one or both methods, depending on the complexity of the child's SSD, the information you need, and the time and resources you have available. The first and more accurate method is to calculate the overall PCC (Shriberg & Kwiatkowski, 1982c) and percentages of early-, middle-, and late-8 consonants correct (Shriberg, 1993), specifically:

$$\text{PCC} = \frac{\text{number of correct consonants}}{\text{number of correct plus incorrect consonants}} \times 100$$

FIGURE 9-8 **(7) Consonants correct for Luke (4;3 years)**

(a) CHIRPA template

(7) Consonants correct
- Calculate + report percentage of consonants correct
- Highlight consonants that are frequently or always accurate
- Parentheses ( ) around consonants sometimes accurate

Percentage of consonants correct

^Early-8   [m   b   j   n   w   d   p   h]

^Middle-8 [t   ŋ   k   g   f   v   tʃ   dʒ]

^Late-8   [ʃ   θ   s   z   ð   l   ɹ   ʒ]

^Based on Shriberg (1993)
Comments

Problem area ☐ yes ☐ no

(b) CHIRPA based on Luke's speech sample

(7) Consonants correct
- Calculate + report percentage of consonants correct
- Highlight consonants that are frequently or always accurate
- Parentheses ( ) around consonants sometimes accurate

Percentage of consonants correct
48.4% conversational speech; 38.6% single words

^Early-8   [m   b   (j) n   w   d   (p) h]

^Middle-8 [(t)(ŋ)(k)(g) f   v   tʃ   dʒ]

^Late-8   [ʃ   θ   s   z   ð   (l)   ɹ   ʒ]

^Based on Shriberg (1993)
Comments
- *Early-8 better than the middle-8 better than the late-8*
- *Luke's percentage of consonants correct better in conversational speech than single words*

Problem area ■ yes ☐ no

Source: Used by permission from Elise Baker.

The rules for calculating PCC (and other variants of the PCC measure) are described later in this chapter in the section on speech production measures. The second method complements the quantitative measures. It simply involves scanning a child's speech sample and (1) highlighting consonants on the CHIRPA that are consistently accurate—that is, accurate most if not all of the time, (2) putting parentheses around consonants that are sometimes accurate, and (3) leaving consonants that are never accurate (typically, consonants excluded from a phonetic inventory) unmarked. It is important to remember that even if a child overuses a particular consonant, such as /d/, overuse does not automatically imply incorrect. Remember, you are comparing intended productions with actual productions. If a child's intended consonant was /d/, and the child produced [d], then it would be scored as correct. If the intended consonant was /s/ and the child produced [d], then /s/ would be scored as incorrect. In Luke's case five of the early-8 consonants were consistently accurate. Four of the middle-8 consonants were sometimes accurate, while only one of the late-8 consonants (/l/) was sometimes accurate. For a child with a **developmental** (as opposed to **disordered**) SSD, this type of pattern is common—decreasing consonant accuracy from the early to later acquired consonants. Consonants with positional constraints (identified in Box 1), would be identified as sometimes accurate. Luke's case is a good example. Luke's production of /k/ is sometimes accurate because although word-final productions are correct, his word-initial productions of /k/ are not.

(8) Vowels correct

In keeping with the procedure for describing consonant accuracy, Box 8 (Figure 9-9) of the CHIRPA is used to record your observations about the child's ability to produce vowels correctly. As shown in Figure 9-9, Luke's percentage of vowels correct was 85.5%. Most of Luke's monophthongs were highlighted, because they were frequently or always accurate. The rhotic vowels and diphthongs are unmarked, because they were not in his

■ ■

 APPLICATION: *Accuracy of early-, middle-, and late-8 consonants*

1. Review Luke's production of the following words and complete the table.

Target word	Adult pronunciation	Luke's production	Initial consonant	Correct or incorrect?	Final consonant	Correct or incorrect
1. sun	/sʌn/	[dʌn]	/s/		/n/	
2. fan	/fæn/	[bæn]	/f/		/n/	
3. light	/laɪt/	[laɪt]	/l/		/t/	
4. fat	/fæt/	[bæt]	/f/		/t/	
5. zip	/zɪp/	[dɪp]	/z/		/p/	
6. meat	/mit/	[mit]	/m/		/t/	
7. like	/laɪk/	[laɪk]	/l/		/k/	
8. bite	/baɪt/	[baɪt]	/b/		/t/	
9. seat	/sit/	[dit]	/s/		/t/	
10. chip	/tʃɪp/	[dɪp]	/tʃ/		/p/	
11. ship	/ʃɪp/	[dɪp]	/ʃ/		/p/	
12. thin	/θɪn/	[dɪn]	/θ/		/n/	
13. feet	/fit/	[bit]	/f/		/t/	
14. bike	/baɪk/	[baɪk]	/b/		/k/	
15. that	/ðæt/	[dæt]	/ð/		/t/	
16. fun	/fʌn/	[bʌn]	/f/		/n/	

(Continued)

Answers:

Target word	Adult pronunciation	Luke's production	Initial consonant	Correct or incorrect?	Final consonant	Correct or incorrect
1. sun	/sʌn/	[dʌn]	/s/	✗	/n/	✓
2. fan	/fæn/	[bæn]	/f/	✗	/n/	✓
3. light	/laɪt/	[laɪt]	/l/	✓	/t/	✓
4. fat	/fæt/	[bæt]	/f/	✗	/t/	✓
5. zip	/zɪp/	[dɪp]	/z/	✗	/p/	✓
6. meat	/mit/	[mit]	/m/	✓	/t/	✓
7. like	/laɪk/	[laɪk]	/l/	✓	/k/	✓
8. bite	/baɪt/	[baɪt]	/b/	✓	/t/	✓
9. seat	/sit/	[dit]	/s/	✗	/t/	✓
10. chip	/ʧɪp/	[dɪp]	/ʧ/	✗	/p/	✓
11. ship	/ʃɪp/	[dɪp]	/ʃ/	✗	/p/	✓
12. thin	/θɪn/	[dɪn]	/θ/	✗	/n/	✓
13. feet	/fit/	[bit]	/f/	✗	/t/	✓
14. bike	/baɪk/	[baɪk]	/b/	✓	/k/	✓
15. that	/ðæt/	[dæt]	/ð/	✗	/t/	✓
16. fun	/fʌn/	[bʌn]	/f/	✗	/n/	✓

2. Using the above sample and the example provided, calculate the percent correct production of the following three consonants: /n, f, l/ (/b/ already has been calculated as an example).

Consonant	Number of opportunities*	Number of correct productions*	% correct [correct/opportunities]
Early: /b/	2	2	100%
Early: /n/			
Middle: /f/			
Late: /l/			

*If you used a larger sample, you would have more opportunities to determine a more valid and accurate percentage of correct productions for each consonant.

FIGURE 9-9 **(8) Vowels correct for Luke (4;3 years)**

(a) CHIRPA template

(8) Vowels correct
- Calculate + report percentage of vowels correct
- Highlight vowels that are frequently or always accurate
- Parentheses ( ) around vowels sometimes accurate

Percentage of vowels correct

Monophthongs [i ɪ e ɛ æ u ʊ o ɔ ɑ ɒ ə ʌ ɜ ɝ ɚ]

Diphthongs [ɪɹ ɛɹ ʊɹ ɔɹ ɑɹ aɪ aʊ ɔɪ]

Comments

Problem area ☐ yes ☐ no

(b) CHIRPA based on Luke's speech sample

(8) Vowels correct
- Calculate + report percentage of vowels correct
- Highlight vowels that are frequently or always accurate
- Parentheses ( ) around vowels sometimes accurate

Percentage of vowels correct *85.5% conversational speech*

Monophthongs [i ɪ e ɛ æ u ʊ o ɔ ɑ ɒ ə ʌ ɜ ɝ ɚ]

Diphthongs [ɪɹ ɛɹ ʊɹ ɔɹ ɑɹ aɪ aʊ ɔɪ]

Comments *Vowels adequate apart from rhotic vowels and diphthongs such as [ɛɹ]→[ɛə], [aɪ]→[a] and [ɔɹ]→[ɔ]*

Problem area ■ yes ☐ no

Source: Used by permission from Elise Baker.

phonetic inventory. In contrast with Box 3, notice the comment in Box 9 about Luke's vowel errors (e.g., [ɛɹ]→[ɛə]). This annotation simply provides a way of summarizing the nature of the child's error—in this example, the substitution of [ɛə] for /ɛɹ/. Given that a vowel error analysis table is not included with the CHIRPA, more in-depth analyses may be needed to examine a child's pattern of vowel errors, if one or more vowels are incorrect. For instance, if a child says *shirt* /ʃɝt/ as [ʃɔt], it would be helpful to analyze the child's speech sample more carefully to describe and better understand any error patterns.

(9) Syllable shapes correct

Descriptive analysis of a child's inventory of syllable shapes correct is completed in Box 9 (Figure 9-10). Highlight syllable shapes frequently or always correct, with parenthesis for syllable shapes sometimes correct. As shown in Figure 9-10, Luke's inventory of syllable shapes correct was limited to singleton consonant-vowel combinations (e.g., CV, CVC, VC). His limited use of word-final consonant clusters is shown using parentheses.

(10) Word lengths correct

A child's inventory of correct word lengths is described in Box 10 (Figure 9-11). For some children, this box can be relatively quick to complete based on your review of the data when completing Box 5 (independent inventory of word length). Specifically, if it is readily apparent that a child can produce words of varying lengths without syllable omission (e.g., *cat*, *caterpillar*), those word lengths would be highlighted to show that they were frequently or always accurate. This was the case for Luke. His reduced speech intelligibility was primarily associated with a limited inventory of singleton consonants and consonant clusters (see Figure 9-11). However, if a child omits syllables from words, you will need

---

FIGURE 9-10 **(9) Syllable shapes correct for Luke (4;3 years)**

(a) CHIRPA template

(9) Syllable shapes correct
• Highlight syllable shapes frequently or always accurate
• Parentheses ( ) around syllable shapes sometimes accurate
V CV VC CVC CCV[C+] [C+]VCC
CCCV[C+] [C+]VCCC
Others
Comments
Problem area ☐ yes ☐ no

(b) CHIRPA based on Luke's speech sample

(9) Syllable shapes correct
• Highlight syllable shapes frequently or always accurate
• Parentheses ( ) around syllable shapes sometimes accurate
V CV VC CVC CCV[C+] ([C+]VCC)
CCCV[C+] [C+]VCCC
Others
Comments *Difficulty with consonant clusters*
Problem area ■ yes ☐ no

Source: Used by permission from Elise Baker.

FIGURE 9-11 **(10) Word lengths correct for Luke (4;3 years)**

(a) CHIRPA template

(10) Word lengths correct	
• Highlight word lengths frequently or always accurate	
• Parentheses ( ) around word lengths sometimes accurate	
Monosyllables	4-syllables
Disyllables	5+ syllables
3-syllables	Evidence of syllable and/or consonant addition? ☐ yes ☐ no
Comments	
Problem area ☐ yes ☐ no	

(b) CHIRPA based on Luke's speech sample

(10) Word lengths correct	
• Highlight word lengths frequently or always accurate	
• Parentheses ( ) around word lengths sometimes accurate	
Monosyllables	4-syllables
Disyllables	5+ syllables
3-syllables	Evidence of syllable and/or consonant addition? ☐ yes ■ no
Comments *No obvious difficulty matching word length*	
Problem area ☐ yes ■ no	

Source: Used by permission from Elise Baker.

COMMENT: *Syllable stress patterns in CAS*

A common feature of CAS is **dysprosody**. Dysprosody can manifest in a variety of ways, such as the omission of weak syllables (w), weak syllables being produced as strong syllables (S) or stress being unusually equal across syllables, and syllable segregation (i.e., pausing between syllables so that there is no smooth transition from one syllable to the next) (Ballard et al., 2010; Shriberg et al., 2012). So, when you suspect that a child may have CAS, pay particular attention to the child's inventory of correct syllable stress patterns (as you did with their inventory of syllable and word shapes). According to Velleman and Shriberg (1999), children with phonological impairment tend to stop omitting weak syllables by around 6 years, while children with CAS may continue to omit weak syllables. Children with CAS may also show stress equalization (e.g., SS instead of wS). As discussed later in this chapter, acoustic analyses can be a helpful complement to independent and relational phonological analyses derived from a phonetically transcribed speech sample when there is a need to better understand the nature of a child's difficulty with syllable stress.

to spend a little more time completing Box 10. For instance, a toddler who is late to talk may be limited to producing mono- and disyllabic words. As noted earlier, look out for children's attempts at polysyllabic words. If necessary, calculate the percentage of correct word lengths for each word including two-, three-, four-, and five-plus-syllable words. As noted earlier in this chapter, children with CAS can find it difficult to sequence words of increasing length. If you suspect that a child has CAS, spend a little more time completing Box 10, calculating a child's percent correct production for each word length.

(11) Syllable stress patterns correct

An understanding of a child's inventory of syllable stress patterns correct will be guided by your observations about the child's independent inventory of syllable stress patterns (Box 6). If you noticed that a particular stress pattern was infrequent, consider why. Was it infrequent because the sample was limited (e.g., only two opportunities to produce a weak onset in the words *banana* and *giraffe*), or was it infrequent because the child had difficulty matching the adult stress pattern despite being given adequate opportunity? If the sample was inadequate, you can note this in Box 18 and collect more words before completing Box 11 (Figure 9-12). If the sample was adequate, calculate a child's percentage of syllable stress patterns correct. Pay particular attention to children's use of **iambic** stress patterns, where a weak syllable is followed by a strong syllable (e.g., wS, wSw/wSs). These are more difficult than **trochaic** stress patterns, which occur when a strong syllable is followed by a weak syllable (e.g., Sw). In Luke's case, he was frequently able to match stress across all the patterns listed in Box 11 (see Figure 9-12).

FIGURE 9-12   **(11) Syllable stress patterns correct for Luke (4;3 years)**

(a) CHIRPA template

(11) Syllable stress patterns correct
- Highlight stress patterns frequently or always accurate
- Parentheses ( ) around stress patterns sometimes accurate

| SS | Sw | wS | Sww | Sws | wSw / wSs | Swsw |

Other(s):
Is stress unusually equal across syllables? ☐ yes ☐ no
Comments
Problem area ☐ yes ☐ no

(b) CHIRPA based on Luke's speech sample

(11) Syllable stress patterns correct
- Highlight stress patterns frequently or always accurate
- Parentheses ( ) around stress patterns sometimes accurate

| SS | Sw | wS | Sww | Sws | wSw/wSs | Swsw |

Other(s): *Swsww (sampled once in hippopotamus)*
Is stress unusually equal across syllables? ☐ yes ■ no
Comments *No obvious difficulty matching word stress*
Problem area ☐ yes ■ no

Source: Used by permission from Elise Baker.

(12) Singleton consonant error analysis

Error pattern analysis of singleton consonants (Box 12, Figure 9-13) is a relational analysis, where intended consonants in word-initial, within word, and word-final positions are compared with a child's attempt. The steps involved are similar to SODA analysis, phoneme and cluster realization analysis by Grunwell (1985), and voice-place-manner error pattern analysis by Williams (2003). First, identify all instances of an intended consonant in relevant word positions in the sample (e.g., identify all opportunities to produce /f/ in the word-initial position). Second, review the child's realizations of the intended consonant and note the child's rendition. If the child's attempts at the consonant were frequently or always correct, highlight the consonant in the box. However, if the child's attempts were incorrect, use superscript notation to show the nature of the substitution, omission, or distortion error. (Errors of addition are noted in Box 10.) For instance, Luke's substitution of [b] for /f/ in the word *feet* /fit/ → [bit] would be noted as a superscript [b] in word-initial position for the fricative /f/. For Luke's omission of /h/ in *helicopter* /hɛlikɑptɚ/ → [ɛlidɑpə], the symbol ø would be placed as a superscript next to [h] (see Figure 9-13). Finally, summarize a child's errors according to place, voice, and manner (Williams, 2003). This analysis is a helpful prequel to phonological process analysis (Box 14) and the identification of a child's loss of phonemic contrast (Box 15).

FIGURE 9-13 | (12) Singleton consonant error analysis for Luke (4;3 years)

(a) CHIRPA template

(12) Singleton consonant error analysis
- Highlight consonants that are frequently or always correct
- Parentheses ( ) around consonants sometimes accurate
- If incorrect, note substituted phone(s) in cell or ∅ if omitted

WORD-INITIAL POSITION   Problem area ☐ yes ☐ no

Plosives	p	b			t	d			k	g	
Nasals		m				n					
Fricatives	f	v	θ	ð	s	z	ʃ				h
Approximants		w				ɹ		j			
Lat. Approx.						l					
Affricates							tʃ	dʒ			

WITHIN-WORD POSITION   Problem area ☐ yes ☐ no

Plosives	p	b			t	d			k	g	
Nasals		m				n				ŋ	
Fricatives	f	v	θ	ð	s	z	ʃ	ʒ			h
Approximants		w				ɹ		j			
Lat. Approx.						l					
Affricates							tʃ	dʒ			

WORD-FINAL POSITION   Problem area ☐ yes ☐ no

Plosives	p	b			t	d			k	g	
Nasals		m				n				ŋ	
Fricatives	f	v	θ	ð	s	z	ʃ	ʒ			h
Approximants						ɹ					
Lat. Approx.						l					
Affricates							tʃ	dʒ			

Observations:

(b) CHIRPA based on Luke's speech sample

(12) Singleton consonant error analysis
- Highlight consonants that are frequently or always correct
- Parentheses ( ) around consonants sometimes accurate
- If incorrect, note substituted phone(s) in cell or ∅ if omitted

WORD-INITIAL POSITION   Problem area ■ yes ☐ no

Plosives	p ᵇ	b			(t) ᵈ	d			k ᵈ	g ᵈ	
Nasals		m				n					
Fricatives	f ᵇ	v ᵇ	θ ᵈ	ð ᵈ	s ᵈ	z ᵈ	ʃ ᵈ				h ∅
Approximants		w				ɹ ʷ		(j) ∅			
Lat. Approx.						l					
Affricates							tʃ ᵈ	dʒ ᵈ			

WITHIN-WORD POSITION   Problem area ■ yes ☐ no

Plosives	(p) ᵇ	b			(t) ᵈ	d			(k) ᵈ	(g) ᵈ	
Nasals		m				n				ŋ	
Fricatives	f ᵇ	v ᵇ	θ ∅	ð ᵇ	s ᵈ	z	ʃ ᵈ	ʒ *			h ∅
Approximants		w				ɹ ʷ		j ∅			
Lat. Approx.						l					
Affricates							tʃ ᵗ	dʒ ᵈ			

WORD-FINAL POSITION   Problem area ■ yes ☐ no

Plosives	p	b			t	d			k	g ᵏ	
Nasals		m				n				ŋ	
Fricatives	f ᵖ	v ᵖ	θ ᵖ	ð *	s ᵗ	z ᵗ	ʃ ᵗ	ʒ *			
Approximants						ɹ ᵊ					
Lat. Approx.						l					
Affricates							tʃ ᵗ	dʒ *			

Observations: *voiceless → voiced word-initial position; word-initial velars → alveolars; fricatives and affricates→ homorganic (or near) plosive; alveolar approximant →labiovelar approximant; derhoticization of /ɹ/ in word-final; palatal approximant → ∅*
*= not sampled during assessment

■ ▨ ■ ▨ ■ ▨ ■ ■ ▨ ■ ▨ ■ ▨ ■ ▨ ■ ▨ ■ ▨ ■ ▨ ■ ■ ▨ ■ ▨ ■ ▨ ■ ▨ ■ ■ ▨ ■ ▨ ■

 APPLICATION: *Voice, place, and manner analysis of Luke's speech sample*

Using the error analysis results for consonant singletons (shown in Figure 9-13), summarize Luke's errors for singleton consonants with respect to voice, place, and manner across word-initial, within word, and word-final positions.

Answer: In Luke's case all word-initial and some within-word velar consonants were substituted with the alveolar plosive /d/. Word-initial voiceless obstruents were usually voiced. All fricatives and affricates were replaced with homorganic (or near) plosives, except for /h/, which was omitted. The palatal approximant was usually omitted in word-initial position and always omitted in within-word position. The alveolar approximant /ɹ/ was substituted with the labiovelar approximant /w/ in word-initial and within-word positions and replaced with a derhotacized vowel /ə/ in word-final positions.

Typical variability, inconsistency, or unique phonological patterns?
If a child's errors are consistent (e.g., Luke always substituted /f/ with [b] in word-initial position, always omitted /h/ in word-initial position, and always substituted /k/ with [d] in word-initial position), completion of Box 12 is relatively straightforward. Notice that we did not say quick. Of all the boxes in the CHIRPA, Box 12 will take the most time to complete. Do not rush your completion of this box. If you complete it carefully, then Boxes 14 (phonological process analysis) and 15 (analysis of loss of phonemic contrast) and goal setting will be easier to complete. If a child's errors are variable, you need to consider why. The first and most obvious reason is that your sample is too small to identify error patterns. As discussed in Chapter 8, if you only have two or three instances of a particular consonant and each instance is different and in error, further strategic sampling is needed to better understand the nature of a child's difficulty. Assuming you have an adequate sample, variable realizations of a particular phoneme could be indicative of:

- **Acquisition:** As discussed in Chapter 6, increasingly correct productions can be a sign that a child is in the process of acquiring a specific phoneme. If you suspect this to be the case, you might decide to monitor a child's acquisition of such phonemes over the course of intervention targeting other goals.
- **Phonological idioms and/or frozen forms:** A child might say a particular word in a more advanced form relative to the rest of his or her phonological system (i.e., phonological idiom) (Moskowitz, 1973) or produce a word using an earlier version despite his or her system being more advanced (i.e., frozen form), such as a child saying [lɛlo] for *yellow* despite the child using /j/ correctly in words such as *yes, yo-yo,* and *yoghurt* (Smit, 2004). If the speech sample you collect is limited, it might appear that the child has variable realizations of the consonants in the phonologically advanced word or frozen form. Additional samples will help differentiate phonological idioms and frozen forms from the rest of a child's phonological system.
- **Difference due to sampling context:** As discussed in Chapter 8, children can show variation in their production of the same word (and indeed consonants or vowels in words) depending on the sample context, such as single words versus connected speech.
- **A constraint-based rule in a child's phonological system:** An example of a constraint-based rule system could be a consonant-vowel sequencing constraint whereby velars /k, g/ → [t, d] except when produced with a back vowel [u]. If you suspect an interaction between different aspects of a child's phonological system (e.g., between consonants and vowels; consonants and stress patterns; consonants and syllable shapes), we recommend that you conduct more in-depth analysis to identify the constraints (e.g., Bernhardt & Stemberger, 2000; Velleman, 2003).

■ **Inconsistent speech disorder *or* CAS:** Inconsistent speech disorder occurs when there are variable realizations of the same word, such as *skip* /skɪp/ → [sɪp], [dɪp], [kɪ], and it can be differentiated from CAS. Refer to Chapters 2 and 8 for further information about differential diagnosis of inconsistent speech disorder, CAS, and phonological impairment.

(13) Consonant cluster error analysis

Error analysis of consonant clusters is similar to the error analysis of singleton consonants. First, identify all instances of a child's attempts to produce words containing consonant clusters. Start by focusing on two-element word-initial /w/ consonant clusters, followed by two-element word-initial /j/, /l/, /ɹ/, and /s/ consonant clusters, then three-element word-initial consonant clusters, and finally word-final consonant clusters. Highlight a consonant cluster if the child's attempt is frequently or always correct. Otherwise, using superscripts, note the entire cluster was omitted (ø), reduced to one consonant, or simplified. Recall that an asterisk is used to indicate any consonant clusters not sampled during an assessment. As shown in Figure 9-14, Luke did not produce any word-initial clusters correctly—[d] and [b] feature prominently as the consonant cluster substitutes. Also notice that for some consonant clusters, Luke had up to two possible realizations (e.g., /θɹ/→ [d, b]).

In contrast with word-initial consonant clusters, error analysis of word-final clusters requires you to list any nasal, liquid, or fricative consonant clusters correctly produced. Productions in error are simply listed (e.g., /st/ → [t]) as shown in Figure 9-14. Once you have completed your overview of a child's consonant cluster errors, indicate whether the errors constitute a problem in light of the child's age. As with Box 12, careful, methodical review of a child's speech sample will not only help you complete Box 13 (Figure 9-14) but will contribute to the completion of Box 15.

(14) Phonological processes

Recall from Chapter 5 that phonological processes are descriptive terms for error patterns evident in children's speech (e.g., *sleep* /slip/ → [lip] is **cluster reduction**). Phonological

---

FIGURE 9-14 **(13) Consonant cluster error analysis for Luke (4;3 years)**

(a) CHIRPA template

(13) Consonant cluster error analysis
- Highlight consonant clusters frequently or always correct
- Parentheses ( ) around clusters sometimes accurate
- If incorrect, note reduced or substituted phone, simplified cluster or ∅ if omitted

WORD-INITIAL POSITION

tw	kw	sw						
pj	bj	kj	mj	fj	vj			
pl	bl	kl	gl	fl	sl			
pɹ	bɹ	tɹ	dɹ	kɹ	gɹ	fɹ	θɹ	ʃɹ
sp	st	sk	sm	sn	sf			
spɹ	stɹ	skɹ	spl	skw				

WORD-FINAL POSITION

Nasal clusters: Fricative clusters:
Liquid clusters: Errors:

Observations:

Problem area ☐ yes ☐ no

(b) CHIRPA based on Luke's speech sample

(13) Consonant cluster error analysis
- Highlight consonant clusters frequently or always correct
- Parentheses ( ) around clusters sometimes accurate
- If incorrect, note reduced or substituted phone, simplified cluster or ∅ if omitted

WORD-INITIAL POSITION

tw ᵈ	kw ᵈ	sw ᵈ						
pj ᵇ	bj ᵇ	kj ᵈ	mj ᵐ	fj *	vj *			
pl ᵇ	bl ᵇ	kl ᵈ	gl ᵈ	fl ᵇ	sl ᵈ,ˡ			
pɹ ᵇ	bɹ ᵇ	tɹ ᵈ	dɹ ᵈ	kɹ ᵈ	gɹ ᵈ	fɹ ᵇ	θɹ ᵇ,ᵈ	ʃɹ ᵈ
sp ᵇ	st ᵈ	sk ᵈ	sm ᵐ	sn ⁿ	sf *			
spɹ ᵇ	stɹ ᵈ	skɹ ᵈ	spl ᵇ	skw ᵈ				

WORD-FINAL POSITION

Nasal clusters: [nt, ŋk, mp]   Fricative clusters: *Nil*
Liquid clusters: *Nil*   Errors: /st/→[t];/nd/→[n];/lz/→[lt,t]; /nts/→[nt]; /vz/→[b]; /ndʒ/→ [nt]

Observations: *Word-initial clusters usually reduced to a voiced plosive except nasal clusters (which were reduced to nasal). Correct final consonant clusters limited to homorganic nasal+plosive.*
*= not sampled during assessment

Problem area ■ yes ☐ no

Source: Used by permission from Elise Baker.

processes do not have a psychological reality. They are merely helpful terms for summarizing error patterns in children's speech. Phonological process analysis can be completed in one of three ways:

1. Analysis in accordance with the instructions in a standardized test, such as:
   - Bankson-Bernthal Test of Phonology (BBTOP) (Bankson & Bernthal, 1990);
   - Clinical Assessment of Articulation and Phonology (CAAP) (Secord & Donohue, 2002);
   - Diagnostic Evaluation of Articulation and Phonology: Phonology Assessment (DEAP) (Dodd, Hua, et al., 2002, 2006);
   - Hodson Assessment of Phonological Patterns: Third Edition (HAPP-3) (Hodson, 2004); and
   - Smit-Hand Articulation and Phonology Evaluation (SHAPE) (Smit & Hand, 1997).
2. Computer-based analyses (see the list of relevant software earlier in this chapter).
3. Informal manual analysis of a child's speech sample, such as:

   - identifying the presence or absence of processes from a predetermined list of common processes;
   - calculating the percent occurrence of those processes; and
   - describing any additional less common or idiosyncratic process in a child's speech sample.

Box 14 (Figure 9-15) of the CHIRPA is consistent with the third option: manual analysis in the form of a checklist for noting the presence or absence of common processes in a child's speech, description of a child's particular pattern for a process (should a child have one), and calculation of the percent occurrence for processes with less than 100% occurrence. This calculation is important, because a common mistake for beginning clinicians is to assume that all children use phonological processes in the same way, and that the occurrence of a process simply diminishes over time. Not true. For instance, two children (Caleb and Zak) might show evidence of final consonant deletion. Caleb might delete all final

COMMENT: *Malapropisms, eggcorns, and mondegreens*

Not every mispronunciation is the result of difference between a child's phonological system and the adult system. Sometimes children's mispronunciations can be innocuous instances of a malapropism, eggcorn, or mondegreen. A malapropism is an inadvertent use of a similar-sounding word for another. For instance, the *Cystic Fibrosis Association* holds an annual fund-raising event called *65 Roses*, after this mispronunciation of the disease by the younger brother of a child with cystic fibrosis. Vihman (1981) reports a similar example of a 3-year-old child using *ammonia* for *pneumonia*. An eggcorn occurs when one word is replaced by a near-homophone considered semantically reasonable to the speaker (Ching, 2008). For instance, the phrase *spread like wildflower* (as opposed to *wildfire*) is an eggcorn (Ching, 2008). One of our own children thought the *linen cupboard* was the *lemon cupboard*. This was an eggcorn because he was puzzled by the fact that bed linen rather than lemons were kept in the cupboard. A mondegreen is a misheard phrase, verse, or lyric (Aronson, 2009). For instance, on repeating the Pledge of Allegiance, children have been known to mishear and subsequently repeat *liberty and justice* as *liver tea and just us*. You may have your own example of a malapropism, eggcorn, or mondegreen from childhood. While they are usually innocuous (and sometimes entertaining!), repeated instances of malapropisms, eggcorns, or mondegreens suggest that more detailed assessment and analysis of a child's auditory and phonological processing skills is warranted.

FIGURE 9-15   **(14) Phonological process analysis for Luke (4;3 years)**

(a) CHIRPA template

(14) Phonological processes
- Shade box ■ for processes evident in the child's speech
- Comment on specific application of a process such as velar fronting word-initial only, and gliding only on /ɹ/
- Describe atypical, idiosyncratic processes
- Calculate percent occurrence as necessary

Syllable structure processes
☐ Weak syllable deletion

☐ Reduplication

☐ Final consonant deletion

☐ Initial consonant deletion

☐ Cluster reduction

Substitution processes
☐ Velar fronting

☐ Palatal fronting

☐ Stopping of fricatives

☐ Stopping of affricates

☐ Deaffrication
☐ Gliding of liquids

☐ Context sensitive voicing

☐ Consonant cluster simplification

☐ Fricative simplification

☐ Glottal insertion

☐ Backing

Assimilation processes
☐ Velar

☐ Labial

☐ Alveolar
Other processes

Problem area ☐ yes ☐ no

(b) CHIRPA based on Luke's speech sar

(14) Phonological processes
- Shade box ■ for processes evident in the child's speech
- Comment on specific application of a process such as velar fronting word-initial only, and gliding only on /ɹ/
- Describe atypical, idiosyncratic processes
- Calculate percent occurrence as necessary

Syllable structure processes
☐ Weak syllable deletion

☐ Reduplication

☐ Final consonant deletion

☐ Initial consonant deletion

■ Cluster reduction *(All word-initial clusters reduced to one element – 100%. Nasal + plosive final consonant cluster reduction only 28% occurrence.)*

Substitution processes
■ Velar fronting *(All word-initial velars in singleton and clusters contexts fronted to alveolar plosive /d/ - 100%. Velar fronting not prominent in within-word or word-final position.)*
■ Palatal fronting *(Indirectly evident as post-alveolar fricatives and affricates were stopped to an alveolar plosive.)*
■ Stopping of fricatives *(All fricatives stopped to homorganic plosive – 100%, except /h/ which was consistently omitted.)*
■ Stopping of affricates *(All affricates stopped to an alveolar plosive – 100%.)*
☐ Deaffrication
■ Gliding of liquids *(Gliding only present on /ɹ/ not /l/. Word-final /ɹ/ substituted with schwa.)*

■ Context sensitive voicing *(Voicing of voiceless consonants in word-initial position, and tendency for devoicing of voiced consonants in word-final position.)*
■ Consonant cluster simplification *(Not evident for word-initial clusters, as they were reduced. However, some simplification of final consonant clusters was evident due to other substitution processes.)*
☐ Fricative simplification

☐ Glottal insertion

☐ Backing

Assimilation processes
☐ Velar

☐ Labial

☐ Alveolar
Other processes

Problem area ■ yes ☐ no

Source: Used by permission from Elise Baker.

consonants. Zak might appear to delete some but not all final consonants. If you determine that Zak has 64% occurrence of final consonant deletion, you could be misled to think that Zak is learning to use final consonants and therefore that you will simply monitor the disappearance of the process. With more careful inspection of the data, you might find that Zak deletes fricatives and affricates only. This translates as 100% occurrence of final consonant deletion of fricatives and affricates. Luke's case is another good example (see Chapter 16). If you calculated Luke's percent occurrence of velar fronting from his comprehensive speech sample, you could be misled to think that the process is disappearing, because overall it was 40%. It was not disappearing. Luke had 100% occurrence of velar fronting of velar plosives in singleton and cluster contexts in word-initial position. The more specific your description of a child's particular pattern, the better you can tailor a child's intervention. Remember, if your percentage of occurrence calculation is < 100%, make sure that you have not missed a specific constraint in the child's phonological system.

The phonological processes listed on the CHIRPA (described in Chapter 5) are in keeping with terms used by Edwards and Shriberg (1983), Grunwell (1982, 1987, 1997), Ingram (1976), Stoel-Gammon and Dunn (1985), and Weiner (1979). If you have not already done so, complete the clinical application exercises in Chapter 5 on the identification and application of phonological processes. You need to be competent (and confident) at identifying and applying phonological processes in samples of children's speech to complete the phonological process checklist on the CHIRPA. Do this now before noting down the phonological processes evident in Luke's speech sample (Chapter 16).

As shown on Figure 9-15, the only syllable structure process evident in Luke's speech was cluster reduction (e.g., *blue* /blu/ → [bu]). Substitution processes were more common, with some processes, such as velar fronting (e.g., *key* /ki/ → [ti]) always evident in word-initial position. Notice that assimilation processes (e.g., *dig* /dɪg/ → [dɪd]) were not evident in Luke's speech sample.

(15) Loss of phonemic contrast

Relational analysis of a child's loss of phonemic contrast is based on a component of Williams' (2003) Systemic Phonological Analysis of Child Speech (SPACS) and Grunwell's (1985) Phonological Assessment of Child Speech (PACS). The analysis involves the identification and description of a child's system of phonemic contrasts relative to the adult

---

 APPLICATION: *Describing unique phonological patterns*

In Chapter 5 we described many common and unusual phonological processes. The names for these patterns are based on observations of children's speech. What if you come across an error pattern in a child's speech sample that does not have an existing name? You simply describe the pattern. Consider the following sample from James (2;8 years). Describe the pattern with respect to James' production of word-final consonants.

cat /kæt/ →[kæt]	*sheep* /ʃip/ → [sip]	*teeth* /tiθ/ →[tif]
cat bed /kæt bɛd/ → [kæ bɛd]	*sheep big* /ʃip bɪg/ → [si bɪg]	*teeth clean* /tiθ klin/ → [tif kin]
cat in /kæt ɪn/ → [kæt ɪn]	*sheep in* /ʃip/ → [sip ɪn]	*teeth out* /tiθ aʊt/ → [tif aʊt]

Hint: Sort all of James' productions according to whether the final consonant is retained or deleted. For the two word utterances, compare the initial segment of the second word in relation to the presence or deletion of the final consonant of the first word. What do you notice?

Answer: James has difficulties with juncture. He deletes final voiceless plosive consonants, only in connected speech, and only if the succeeding word begins with a consonant. If the succeeding word begins with a vowel, the final consonant is retained.

■ ■

APPLICATION: So what phonological process is it—alveolar assimilation or velar fronting?

Recall from Chapter 5 that multiple phonological processes can apply to one word. Sometimes it is also possible that two different processes can result in the same realization of a word. Revisit Molly's case in Chapter 5, and then consider Bethany's (3;8 years) speech sample below.

cape /kep/ → [tep]	*key* /ki/ → [ti]	*meat* /mit/ → [mit]
cake /kek/ → [tet]	*spoon* /spun/ → [pun]	*skate* /sket/ → [tet]
book /bʊk/ → [bʊt]	*look* /lʊk/ → [wʊt]	*Kay* /ke/ → [te]
sack /sæk/ → [tæt]	*sheep* /ʃip/ → [tip]	*foot* /fʊt/ → [pʊt]

At first glance you might suppose that Bethany's production of *skate* /sket/ → [tet] shows complete regressive alveolar assimilation. However, another explanation is possible. Bethany's production of *skate* /sket/ → [tet] could be described as a combination of velar fronting and cluster reduction. How do you find out the most likely answer to such phonological riddles?

1. Select one of the possible processes and identify words where only that process could apply. In Bethany's case, only velar fronting could be used to describe *key* /ki/ → [ti].
2. Search the rest of a child's speech sample for other opportunities for that process, to confirm whether this pattern is indeed present. For instance, Bethany's production of *cape* /kep/ → [tep]; *cake* /kek/ → [tet]; *book* /bʊk/ → [bʊt]; *sack* /sæk/ → [tæt] could all, in part, be described as velar fronting.
3. Search for instances of the alternate explanation. In Bethany's case, the alternate explanation for *skate* /sket/ → [tet] is complete regressive alveolar assimilation. Look through the sample for words ending in alveolars (e.g., *foot*, *meat*). Did alveolar assimilation occur? No. *Meat* was correct, and Bethany's production of *foot* /fʊt/ → [pʊt] shows stopping of fricatives. Having excluded alveolar assimilation and identified other instances of velar fronting, the riddle is solved. Bethany's production of *skate* /sket/ → [tet] best reflects velar fronting in combination with cluster reduction.

> **COMMENT:** *Matching phonological analysis approaches with intervention approaches: A word on Hodson's (2007) phonological patterns and cycles intervention*
>
> If you intend to use Hodson's (2007) cycles approach for intervention with a child who has a phonological impairment (see Chapter 13), you will need to complete Hodson's analysis of phonological patterns (see Hodson, 2003) and calculate the percent occurrence of each pattern. In Chapter 10 we provide an overview of Hodson's patterns and recommended order for targeting those patterns.

system. This is the last relational analysis box (Box 15, Figure 9-16) on the CHIRPA. Consider Luke's production of *chip* /tʃɪp/ → [dɪp] and *zip* /zɪp/ → [dɪp]. Both *chip* and *zip* are produced as homonyms. Review Luke's speech sample in Chapter 16 and count how many words he produced with word-initial [d] (that should not have started with [d]). Once you have done that, review Luke's consonant singleton and consonant cluster error analysis (depicted in Figures 9-13 and 9-14). What do you notice? Clearly, Luke's favorite sound is [d]. Many singleton consonants and consonant clusters are substituted with [d]. What follows is a

FIGURE 9-16 **(15) Loss of phonemic contrast for Luke (4;3 years)**

(a) CHIRPA template

(15) Loss of phonemic contrast
- Using error analysis (box #12 and #13), list singleton consonants and consonant clusters with the same substitute (consonant or ∅) in the same word position.
- Describe loss of phonemic contrast according to major class features (obstruents/sonorants), natural classes (plosives, nasals, glides, liquids, fricatives and affricates) and consonant clusters (Williams, 2003). For example, non-labial singleton obstruents (including plosives, fricatives and affricates) and clusters /t, k, g, s, z, ʃ, θ, ð, tʃ, dʒ, ɹ, st, stɹ, sk, skɹ, skl, skw, kɹ, dɹ, gɹ, kl, gl/ are all substituted with [d] word-initially.

Word initial	Word final

Problem area ☐ yes ☐ no

(b) CHIRPA based on Luke's speech sample

(15) Loss of phonemic contrast
- Using error analysis (box #12 and #13), list singleton consonants and consonant clusters with the same substitute (consonant or ∅) in the same word position.
- Describe loss of phonemic contrast according to major class features (obstruents/sonorants), natural classes (plosives, nasals, glides, liquids, fricatives and affricates) and consonant clusters (Williams, 2003). For example, non-labial singleton obstruents (including plosives, fricatives and affricates) and clusters /t, k, g, s, z, ʃ, θ, ð, tʃ, dʒ, ɹ, st, stɹ, sk, skɹ, skl, skw, kɹ, dɹ, gɹ, kl, gl/ are all substituted with [d] word-initially.

Word initial	Word final
• /t, k, g, θ, ð, s, z, ʃ, tʃ, dʒ, tw, ɹ, dɹ, θɹ, sw, sl, st, sk, stɹ, skw, skɹ, ʃɹ, kw, kl, gl, kɹ, gɹ, kj/→ [d]	• /s, z, ʃ, tʃ, lz, st/ → [t]
• /p, f, v, pj, bj, pl, bl, fl, pɹ, bɹ, fɹ, θɹ, sp, spɹ, spl/ → [b]	• /f v θ/ → [p]
• /ɹ, j/ → [w]	
• /h, j/ → [∅]	

Problem area ■ yes ☐ no

Source: Used by permission from Elise Baker.

brief description of the steps involved in the identification of Luke's loss of phonemic contrast in his speech sample. For further information about systemic phonological analysis and the identification of phoneme collapses, see Williams (2003). For further information about Grunwell's contrastive assessment, see Grunwell (1985).

1. Review the child's speech sample and complete an analysis of consonant singleton and cluster errors (see Figures 9-13 and 9-14).
2. Inspect the error analysis results in word-initial position (for singleton and consonant clusters), identifying a common substitute sound (e.g., /ʃ/ → [d]).
3. Create a list of all the singleton consonants and consonant clusters substituted with that sound (e.g., /t, k, g, θ, ð, s, z, ʃ, tʃ, dʒ, tw, tɹ, dɹ, θɹ, sw, sl, st, sk, stɹ, skw, skɹ, ʃɹ, kw, kl, gl, kɹ, gɹ, kj/ → [d]). Williams (2003) refers to a child's use of one speech sound for many speech sounds as a **collapse of contrast** and uses a numeric ratio to capture the number of sounds (singletons and consonant clusters) reduced to one speech sound. In Luke's case his collapse of contrast to [d] would have a ratio of 28:1.
4. Review the sample again, repeating steps 2 and 3, until speech sounds (consonant singletons and clusters) substituted by another speech sound (or omitted) have been described, including 1:1 substitutions (e.g., /ɹ/ → [w]). It is important that you identify all favorite speech sounds, and all the consonants and vowels replaced by each favorite speech sound (i.e., all phoneme collapses and each member of a phoneme collapse) in word-initial and word-final positions, so that you can make well-informed decisions about the goals of intervention (see Chapter 10). The identification and description of a child's loss of phonemic contrast within words is not routinely done.
5. Summarize each group of speech sounds realized as the same sound using distinctive features, including the major class features of obstruent and sonorant (Williams, 2003). As noted in Figure 9-16, Luke realized many singleton consonants

and consonant clusters as [d] in word-initial position. This could be summarized as non-labial (i.e., coronal and dorsal) singleton obstruents and consonant clusters were realized as [d]. Remember that Luke's CHIRPA, described in this chapter, was based on a comprehensive single-word and connected speech sample. Chapter 16 provides portions of this sample.

(16) Additional observations: Suprasegmentals and beyond (prosody, phonation, resonance, and respiration)

Boxes 1 through 15 of the CHIRPA comprise the independent and relational analyses. Three additional boxes are included on the CHIRPA template to capture:

- additional observations about a child's speech production skills;
- speech ratings; and
- comments about the adequacy of the speech sample used to complete the CHIRPA.

Box 16, the additional observations box (Figure 9-17), provides an opportunity for you to note whether prosodic (e.g., stress and intonation), phonation, resonance, and respiratory aspects of a child's speech are natural or unnatural.

As shown in Figure 9-17, no calculations are required for this box. It is simply based on your perceptual judgment with respect to:

1. **Stress:** Using both a single-word and connected speech sample, consider the child's ability to signal stress appropriately in words and sentences. Specifically:
   - **Lexical (word) stress:** As you listen to a child's speech, ask yourself whether the child produces a natural contrast between Sw (e.g., paper) and wS (e.g., giraffe) stress patterns in words. Is the child's production of spondees (i.e., compound words containing a strong-strong stress pattern) different from words with iambic and trochaic stress? This is important to observe if you suspect that a child has a motor speech disorder rather than phonological impairment, because the presence of stress equalization has been associated with CAS (Ballard et al., 2010).
   - **Sentence stress:** Does the child use stress appropriately in sentences and connected speech? Consider whether a child uses excess, equal, or misplaced stress. Again, this is important to consider if you suspect that a child has CAS. In a study of 53 children with CAS, around one in two (52%) were perceived as having unnatural (excess, equal, or misplaced) stress in connected speech (Shriberg,

FIGURE 9-17   **(16) Suprasegmentals and prosody for Luke (4;3 years)**

(a) CHIRPA template

(16) Additional observations: prosody/phonation/resonance/respiration
☑ natural or ☒ unnatural/problematic
☐ **Stress**
　Lexical stress　　　☐ Sw　☐ wS
　Sentence stress　　☐
　Emphatic stress　　☐
☐ **Words of increasing length** (e.g., *hip, hippo, hippopotamus*)
Is syllable segregation evident? ☐ yes ☐ no
☐ **Speech rate** ☐ Too slow ☐ Too fast ☐ Poorly regulated
☐ **Intonation**
☐ **Phonation**
☐ **Resonance**
☐ **Respiration / speech breathing**
Problem area ☐ yes ☐ no

(b) CHIRPA based on Luke's speech sample

(16) Additional observations: prosody/phonation/resonance/respiration
☑ natural or ☒ unnatural/problematic
☑ **Stress**
　Lexical stress　　　☑ Sw　☑ wS
　Sentence stress　　☑
　Emphatic stress　　☑
☑ **Words of increasing length** (e.g., *hip, hippo, hippopotamus*)
Is syllable segregation evident? ☐ yes ☑ no
☑ **Speech rate** ☐ Too slow ☐ Too fast ☐ Poorly regulated
☑ **Intonation**
☑ **Phonation**
☑ **Resonance**
☑ **Respiration / speech breathing**
Problem area ☐ yes ■ no

Source: Used by permission from Elise Baker.

Aram, & Kwiatkowski, 1997b). Be careful not to assume that difficulty with stress is a clear and convincing diagnostic sign of CAS, because in the same study by Shriberg, Aram, and Kwiatkowski (1997b), around 10% of children with phonological impairment were perceived as having unnatural stress.

■ **Emphatic stress:** Consider whether the child is able to use stress emphatically to emphasize a point (e.g., "I said it was GREEN!") or to contrast a word in an utterance with a prior utterance (e.g., "I have a red book"; "I have a BLUE book").

2. **Articulation of words of increasing length:** Consider whether a child has difficulty producing words of increasing length such as *but, butter, butterfly*; *hip, hippo, hippopotamus*. A decrease in accuracy as the word length increases can be characteristic of CAS (Velleman, 2003).

3. **Syllable segregation:** As you listen to a child's connected speech, take note of his or her ability to naturally sequence syllables. By naturally, we mean move smoothly from one syllable to the next in a word without syllable segregation (i.e., brief pausing between syllables). Syllable segregation is considered another characteristic of CAS (Shriberg et al., 2012; Ballard et al., 2010).

4. **Speech rate:** Is the child's speech rate adequate, too slow, or too fast? An unnaturally slow speech rate can be indicative of motor speech disorders such as childhood dysarthria (Marchant, McAuliffe, & Huckabee, 2008) and CAS (Shriberg et al., 2012), while a fast speech rate can be indicative of cluttering (Van Zaalen-op't Hof, Wijnen, & De Jonckere, 2009).

5. **Intonation:** Consider the child's ability to use intonation appropriately, with respect to chunking, affect, interaction, and focus (Wells & Peppé, 2001):

■ **Chunking:** Can you perceive a difference between a child's production of compound nouns versus a list of nouns (e.g., "chocolate cake and pumpkin pie" versus "chocolate, cake, and pumpkin pie")?

■ **Affect:** Does a child use prosody to communicate affective or attitudinal meaning (Wells & Peppé, 2001)? For instance, do you hear a rise-fall when a child expresses a liking for something (e.g., "Mmm!")?

■ **Interaction:** Does the child use intonation appropriately during conversational speech? For instance, does the child use intonation to mark the end of his or her conversational turn (Wells & Peppé, 2001)? Do questions and statements have an appropriate intonation contour (e.g., rising contour for yes-no questions such as "Do you like chocolate?")?

■ **Focus:** Does the child use intonation to draw a conversation partner's attention to a particular word in an utterance (e.g., "I saw elephants, tigers, and a polar bear!")? If you suspect intonation to be problematic, then conduct a more detailed assessment and analysis using a tool such as the Profiling Elements of Prosody in Speech-Communication (PEPS-C) (Peppé & McCann, 2003; Peppé 2015), as described in Chapter 8.

6. **Phonation:** Consider the quality of a child's phonation—is it natural or unnatural? Children with childhood dysarthria may have difficulty regulating pitch (e.g., pitch breaks or tremor), speaking at an appropriate pitch (e.g., too high or too low) or loudness (e.g., too loud or soft), managing the demands of voicing (e.g., continuous voicing rather than having contrasts between voiced and voiceless consonants), and/or may have an abnormal voice quality (e.g., breathy, strain-strangled, occasional dysphonia) (Hodge & Wellman, 1999).

7. **Resonance:** As you listen to a child's speech, notice the quality of his or her resonance. Do you hear nasal emission? Is the child's speech hyper- or hyponasal or a combination of both (i.e., mixed nasality)? Children with childhood dysarthria can have muffled resonance (Hodge & Wellman, 1999). Children with an SSD secondary to cleft palate velopharyngeal dysfunction can have difficulty with resonance, typically hypernasality and nasal emission (Kummer, 2011).

8. **Respiration:** Notice the child's speech breathing ability. Is the child able to manage the demands of speech breathing (e.g., variable breath group lengths)? Do you notice inappropriate inspiration and/or expiration? Children with childhood dysarthria may struggle to regulate their vocal loudness because their breath runs out before the end of an utterance (Hodge & Wellman, 1999).

> **COMMENT:** *Syllable segregation and connected speech processes*
>
> If you hear syllable segregation in connected speech, it can be helpful to analyze a child's speech sample by taking a closer look at how the child deals with juncture. What might initially sound like all syllables being segregated could in fact be a specific difficulty with juncture. Consider whether the child is capable of assimilation, elision, and/or liaison, and whether some juncture contexts are easier than others (Pascoe, Stackhouse, & Wells, 2006). See Chapter 8 for further information about the assessment of juncture.

As shown in Figure 9-17, Luke was perceived to have natural lexical, sentence, and emphatic stress. Syllable segregation was not perceived. His intonation and speech rate was appropriate. He was also able to produce words of increasing length, albeit with segmental errors irrespective of length. His phonation, resonance, and respiration for speech were also perceived to be natural. Contrast Luke's case with Michael (4;2 years). Michael was diagnosed with CAS. His prosody was unnatural. When Michael produced a polysyllabic word, there was evidence of stress equalization and syllable segregation. He had difficulty moving from one syllable to the next. During conversation, Michael's speech sounded robotic. Lian's case also contrasts with Luke's. Lian (14;2 years) has spastic dysarthria. Her speech rate was slow. Her pitch and loudness was poorly regulated. Her speech could be too high or too low and/or too loud or too soft. Pitch breaks were also evident in her speech. Lian's voice quality was strained-strangled. Her resonance was unnatural—her speech was mildly hypernasal, with nasal air emission on vowels in words containing nasal consonants. Lian also had difficulty regulating her breath during speech, opting for short, brief utterances.

Read more about Luke (4;3 years), Michael (4;2 years), and Lian (14;2 years) in Chapter 16.

(17) Speech ratings

Box 17 is the speech ratings box (Figure 9-18). This section provides you with an opportunity to rate a child's speech with respect to consistency, severity, and intelligibility.

1. **Consistency:** Observation about a child's speech consistency will be based on findings from the error pattern analysis of singleton consonants and consonant clusters. As discussed earlier, it can be difficult to separate acceptable variable speech errors from inconsistent speech. If you suspect that a child has inconsistent errors that cannot be explained by other possibilities, indicate your concerns about the consistency of the child's speech on the CHIRPA form, and conduct further analysis. For instance, Dodd (2005) recommends calculating an index of inconsistency by determining the

FIGURE 9-18   **(17) Speech ratings for Luke (4;3 years)**

(a) CHIRPA template

(17) Speech ratings
Consistency rating
☐ Consistent   ☐ Inconsistent – further assessment and analysis needed
Severity rating
☐ Mild   ☐ Moderate-severe
☐ Mild-moderate   ☐ Severe
Intelligibility rating
☐ Intelligible   ☐ Mainly unintelligible
☐ Mainly intelligible   ☐ Unintelligible
☐ Partially intelligible

(b) CHIRPA based on Luke's speech sample

(17) Speech ratings
Consistency rating
■ Consistent   ☐ Inconsistent – further assessment and analysis needed
Severity rating *based on conversational speech sample*
☐ Mild   ☐ Moderate-severe
☐ Mild-moderate   ■ Severe
Intelligibility rating
☐ Intelligible   ■ Mainly unintelligible
☐ Mainly intelligible   ☐ Completely unintelligible
☐ Partially intelligible

Source: Used by permission from Elise Baker.

percentage of words with variable pronunciations from a group of words (e.g., 25 words) spoken by a child. A word is considered variable when two of three elicitations of the same word in the same sampling context (typically, single-word picture-naming task) are different. Dodd (2005) uses the value of > 40% variable words (e.g., 10 of 25 words show different productions on two of three occasions) as indicative of inconsistent speech. The Diagnostic Evaluation of Articulation and Phonology (Dodd, Hua, et al., 2002, 2006) contains an inconsistency subtest designed specifically to explore this aspect of children's speech. In Luke's case, his speech errors were consistent, so no further analysis of consistency was conducted. See Jarrod's case (Chapter 16) for further information and examples of inconsistent speech.

2. **Severity:** Severity adjectives capture the degree or severity of involvement of a problem. The most widely used system was developed by Shriberg and Kwiatkowski (1982c). It involves the calculation of the PCC from a conversational speech sample and assigning a severity adjective to a numerical score (see Table 9-3). In Luke's case, his PCC during conversational speech was 48.4%, consistent with a severe severity rating. There is a range of severity scales for describing the degree of a child's SSD. Table 9-2 provides a summary of three different systems. Rules and methods for calculating PCC are described later in this chapter.

3. **Intelligibility:** The final rating on the CHIRPA form refers to the child's speech intelligibility. Intelligibility captures the degree to which a listener understands a person's speech. There are many different methods (quantitative and qualitative) for assessing a child's speech intelligibility (see Chapter 8 for further information). The CHIRPA uses a simple and brief qualitative 5-point rating scale, including:

> 1 = intelligible
> 2 = mainly intelligible
> 3 = partially intelligible
> 4 = mainly unintelligible
> 5 = completely unintelligible

As shown in Figure 9-18, Luke's speech was rated by his SLP as mainly unintelligible.

(18) Sampling constraints

The eighteenth and final box of the CHIRPA prompts you to think about the representative nature of the speech sample you have analyzed. Ideally, phonological analysis begins once you have gathered a comprehensive speech sample. However, not all published assessment

---

TABLE 9-2 **Severity systems used to describe the degree of a child's speech sound disorder**

Severity ratings based on PCC from conversational speech* (Shriberg et al., 1986)	Total Occurrence of Major Phonological Deviations (TOMPD) rating** (Hodson, 2004)	4-point clinical judgment scale (Bleile, 1996)
■ Mild = 85–100%	■ Mild = 1–50	1 = no disorder
■ Mild-moderate = 65–84.9%	■ Moderate = 51–100	2 = mild disorder
■ Moderate-severe = 50–64.9%	■ Severe = 101–150	3 = moderate disorder
■ Severe = < 50%	■ Profound = > 150	4 = severe disorder

*If a PCC score is within 4 percentage points of another severity category, and the child is older than 6 years or the conversational speech sample contains fewer than two-thirds glossable utterances, or there is a noticeable difference on one or more suprasegmental features (pitch, loudness, voice quality, phrasing, stress, and rate) on more than 15% of utterances in a conversational speech sample, then the next more severe severity adjective is used (Shriberg, Kwiatkowski, Best, Hengst, & Terselic-Weber, 1986). As discussed later in this chapter, it is inappropriate to calculate PCC if a child primarily displays errors of distortion. In such cases, the PCC should be adjusted (PCC-A) or revised (PCC-R) to account for the errors of distortion.

** The TOMPD is based on a child's performance on the Hodson Assessment of Phonological Patterns-3 (HAPP-3) (Hodson, 2004).

FIGURE 9-19   **(18) Sampling constraints for Luke (4;3 years)**

(a) CHIRPA template

(18) Sampling constraints? ☐ More sampling required	
☐ Polysyllables	☐ Words with weak-onset stress
☐ Consonant clusters	☐ Other

(b) CHIRPA based on Luke's speech sample

(18) Sampling constraints? ■ More sampling required	
☐ Polysyllables	☐ Words with weak-onset stress
☐ Consonant clusters	■ Other
Sample more instances of /θ, ʒ, ʤ, j/	

Source: Used by permission from Elise Baker.

tools sample all aspects of speech. Some articulation tests focus primarily on consonants, with less attention given to phonotactics (e.g., consonant clusters and polysyllabic words). As discussed in Chapter 8, the speech sample that you analyze is often dependent on your preliminary observations about a child's SSD and your strategic sampling of a particular problematic skill (e.g., elicit additional polysyllabic words beginning with weak onsets; sample more words containing a wider range of consonant clusters). Despite your best efforts to collect a comprehensive speech sample, the need to collect additional samples of a specific skill can become apparent once you start to analyze a speech sample. In such instances, complete as much of the CHIRPA as you can between sessions, and then finalize the analysis once the additional samples have been gathered. As shown in Figure 9-19, additional instances of word-initial and within word /θ, ʒ, ʤ, j/ were required to better understand Luke's error patterns.

■ ▦ ▥ ■ ▦ ▤ ■ ▦ ▣ ■ ▦ ▤ ■ ▦ ▣ ■ ▦ ▤ ■ ▦ ▣ ■ ▦ ▤ ■ ▦ ▣ ■ ▦ ▤ ■ ▦ ▣ ■ ▦ ▤ ■ ▦ ▣ ■ ▦ ■

 APPLICATION: *Distinctive feature analysis*

Recall from Chapter 5 that distinctive features capture acoustic and articulatory similarities and differences among phonemes and that phonemes can be described according to their unique bundle of features. While traditional distinctive feature analysis (e.g., Costello, 1975) is not routinely completed by practicing SLP, it is helpful to have an understanding of distinctive features for two reasons. First, knowledge of feature terminology is essential when you conduct a constraint-based nonlinear analysis (e.g., Bernhardt & Stemberger, 2000). Second, distinctive feature analysis can offer insight into uncommon and unusual error patterns. Consider the following speech sample from a child (Ben, 4;11 years).

look /lʊk/ → [nʊk]	*lip* /lɪp/ → [nɪp]	*pillow* /pɪlo/ → [pɪno]	*Billy* /bɪli/ → [bɪni]
lamb /læm/ → [næm]	*leaf* /lif/ → [nif]	*loud* /laʊd/ → [naʊd]	*leg* /lɛg/ → [neg]

What underlies Ben's nasalization of the lateral /l/? Review the table of distinctive features in Chapter 5, and describe Ben's error pattern using those features.

Answer: Although the consonants /l/ and /n/ have many features in common (particularly with regards to voice and place), Ben is not using the major class feature [+ approximant] in combination with [+ continuant], [+ lateral] and [– nasal] to contrast liquid /l/ from the nasal /n/.

	[n]	**[l]**
Major class features	– [approx]	+ [approx]
Manner features	– [cont]	+ [cont]
	+ [nasal]	– [nasal]
	– [lat]	+ [lat]

SPEECH MEASURES

There are various methods for measuring speech accuracy. These measures have emerged out of a need to capture different aspects of speech acquisition and SSD within and across languages, and across children. Consider the following speech samples derived from a conversation with two typically developing toddlers.

- George (18 months) says *baby* /bebi/, *hat* /hæt/, *dad* /dæd/, *me* /mi/, and *no* /no/ correctly. He does not produce words longer than two syllables.
- James (19 months) says *dad* /dæd/, *me* /mi/, and *no* /no/ correctly but *butterfly* /bʌtɚflaɪ/ as [bʌtəbaɪ] and *caterpillar* /kætɚpɪlɚ/ as [dætəbɪwə].

If we were to measure the accuracy of the toddlers' speech samples by calculating the PCC, George would achieve 100%. He produced all eight consonants across the five words correctly. James produced 7/12 consonants correctly, yielding a PCC of 58%. Do you think this is a valid measure of George's and James' speech production abilities? Clearly, this relatively simple measure of consonant accuracy does not capture the fact that James produced a three-syllable and four-syllable word. What follows is a brief description of a range of segmental and whole-word measures from literature on speech acquisition and SSD. Where relevant, we summarize the rules for calculating specific measures and offer suggestions regarding their clinical relevance.

■ Measures of segments

You can quantitatively measure the accuracy of speech segments, consonants and vowels, in a few different ways. The method you choose will be guided by the errors you observe in a child's speech sample.

Percentage of Consonants Correct (PCC) (Shriberg & Kwiatkowski, 1982c)

The most frequently used and universal measure of children's speech accuracy is the PCC. This measure was first described by Shriberg and Kwiatkowski (1982c) and later expanded (Shriberg, Austin, Lewis, McSweeny, & Wilson, 1997b). It involves working out the percentage of consonants produced correctly in a speech sample, relative to the total number of consonants sampled. PCC is based on narrow phonetic transcription (particularly to capture common clinical distortions such as [s]). Rules for calculating PCC are listed in Table 9-3.

Variations on PCC

Shriberg and colleagues (e.g., Shriberg, 1993; Shriberg, Austin, et al., 1997a) developed a range of additional segmental measures to address some of the limitations of the PCC measure. These measures and the methods for calculating them are summarized in Table 9-4. Six of the measures are minor variations of the original PCC metric (Shriberg & Kwiatkowski, 1982c), addressing distortions (PCC-A; PCC-R), vowel accuracy (PVC, PVC-R), and total phonemes correct (PPC; PPC-R). The relative distortion index (RDI), the articulation competence index (ACI), and the percentage of consonants in the inventory (PCI) offer additional insights into children's speech accuracy.

The RDI quantifies the proportion of distortion errors in a sample relative to the total number of errors. The ACI uses a child's RDI and PCC to yield a measure that accounts for distortion errors (Shriberg, 1993). It requires calculation of the PCC and RDI from a sample. To calculate the ACI, PCC and RDI are added, and then divided by two.

PCI is a quantitative measure of a child's relational inventory of consonants mastered (Shriberg, Austin, et al., 1997a). The denominator is the number of intended consonants (belonging to the child's language) in a sample. A single attempt is worth 0.5 points. Two or more attempts are worth 1 point. In English the total number of points from an exhaustive sample is 24. The numerator is simply the total number of different consonants correct. One correct instance is worth 0.5 points, while two or more are worth 1 point. Distortions are considered correct. When converted to a percentage, two or more correct instances of every type of consonant in the sample yields a PCI of 100%.

■ Measures of whole words

In this section we describe four different strategies for measuring whole words, with respect to correctness, complexity, intelligibility, and variation (Ingram, 2002; Ingram & Ingram, 2001). We have used the term *proportion* for the whole-word measures, in keeping with terminology used by Ingram and Ingram (2001). For ease of consistency with the segmental measures, you could convert the proportions to a percentage measure. A summary of the different types of measures is provided in Table 9-5.

TABLE 9-3 **Guidelines and rules for calculating Percentage of Consonants Correct (PCC) on a conversational speech sample**

1. Count the total number of consonants and the total number of consonants produced correctly.
2. Exclude:
   (i)   all vowels including rhotic vowels;
   (ii) consonants added before a vowel;
   (iii) consonants that are partially or completely unintelligible;
   (iv) consonants in the second or subsequent repetitions of a syllable (e.g., *bunny* /bʌni/ → /bʌ bʌni/—only score one instance of [b]); and
   (v)   consonants in the third or subsequent consistent repetition of a word, unless the child's productions of that word are variable.

2. Consonants are incorrect[a] if they are:
   (i)   deleted (except for word-initial /h/ in unstressed syllables in connected speech);
   (ii) substituted with another consonant, or in the case of word-initial consonants, show evidence of partial-voicing;
   (iii) distorted (no matter how subtle); and
   (iv) added to (whether the target consonant is correct or incorrect) (e.g., *spoon* /spun/ → [spunt]).

3. Consider if the following apply:
   (i)   Dialectical variations should be analyzed according to the child's dialect (e.g., *ask* /ask/ → [aks] is acceptable in African-American English) (Stockman, 2007).
   (ii) Casual productions from connected speech should be analyzed according to what is acceptable and intended (e.g., *don't know*→*dunno*).
   (iii) Acceptable allophonic variations are scored as correct (e.g., alveolar flap is acceptable in casual connected speech, such as "She's *cutting* [kʌɾɪŋ] the carrot").

Source: Adapted from Shriberg & Kwiatkowski (1982c).

[a] Exceptions to the rule: word-initial /h/ deletion (i.e., productions such as *"see him"* /si hɪm/ → [si əm]) is not considered incorrect if it occurs in an unstressed syllable in connected speech; word-final substitution of /n/ for /ŋ/ (i.e., *running* /ɹʌnɪŋ/ → [ɹʌnən]) is not considered incorrect in an unstressed syllable in connected speech.

COMMENT: *What are common and uncommon clinical distortions?*

It is possible for two children to have a similar PCC yet different types of SSD (e.g., phonological impairment characterized by substitutions, and articulation impairment characterized by distorted sibilants /s, z/). The PCC-A and PCC-R metrics (see Table 9-4) were developed to separate phonetic errors of distortion from other types of speech errors. Calculation of PCC-A and PCC-R requires an understanding of common and uncommon clinical distortions. Common clinical distortions include labialized, velarized, and derhotacized /ɹ/, /ɝ/, and /ɚ/, labialized and velarized /l/ in addition to dentalized and lateralized /s/, /z/, /ʃ/, /ʒ/, /tʃ/, and /dʒ/ (Shriberg, Austin, et al., 1997a). All other distortions are considered uncommon. The appendix of Shriberg (1993) provides a helpful, detailed description of common and uncommon clinical distortions.

TABLE 9-4 Measures of segmental accuracy

Measure of segment accuracy	What is counted?*	How it is calculated?
Percentage of consonants correct (PCC)	▪ Accurate consonants (= correct) ▪ All errors of substitution, omission, distortion, and addition (= incorrect)	$\dfrac{\text{correct consonants}}{\text{correct + incorrect consonants}} \times 100 = \%$
Percentage of consonants correct – adjusted (PCC-A)	▪ Accurate consonants, and consonants showing common clinical distortions (= correct) ▪ Errors of substitution, omission, addition, and uncommon clinical distortions (= incorrect)	$\dfrac{\text{correct consonants + common distortions}}{\text{correct + incorrect consonants}} \times 100 = \%$
Percentage of consonants correct – revised (PCC-R)	▪ Accurate consonants, and consonants showing common or uncommon clinical distortions (= correct) ▪ Errors of substitution, omission, and addition (= incorrect)	$\dfrac{\text{correct consonants + common + uncommon distortions}}{\text{correct + incorrect consonants}} \times 100 = \%$
Percentage of phonemes correct (PPC)	▪ Accurate phonemes (i.e., consonants and vowels) (= correct) ▪ All errors of substitution, omission, and distortion (= incorrect)	$\dfrac{\text{correct phonemes}}{\text{correct + incorrect phonemes}} \times 100 = \%$
Percentage of phonemes correct – revised (PPC-R)	▪ Accurate phonemes, and phonemes showing clinical distortions (= correct) ▪ Errors of substitution or omission (= incorrect)	$\dfrac{\text{correct phonemes + phonemes distortions}}{\text{correct + incorrect phonemes}} \times 100 = \%$
Percentage of vowels correct (PVC)	▪ Accurate vowels (= correct) ▪ All vowel errors of substitution, omission, and distortion (= incorrect)	$\dfrac{\text{correct vowels}}{\text{correct + incorrect vowels}} \times 100 = \%$
Percentage of vowels correct – revised (PVC-R)	▪ Accurate vowels, and vowels showing clinical distortions (= correct) ▪ Errors of substitution or omission (= incorrect)	$\dfrac{\text{correct vowels + vowel distortions}}{\text{correct + incorrect vowels}} \times 100 = \%$
Percentage of consonants in the inventory (PCI)	▪ Number of different types of consonants correct ▪ Number of different types of intended consonants	$\dfrac{\text{number of different types of consonants correct}}{\text{number of different types of intended consonants}} \times 100 = \%$
Relative distortion index (RDI)	All errors, divided into two groups: (i) distortions (common and uncommon) (ii) all other errors (e.g., substitutions, omissions)	$\dfrac{\text{number of common + uncommon distortion errors}}{\text{total number of consonant errors}} \times 100 = \%$
Articulation competence index (ACI)	PCC and RDI need to be calculated (see previous row)	$\dfrac{\text{PCC + RDI}}{2} \times 100 = \%$

Source: Adapted from Shriberg (1993); Shriberg & Kwiatkowski (1982c); Shriberg, Austin, Lewis, McSweeny, & Wilson (1997b).

*See Table 9-3 for further guidelines about how to calculate PCC, as these guidelines also apply to variants of the PCC metric.

TABLE 9-5 Measures of whole-word accuracy

Measure of whole-word accuracy	What is counted?	How it is calculated?
Proportion of whole-word correctness (PWC)	■ Correct words (= correct) ■ Words containing speech errors (= incorrect)	$$\frac{\text{number of correct words}}{\text{number of correct words} + \text{words containing speech errors}}$$
Phonological mean length of utterance (pMLU)	■ Phonological length of each word (based on rules in Table 9-6)	$$\frac{\text{sum of the phonological length of each word}}{\text{total number of words in the sample}}$$
Proportion of whole-word proximity (PWP)	■ pMLU of the child's sample ■ pMLU of the intended sample	$$\frac{\text{child pMLU}}{\text{adult (target) pMLU}}$$
Proportion of whole-word variability (PWV)	■ Number of different forms of a word. (If a word is consistently said the same way, the number of different forms = 0) ■ Number of instances of a word	$$\frac{\text{number of different forms of a word}}{\text{number of instances of a word}} \text{ then}$$ $$\frac{\text{sum of PWV ratios}}{\text{number of words in sample with PWV ratio}}$$

Source: Adapted from Ingram (2002); Ingram & Ingram (2001).

Proportion of Whole-Word Correctness (PWC) (Ingram, 2002)

PWC is a measure of whole-word correctness. PWC is a simple measure of the proportion of whole words produced correctly by a child relative to the total number of words said by a child in a given sample. For instance, if a child said 11 words correctly in a sample of 20, the PWC would be 0.55 (or 55%). The PWC was originally described by McCabe and Bradley (1973) as a measure of whole-word accuracy (WWA) and is calculated as part of the Bankson-Bernthal Test of Phonology (BBTOP, Bankson & Bernthal, 1990).

Phonological Mean Length of Utterance (pMLU) (Ingram & Ingram, 2001)

pMLU is a measure of whole-word complexity. pMLU was developed to examine the phonological complexity of children's words, with regards to length and number of consonants. Conceptually it is similar to the traditional mean length of utterance (MLU) calculation (Brown, 1973) and Shriberg and Kwiatkowski's (1982c) measure of the mean number of consonants per word. Unlike the relatively simple PWC measure, calculation of pMLU is more complicated. Specifically, a word is assigned a point for each segment (consonant or vowel) regardless of accuracy, and one point for each consonant correct. For example, the word *sun* /sʌn/ correctly produced as /sʌn/ is equivalent to 5 points (3 for each segment, and 2 for each consonant correct). *Sun* said as [dʌn] would be equivalent to 4 points (3 for each segment, and 1 for the correct consonant /n/). pMLU is based on the mean score in sample. Table 9-6 summarizes the rules for calculating pMLU (Ingram & Ingram, 2001; Ingram, 2002).

Proportion of Whole-Word Proximity (PWP) (Ingram, 2002; Ingram & Ingram, 2001)

Proportion of whole-word proximity (PWP) is a measure of the intelligibility of whole words. PWP captures the proximity of a child's production to the adult production. Presumably, the closer a child's production of a word is to the adult target, the more intelligible the child's speech. To calculate PWP, you divide the pMLU of the target words into the pMLU of the child's productions of those words (Ingram, 2002). For example, using three words from Luke's single-word sample in Chapter 16 (*sheep, elephant, present*), his average PWP for these three words would be 0.79 (see Table 9-7 for formula).

TABLE 9-6	Rules for calculating phonological Mean Length of Utterance (pMLU)
Rule type	**Rule**
Sample size	50 different words (recommended minimum of 25 words)
Lexical class rule	Count single words from common linguistic categories (e.g., nouns, verbs, adjectives, prepositions, and adverbs) present in everyday adult conversation. Ingram (2002) excludes children's reduplicated word forms (e.g., *mommy, daddy, baba*), because the inclusion of such forms can inflate a child's pMLU.
Compound rule	Count closed compound words only as single words (e.g., *rainbow, watermelon,* and *shoelace*). Open compound words (e.g., *post office, swimming pool, washing machine*) are not counted as a single word.
Variability rule	All words in a sample are to be different (i.e., no repetitions allowed). If you are creating a list of 50 words from a larger conversational speech sample, and the child produces variable productions of one word (e.g., *key* /ki/ → [ti, di, ki, di]), use the most frequent variable production (e.g., *key* /ki/ → [di]). If all the productions are different (e.g., *key* /ki/ → [ti, di, ki]), use the last production of the word in the sample (e.g., *key* /ki/ → [ki]).
Production rule	One point is assigned for each segment (consonant or vowel) in a word (e.g., *blue* /blu/ → [bwu] = 3 points), except for consonant additions. Consonant additions are not assigned a point (e.g., *blue* /blu/ → [bəlu] = 3 points) to avoid giving an incorrect production a high score. Syllables containing a syllabic consonant are counted as one consonant, rather than a vowel followed by a consonant (e.g., *button* /bʌtn̩/ = 4 segments, rather than /bʌtən/).
Consonants correct rule	Each correct consonant is assigned an additional point. According to Ingram and Ingram (2001, p. 273), "vowels correct are not scored because transcribers vary more greatly in their transcriptions of vowels."

Source: Adapted from Ingram & Ingram (2001); Ingram (2002).

TABLE 9-7	Example calculation of the Proportion of Whole-Word Proximity (PWP) for the words *sheep, elephant,* and *present*

Adult word	pMLU	Child's word	pMLU	Proportion of whole-word proximity (PWP) calculation
sheep /ʃip/	5	[dip]	4	$\frac{4}{5} = 0.80$
elephant /ɛləfənt/	11	[ɛləbənt]	10	$\frac{10}{11} = 0.91$
present /pɹɛzənt/	12	[bɛdənt]	8	$\frac{8}{12} = 0.67$
				Average = 0.79

> **COMMENT** *Capturing the effect of intervention using whole-word measures*
>
> Whole-word measures can be helpful for capturing positive changes in children's phonological abilities over the course of intervention. For example, Martikainen and Korpilahti (2011) calculated pMLU, PWP, and PWC to measure the effect of two different interventions (Melodic Intonation Therapy [MIT] and the Touch-Cue method) for a child who had CAS. Martikainen and Korpilahti (2011) commented that the whole-word measures complemented the segmental (PCC and PVC) measures, providing insight into the gradual improvement in speech intelligibility.

TABLE 9-8	Calculation of a child's proportion of Whole-Word Variability (PWV) for the words *spoon, snow, elephant,* and *sheep*		
Child's production	**Total number of different forms**	**Total number of productions**	**Proportion of whole-word variability (PWV)**
spoon /spun/ → [pun], [bun], [fun], [pun], [bun]	3	5	$\frac{3}{5} = 0.60$
snow /sno/ → [no], [no], [so], [θno], [θo]	4	5	$\frac{4}{5} = 0.80$
elephant /ɛləfənt/ → [ɛləbənt], [ɛbələnt], [ɛbələnt], [ɛləbənt], [ɛbənt]	3	5	$\frac{3}{5} = 0.60$
sheep /ʃip/ → [dip], [dip], [dip], [dip], [dip]	0	5	$\frac{0}{5} = 0.00$
		Average	0.5

Proportion of Whole-Word Variability (PWV) (Ingram, 2002; Ingram & Ingram, 2001)

PWV is a measure of the variability of a child's production of whole words. This measure provides additional insight into a child's speech intelligibility because it helps to differentiate children who produce words in consistently the same way from children who produce the same word differently. Presumably, you have a better chance of understanding children's speech if their errors are predictable and consistent rather than inconsistent and unpredictable. PWV is calculated on a speech sample containing multiple productions of the same words (e.g., four instances of the word *spoon*). To calculate PWV you divide the total number of different forms for a word into the total number of productions of that word, then calculate the average variability of all the words with multiple attempts (Ingram, 2002), as shown in Table 9-8.

INSTRUMENTAL ANALYSES OF CHILDREN'S SPEECH

So far in this chapter, your analyses have relied on impressionistic transcription based on your perception of children's speech. However, as indicated in Chapter 4, impressionistic transcription cannot capture all of the articulatory and acoustic details of speech. Ball, Manuel, and Müller (2004) suggest that instrumental images are helpful when there is uncertainty about the impressionistic transcription of an individual's speech. Instrumental analyses are useful for when you need to visualize speech, when children's speech difficulties are complex, when you need an objective and quantifiable measure of change, or when you need a biofeedback device during assessment and intervention to enable children (and yourself) to see what they are doing when they produce consonants and vowels. There is a range of instrumental analyses that have been developed for seeing speech to capture articulatory and acoustic information that can be used in real time or as delayed capture tools (see Table 9-9). For additional information, the book by Ball and Code (1997) contains a chapter on the application of each of these to the field of clinical phonetics, which is relevant to speech-language pathology.

Most clinical SLPs will not have ready access to many of the instruments outlined in Table 9-9 and, if considered to be necessary, will collaborate with specialists or researchers in universities to undertake instrumental analysis of children's speech. The remainder of this chapter will provide information about acoustic analyses that can be undertaken by all SLPs who have a computer and the ability to download free software. Additionally, a brief description of how to interpret acoustic images in addition to information provided by ultrasound and electropalatography (EPG) will be provided, since these are among the more common instrumental analyses used for children with SSD.

TABLE 9-9	Instrumental techniques for seeing speech, loosely arranged from the least to most invasive	
Instrument and area of focus	**Method**	**Example analyses**
Photography and video	The child is photographed or videoed with a standard camera.	Use a photo to study oral facial structures (e.g., dentition, lingual frenulum) and symmetry. Use video recordings to analyze child's lip movement during production of /ɹ/ and tongue protrusion during interdentalized /s, z/.
Acoustic analysis: spectrogram, waveform	The child speaks into a microphone and the acoustic signal is transferred (either immediately or later) to an acoustic analysis program to analyze aspects of the speech signal via a computer.	Visually inspect a spectrogram to determine whether a child's apparent dental lisp contains stridency or is indeed a true interdental /θ/ (Shine, 2007). Measure syllable duration, intensity, or fundamental frequency (F0) from a spectrogram to help determine whether a child's attempts at Sw and wS words exhibit stress equalization (Ballard et al., 2010).
Ultrasound	An ultrasound probe is held under the child's chin (or anchored under the chin via a helmet), and the child's tongue movement is observed on screen. Still and video images can be captured for later analysis.	Visually inspect coronal and sagittal ultrasound video/still images of a child's tongue shape, position, or movement during the articulation of lingual stops, vowels, sibilants, or liquids, to determine whether they are typical or atypical (Bernhardt et al., 2006).
Nasometry	The child wears a helmet that has a baffle plate that sits under the nose to measure nasal versus oral airflow.	Quantify nasalance (i.e., the acoustic correlate of the perceptual term *nasality*) to differentially diagnose hyper- from hyponasality (Brunnegård, Lohmander, & van Doorn, 2012).
Dynamic magnetic resonance imaging (MRI)	The child lies still within an MRI machine so that structure and movement of the articulators can be observed and recorded during speech. Still and video images can be captured for later analysis.	Examine pattern and degree of velopharyngeal closure during the production of oral consonants, using coronal and sagittal MRI images (Tian et al., 2010).
Electropalatography (EPG)	The child wears a custom-made dental plate that covers the hard palate and is fitted with electrodes. Multiple images (e.g., 1 per 10 ms) of tongue/palate contact are captured and displayed on screen.	Analyze articulatory timing and precision of tongue/palate contact for lingual consonants. Determine presence of undifferentiated gestures (Gibbon, 1999).
Speech video nasendoscopy	A flexible fiberoptic endoscope (long flexible tube) with special audio and video recording equipment is carefully inserted into the child's nose through to the pharynx, until the velopharyngeal port can be seen (Karnell, 2011).	Using video footage, analyze the size, shape, and possible cause of identified velopharyngeal insufficiency, and examine the movement of the velum and pharyngeal wall during attempts to close the velopharyngeal port (Karnell, 2011).
Electromagnetic articulography (EMA)	Sensor coils are attached to the lips and tongue and movement is recorded while wearing a purpose-built helmet. Data are recorded and displayed as graphs for later kinematic analysis.	Examine images of the motion path of the tongue or lips during speech production, considering patterns of movement, duration, distance travelled, velocity, and acceleration. EMA predominantly is used for research, although it has been used clinically with adults (e.g., Katz, McNeil, & Garst, 2010).

■ Acoustic analysis of children's speech

Most acoustic analyses use waveforms and spectrograms that are generated via an acoustic signal (often an audio recording). Acoustic analyses have been available for many years; however, it has only been in the last two decades that acoustic analysis no longer requires expensive equipment, but is available for free to download to your own computer (see "Acoustic Analysis Software"). Using acoustic analysis software you can create spectrograms, LPC (linear predictive coding) spectrums, and waveforms of speech from acoustic recordings to analyze aspects of speech such as pitch contour, vowel and syllable duration, voice onset time, vowel formants and formant patterns, fundamental frequency, vocal intensity, and the spectral mean and variance of fricatives (e.g., Ballard et al., 2010; Glaspey & MacLeod, 2010; McAllister Byun & Hitchcock, 2012). Spectrograms and LPC spectra both show formants. A spectrogram shows formants as horizontal bars, while LPC spectra show them as vertical peaks (McAllister Byun & Hitchcock, 2012).

Figure 9-20 was created using standard settings on the freely available program Praat (Boersma & Weenink, 2013) for the sentence "Say *buzzy* again" /seɪ bʌzi əgen/. The consonants and vowels are displayed from left to right. Each consonant and vowel has a

---

FIGURE 9-20   **Waveform and spectrogram of the sentence "Say *buzzy* again" created using Praat**

(a) The initial /s/ is segmented, highlighted, and labeled; (b) the display using the "show formants" feature; (c) using the "show pulses" feature (vertical lines); (d) using the "show pitch contour" feature (horizontal line).

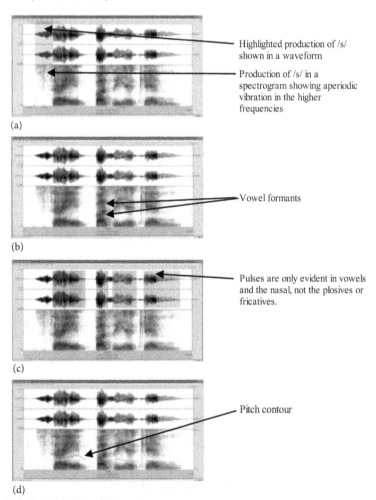

Source: Used by permission from Sharynne McLeod. Created using Praat (Boersma & Weenink, 2013).

COMMENT: *Acoustic analysis software*

There are many different programs that can be used to undertake acoustic analysis. Some are free and some are commercially available. The most commonly used programs include:

- Praat (Boersma & Weenink, 2013): Free software for recording and analysis on Windows and Macintosh computers.[1]

- WaveSurfer (X waves) (Sjölander & Beskow, 2006): Free software for acoustic analysis on Windows, Macintosh, and Linux computers.[2]

- EMU (Cassidy & Harrington, 2010): Free software for acoustic analysis on Windows, Macintosh, and Linux computers.[3]

- Speech Filing System (Huckvale, 2009): Free software for recording and analysis on Windows computers.[4]

- Computerized Speech Lab (CSL): Hardware and software purchased from PENTAX Medical typically used in research laboratories or specialist clinics for recording and analysis.[5]

- TF32 (Milenkovic, 2001): Commercially available software for acoustic analysis on Windows computers (an older version is free).[6]

- Articulate Assistant Advanced (AAA) (Wrench, 2013): Commercially available hardware and software for recording and analyzing acoustic data combined with data from other instruments including electropalatography, ultrasound, and MRI.[7]

[1] http://www.fon.hum.uva.nl/praat/
[2] http://www.speech.kth.se/wavesurfer/index2.html
[3] http://emu.sourceforge.net/
[4] http://www.phon.ucl.ac.uk/resource/sfs/
[5] http://pentaxmedical.com/pentax/en/99/1/ENT-Speech/
[6] http://userpages.chorus.net/cspeech/
[7] http://www.articulateinstruments.com/

different configuration on a spectrogram. The label on Figure 9-20 (a) shows /s/. You will notice by comparing the labeled section in (a) with the spectrogram in (b) that there are no formants during the production of /s/. This is because /s/ is a voiceless consonant. The spectrogram for /s/ shows the frication or noise from the sibilant air. The vowels are shown as the darkest sections of the spectrogram and are depicted by formants. In (a) formants look like darker horizontal bars and in (b) the formants are identified by the three layers of faint dots. Formants are important acoustic cues for the identification of consonants and vowels. For example, a hallmark of American English /ɹ/ is that formant 3 (F3) is often so low that it is merged with formant 2 (F2) (Boyce & Espy-Wilson, 1997). The formant transitions from consonant to vowel signify important perceptual cues; for example, formant 1 (F1) will always increase from a plosive to a vowel, but the transitions for formants 2 and 3 are less clear-cut (Kent & Read, 2002). Each vowel has a different formant pattern. The first vowel in Figure 9-20 is the diphthong /eɪ/, and you can see the transition of the formants from /e/ to /ɪ/. If you count the number of vowels in Figure 9-20, you will see that the formant for the unstressed vowel /ə/ is very short because schwa is an unstressed vowel. The section of white space followed by the straight line half of the way along the spectrogram shows the closure then release for /b/ that corresponds to the lip closure then plosive expulsion of air when producing /b/. There is a shorter closure phase later for /g/ with a clearly marked release (straight vertical line through the spectrogram). The /n/ at the end of the sentence is represented by the less intense section at the end of the waveform and the low horizontal bar at the end of the spectrogram.

From the pulses in Figure 9-20 (c), you can see that the consonants and vowels are differentiated. While the vowels are identified by the vertical lines, almost all of the

COMMENT: *Creating a high-quality sound recording for analysis*

Acoustic analyses cannot be performed unless the sound recording is of a high quality. You will recall from Chapter 7 that Vogel and Morgan (2009) indicated that high-quality recordings can be achieved in an anechoic chamber or soundproof room along with a good quality microphone, a hard disk recorder, and an independent mixer that can attenuate the incoming signal. Issues such as availability, portability, cost, and expertise mediate the actual recording equipment that can be and is used. Consequently, consider these factors, identified by Vogel and Morgan (2009), when making sound recordings:

■ **Hardware**: varies in quality (e.g., hard disk recorder, digital audio tape [DAT], MP3 recorder, computer)

■ **Software**: varies regarding sampling rate, mono or stereo input, and file format

■ **Microphone**: varies in quality and range (e.g., unidirectional, omnidirectional, bidirectional)

■ **Environmental noise**: signal-to-noise ratio can be reduced as a result of the environment (e.g., air conditioning), wiring, moving parts in recording devices, and the microphone

■ **Analogue-to-digital conversion**: "sampling rate (number of samples per second) and quantization level (the number of discrete levels of sound amplitude as defined by the number of binary bits in each number) of a recording determine how much of the signal is captured" (Vogel & Morgan, 2009, p. 435)

■ **File format**: .avi or .wav formats are recommended because they store uncompressed signals

Vogel and Morgan (2009) provide helpful tables for weighing up the options. However, it is important to know that if a recording is not of high enough quality, then many acoustic analyses cannot be undertaken. For example, if there is too much background noise (including the almost inaudible hum of the fan on a laptop computer), then an audio sample may not be able to undergo acoustic analysis. In fact, it is good practice to use high-quality recording equipment for checking the accuracy of your impressionistic transcriptions, and for having a historical record of progress, even if you do not intend to use the sample for acoustic analysis.

---

consonants—/s/, /b/, /z/, /g/—are not. The exception is /n/. Although /n/ is not a vowel, pulses are shown for the production of /n/ in (c) because it is a sonorant consonant (see Chapter 5). Finally, by using the "show pitch contour" feature, as shown in Figure 9-20 (d), you can see the contour of the utterance. Notice how the pitch decreases or falls towards the end of the utterance.

When undertaking acoustic analyses, there are standard protocols for segmenting and measuring each consonant and vowel. The classic study by Peterson and Lehiste (1960) suggests that to identify the beginning and end of the vowel and syllable, use pitch and intensity contours and formant trajectories. Syllable and vowel duration is measured in milliseconds. Vowel duration can be measured by identifying the onset and offset of each vowel. Syllable duration is easier to measure if plosive consonants are produced either side of the vowel. For example, Ballard et al. (2010) measured syllable duration from the onset of the burst for the first plosive to the onset of the burst for the next plosive.

Acoustic analyses have been used to supplement impressionistic transcription in clinical and research settings. For example, acoustic analyses have been used to:

■ Differentiate between 9- to 17-year-old speakers who had histories of phonological impairment versus histories of articulation impairment on rhotics /ɹ/, /ɝ/, and /ɚ/. An acoustic analysis of **formants** 2 and 3 in the words *bird, burg,* and *burr* showed differences of greater than 6.0 between groups for a *z* score calculated by subtracting formant 2 from formant 3 (Shriberg, Flipsen, Karlsson, & McSweeny, 2001).

■ Differentiate between 9- to 17-year-old speakers who had histories of phonological impairment versus histories of articulation impairment on sibilants including /s/. A **spectral moment analysis** of perceptually correct productions of /s/ in the words *skin*, *spin*, and *spoon* showed differences between mean spectral frequency (moment 1) and spectral variance (moment 2) (Karlsson, Shriberg, Flipsen, & McSweeny, 2002).

■ Identify covert contrasts in children's productions of words that sounded like homonyms. For example, McGregor and Schwartz (1992) described a child aged 4;6 who had difficulty producing liquids, fricatives, and affricates. When this child produced words such as *wish* /wɪʃ/ and *witch* /wɪtʃ/, they both were perceived as homonyms [wɪθ]; however, acoustic analyses demonstrated a significant difference between fricative versus affricate productions, with vowel-to-affricate latencies being approximately 190 ms longer than for vowel-to fricative latencies. In another example, a 5-year-old child with a phonological impairment was perceived to produce homonyms for *yes/less* [jes], *yuck/luck* [jʌk], *yacht/lot* [jot]; however, using acoustic analysis it was evident that he consistently produced a sound of greater **intensity** and longer **duration** for /j/ than /l/ (McLeod & Isaac, 1995). Additionally, covert contrasts have been identified via acoustic differences in **voice onset time** (VOT) in children's homonyms. For example, typically developing 2-year-old children produced the VOT for the stop (e.g., /p, t, k/) in the homonym containing a consonant cluster (e.g., *ski* /ski/ → [ki]) as significantly shorter than the VOT for the stop in the target word containing a singleton (e.g., *key* /ki/ → [ki]) (McLeod, Van Doorn, & Reed, 1996).

■ Document increased skill of children with CAS in the production of strong-weak (Sw) and weak-strong (wS) stress patterns in three-syllable nonwords (Ballard et al., 2010). The following acoustic measures were made by Ballard et al. on the test words: syllable and vowel duration (ms), peak vocal intensity (dB), and peak fundamental frequency (F0 in Hz). A pairwise variability index (PVI) (Low, Grabe, & Nolan, 2000):

> was calculated to determine the degree of asymmetry across the first two syllables of a string ... A positive PVI is consistent with an SW pattern (i.e., greater duration, intensity, or F0 on the first syllable), and a negative PVI is consistent with a WS pattern (i.e., greater duration, intensity, or F0 on the second syllable), with increasing values indicating more pronounced contrast. A zero PVI value indicates equal stress over both syllables". (Ballard et al., 2010, p. 1233)

The formula for calculating the PVI is as follows:

$$PVI\,(dur) = 100 \times (d_k - d_{k+1})/[(d_k - d_{k+1})/2]\}$$

where *d* is the duration of the *k*th syllable.

Acoustic analyses have many different uses for analyzing the speech of children with articulation impairment, phonological impairment, inconsistent speech disorder, CAS, dysarthria, or SSD due to variation in craniofacial structure or hearing loss. Shriberg and Kent (2013) provide additional information regarding acoustic analysis of English consonants and vowels. As you will learn in Chapter 14, instrumental images of speech can also be used in intervention as a form of biofeedback.

■ Electropalatography (EPG)

An early technique for seeing speech was to paint black chalk on the palate, then look at the shape of the tongue contact after the production of a consonant (e.g., Moses, 1939; Shohara & Hanson, 1941). Over time, use of this technique has become much more sophisticated, but the same principle applies in electropalatography (EPG). Currently there are two main companies that make electropalatography equipment: Articulate Instruments[3] and CompleteSpeech.[4] The Reading EPG palate (available from Articulate Instruments) is the most commonly used electropalatograph instrument in research for

---

[3]http://www.articulateinstruments.com/
[4]http://www.completespeech.com/

children with SSD to date. The Reading EPG palate is shown in Chapter 4, and you will see that that palate contains 68 electrodes spread across the hard palate with wires extending out of the mouth that are linked to a multiplexer (white box) and computer. The margins of the EPG palate extend around the teeth, then across the juncture between the hard and soft palate. In Chapter 4, images created using the Reading EPG palate were provided to demonstrate typical tongue/palate contact for the production of English consonants. The figures in Chapter 4 are taken from a printout that has multiple frames of tongue/palate (1 frame per 10 ms). Figure 9-21 shows a printout of all of the EPG frames during the production of the word *cat* /kæt/. You will notice that from frames 471 to 487 there is complete closure across the back of the hard palate during the /k/; this complete closure lasts for 170 ms. The transition from the /k/ through the vowel /æ/ to the /t/ occurs from frames 488 through 531. This transition involves increasing contact along the margins of the palate, the back of the tongue no longer contacting the midline at the back of the palate, and increasing tongue tip contact on the alveolar ridge. Frames 531 to 548 show the classic horseshoe production of /t/, followed by frames 549 to 562, where the tongue transitions to a resting position.

Each consonant in Chapter 4 is accompanied by a description of errors made by children with SSD that can be identified using EPG. For example, when a child produces /k/ → [t], the [t] typically looks like a production of /t/ as shown in frames 531 to 548 above. Different productions of /s/ are markedly different from one another, as demonstrated in Chapter 4. Figure 4-24 in Chapter 4 provides a comparison between stylized transverse images of four productions of /s/: typical, interdental, lateral, and stopped. The usefulness of EPG to identify and provide biofeedback on these different productions of /s/ is clear.

FIGURE 9-21 **Electropalatographic (EPG) printout of tongue/palate contact during the first author's production of the word *cat***

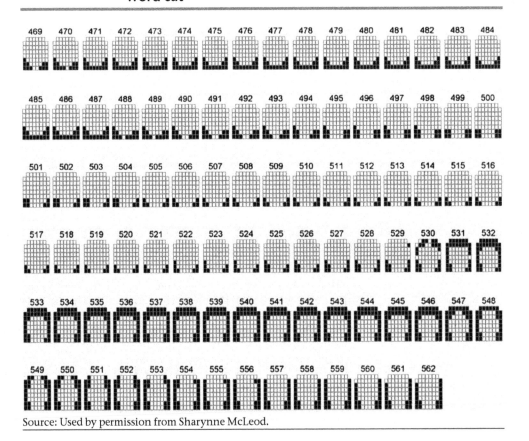

Source: Used by permission from Sharynne McLeod.

■ ■

 APPLICATION: *Spot the difference between the EPG images*

In Chapter 4, there is an EPG image of a child producing an undifferentiated gesture during the production of [d] (Figure 4-18). There is also an EPG image of [d] produced by an adult with typical speech (Figure 4-17). Compare the child's image with the typical speaker's image.

Question: What is the main difference between the child's image and the adult's image? How could the two EPG images be used in intervention with the child?

Answer: The child covered the entire palate with the tongue, while the typical speaker's production shows a horseshoe shape. The EPG could be used as biofeedback to show the child that the tongue's contact with the palate needed to be in a horseshoe shape for the production of /d/.

■ Ultrasound

Many of you will have seen images that are created by ultrasound (e.g., of unborn babies during pregnancy). Ultrasound technology is available in most hospitals. You could collaborate with your local sonographers to view tongue position and movement, especially if they have ultrasound probes that are suited to viewing tongue movement (these are typically smaller than the ones used for other parts of the body). Alternatively, as we describe further in Chapter 14, you could turn your computer into an ultrasound machine using a special probe and accompanying software. The probe is placed in the middle of the curve of the mandible on the tissue under the chin (in Figure 4-14 the ultrasound probe is attached to the base of the helmet in order to keep the probe in the same place to create comparative images for research). In Chapter 4, the sagittal (midline) diagrams of placement of the articulators were generated by tracing over ultrasound images. Examples of an ultrasound image used for creating the sagittal diagrams in Chapter 4 are shown in Figure 9-22. You will notice that there is a white curve in the middle of the image. This represents the air immediately above the tongue surface. The sharp white diagonal lines towards the base of the image depict the hyoid bone. You can see that in the ultrasound image of /p/ the tongue is at rest, with the front of the tongue slightly lowered compared with the ultrasound image of /t/. The tongue tip for /t/ is obscured by the jaw shadow. Unfortunately, this is a limitation of using ultrasound to view the tongue; the tongue tip for alveolar sounds cannot be seen. The ultrasound image of /k/ in Figure 9-22 is quite different from /p/ and /t/. The tongue tip is down, and the back of the tongue is rounded. For additional information, Stone (2005) provides greater detail about how to interpret ultrasound images. In Chapter 14 we describe how ultrasound technology has been used in the remediation of lingual stops, vowels, sibilants, and liquids, particularly /ɹ/, for children and adolescents who benefit from visual cues (e.g., those with hearing loss) (Bernhardt, Gick, Bacsfalvi, & Adler-Bock, 2005).

FIGURE 9-22 **Ultrasound images of /p/, /t/, /k/**

The white curve in the middle of each screen is the air above the tongue surface. The tongue tip is on the right.

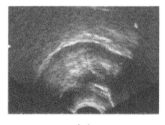 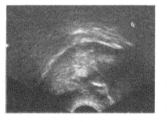 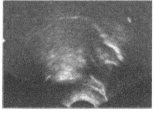

/p/ /t/ /k/

Source: Used by permission from Sharynne McLeod.

> **COMMENT:** *Different approaches to analysis can yield different insights into SSD in children*
>
> In this chapter we have described common methods for analyzing children's speech. Other approaches exist in the literature. You are encouraged to learn more about these methods in the years to come, as a broad theoretical knowledge base will help you problem-solve more cases. Other analysis frameworks to investigate include:
>
> ■ **Nonlinear phonology**: Bernhardt and Stemberger (2000) offer a series of helpful templates and case-based examples in their *Workbook in Nonlinear Phonology for Clinical Application*. Online tutorials exist by Barbara May Bernhardt and Joseph Stemberger on nonlinear phonological analysis.[1] Additionally, the Computerized Articulation and Phonology Evaluation System (CAPES) (Masterson & Bernhardt, 2001) is analysis software designed to help clinicians complete segmental and prosodic (syllable, stress) constraint-based nonlinear analyses.
>
> ■ **Psycholinguistics**: Stackhouse and Wells (1997) offer a broad-based approach for profiling (rather than explicitly analyzing) children's speech and literacy difficulties. Assessment from a psycholinguistic perspective creates a profile of a child's areas of strength and difficulty with respect to input processing, representation, and output processing. Analysis methods discussed in this chapter (e.g., independent and relational analysis) can be used to build one aspect of a child's overall profile. We recommend that you consult Stackhouse and Wells (1997) for further information about profiling children's speech and literacy abilities from a psycholinguistic perspective.
>
> [1]http://phonodevelopment.sites.olt.ubc.ca/

Chapter summary

In this chapter you learned about two common approaches for analyzing phonetically transcribed speech samples: SODA analysis, and independent and relational phonological analysis. Methods for quantifying speech accuracy were also described. You also learned about acoustic analysis of a spectrogram and waveform, EPG recordings, and ultrasound images. Having reaching the end of this chapter, you have the knowledge (but not necessarily the many hours of experience) to carefully study a speech sample, analyze it, and list the skills requiring intervention.

Suggested reading

■ Bernhardt, B. H., & Stemberger, J. P. (2000). *Workbook in nonlinear phonology for clinical application.* Austin, TX: Pro-Ed.

■ Shriberg, L. D., & Kent, R. D. (2013). *Clinical phonetics* (4th ed.). Boston, MA: Pearson.

■ Stackhouse, J., & Wells, B. (1997). *Children's speech and literacy difficulties: A psycholinguistic framework.* London, UK: Whurr.

■ Velleman, S. L. (1998). *Making phonology functional: What do I do first?* Boston, MA: Butterworth-Heinemann.

Application of knowledge from Chapter 9

If you have worked through the application questions in this chapter, you will have developed a range of skills to analyze children's speech. To further develop your skills, complete the following tasks.

1. Using the speech samples for Michael (4;2 years) in Chapter 16, complete an independent and relational analysis of Michael's speech. (In reality, your speech sample would be considerably larger than the sample offered in Chapter 16.) Summarize Michael's strengths and areas of difficulty.

2. Select a standardized assessment of articulation and/or phonology suitable for children. (Refer to Chapter 8 for further information and examples.) What types of analyses are needed to calculate a child's standard score or percentile rank? Do you think this type of analysis would be adequate for a child like Luke (4;3 years), who has a severe phonological impairment (Case 1 in Chapter 16)? Why or why not?

3. In a small group, discuss the advantages and disadvantages of analyzing children's speech samples. As part of your discussion, consider the consequences of inadequate analysis.

Appendix 9-1 Children's Independent and Relational Phonological Analysis (CHIRPA) Template

Children's Independent and Relational Phonological Analysis: General American English (CHIRPA: GAE)[1]

CLIENT NAME _____ DATE OF BIRTH_____ AGE_____

SPEECH SAMPLE ☐ single words ☐ connected speech   DESCRIPTION OF SAMPLE: _____

INDEPENDENT ANALYSIS

(1) Phonetic inventory: singleton consonants
- Highlight consonants produced more than once
- Parentheses ( ) around consonants produced once
- Circle if most consonants in a sound class are present and use ( ) if only one or few sounds in a sound class are present

[p b t d k g m n ŋ f v θ ð s z ʃ ʒ h tʃ dʒ ɹ j l w]

Sound classes present
nasals plosives glides liquids fricatives affricates
Positional constraints ☐ yes ☐ no
Comments

Problem area ☐ yes ☐ no

(2) Phonetic inventory: consonant clusters
- Highlight consonant clusters produced more than once
- Parentheses ( ) around consonant clusters produced once

Initial	Final
[tw kw sw]	[s] + consonant
	e.g.,
[pj bj kj mj fj vj]	consonant + [s] or [z]
	e.g.,
[pl bl kl gl fl sl]	[l] + consonant
	e.g.,
[pɹ bɹ tɹ dɹ kɹ gɹ fɹ θɹ ʃɹ]	[ɹ] + consonant
	e.g.,
[sp st sk sm sn sl sw sf]	nasal + consonant
	e.g.,
[spɹ stɹ skɹ spl skw]	

Additional consonant clusters
Sequence constraints ☐ yes ☐ no
Comments

Problem area ☐ yes ☐ no

(3) Phonetic inventory: vowels
- Highlight vowels produced more than once
- Parentheses ( ) around vowels produced once

Monophthongs [i ɪ e ɛ æ u ʊ o ɔ ɑ ə ʌ ɜ ɝ]

Diphthongs [ɪɹ ʊə ɪə eɹ ʊɹ ɔɹ ɑɹ aɪ aʊ ɔɪ]
Comments

Problem area ☐ yes ☐ no

(4) Syllable shape inventory
- Highlight syllable shapes produced more than once
- Parentheses ( ) around syllable shapes produced once
- [C+] = 0 or more consonants

V   CV   VC   CVC   CCV[C+]   [C+]VCC
CCCV[C+]   [C+]VCCC
Others
Comments

Problem area ☐ yes ☐ no

(5) Word length inventory
- Highlight word lengths produced more than once
- Parentheses ( ) around word lengths produced once
- List common and most complex syllable shape for each word length such as monosyllables CV and CVCC; disyllables CVCV and CVC,CV; 3-syllables CVCVCV and CVCVCVC

Monosyllables e.g.,

Disyllables e.g.,

3-syllables e.g.,

4-syllables e.g.,

5+ syllables e.g.,

Sequence constraints ☐ yes ☐ no
Comments

Problem area ☐ yes ☐ no

(6) Syllable stress inventory
- Highlight syllable stress patterns produced more than once
- Parentheses ( ) around stress patterns produced once

SS e.g., *rainbow*   **Swsw** e.g., *watermelon*
Sw e.g., *carrot*   **Other polysyllabic words**
wS e.g., *giraffe*   e.g., *hippopotamus*
Sww e.g., *elephant*
Sws e.g., *dinosaur*
wSw / wSs e.g., *potato*
Comments

Problem area ☐ yes ☐ no

[1]Baker, E. (2016). *Children's Independent and Relational Phonological Analysis: General American English*. Sydney, Australia: Author. Copyright ©2016 Elise Baker

Appendix 9-1 (*Continued*)

RELATIONAL ANALYSIS

(7) Consonants correct
- Calculate + report percentage of consonants correct
- Highlight consonants that are frequently or always accurate
- Parentheses ( ) around consonants sometimes accurate

Percentage of consonants correct

^Early-8   [m b j n w d p h]

^Middle-8 [t ŋ k g f v tʃ dʒ]

^Late-8   [ʃ θ s z ð l ɹ ʒ]

^Based on Shriberg (1993)

Comments

Problem area ☐ yes ☐ no

(8) Vowels correct
- Calculate + report percentage of vowels correct
- Highlight vowels that are frequently or always accurate
- Parentheses ( ) around vowels sometimes accurate

Percentage of vowels correct

Monophthongs [i ɪ e ɛ æ ʊ u o ɔ ɑ ə ʌ ɜ˞ ɚ]

Diphthongs [ɔɪ oʊ aɪ aɪ ɔɪ ɪɔ eɪ aɪ aʊ ɔɪ]

Comments

Problem area ☐ yes ☐ no

(9) Syllable shapes correct
- Highlight syllable shapes frequently or always accurate
- Parentheses ( ) around syllable shapes sometimes accurate

V   CV   VC   CVC   CCV[C+]   [C+]VCC

CCCV[C+]   [C+]VCCC

Others

Comments

Problem area ☐ yes ☐ no

(10) Word lengths correct
- Highlight word lengths frequently or always accurate
- Parentheses ( ) around word lengths sometimes accurate

Monosyllables   4-syllables

Disyllables   5+ syllables

3-syllables   Evidence of syllable and/or consonant addition? ☐ yes ☐ no

Comments

Problem area ☐ yes ☐ no

(11) Syllable stress patterns correct
- Highlight stress patterns frequently or always accurate
- Parentheses ( ) around stress patterns sometimes accurate

SS   Sw   wS   Sww   Sws   wSw / wSs   Swsw

Other(s):

Is stress unusually equal across syllables? ☐ yes ☐ no

Comments

Problem area ☐ yes ☐ no

(12) Singleton consonant error analysis
- Highlight consonants that are frequently or always correct
- Parentheses ( ) around consonants sometimes accurate
- If incorrect, note substituted phone(s) in cell or ⊘ if omitted

WORD-INITIAL POSITION   Problem area ☐ yes ☐ no

Plosives	p	b			t	d			k	g	
Nasals		m				n					
Fricatives	f	v	θ	ð	s	z	ʃ				h
Approximants		w				ɹ		j			
Lat. Approx.						l					
Affricates							tʃ	dʒ			

WITHIN-WORD POSITION   Problem area ☐ yes ☐ no

Plosives	p	b			t	d			k	g	
Nasals		m				n				ŋ	
Fricatives	f	v	θ	ð	s	z	ʃ	ʒ			h
Approximants		w				ɹ		j			
Lat. Approx.						l					
Affricates							tʃ	dʒ			

WORD-FINAL POSITION   Problem area ☐ yes ☐ no

Plosives	p	b			t	d			k	g	
Nasals		m				n				ŋ	
Fricatives	f	v	θ	ð	s	z	ʃ	ʒ			
Approximants						ɹ					
Lat. Approx.						l					
Affricates							tʃ	dʒ			

Observations:

(13) Consonant cluster error analysis
- Highlight consonant clusters frequently or always correct
- Parentheses ( ) around clusters sometimes accurate
- If incorrect, note reduced or substituted phone, simplified cluster or ⊘ if omitted

WORD-INITIAL POSITION

tw	kw	sw						
pj	bj	kj	mj	fj	vj			
pl	bl	kl	gl	fl	sl			
pɹ	bɹ	tɹ	dɹ	kɹ	gɹ	fɹ	θɹ	ʃɹ
sp	st	sk	sm	sn	sf			
spɹ	stɹ	skɹ	spl	skw				

WORD-FINAL POSITION

Nasal clusters: Fricative clusters:

Liquid clusters: Errors:

Observations:

Problem area ☐ yes ☐ no

Appendix 9-1 (*Continued*)

RELATIONAL ANALYSIS continued

(14) Phonological processes
- Shade box ■ for processes evident in the child's speech
- Comment on specific application of a process such as velar fronting word-initial only, and gliding only on /ɹ/
- Describe atypical, idiosyncratic processes
- Calculate percent occurrence as necessary

Syllable structure processes
- ☐ Weak syllable deletion
- ☐ Reduplication
- ☐ Final consonant deletion
- ☐ Initial consonant deletion
- ☐ Cluster reduction

Substitution processes
- ☐ Velar fronting
- ☐ Palatal fronting
- ☐ Stopping of fricatives
- ☐ Stopping of affricates
- ☐ Deaffrication
- ☐ Gliding of liquids
- ☐ Context sensitive voicing
- ☐ Consonant cluster simplification
- ☐ Fricative simplification
- ☐ Glottal insertion
- ☐ Backing

Assimilation processes
- ☐ Velar
- ☐ Labial
- ☐ Alveolar

Other processes

Problem area ☐ yes ☐ no

(15) Loss of phonemic contrast
- Using error analysis (box #12 and #13), list singleton consonants and consonant clusters with the same substitute (consonant or ∅) in the same word position.
- Describe loss of phonemic contrast according to major class features (obstruents/sonorants), natural classes (plosives, nasals, glides, liquids, fricatives and affricates) and consonant clusters (Williams, 2003). For example, non-labial singleton obstruents (including plosives, fricatives and affricates) and clusters /t, k, g, s, z, ʃ, θ, ð, tʃ, dʒ, tɹ, st, stɹ, sk, skɹ, skl, skw, kɹ, dɹ, gɹ, kl, gl/ are all substituted with [d] word-initially.

Word initial	Word final

Problem area ☐ yes ☐ no

(16) Additional observations: prosody/phonation/resonance/respiration
☑ natural or ☒ unnatural/problematic
- ☐ **Stress**
  - Lexical stress ☐ Sw ☐ wS
  - Sentence stress ☐
  - Emphatic stress ☐
- ☐ **Words of increasing length** (e.g., *hip, hippo, hippopotamus*)
- **Is syllable segregation evident?** ☐ yes ☐ no
- ☐ **Speech rate** ☐ Too slow ☐ Too fast ☐ Poorly regulated
- ☐ **Intonation**
- ☐ **Phonation**
- ☐ **Resonance**
- ☐ **Respiration / speech breathing**
- **Problem area** ☐ yes ☐ no

(17) Speech ratings
Consistency rating
- ☐ Consistent
- ☐ Inconsistent – further assessment and analysis needed

Severity rating
- ☐ Mild
- ☐ Mild-moderate
- ☐ Moderate-severe
- ☐ Severe

Intelligibility rating
- ☐ Intelligible
- ☐ Mainly intelligible
- ☐ Partially intelligible
- ☐ Mainly unintelligible
- ☐ Unintelligible

(18) Sampling constraints? ☐ More sampling required
- ☐ Polysyllables
- ☐ Consonant clusters
- ☐ Words with weak-onset stress
- ☐ Other

Appendix 9-2 Children's Independent and Relational Phonological Analysis (CHIRPA) Template: Worked example for Luke (4;3 years)

Children's Independent and Relational Phonological Analysis: General American English (CHIRPA: GAE)[1]

CLIENT NAME: *Luke*   **DATE OF BIRTH**: *10th November 2011*   **AGE:** *4;3 years*

SPEECH SAMPLE ■ single words ■ connected speech   **DESCRIPTION OF SAMPLE:** *Words from standardized phonology assessment*
(Dodd, Hua, Crosbie, Holm, & Ozanne, 2006), single-word samples (clusters, polysyllables), and two x 10-minute conversational speech samples.

INDEPENDENT ANALYSIS

(1) Phonetic inventory: singleton consonants
- Highlight consonants produced more than once
- Parentheses ( ) around consonants produced once
- Circle if most consonants in a sound class are present and use ( ) if only one or few sounds in a sound class are present

[p b t d k g m n ŋ f v θ ð s z ʃ ʒ h tʃ dʒ ɹ j l w]

Sound classes present
(nasals) (plosives) (glides) (liquids) fricatives affricates
Positional constraints ■ yes ☐ no
Comments
- *Velar [k, g] limited to medial and final position*
- *[j] limited to word-initial position*
- *[p] limited to word-final position*
- *Tendency for [+ voice] in word-initial position only*

Problem area ■ yes ☐ no

(2) Phonetic inventory: consonant clusters
- Highlight consonant clusters produced more than once
- Parentheses ( ) around consonant clusters produced once

Initial	Final
[tw kw sw]	[s] + consonant e.g.,
[pj bj kj mj fj* vj*]	consonant + [s] or [z] e.g.,
[pl bl kl gl fl sl]	[l] + consonant e.g., ([lt])
[pɹ bɹ tɹ dɹ kɹ gɹ fɹ θɹ ʃɹ]	[ɹ] + consonant e.g.,
[sp st sk sm sn sl sw sf*]	nasal + consonant e.g., [nt, ŋk, mp]
[spɹ stɹ skɹ spl skw]	

Additional consonant clusters
Sequence constraints ■ yes ☐ no
Comments
- *Limited to nasal + plosive and lateral+ plosive word-final clusters*
- *No word-initial consonant clusters*
- ** = not sampled during assessment*

Problem area ■ yes ☐ no

(3) Phonetic inventory: vowels
- Highlight vowels produced more than once
- Parentheses ( ) around vowels produced once

Monophthongs [i ɪ e ɛ æ u ʊ o ɔ ɑ ə ʌ ɜ˞ ɚ]

Diphthongs [ɪɹ ɛɹ ʊɹ ɔɹ ɑɹ aɪ aʊ ɔɪ] Also [ɛə]
Comments
- *No rhotic vowels*

Problem area ■ yes ☐ no

(4) Syllable shape inventory
- Highlight syllable shapes produced more than once
- Parentheses ( ) around syllable shapes produced once
- [C+] = 0 or more consonants

V   CV   VC   CVC   CCV[C+]   [C+]VCC
CCCV[C+]   [C+]VCCC
Others
Comments
- *Mostly CV and CVC syllables*
- *[C+]VCC included CVCC and VCC syllable shapes*
- *No evidence of CCV[C+], CCCV[C+], or [C+]VCCC*

Problem area ■ yes ☐ no

(5) Word length inventory
- Highlight word lengths produced more than once
- Parentheses ( ) around word lengths produced once
- List common and most complex syllable shape for each word length such as monosyllables CV and CVCC; disyllables CVCV and CVC,CV; 3-syllables CVCVCV and CVCVCVC

Monosyllables e.g., v; cv; vc; cvc; cvcc

Disyllables e.g., cvcv; cvcvc; cvcvcc; cvc,cv; cvc,cvc ; vcvcc

3-syllables e.g., cvcvcv; cvcvcvc ; cvc,cvcv ; vcvcvcc; cvvcvc

4-syllables e.g., vcvcvcv; cvcvcvcv

(5+ syllables) e.g., vcvcvcvcvc

Sequence constraints ■ yes ☐ no
Comments
- *Sequence constraint due to small phonetic inventory as no sequences involving postalveolar place of articulation*
- *Overall, word length does not appear to be a problem*

Problem area ☐ yes ■ no

(6) Syllable stress inventory
- Highlight syllable stress patterns produced more than once
- Parentheses ( ) around stress patterns produced once

SS e.g., *rainbow*   **Swsw** e.g., *watermelon*
Sw e.g., *carrot*   **Other polysyllabic words**
wS e.g., *giraffe*   e.g., (Swsww) *hippopotamus*
Sww e.g., *elephant*
Sws e.g., *dinosaur*
wSw / wSs e.g., *potato*
Comments
- *No obvious difficulties with stress*

Problem area ☐ yes ■ no

[1]Baker, E. (2016). *Children's Independent and Relational Phonological Analysis: General American English.* Sydney, Australia: Author. Copyright ©2016 Elise Baker

Appendix 9-2 (*Continued*)

RELATIONAL ANALYSIS

(7) Consonants correct
- Calculate + report percentage of consonants correct
- Highlight consonants that are frequently or always accurate
- Parentheses ( ) around consonants sometimes accurate

Percentage of consonants correct
48.4% conversational speech; 38.6% single words

^Early-8 [m b (j) n w d (p) h]

^Middle-8 [(t)(ŋ)(k)(g) f v tʃ dʒ]

^Late-8 [ʃ θ s z ð (l) ɹ ʒ]

^Based on Shriberg (1993)

Comments
- Early-8 better than the middle-8 better than the late-8
- Luke's percentage of consonants correct better in conversational speech than single words

Problem area ■ yes □ no

(8) Vowels correct
- Calculate + report percentage of vowels correct
- Highlight vowels that are frequently or always accurate
- Parentheses ( ) around vowels sometimes accurate

Percentage of vowels correct *85.5% conversational speech*

Monophthongs [i ɪ e ɛ æ ʊ u o ɔ ɑ ə ʌ ɜ˞ (ɚ)]

Diphthongs [ɔɪ oʊ aɪ ɪɚ ɛɹ ɔɹ ɑɹ]

Comments *Vowels adequate apart from rhotic vowels and diphthongs such as [ɛɹ]→[ɛə], [aɪ]→[a] and [ɔɹ]→[ɔ]*

Problem area ■ yes □ no

(9) Syllable shapes correct
- Highlight syllable shapes frequently or always accurate
- Parentheses ( ) around syllable shapes sometimes accurate

V CV VC CVC CCV[C+] ([C+]VCC)

CCCV[C+] [C+]VCCC

Others

Comments *Difficulty with consonant clusters*

Problem area ■ yes □ no

(10) Word lengths correct
- Highlight word lengths frequently or always accurate
- Parentheses ( ) around word lengths sometimes accurate

Monosyllables	4-syllables
Disyllables	5+ syllables
3-syllables	Evidence of syllable and/or consonant addition? □ yes ■ no

Comments *No obvious difficulty matching word length*

Problem area □ yes ■ no

(11) Syllable stress patterns correct
- Highlight stress patterns frequently or always accurate
- Parentheses ( ) around stress patterns sometimes accurate

SS Sw wS Sww Sws wSw/wSs Swsw

Other(s): *Swsww (sampled once in hippopotamus)*

Is stress unusually equal across syllables? □ yes ■ no

Comments *No obvious difficulty matching word stress*

Problem area □ yes ■ no

(12) Singleton consonant error analysis
- Highlight consonants that are frequently or always correct
- Parentheses ( ) around consonants sometimes accurate
- If incorrect, note substituted phone(s) in cell or ∅ if omitted

WORD-INITIAL POSITION Problem area ■ yes □ no

Manner	Bilabial	Labiodental	Dental	Alveolar	Post-alv	Palatal	Velar	Glottal
Plosives	p^b b			(t)^d d			k^d g^d	
Nasals	m			n				
Fricatives		f^b v^b	θ^d ð^d	s^d z^d	ʃ^d			h^∅
Approximants	w			ɹ^w		(j)^∅		
Lat. Approx.				l				
Affricates					tʃ^d dʒ^d			

WITHIN-WORD POSITION Problem area ■ yes □ no

Manner	Bilabial	Labiodental	Dental	Alveolar	Post-alv	Palatal	Velar	Glottal
Plosives	(p)^b b			(t)^d d			(k)^d (g)^d	
Nasals	m			n			ŋ	
Fricatives		f^b v^b	θ^∅ ð^b	s^d z	ʃ^d ʒ^*			h^∅
Approximants	w			ɹ^w		j^∅		
Lat. Approx.				l				
Affricates					tʃ^t dʒ^d			

WORD-FINAL POSITION Problem area ■ yes □ no

Manner	Bilabial	Labiodental	Dental	Alveolar	Post-alv	Palatal	Velar	Glottal
Plosives	p b			t d			k g^k	
Nasals	m			n			ŋ	
Fricatives		f^p v^p	θ^p ð^*	s^t z^t	ʃ^t ʒ^*			
Approximants				ɹ^ə				
Lat. Approx.				l				
Affricates					tʃ^t dʒ^*			

Observations: *voiceless → voiced word-initial position; word-initial velars → alveolars; fricatives and affricates→ homorganic (or near) plosive; alveolar approximant →labiovelar approximant; derhoticization of /ɹ/ in word-final; palatal approximant → ∅*
*= not sampled during assessment

(13) Consonant cluster error analysis
- Highlight consonant clusters frequently or always correct
- Parentheses ( ) around clusters sometimes accurate
- If incorrect, note reduced or substituted phone, simplified cluster or ∅ if omitted

WORD-INITIAL POSITION

tw^d	kw^d	sw^d			
pj^b	bj^b	kj^d	mj^m	fj^*	vj^*
pl^b	bl^b	kl^d	gl^d	fl^b	sl^d,l
pɹ^b	bɹ^b	tɹ^d	dɹ^d	kɹ^d	gɹ^d	fɹ^b	θɹ^b,d	ʃɹ^d
sp^b	st^d	sk^d	sm^m	sn^n	sf^*
spɹ^b	stɹ^d	skɹ^d	spl^b	skw^d	

WORD-FINAL POSITION

Nasal clusters: [nt, ŋk, mp]   **Fricative clusters:** *Nil*

Liquid clusters: *Nil*   **Errors:** /st/→[t]; /nd/→[n]; /lz/→[lt,t]; /nts/→[nt]; /vz/→[b]; /ndʒ/→ [nt]

Observations: *Word-initial clusters usually reduced to a voiced plosive except nasal clusters (which were reduced to nasal). Correct final consonant clusters limited to homorganic nasal+plosive.*
*= not sampled during assessment

Problem area ■ yes □ no

[1]Baker, E. (2016). *Children's Independent and Relational Phonological Analysis: General American English*. Sydney, Australia: Author. Copyright ©2016 Elise Baker

Appendix 9-2 (*Continued*)

RELATIONAL ANALYSIS continued

(14) Phonological processes
- Shade box ■ for processes evident in the child's speech
- Comment on specific application of a process such as velar fronting word-initial only, and gliding only on /ɹ/
- Describe atypical, idiosyncratic processes
- Calculate percent occurrence as necessary

Syllable structure processes
☐ Weak syllable deletion

☐ Reduplication

☐ Final consonant deletion

☐ Initial consonant deletion

■ Cluster reduction (*All word-initial clusters reduced to one element – 100%. Nasal + plosive final consonant cluster reduction only 28% occurrence.*)

Substitution processes
■ Velar fronting (*All word-initial velars in singleton and clusters contexts fronted to alveolar plosive /d/ - 100%. Velar fronting not prominent in within-word or word-final position.*)
■ Palatal fronting (*Indirectly evident as post-alveolar fricatives and affricates were stopped to an alveolar plosive.*)
■ Stopping of fricatives (*All fricatives stopped to homorganic plosive – 100%, except /h/ which was consistently omitted.*)
■ Stopping of affricates (*All affricates stopped to an alveolar plosive – 100%.*)
☐ Deaffrication
■ Gliding of liquids (*Gliding only present on /ɹ/ not /l/. Word-final /ɹ/ substituted with schwa.*)
■ Context sensitive voicing (*Voicing of voiceless consonants in word-initial position, and tendency for devoicing of voiced consonants in word-final position.*)
■ Consonant cluster simplification (*Not evident for word-initial clusters, as they were reduced. However, some simplification of final consonant clusters was evident due to other substitution processes.*)
☐ Fricative simplification

☐ Glottal insertion

☐ Backing

Assimilation processes
☐ Velar

☐ Labial

☐ Alveolar
Other processes

Problem area ■ yes ☐ no

(15) Loss of phonemic contrast
- Using error analysis (box #12 and #13), list singleton consonants and consonant clusters with the same substitute (consonant or ∅) in the same word position.
- Describe loss of phonemic contrast according to major class features (obstruents/sonorants), natural classes (plosives, nasals, glides, liquids, fricatives and affricates) and consonant clusters (Williams, 2003). For example, non-labial singleton obstruents (including plosives, fricatives and affricates) and clusters /t, k, g, s, z, ʃ, θ, ð, tʃ, dʒ, ɹ, st, stɹ, sk, skɹ, skl, skw, kɹ, dɹ, gɹ, kl, gl/ are all substituted with [d] word-initially.

Word initial	Word final
• /t, k, g, θ, ð, s, z, ʃ, tʃ, dʒ, tw, tɹ, dɹ, θɹ, sw, sl, st, sk, stɹ, skw, skɹ, ʃɹ, kw, kl, gl, kɹ, gɹ, kj/→ [d]	• /s, z, ʃ, tʃ, lz, st/ → [t]
• /p, f, v, pj, bj, pl, bl, fl, pɹ, bɹ, fɹ, θɹ, sp, spɹ, spl/ → [b]	• /f v θ/ → [p]
• /ɹ, j/ → [w]	
• /h, j/ → [∅]	

Problem area ■ yes ☐ no

(16) Additional observations: prosody/phonation/resonance/respiration
☑ natural or ☒ unnatural/problematic
☑ **Stress**
   Lexical stress   ☑ Sw ☑ wS
   Sentence stress   ☑
   Emphatic stress   ☑
☑ **Words of increasing length** (e.g., hip, hippo, hippopotamus)
Is syllable segregation evident? ☐ yes ☑ no
☑ **Speech rate** ☐ Too slow ☐ Too fast ☐ Poorly regulated
☑ **Intonation**
☑ **Phonation**
☑ **Resonance**
☑ **Respiration / speech breathing**
Problem area ☐ yes ■ no

(17) Speech ratings
Consistency rating
■ Consistent   ☐ Inconsistent – further assessment and analysis needed

Severity rating *based on conversational speech sample*
☐ Mild   ☐ Moderate-severe
☐ Mild-moderate   ■ Severe

Intelligibility rating
☐ Intelligible   ■ Mainly unintelligible
☐ Mainly intelligible ☐ Completely unintelligible
☐ Partially intelligible

(18) Sampling constraints? ■ More sampling required
☐ Polysyllables   ☐ Words with weak-onset stress
☐ Consonant clusters ■ Other
Sample more instances of /θ, ʒ, dʒ, j/

[1]Baker, E. (2016). *Children's Independent and Relational Phonological Analysis: General American English.* Sydney, Australia: Author. Copyright ©2016 Elise Baker

10

Goal Setting

OVERVIEW

In this chapter you will learn evidence-based strategies for identifying, writing, and prioritizing goals for children with SSD. It is important that you understand how to develop goals, because intervention is a goal-directed activity. Clearly specified goals are like a map towards a destination. They serve as the starting point for intervention. They guide your program of intervention and signify when you have come to your end point. Intervention without well-defined goals is like driving without a map—you might begin intervention by working on an obvious error, but after a while you wonder where you are going and where you need to get to.

In this chapter you will learn how to write long-term goals for children with SSD and how to develop a hierarchy of short-term goals that contribute towards long-term goals. You will also learn about the fundamental concept of **generalization**. It is important that you understand this concept before learning about different approaches to intervention, because a common goal of most approaches is to facilitate generalization. Your understanding and application of the information in this chapter serves as a foundation for Chapters 11 through 14 on intervention.

WHAT ARE INTERVENTION GOALS?

A goal is an ambition that an individual aspires to achieve. The identification and prioritization of an individual child's goals requires careful consideration of the child's assessment results in conjunction with research evidence and child and family preferences. An obvious goal for a child with SSD would be intelligible speech. Given that different types of SSD exist and that children can be affected in unique and individual ways, intervention goals can vary. For example:

- improving a child's speech intelligibility,
- surgical repair of a cleft of the soft palate,
- developing a child's emergent literacy skills to ameliorate future risk of literacy difficulties,
- developing a child and communication partner's competence to use an alternative or augmentative form of communication,
- increasing a child's verbal interaction with peers at preschool or school,
- reducing immediate consequences of SSD such as bullying,
- equipping families with strategies for resolving communication breakdown,
- increasing family members' and relevant professionals' knowledge about SSD to dispel false beliefs and myths, and
- improving communication partners' abilities to listen to a child with SSD so that the child's messages are understood.

As these examples show, goals are not always limited to the child who has the SSD but can include other people in a child's life. The types of goals you identify emerge from your perspective about SSD in children.

IDENTIFYING GOALS FOR CHILDREN WITH SSD FROM DIFFERENT PERSPECTIVES

There are three perspectives or ways of thinking about how to manage SSD in children. These perspectives include:

1. Impairment-based perspective
2. Social-based perspective
3. Biopsychosocial perspective using the ICF-CY (WHO, 2007)

Traditionally, SLPs relied on the impairment-based perspective for specifying goals. This perspective is consistent with the medical model. According to Duchan (2001), an

Read more about
Susie (7;4 years),
a girl with an articulation
impairment (lateral lisp),
in Chapter 16 (Case 2).

impairment-based perspective assumes that communication difficulty is in the child and that the difficulty can be treated by giving the child the missing processing skills or knowledge. Improving Susie's articulation of /s/ in everyday conversational speech is an example of an impairment-based articulation goal. Increasing the accuracy of a child's production of consonant clusters is an example of an impairment-based phonology goal.

An alternative to the impairment-based perspective is the social perspective. According to Duchan (2001), the social-based perspective considers the impact of a child's communication differences (as opposed to impairment) within society. For example, a goal for a child with SSD who avoids playing with other children at preschool might be to interact with one other child in the sandpit playground at preschool.

The third perspective—the biopsychosocial perspective—uses the ICF-CY framework (WHO, 2007) and integrates both impairment and social perspectives. Recall from Chapter 2 that the ICF-CY framework was developed by the World Health Organization (2007) for considering the health and wellness of children and young people. The framework comprises two broad parts, with components and domains within each part, including:

Part 1: Functioning and disability:

1. Body Structures[1] (e.g., b3 Voice and speech function)
2. Body Function (e.g., s3 Structures involved in voice and speech function)
3. Activities and Participation (e.g., d3 Communication, d7 Interpersonal interactions and relationships)

Part 2: Contextual factors:

1. Environmental Factors (e.g., e4 Societal attitudes and norms)
2. Personal Factors (e.g., sex and age of the child)

As you learned in Chapters 7 and 8, most SLP assessments for children with SSD focus on Body Function, particularly articulation (including phonology) function. However, an assessment that accounts for the impact of SSD on a child's Activities and Participation and relevant Contextual Factors can provide a rich understanding about a child, his or her SSD, and the impact of the SSD on the child and family's life. A template for you to structure your assessment plan for a child with SSD using the ICF-CY framework was provided in Appendix 8-1. Appendix 10-1 provides a template for you to identify potential goals for a child with SSD, based on the assessment template. Figure 10-1 provides an example of a completed template for Luke's case.

Let's first consider the results from an assessment of functioning and disability using the ICF-CY framework based on a biopsychosocial perspective. If you identify problems with **Body Structure**, then a goal would be to address the Body Structure. For example, if you identified repeated episodes of glue ear accompanied by fluctuating conducting hearing loss, a goal may be to eliminate repeated episodes of glue ear. An ear, nose, and throat (ENT) specialist may prescribe a course of antibiotics, or perform a myringotomy and insert pressure equalization (ventilation) tubes, to achieve this goal. If you identified a structural problem with a child's hard or soft palate during assessment, a goal might be to repair the child's cleft. For the majority of children referred to an SLP with suspected SSD, the problem will be associated with one or more aspects of **Body Function**, particularly b320 Articulation Function. As shown in Appendix 10-1, Body Function goals for children with SSD can be divided into articulation function and other relevant functions such as auditory perception, receptive and expressive language, and memory functions.

Assessment using the ICF-CY framework also includes the components of **Activities and Participation**. Goals targeting one or both of these components will depend on the information gathered from an individual child and his or her family during the assessment. For example, Mark (4;7 years) had a moderate-severe phonological impairment (PCC = 54%). A case history interview with Mark's parents revealed that Mark was experiencing significant social isolation at preschool. Mark was also reported to be sensitive to communication failure. Assessment using the SPAA-C (McLeod, 2004) found that Mark did

---

[1]Capitalization has been used to be consistent with usage in the ICF-CY and to differentiate between everyday usage of these terms.

| FIGURE 10-1 | Goal identification template for Luke |

Name: _____ Date of birth: _____ Age: _____

Reason for referral: _____ Language(s) spoken: _____

Diagnosis: _____

		Areas requiring consideration in intervention
Function and disability	Body functions	☒ b320 Articulation functions (includes phonology)
		☒ b1560 Auditory perception
		☐ b230 Hearing functions
		☒ b144 Memory functions (including phonological processing)
		☐ b1670 Reception of language
		☐ b1671 Expression of language
		☐ b310 Voice functions
		☐ b330 Fluency and rhythm of speech functions
		☐ b117 Intellectual functions
	Body structures	☐ b126 Temperament and personality functions
		☐ s320 Structure of mouth
		☐ s1 Structure of nervous system, s240–260 Structure of ear, s310 Structure of nose, s330 Structure of pharynx, s340 Structure of larynx, s430 Structure of respiratory system
	Activities and participation	☐ d3 Communication
		☐ d1 Learning and applying knowledge (including d115 Listening, d140 Learning to read, d145 Learning to write)
		☐ d7 Interpersonal interactions and relationships
		☐ d810–820 Education
		☐ d9 Community, social and civic life
Contextual factors	Environmental	☒ e3 Support and relationships
		☐ e4 Attitudes
		☐ e1 Products and technology,
		☐ e5 Services, systems and policies
	Personal	*Luke circled ⊗ when asked how he felt about people not understanding him. He shrugged his shoulders and circled "?" (don't know) in response to questions about talking with friends and teachers. Monitor Luke's personal experience with living with SSD over the course of intervention.*

not like being misunderstood. He preferred to not communicate with his peers rather than face repeated episodes of miscommunication. At preschool, Mark's strategy was to select activities or toys that no other child played with. If another child approached or wanted to share the activity or toy, Mark would leave the activity in search of another. While this strategy meant that Mark successfully avoided talking, he missed out on the opportunity to develop friends and social skills. Based on the information gathered from the SPAA-C (McLeod, 2004), Mark reported feeling sad about the way he talked, and happiest when he was playing on his own. The findings from this assessment translated into goals targeting Mark's Activities and Participation (e.g., Mark's parents wanted Mark to enjoy talking with

━━━

✅ **APPLICATION:** *Identifying areas requiring goals for Susie, Jarrod, Michael, and Lian*

Using Appendix 10-1 and the case-based information in Chapter 16, complete a goal identification template for Susie (7;4 years), Jarrod (7;0 years), Michael (4;2 years), and Lian (14;2 years). Review the children's assessment results in Chapter 16 to guide your completion of the template. Using the template, identify the problem areas requiring goals.

━━━

and playing alongside another child at preschool) and Personal Factors (e.g., Mark wanted to feel happier about the way he talked).

Assessment using the ICF-CY framework can also reveal Contextual Factors (Environmental and Personal) that act as facilitators or barriers for a child with SSD. Consider Sam's case, described by McLeod and Threats (2008). Sam is a 6-year-old boy who has a lisp and concomitant language and fluency difficulties. Using environmental domains of the ICF-CY (WHO, 2007), McLeod and Threats (2008, p. 100) described Sam's contextual factors as follows:

> He is the second son of single mother (who is divorced) (e310). His mother works long hours, yet receives a low income (d8700). His grandmother (e315) often takes care of the children while their mother is at work. Sam has a few close friends (e320), but others at school tease him about his speech (e425). Sam's brother (e310) goes to the same school and protects and supports (e410) him in the playground. Sam lives in a small rural town (e2151) that has intermittent SLP services (e580). (McLeod & Threats, 2008, p. 100)

While some contextual factors may be translated into goals, others may simply be identified as barriers or facilitators and worked with or around in the development of an intervention plan. In Sam's case, contextual goals could be for Sam's school to develop an anti-teasing and anti-bullying program to change the attitudes of Sam's peers about individual differences and abilities and for Sam's SLP to lobby relevant governing bodies about the need for SLP services in rural areas for children like Sam.

Given that all children are unique individuals, goals will be unique from one child to another. Some children primarily have impairment-based goals targeting speech function, because the impact of their SSD on their Activities and Participation may be minimal. For others the impact of their SSD on their Activities and Participation or barriers in their environment may mean that socially based goals are of prime importance. Use the ICF-CY framework to think about the children on your caseloads from both impairment-based and socially based perspectives to generate goals on a case-by-case basis. As children learn and change, so will the goals. As one goal is achieved, other goals may be realized and new goals may be identified.

OPERATIONALLY DEFINED GOALS

Goals need to be realistic, achievable, and measurable. To be measurable, goals need to be operationally defined. Based on descriptions by Hegde (1985) and Klein and Moses (1999), most operationally defined long-term goals include:

- the behavior or attitude to be learned (e.g., intelligible speech during conversation, interaction with a peer at preschool, positive rating ☺ about speech);
- the task that will be used to measure the behavior or attitude (e.g., standardized single-word assessment tool, conversational speech sample);
- who will conduct the measurement (e.g., the SLP, the child's caregiver, the child's preschool teacher);
- setting(s) where measurement will take place (e.g., in the clinic, in the home, in the preschool, via telehealth);
- criterion (e.g., with 90% accuracy from a conversational sample containing at least 100 different words; with 70% accuracy in conversation for a 15-minute play-based period; intelligibility rating of "usually understood" or "always understood" over a month; score within normal limits on a standardized test); and

- the total expected duration of intervention (e.g., within 6 months of starting intervention, within 12 months of regular weekly SLP intervention combined with daily home practice).

Consider the wording of the following long-term goal for Luke: "Luke's speech will be age appropriate and intelligible with a variety of speakers in a variety of environments." Although this goal is aspirational, it is not measurable. How will you know if his speech is age appropriate and intelligible? What type of speech sample will the goal be based on? Who will be the variety of speakers and what are the speaking environments? Consider the following rephrased long-term goal for Luke:

Luke will have age appropriate and intelligible speech based on: (a) Diagnostic Evaluation of Articulation and Phonology: Phonology Assessment (Dodd, Hua, et al., 2006) standard score being within normal limits (administered and scored by the SLP), (b) a 10-minute conversational speech sample percentage of consonants correct (PCC) being > 80% (based on Austin & Shriberg, 1997) (collected and scored by the SLP), and (c) intelligibility rating from the Intelligibility in Context Scale (ICS) (McLeod, Harrison, & McCormack, 2012a) being 4.5–5.0 (usually to always understood by a range of communicative partners), as completed by Luke's parent/caregiver, within 12 months of starting intervention.

COMMENT: *Long-term goals for Luke*

The assessment results for Luke identified four areas to be addressed in intervention. These areas can be transformed into long-term goals addressing (1) speech production, (2) speech perception, (3) emergent literacy including phonological awareness and letter knowledge, in addition to (4) Luke's own feelings about the way he talks. Suggested long-term goals for Luke include:

1. **Luke will have age appropriate and intelligible speech** based on: (a) Diagnostic Evaluation of Articulation and Phonology: Phonology Assessment (Dodd, Hua, et al., 2006) standard score being within normal limits (administered and scored by the SLP), (b) a 10-minute conversational speech sample percentage of consonants correct (PCC) being > 80% (based on Austin & Shriberg, 1997) (collected and scored by the SLP), and (c) intelligibility rating from the Intelligibility in Context Scale (ICS) (McLeod, Harrison, & McCormack, 2012a) being 4.5–5.0 (usually to always understood by a range of communicative partners), as completed by Luke's parent/caregiver, within 12 months of starting intervention.

2. **Luke will have adequate speech perception skills** based on identification of words containing /s/ and /ʃ/ on an informal speech perception task comprising 24 items (Locke, 1980b) with the clinician in the clinic with ≥ 90% accuracy, within 12 months of starting intervention.

3. **Luke will develop age-appropriate phonological awareness and letter knowledge** based on a phonological awareness composite from the Comprehensive Test of Phonological Processing 2 (CTOPP-2) (Wagner, Torgesen, Rashotte, & Pearson, 2013) being within the average range; and a score for letter recognition (i.e., can point to a lowercase letter when the letter sound is given) and recall (i.e., can say a letter name and sound when a letter is pointed to) being 26 and 23 respectively out of 32 letters, based on an informal task reported by Dodd and Carr (2003) with the clinician in the clinic, within 12 months of starting intervention.

4. **Luke will rate that he feels ☺ happy about the way he talks**, based on conversation throughout a week with family at home and conversation throughout a week with teachers and peers at preschool, using the Speech Participation and Activity Assessment of Children (SPAA-C) (McLeod, 2004) questions for children, including, "How do you feel about the way you talk?" "How do you feel when you talk to your [pre]school teachers?" and "How do you feel when you talk to the whole class?" administered by the clinician in the clinic, within 12 months of starting intervention.

Read more about Luke (4;3 years), a boy with a phonological impairment, in Chapter 16 (Case 1).

■ ■

 APPLICATION: *Long-term goals for Susie, Michael, Jarrod, and Lian*

Read more about Susie (7;4 years), Jarrod (7;0 years), Michael (4;2 years), and Lian (14;2 years) in Chapter 16.

Using the assessment results (in Chapter 16) and the goal identification templates that you completed for Susie (7;4 years), Jarrod (7;0 years), Michael (4;2 years), and Lian (14;2 years), generate realistic, achievable, and measurable long-term goals. Your long-term goals could focus on articulation function, in addition to other problems areas (e.g., social interaction, emergent literacy skills, child and/or parent satisfaction). Refer to Appendix 10-1 for the goal identification template and to the previous application box related to this task.

Although Luke's long-term speech goal seems detailed, you know who will be involved in collecting data and measuring the goal (clinician and parent/caregiver), you know what measures will be used to determine if and when Luke's speech is intelligible (standard score, PCC, intelligibly rating), the criterion for those measures (performance within the normal range on a standardized test, PPC > 80%, and intelligibility ratings of 4 or 5), how the information for the measures will be gathered (formal test, 10-minute conversational speech sample, and general conversation at home over a 1-month period), and in what time frame the goal could be expected to be achieved (within a year of starting intervention).

GOAL FRAMEWORKS AND HIERARCHIES

Intervention goals need to be contextualized within a goal framework. A goal framework is a hierarchically organized network of goals designed to achieve a basic or long-term goal. The number of goals and levels within a hierarchy reflects both the nature of the problem and the impact of the problem on a child's activity and participation. A variety of generic goal hierarchies have been described in the literature (e.g., Fey, 1986; Klein & Moses, 1999). Klein and Moses (1999) describe a three-level goal hierarchy:

1. **Long-term goals**
2. **Short-term goals**
3. **Session goals**

Long-term goals typically summarize what needs to be achieved before a child and his or her family can be dismissed from intervention services. **Short-term goals** describe the specific behavior or skill being targeted to achieve the long-term goal. Sometimes a long-term goal can be divided into multiple short-term goals. Sometimes you may only have a few short-term goals to achieve a long-term goal. For example, an important long-term goal for Luke (4;3 years) is that he will have age-appropriate and intelligible speech. (Refer to the "Long-Term Goals for Luke" box.) This goal could be achieved by working on a range of skills identified from your analysis of Luke's speech. For example, in Chapter 9 we identified Luke's largest phoneme collapse, or group of singleton consonants and consonant clusters reduced to one consonant, in word-initial position: /t, k, g, θ, ð, s, z, ʃ, tʃ, dʒ, tw, tɹ, dɹ, θɹ, sw, sl, st, sk, stɹ, skw, skɹ, ʃɹ, kw, kl, gl, kɹ, gɹ, kj/ → [d]. This loss of phonemic contrast could be transformed into a short-term goal: Luke will contrast /d/ with each of the following singleton consonants and consonant clusters including /t, k, g, θ, ð, s, z, ʃ, tʃ, dʒ, tw, tɹ, dɹ, θɹ, sw, sl, st, sk, stɹ, skw, skɹ, ʃɹ, kw, kl, gl, kɹ, gɹ, kj/ in word-initial position during 20 minutes of conversational speech with the clinician in the clinic with 50% accuracy within approximately 6 months of targeting the goal. The five other collapses that were identified from the analysis could form his other short-term goals. As you will learn later in this chapter, the largest collapse in a child's system is prioritized over smaller collapses, in the hope that an improvement in the largest collapse will automatically lead to improvements (i.e., generalize) to smaller collapses (Williams, 2003). Achievement of short-term goals is routinely monitored through generalization probes. As discussed in Chapter 12, generalization probes are one type of data collected over the course of intervention, to evaluate intervention efficacy. Briefly, short-term goals specify:

- the response behavior to be monitored for generalized learning or the attitude to be monitored for change;
- the task that will be used to measure the skill, behavior, or attitude;
- who will conduct the measurement;
- the setting(s) where measurement will take place;
- criterion (e.g., 70% accuracy); and
- expected duration to achieve the short-term goal (e.g., with 3 months of starting intervention on the goal).

Short-term goals are transformed into **session goals**—the behaviors, skills, or knowledge taught through intervention procedures (see Chapter 12) within an activity during intervention sessions with an intervention agent. Session goals typically specify:

- the child's observable behavior (e.g., production of multiple opposition treatment word sets including word-initial /d/ contrast with word-initial /k, ʃ, sl, ʧ/ at word level),
- the response mode (e.g., with a model for delayed imitation),
- the response level (e.g., at word level, phrase level),
- the teaching and learning procedure(s) (e.g., metaphor, auditory models of treatment words for delayed imitation),
- dose (e.g., two treatment sets or approximately 40 trials),
- criterion (e.g., 70% accuracy),
- the intervention agent (e.g., the clinician, computer), and
- the context (e.g., drill- or play-based activities in the clinic).

For example, if we were to use Williams' (2003) multiple oppositions intervention with Luke (see Chapter 13 for further information about multiple oppositions intervention), a session goal could include: "Luke will contrast /d/ with /k, ʃ, sl, ʧ/ in word-initial position, at word level, given a metaphor and an auditory model for delayed imitation, across two treatment sets (comprising 40 trials) with 70% accuracy, during drill-play activities (e.g., bowling, fishing) with the clinician in the clinic." The session goals vary within a session and from one session to the next, depending on a child's progress.

The hierarchical organization of goals means that realization of one goal may lead to the realization of other goals. Usually, session goals contribute to the realization of short-term goals, and short-term goals contribute to the realization of a long-term goal. Sometimes, the realization of one goal facilitates realization of another different goal, without direct intervention on that goal. When a speech production goal facilitates the realization of other speech production goals, the phenomenon of generalization is at work.

COMMENT: *What's the difference between three- and four-tiered goal frameworks?*

Fey (1986) proposed four levels of goals intertwined with procedures and activities. The four levels include basic goals (long term), specific goals (short term), subgoals, and session goals. As with the Klein and Moses (1999) hierarchy, basic goals are commensurate with long-term goals and specify the main objective of intervention. Specific goals are commensurate with short-term goals, and subgoals are the steps required to achieve a specific goal. Session goals, within the Fey (1986) four-tiered framework, refer to the compilation of subgoals targeted within a session. In any one session (whether it be with a clinician in a clinic, with a child's carer at home, or with a child's teacher at preschool), one or more subgoals may be targeted. In Klein and Moses' (1999) hierarchy, session goals are equivalent to Fey's (1986) subgoals.

GENERALIZATION

According to Elbert (1989) "the occurrence of generalization is often viewed as rather wondrous" (p. 31). Generalization (sometimes called transfer) is the process by which desired change in a behavior in an intervention context facilitates change in the same behavior and/or different but related behaviors in other non-intervention contexts (Gordon-Brannan & Weiss, 2007; Stokes & Baer, 1997). Essentially, the occurrence of generalization means that clinicians do not have to teach every child every speech behavior, such as all speech sounds across all word positions, in every word spoken in the language they are learning, in every setting they speak in, with everyone they speak with. Rather, clinicians need to provide intervention that facilitates generalization. It is a fascinating yet essential phenomenon if intervention is to work efficiently. The occurrence of generalization is one of the most important outcomes of intervention for a child with SSD. For example, if a child was referred for speech-language pathology services because he or she was gliding /ɹ/ → [w], intervention would no longer be required once the child showed *generalized* acquisition of the correct production of /ɹ/ during everyday conversational speech.

Historically, generalization was considered once intervention had started. In the past, a speech sound was targeted for intervention, and if progress was slow or not evident in everyday speech, procedures may have been adopted to facilitate generalization. In this context, it would seem at odds to discuss generalization in a chapter on goal setting. However, the shift from articulation to phonology during the mid-1970s saw generalization as a phenomenon to plan for from the outset of intervention, at the point when goals are being identified and prioritized. For this reason, the two types of generalization (stimulus and response) are reviewed briefly before examining the literature on different approaches for identifying and prioritizing intervention speech production goals for different types of SSD in children.

■ Stimulus generalization

Stimulus generalization occurs when a trained behavior is evoked with different stimuli (Bernthal, Bankson, & Flipsen, 2013). An example illustrates this phenomenon. A trained context might be a child saying the affricate /ʧ/ in the word *chicken* to the SLP (audience stimuli) in response to being shown a photo of a chicken (physical stimuli), the SLP saying, "What is this?" (verbal stimuli), in a clinic room (setting stimuli). Stimulus generalization occurs when the child says the affricate /ʧ/ in the word *chicken* to his father (audience stimuli), in response to the child seeing a picture of a chicken in a book (physical stimuli), the father pointing to the chicken and saying, "What type of animal live on this farm?" (verbal stimuli), at home (setting stimuli). Figure 10-2 summarizes the types of stimulus generalization observed during intervention for SSD in children.

■ Response generalization

Response generalization refers to "the process in which responses that have been taught carry over to other behaviors that are not taught" (Bernthal, Bankson, & Flipsen, 2013, p. 255). For children with an articulation impairment, response generalization is thought to occur when the targeted speech skill improves across untreated word positions, in untreated words during conversational speech. For children with a phonological impairment, response generalization is thought to occur when there is an increase in a child's productive phonological knowledge (i.e., what a child knows about the phonological system of the language that he or she is learning). Figure 10-3 provides a summary of the different types of phonological response generalization associated with an increase in children's productive phonological knowledge.

Using Figure 10-3 as a guide, a child who is taught to say /ʧ/ in *chicken* shows phonological response generalization when the child says *cheese* (i.e., generalization to other words not used in intervention), *catching* and *watch* (i.e., generalization across word positions not targeted during intervention), "I had *chicken* for dinner" (i.e., generalization of

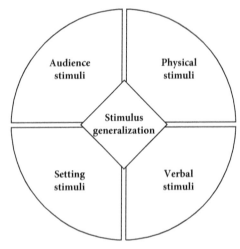

FIGURE 10-2   Categories of stimulus generalization

Source: Based on concepts from Bernthal, Bankson, & Flipsen (2009).

FIGURE 10-3   Categories of response generalization

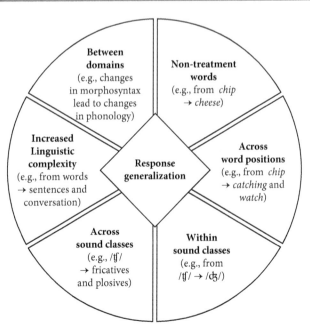

Source: Based on Elbert & Gierut (1986).

the trained sound to more complex linguistic units such as sentences and conversation), /ʤ/ in *jump* (i.e., generalization of the trained sound to sounds within the same class—in this case, affricates), and /ʃ/ in *shop* (i.e., generalization of the trained sound to sounds across other sound classes—in this case, fricatives). This later production also reflects generalization based on implicational relationships—in this case, affricates implying fricatives (Schmidt & Meyers, 1995). Tyler (2005a) adds that between-domain generalization is also possible, such as morphosyntax intervention targeting children's production of finite morphemes indirectly facilitating change in children's phonological abilities.

APPROACHES TO GOAL SETTING FOR CHILDREN WITH SSD

The task of selecting an intervention goal to work on can seem quite simple. If a child has difficulty with a particular speech sound, then work on it. However, most children who have SSD have more than one issue requiring intervention. Your assessment may have identified one or more Body Functions (e.g., articulation function, auditory perception), in addition to issues regarding Activities and Participation. Whether a child has a phonological impairment, inconsistent speech disorder, an articulation impairment, CAS, or childhood dysarthria, you need to consider both research evidence and family preferences to prioritize which goals you will work on in what order, or indeed whether there are some goals that you can work on concurrently.

For the remainder of this chapter, we examine goal setting for the different types of SSD. We dedicate more space to phonological impairment, because the research evidence suggests *"what is treated may be more important than how it is taught"* (Gierut, 2005, p. 203). This is because some intervention targets (i.e., goals focused on children's speech) can induce more widespread and efficient change in children's phonological systems than others. Your job is to learn about the different approaches to target selection and consider the evidence with each approach.

GOAL SETTING FOR CHILDREN WITH PHONOLOGICAL IMPAIRMENT: THE IMPORTANCE OF THE TARGET

The selection and prioritization of intervention targets for children with a phonological impairment represents a critical link between comprehensive analysis and intervention (Kamhi & Pollock, 2005). At first glance, it would seem intuitive to start working on easy, stimulable, early developing speech sounds or word shapes that are problematic and help children build their phonological systems as one would build a house, from the ground up. However, target selection for children with phonological impairment is not that straightforward. Since the work by Elbert and McReynolds (1979) on generalization, six target selection approaches have been reported in the literature:

1. **Traditional developmental approach** (e.g., Rvachew & Nowak, 2001).
2. **Complexity approach** (e.g., Gierut, 2007).
3. **Cyclical approach** (e.g., Hodson, 2007).
4. **Systemic approach** (e.g., Williams, 2003).
5. **Nonlinear approach** (e.g., Bernhardt & Stemberger, 2000).
6. **Neuro-network approach** (e.g., Norris & Hoffman, 2005).

The disparate theoretical orientations across the approaches make it a controversial area (Baker & McLeod, 2011a). For instance, while some authors suggest that the complexity approach may be better for facilitating widespread phonological change (e.g., Gierut, 2007), others do not support this position, pointing to evidence that suggests that similar or even better outcomes can be achieved with a developmental approach (Rvachew & Nowak, 2001; Rvachew & Bernhardt, 2010). To date, no single approach has been reported to be the most ideal. Adequate comparative research simply has not been done. Additionally, what may be best for one child at a particular time may not be the best for another. What follows is a brief description of the six different target selection approaches, an overview of the evidence base associated with an approach, and comment on the types of SSD and child characteristics suited to each approach.

■ Traditional developmental approach

Prior to the paradigm shift from articulation to phonology, most SLPs tended to select an early developing, stimulable speech sound from a list of options derived from **SODA analysis**, and worked through that list developmentally, sound by sound. Although the shift to a phonological emphasis saw patterns or rules being targeted (rather than individual sounds), developmental norms regarding the age of acquisition of speech sounds still applied (Williams, 2005b).

What are traditional developmental intervention targets?

According to Dyson and Robinson (1987), the following four criteria characterize phonological processes that align with a developmental approach to target selection:

1. Phonological processes that occur frequently but are optional (i.e., targets that the child has some phonological knowledge of).
2. Phonological processes that affect sounds that are stimulable or sounds that are within a child's phonetic inventory.
3. Phonological processes that affect intelligibility, such as idiosyncratic processes or extensive harmony.
4. Phonological processes that affect early developing sounds.

Rvachew and Nowak (2001) suggest that such traditional or developmental guidelines to target selection are based two underlying assumptions: (1) children should not be discouraged or frustrated by the intervention process, and (2) the acquisition of earlier developing sounds and syllable/word shapes serves as a prerequisite for the acquisition of later developing sounds and syllable/word shapes. For a long time, these assumptions (rather than research evidence) guided SLPs' clinical decision-making.

Let's take a look at the evidence associated with the developmental approach to target selection. In a group study of 48 children with a moderate or severe phonological impairment, Rvachew and Nowak (2001) compared the efficacy of intervention for children assigned to either early developing phonemes associated with most productive phonological knowledge (ME group) or late developing phonemes associated with least productive phonological knowledge (LL group). Rvachew and Nowak (2001) reported significant differences between the two groups, with the children in the ME group showing better progress on their target sounds during intervention sessions. Measures of the children's conversational speech skills post-intervention showed no difference between the groups, with both groups adding "approximately 2.5 phonemes to their inventories (with a range of 0 to 7 new phonemes for both groups)" (Rvachew & Nowak, 2001, p. 619). One child's performance in the ME group was particularly intriguing. Before intervention his phonetic inventory comprised: [w, j, m, n, p, b, t, d, g, l]. Intervention targeted /p, h, k, f/. Following 12 weeks of intervention, six new phonemes had been added to his phonetic inventory /dʒ, f, v, θ, ð, ʃ/ and final consonants were consistently being used. In a rarely reported outcome of intervention, Rvachew and Nowak (2001) also explored measures of both parent and child satisfaction with the intervention. Rvachew and Nowak reported no difference in child enjoyment between the groups, but that the parents were more satisfied if their child was in the traditional group compared to the nontraditional group. In light of the results of their investigation, Rvachew and Nowak (2001) recommend that early developing sounds associated with more productive phonological knowledge be prioritized for intervention over later developing sounds associated with less productive phonological knowledge. They further stated that although their study did not support the use of nondevelopmental targets (i.e., speech sounds that are late developing or associated with no productive phonological knowledge), they would not avoid such targets if there was a particular motivation for selecting such targets for a child. In an interesting commentary on Rvachew and Nowak's (2001) study, Morrisette and Gierut (2003) suggest that Rvachew and Nowak's (2001) findings provide support for their alternative approach to target selection—the complexity (nondevelopmental) approach.

Who is suited to the traditional developmental approach?

The developmental approach is potentially suitable for any child who has SSD. It may be particularly useful with children who have a reactive temperament, or who have a fear of failure and would benefit from the experience of early success in intervention.

■ Complexity approach to target selection

Since the recognition of the importance of response generalization, careful selection of one or two complex phonological targets has been suggested as a way to induce widespread change in children's phonological systems (Gierut, 2007). An understanding of this idea requires an understanding of two concepts: **complexity** and **learnability**.

APPLICATION: *Short-term goals for Luke from a developmental perspective*

Luke (4;3 years) has a severe phonological impairment. In Chapter 9, you completed an independent and relational phonological analysis of Luke's speech sample. To help you understand, compare, and contrast the different types of target selection approaches for children with phonological impairment, write a series of short-term goals for Luke targeting the phonological processes identified for Luke from a developmental perspective. Each short-term goal will focus on a specific phonological process evident in his speech. For example, you could target the phonological process of velar fronting in word-initial position as a goal. To complete this exercise, you will need to refer to Chapter 6 on typical speech acquisition, so that you can use general developmental sequence to order the phonological processes in Luke's speech that require intervention.

Read more about
Luke (4;3 years),
a boy with a phonological
impairment,
in Chapter 16 (Case 1).

What is complexity?

Complexity is a useful yet somewhat abstract concept for studying systems, the constituents or parts of systems, and how they interrelate with one another in organized hierarchies (Baker, 2015). Recall that all phonological systems across languages are in fact systems. A phonological system contains parts such as speech sounds, distinctive features, syllable shapes, tones, word lengths, and stress patterns. The parts are hierarchically arranged, with each part within a system having a complexity status. Parts higher in the system are considered more complex, as they carry more information about the system and dominate parts lower in the system. This idea is best illustrated by the theoretical concept of implicational relationships. Recall from Chapter 5 that the existence of one group of phonemes in a system can imply the existence of another, but not vice versa. The relationships are unidirectional. For example, fricatives imply the presence of plosives, but the existence of plosives in a system does not imply that fricatives will be present. Using this example, fricatives are more complex than plosives. Implicational relationships are further discussed in Chapter 5 and listed in Table 5-3.

Complexity and learnability

The process by which children's phonological systems change is believed to be guided by principles of **learnability**. Put simply, what a child knows about a phonological system is a subset of what an accomplished speaker of the language knows (Gierut, 2007). The child's task is to learn more and more about the phonological system and the complexities of the system (such as the parts and the rules governing the relationships among the parts) to become an intelligible, adultlike speaker.

Figure 10-4 provides a diagram illustrating phonological learning over time. At time 1, a child may have knowledge of early developing phonemes, word shapes, and stress patterns. As a child is exposed to relatively more complex parts of the phonological system, the child learns about the system and his or her subset of phonological knowledge expands (time 2). The goal for a child is expand or grow his or her phonological system so that it matches that of the adult speakers in the child's community.

Using this basic tenet of learnability, Gierut (2007) suggests that more complex input beyond or outside children's existing knowledge facilitates children's learning of the phonological system they are trying to learn. So, what makes for complex input? What makes a phonological intervention target complex? Gierut (2001) proposed four categories for describing the complexity of targets:

1. complex articulatory phonetic factors
2. complex linguistic structures
3. complex clinical factors
4. complex psycholinguistic structures

| **FIGURE 10-4** | **The relationship between a child's phonological system and the adult phonological system over time** |

At time 1, the child's system is a subset of the adult system. At time 2, following exposure to more complex aspects of the phonological system, the child's phonological system has expanded.

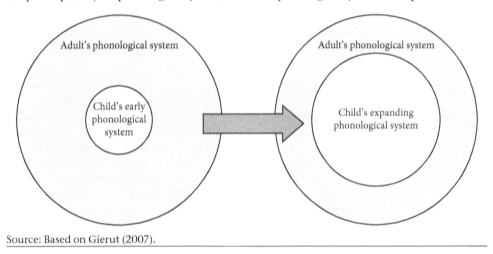

Source: Based on Gierut (2007).

Table 10-1 provides a description of each category and corresponding research evidence. As you read through the information in Table 10-1, reflect on what Luke (4;3 years) knows about the phonological system and what he needs to learn.

What are complex intervention targets?

Complex targets are non-stimulable, phonetically more complex segments or true consonant clusters that are associated with least productive phonological knowledge for an individual child (and therefore consistently in error). They are marked (i.e., their existence implies the existence of less marked targets) and are later developing.

Why select complex targets? Intervention that prioritizes more complex phonological targets is thought to trigger greater phonological learning relative to intervention that starts with less complex targets. See Gierut (2001, 2005, 2007) for helpful reviews. You are also encouraged to read Rvachew and Bernhardt (2010) and Rvachew and Brosseau-Lapré (2012) for an opposing view of this literature.

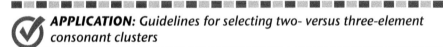

✅ APPLICATION: *Guidelines for selecting two- versus three-element consonant clusters*

Complex onsets can include two- and three-element consonant clusters. Morrisette, Farris, and Gierut (2006) provide helpful suggestions for deciding when to select two- versus three-element consonant clusters for children with phonological impairment. Briefly, you need to work out the whether a child has /s/ (C_1, that is, the first consonant in a three-element cluster), /p, t, k/ (C_2), and /l, ɹ, w/ (C_3) as phonemes in their phonological system. If a child has C_1 but not C_2 or C_3, consider two-element clusters with small sonority different scores. (Refer to Chapter 5 for further information about sonority and examples of true consonant clusters according to their sonority difference score.) However, if C_2 and C_3 are singleton phonemes in a child's phonological system, then consider three-element clusters (Morrisette et al., 2006). Monitor two-element consonant clusters to see if they are changing by implication. Refer to Chapter 12 for further information about the different types of data use to monitor children's progress during intervention.

TABLE 10-1	Phonological intervention research supporting the complexity approach to target selection
Complexity category	**Intervention target recommendation and supporting research evidence example**

Articulatory phonetic factors

Stimulability	**Intervention target recommendation:** Intervention targeting non-stimulable sounds is associated with more widespread system change relative to intervention targeting only stimulable sounds.
	Example of research evidence: Powell, Elbert, and Dinnsen (1991) conducted an intervention study with six children (aged 4;11–5;6 years) and examined the role of speech sound stimulability on phonological learning. Powell et al. discovered that even though the non-stimulable sounds were slower to generalize or learn than the stimulable sounds, intervention targeting the non-stimulable sounds led to the greatest changes in the children's phonological systems overall. Powell et al. noted that "for 86% of the 28 monitored sounds, generalization was consistent with pre-treatment stimulability skills; production of stimulable sounds tended to improve regardless of treatment target" (p. 1318). They concluded that stimulable speech sounds would be more likely to improve without intervention compared to non-stimulable speech sounds.
Phonetic complexity	**Intervention target recommendation:** Complex phonetic distinctions seem to be associated with more widespread change relative to less complex phonetic distinctions.
	Example of research evidence: Tyler and Figurski (1994) explored the effect of intervention on more complex targets in two children aged 2;8 and 2;10 years using the Dinnsen, Chin, Elbert, and Powell (1990) implicational hierarchy of feature distinctions (levels A–E, with A associated with less phonetic complexity, and E the most phonetic complexity). Both children were still at the single-word stage of language development. Tyler and Figurski reported that one participant (2;8 years) with knowledge of levels A and B, increased his phonetic inventory from 9 to 21 sounds (added 12 sounds), given two 9-week blocks of intervention separated by a 5-week break targeting /l/, associated with level D distinction. Such widespread change was not observed for the other participant given intervention targeting level C distinction. Tyler and Figurski (1994) suggested that greater change might occur when intervention focuses on more complex phonetic distinctions.

Complex linguistic structures

Phonological knowledge	**Intervention target recommendation:** Intervention targets associated with least productive phonological knowledge for a child may induce greater system-wide change relative to targets of which a child has most or more knowledge.
	Example of research evidence: Gierut, Elbert, and Dinnsen (1987) proposed six levels of productive phonological knowledge (1 = most, and 6 = least). In an experimental study with six children, they reported that more widespread phonological change occurred for participants given targets associated with less productive phonological knowledge.
Implicational relationships for syllable structures	**Intervention target recommendation:** More marked syllable structures (consonant clusters) may induce more system-wide change relative to less marked syllable structures (consonant clusters and singletons).
	Example of research evidence: Gierut (1999) examined patterns of generalization across 11 children and found that clusters with a small sonority difference implied clusters with a greater sonority difference. Gierut and Champion (2001) found that three-element clusters (e.g., /spl/) implied two-element clusters and singletons, with specific patterns of generalization being influenced by participants' phonological knowledge pre-intervention. Elbert, Dinnsen, and Powell (1984) reported that fricative-liquid clusters implied stop-liquid clusters.
Implicational relationships for phonemes	**Intervention target recommendation:** Marked phonemes may induce more system-wide change relative to less marked phonemes.
	Example of research evidence: Robb, Bleile, and Yee (1999) observed that intervention targeting consonants facilitated an improvement in vowels (i.e., consonants imply vowels); Dinnsen and Elbert (1984) reported that the existence of fricatives implies stops; McReynolds and Jetzke (1986) observed in children with a hearing impairment, that voiced obstruents implied voiceless obstruents.

(Continued)

| TABLE 10-1 | *Continued* |

Complexity category	Intervention target recommendation and supporting research evidence example
Implicational relationship among distributional properties	**Intervention target recommendation**: Marked word positions may induce more widespread generalization across word positions relative to less marked word positions. **Example of research evidence**: Based on observations from speech acquisition studies, Gierut (2007) noted that fricatives in initial position imply fricatives in final position, stops in final position imply stops in initial position, and word-initial /ɹ/ implies postvocalic /ɹ/.

Complex clinical factors

Consistency of error	**Intervention target recommendation**: Speech sounds consistently in error may induce more widespread change in children's phonological systems because they are associated with less phonological knowledge relative to speech sounds that are occasionally not in error. **Example of research evidence**: Gierut (2001) recommends that speech sounds excluded from a child's phonetic and phonemic inventories and consistently in error (associated with least productive phonological knowledge) be prioritized over those sounds of which a child has some productive phonological knowledge. Using Case 6 as an example from Gierut, Elbert, and Dinnsen (1987), the target was /v/ (consistently in error) and it resulted in improved production of other non-treatment sounds that were in error inconsistently or consistently (Gierut, 2001).
Developmental norms	**Intervention target recommendation**: Later developing speech sounds seem to be more complex and therefore associated with more widespread change relative to earlier developing speech sounds. **Example of research evidence**: Gierut, Morrisette, Hughes, and Rowland (1996, p. 227) reported that intervention targeting later-acquired speech sounds promoted greater widespread change in children's sound systems because of across-class generalization. Gierut et al. noted that intervention targeting earlier-acquired speech sounds did not have the same system-wide effect.
Number and nature of errors to be treated	**Intervention target recommendation**: Pairing two or more phonemes that differ by major class and maximal feature distinctions is more complex, because they may facilitate greater system-wide changes in intervention compared with targeting one sound. **Example of research evidence**: Targeting two unknown phonemes in a pair resulted in more widespread change than using a conventional minimal opposition contrast that targeted a child's production with the intended adult target, or intervention targeting one known with one unknown phoneme (e.g., Gierut, 1991, 1992).

Complex psycholinguistic structures

Treatment words	**Intervention target recommendation**: High-frequency words seem to be more complex because they facilitate more change in children's phonological systems compared with low-frequency words. Recommendations regarding other characteristics such as neighborhood density, age of acquisition, and lexicality (i.e., real versus nonwords) remain to be determined, given unclear findings across the research (Baker, 2015). **Example of research evidence**: Morrisette and Gierut (2002) studied the relationship between word characteristics (word frequency and neighborhood density) and patterns of phonological generalization with eight children with a phonological impairment. They found that intervention using high (rather than low) frequency words was associated with more change in treated and untreated speech sounds within and across sound classes. They added that words from high-density neighborhoods may need to be avoided, as generalization is to be induced. More recent research partly contradicted reports about neighborhood density, as Gierut and Morrisette (2012b) suggest that "frequent words from dense neighborhoods" were "optimal for generalization" (p. 804). Further research is needed to unravel the relationships between lexical characteristics and phonological learning (Baker, 2015).

Source: Adapted from Gierut (2001, 2007).

> **COMMENT:** *Relationships between phonological and lexical characteristics in intervention*
>
> Words are part of the lexical system, and like phonemes, they have a complexity status. Four different yet related lexical characteristics have been studied: age of acquisition, lexicality (i.e., nonwords versus real words), neighborhood density, and word frequency (e.g., Bellon-Harn, Credeur-Pampolina, & LeBoeuf, 2013; Cummings & Barlow, 2011; Gierut & Morrisette, 2010, 2012a, b; Gierut, Morrisette, & Champion, 1999; Gierut, Morrisette & Ziemer, 2010; Morrisette & Gierut, 2002). Although high-frequency words are thought to be better for facilitating phonological change in intervention compared to low-frequency words (Morrisette & Gierut, 2002), nonwords (by definition, low-frequency words) have been reported to be better than real words (Gierut & Morrisette, 2010). Later acquired words have also been reported to be better than earlier acquired words for facilitating phonological change (Gierut & Morrisette, 2012a). Further research is needed to clarify the individual and combined effects of lexical characteristics on phonological learning. Until such time, if an intervention approaches calls for real words, consider using high-frequency words from both high- and low-density neighborhoods.

APPLICATION: *Short-term goals for Luke from a complexity perspective*

Write a series of short-term goals for Luke from a complexity perspective. Your short-term goals might target complex singleton consonants such as an obstruent /tʃ/ and sonorant /l/ via treatment of the empty set intervention. (You will learn more about this intervention approach in Chapter 13.) Alternatively, you might prioritize consonant clusters with small sonority difference scores in an effort to expand Luke's phonetic and phonemic inventories. A third option could be to target the elimination of the phonological processes evident in Luke's speech, beginning with phonological processes that are more complex and later to disappear in typical development.

Who is suited to the complexity approach?

The complexity approach is potentially suitable for most, if not all, children who have SSD. Some commentators have suggested that the approach is more suited to children who have no confounding difficulties and appear to be confident risk-takers (Bernhardt, Stemberger, & Major 2006), or have no concomitant cognitive or attention limitations (Bleile, 1996). The intervention research on the approach has also focused on segmental rather than word-length and prosodic difficulties (e.g., Gierut, 1992), suggesting that children with small phonetic inventories only, as opposed to small phonetic *and* syllable structure, stress, and word length inventories, may be more suited to this target selection approach. The children involved in the published research on the approach have also had typical receptive language and no other concomitant difficulties (e.g., Gierut, 1999).

■ Cycles approach to target selection

The cycles approach to target selection is one aspect of Hodson and Paden's unique Cycles Phonological Remediation Approach for treating severe to profound phonological impairment in children (Hodson & Paden, 1983, 1991; Hodson, 2006, 2007) (see Chapter 13). As part of the cycles approach, patterns (or processes) evident in children's speech are identified then targeted in a predetermined order, with primary target patterns being selected prior to secondary target patterns, which are in turn selected prior to advanced target patterns.

What are cycles intervention targets?

There are three types of cycles-based targets: primary, secondary, and advanced patterns. Primary patterns are listed in Table 10-2. These patterns are targeted first. The actual sequence of primary patterns targeted for an individual child is dependent on the patterns exhibited by the child following a comprehensive phonological analysis. Of the patterns present in a child's speech, intervention begins with patterns that show a readiness to change (Hodson, 2007). In this context, readiness refers to stimulability or ease with which a child can produce an intervention target associated with a pattern and can achieve the most immediate success. Subsequent primary target patterns are prioritized in a similar fashion—according to their stimulability (or readiness) status. Secondary target patterns are only targeted once children meet predetermined criteria. Specifically, Hodson (2007) suggests that children must produce syllables and basic word structures, anterior-posterior contrasts, and show signs of stridency in conversational speech before starting on secondary target patterns. In addition, children must have the ability to produce a liquid (e.g., /l/) at least within production practice words. Advanced target patterns are targeted in children above the age of 8 years who experience difficulty with complex multisyllabic words and complex sequences. As shown in Table 10-2, Hodson (2007) also suggests that some patterns are inappropriate intervention targets for preschool children (e.g., targeting weak syllable deletion in multisyllabic words).

Unlike most other approaches to target selection, performance-based criteria for a treated target are not needed to move onto another target. Rather, a time-based criterion applies whereby each stimulable phoneme within a pattern is targeted for 60 minutes (e.g., one 60-minute session, two 30-minute sessions), with most patterns being targeted for 2 to 6 hours (Hodson, 2007). You will learn more about these different aspects of service delivery in Chapter 11. The total duration of a cycle (period of time in which phonological patterns are targeted) depends on the number of phonemes within the number of patterns

---

TABLE 10-2 **Prioritization of primary, secondary, and advanced target patterns for intervention, according to Hodson's cycles approach**

Pattern type	Pattern subtypes
Primary target patterns	1. Word structures (two-syllable and three-syllable word combinations and singleton consonants within CV, VC, CVC, VCV shapes) 2. /s/ clusters (e.g., initial /sp, st, sm/ and final /ts, ps/) 3. Anterior-posterior contrasts (e.g., word-final and word-initial /k/, initial /h/, alveolars/labials for "backers") 4. Liquids (e.g., word-initial /l, ɹ/, /word-initial /kɹ, gɹ/ once the child produces singleton velars, word-initial /l/ clusters once the child produces prevocalic /l/)
Secondary target patterns	1. Palatals (e.g., glide /j/, postalveolar sibilants /ʃ, ʒ, tʃ, dʒ/ identified as palatals by Hodson, 2007), vocalic /ɝ, ɚ/ (unless dialectal), and medial /ɹ/ 2. Other consonant sequences (e.g., /s/ + C in medial and final position, CC containing sonorants including glides such as /kw, gj/ and liquids such as /pr, bl/, three-element clusters such as /spl, stɹ/) 3. Singleton stridents (e.g., /f, s/) 4. Prevocalic voicing 5. Non-dialectal vowel contrasts 6. Assimilations 7. Any remaining idiosyncratic deviations
Advanced target patterns	1. Complex multisyllabic words (e.g., *thermometer, hippopotamus, rhinoceros*) 2. Complex consonant sequences (e.g., *strengths, excuse, extra*)
Inappropriate targets for preschool children	1. Voiced word-final obstruents (e.g., /d/ in *bed*) 2. Postvocalic/syllabic /l/ (e.g., *ball, apple, doll*) 3. Word-final /ŋ/ (e.g., *going, doing, coming*) 4. /θ, ð/ (e.g., *earth, with*) 5. Unstressed (weak) syllables (e.g., *refrigerator*)

Source: Adapted from Hodson (2007).

to be targeted for intervention. The only instance when performance-based criteria do apply is the transition from primary to secondary target patterns.

The gradual acquisition of speech sounds, syllable/word shapes, and stress patterns in typically developing children underlies the basic premise of cycling intervention targets (Hodson, 2006). Although there is empirical evidence supporting the efficacy of a modified format of the cycles approach (e.g., Almost & Rosenbaum, 1998), in conjunction with numerous case-study reports (e.g., Hodson, Nonomura, & Zappia, 1989), there has been little research investigating the primary versus secondary versus advanced order in which intervention targets are cycled. Furthermore, it is unknown whether the exclusion of particular intervention targets for preschoolers is efficacious. For instance, Hodson (2007) does not recommend targeting weak syllable deletion in preschool children. However, acquisition research suggests that typically developing children have the ability to produce weak syllables during the preschool years. Indeed, Kehoe (2001) suggests that the deletion of stressed syllables is infrequent from 2 years of age, and that the deletion of unstressed syllables is less frequent from 3 years of age. Moreover, Kehoe suggests that ongoing syllable deletion in children aged 3½ years or older age may be a sign of prosodic difficulties. Given the relationship between difficulty with polysyllable production and literacy difficulties (James, Van Doorn, & McLeod, 2008), exclusion of potential intervention targets such as the deletion of weak syllables for preschoolers is questionable. Although the cycles approach (as an intervention package that includes the cyclical target selection of primary patterns followed by secondary patterns and then advanced patterns) has empirical support, it would seem that further research is needed to support some of the specific recommended target selection guidelines.

Who is suited to the cycles approach?

Hodson's (2007) cycles approach to target selection is suitable for all children who have SSD characterized by:

1. primary target patterns (e.g., word structures; anterior-posterior contrasts; reduction of /s/ consonant clusters such as initial /sp, st, sm/ and final /ts, ps/);
2. secondary target patterns (e.g., difficulty with palatals; prevocalic voicing; assimilation); and
3. advanced target patterns (e.g., deletion of syllables in complex multisyllabic words).

■ Systemic (functional) approach to target selection

The systemic or functional approach to target selection, developed by Williams (2003), considers the function of sounds within children's phonological systems as opposed to the characteristics of individual sounds. The approach emerged out of Williams' work on the Systemic Phonological Analysis of Child Speech (SPACS, Williams, 2003, 2005c) and the multiple opposition intervention approach (Williams, 2000a,b, 2005b).

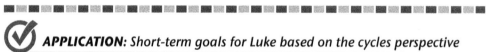

✓ *APPLICATION: Short-term goals for Luke based on the cycles perspective*

Write short-term goals for Luke in keeping with Hodson's (2007) cycles approach. To do this, you need to identify the primary, secondary, and advanced phonological patterns evident in Luke's speech. Use Luke's speech samples in Chapter 16 and Table 10-2, listing the phonological patterns, as a guide. An example goal cycles goal for Luke would be: "Luke will produce appropriate anterior and posterior contrasts (specifically /k/ versus /t/, and /g/ versus /d/ and /h/) in initial position in words during 10 minutes of conversational speech with the clinician in the clinic, with 70% accuracy." Note, although you could order Luke's short-term goals into primary, second, and advanced, the final order for targeting each pattern within a group (particularly the order for targeting all relevant primary patterns) will be dependent on Luke's stimulability and readiness from one session to the next.

What are systemic intervention targets?

The systemic approach is unique in that a specific sound is not targeted. Rather, the phonological function of a carefully selected group of sounds is targeted. The group of sounds is identified from a child's collapse of contrast (Williams, 2005b). In Chapter 9, we identified Luke's limited contrastive system. He realized words beginning with the following phonemes /t, k, g, θ, ð, s, z, ʃ, tʃ, dʒ, tw, tɹ, dɹ, θɹ, sw, sl, st, sk, stɹ, skw, skɹ, ʃɹ, kw, kl, gl, kɹ, gɹ, kj/ as [d], equivalent to 28 phonemes being realized as one phoneme. This means that words like *core, tore, sore, store, score, shore, chore, jaw* would all be pronounced as *door*. When a child collapses several phonemes to one sound, not all are selected for intervention. Rather, Williams (2005b) suggests that a distance metric incorporating the two parameters of maximal classification and maximal distinction are used to select three or four targets. According to Williams (2005b), "maximal classification involves selection of sound members from different manner classes, different places of production, and different voicing," and maximal distinction refers to the "selection of target sounds that are maximally distinct from the child's error in terms of place, voice, manner and linguistic unit (singleton versus cluster)" (pp. 103–104). In Luke's case, maximally classified and maximally distinct targets to contrast with [d] could be [k, tʃ, sl, ʃ]. Between /d/ and the four selected phonemes, there is:

- a voice [d] versus voiceless [k, tʃ, ʃ] distinction;
- contrasting places of articulation including alveolar [d, sl], postalveolar [ʃ, tʃ], and velar [k];
- contrasting manners of articulation including plosive [d, k], fricative [sl, ʃ], and affricate [tʃ]; and
- contrasting linguistic units including singletons [d, k, tʃ, ʃ] and a consonant cluster [sl].

In doing so, the systemic approach moves aside from the debate between developmental versus complex targets, as the stimulability status, developmental order, markedness, and phonological knowledge (most or least) of potential targets is not considered (although, the final group of sounds may contain stimulable and/or non-stimulable sounds, early and/or later developing sounds, and sounds associated with most or least phonological knowledge for an individual child) (Williams, 2005b). The ultimate goal of selecting multiple targets that are maximally different from each other and different from the child's substituted sound is to induce phonemic contrasts in the child's system and reduce the homonymy (Williams, 2000b).

Who is suited to the systemic approach?

The systemic approach is most suited to children who have large collapses of contrast in their phonological system. That is, they may use one consonant in the place of many different consonants. You will find that children with moderate or severe phonological impairment who have relatively good syllable structures but limited phonetic inventories have collapses of contrast.

 APPLICATION: *Short-term goals for Luke based on the systemic approach*

Write a series of short-term goals for Luke (4;3 years) using Williams' (2003) systemic approach for targeting multiple collapses of contrast. Luke would seem to be a particularly ideal candidate for this approach given his large collapses of contrast, particularly to /d/ in word-initial position. To complete this exercise, review Luke's CHIRPA analysis in Chapter 9 and the example short-term goal for his largest collapse earlier in this chapter. Identify each phoneme collapse in word-initial and word-final positions as a short-term goal. Over the course of intervention you might not need to target some of the small collapses, because intervention on the larger collapse should hopefully generalize and develop the contrasts in his system.

■ Constraint-based nonlinear approach to target selection

Historically, SLPs have focused on the selection and treatment of speech sounds for children with SSD (Velleman, 2002). Some of the target selection approaches reviewed in this chapter (e.g., developmental approach, complexity approach, systemic approach) reflect this focus. According to Velleman (2002), speech sounds serve as the content of spoken words. Velleman argues that the frame (word and syllable structures, timing units, stress patterns) within which consonants and vowels are placed has received relatively less attention. Bernhardt and colleagues (e.g., Bernhardt, 2003, 2005; Bernhardt & Stemberger, 2000; Bernhardt, Bopp, Daudlin, Edwards, & Wastie, 2010) advocate an alternative approach to target selection founded on the theoretical principles of constraint-based nonlinear phonology.

What are constraint-based nonlinear intervention targets?

Unlike the target selection approaches that focus on which sound(s) to select, Bernhardt and Stemberger (2000) consider the content and frame of a child's phonological system for target selection. Chapter 5 provided a brief introduction to some of the key theoretical concepts associated with **constraint-based nonlinear phonology**. Briefly, Bernhardt and Stemberger (2000) use a collection of nonlinear theories to guide the analysis of children's speech to identify:

- what a child knows about the phonological system, according two hierarchically arranged tiers: **segmental tier** (i.e., sounds segments and features) and **prosodic tier** (i.e., phrase stress and intonation, word length, word stress, word shape/sequences);
- how a child's knowledge of each tier interacts between tiers; and
- what phonological knowledge is missing that a child still needs to learn.

Bernhardt and Stemberger (2000) suggest that you organize this information into a framework of four goal types, specifically:

1. **New word and phrase structures**, including:
   (a) **phrasal stress and intonation**, such as producing unstressed grammatical morphemes in phrases or using appropriate intonation chunking in phrases (e.g., "chocolate cake and apple pie" versus "chocolate, cake, and apple pie");
   (b) **word lengths**, such as producing di- and polysyllabic words (e.g., from *but* to *butter* and then *buttercup*);
   (c) **word stress patterns**, such as producing words with weak onsets (e.g., wS in *giraffe*, and wSs in *potato*) or using a variety of lexical stress patterns (e.g., Sws, Ssw, Sww, wS, wSw, wSs); and
   (d) **word shapes** involving consonant and vowel sequences, such as producing final consonants (e.g., *bus* /bʌs/) or consonant clusters (e.g., *sleep* /slip/).
2. **New segments involving new features** such as new manners or places of articulation that a child has never produced (e.g., producing velar consonants identified as absent from a phonetic inventory).
3. **New combinations of existing features** to create new segments (e.g., if a child only uses labiodental fricatives [f, v], combining the fricative feature of the labiodental fricative [f] with the place feature of the voiceless alveolar plosive [t] to introduce the voiceless alveolar fricative [s]).
4. **New sequences of structures and segments**, such as learning to use a known feature in a new word position (e.g., copying word-final velars to word-initial position) or in a new sequence (e.g., copying word-final /st, sp/ clusters to word-initial position; learning to produce consonant clusters with different place sequences such as [pɹ, gl, fl] rather than being constrained to one place of articulation for all consonants in cluster sequences such as [pw, fw]).

Bernhardt and colleagues (e.g., Baker & Bernhardt, 2004; Bernhardt, 2003, 2005; Bernhardt & Major, 2005; Bernhardt & Stemberger, 2000; Major & Bernhardt, 1998) provide a series of guiding principles for prioritizing nonlinear goals. First, new features or segments are targeted using established word structures, and new word structures are targeted using established segments. In this way, a child's strengths support the development of his or her areas of difficulty. In a follow-up of a nonlinear phonological intervention study of 19 children, Bernhardt and Major (2005, p. 24) reported that "when a child was not immediately stimulable for a structure or segment, shaping from an existing structure or segment was used to approximate the new target." Second, selection of a goal or target from each of the four categories is recommended within intervention blocks that use a cyclical-goal attack strategy. (You will learn more about goal attack strategies later in this chapter.) Third, while non-default marked goals are preferred, Bernhardt (2005) stipulates that other factors such as **cognitive-linguistic**, **personal-social**, **perceptual**, and **articulatory** abilities are important to consider when planning goal selection. For example, Bernhardt (2005) described how challenging non-default targets (consonant clusters rather than singletons) were prioritized for two children (Brandy, 3 years, and Bill, 5 years) during their first block of intervention. In an effort to facilitate their relatively slow progress, Bernhardt considered negative personal-social factors (lack of motivation and confidence) when prioritizing goals for their second block of intervention. So in the second block of intervention Bernhardt (2005) selected more attainable, less challenging, less marked targets so as to facilitate more immediate success and bolster the children's confidence. Having achieved success, the more challenging targets were re-trialed. Fourth, consider selecting targets that would enhance a child's speech intelligibility (Bernhardt & Stemberger, 2000). Finally, consider selecting more than one exemplar for each goal type. For example, Bernhardt and Major (2005) suggest that if targeting the feature [+ **continuant**], then two or three fricatives contrasting in voice and place characteristics should be selected. If targeting the word shape CCVC, then a variety of consonant clusters incorporating segments a child already can produce should be selected (e.g., /tw, bj, kw/). If you would like to extend your knowledge in this area, Bernhardt and Stemberger (2000) provide a detailed account of constraint-based nonlinear analysis and goal selection. Online tutorials on nonlinear target selection are also available.[2]

 APPLICATION: *Short-term goals for Luke based on constraint-based nonlinear perspective*

Write a series of short-term goals for Luke (4;3 years) using Bernhardt and Stemberger's (2000) constraint-based nonlinear phonology perspective. To begin this exercise, review your findings from your CHIRPA analysis in Chapter 9. Consider what (if anything) Luke needs to learn about each of the potential four goal types: (1) new word and phrase structure, (2) new segments using new features, (3) new segments using combinations of existing features, and (4) new sequences of structures and segments. You could refer to Bernhardt and Stemberger (2000) and use their Nonlinear Scan Analysis Form to complete this exercise.

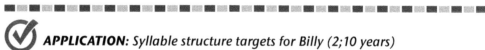 **APPLICATION:** *Syllable structure targets for Billy (2;10 years)*

Billy (2;10 years) articulates the following words correctly: *mommy, daddy, puppy, nanny, poppy, dinner, Wippy* (his dog). By contrast, Billy says *potty* as [pɒ:], *beanie* as [bibi], *tummy* as [ta], and *water* as [wʌwʌ].

1. What pattern best describes Billy's ability to produce CVCV words?

   Answer: Billy's production of CVCV is limited to the consonant sequences involving the same place of articulation. He can produce different manners of articulation, as long as the two consonants belong to the same place.

2. In light of Billy's sequencing constraint, write a specific goal that targets Billy's CVCV constraint.

---

[2]http//:phonodevelopment.sites.olt.ubc.ca

Who is suited to the constraint-based nonlinear approach?

The constraint-based nonlinear approach is suitable for most if not all children who have an SSD, whether they have segmental or prosodic difficulties. Bernhardt, Stemberger, and Major (2006) suggest that more complex segmental and/or prosodic targets could be prioritized for intervention with children who have good language skills and are described as confident risk-takers.

■ Neuro-network approach to target selection

According to Norris and Hoffman (2005), phonology is an integral component of the language system. A child with a phonological impairment therefore does not present with individualized phonological problems to be targeted but rather a system or network that can be facilitated to induce change in a child's phonological ability.

What are neuro-network intervention targets?

The neuro-network approach to target selection contrasts with the other approaches described in this chapter in that specific targets such as velars or consonant clusters are not selected. Instead, more general goals are identified, such as increase a child's PCC in conversational speech or add six new phonemes to a child's phonemic inventory (Norris & Hoffman, 2005). The only time in which specific targets may be identified is when a child has residual distortion errors of later developing phonemes such as /s/ or /ɹ/ (Norris & Hoffman, 2005). In such cases, the targets are obvious and prioritization of one target over another would seem to be irrelevant. For children with moderate or more severe phonological difficulties, the rationale underlying a long-term goal (as opposed to short-term intervention target) is based on Norris and Hoffman's (2005) constellation model of language processing.

    The constellation model of language processing includes nine different levels of processing (e.g., referential units or words, auditory and visual perceptual features that make up words, categorical units comprising the phonemes that make up spoken words and the letters that make up written words, canonical units comprising the auditory sequence of consonants and vowels that make up spoken words). All the levels interact with one another by receiving and sending input to all other levels, assimilating new input within a level, and accommodating this new input throughout all levels within the constellation system over time (Norris & Hoffman, 2005). This process of assimilating and accommodating new input has been described as self-organization of the neuro-network. Phonological change such as the addition of a new phoneme takes place through facilitating the system as a whole. According to Norris and Hoffman (2005),

> because the system will naturally reorganize itself to more closely approximate input received from the environment, it is unnecessary for the intervention to select target phonemes or control the stimuli to focus on specific phonemes when the child's inventory of correct productions is small. (p. 78)

Intervention based on the principles of language processing and self-organizing networks induces change in a child's phonological system, making specific target selection from the outset of intervention inappropriate.

Who is suited to the neuro-network approach?

The neuro-network approach could be suitable for children with concomitant speech and language difficulties. Given the limited comparison research on the approach, you would need to gather your own evidence and compare it with other options for children with concomitant speech and language difficulties, such as targeting specific speech and language skills using an alternating goal attack strategy (e.g., Tyler, Lewis, Haskill, & Tolbert, 2003).

> **COMMENT:** *Which target selection approach is the best for children with phonological impairment?*
>
> There are no quick and easy answers to this question. In Tyler's (2005b) reflection on her approach to target selection and intervention for children with phonological impairment, she remarked, "my initial focus on error patterns reflects my early training in natural phonological theory and phonological processes; however, my target selection approach is both developmental and complexity based, reflecting my consideration of constraint-based theory and complexity in learning" (p. 68). As an SLP engaging in EBP, integrate peer-reviewed published evidence with child characteristics and preferences. Think about what you know about the child with respect to his or her personal and social contexts as well as language, cognitive, perceptual, and motor abilities as you prioritize goals (Bernhardt, 2005). Remember, you are working with a real child in that child's context, not rearranging a phonological system through a computer.

GOAL SETTING FOR CHILDREN WITH ARTICULATION IMPAIRMENT

The goals you identify for children with articulation impairment typically involve (1) target sounds and (2) activities and participation. The identification and selection of the target sound(s) is usually straightforward. If a child presents with an incorrect production of a particular sound, then that is the sound to be targeted. Typically, articulation goals focus on rhotics and/or sibilants. When more than one sound or pair of cognates (e.g., /s, z/) is in error, Gordon-Brannan and Weiss (2007) suggest that the sound(s) selected should ideally be correct in one or more phonetic contexts, be the most stimulable, be relatively earlier in development, motivating for a child to practice, and have the potential to impact speech intelligibility. You would also consider the views (and needs) expressed by a child and his or her family, and the impact of the child's articulation difficulty on his or her Activities and Participation.

APPLICATION: *Short-term goals for Susie's articulation impairment*

Earlier in this chapter you wrote a long-term goal for Susie. Draft a short-term goal for Susie, targeting her production of /s/ and /z/ in non-treatment words, as measured by a single-word generalization probe and two 10-minute samples of conversational speech collected. As you draft the goal, consider the following questions:

- How many and what types of words will you sample in your single-word probe?
- What word positions will you examine in the single-word probe and conversational speech?
- What will be the performance criterion for the single-word probe and the sample of conversational speech?
- Who will administer the single-word generalization probe?
- Who will collect the conversational speech samples?

Hint: The samples could be collected by an SLP and parent/caregiver to consider both stimulus and response generalization.

Review your short-term goal once you have finished reading Chapter 14 on intervention approaches suitable for children like Susie.

■ ■

 APPLICATION: *Short-term goals for Jarrod's inconsistent speech disorder*

Earlier in this chapter you wrote long-term goals for Jarrod. Ideally, one of these goals should focus on Jarrod's speech—that he needs to be intelligible and have lexically consistent productions during conversation with a variety of speakers in a variety of speaking environments. (Your goal would of course contain more details about how you will determine if this has been achieved). Draft a short-term goal for Jarrod specifically targeting lexical consistency, as measured using a single-word probe of non-treatment words. Remember to note your performance criteria, the number of words in the single-word probe, and who will administer the probe. Review your short-term goal once you have read about core vocabulary intervention for children with inconsistent speech disorder (in Chapter 13).

Read more about Jarrod (7;0 years), a boy with inconsistent speech disorder, in Chapter 16 (Case 3).

■ Goal setting for children with inconsistent speech disorder

Children with inconsistent speech disorder require a unique approach to target selection. Given that a feature of their difficulty is inconsistent productions of the same lexical item, selecting specific consonants, syllable shapes, word lengths, or stress patterns is not appropriate. Children with inconsistent speech disorder need to learn how to say a word in the same way each time it is said (Dodd, Holm, Crosbie, & McIntosh, 2010). As discussed in Chapters 8 and 9, if you have completed an in-depth analysis of a child's speech sample and your assessment reveals a score of at least 40% inconsistency on the Inconsistency subtest of the Diagnostic Evaluation of Articulation and Phonology (Dodd, Hua, et al., 2002, 2006), then your intervention goal will be to establish lexical consistency. Your target will be consistent productions of a core vocabulary of words, selected by the child and his or her family in collaboration with the child's SLP and teacher. Additional goals addressing Activities and Participation and Contextual Factors should be identified and addressed on a case-by-case basis.

■ Goal setting for children with CAS

Goal setting for children with CAS depends on a number of factors: the child's age, the nature and severity of the child's impairment, presence of concomitant conditions, and motivation. You might have a broad range of goals addressing speech intelligibility in addition to Activity and Participation. In this section we will focus on target selection for improving speech intelligibility, knowing that what you work on could in fact be influenced by what a child needs to say in everyday conversation to participate in day-to-day activities.

Intervention targets for children with CAS

The targets that you select for children with CAS differ from those you would select for a child with phonological impairment because of the inherent differences underlying the two problems (see Chapter 2 for further information). Although the long-term goals will be similar (e.g., the child will develop functional and intelligible communication based on a period of conversation with specified communication partners in specified contexts in a designated period of time, as measured by a specified functional communication outcome measurement tool), the nature of what you target and how you work on those targets varies.

For children with CAS, their difficulty is typified by "(a) inconsistent errors on consonants and vowels in repeated productions of syllables or words, (b) lengthened and disrupted coarticulatory transitions between sounds and syllables, and (c) inappropriate prosody, especially in the realization of lexical or phrasal stress" (American Speech-Language-Hearing Association, 2007b, p. 4). Intervention therefore needs to target these three areas of difficulty, knowing that they are related to an underlying difficulty with planning, programming, and executing sequential movement gestures (Strand & Skinder, 1999). As Fish (2011) points out, "children with CAS demonstrate challenges with phoneme sequencing due to their difficulty establishing an initial articulatory gesture and then transitioning smoothly into the next articulatory gesture" (p. 57). They need to practice "movement transitions, in the context of speech" (Yorkston et al., 2010, p. 387). As part of this problem, they also need to develop appropriate intonation and prosody. What might intervention targets look like, then, for a child with CAS?

Intervention goals for young children with CAS: Establishing phonetic inventories and basic movement sequences

For young children with limited speech (particularly limited syllable structure and segments), short-term goals might be to establish movement sequences involving simple syllables such as CV and VC, and simple (meaningful) two- and three-word phrases (Strand & Skinder, 1999). Velleman (2003) offers a helpful hierarchy of phonotactic (i.e., syllable and word shape) difficulty to guide your target selection for young children with CAS. It includes:

- simple CV open syllables beginning with glides for a child who has no true consonants (e.g., *hi, yeah, whee!*) followed by other sonorants and obstruents (e.g., *more, no, me, see*);
- complete replicated open syllables (e.g., *bye bye; baa baa*);
- partially reduplicated open syllables involving either consonant harmony with different vowels (e.g., *mommy, daddy, baby*) or vowel harmony with different consonants (e.g., *beanie, TV*);
- non-reduplication forms with no harmony/assimilation (e.g., *teddy, honey, kitty, happy, funny, pillow*);
- harmonized closed monosyllable CVC where the first and last consonant is the same (e.g., *mom, dad, pop, pup, bib*);
- non-harmonized closed syllables CVC where the consonants are different (e.g., *cat, dog, bed, look*);
- CVCVC words including words with the same consonants and vowels, different consonants, different vowels, and different consonants and vowels (e.g., *button, donut, sausage*); and
- words with consonant clusters beginning with open syllables, such as VCC (e.g., *ant, and, ask*) and CCV (e.g., *play, blue, fly*) to closed syllables such as CVCC (e.g., *hand, jump, toast*) and CCVC (e.g., *sleep, spoon, black*) and then medial clusters (e.g., *monster, handstand*).

Williams and Stephens (2010) suggest a similar developmental approach, starting with "CV words, followed by CVCV words, CVC words, multisyllabic words, consonant cluster words, phrases and sentences" (Williams & Stephens, 2010, p. 161). Williams and Stephens (2010) also suggest that you could start with sounds in isolation, although other authors recommend that you start with syllables, because "although there are anecdotal reports that it is easier for children with apraxia to learn sounds in isolation, this does not appear to carry over to the use of the same sounds in syllables and words" and is therefore "not the best use of therapy time" (Velleman, 2003, p. 54).

COMMENT: *Targets and stimuli for young children with CAS*

Given that young children with CAS can be frustrated by their unsuccessful attempts to communicate, Strand and Skinder (1999) suggest that meaningful and communicatively powerful words be selected as stimuli to address your intervention targets, because they can help increase a child's motivation. In Chapter 14 we address this need to carefully consider the stimuli that you use during intervention to target speech production goals for children with CAS.

■ ■■ ■■ ■■ ■■ ■ ■■ ■■ ■ ■■ ■ ■ ■■ ■ ■■ ■ ■ ■■ ■ ■ ■■ ■ ■ ■ ■■ ■ ■ ■ ■ ■■ ■ ■■ ■ ■ ■ ■

 APPLICATION: *Goals for Naomi (2;11 years)*

Naomi (2;11 years) has suspected CAS. Based on an independent and relational analysis of a conversational speech sample, Naomi's phonetic repertoire includes the consonants [d, n, h, w] and vowels [i, ɑ, ʌ], and the syllable structure CV. Naomi's mother reported that Naomi was quiet as a baby and late to talk. It was difficult to determine how many words Naomi has because of her limited intelligibility. Naomi also has difficulty initiating speech motor movements. A long-term goal for Naomi could be to speak clearly and communicate independently in a variety of situations with a variety of communication partners (including family, friends, and unfamiliar adults) as measured by the Focus on Communication Outcomes Under Six (FOCUS) outcome measure (Thomas-Stonell, Robertson, Walker, Oddson, Washington, & Rosenbaum, 2012), as completed by Naomi's parents, within approximately 2 years of starting intervention. Your task is to identify and generate beginning short-term goals for Naomi.

Possible beginning short-term goals:

■ Naomi will expand her phonetic inventory to include two new consonants [m, b] and the vowels [u] and [o] in V and CV syllables in real words (e.g., *me, ma, bee, baa, oh!, no, dough, moo!*) during 10 minutes of conversational speech, and a 12-item single-word generalization probe with the clinician in the clinic with 70% accuracy.

■ Naomi will learn to plan and produce movement sequences comprising two-syllable words using the syllable shape CVCV using known consonants [d, n, h, w] and developing consonants [m, b] in words with natural speech rate and prosody (i.e., no evidence of syllable segregation), during 10 minutes of conversational speech, in the clinic with the clinician and at home with parent/caregiver, with 70% accuracy.

Note: Your session goals could begin with CVCV words involving complete reduplicated open syllables (e.g., [nɑnɑ] for *banana, mama*) followed by partially reduplicated open syllables with either consonant harmony (e.g., *mommy, bobby*) or vowel harmony, then finally non-reduplication forms with no harmony/assimilation (e.g., *honey, bunny, money, beanie*).

Intervention goals for children with CAS: Increase word length, develop lexical stress, smooth transitions, and use appropriate intonation

Children with CAS can vary in their clinical presentation. For some children you will need to focus on consonants and vowels in simple syllable structures. For other children, your short-term goals will focus on more complex aspects of speech such as:

■ increasing word lengths from monosyllables to di- and polysyllables comprising a variety of lexical stress patterns;

■ developing accurate lexical stress, marking natural contrasts between Sw and wS stress patterns in words;

■ developing natural sentence stress in everyday conversation, eliminating excessive, equal, or misplaced stress in sentences and everyday conversational speech;

■ developing emphatic stress needed to emphasize a point or to contrast a word in an utterance with a prior utterance;

■ producing utterances with smooth transitions between syllables in words, and smooth transitions between words in phrases (i.e., eliminating syllable segregation);

■ using a natural speech rate during a period of conversational speech; and

■ using intonation appropriately, with respect to chunking, affect, interaction, and focus (Wells & Peppé, 2001).

These goals could be identified using your analysis of the child's suprasegmental skills. See Chapter 9 for further information.

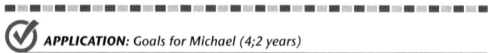

 APPLICATION: *Goals for Michael (4;2 years)*

Read more about Michael (4;2 years), a boy with childhood apraxia of speech (CAS), in Chapter 16 (Case 4).

Michael (4;2 years) has CAS. As shown in Table 16-15, the syllables that comprised Michael's attempted production of polysyllables were strong and equally timed, with evidence of segregation. Words beginning with weak onset syllables were particularly challenging. Although Michael's phonetic inventory was almost complete, his articulation accuracy during polysyllables was also reduced. Write a short-term goal for Michael targeting his production of two- and three-syllable words with weak onset stress and smooth transitions between syllables.

 APPLICATION: *Goals for Lian (14;2 years)*

Read more about Lian (14;2 years), a girl with childhood dysarthria, in Chapter 16 (Case 5).

Lian (14;2 years) has spastic dysarthria. As shown in Tables 16-17 and 16-18, one area of difficulty for Lian is her imprecise articulation of the affricates /tʃ, dʒ/.

1. Write a short-term goal for Lian targeting her production of these two consonants.
2. Identify another area of need from the assessment and translate that into a measurable and achievable goal.

■ Goal setting for children with childhood dysarthria

The goals you establish for children with childhood dysarthria will be highly dependent on the type and severity of their dysarthria and the presence of concomitant conditions. In this book we use the systems approach (e.g., Pennington, Miller, Robson, & Steen, 2010) to guide assessment, analysis, goals, and intervention. Briefly, based on your assessment you will have identified areas of difficulty for a child associated with one or more speech subsystems: articulation, phonation, resonance, and respiration. Based on these four subsystems, common generic short-term goals for children with childhood dysarthria who have the potential to use spoken communication include:

- improve articulation accuracy of problematic consonants and/or vowels, syllable shapes, or word lengths;
- encourage respiratory support and breath control for speech, therefore improving speech intelligibility;
- reduce hypernasality; and
- increase the naturalness of a child's phonation through increasing a child's awareness of and use of appropriate pitch and vocal loudness. (Note: Loudness could in part be addressed via goals targeting respiration, as a breathy voice quality can be symptomatic of a difficulty managing the demands of speech breathing.)

GOAL SETTING CONSIDERATIONS FOR CHILDREN WITH HIGHLY UNINTELLIGIBLE SPEECH

The goals that you identify for children who have highly unintelligible speech, whether due to phonological impairment, inconsistency, CAS, or childhood dysarthria, need to be a combination of both impairment-based and socially based goals. The impairment-based goals may target any one of a number of areas of speech (e.g., segments, syllable structure, prosody, word stress, phrase stress, sentence stress, juncture in connected speech) (Velleman, 2003). Given the impact of severe motor speech disorders on children's activities and participation, socially based goals may need to take precedence in order to get a child communicating and reduce the child's day-to-day frustration from not being understood. For example, goals for a child with highly unintelligible speech could include:

- teaching the child to use an alternative or augmentative form of communication (e.g., gesture, sign, electronic communication device) as a bridging step to supplement speech,
- targeting the child's speech intelligibility of a small vocabulary of phonologically simple, meaningful words (e.g., *no, yes, bye, mine, more*, the child's name, names of significant others), and
- teaching others in the child's environment to understand the child's productions (cf. McCormack, McLeod, Harrison, & McAllister, 2010).

Obviously, the social goals for children with highly unintelligible speech need to be generated by the children and their families, with your support.

GOAL ATTACK STRATEGIES

Having identified potentially suitable intervention targets and prioritized the order in which selected targets will be worked on, you need to think through one more decision with respect to goal setting. You need to schedule the goals. According to Tyler, Lewis, Haskill, and Tolbert (2003), the way in which multiple goals are scheduled is known as the goal attack strategy. Fey (1986) proposed three contrasting goal attack strategies, including:

1. vertical
2. horizontal
3. cyclical

A **vertical goal attack strategy** typically involves the targeting of one or two speech targets (e.g., phonemes, phonological processes, word shapes, stress patterns, prosodic pattern) at a time. The target is worked on until a predetermined performance criterion is met. Elbert and Gierut (1986) refer to this strategy as **training deep**. A vertical goal attack strategy is often recommended for children who have an articulation impairment characterized by one or two speech sounds in error. It can also be used with children who have a phonological impairment (e.g., Powell, 1991; Tyler, 1995). The vertical goal attack strategy simply provides a child with multiple opportunities to learn one or two targets over a period of time before learning additional targets.

A **horizontal goal attack strategy** involves working on several speech production targets within a session (Tyler, Lewis, Haskill, & Tolbert, 2003). Elbert and Gierut (1986) describe this approach as **training wide**. According to Bleile (2004), the opportunity to work on three or more targets per session helps children with a phonological impairment to discover the relationships among the targets in the phonological system they are trying to learn. For children with motor speech difficulties, a horizontal goal attack strategy may enhance motor learning (Maas et al., 2008).

The **cyclical goal attack strategy** involves working on several speech production targets within a specified period of time, independent of accuracy (Tyler, Lewis, Haskill, & Tolbert, 2003). The approach was developed by Hodson and Paden (1991) as part of their unique cycles approach to phonological intervention (discussed in Chapter 13). Like the vertical approach, one speech production target or phonological process or pattern is targeted per session. However, unlike the vertical approach, the selected target or phonological process is targeted for a limited period of time (e.g., 2 to 6 hours) rather than until a predetermined performance criterion is met (Hodson, 2007). The cyclical goal attack strategy has been used successfully as part of the cycles approach to intervention (e.g., Almost & Rosenbaum, 1998; Mota, Keske-Soares, Bagetti, Ceron, & Filha, 2007; Tyler, Edwards, & Saxman, 1987).

COMMENT: *Goal attack strategies for children with SSD and expressive language impairment*

What about children who have more complex communication disorders, such as concomitant SSD and expressive language impairment? Clearly such children need multiple goals to be targeted, but how are such goals best scheduled? Tyler, Lewis, Haskill, and Tolbert (2003) offer three ideas for scheduling intervention goals for children who have concomitant speech and language difficulties. The three schedules include:

1. **Block scheduling**: intervention targeting goals for one domain for a period of time followed by the goals for another domain for a similar length of time (e.g., 10 weeks of SSD intervention followed by 10 weeks of language intervention).
2. **Alternating sequencing**: intervention targeting goals in the respective domains every other session (e.g., SSD intervention on even weeks and language intervention on odd weeks).
3. **Simultaneous scheduling**: intervention targeting goals across two or more domains each session (e.g., SSD intervention and language intervention conducted within the same session activity).

In a study comparing different types of goal attack strategies (block versus alternating versus simultaneous) for children with concomitant phonological impairment and morphosyntactic impairment, Tyler, Lewis, Haskill, and Tolbert (2003) reported that although no particular goal attack strategy was superior for achieving the phonological goals, there were significant differences with respect to the morphosyntactic goals. In particular, improvements in morphosyntax were the greatest for the children who received the alternating goal attack strategy. Tyler et al. concluded that the alternating goal attack strategy might be the preferred scheduling option for children with concomitant phonological and language impairments. To date, there is no consensus on which goal attack strategy might be the best for children with concomitant motor speech and language learning difficulties.

Chapter summary

In this chapter you learned about goal identification and prioritization for children with SSD. You learned that goals can be impairment-based, socially based, or a combination of the two, structured using the ICF-CY framework (Duchan, 2001; WHO, 2007). Goals need to be operationalized and organized in a hierarchical framework, to help you navigate your way from the first intervention session with a child and his or her family through to the point of dismissal. You learned that session goals define what will be worked on, when, where, and with whom during intervention sessions. The realization of session goals

contributes to the realization of short-term goals, which ultimately contribute to the realization of long-term goals. You learned that the selection and prioritization of intervention goals (whether they be impairment-based or socially based) require careful consideration of peer-reviewed published evidence in conjunction with child and family characteristics and preferences. This chapter has been about *what* to work on in intervention. Over the next four chapters, you will learn about intervention principles, procedures, and approaches, so you know *how* to work on intervention goals.

Suggested reading

The following book contains further information about goal setting from different theoretical perspectives for children with phonological impairment.

■ Kamhi, A. G., & Pollock, K. E. (Eds.). (2005). *Phonological disorders in children: Clinical decision making in assessment and intervention*. Baltimore, MD: Paul H. Brookes.

Application of knowledge from Chapter 10

Over the course of this chapter you have completed numerous application tasks for the five children featured throughout this book: Luke (4;3 years), Susie (7;4 years), Jarrod (7;0 years), Michael (4;2 years), and Lian (14;2 years) (Chapter 16). Extend your knowledge about goal setting by completing the following questions.

1. In a small group, compare and contrast short-term goals for Luke (4;3) from two or more of the different target selection frameworks addressed in this chapter.
2. How long do you think it would take to help a child like Luke (4;3) become intelligible? We suggest

approximately 12 months, given an effective intervention at the recommended intensity. In reality not all children will require the same amount of intervention or the same number of sessions to achieve the same goals (Baker & McLeod, 2004). However, time-bound goals provide SLPs and families with a useful estimate against which progress can be monitored, compared, and addressed. Compare your suggested time frame with comments and reports from published literature. Suggested readings to complete this task include Baker and McLeod (2011a), Hodson (2007), Jacoby, Lee, Kummer, Levin, and Creaghead (2002), and Williams (2012).

Appendix 10-1. Goal identification template

Name: _____ Date of birth: _____ Age: _____

Reason for referral: _____ Language(s) spoken: _____

Diagnosis: _____

		Areas requiring consideration in intervention
Function and disability	**Body Functions**	☐ b320 Articulation functions (includes phonology)
		☐ b1560 Auditory perception
		☐ b230 Hearing functions
		☐ b144 Memory functions (including phonological processing)
		☐ b1670 Reception of language
		☐ b1671 Expression of language
		☐ b310 Voice functions
		☐ b330 Fluency and rhythm of speech functions
		☐ b117 Intellectual functions
	Body Structures	☐ b126 Temperament and personality functions
		☐ s320 Structure of mouth
		☐ s1 Structure of nervous system, s240–260 Structure of ear, s310 Structure of nose, s330 Structure of pharynx, s340 Structure of larynx, s430 Structure of respiratory system
	Activities and Participation	☐ d3 Communication
		☐ d1 Learning and applying knowledge (including d115 Listening, d140 Learning to read, d145 Learning to write)
		☐ d7 Interpersonal interactions and relationships
		☐ d810–820 Education
		☐ d9 Community, social and civic life
Contextual factors	**Environmental**	☐ e3 Support and relationships
		☐ e4 Attitudes
		☐ e1 Products and technology
		☐ e5 Services, systems and policies
	Personal	

The goal identification template can be freely copied with acknowledgment of the source being McLeod & Baker (2017)

11

Intervention Principles and Plans

LEARNING OBJECTIVES

1 State the difference between intervention goals, principles, plans, and procedures.

2 Describe principles of intervention across six areas: phonology, speech perception, motor learning, cognition and meta-awareness, behavior, and neurology.

3 Explain how principles of intervention influence plans and procedures.

4 List the components of intervention management plans and session plans for children with SSD.

5 Compare and contrast different methods of service delivery for children with SSD.

6 Describe intervention discharge criteria.

KEY WORDS

Principles of intervention: phonology, speech perception, motor learning, cognition and meta-awareness, behavioral learning, and neurological experience

Plans: management plans and session plans; service delivery options including setting, agent, intensity, format, and continuity (ongoing and block formats)

Progress and discharge planning: short-term and long-term goal criteria

OVERVIEW

This chapter is about intervention principles and plans for children with SSD. It is essential for understanding the different **approaches** to intervention described in Chapters 13 (for phonological impairment) and 14 (for motor speech difficulties). You will learn what intervention is and appreciate the phonological, speech perception, motor learning, cognitive, behavioral, and neurological principles that underlie different approaches to intervention. You will learn about the basic components of an intervention management plan and session plan. Information is also provided to guide clinical decisions such as who will provide intervention, when, where, how often, and in what format (individual and/or group). You will also learn how to decide when intervention is no longer necessary.

This chapter complements Chapter 12 on intervention procedures and evaluation. Together Chapters 11 and 12 are like a must-read travel guide—the more familiar you are with these chapters, the better equipped you will be to understand the different intervention approaches described in Chapters 13 and 14.

WHAT IS INTERVENTION?

Intervention is a goal-directed activity based on plans and procedures designed to improve a presenting problem. Unlike a relatively simple plan for managing a mild insect bite (e.g., apply suitable ointment/cream twice daily until the itching stops), intervention plans for managing SSD in children can be complex. Many decisions need to be made, such as deciding what to work on, choosing teaching procedures suited to a child's SSD, identifying strategies that will maximize generalization, deciding how you will monitor progress, determining who will provide intervention, deciding on the frequency and duration of intervention sessions, considering whether intervention will be conducted in an individual or group format, determining how children and their families will be cared for and involved in the decision-making process, and considering how the impact of an SSD on children's day-to-day activity and participation could be addressed. Principles of intervention influence your decisions. Those decisions are then compiled into a plan.

■ Intervention Principles, Plans, and Procedures

Intervention principles lead to intervention plans and procedures (see Figure 11-1). What you think will help address a problem (principles) influences your plans to do something

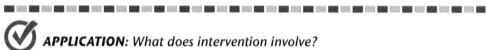

✓ APPLICATION: What does intervention involve?

1. Talk with a peer about what you think intervention involves. Use the questions below to guide your discussion. As you listen to one another's answers, reflect on the similarities and differences in your answers.
   - What do you think an SLP would do to work with a child similar to Luke (4;3), who has a phonological impairment, and why?
   - What do you think an SLP would do to work with a child similar to Susie (7;4), who has a lateral lisp, to improve her production of /s/, and why?
2. Interview friends or family members who are not studying SSD in children and have little background or training in the area. Ask them what they think an SLP would do to help a child like Luke (4;3), who has a phonological impairment and who says *bike* /baɪk/ as [baɪk] but *cat* /kæt/ as [dæt]. What do you think their answers suggest about their understanding of the nature of a phonological impairment, and therefore the principles of intervention?

Read more about Luke (4;3 years) and Susie (7;4 years) in Chapter 16.

| FIGURE 11-1 | Principles, plans, and procedures in intervention |

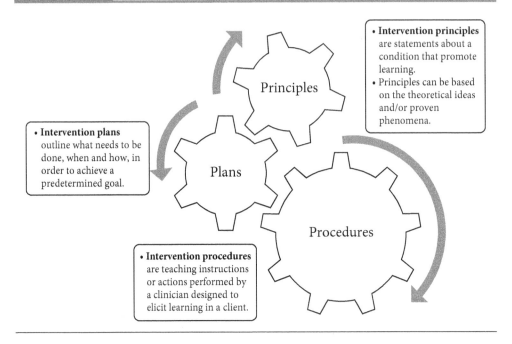

- **Intervention principles** are statements about a condition that promote learning.
- Principles can be based on the theoretical ideas and/or proven phenomena.

- **Intervention plans** outline what needs to be done, when and how, in order to achieve a predetermined goal.

- **Intervention procedures** are teaching instructions or actions performed by a clinician designed to elicit learning in a client.

about a problem and the procedures or actions you will take to implement your plan. By definition, an **intervention principle** is a statement about a condition that promotes learning. Principles can be based on theoretical ideas and/or proven phenomena. An **intervention plan** is a proposal outlining what needs to be done, and when and how it should be done, in order to achieve a predetermined goal. An **intervention procedure** is a teaching instruction or action performed by a clinician designed to elicit learning in a client.

We will use Susie's case (case 2 in Chapter 16) to illustrate the difference between principles, plans, and procedures. Recall from your analysis of Susie's speech (Chapter 9) that you identified that the long-term goal was for Susie was to articulate /s, z/ clearly (without lateralization) in everyday conversational speech, with a variety of partners in a variety of contexts (Chapter 10). In principle, motor skills are learned through a period of pre-practice followed by practice (Maas et al., 2008). During the practice phase, **variable random practice** (i.e., practicing skills in different ways and contexts) can help promote generalization (Maas et al., 2008; Skelton, 2004a). Knowing these principles, your intervention **plan** would include opportunities for Susie to first learn how to produce a clear [s] followed by a variable random practice schedule involving a range of different [s] exemplar types such as [s] in word-initial, within word, and word-final contexts (including imitated and spontaneous productions) practiced in random order (Skelton, 2004a). Your plan would of course adopt other principles of motor learning and include information such as the frequency (i.e., how often), location (i.e., where), format (i.e., individual or group), and duration of Susie's intervention sessions (e.g., 30 minutes), a schedule of the data that you will collect (e.g., treatment data, generalization probe data), a list of motivating activities or games you might use with Susie, a homework schedule consistent with the principles of motor learning, and a list of relevant materials and resources that you would need during a session. To help Susie learn how to articulate a clear /s/, your teaching **procedures** could include an auditory model of /s/ for Susie to imitate, verbal cues about the placement of the articulators (Secord, Boyce, Donohue, Fox, & Shine, 2007), and a shaping technique such as the long [t] (Shine, 2007). You will learn more about the elements of this plan for Susie through this chapter and Chapter 12.

To understand the many different intervention approaches in Chapters 13 and 14, you need to understand the range of principles, plans, and procedures that make up interventions. In doing so, you will be able to appreciate the similarities and differences among

Read more about Susie (7;4 years), a girl with an articulation impairment (lateral lisp), in Chapter 16 (Case 2).

the approaches, decide which approach(es) are suitable for different children with different problems, and most importantly, have the knowledge (and given opportunity, the skill) to faithfully implement approaches in accordance with developers' intentions (Sanetti & Kratochwill, 2009).

PRINCIPLES OF INTERVENTION

Speech is a complex ability acquired through different types of learning. As shown in Figure 11-2, speech involves:

- phonology: knowledge about the sound system of a language;
- speech perception: sound that can be detected with the ear and perceived by the brain;
- motor learning: carefully timed sequences of physical movement developed through practice;
- cognition and meta-awareness abilities: processes that code, store, remember, retrieve, and reflect upon information;
- behavioral learning: actions that can be elicited with a stimulus and modified via consequences; and
- neurological experience: information learned by an adaptive brain.

In this section we describe principles of intervention for children with SSD based on these six different perspectives on speech. After reading the principles, you will appreciate why certain teaching and learning procedures are used in different intervention approaches for different types of SSD.

◼ Principles of intervention: Phonology

In Chapter 5 you learned about phonological concepts and theories. You learned that speech is more than a string of unrelated sounds—it is part of an organized linguistic system comprising rules and relationships. In this section we provide an overview of phonological principles that influence intervention.

- Phonological acquisition is systematic.
  Principle: Phonological intervention should focus on children learning phonological *systems* rather than the articulation of individual phonemes (Stoel-Gammon & Dunn, 1985).

FIGURE 11-2 Types of learning involved in speech acquisition and intervention

Speech is a complex ability acquired through the phonology system, speech perception, motor learning, cognition and meta-awareness, behavioral learning, and neurological experience.

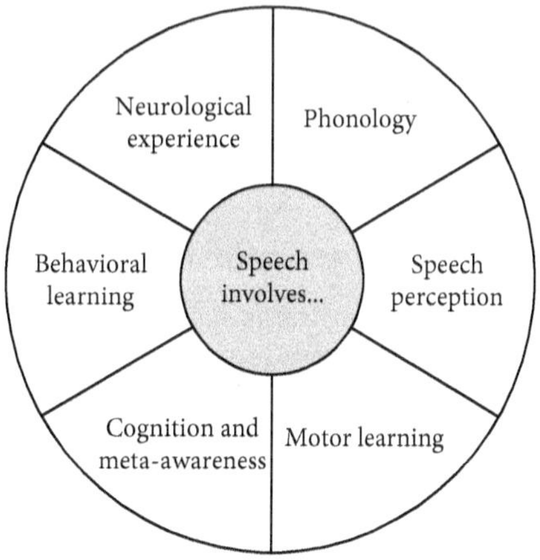

■ Phonological systems are hierarchically organized, with the constituent parts having implicational relationships (Gierut, 2001, 2005).
Principle: Phonological intervention targets can be carefully selected to facilitate generalization or widespread change in children's phonological systems (Gierut, 2001, 2005, 2007; Stoel-Gammon & Dunn, 1985).

■ Phonological systems are rule governed.
Principle: Phonological intervention should help children discover and learn the rules of a phonological system (Lowe, 1994).

■ Phonemes serve a communicative function in speech.
Principle: Phonological intervention procedures should be meaning-based (Lowe, 1994; Weiner, 1981).

■ Speech is meaningful and bound by pragmatic principles of informativeness—speakers can accommodate to listeners' needs by resolving uncertainties and miscommunication by modifying their speech in conversational repair sequences (Greenfield & Smith, 1976).
Principle: Phonological intervention can include conversational repair sequences (e.g., listener requests for clarification) to facilitate improved speech intelligibility (Weiner, 1981).

■ Principles of intervention: Speech perception

The ability to listen to speech influences your ability to produce speech. It is reasonable to suggest, therefore, that principles about how we perceive speech might influence therapeutic techniques used to help children better perceive and produce speech.

■ The ability to perceive speech both shapes and is shaped by the acquisition of language-specific phonological systems (Munson et al., 2011).
Principle: Intervention should incorporate opportunities for listening to spoken language.

■ Detailed and robust auditory-perceptual representations are based on acoustic variance within and across speakers (e.g., men versus women versus children with accurate versus inaccurate speech), speaking contexts (e.g., slow versus rapid speech rate), and phonetic contexts (e.g., consonants adjacent to different vowels in words) (e.g., Bradlow & Bent, 2008; Creel & Jimenez, 2012; Lively, Logan, & Pisoni, 1993).
Principle: Intervention targeting speech perception should exploit varied speakers and contexts (e.g., Rvachew, 1994).

■ Good speech perception is characterized by distinct perceptual boundaries between phonemes (Samuel, 2011).
Principle: Intervention targeting speech perception should facilitate children's abilities to perceive differences between phonemes in words (e.g., Rvachew, 1994).

■ Children who have an SSD can have perceptual boundaries that are too broad—accepting inaccurate productions of speech sounds in words as correct (Rvachew & Brosseau-Lapré, 2012).
Principle: Intervention targeting speech perception should include opportunities for children to make judgments about the accuracy of the speech sounds they hear in words (Rvachew, 1994).

■ Principles of intervention: Motor learning

Speech is a motor skill acquired through practice. In this section we provide an overview of principles and supporting research on motor learning. Compared to the other sections about principles of learning in this chapter, this section on principles of motor learning is presented in more depth, because there are relatively more principles and because many intervention decisions are influenced by these principles. We begin with five broad principles of motor learning, and then explore specific principles that help guide the decisions that you make when you ask children to engage in speech production practice.

- **Motor learning** refers to "a set of internal processes associated with practice or experience leading to relatively permanent changes in the capability for motor skill" (Schmidt & Lee, 2005, p. 466).

  Principle: During intervention, performance during practice (*acquisition* of a skill) should be measured separately from performance after the completion of practice to determine whether practice has led to *learning* or permanent retention of a motor skill (Maas et al., 2008).

- Using the basic tenets of Guadagnoli and Lee's (2004) **challenge point framework**, motor learning is closely related to the information available and interpretable when completing a task, and the difficulty of the task. No learning occurs without information. Too little or too much information can hamper learning.

  Principle: During intervention, an optimal amount of information should be provided to challenge a child to learn. This information should be tailored to both the skill level of the child and the task difficulty (Guadagnoli & Lee, 2004).

- What you practice should mirror what you want to learn. Although speech uses some of the same muscles as non-speech oromotor movements (e.g., blowing, repeatedly lifting the tongue to the alveolar ridge), movements for speech are different from non-speech movements—they are task specific (Lof, 2015; Weismer, 2006). Research by Forrest and Iuzzini (2008) also suggests that non-speech oromotor exercises do not necessarily improve children's speech production skills.

  Principle: During intervention-focused speech motor learning, consider the specificity of practice and focus on speech rather than non-speech oromotor mouth exercises (Lof, 2015).

- Motor learning can be divided into phases. Based on Fitts' (1964) three-phase view of motor learning, a learner first figures out what needs to be done to perform a particular skill (the cognitive or thinking stage). Next, a learner refines or fine-tunes the skill via practice (the associative stage). Finally, the skill can be performed with little conscious effort or attention (the autonomous phase) (Fitts, 1964; Schmidt & Lee, 2005). In an intervention context, learning can be divided into a period of **pre-practice** (figuring out what needs to be done and how) followed by **practice** (repetitively engaging in tasks to refine the skill), so that the skill becomes automatic or permanently learned. Practice conditions influence how well a new skill is acquired, generalized to other related skills, and retained over the long term. Practice conditions include practice amount, the distribution of practice, practice variability, practice schedule, the complexity of the task being practiced, practice fraction, the degree of accuracy expected during practice, and the learner's attentional focus. The type, frequency, and timing of the feedback given to a learner during practice can also influence generalization and transfer. Figure 11-3 depicts the conditions of practice and feedback influenced by the principles of motor learning.

  Principle: During the **pre-practice phase of intervention**, individuals should be provided with information about the skill to be developed (including what constitutes a correct response) and taught how to produce a correct response (Maas et al., 2008).

  Principle: During the **practice phase of intervention**, conditions of practice and feedback should be guided by empirical research on speech motor learning.

In the following section, we explore the concepts and evidence associated with conditions of practice and feedback.

Principles of motor learning: Conditions of practice

When we ask children to engage in speech production practice, we need to be mindful of the types of practice conditions that help facilitate generalized learning. These conditions include: **practice amount** (small versus large), **distribution of practice** (massed versus distributed), **practice variability** (constant versus variable), **practice schedule** (blocked versus random), the type of task being practiced (complex versus simple), **practice fraction** (whole versus part), the **accuracy of practice** (errorless versus errorful), and the **learner's attentional focus** (internal versus external).

FIGURE 11-3 Conditions of practice and feedback influenced by the principles of motor learning

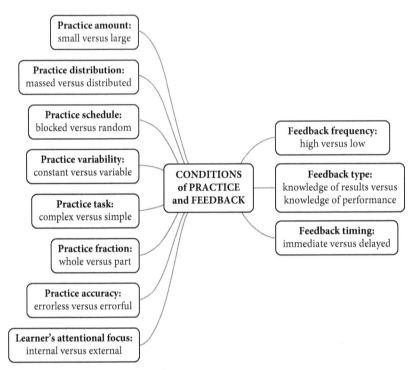

Source: Adapted from Maas et al. (2008); Schmidt & Lee (2005); Skelton (2004a); Utley & Astill (2008).

Practice amount: Small versus large

Practice amount or **dose** in a session can be large or small. Although it seems obvious to state, more learning occurs when more practice occurs (Schmidt & Lee, 2005). This of course assumes that other conditions of practice and feedback are optimal. If more is better, how much more? We suggest that you be guided by evidence-based dosage recommendations associated with specific intervention approaches. For example, Edeal and Gildersleeve-Neumann (2011) compared a high dose (referred to as high-frequency practice) of 100 to 150 productions in a 15-minute period with a moderate dose of 30 to 40 productions in the same time period using the Dynamic Temporal and Tactile Cueing (DTTC) approach with two children with CAS. They reported that the high-frequency condition was associated with more rapid acquisition of the targets, superior performance in intervention sessions, and better generalization to non-treatment probe words when compared to the low-frequency condition. In an investigation of the intensity of phonological intervention (specifically, multiple oppositions and minimal pairs therapy approaches), Williams (2012) noticed that a minimum dose of 50 trials in a 30-minute session conducted twice weekly for a total of at least 30 sessions was required for phonological intervention to be effective. A higher dose (at least 70 trials per session) for approximately 40 sessions was suggested for children with more severe SSD (Williams, 2012). The importance of dose aside, do not assume that you can help children become more intelligible if you simply get them to do the same thing over and over again. Other conditions of practice and feedback interact with practice amount to influence how well and quickly a skill is generalized to everyday speech.

Practice distribution: Massed versus distributed

Practice distribution is about how a particular amount of intervention, such as 3,000 production practice trials, is dispersed over time (Maas et al., 2008). If the amount is dispersed with less time between trials and/or sessions, practice is massed. If there is more time between trials and/or sessions, practice is distributed. There are pros and cons associated with each practice distribution. Although massed practice can be helpful for initial skill acquisition, distributed practice would seem to be better for long-term retention and transfer (Caruso & Strand, 1999). With that said, overly massed practice (e.g., excessively long sessions) may not be tolerated by some children and/or could lead to boredom and lack of motivation, while infrequent distributed practice (e.g., sessions scheduled once a month) could lead to skills being forgotten or learned over an unreasonably long period of time. You need to be guided by the available empirical evidence regarding session dose, duration, and frequency (concepts discussed later in this chapter) for specific intervention approaches. For example, in a randomized controlled trial of the multiple oppositions approach (see Chapter 13), Allen (2013) reported that more frequent intervention (three 30-minute sessions per week for 8 weeks) was associated with significantly better outcomes than less frequent (one 30-minute session per week for 24 weeks) for children with phonological impairment. Pennington et al. (2010) found that intensive intervention (three 30- to 45-minute sessions per week for 6 weeks) using the systems approach (see Chapter 14) was associated with improvements in speech intelligibility for older children with cerebral palsy and dysarthria. Namasivayam et al. (2015) reported that for children with CAS, twice weekly SLP sessions for 10 weeks were associated with better performance on measures of articulation and functional communication compared to weekly SLP sessions for the same time period, even when regular home practice was encouraged between sessions. Namasivayam et al. (2015) did note that measures of word- and sentence-level intelligibility did not show a significant improvement for either intervention intensity. In a study involving 91 children with an articulation impairment involving /s/ or /ʃ/, significantly more children who regularly completed home practice between sessions finished intervention after eight sessions compared with children who did not practice between sessions (Günther & Hautvast, 2010). Caruso and Strand (1999) suggest that clinicians tend to do massed practice for more severe SSD and shift towards distributed practice as the severity decreases.

Practice variability: Constant versus variable

Practice can be **constant** (practicing a specific speech skill in the same way in the same context) or **variable** (practicing the same skill with variations in parameters such as changes in rate, pitch, intensity, and force) (Preston et al., 2014). Practice variability can also be interpreted as practicing a specific speech sound in varying linguistic contexts (Skelton & Hagopian, 2014). For example, think about all the various ways that the phoneme /s/ is produced when you say the following utterance: "Susie saw six spotted seals in the sea as she sorted sixty-seven saxatile seashells on the shore." Did you produce the /s/ in the exact same position in words every time? No. The phoneme /s/ was produced in various linguistic contexts—different word positions (initial, medial, and final), in singleton and consonant cluster contexts, in strong and weak stressed syllables, in mono- and bimorphemic words, in nouns, verbs, and adjectives, in a sentence, and (if you have not come across *saxatile* before) a new word. You could also vary your production of /s/ in those different linguistic contexts by loudness and speech rate, using different intonation patterns and stress. In addition, you could produce /s/ in various communicative contexts, in an imitation or spontaneous speech context, with an individual or in a group, using an electronic medium or in a face-to-face context. You could elicit /s/ using various stimuli—printed pictures, electronic pictures on a screen, real or toy objects, written words, a game, or conversation. You have developed the ability to produce /s/ in a variety of words and utterances in different speaking conditions. Aside from focusing on variable ways of practicing one specific target, variable practice could also be conceptualized as practicing different targets, such as plosives and fricatives in different contexts (Maas et al., 2008). Both variable and constant practices have merits and are useful for different purposes.

Constant practice is considered helpful when first acquiring a new skill, whereas variable practice is thought to be helpful for promoting learning or permanent retention of a skill (Preston et al., 2014). As you read the intervention research studying this issue, notice the way researchers have realized the concept of variable practice. For instance, Preston et al. (2014) compared speech production accuracy in practice with and without prosodic variations (e.g., asking questions, making exclamations, and saying statements) with eight children with residual speech sound errors. Preston et al. (2014) reported improvements in target sound accuracy in words, irrespective of the prosodic variation conditions. Skelton

> **COMMENT:** *"Quiet, or the butterflies will hear us!": The role of GMPs, schemas, and practice variability*
>
> Using Schmidt's (1975) schema theory (see Chapter 5), **a generalized motor program** (GMP) is an abstract motor program that can be expressed in different ways, depending on the **parameters** supplied to the program. It can be helpful to think of a GMP like a mathematical formula and the parameters like the numbers supplied to the formula (Schmidt & Lee, 2005). Once you have selected a GMP and executed (or even started to execute) a movement by adding relevant parameters, Schmidt (1975) suggests that you learn **schemas** (rules) about relationships between four sources of information to refine the current movement and/or inform future movement. This information (stored temporarily in short-term memory) includes: (1) what the conditions were before making the movement, (2) the parameters assigned to the GMP such as the duration, force, and specific muscles used to produce movement, (3) the sensory experience such as how it felt or sounded, and (4) the outcome—whether the intended goal was achieved (Schmidt & Lee, 2005). There are two types of schemas in Schmidt's (1975) theory (1) **recall schema**—rules about relationships between initial conditions, the parameters used to execute a movement, and the outcome, and (2) **recognition schema**—rules about relationships between initial conditions, the sensory consequences, and the outcome.
>
> What does this have to do with speaking quietly so butterflies do not hear? Adelaide (4;0 years) was observing butterflies in the garden when she said to Elise, *"Quiet, the butterflies will hear us!"* This utterance was said with a quiet voice. Adelaide was also observed to say the word *butterfly* in a loud voice, and with rising intonation in a question (*"Did you see the butterfly?"*). Adelaide was capable of saying the word *butterfly* in different ways because of variable practice. Through variable practice children develop schemas that allow them to select relevant GMPs and apply parameters based on the speaking conditions (e.g., whispering in a cinema, raising their voice to be heard across a playground).

and Hagopian (2014) used a variable-random practice schedule with three children with CAS, whereby variability involved practicing intervention targets in different response modes (imitation and spontaneous production) and response lengths (e.g., syllables, words, two-word phrases, three-word phrases). They reported improved accuracy during treatment and generalization probes (words and phrases) for all children. In Chapter 14, you will learn about concurrent treatment (Skelton, 2004a)—an intervention approach characterized by a variable-random practice schedule for treating articulation errors such as an interdental lisp.

Practice schedule: Blocked versus random

A schedule of practice can be blocked or random. Blocked practice involves practicing a skill or speech target a number of times before moving on to another (e.g., if targeting word-initial consonant clusters you might have a child say *glass* 10 times, then *snake* 10 times, and then *frown* 10 times). Random practice involves different movements being produced on successive trials, so that a learner cannot predict what trial follows another (e.g., randomly saying words containing word-initial consonant clusters one after another: *glass, frown, snake, frown, snake, glass*) (Maas & Farinella, 2012).

Clinical research examining the effect of random versus blocked practice schedules with children has produced mixed results. Skelton (2004a) found that a variable-random sequence facilitated learning in four school-age children who had an interdental lisp. The sequence was variable, because different contexts for producing /s/ were practiced (e.g., syllables, words, phrases, sentences). It was random because the order of practice for the stimuli for those contexts changed throughout the session (e.g., syllable, sentence, word, phrase, syllable, word). By contrast, Maas and Farinella (2012) reported mixed results for four children with CAS. Of the four children in their study, two showed a blocked practice advantage, one benefitted more from random practice, while the other showed no clear improvement with either schedule. Maas and Farinella (2012) also pointed out that it was difficult to strictly adhere to a random schedule during practice. If a child made an error, the child was encouraged to make another attempt of the same target (with additional support from the clinician), in an effort produce an accurate response (Maas & Farinella, 2012). Until further research is conducted, it would seem that for some children, particularly those with CAS, blocked practice might be useful to establish basic motor patterns early on in intervention, with random practice being introduced at a later point, in an effort to facilitate generalization and transfer (Maas & Farinella, 2012). It may also be that a combination of blocked-random practice is preferable (e.g., 10 trials of one target followed by 10 trials of another randomly selected target and so on). As an evidence-based clinician, be guided by the emerging research in this area.

Practice task: Complex versus simple learning

Learning can involve complex or simple tasks. As discussed in Chapter 10, intervention targeting a phonologically complex target (e.g., consonant clusters with small sonority differences such as /sl/) could facilitate learning of simpler targets (e.g., singleton fricatives such as /s/ and /f/) (Gierut, 1999). While preliminary evidence suggests that adults who have a motor speech disorder benefit more from practicing complex skills (e.g., Schneider & Frens, 2005), the effect of prioritizing complex over simple skills with children who have a motor speech disorder has received little experimental attention. It is conceivable that children with CAS benefit more from practicing complex syllable sequences such as di- and polysyllables rather than simple CV syllables, because such sequences mirror whole rather than part practice (a concept discussed next in this chapter) and help address one of the core features of CAS—difficulty with movement sequences. That aside, across intervention literature focused on children with severe CAS, experts recommend starting with simple stimuli and progressing to more complex (e.g., Strand & Skinder, 1999; Velleman, 2003; Williams & Stephens, 2004). Easier targets are thought to provide young children with opportunities for early success. Success can help to build trust between a child and a clinician and can increase a child's motivation (Strand & Skinder, 1999). Presumably you would trial more complex tasks with children when they are ready, bearing in mind the principle that children should be optimally challenged in order to learn. You will learn more about practice tasks for children with motor speech disorders in Chapter 14.

Practice fraction: Whole versus part practice

A motor skill can be practiced as the **whole** movement or the constituent **parts** of the whole. Movements that are not too complex but are highly organized (e.g., catching a ball) are best suited to whole-task practice (Utley & Astill, 2008). Other movements can be divided and practiced in parts. Think about the word *butterfly*. Can you divide the word into parts? Yes, you can say the three syllables. You can also say each phoneme separately. You could say *fly* as [f], [l], [aɪ]. This means that part practice of some speech movements is possible (Skelton, 2004b). Review the box titled "What Is OK and Not OK When Engaging in Part Practice?" and think when and how part practice for speech might be done.

Practice accuracy: Errorless versus errorful learning

In errorless practice, mistakes are discouraged. Errorless learning is designed to encourage and strengthen accurate acquisition of a motor skill (Bergan, 2010). By contrast, errorful practice permits and includes opportunities for errors, to allow the learner to define and refine a motor skill (Bergan, 2010; Middleton & Schwartz, 2012). Errors are thought to give a learner the chance to develop more precise error detection and correction skills (Maas et al., 2008).

Across interventions for SSD, authors vary in their position on errorless versus errorful learning. For example, cycles therapy (Hodson, 2007; see Chapter 13) prioritizes only stimulable sounds or patterns to encourage accurate practice. By contrast, minimal pairs therapy (Weiner, 1981; see Chapter 13) includes a period of rule discovery in which children are encouraged to determine what is a correct response via episodes of communication breakdown and repair. Parents and Children Together (PACT) therapy (Bowen, 2015; see Chapter 13) is another approach that allows children to learn from errors through the use of "fixed-up-one" routines—a meta-linguistic self-monitoring and correction technique.

COMMENT: *What is OK and not OK when engaging in part practice?* **But** *to* **butter** *to* **butterfly,** *but not isolated lip movements*

For some children (especially children who have CAS), polysyllables can be challenging. One technique for helping children develop the ability to produce (but not necessarily permanently learn) the sequencing of multiple syllables during the **pre-practice phase of intervention** is part practice. According to Wightman and Lintern (1985), there are three types of part practice. When targeting speech production, simplification and additive segmentation are preferred over fractionation.

- **Simplification:** modifying the movements of a skill to make it easier (e.g., saying a word more slowly) (Skelton, 2004b). Simplification of a task during the **pre-practice** phase of intervention can help a child learn how to produce the whole skill.

- **Segmentation:** dividing a skill along a temporal dimension into parts and then practicing them in an additive manner. For example, to develop the ability to sequence syllables in a word such as *butterfly*, start by saying the first syllable *bu* [bʌ] then adding the next syllable to get *butter* [bʌtɚ] until the whole word is said: *butterfly* [bʌtɚflaɪ]. Take care doing this with children with CAS, as they can have prosodic distortions. Ensure that if you use additive segmentation, normal prosody is modelled as the syllables are put together. Segmentation is also known as additive segmentation (Skelton, 2004b) or the **progressive parts method** (Utley & Astill, 2008).

- **Fractionation:** dividing simultaneously produced movements in a skill into independent components, then practicing each movement (Forrest, 2002). For example, learning how to articulate [t] by separating all of the different mouth movements used to produce [t], such as anchoring the tongue along the lateral margins of the palate and moving the tongue tip to the alveolar ridge. Fractionation of the movements used to produce a speech sound, syllable, or word results in non-speech oromotor movements (e.g., raising and lowering of the jaw; elevation of the tongue to the alveolar ridge; elevation of the velum). Practice of such isolated movements is not recommended for children who have an SSD (Forrest, 2002). This is because an isolated movement can become so dissimilar to the way it is used in the whole skill being learned, that it disregards the principle of the specificity of practice (Skelton, 2004b).

Interventions for motor speech disorders based on principles of motor learning also allow errors (e.g., Rapid Syllable Transition Treatment [ReST]; McCabe and Ballard, 2015; see Chapter 14) and encourage learners to develop and refine their own error-detection abilities. What is undetermined is the extent to which you allow children to make errors. As an evidence-based clinician, you could take some direction from the growing body of research on the effect of different principles of motor learning with children who have an SSD. The study by Edeal and Gildersleeve-Neumann (2011) is a good example. The focus of their study was on the effect of a high or moderate dose in a session for children who have CAS. Using the dynamic temporal and tactile cueing (DTTC) approach (Strand, Stoeckel, & Baas, 2006), they modified a child's practice schedules (blocked or random practice) in response to a child's errors. Blocked practice was used when a child was first learning how to accurately produce a new skill (i.e., during pre-practice). Random practice was used during the practice phase until an error occurred. Blocked practiced was reintroduced to better establish a correct response. In this study, although accuracy was emphasized, errors were allowed. Murray, McCabe, and Ballard (2015) used a similar strategy, reverting back to a period of pre-practice to avoid excessive practice of errors in the practice phase of intervention for children with CAS.

Like many of the principles of motor learning, further research is needed with children who have an SSD to understand the optimal balance between errorless and errorful practice. We would add that the role of children's individual temperament (particularly their resilience) needs to be considered when children engage in errorful practice. Some children might cope with being told that they have not been understood or that they have made a mistake. Some children might also cope with a reduced frequency of feedback during practice and not being told whether or not they have made an error. Some children, however, may be discouraged and frustrated by such practice and may instead need further support to engage in practice that is errorless.

Attentional focus: Internal versus external

Attentional focus during pre-practice and practice can be **internal** or **external**. Instruction and feedback that focuses children's attention on mouth movements is internal (e.g., "Focus on what your tongue is doing when you say [s]. Try and keep your tongue behind your teeth"). Maas et al. (2008) suggest that instruction and feedback that focuses a learner's attention on the acoustic effect or sound of those movements is external (e.g., "Listen to the [s] sound and focus on whether it is clear and snake-like [s] or muffled like [θ]"). During pre-practice, when you are helping children to figure out what is a correct response, your instruction and feedback might be both internal and external—you might ask children to focus on the movement of their articulators and the acoustic output (i.e., did it *sound* correct?). However, once a child understands and is capable of producing a correct response, it may be helpful to encourage an external (rather than internal) attentional focus in an effort to facilitate generalization (Lisman & Sadagopan, 2013). Why? Based on the **constrained action hypothesis** by Wulf, McNevin, and Shea (2001), an internal focus of attention on a behavior that is becoming an unconscious automatic movement (such as speech) derails the process of the behavior becoming automatic (Lisman & Sadagopan, 2013). That is, if you continually focus children's attention on what their articulators are doing, you hamper the development of automaticity—the very thing you are working towards! Therefore, once children can produce a correct response and are in the **practice** phase of intervention, encourage them to self-monitor by listening to and judging the accuracy of their speech, rather than focusing on what their tongue, mouth, or lips are doing.

Principles of motor learning: Conditions of feedback

Feedback helps children figure out what are successful and unsuccessful attempts and how their attempts can be modified so that future attempts are successful (Maas, Butalla, & Farinella, 2012). Feedback can be both **intrinsic** (i.e., information children experience about an attempt, such as how it feels or sounds) and **extrinsic** or **augmented** (i.e., supplementary information about an attempt). Augmented feedback can be from another person or technology (e.g., spectrogram, electropalatography). The type, frequency, and timing of augmented feedback can vary. Each of these concepts is considered in turn.

Feedback type: Knowledge of results versus knowledge of performance

There are two types of augmented feedback—**knowledge of results (KR)** and **knowledge of performance (KP)**. KR tells children whether their responses are correct or incorrect. For example, "That was great!" KP tells children why their responses are correct or incorrect. For example, "You didn't round your lips enough" (Maas et al., 2012, p. 247); "Emphasis and fluency were spot on, but your voice was too loud" (Ballard et al., 2010, p. 1232). Both KR and KP are helpful during pre-practice. Together they help children understand why their responses are correct or incorrect. KP also helps shape incorrect responses towards accurate responses. During the practice phase of intervention, however, generalization is enhanced when feedback is limited to KR only—telling learners if their responses are correct or incorrect (Maas et al., 2008). By limiting your feedback to KR only, you encourage learners to use and rely on their own intrinsic feedback. Although there is extensive research to support this idea in the wider body of literature on motor learning (e.g., Salmoni, Schmidt, & Walter, 1984), there is limited experimental research about the benefit of providing children with SSD with KR only during the practice phase of intervention. Presumably, if a child is struggling during the practice phase and seems to have forgotten what constitutes a correct response and why/how to produce a correct response, you would revert back to the pre-practice phase and provide both KR and KP. This is precisely what Murray,

■ ■

 APPLICATION: *What type of feedback will help Susie produce a clear /s/ during everyday conversational speech?*

Imagine you will see Susie for intervention. Write down examples of feedback that you think might help Susie during the pre-practice and practice phases of intervention based on principles of motor learning. Your feedback during pre-practice should include knowledge of results (KR) and knowledge of performance (KP). Your feedback during practice should primarily focus on KR. Remember to consider the attentional focus of your feedback. Compare your feedback examples with a peer.

Read more about Susie (7;4 years), a girl with an articulation impairment (lateral lisp), in Chapter 16 (Case 2).

McCabe, and Ballard (2015) did, as a period of pre-practice was reinstated when a child with CAS struggled to provide an accurate response within two 20-item blocks of practice that included KR feedback only. Like the application of other principles of motor learning, we suggest that you guide your clinical decisions based on the latest evidence and your own clinical data and modify your procedures to facilitate individual children's learning.

Feedback frequency: High versus low
Feedback frequency refers to how often children receive augmented (extrinsic) feedback on their attempts (Maas et al., 2012). Feedback on every attempt would be considered high, while reduced feedback (e.g., feedback on 50% or fewer of attempts) would be considered low (Maas et al., 2012). High- and low-frequency feedback each serve a purpose. High-frequency feedback is helpful in the early stages of intervention (e.g., pre-practice), when children are figuring out what constitutes a correct response—it enhances performance (Maas et al., 2008). By contrast, low frequency is thought to be helpful during the practice phase of intervention because it encourages learners to rely on their own intrinsic forms of feedback. Based on **the guidance hypothesis** (Salmoni et al., 1984), too much feedback is thought to impede children's development of internal response evaluations and error correction mechanisms. By contrast, less frequent feedback encourages children to develop and use their own feedback mechanisms. The challenge is to find the right high-low balance.

In a study of four children with CAS, Maas et al. (2012) experimentally examined the benefit of high and low feedback conditions. Low-frequency feedback was operationalized as feedback on approximately 60% of a child's responses during practice. Maas et al. (2012) did this by marking six of 10 index cards for each intervention target—if the card was marked, the child received feedback; if the card was not marked, the child did not receive feedback. Feedback included both KR and KP, in the context of DTTC intervention (described in Chapter 14). Their results were mixed. Two children showed an advantage for low-frequency feedback, one for high-frequency feedback, and one child made minimal progress. The two children who showed an advantage for low-frequency feedback were older and showed evidence of self-correction attempts—they had an emerging ability to detect and correct errors. Maas et al. (2012) suggested that the ability to self-correct might be an important prerequisite for children to take advantage of low-frequency feedback. Severity and age may be other factors to take into consideration. Like other principles of motor learning, you need to think through how you will apply them, take data, and tailor your procedures to facilitate learning.

Feedback timing: Immediate versus delayed
Augmented feedback can be given concurrently with a response, immediately after a child's response, or following a short delay (e.g., 3 seconds) (Maas et al., 2008). During intervention sessions with children, it feels intuitive to immediately follow up their attempts with feedback—you want to tell them that their attempt was great, or you might want to provide an encouraging remark if they tried hard (e.g., "That was a very clear /s/!"). While concurrent and immediate feedback certainly help improve children's performance during practice, a short delay is thought to be better for learning (Ballard et al., 2010; Murray, McCabe, & Ballard, 2015). The delay encourages children to detect and self-correct errors—it gives them time to evaluate their own responses and figure out how to revise or improve their next attempt. The delay also means that when children receive feedback from a clinician, they get the chance to determine if and how their judgment compares to their clinician's judgment.

Delayed feedback has been included in intervention studies with children who have CAS (e.g., Ballard et al., 2010; Maas et al., 2012; Murray, McCabe, & Ballard, 2015); however, the effect remains to be experimentally examined. Like other principles of motor learning, you will need to consider children's age and severity of impairment, in addition to how they are responding to intervention.

■ Principles of intervention: Cognition and meta-awareness

Cognition is about the acquisition, storage, retrieval, and use of knowledge (Reed, 2013). Various mental processes (attention, perception, short- and long-term memory) transform incoming sensory information into knowledge (Reed, 2013). Consider speech—it starts out as sound (i.e., acoustic information) that our ears hear. With repeated experience we learn to perceive it, create abstract stored representations of words in our head, and later retrieve it as spoken words. We use our cognitive abilities to transform sound into meaning. We also have the ability to think about and reflect on our thoughts, our knowledge, and the processes involved in creating knowledge—a concept broadly described as meta-awareness. Different types of meta-awareness are possible, such as **metacognition** (the ability to think about and reflect on your cognitive abilities) and **metalinguistic awareness** (the ability to think about and reflect on your linguistic knowledge) (Gillon, 2004). Just as there are different branches of linguistics, there are also different branches of metalinguistics, such as syntactic awareness, morphological awareness, semantic awareness, pragmatic awareness, and phonological awareness. During intervention you can use principles of cognition and meta-awareness to help children learn.

- Meta-awareness abilities can be used to:
  - think about what the articulators are doing as you speak (**phonetic awareness**). For example, "Great your tongue is touching behind your front teeth" (Shine, 2007, p. 180).
  - become aware of and think about different properties of a phonological system such as how fricative speech sounds are long and plosives are short (**metaphonology**). For example, Howell and Dean (1987) reported of a child who was observed to cough in an SLP waiting room, in an effort to clear his throat. The child then gained his mother's attention and coughed again, deliberately. He then said to his mother, "I think that's a back sound" (Howell & Dean, 1987, p. 265).
  - reflect on, detect, categorize, match, isolate, blend, segment, or manipulate the phonological structure of spoken words (**phonological awareness**) (Gillon, 2004). For example: "You've chosen the [g] picture. If *soap* had a [g] at the beginning, it would sound like this, [gəʊp]. Let's listen again" (Hesketh, 2010, p. 267). (Note: We consider metaphonology to be similar to but distinct from phonological awareness, as metaphonological abilities require children to reflect on properties of a phonological system, whereas phonological awareness requires a child to reflect on then do something to the structural elements of words such as blend, segment, or manipulate phonemes or syllables).
  - identify prosodic characteristics in speech (e.g., loudness, fluency, intonation, and stress) (**prosodic awareness**). For example, "Emphasis and fluency were spot on, but your voice was too loud." (Ballard et al., 2010, p. 1232).
  - liken speech sounds to other concepts and ideas (**metaphor**). For example: "/ɹ/ is a roaring lion sound; /ʧ/ is a choo-choo train; /f/ is a bunny rabbit sound, because it is made with teeth like a bunny" (Bowen, 2009, p. 309).
  - consciously monitor and evaluate the accuracy of speech (**self-monitoring and self-evaluation**). For example, children's revisions of inaccurate productions during conversational speech show instances of self-monitoring and self-evaluating (Shriberg & Kwiatkowski, 1990).
  - become aware of and repair breakdowns in communication (**pragmatic/ communication awareness**). For example:

    "Ben: [tændəwu] (target *kangaroo*);
    Researcher: did you say /tæmbəlu/?
    Ben: no, [kæŋgəwu]" (Masso, McCabe, & Baker, 2014, p. 377)

■ make sense of visual feedback to increase **phonetic awareness** about where and/or how the articulators move during speech production. For example, when using ultrasound feedback, the clinician could say, "Yes. That's /s/. Now make that tongue shape/movement again," to encourage children to think how the display relates to their tongue movement (Bernhardt, Gick, Bacsfalvi, & Alder-Bock, 2005, p. 611).
Principle: During intervention, utilize children's meta-awareness abilities (including phonetic, phonological, prosodic, and pragmatic awareness, self-monitoring/evaluation, and understanding of metaphor) to facilitate learning.

■ Children with SSD can have difficulty with the cognitive processing of speech including the perception, creation, storage, and/or retrieval of phonological representations (Anthony et al., 2011; Munson, Baylis, Krause, & Yim, 2010; Sutherland & Gillon, 2005).
Principle: Intervention should include opportunities for children to improve how they perceive, create, store, and retrieve more robust underlying phonological representations.

■ Children with SSD can have difficulty with phonological awareness (Gillon 2005; Gillon & Moriarty, 2007; Hesketh, 2010; Moriarty & Gillon, 2006).
Principle: During intervention include opportunities to develop children's phonological awareness, as part of an integrated approach to improving their speech and emergent literacy abilities.

 APPLICATION: *"Great snake sound!": Meta-talk in intervention dialogue*

Review the following utterances spoken by clinicians during intervention. State the different types of awareness required to understand each utterance: metaphonological awareness, phonological awareness, phonetic awareness, prosodic awareness, pragmatic awareness, metaphor, and/or self-monitoring. Some utterances contain more than one type of awareness.

1. "The word *sea* has /s/ at the beginning. What word do we make when we take away the /s/ and put /m/ at the beginning?"
2. "You forgot to use the snake sound /s/ when you said *spoon*. Say it again and remember to use /s/ at the beginning of the word."
3. "I'm not sure what you mean?"
4. "Where is the tip of your tongue?"
5. "When you make the long /f/ sound, you bite your bottom teeth and blow."
6. "How would you rate the fluency of your word that time?"

Answers:

1. "The word *sea* has /s/ at the beginning. What word do we make when we take away the /s/ and put /m/ at the beginning?"	Phonological awareness
2. "You forgot use the snake sound /s/ when you said *spoon*. Say it again and remember to use /s/ at the beginning of the word."	Phonological awareness, metaphor, self-monitoring
3. "I'm not sure what you mean?"	Pragmatic awareness
4. "Where is the tip of your tongue?"	Phonetic awareness
5. "When you make the long [f] sound, you bite your bottom teeth and blow."	Metaphonological and phonetic awareness
6. "How would you rate the fluency of your word that time?"	Prosodic awareness, self-evaluation

CHILDREN'S INSIGHTS: *Children's understanding of the purpose of intervention*

When you work with children, it is important that they understand the metalinguistic talk used during intervention. It can also be helpful that they understand the purpose of intervention (Howell & Dean, 1994). Consider the following conversation between an adult and a child. What do you think this child's understanding is of the purpose of intervention?
Adult: What do you usually do in therapy?
Child: Well I'm supposed to make the bad r sounds and Mrs Smith is supposed to make the good r sounds.
Adult: Don't you ever make the good r sounds?
Child: No I'm supposed to make the bad r's. (Ripich & Panagos, 1985, p. 343)

CHILDREN'S INSIGHTS: *"I'm thinking of a word starting with the letter Y ... it's rhinoceros!"*

Harrison, aged 3;5, said to Elise, "I'm thinking of a word starting with the letter Y ... it's *rhinoceros* [waɪnɑsəwəs]!" This statement shows Harrison's emerging metacognitive abilities. His mispronunciation of /ɹ/ → [w] in the word *rhinoceros* meant that the first syllable of the word sounded like the letter Y. Consequently, he thought that the word *rhinoceros* began with the letter Y. Children's metacognitive abilities develop with time. As a clinician working with young children, it is important that you know if a child has the cognitive and/or meta-awareness abilities to understand your instruction and feed-back during intervention. For instance, typically developing 2- and 3-year-olds can be pragmatically aware—they are capable of revising their speech when they have not been understood (Gallagher, 1977). However, most 2- and 3-year-olds do not understand the relationship between phonemes and graphemes (including the difference between letter names and letter sounds) so could probably not tell you a word starting with the letter Y.

■ Principles of intervention: Behavioral learning

Learning occurs when a new behavior emerges, when there is a change in a behavior, when a behavior increases or decreases, and/or when an existing behavior disappears (Domjan, 2015). Specific speech skills that you work on with children can be taught and/or modified through behavioral principles. The principles in this section are influenced by basic behavioral concepts (e.g., modelling and imitation), and one of the most enduring theories of behavioral learning—**operant conditioning** (Skinner, 1938).

- Humans have the capacity to imitate others' behavior. This ability is thought to be the result of mirror neurons (special cells in the cerebral cortex) that activate and simulate another person's behavior that can be seen and/or heard (Rizzolatti & Craighero, 2004). A behavior provided as an example to **imitate** is a **model**.
  Principle: During intervention when children are first learning a new speech behavior, provide spoken models for children to imitate.
- Skinner (1938) proposed that behaviors can be trained with operant conditioning—they can be elicited with an **antecedent stimulus** or event and then shaped (increased, strengthened, decreased, or extinguished) via **consequences** such as reinforcement, punishment, and/or extinction. This sequence for training a behavior (antecedent stimuli/event–response–consequence) is the basic structure of most teaching moments in intervention. For example:

Clinician: "What is the girl watering?" (antecedent stimuli—verbal request and picture)
Child: "A *seed*." [sid] (response—child said targeted behavior /s/)
Clinician: "That's right. You said *seed* with a perfectly clear /s/! You can put another tick on your chart for that lovely /s/." (consequence—verbal and tangible reinforcement)

Principle: During intervention, antecedent stimuli (e.g., picture and verbal request) and consequences (e.g., verbal praise, correction, feedback, and tangible reward) can be used to increase, strengthen, decrease, or eliminate targeted speech behaviors (e.g., production of a particular speech consonant or vowel, stress pattern, loudness, speech rate, and fluency).

Types of consequences

There are two types of consequences in intervention—pleasant and unpleasant. Pleasant consequences are reinforcers and unpleasant consequences are punishers (Skinner, 1938). Consequences can also be positive or negative. A **positive reinforcer** occurs after a behavior—something you enjoy happens (e.g., you receive verbal praise for your amazing singing at a karaoke event; at the next karaoke event, you sing because you enjoyed the praise from the previous event and you anticipate receiving praise again). A **positive punisher** also occurs after a behavior, but the consequence is not something that you enjoy (e.g., you are told that your singing was terrible at a karaoke event; at the next karaoke event, you don't sing because you don't want to be told that your singing isn't very good). A **negative reinforcer** stops once a behavior occurs—something you are not enjoying comes to an end (e.g., your friends nag you until you agree to sing karaoke; at the next karaoke event you sing to avoid being nagged). Finally, a **negative punisher** stops once a behavior occurs—something you were enjoying comes to an end (e.g., your friends leave karaoke when you start singing; at the next karaoke event you don't sing because you would rather enjoy the company of your friends than have them leave when you sing). Reinforcers increase or strengthen a behavior, while punishers decrease or weaken a behavior (Cartwright, 2002). The most common type of consequence used during intervention with children who have an SSD is positive reinforcement (e.g., verbal praise accompanied by a smile, such as "Fantastic /s/ sound when you said *sun*!"). Positive punishment (often described as correction) is also used to shape a behavior (e.g., verbal correction such as "Oops, that was a slushy /s/ that time. Try again," accompanied by an appropriate facial expression).

Types of positive reinforcement

There are different types of positive reinforcers—primary, social, conditioned, informative, and self-reinforcers (Hegde & Davis, 2010; Mowrer, 1989; Peña-Brooks & Hegde, 2015; Skinner, 1938). They can be used on their own (e.g., social reinforcement only) or combined with one another (e.g., social, conditioned, and informative reinforcement) (Peña-Brooks & Hegde, 2015). **Primary reinforcers** are naturally occurring or biological in nature and do not need to be taught or conditioned as reinforcers (e.g., food and water). Powell et al. (1991) reported successfully using candy as a primary reinforcer for correct responses in an intervention study with children who had an SSD. Mowrer (1989) suggested that you should probably rule out food items as reinforcers, particularly when working in school settings. If you do use them, Hegde and Davis (2010) suggest that primary reinforcers should only be used with parent/caregiver permission and, when food is involved, that healthy options be considered. **Social reinforcers** will be familiar to you. They include any kind of verbal or nonverbal social response that a child would find pleasant (e.g., verbal praise, attention, a smile, encouraging facial expression, a high five, a gentle pat on the shoulder, or verbal approval) (Hedge & Davis, 2010). **Conditioned reinforcers** (also referred to as secondary reinforcers) are conditioned or taught to children as reinforcing. There are three different types—tangible reinforcement, activity reinforcement, and tokens. A **tangible reward** is a concrete reward that a child finds pleasant (e.g., stamp, sticker, check mark on a chart, a bead to make a bracelet, or a piece of craft that contributes to a collage). We recommend that you keep your tangible rewards inexpensive and simple, such as stamps and stickers. A **reinforcing activity** is an activity that a child enjoys doing (e.g., using an electronic device, taking a turn in a game, or gluing a piece of craft on a collage). A **token** is something that a child can exchange for another type of positive reinforcer. Tokens acquire value when children learn that they can be exchanged for something else (e.g., 10 tokens = 1 minute playing an electronic game). Mowrer (1989) described an interesting token economy system, whereby children could redeem tokens for reinforcers from what he calls a reinforcement menu. Using Mowrer's idea, the menu could include a wide range of reinforcers, each with their own cost (e.g., stamp = 10 tokens; a small toy car = 100 tokens; a small plastic insect = 80 tokens; opportunity to play a game on an electronic device = 50 tokens). These reinforcers could be used as part of a token economy system. Table 11-1 provides a list of tangible and activity reinforcers that you could use with children. The list of ideas in Table 11-1 is not exhaustive—as you work with children, you will discover what individual children enjoy and what might work as reinforcement.

An **informative reinforcer** is verbal or nonverbal information that individuals receive about their performance (Peña-Brooks & Hegde, 2015). Informative verbal reinforcement could be a comment about how the child has improved and how he or she is on track to achieving a predetermined goal (e.g., "In the first session when we started working on the /s/ sound, you could produce the sound correctly about 20% of the time. Today you achieved 80% correct. You've really improved!"). Informative nonverbal reinforcement could be a graph that depicts improvement over time. It could also be images from biofeedback devices such as an ultrasound, electropalatogram, or spectrograph from the beginning of intervention to a later point in time.

Self-reinforcement can involve children simply taking pleasure in their own correct or improved performance—they become intrinsically motivated to do well. Self-reinforcement can also involve children administering their own reinforcement (e.g., stamp on a page, selecting a token for each correct response) contingent upon their own judgment of success (Blount & Stokes, 1984).

Schedules of reinforcement

Reinforcement can be helpful for establishing a new behavior. However, given that one of the goals of intervention is to facilitate generalized acquisition of a behavior, you do not want children to only use targeted behaviors when reinforcers are present. To help strengthen and sustain behaviors, it is important that you use a reinforcement schedule—a

TABLE 11-1 Suggested tangible and activity reinforcers to use during intervention with children with SSD

Tangible reinforcers	Activity reinforcers
■ stamp	■ turn of a game
■ sticker	■ play a favorite electronic game
■ check mark on a chart	■ brief ball game
■ a small bead to form a bracelet	■ draw on a whiteboard
■ trading card	■ listen to more of a story
■ marbles that can be used in a game	■ turn of a pop-up toy
■ portions of modelling dough used to create an object	■ turn of a spinning top
■ puzzle pieces used to create a puzzle	■ turn of a windup toy
■ toy building blocks to create a tower	■ look through a kaleidoscope
■ pieces of a picture to create a poster of a child's favorite animal or superhero	■ take a funny photo
■ items of doll's clothing used to dress a doll	■ blow and pop some bubbles
■ craft pieces (e.g., feather, piece of fabric, cardboard shape, button, straw) used to create a collage	■ throw a ball at a tower of blocks
■ tea party pieces used to create a tea party activity	

schedule that describes how often or when reinforcement is provided. Based on Skinner's (1938) original ideas, five types of schedules are possible:

- **Continuous schedule:** reinforcement is given immediately following every response.
- **Fixed ratio:** reinforcement is given after a predetermined number of responses (e.g., every fifth response is reinforced).
- **Variable ratio:** reinforcement is given after an average number of responses (e.g., reinforce the third response, then the seventh response, making an average of five responses until reinforcement is provided).
- **Fixed interval:** reinforcement is given after a predetermined period of time (e.g., every 2 minutes during a conversational speech task).
- **Variable interval:** reinforcement is given after an average period of time (e.g., reinforce at 1 minute, then 3 minutes, making an average of 2 minutes until reinforcement is provided).

A continuous schedule may be used early on in intervention, to help establish a behavior. Paradoxically, behaviors are strengthened, more resistant to extinction, and more likely to generalize when they are reinforced intermittently (via a fixed or variable ratio/interval) rather than continuously (Miltenberger, 2016).

CHILDREN'S INSIGHTS: *Reinforcement plans and schedules for individual children with SSD: "Stickers are a bit too boring ..."*

When Elise's son was 11 years old, stamps and stickers had clearly lost their positive reinforcing power when he commented that "Stickers are a bit too boring for me now." Although reinforcement can do wonders to motivate children during intervention, you need to think about the type of reinforcement(s) that you will use. You also need to have a schedule for how your reinforcement will be delivered. In a study of the concurrent approach with school-age children who had an interdental lisp, Skelton (2004a) used a variety of positive reinforcers including verbal praise, a token economy system, and tangible reinforcement (e.g., stickers, pens, and small toys). Initially a continuous schedule was used. Once the children achieved 90% correct productions, the reinforcement scheduled changed to a fixed ratio of two. After another 90% correct productions, a fixed ratio of three was used. The schedule was eventually changed to a fixed ratio of six. If a child's performance dropped to below 50% correct, the reinforcement schedule was changed to the previous fixed ratio (Skelton, 2004a).

APPLICATION: *Create a suitable reinforcement plan for Susie*

Review Susie's background history (Chapter 16) and create a suitable reinforcement plan. As part of your plan, describe the type(s) of reinforcement and the schedule that you could use. Your answers to the following questions will help you devise a plan.

- What are Susie's interests?
- What type(s) of reinforcement might motivate Susie to practice accurate articulation of /s/ during intervention with an SLP?
- What type of reinforcement schedule could you use during the first two sessions? How could you vary the schedule in subsequent sessions, and why?

Read more about Susie (7;4 years), a girl with an articulation impairment (lateral lisp), in Chapter 16 (Case 2).

> **COMMENT:** *Principles of behavioral learning and principles of motor learning*
>
> Principles of behavioral learning influenced the principles of motor learning. For instance, Skinner's (1936) work with rats on the effect of different intervals of time between a behavior and reinforcement of that behavior influenced Schmidt and colleagues' research on the effect of delayed feedback on motor learning in humans (e.g., Salmoni et al., 1984). This is why you find some similarity in terms and ideas between the principles of behavioral learning and the principles of motor learning.

■ Principles of intervention: Neurological experience

The brain can change its structure and function as a result of activity or experience (Doidge, 2010). The term used to describe this change is **experience-dependent neural plasticity** (Kleim & Jones, 2008). However, lasting neural change does not happen instantly—you cannot change your brain simply by doing something once. In this section we consider principles of experience-dependent neural plastic change as they relate to intervention for children with SSD. You will notice that some of these principles are similar to the principles of motor learning.

- If you use a new skill you can improve it; if you do not use it, you can lose it (Kleim & Jones, 2008).
  Principle: When helping children learn a new speech skill, regular practice can help improve that skill; without any practice, a new skill can be forgotten. An extreme example of this principle occurs in children born profoundly deaf. Without any practice at processing sound, the auditory cortex (section of the brain that was set up to process speech) can be taken over or recruited by the visual system through lack of auditory input (Cardon, Campbell, & Sharma, 2012).
- Younger brains are more plastic and have sensitive periods or windows of time during which neural development more readily takes place (Gollin, 1981).
  Principle: Intervention for children with SSD needs to take place at an optimal time—earlier being better than later. For instance, Fulcher, Purcell, Baker, & Munro (2012) found that timing was crucial for children with hearing loss to learn to speak clearly and intelligibly. They studied the speech and language abilities of children with early- versus late-identified hearing loss who had been enrolled in the same oral auditory-verbal early intervention program. The children with early-identified hearing loss (< 12 months) significantly outperformed the children with late-identified hearing loss (> 12 months but < 5 years), with 96% of the early-identified children having age-appropriate intelligible speech by 5 years of age.
- Experience-dependent neural plastic change requires sufficient repetition and intensity of practice (Kleim & Jones, 2008).
  Principle: For neural plastic change to occur, intervention for children with SSD needs to involve opportunities for repetitive practice (i.e., an adequate dose both within and across sessions) and an optimal intervention intensity (e.g., Allen, 2013; Williams, 2012). Insufficient repetition of a new skill and an inadequate intensity (e.g., low dose, relatively short session duration, frequency, or total intervention duration or time) has been associated with inadequate improvement (e.g., Glogowska, Roulstone, Enderby, & Peters, 2000).
- The salience of an experience can influence the extent of experience-dependent neural plastic change, with highly salient experiences being associated with greater neural change (Kleim & Jones, 2008).
  Principle: During intervention for children with SSD, ensure that practice is salient and important. Salience is evident when children are focused (i.e., attentive, motivated, and making an effort). As Kwiatkowski and Shriberg (1998) point out, lack of motivation in a child can be a reason why a child fails to learn.

COMMENT: *Intelligible speech is still possible after a hemispherectomy*

Hemispherectomy is a rare and radical surgical procedure for children needing relief from drug-resistant epilepsy (Liégeois et al., 2010). In a study of the speech production skills of 13 speakers (aged 9;7 to 23;11 years) who had undergone childhood hemispherectomy 1 to 13 years prior to the study, Liégeois et al. (2010) reported that 12 of the 13 speakers had intelligible speech. They did, however, show symptoms of mild flaccid-ataxic dysarthria, suggesting considerable but not necessarily complete neural reorganization of the control of fine speech motor movements. It is important to note that prior to the hemispherectomy, all speakers had hemiplegia associated with different pathologies (e.g., cyst, cerebrovascular accident of the middle cerebral artery, Rasmussen's encephalitis), and that they had varied verbal IQ scores (from extremely low to average). Vargha-Khadem et al. (1997) reported a similarly remarkable case of a 9-year-old boy (Alex) with Sturge-Weber syndrome. Alex learned to speak following a hemispherectomy and the withdrawal of anticonvulsant medication. These cases are remarkable examples of the plasticity of children's brains.

COMMENT: *Experience-dependent neural plastic change observed in children's brains after intervention*

Kadis et al. (2014) assessed the cortical thickness of nine children's brains using magnetic resonance imaging (MRI) before and after PROMPT intervention. (PROMPT intervention is discussed in Chapter 14). The children had been diagnosed as having CAS. Through the use of magnetic resonance imaging (MRI), Kadis et al. (2014) discovered that an area of the children's brains, the left posterior superior temporal gyrus (also known as Wernicke's area), showed significant thinning after 8 weeks of PROMPT intervention. Kadis et al. suggested that the thinning reflected possible neural pruning. This is one of the first papers to publish evidence of experience-dependent neural plastic change in children with SSD.

APPLICATION: *What do children find motivating?*

Read more about Jarrod (7;0 years), Michael (4;2 years), and Lian (14;2 years) in Chapter 16.

Review the background information for the clinical cases discussed in Chapter 16 of this book. In light of Jarrod, Lian, and Michael's interests, what could you do to foster their motivation during intervention?

INTERVENTION PLANS

Intervention plans are an important part of your day-to-day work—they help you navigate a course of action to achieve a goal. Plans outline what needs to be done, when, how, and by whom. They are influenced by your model of intervention practice. In this section we describe four different models of intervention practice. We then provide an overview of two types of plans (management plans and session plans) and the service delivery options involved in making those plans.

■ Models of intervention practice: Therapist-centered, parent-as-therapist aide, family-centered, and family-friendly practice

There are four different models of practice that influence how practice is conducted and who is responsible for making clinical decisions and plans: therapist-centered, parent-as-therapist aide, family-centered practice, and family-friendly practice (Watts Pappas & McLeod, 2009).

- **Therapist-centered practice:** Traditionally, SLPs used therapist-centered practice. In this model of practice, the SLP is considered the expert who directs and controls the planning and delivery of intervention, as well as how parents may or may not be involved in the therapeutic process (Watts Pappas, McLeod, McAllister & McKinnon, 2008). The child is the client, not the child and his or her family. Historically, this approach to management was adopted for children with SSD because families (particularly parents) were believed to underlie the problem. Consider the following comment from Wood (1946): "Functional articulatory defects of children are definitely and significantly associated with maladjustment and undesirable traits on the part of the parents, and such factors are usually maternally centered" (p. 272). There is no evidence to support this belief. However, in modern Western contexts, families may be less likely to advocate for a therapist-centered approach because they have access to a wide range of information via the Internet and may prefer to have more involvement in the planning and delivery of intervention, so will opt for one of the approaches below.
- **Parent-as-therapist aide:** Parent-as-therapist aide is a variation on therapist-centered practice where the family is involved in intervention provision but not in intervention planning (Watts Pappas & McLeod, 2009). The primary decision-maker is still the SLP, and the primary client is still the child. There is a substantial evidence base to support the involvement of parents in intervention (e.g., Law, Garrett, & Nye, 2010).
- **Family-centered practice:** Family-centered practice considers the whole family to be the client, not just the child. The family is actively involved in intervention planning. Families (not clinicians) are the primary decision-makers—with their decisions being supported and accepted by clinicians even if clinicians do not agree with them (King, Rosenbaum, & King, 1997). Positive relationships between parents and clinicians are a hallmark of family-centered practice, with parents acknowledged as capable rather than being dependent on clinicians (Dunst, 2002). This model of practice is frequently used with families who have a child with long-term or lifelong complex disorders requiring input from many different professionals (e.g., cerebral palsy).
- **Family-friendly practice:** Family-friendly practice is a model developed by Watts Pappas (2010). It is a combination of therapist- and family-centered practice: families are the client (rather than the child) and are involved in intervention planning; however, in this approach SLPs use their expertise to guide intervention, fulfilling their responsibility to provide effective, empirically supported intervention (Watts Pappas, 2010). Families are also supported to be involved in intervention, if required.

Both family-centered and family-friendly practices are the preferred models of practice. They align with legislation (e.g., IDEA 2004) mandating family involvement. In Chapters 13 and 14 you will learn about intervention approaches that adopt a family-friendly model of practice, such as Bowen and Cupples' (1999a) Parents and Children Together (PACT) approach for children who have phonological impairment, and the core vocabulary approach by Dodd et al. (2010) for children who have inconsistent speech disorder. What follows is an overview of the types of plans and the service delivery options that make up those plans.

■ Management plans

Management plans outline your broad plan or program for managing an individual case. The level of detail and the range of areas addressed in a management plan are usually influenced by your place of work (e.g., school and local education agency, early intervention service, health care setting, private practice), relevant public laws and/or policies, and guiding model of practice. As depicted in Figure 11-4, most management plans cover six areas:

FIGURE 11-4 Areas addressed in management plans for children with SSD

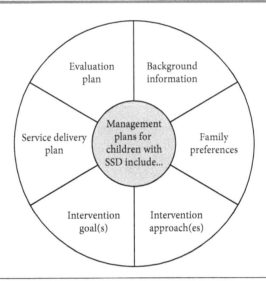

■ **Background information:** This section includes the child and family's demographic details, a description of the children's interests, diagnostic and prognostic statements, in addition to an empirically supported estimate of the total intervention duration required to achieve the long-term goal (e.g., number of anticipated SLP hours; anticipated period of time in weeks, months, years, or school terms).

■ **Family preferences and a plan for family involvement in intervention:** This section includes an overview of the family structure, family's preferences for management (including service delivery), and parent/caregiver roles, that may include one or more of the following:
  ■ parent/caregiver training for the parent/caregiver to be the primary provider of intervention;
  ■ parent/caregiver training for the parent/caregiver to provide home activities;
  ■ parent/caregiver attendance at intervention sessions;
  ■ parent/caregiver participation in intervention sessions;
  ■ parent/caregiver involvement in home activities.

■ **Intervention goals:** This section includes your target selection approach and a relevant evidence-based rationale, in addition to the long-term, short-term, and anticipated session goals based on assessment and analysis. (Refer to Chapters 9 and 10 for information on analysis and goal setting.)

■ **Intervention approach:** This section identifies your intervention approach and relevant evidence-based rationale.

■ **Service delivery plan:** This section outlines the intervention setting (pull-out session in a school, session within a classroom, early childhood setting, public speech-language pathology clinic, private speech-language pathology practice, telehealth or other), intervention agent (SLP, SLP assistant, teacher's assistant, teacher, parent/caregiver, computer, or other), session duration and session frequency, intervention format (individual and/or group intervention, parent training), and intervention continuity (continuous or block for a specified duration).

■ **Evaluation plan:** Your evaluation plan specifies the type of data that will be collected, how it will be collected, who will collect the data, and how often. As you will learn in Chapter 12, five different types of data need to be considered to evaluate intervention—assessment data, baseline data, treatment data, generalization data (stimulus and response), and control data.

Appendix 11-1 provides a generic management plan template that you could use to plan intervention with children and their families.

Management plans: IEPs and IFSPs

A management plan for a child with a diagnosed disability is referred to as an **Individual Education Program (IEP)**. It is a plan developed in consultation with relevant health and/or education professionals and the child's family. It typically contains information about a child's current levels of academic achievement and functional performance (including strengths and areas of need), measurable annual goals and short-term goals or objectives, statements about any special factors requiring consideration (e.g., child has limited English proficiency), the service(s) and supplementary aids to be provided that will help a child progress in the education curriculum, in addition to an outline of how and when a child's progress will be evaluated (Ellis & Hodson, 2013). An IEP is reviewed at least every year to determine if any changes to the plan are needed (Ellis & Hodson, 2013). A plan for a younger child (birth to under three years of age) receiving early intervention services is referred to as an **Individual Family Service Plan (IFPS)**. In the United States, both plans (IEPs and IFSPs) are provided under the Individuals with Disabilities Education Act (2004) (IDEA 2004). It is important to realize that not all children living in the United States who have an SSD will be eligible for special education services under IDEA 2004. This is because eligibility for special education for "impaired articulation" under CFR (Code of Federal Regulations) 34 Section 300.8(c)(11) of the law specifies that a child's speech difficulty "adversely affects a child's educational performance." When it cannot be reasonably established that a child's SSD negatively affects a child's educational performance (e.g., children who have a mild SSD associated with one or two later developing sounds such as interdental /s/ or distorted /ɹ/), they could receive **early intervening services (EIS)** using a **response to intervention** framework (Mire & Montgomery, 2009). We encourage you to become familiar with the laws and policies that guide clinical services for the children with SSD in the state or country in which you work, so that you are familiar with the types of plans needed. See Chapter 15 for further information about different types of laws and policies influencing speech-language pathology services.

Response to intervention

Response to intervention (RTI) is a three-tiered process through which children can be provided with intervention before receiving an assessment to determine if they are eligible for special education services under IDEA (2004) (Power-de Fur, 2011). Tier 1 consists of evidence-based educational instruction in the classroom. If data suggest that a child is not responding to Tier 1 instruction, the child could be provided with Tier 2 instruction (e.g., increased intensity and intervention in a small group) (Mire & Montgomery, 2009). Finally, if a child does not maintain progress given Tier 2 intervention, then the child may be assessed to determine whether he or she meets IDEA and state eligibility criteria for Tier 3 (i.e., special education services) (Mire & Montgomery, 2009). Although Tier 1 and Tier 2 early intervening services for children with more mild SSD may not be linked to special education and an IEP, you will still need to write a management plan—you will still need to identify goals, understand family preferences, specify an intervention approach, select a suitable service delivery option, and identify strategies for evaluating progress (i.e., evaluate the child's response to intervention). Kuhn (2006) and Mire and Montgomery (2009) provide helpful practical examples of programs used to manage children with SSD in early intervening services, using a response to intervention framework.

■ Session plans

A session plan (also known as a lesson plan or remediation plan) outlines what will occur during an intervention session. Think of session plans as practical step-by-step guides for implementing management plans. As shown in Figure 11-5, a session plan usually includes some brief background information, the goals to be targeted during the session, a summary of the service delivery plan (setting, agent, intensity, format, continuity), the intervention approach(es) to be used, a description of the dialogue to be used during a typical teaching and learning moment (including antecedent event, response and consequent event), the intervention stimulus (types of intervention words, phrases, sentences, or conversation topics that you will use), your plan of activities (including a description of the

FIGURE 11-5   Areas addressed in session plans for children with SSD

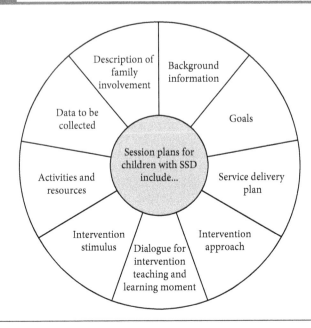

resources/materials required during the session), an outline of the type of data to be collected during the session, and a statement about how the family/significant others may be involved, including a description of the home activities. A generic intervention session plan template is provided in Appendix 11-2. You will learn more about data collection plans in Chapter 12, and the types of intervention approaches that you can use with children in Chapters 13 and 14. What follows is an overview of service delivery options that are used when working with children with SSD.

■ Service delivery options

Intervention plans for children with SSD require various decisions to be made regarding the delivery of the service. These decisions include:

- intervention setting: where will the session be conducted;
- intervention agent: who will provide intervention;
- intensity: the duration, frequency, and total number of anticipated intervention sessions;
- continuity: whether intervention will be conducted in continuous or block mode; and
- format: whether intervention will be provided in an individual or group format.

Intervention settings

Intervention can be conducted in a range of settings; however, the setting is usually influenced by SLPs' places of work and/or where the clients live. As a student clinician, your first clinical practicum may be at a university clinic. Other settings for working with children with SSD and their families can include schools, preschools, early childhood centers, hospitals, community health clinics, specialist centers, private practice clinics, and homes. In schools, preschools, and early childhood centers, a **pull-out model** (seeing students for an assessment and/or intervention in an SLP's office or clinical room set aside for that purpose) or a **push-in model** (seeing one or more students in a separate area of the classroom while the rest of the class completes other activities) may be used (Hegde & Davis, 2010). SLPs can also work alongside a teacher with the whole class, coordinating and running lessons together—this is an example of **collaborative consultation**. For children with SSD, whole-classroom activities may focus on emergent literacy abilities including phonemic awareness (Gillon, 2005). Collectively, these settings reflect a **side-by-side** or **in-person model** of service delivery—you and the child and his or her family or significant others meet together in the same location (Grogan-Johnson et al., 2013).

Telepractice (also known as telehealth, telemedicine, telerehabilitation, tele-speech, speech teletherapy) offers an alternate setting in which telecommunication technology is used to provide speech-language pathology services at a distance—the clinician is in one location and the child and his or her family or significant other are in another location (ASHA, 2010d). The service can be provided in **real time** (i.e., synchronous) involving a live audio and visual connection between the clinician and the client, in a **store-and-forward** manner (i.e., asynchronous), or a **hybrid** of the two (Stewart Keck & Doarn, 2014). In a study comparing outcomes for 13 children with SSD (aged between 6 and 11 years) receiving traditional articulation therapy delivered in-person or via telepractice, Grogan-Johnson et al. (2011) reported that the children in both groups significantly improved their scores on the Goldman-Fristoe Test of Articulation-2 (Goldman & Fristoe, 2000). The children receiving the telepractice option also received support from an e-helper—to provide adult supervision and ensure that any problems with the technology could be solved. In a similar study, Grogan-Johnson et al. (2013) compared in-person and telepractice-delivered intervention for 14 children (aged between 6 and 11 years) with SSD. The children in this study were randomly assigned to one condition, receiving traditional articulation therapy in 30-minute sessions twice weekly for 5 weeks. Children in both groups improved their speech production skills. Given that telepractice delivery is a relatively new option and that technology continues to improve, further research would be needed to identify the types of children and families, SSD, and intervention approaches suited to delivery via telepractice.

Intervention agents: Direct and indirect intervention

Intervention can be provided directly by the SLP or indirectly by other personnel such as parents and caregivers, teachers, and SLP assistants trained and supervised by SLPs. Most of the published intervention research is based on outcomes associated with direct intervention by SLPs, with other personnel serving a supplementary role (e.g., completing homework activities, participating in sessions) (e.g., Bowen & Cupples, 1999a; Strand et al., 2006). Of the small number of studies reporting outcomes for children with SSD when treated by other personnel as the primary agent, improvements in children's speech have been reported. Across these studies, it would seem that the type and amount of training provided to parents and other personnel is an important consideration. For example, Costello and Schoen (1978) reported that trained paraprofessionals achieved outcomes as good as those achieved by SLPs when using a prescriptive program (S-Pack by Mowrer, 1968) with school-age children who had an interdental lisp. Eiserman, McCoun, and Escobar (1990) compared SLP and parent-delivered intervention. The SLP intervention was delivered in small groups (each comprising two preschoolers) for 1 hour once a week over 7 months. The parent-delivered intervention consisted of 40-minute individual parent-training sessions at home twice a month over 7 months and their preschoolers receiving parent-delivered intervention for 20- to 30-minute sessions four times per week. Eiserman et al. (1990) reported that the children who received intervention from their parents at home performed at least as well as the children who received small group intervention from their SLP in the clinic, based on measures of speech, language, and general development. Broen and Westman (1990) reported similar positive findings for preschoolers who had phonological impairment. Their parent-delivered intervention (1½ hour weekly parent classes over 17 weeks) was associated with significantly greater improvement over time compared to a control group. By contrast, a community-based study of eclectic intervention (intervention comprising an informal mix or assortment of intervention methods) reported strongly significant gains for children receiving intervention provided by an SLP, with lesser but still significant gains being made by children receiving intervention from parents, and no change apparent in a group of untreated children (Lancaster, Keusch, Levin, Pring, & Martin, 2010). In the study by Lancaster and colleagues, the parents received 2 hours of parent training in a group, resources, and six weekly review appointments with an SLP.

The type of SSD also seems important to consider when deciding on primary and/or supplementary intervention agents. Across the SSD intervention literature, parents or SLP assistants have been the primary intervention agent for children who had an interdental lisp (Costello & Schoen, 1978) or phonological impairment (e.g., Broen & Westman, 1990; Lancaster et al., 2010). The role of parents and paraprofessionals as the primary agent for children with motor speech disorders such as CAS and childhood dysarthria has received less attention. However, this does not mean that involvement from parents or other personnel with these children is not valuable. On the contrary, given that motor speech disorders require regular practice over a long period of time, parents and others as supplementary intervention agents can be very valuable (e.g., Strand et al., 2006). As Fish (2011) highlights, parents are in the ideal position to help their children to practice targeted speech skills in naturalistic ways in everyday activities as well as in extra practice sessions at home.

COMMENT: *How can I encourage parents to complete effective home practice?*

According to Watts Pappas (2010), two components help to ensure successful home practice: motivation and effective parent training.

1. **Motivation:** Both parents and their children need to be motivated to complete home practice. In a study of eight children with severe motor speech disorders, Nordness and Beukelman (2010) discovered that the act of asking parents to write down how much practice is being done meant that more practice occurred (or if none was being done in the first place, it actually was done)! Günther and Hautvast (2010) also discovered that contingency management strategies (e.g., a child receiving a token for achieving a predetermined goal, then being able to exchange the token for a motivating tangible or social reward such as stickers, candy, coloring books, or activities) increased the amount of home practice done between speech-language pathology sessions. They also noted that regular home practice can improve intervention outcomes.

2. **Effective parent training:** A variety of methods can be used to provide clear and effective training for parents, such as:

   ■ SLPs providing parents with standardized written and verbal information;
   ■ parents observing and participating in sessions;
   ■ SLPs and parents engaging in role play;
   ■ parents observing videos of clinicians and other parents conducting intervention;
   ■ SLPs providing parents with both encouraging and constructive verbal, written, and graphic feedback; and
   ■ parents watching then reflecting on videos of themselves conducting intervention with their child and evaluating their child's progress (Scherer & Kaiser, 2010).

Bowen (1998) provided helpful information for parents about a range of teaching and learning techniques including modelling, recasting, encouraging children to self-monitor and self-correct, auditory input, and praise. A website developed and maintained by SLP Dr. Caroline Bowen contains a wealth of parent-training resources targeted towards phonological impairment.[1] Fish (2011) provides helpful information for clinicians partnering with parents with children who have CAS, such as providing parents with comprehensive sources of information about CAS, allowing parents to observe and participate in sessions, encouraging parents to develop their own games and activities for home practice, helping parents recognize their child's gains even when they may be small or slow in coming, and being sensitive to parents' emotions and growing understanding about the nature and extent of their child's difficulties.

[1]http://speech-language-therapy.com

Computers can be another agent of intervention. Although they do not completely replace personnel, computer-delivered practice has some advantages. Children can find computer-delivered intervention more engaging than traditional tabletop activities (Jamiseon, 2004). Depending on the speed and type of computer program, computer-delivered intervention can engage children in repetitive practice of a newly learned skill. For example, Nordness and Beukelman (2010) discovered that computer-led practice (in the form of pictures and animations in a PowerPoint presentation), increased the amount of home practice completed by children working on a motor-based intervention, relative to parent-led practice.

Intervention intensity: Dose, frequency, session duration, and total intervention duration

Based on the principles of motor learning and neural plasticity, learning requires practice—and practice requires sufficient repetition or intensity (Kleim & Jones, 2008). Warren, Fey, and Yoder (2007) provide a helpful framework capturing all the different ways that the intensity of intervention for children with SSD can be measured and manipulated. Based on their framework, intervention intensity includes:

- **Dose form:** the activity in which episodes of teaching are delivered (Warren et al., 2007). For children with SSD, this could mean providing intervention during a drill, drill play, structured play, or unstructured play activity (Shriberg & Kwiatkowski, 1982b). You will learn more about these different types of activities in Chapter 12.
- **Dose:** the total number of teaching episodes in an intervention session (Warren et al., 2007). For children with SSD, this could mean the number of times a particular skill is practiced during a session, such as 100 production practice trials of minimal pair words targeting /s/ cluster reduction during a 45-minute intervention session (Baker & McLeod, 2004).
- **Session duration:** the period of time taken to run a session. Using dose and session duration, you can also calculate dosage rate or the density of teaching episodes per unit of time (Warren et al., 2007). For example, Dodd et al. (2010) recommend a high dosage rate (150 to 170 trials in a 30-minute session, equivalent to approximately 5 trials per minute) for core vocabulary intervention.
- **Dose frequency:** the number of intervention sessions in a given period of time such as per week or month (Baker, 2012a). For children with SSD, this could mean attending intervention sessions three times per week (Allen, 2013).
- **Total intervention duration:** the period of time during which intervention is provided. Intervention can be provided for a predetermined period of time, or the total period of time from referral to dismissal. It can be measured in number of sessions, number of SLP hours, or calendar time (weeks, months, or years). For example, Williams (2012) recommended that for children with severe phonological impairment receiving multiple oppositions intervention, they receive a dose of at least 70 trials in 30-minute sessions for approximately 40 sessions (Williams, 2012).

 APPLICATION: *Intervention intensity plan for Susie*

Susie's case is outlined in Chapter 16. Suppose you are a school-based SLP and you are going to work with Susie on production practice of clear /s/, using a variable random practice sequence, in keeping with Skelton's (2004a) concurrent approach to intervention (as described in Chapter 14).

1. Develop an intervention intensity plan for Susie, deciding on session dose, duration, frequency, and total intervention duration.
2. Calculate the anticipated dosage rate and cumulative intervention intensity.
3. Compare and contrast your intervention intensity plan with a peer, in addition to the information about Skelton's (2004a) concurrent intervention approach in Chapter 14.

Read more about
Susie (7;4 years),
a girl with an articulation
impairment (lateral lisp),
in Chapter 16 (Case 2).

■ **Cumulative intervention intensity:** a quantitative measure summarizing the amount of practice in a session (dose) times (×) the session or dose frequency and total intervention duration (e.g., 70 trials × twice weekly × 20 sessions = 2,800 production practice trials). You will learn more about the intervention intensity recommendations for different approaches to intervention for different types of SSD in Chapters 13 and 14.

Continuity: Ongoing intervention and block formats

Intervention can be provided in an ongoing, continuous manner (e.g., weekly until a particular goal is achieved) or in blocks and breaks (e.g., two 9-week blocks separated by a 5-week break) (Tyler & Figurski, 1994). Like individual and group formats, they each have advantages and disadvantages. In a continuous format, practice can be regular and children and their families can be motivated to work towards a goal. Without a break, however, some children can lose motivation and interest. In contrast, planned blocks and breaks can provide children with a period of time to consolidate newly learned skills and allow phonological generalization to occur (Bowen, 2009; Hodson & Paden, 1991; Tyler & Figurski, 1994). Blocks interspersed with breaks also offer a convenient and efficient method for scheduling intervention (Tyler & Figurski, 1994; Tyler, Lewis, Haskill, & Tolbert, 2003). In addition, planned blocks and breaks can provide families with a period for respite and an opportunity to refresh before another block (Bowen, 2009). Blocks and breaks can be scheduled around school terms and school holidays (e.g., 10-week school term followed by a 2-week school holiday). As an evidence-based clinician, decisions regarding the provision of ongoing intervention versus blocks and breaks should be guided by empirical evidence and workplace policy, in addition to child and family preference.

Intervention format: Individual and groups

Intervention can be provided in a few different formats: **individually** (i.e., 1:1), in a **group**, or in a **combination** of individual and group. The formats used are often influenced by your place of work. For instance, in a survey of 489 SLPs working in the United States (working in preschools and schools, early childhood centers, private practice, or university clinics), Brumbaugh and Smit (2013) reported that SLPs provided intervention in individual, group, or a combination of individual and group formats, with more SLPs providing intervention in an individual format. Reports from the American Speech-Language-Hearing Association National Outcome Measurement System (NOMS) found that of the majority of SLPs working on articulation/intelligibility with pre-kindergarten children, 92.1% reported using individual pull-out intervention, with 5.6% providing intervention in groups, 1% providing intervention in the classroom, and 1% in a self-contained classroom (American Speech-Language-Hearing Association, 2011). A similar finding was reported in a survey about 231 SLPs working in Australia (private practice: 38.1%, education: 37.7%, or community health: 29.0%). In this study, participants could check as many different setting types and intervention options as they used within their clinical setting. The majority (95.7%) provided individual intervention, with group intervention only being used by 36.7% of participants (McLeod & Baker, 2014).

■■■

✅ **APPLICATION:** *Should children with SSD be seen individually or in a group format?*

1. What do you think are the advantages and disadvantages of conducting intervention for Luke (4;3 years) in an individual format versus a group format? For the group format, assume that Luke is one of three preschoolers with a severe phonological impairment. Compare your list of advantages and disadvantages with a peer and the list offered in Table 11-2. (See Chapter 16 for further information about Luke.)

2. If you had to work with Luke in a group format, what practical steps could you take to overcome some of the disadvantages of a group format?

Read more about Luke (4;3 years), a boy with a phonological impairment, in Chapter 16 (Case 1).

Individual and group intervention each has advantages and disadvantages; however, is one format superior to another? The majority of intervention research has been conducted using an individual format. For example, in a narrative review of 134 peer-reviewed intervention studies for children with phonological impairment, most interventions were conducted in a one-to-one format (78.7%), with some in groups (10.3%) or combinations of individual and group (7.4%) (Baker & McLeod, 2011a). A systematic review of 23 peer-reviewed published studies for children with CAS reported that all interventions were delivered individually (Murray, McCabe, & Ballard, 2014). Relatively little is known empirically if one format is better than another (Cirrin et al., 2010). One study (Sommers et al., 1966) reported no difference in the outcomes for 240 children receiving approximately 8½ months of weekly traditional articulation therapy (discussed in Chapter 14) in an individual versus group format. However, the children in the individual format received 30-minute sessions while the children in the group format (each comprising three to six children) received 45-minute sessions. It seems that some attempt was made to ensure that the children in the group condition had similar numbers of opportunities to practice (i.e., dose). In addition, the authors noted that each child receiving group therapy received at least 5 minutes of one-to-one instruction from the SLP during each 45-minute session in an effort to motivate the

| TABLE 11-2 | Advantages and disadvantages of individual versus group intervention for children with SSD |

Individual intervention	Group intervention
Advantages	**Advantages**
■ Easier to achieve recommended optimum dose.	■ More children can be seen in the same time period—resulting in economic benefits for a service and reduced waiting lists.
■ Sessions (including speech perception and/or production targets, activities, and reinforcement) can be planned according to an individual child's needs, interests, and motivation.	■ Groups create opportunities for parents of children with SSD to meet and support one another.
■ Sessions can be modified given an individual child's response to intervention.	■ Multiple speakers (including children and adults) can provide opportunities for targeting speech perception skills (particularly judgment of correctness tasks) in an effort to refine underlying perceptual representations of words.
■ Children who are self-conscious and shy may be more willing to participate and talk in an individual session.	■ Competition during an activity can increase motivation to practice for some children.
■ Appointment schedules can be more flexible.	■ Children may not feel singled out when participating in a small group.
■ Data collection (including treatment, generalization, and control data) can be easier and more efficient.	■ Groups create opportunities for developing turn taking and listening skills.
■ Confidentiality is easier to maintain in an individual context.	■ Activities requiring naturalistic conversation (including opportunities to respond to requests for clarification) are readily available in a group format.
■ Outcomes for individual intervention can be better than group intervention.	**Disadvantages**
Disadvantages	■ Children need to wait for their turn, making it more challenging to achieve each individual child's optimum dose for the session.
■ It can be more expensive to provide intervention in an individual format.	■ Time can be occupied by managing other children's off-task behaviors and group dynamics.
■ Relative to a group context, there are fewer opportunities to work on stimulus generalization and naturalistic conversation.	■ Some children can be easily distracted by other children in a group format.
■ Parents/caregivers miss out on the opportunity to meet other parents with children who have SSD.	■ Children can spend time listening to unusual or distorted productions of target sounds, which (without time spent on judgment of correctness tasks) could interfere with the development of their perceptual boundaries for sounds in words.

Adapted from: American Speech-Language-Hearing Association (2011); Boyle et al. (2007); Masterson (1993); Reilly (2012).

child, improve speech, facilitate carryover, and set specific goals (Sommers et al., 1966). Thus, although the children in the group condition showed similar outcomes, their outcome could have been influenced by the period of individual intervention received. In a report based on pre-kindergarten NOMS data by the American Speech-Language-Hearing Association, it was noted that the children who received individual sessions were much more likely to show measurable improvements in their speech compared to the children who received group intervention (American Speech-Language-Hearing Association, 2011). Given the limited empirical and practice-based evidence to date, it would seem that clinicians favor individual intervention and that outcomes may be better with an individual format.

PROGRESS AND DISCHARGE PLANNING

Intervention plans include a starting point (the date of the first intervention session) and an anticipated end point when a child can be dismissed or discharged from intervention. In an ideal world, that end point occurs when a long-term goal has been achieved and a child's speech is intelligible and he or she no longer qualifies for services (Baker, 2010a). This sounds simple. In reality, however, progress and discharge planning is a little more complicated. For children with more than one short-term goal, you need to specify criteria for moving on from one goal to the next. You also need to specify the conditions under which a child will be discharged from speech-language pathology services.

■ Short-term goal criteria: When do I move on to a new goal?

There are three approaches for moving on from one short-term goal to another (Bleile, 1996).

- ■ **Performance-based criteria** specify a level of performance that a child must achieve. A variety of criteria have been reported in the literature. Most suggest that children do not need to reach 100% or even 90% accuracy on a generalization probe to advance to another goal. For example, Baker and McLeod (2004) found that children continued to improve without intervention when they achieved 70% correct production of /s/ consonant clusters (in non-treatment words in trained /sp, st, sn/ and untrained /s/ clusters /sl, sw, sk, sm/) in conversational speech. McKercher, McFarlane, and Schneider (1995) recommend 75% accuracy on a single-word probe for targeted sounds. Olswang and Bain (1985) reported that performance between 30% and 74% accuracy of the targeted sound in a probe of untrained single words across three sessions was sufficient for children to continue to improve without further information on the targets. For children with phonological impairment, Williams (2000a) recommends that intervention on a particular target can be discontinued when a child shows 50% accuracy of the targeted sound during conversational speech.
- ■ **Time-based criteria** specify a time during which a particular skill is worked on. For example, "Each phoneme (or consonant cluster) within a pattern is targeted for approximately 60 minutes per cycle (i.e., one 60-minute session, two 30-minute, or three 20-minute sessions) before progressing to the next phoneme in that pattern and then onto other deficient phonological patterns" (Hodson, 2007, p. 90).
- ■ **Flexible criteria** accommodate child factors, changing to new target(s) if a child becomes disinterested or overly frustrated with current target(s) (Bleile, 2006).

■ Long-term goals: When is a child discharged from intervention?

Criteria for discharging a child from intervention center on when the problem is no longer apparent or when a child no longer meets a service's eligibility criteria. For example, for children with an individualized education plan, "dismissal occurs when a student no longer needs special education or related services to take advantage of educational opportunities" (ASHA, 2000, p. 50). Criteria used to determine when intervention is no longer needed have included:

> **CHILDREN'S INSIGHTS:** *When is the right time to finish intervention?*
>
> Sometimes children (particularly school-age children and teenagers) will have their own criteria for when to stop intervention. For example, Jarvis (1989) reported that Luke decided to stop intervention: "I ain't coming to speech no more. My talking's alright" (p. 28). In this situation the SLP agreed because "he was intelligible to unfamiliar adults and children, and his class teacher reported that he did not stand out in the class as a child with a speech problem" (Jarvis, 1989, p. 28).

- children's speech being largely intelligible in conversational speech and any remaining phonological patterns being below 40% occurrence (Hodson & Paden, 1991);
- children's speech being considered appropriate for their chronological age, based on speech intelligibility ratings by an SLP (Montgomery & Bonderman, 1989); and
- intervention targets being produced correctly in spontaneous speech 75% to 90% of the time, with the higher percentage being used if the SLP is concerned that the child might regress once intervention has finished (Bleile, 2004).

Authors also recommend that children's speech be probed in a follow-up appointment (usually about 6 months after stopping intervention), to confirm that generalization did continue as anticipated and that there are no issues requiring intervention (Smit, 2004).

For children with a complex or persistent SSD associated with a concomitant condition (e.g., childhood dysarthria associated with cerebral palsy—as was Lian's case in Chapter 16), discharge criteria may focus on the child developing functional communication skills in accordance with his or her physical capability (ASHA, 2000). Sometimes a child may be discharged for other reasons, such as a plateau in progress (i.e., little documented change over a period of time), poor motivation and attendance, or cessation of intervention at the parent/caregiver request (Steppling, Quattlebaum, & Brady, 2007).

Chapter summary

In this chapter you learned about intervention principles and plans. You learned about phonological, auditory-perceptual, motor, neurological, behavioral, and cognitive principles that underlie interventions for children with SSD. You also learned about models of intervention, management plans, and session plans.

The evidence associated with various service delivery options was covered. Now that you understand principles and plans, you are ready to learn about intervention procedures and how to measure the effect of plans on children's outcomes.

Suggested reading

The following readings contain helpful information about intervention principles and plans.

- Hegde, M. N., & Davis, D. (2010). *Clinical methods and practicum in speech-language pathology* (5th ed.). Clifton Park, NY: Delmar Learning.

- Maas, E., Robin, D. A., Hula, S. N. A., Freedman, S. E., Wulf, G., Ballard, K. J., & Schmidt, R. A. (2008). Principles of motor learning in treatment of motor speech disorders. *American Journal of Speech-Language Pathology, 17,* 277–298.

- Paul, R. (Ed.). (2014). *Introduction to clinical methods in communication disorders* (3rd ed.). Baltimore, MD: Paul H. Brookes.

Application of knowledge from Chapter 11

1. Explain how the principles of motor learning could inform a practice phase of intervention for Michael (4;2 years) (Chapter 16), considering conditions of practice and feedback.

2. In a small group, debate the pros and cons of the four different models of intervention: therapist-centered, parent-as-therapist aide, family-centered practice, and family-friendly practice.

3. Prepare a list of tangible and activity reinforcers for children of different ages, including toddler, preschooler, school-age child, and adolescent with SSD.

4. Compare and contrast different service delivery settings including:

- pull-out versus push-in model
- telepractice versus in-person

5. Suppose a school-age child (8;2 years) with a lateral lisp decides that he no longer wants to come to therapy. What would you do?

6. Draft a management plan and session plan for Luke and Susie, completing background information, diagnosis and prognosis, your hypothetical plan regarding family preferences and plan for family involvement, long-term, short-term, and session goals, and service delivery options. You will complete your plans for Luke and Susie once you have read about intervention relevant to Luke's case (Chapter 13) and Susie's case (Chapter 14).

Appendix 11-1 Speech Sound Disorder Management Plan

(1) BACKGROUND INFORMATION, DIAGNOSIS, AND PROGNOSIS

Background information		
Child's name:	Date of birth:	
Parents/caregivers:	Phone:	Email:
Name of school / clinic:	Clinician:	
Child's interests:		
Diagnosis (including severity):		
Prognosis (for achieving long term goal):		
Date of first intervention session:	**Anticipated total intervention duration** (number of sessions, hours, time):	

(2) FAMILY PREFERENCES AND PLAN FOR FAMILY INVOLVEMENT

Family members to be involved in intervention:	**Family preferences** (e.g., service delivery, intervention role):

Plan for family involvement

☐ parent/caregiver training for the parent/caregiver to be the primary provider of intervention

☐ parent/caregiver training for the parent/caregiver to provide home activities

☐ parent/caregiver attendance at intervention sessions

☐ parent/caregiver participation in intervention sessions

☐ parent/caregiver involvement in home activities

☐ involvement of siblings

☐ involvement of grandparents

☐ involvement of friends

(Continued)

Appendix 11-1 *Continued*

(3) LONG-TERM, SHORT-TERM, AND SESSION GOALS

Target selection approach:	Evidence-based rationale:

Long-term goal *(including anticipated time to realize the goal):*		
1. Short-term goal (objective)	1. Short-term goal (objective)	2. Short-term goal (objective)
1d. Session goal	2d. Session goal	3d. Session goal
1c. Session goal	2c. Session goal	3c. Session goal
1b. Session goal	2b. Session goal	3b. Session goal
1a. Session goal	2a. Session goal	3a. Session goal

Note: A child may have more or fewer short-term goals and/or session goals. Add or delete goals based on the results of your assessment and analysis, individual child's needs, and family preferences.

(4) INTERVENTION APPROACH(ES)

Intervention approach:	Evidence-based rationale:

(Continued)

Appendix 11-1 *Continued*

(5) SERVICE DELIVERY

Intervention setting	Intervention agent	Intervention intensity		Format	Continuity
☐ School (pull-out) ☐ School (classroom) ☐ Early childhood setting ☐ Public SLP clinic (e.g., hospital, health care setting) ☐ Private SLP practice ☐ Other _____	☐ Clinician ☐ SLP assistant ☐ Teaching assistant ☐ Teacher ☐ Parent/caregiver ☐ Computer ☐ Other _____	**Session duration** ☐ 20 minutes ☐ 30 minutes ☐ 45 minutes ☐ 60 minutes ☐ Other _____	**Session frequency** ☐ Daily ☐ 5 x week ☐ 4 x week ☐ 3 x week ☐ 2 x week ☐ 1 x week ☐ Fortnightly ☐ Monthly ☐ Other _____	☐ Individual ☐ Group ☐ Parent training ☐ Other _____	☐ Continuous ☐ Block duration _____
		Session dose ☐ 50 trials ☐ 100 trials ☐ > 100 trials ☐ Other _____	**Estimated total intervention duration:** _____		

(6) EVALUATION PLAN   (based on Olswang & Bain, 1994; Baker & McLeod, 2004).

Category and type of data to be collected[#]	Who will collect the data?	Where will the data be collected?	How often will the data be collected?

[#]Data category: treatment, response generalization, stimulus generalization, control data.

Data type: qualitative and quantitative

The speech sound disorder management plan can be freely copied with acknowledgment of the source being McLeod & Baker (2017)

Appendix 11-2 Speech Sound Disorder Intervention Session Plan

Speech Sound Disorder Intervention Session Plan

Child's name:	Date of birth:
Diagnosis (including severity):	
Session date:	

SERVICE DELIVERY

Intervention setting	Intervention agent	Intervention intensity		Format	Continuity
☐ School (pull-out) ☐ School (classroom) ☐ Early childhood setting ☐ Public SLP clinic (e.g., hospital, health care setting) ☐ Private SLP practice ☐ Other _____	☐ Clinician ☐ SLP assistant ☐ Teaching assistant ☐ Teacher ☐ Parent/caregiver ☐ Computer ☐ Other _____	**Session duration** ☐ 20 minutes ☐ 30 minutes ☐ 45 minutes ☐ 60 minutes ☐ Other _____	**Session frequency** ☐ Daily ☐ 5 x week ☐ 4 x week ☐ 3 x week ☐ 2 x week ☐ 1 x week ☐ Fortnightly ☐ Monthly ☐ Other _____	☐ Individual ☐ Group ☐ Parent training ☐ Other _____	☐ Continuous ☐ Block duration _____
		Session dose ☐ ≤ 50 trials ☐ 51 - 100 trials ☐ > 100 trials ☐ Other _____	**Estimated total intervention duration:** _____		

INTERVENTION APPROACH(ES):

GOALS

Long term goal	Short term goal/s (objective/s)	Session goal/s (objective/s)

(Continued)

Appendix 11-2 *Continued*

INTERVENTION TEACHING MOMENT

Example dialogue for antecedent instruction, child's response, and consequent event .

---

(1) Antecedent instruction
- *Type of cue* : ☐ auditory cue ☐ production cue
- *Example cue(s):*

- *Example dialogue* :

(2) Child's response
- *Type*: ☐ passive listening ☐ active listening ☐ visual inspection

☐ speech production ☐ speech-related mouth movement ☐ gesture ☐ pragmatic response

☐ reading ☐ metaphonological awareness comprehension or remark about phonological properties

☐ phonological awareness task (detection, categorization, matching, isolating, blending, segmenting or manipulating syllables, rhymes or phonemes)

☐ general meta-awareness ☐ self-correction ☐ other

- *Level* : ☐ isolation ☐ syllable ☐ word ☐ phrase ☐ sentence ☐ conversation

- *Production Mode(s)*
  (based on Rosenbek, Lemme, Ahern, Harris, & Wertz, 1973; Strand & Skinder, 1999)
  ☐ simultaneous imitation ☐ mimed imitation ☐ immediate imitation
  ☐ successive imitation ☐ delayed imitation ☐ spontaneous production

- *Anticipated correct response from child:*

- *Anticipated incorrect / error from child:*

(3) Consequent event

- *Feedback on error*

- *Feedback for correct response*

Stepping down mode/level *(If your teaching and learning moment is too challenging, what could you say and/or do that would be easier?)*	**Stepping up mode/level** *(If your teaching and learning moment is too easy, what will you say or do to make it more challenging?)*

(Continued)

Appendix 11-2 *Continued*

INTERVENTION STIMULUS and RESOURCE

Stimulus (e.g., sound in isolation, syllables, nonwords, real words, phrases, sentences, conversation topic, phonological awareness task, letter knowledge task)	**Resource** (e.g., pictures or objects)

SESSION ACTIVITY PLAN

Sequence of session activities (including type [drill, drill play, play, child-directed] duration and dose for each activity, where relevant)	**Materials required** (e.g., glue, scissors, toy cars, ball, bowling pins, fishing game)

(Continued)

Appendix 11-2 *Continued*

SESSION DATA COLLECTION PLAN

Treatment data	Generalization probe data	Control data

ROLE OF PARENTS / CAREGIVER /SIBLINGS/ SIGNIFICANT OTHERS DURING SESSION AND DESCRIPTION OF HOME ACTIVITY

Person	Role	Home activity

ADDITIONAL COMMENTS

The speech sound disorder intervention session plan can be freely copied with acknowledgment of the source being McLeod & Baker (2017)

12

Intervention Procedures and Evaluation

LEARNING OBJECTIVES

1. Define a teaching and learning moment.

2. Demonstrate auditory and production cues that comprise a teaching and learning moment.

3. Demonstrate responses expected of children during teaching and learning moments.

4. Compare and contrast baseline, treatment, generalization, and control data used to evaluate intervention.

5. Create a data collection plan.

6. Outline a framework for problem-solving slow progress for children with SSD.

KEY WORDS

Procedures: teaching and learning moment, auditory cues, production cues, children's responses

Evaluation: assessment, baseline, treatment, generalization, and control data, data collection plans

Framework for problem-solving slow progress: child-factors, intervention-factors, and clinician-factors

OVERVIEW

This chapter is about intervention procedures—how you work on intervention goals. This chapter complements Chapter 11 on principles and plans and is essential for understanding the different approaches to intervention described in Chapters 13 (for phonological impairment) and 14 (for motor speech disorders). You will learn about the teaching and learning moment—the point in a session when skills are taught and practiced. You will also learn about the importance of planned data collection and what to do when children are making slow progress. By the end of this chapter, you will know how to prepare an intervention management plan and session plan for a child who has an SSD.

INTERVENTION PROCEDURES

Intervention procedures include the teaching cues (i.e., verbal instructions, comments, feedback, or actions), stimuli, resources, and activities that clinicians use to help children learn. They are the courses of action needed to help children achieve session goals, short-term goals, and ultimately long-term goals. Your understanding of the procedures in this chapter will help you appreciate that intervention approaches are unique combinations of intervention procedures.

■ The teaching and learning moment

The teaching and learning moment adopts one of Skinner's (1938) basic behavioral principles of intervention—moments of learning over time can be divided into an antecedent stimulus, a response, and a consequence (as described in Chapter 11). During intervention for children with SSD, this translates into the intervention agent (an SLP, teacher, parent, or indeed a computer) providing an antecedent instruction (i.e., saying and/or doing something), the child responding, and then the intervention agent providing consequent feedback. Over time consequent feedback merges with subsequent antecedent instruction. Consider the following portion of therapy dialogue from a minimal pairs therapy session (Chapter 13) with a 4-year-old preschool child who reduces word-initial /s/ consonant clusters to the least marked member of the consonant cluster.

> Clinician: Tell me a picture to pick up. (Pictures of *snow* /sno/ and *no* /no/ are spread out on the table.)
> Child: *Snow* (pronounced as [no]).
> Clinician: I'm not sure what you mean, did you mean no or *snow* with the snakey /s/ sound at the beginning?
> Child: *Snow* (pronounced as [no]).
> Clinician: Oh, if you want me to pick up the *snow*, you need to use the snakey /s/ at the beginning, listen, *snow*. Let's say *snow* together with the snakey /s/ sound.
> Child/Clinician: *Snow* [sno].
> Clinician: Oh, the *snow* with the /s/ sound, I know what you mean now. Tell me another picture to pick up.

Did you notice that similar types of information or cues can be present in both an antecedent instruction and consequent feedback? In the intervention dialogue you just read, both the antecedent instruction and feedback contained metaphor (*snakey /s/ sound*) and pragmatic information about how phonemes serve to contrast meaning between words ("I'm not sure what you mean"; "I know what you mean now"). Collectively, we refer to any type of information or activity used by a clinician during antecedent instruction and/or consequent feedback as a cue for learning. What follows are descriptions and evidence-based examples of (1) auditory-based cues, (2) production-based cues, and (3) responses expected of children from different approaches to intervention for different types of SSD. We refer to the intervention agent as the clinician; however, the agent could be any of the agents discussed in Chapter 11. As you read over the different types of cues and child responses, consider which principle(s) of intervention they best reflect.

Auditory cues

An auditory cue is an instruction, comment, or action from a clinician that encourages a child to listen to (rather than produce) speech. The cue may involve passive listening or active listening and a metacognitive response.

- **Focused auditory input/auditory stimulation**: The clinician produces carefully selected speech for the child to listen to. For example, "The clinician reads the session's listening list of approximately 20 words that contain the target pattern" (Hodson, 2007, p. 102) or the clinician presents the child with "many exposures to the target phoneme while engaging in a natural conversation about the story and the pictures and placing no pressure on the child to produce the target form" (Rvachew & Brosseau-Lapré, 2012, p. 702).

- **Auditory detection of a target sound or prosodic characteristics**: The clinician asks the child to indicate when he or she hears the clinician produce a target sound in isolation, syllable, word, phrase, sentence, or conversational context, or particular prosodic characteristics. For example, instructing a child, "When I say a word, I want you to show me the happy face if it has your sound in it. If it doesn't, show me the sad face" (Secord, 1989, p. 135). The SLP could ask the child to listen to sentences containing their target sound and identify the sound as it occurs (Secord, 1989). The child could be asked to identify stressed (louder) words in sentences or to determine whether an utterance ends with a rising or falling pitch (Velleman, 2003). For children who struggle with speech rate and prosody, they may be encouraged to identify pauses in spoken sentences (Velleman, 2003).

- **Auditory discrimination**: The clinician asks the child to listen to two spoken words that may or may not be the same, and determine if they sound the same or different. For example, "Listen carefully and decide if you hear the same word twice or two different words" (Bridgeman & Snowling, 1988, p. 248).

- **Auditory identification of a word containing a target sound or prosodic characteristic**: The clinician asks the child to pick up a particular word and then he or she hears it spoken. For example, shown pictures of *rings* and *wings*, the child is asked to pick up a picture of a *ring* (Baker, 2010b).

- **Auditory judgment of correctness tasks**
  a. **Judgment of own speech**: The clinician asks the child to listen to the child's own speech and decide whether target sounds are produced accurately. For example, instructing the child that "each time you read a word which contains your sound I want you to raise your hand if you think you said it correctly" (Engel & Groth, 1976, p. 95).
  b. **Judgment of others' speech**: The clinician asks the child to listen to other people's speech and decide whether target sounds are produced accurately. For example, as part of speech perception intervention, Rvachew and Brosseau-Lapré (2012) offer the following instruction: "You will hear people trying to say the word *shoe*. When you hear a person say the word *shoe* correctly, I want you to point to the picture of *shoe* here on the monitor. (Points to the shoe). Sometimes a person will make a mistake. If the person says the word *shoe* the wrong way, I want you to point the X on the computer screen. (Points to the X). If you hear a word that is *not shoe*, point to the X, OK? Are you ready to listen?" (p. 175).

- **Requests for self-monitoring**
  a. **Elicited self-correction**: The clinician may deliberately misunderstand a child's speech in an effort to encourage the child to reflect on his or her own speech or request that the child revise his or her previous utterance. For example, Bowen (2009, 2015) uses "fixed-up-one" routines as part of PACT intervention to prompt children to correct their speech. She explains the idea as this: "Listen to this. If I accidentally said 'tar' when I wanted to say 'car' it wouldn't sound right. I would have to fix it up and say 'car' wouldn't I. Did you hear that fixed-up-one? I said 'tar' and then I fixed it up and said 'car'" (Bowen, 2009, p. 310). An elicited self-correction focuses on a child's ability to monitor his or her own speech. A pragmatic cue (described in the production cue section) focuses on a child's ability to listen and then revise his or her speech production to resolve a communication breakdown.

b. **Prompted self-correction**: The clinician unintentionally misunderstands a child's speech, which serves as a prompt for the child to reflect on and correct his or her own speech. For example, a child correcting his or her utterance in response to the clinician's comment or gloss of the children's utterance not aligning with what the child was talking about (Shriberg & Kwiatkowski, 1990).

■ **Metaphonological input tasks**: The clinician asks the child to identify specific phonological properties in words. For instance, "The child is required to listen to minimally contrasting words and to judge, for example, whether the word the therapist says begins with a 'noisy' or a 'quiet' sound" (Dean, Howell, Waters, & Reid, 1995, p. 6).

■ **Phonological awareness input tasks**: The clinician asks the child to listen to, reflect on, and silently detect, categorize, match, isolate, blend, segment, or manipulate phonological elements in words. For example, instructing a child that "My friend 'munching monkey' is going to eat the pictures that start with an /m/ sound. Let's help him find the pictures that start with an /m/ sound" (Gillon, 2005, p. 324). There are various types of phonological awareness tasks that require nonverbal/pointing responses. For instance, given four pictures including a *cat, car, fan*, and *comb*, a child is asked, "Which of these words is the odd one out: *cat, car, fan, comb*?" (Hesketh, 2010, p. 264).

Production cues

A production cue is an instruction, comment, or action from a clinician designed to elicit speech from a child, and in some cases, increase understanding about how speech is articulated.

■ **Auditory model for imitation**: The clinician provides an auditory model of a target speech sound, word, or utterance for a child to repeat. The time between when the clinician offers the model and when the child imitates it can vary. Task difficulty is increased when there is more time between the auditory model and the child's imitated response (Strand, Stoeckel, & Baas, 2006). Based on Jakielski (2011), Rosenbek et al. (1973), Strand and Skinder (1999), and Strand et al. (2006), the imitation hierarchy includes:

a. **simultaneous imitation**: The clinician and the child say the word at the same time.

b. **mimed imitation**: The clinician "mouths the target while the child watches the SLP and says the target aloud" (Jakielski, 2011, p. 181).

c. **immediate imitation**: The child repeats the target directly after the clinician's model of the target.

d. **successive repetition**: The child "imitates the SLP's initial model several times successively without being produced an additional model" (Jakielski, 2011, p. 181).

e. **delayed imitation**: The child imitates the clinician's model 2 or 3 seconds after the model has been produced (Strand et al., 2006).

■ **Phonetic cues**: The clinician provides information (using one or more modalities) about how a particular speech sound or word is physically articulated. The different modalities are visual-phonetic, verbal-phonetic, tactile-phonetic, and manual guidance (i.e., motokinesthetic).

a. **Visual-phonetic cue**: A visual-phonetic cue provides a child with information about what the articulators need to do (and in particular where they need to be placed) to articulate speech. Visual information can include:

i. **Looking at mouth placement and/or movement**: For example, "Show the client the exact articulatory position of /f/ in a mirror" (Secord et al., 2007, p. 46).

ii. **Drawings and photos of the mouth**: For example, for the sounds /w/ and /ɪ/, you could demonstrate how "the schematic drawing indicates that both sounds are voiced and have an open velopharynx, while the tongue position is different" (McLeod & Singh, 2009a, p. viii).

iii. **Symbolic drawings about voice, place, manner, and/or lip posture**: For example, "The child is introduced to the articulogram and told he needs to make a 'puff of air' to produce the voiceless plosives" (Williams & Stephens, 2004, p. 197).

    iv. **Instrumental images such as a spectrogram, ultrasound image, or electropalatography (EPG) frame**: For example, using an image generated by an EPG, the child could be told that "to make the sound correctly, you need to place your tongue so that the small green squares (indicated on the screen) turn into large green squares . . ." (Dagenais, 1995, p. 307).

  b. **Verbal-phonetic cue**: The clinician provides a child with spoken information and/or instruction about how to articulate speech sounds. For example, "Tell the client to groove the tongue and then attempt /s/" (Secord, 1989, p. 140), or "Close your jaw a little" (Strand & Skinder, 1999, p. 136). Verbal-phonetic instruction is a common cue used across many intervention approaches.

  c. **Tactile-phonetic cue**: The clinician provides the child with spoken information about what it should feel like in the mouth when articulating particular speech sounds. For example, when learning about alveolar phonemes, "Ask the client to feel the bump on the roof of his or her mouth just behind the two front teeth" (Bleile, 2004, p. 363).

  d. **Manual guidance/motokinesthetic cue**: A child is given assistance to physically articulate speech. That assistance could be in the form of a tool and/or physical guidance from a clinician.

    i. **Use a tool to guide placement**: For example, to produce /l/, you could put a tongue depressor "under the student's tongue tip and then raise the tongue tip behind the upper front teeth" and ask the child to maintain "contact between the tongue tip and the roof of the mouth" while the child attempts to say /l/ (Bleile, 2006b, p. 151). Using a tongue depressor, Secord et al. (2007) suggest that you could "trace a line through the center of his tongue to give the client the idea of a trough" (p. 42).

    ii. **Clinician physically guides child's articulation**: For example, to assist the child in producing /f/, "with latex gloves, the [clinician's] thumb and forefinger are used to move the [child's] lower lip upward until it comes in contact with the upper teeth" (Secord et al., 2007, p. 47). To produce the vowel [o], Dale and Hayden (2013) suggest that "the middle three fingers of the hand are equally distributed on the top lip margin while the thumb and little finger are placed equally on the bottom lip margin and all are slightly pulled forward" (p. 651).

■ **Prosodic cues**: The clinician provides a child with visual and/or verbal information about prosodic aspects of speech such as speech rate, loudness, stress, and fluency.

  a. **Visual-prosodic cue**: The clinician provides visual information about a prosodic aspect of speech. For example, "the visual aids included short and long blocks (representing syllables) on the table" (Ballard et al., 2010, p. 1232). A younger child could be encouraged to reduce his or her speaking rate via picture prompts of turtles or snails (Fish, 2011).

  b. **Verbal-prosodic cue**: The clinician provides verbal information about prosodic aspects of speech. For example, a child is cued reduce his or her speech rate (Fish, 2011). Such cues also rely on children's self-monitoring abilities.

  c. **Manual guidance/motokinesthetic cue**: A child is given assistance to physically articulate movement sequences and/or utterances with appropriate prosody. For example, a child is given manual guidance or a physical prompt to move the articulators from one speech sound to another (Dale & Hayden, 2013).

■ **Orthographic cues**: The clinician uses graphemes or written words corresponding to a spoken phoneme or word to elicit speech and/or facilitate letter-sound knowledge and phonological awareness. For example, given a choice of the letters c and m, the child is instructed that "car starts with a /k/ sound and this letter can make a /k/ sound (pointing to a large poster-size letter of c). Drive the car to the letter c" (Gillon, 2005, p. 324).

■ **Sound-referenced rebuses**: The clinician uses rebuses or pictures representing sounds or parts of sounds in words (also known as pictograms) to make the sounds and syllables visually more salient for children (Young, 1987, 1995). For example, to help a child say the word *tissue*, the child is shown a picture of a *tissue* and a *shoe* and is told that the last syllable or part of the word sounds like *shoe* (Young, 1987). Fish (2011) offers another suggestion for establishing weak syllables—have a picture representing the weak syllable as a reminder to not forget the weak syllable, such as a picture of a person singing for the syllable *le* in *elephant*.

- **Successive approximation/shaping**: The clinician asks the child to produce a particular mouth movement or speech sound with the intent of gradually shaping the child's production towards the target sound, or the clinician asks the child to produce a word or utterance in an easier albeit less natural way in an effort to gradually build up task complexity and naturalness. For example, "Instruct the client to make rapid productions of /t/ and prolong the last one into /s/" (Secord et al., 2007, p. 39). Another example involves encouraging a child to say a target utterance at a reduced speech rate and then gradually increasing the speech rate (while maintaining articulation accuracy) until a normal rate and natural prosody is achieved (Fish, 2011).

- **Facilitating phonetic contexts or key environments**: The clinician has the child produce a speech sound, syllable, or word in particular phonetic contexts with the aim of creating an easier phonetic environment for learning how to articulate a particular speech sound, syllable, or word. For example, producing word-initial /l/ before a high front vowel (Bleile, 2006b). To produce a word-initial consonant, Bernhardt et al. (2010) suggest copying the final consonant in a VC syllable to the initial position through repetitive sequences so that VC becomes CVC (e.g., repeating *up up up* until *pop* is produced). Another suggestion is to use backward chaining, whereby the last part of a word is taught first, with other parts added on, such as saying *key* and then *monkey* or *pot* and then *spot* (Young, 1987).

- **Gestural cues** (hand cues and body motions): The clinician models a hand cue or body movement for the child to imitate and/or associate with a specific speech sound or prosodic characteristic. The gesture could be:
  a. **iconic**: symbolizing an object or action. For example, "pantomime rocking a baby" is associated with the sound /b/ (Miccio & Williams, 2010, p. 192).
  b. **metaphoric**: representing speech sound and/or prosodic characteristics. Example cues for speech segments include placing "four fingertips under chin near throat" as a metaphoric gesture for the back placement of /k, g/, and for the long manner of articulation for /s/ and /z/, sliding "index finger along the length of upper lip or up the length of forearm" (Fish, 2011, p. 109). Examples for prosody include "rhythmic tapping by the clinician and himself . . . to shape appropriate relative durations of syllables without markedly slowed speech rate" (Ballard et al., 2010, p. 1232).

- **Pragmatic cues**: The clinician provides a carefully planned verbal remark designed to highlight communication breakdown associated with the loss of a phonemic contrast or inaccurate production of a target word. For example, the SLP saying, "I'm not sure what you mean. Do you mean *wing* or *ring*? Tell me again" in response to a child say *wing* when it is unclear whether the child has meant *wing* or *ring* (Baker, 2010b, p. 61), or saying "did you say /tæmbəlu/?" in response to the child saying "/tændəwu/ (target *kangaroo*)" (Masso, McCabe, & Baker, 2014, p. 377).

- **Metaphonological cues**: The clinician provides the child with metalinguistic information about a property of the phonological system and the need for the child to use that property. For example, following a child's attempt at saying *shoe*, the clinician says, "I heard you say [tu] with a short sound. Try saying *shoe* again, this time with a long sound /ʃu/."

- **Metaphors**: The clinician assigns metaphors for speech sounds or prosodic features of words as a means for talking about a defining phonetic or prosodic characteristic. For example, explaining that /ɹ/ is the "growling bear sound" and /ʧ/ is the "choo choo train sound" (Fish, 2011, p. 112). You could also use props to represent the metaphor. For example, long sounds or syllables could be represented by a long block, while short sounds or syllables could be represented by a short block. Table 12-1 provides example metaphors for each English consonant and for voice, place, and manner classes and word structures.

TABLE 12-1 Metaphors for speech sounds	
Metaphors for individual sounds	**Metaphors for sound classes, word structures, and error patterns**
/p/ quiet popping sound, lip popping sound	**Voicing**
/b/ noisy popping sound, lip bursting sound	■ voiced sounds—noisy sounds, loud sounds, voice-on sounds
/t/ ticking sound, clock sound	■ voiceless sounds—whisper sounds, quiet sounds, voice-off sounds
/d/ drum sound, jackhammer sound	**Place**
/k/ quiet throat popping sound	■ labial—lip sounds
/g/ noisy throat popping sound	■ alveolar—front sounds
/f/ quiet windy sound, blowing rabbit sound	■ postalveolar—roof-of-the-mouth sounds
/v/ noisy windy sound, noisy rabbit sound	■ velar—back sounds
/θ/ flat snake sound, flat tire sound	**Manner**
/ð/ noisy tongue sound	■ plosives—poppy sounds, short sounds, quick sounds
/s/ snake sound, hissing sound	■ fricatives—windy sounds, long sounds
/ɬ/ slushy sound	■ affricates—train sounds
/z/ buzzing sound, long sleepy sound	■ lateral—singing sound
/ʃ/ quiet sound	■ approximants—wimpy sounds
/ʒ/ vacuum sound	■ nasals—nose sounds
/h/ huffing sound, puppy dog sound	**Word structure**
/tʃ/ train sound	■ initial consonant—beginning sounds, engine sounds, head sounds
/dʒ/ noisy helicopter sound, noisy train sound	■ final consonant—end sounds, carriage sounds, tail sounds
/m/ yummy sound, humming sound	■ monosyllable words—one-tap/one-clap words
/n/ mosquito sound, noisy nose sound	■ polysyllables—tapping or clapping words
/ŋ/ back sound, gong sound	■ words with singleton onsets—lonely words, hungry words
/w/ wimpy sound, whining sound	■ words with consonant cluster onsets—friendly words, buddy words, greedy words
/j/ yo-yo sound	
/ɹ/ growling sound, roaring sound	
/l/ singing sound	

Sources: Based on Bleile (2004); Fish (2011); Klein (1996a); Secord et al. (2007).

Children's responses

During a teaching and learning moment, a range of different responses can be expected of children. Their responses are usually predicated on antecedent auditory or production cues.

■ **Listening**
   a. **Passive listening**: The child listens to focused auditory input/auditory stimulation.
   b. **Auditory discrimination**: The child decides whether two words are the same or different.
   c. **Auditory detection of a target sound or prosodic characteristic**: The child listens for and indicates when he or she hears a particular target sound in isolation, syllables, words, phrases, sentences, or conversation (Secord, 1989), or detects a specific prosodic characteristic such as loudness, word, phrase, or sentence stress, pitch, and fluency, including appropriate and inappropriate pausing (Velleman, 2003).
   d. **Spoken word recognition**: The child points to or picks up a picture of a spoken word (Baker, 2010b).
   e. **Auditory judgment of correctness**
      i. The child decides if his or her own speech is correct or incorrect.
      ii. The child decides if others' speech is correct or incorrect.

■■ ■■

 APPLICATION: *Teaching speech sounds to children*

In Chapter 4 we described the voice, place, and manner characteristics of consonants. We also included coronal and sagittal images. Characteristics of voice, place, manner, coronal and sagittal images help you to appreciate how speech sounds are articulated, as well as explanations for differences between consonants. There are a range of books and resources that offer strategies for teaching speech sounds. For example:

■ *Seeing Speech: A Quick Guide to Speech Sounds* (McLeod & Singh, 2009b)

■ *Eliciting Sounds: Techniques and Strategies for Clinicians* (Secord et al., 2007)

■ *The Late Eight* (Bleile, 2014)

Using the information from Chapter 4 and other resources that you can find in your university library, prepare hypothetical intervention dialogue (i.e., a script comprising a clinician's auditory and production cues accompanied by a child's responses) for one or more of the following children discussed in this book:

1. Susie's lateral /s/: What would you say, do, and/or show Susie to help her perceive and produce a clear /s/?
2. Michael's omission of weak syllables in multisyllabic words: What could you say, do, and/or show Michael to help him perceive and produce multisyllables with all necessary syllables and natural prosody?
3. Lian's difficulty with the affricate /tʃ/: What could you say, do, and/or show Lian to help her perceive and produce the affricate in words?

Read more about Susie (7;4 years), Michael (4;2 years), and Lian (14;2 years) in Chapter 16.

f. **Comprehension of metaphonological cues**: The child listens to and understands metaphonological instruction and feedback. This can be evident in children's pointing or sorting responses, or via comments about the phonological property the child is working on. For example, when a child (3;11 years) was asked what sounds he was talking about in his last therapy session, he remarked, "long sounds like /s/" (Howell & Dean, 1987, p. 264). His remark highlights his comprehension and awareness of the phonological property of frication.

■ **Imitating or spontaneously producing speech**: The child produces speech focusing on:
   a. sounds or sound classes in isolation, syllables, words (real and nonwords), carrier phrases, short phrases, sentences, recountings on a specified topic or conversation, and
   b. prosodic characteristics in syllables, words (real and nonwords), phrases, sentences, and conversation.

■ **Looking at visual information while producing speech**: Visual information could include looking at the clinician's face and/or mouth, drawings and photos of the mouth, or an instrumental image (e.g., spectrogram, ultrasound image, palatogram). For example, using electropalatography, the child is asked to copy the pattern for a velar that they see on the screen (Gibbon & Wood, 2010).

■ **Speech-related mouth movement**: The child makes speech-related mouth movements in response to a model, verbal instruction, or visual information. The mouth movements are typically precursors to speech production (e.g., bite your bottom lip in anticipation of producing /f/).

■ **Gesture**: The child produces an iconic or metaphoric gesture in keeping with the clinician's gestural model or verbal instruction. For example, the child produces the target speech sound and a hand or body gesture for an alliterative character associated with the particular speech sound (Miccio & Elbert, 1996).

■ **Pragmatic response**: The child responds to a request for clarification and attempts to repair a breakdown in communication. For example, the child says "No, not the *tea* /ti/ [ti], the *key* /ki/ [ti]" in response to the clinician picking up a picture of a cup of *tea* when the child intended for the clinician to pick up a picture of a *key*.

- **Reading**: The child is encouraged to read aloud written information containing a target speech sound or prosodic characteristic. For example, Gillon (2005) reported encouraging children to read short words together with the clinician.

- **Phonological awareness**: The child engages in a requested input and/or output phonological awareness task that could include detection, categorization, matching, isolation, blending, segmentation, or manipulation of syllables, rhymes, or phonemes. For example, the child could be asked to blend the sounds /b/ /ɪ/ /g/ to form the word *big*.

- **Metalinguistic comment (solicited or unsolicited)**: The child makes a metaphonetic, metaphonological, or metapragmatic comment about his or her own speech or what the child hears in others' speech. For instance, a child was credited as saying: "I used to say lotta a dotta. That rhymes but it's not the right way to say it" (Bowen & Cupples, 1998, p. 41).

- **Self-correction**: The child reflects on his or her own speech error and then attempts a revised production. Self-corrections may be intentionally elicited, prompted unintentionally by a preceding comment, or be spontaneous and immediate without a preceding question or comment (Shriberg & Kwiatkowski, 1990). For example, "I can see /si/ [ɬi], I mean [si] that."

Stepping up and stepping down during a teaching and learning moment

Teaching and learning moments are dynamic events. You might begin a teaching and learning moment with a young child using a carefully selected group of antecedent cues only to find that the child was unable to produce a correct response. Conversely, a child might respond with ease and accuracy in response to your cues and consequently needs to be further challenged to achieve a predetermined goal. The concepts of stepping up and stepping down are related to the zone of proximal development and scaffolding (Vygotsky, 1978; see Chapter 6) and are used by clinicians to accommodate the dynamic structure of a teaching and learning moment. **Stepping up** involves changing and/or reducing your cues so that a task becomes more challenging for a child. **Stepping down** involves changing and/or increasing your cues so that a task becomes easier for a child. An intervention approach renowned for the dynamic nature of its teaching moment is Dynamic Temporal and Tactile Cueing (DTTC) (Strand & Skinder, 1999; Strand et al., 2006). You will learn more about this approach in Chapter 14.

■ Stimuli, resources, materials, and activities

Intervention procedures are not complete without stimuli to work on and activities in which to conduct teaching and learning moments. **Stimuli** (also referred to as exemplars) refer to what is to be practiced or targeted during a teaching and learning moment (e.g., listening skills; auditory detection, discrimination, or judgment; the production of speech sounds in isolation, syllables, words [real or nonwords], phrases, sentences, or conversational topics; the production of prosodic aspects of speech; phonological awareness skills). **Resources** are the pictures or objects used to elicit stimuli. You do not always need a resource, as you could elicit conversation simply by asking a question. You will learn more about the types of stimuli and resources used in intervention approaches for different types of SSD in Chapters 13 and 14.

Activities refer to the tasks conducted to motivate and engage children during intervention sessions. When preparing a session, it can be helpful to list the **materials** or equipment needed to conduct the session's activities. For instance, if you are going to create a collage of a snowman as an activity targeting minimal pair words *snow* and *no*, you may use cotton wool, glue, and paper. The type and extent of activities you conduct in a session depend on your activity genre. Shriberg and Kwiatkowski (1982b) describe four different activity genres or session management modes that can be used when working with children with SSD: drill, drill play, structured play, and unstructured play. What follows is a brief description of each mode, based on Shriberg and Kwiatkowski (1982b).

■ ■

 APPLICATION: *Stepping down to change* dine-saw *into* dinosaur

Assume you have developed an intervention procedure for Michael (4;2 years) to improve his production (including accuracy and naturalness) of polysyllables. (Refer to Chapter 16 for further information about Michael). Your procedure includes **stimuli** (pictures of polysyllabic real words), an **activity** and **reinforcement schedule** (drill-play bowling game in which Michael gets to stick the pictures of each correctly produced word on toy bowling pins, then bowl over the pins after every 10 trials), and a **list of teaching cues**. You elicit Michael's first attempt at the polysyllabic word *dinosaur* /daɪnɚsɔɹ/ using immediate imitation. Michael's response [daɪn.sɔ] is unnatural and shows weak syllable deletion and syllable segregation.

Question: What cues could you try as a step down in the next teaching and learning moment to help Michael produce the word *dinosaur* with all three syllables?

Answer: You could try one or more of the following teaching cues:

- Use simultaneous or mimed **imitation** instead of immediate imitation (Jakielski, 2011).

- **Shape** Michael's production by having him imitate the word at a reduced speech rate without pauses between syllables (Velleman, 2003).

- Use a **visual-prosodic cue**, representing the strong and weak syllables in the word with long and short blocks (Ballard et al., 2010).

- Provide a **verbal-prosodic cue** including knowledge of performance and an antecedent instruction (e.g., "You said *die* and *saw* clearly but I didn't hear *all* the syllables or parts of the word in *dinosaur*. Try *dinosaur* again after me and say all the parts of the word").

- Provide a sound-referenced **rebus** (series of pictures) depicting the three syllables in the word (e.g., *die* + *no* + *saw*) and ask Michael to repeat his attempt using the rebus as a guide to including all the syllables in the word. This may not help address Michael's syllable segregation; however, you could target his naturalness once he includes all the syllables in the word (see Young, 1995).

- Use **backward chaining** (a facilitating phonetic context designed to provide a child with a strategy for building a word), beginning with *saw* [sɔɹ], then adding *no-saw* [nosɔɹ], then finally *dinosaur* [daɪnɚsɔɹ]) (e.g., Young, 1987).

- Use a **pragmatic cue** by deliberately misunderstanding Michael's production using a request for clarification containing an incorrect production of the target word but with the correct number of syllables and stress pattern (e.g., "You want the *digermore*?")—such a counterintuitive cue improved polysyllable productions of real words in a small number of preschoolers who had a phonological impairment (Masso et al., 2014).

- Use a **metaphoric gestural cue** by rhythmically tapping each syllable on a drum (with natural stress) during Michael's next attempt at *dinosaur* (e.g., Ballard et al., 2010; Shea & Tyler, 2001) .

Read more about Michael (4;2 years), a boy with childhood apraxia of speech (CAS), in Chapter 16 (Case 4).

- **Drill:** high dose or rate of practice with minimal play. That is, the session comprises a series of teaching and learning moments devoid of play but may contain verbal and tangible reinforcement to encourage participation and motivation.
- **Drill play:** relatively high dose or rate of practice during a simple game or activity directed by a clinician. The child may be given a turn at a game or a craft activity during a teaching and learning moment or following a predetermined number of trials or teaching moments. For example, the child sticks stimulus pictures on a bowling pin each time he or she attempts a word, then bowls once all the words have been practiced and the pictures have been stuck on the bowling pins. A drill-play-style

session of 30 minutes duration could contain three or four drill-play activities. Drill play is a frequently used activity genre for preschoolers with SSD.

■ **Structured play:** moderate rate of practice during which an activity is played or craft activity is completed. For example, during a pretend pizza-making activity the clinician and the child take turns to stick the stimulus pictures on a large cardboard pizza. The child is allowed to select the pictures that he or she would like to stick on the pizza, using a predetermined set. Play is structured because the clinician decides what the game will involve and the range of words to be practiced during the play activity.

■ **Unstructured play:** the rate of practice is determined by the child, because the activity is child-directed rather than clinician-directed. Teaching and learning moments are dispersed through play as opportunities arise. For example, the child and the clinician could have a tea party. The tea party objects (rather than pictures) serve as the resource for the stimuli.

EVALUATING INTERVENTION

Once you have selected your goals and started intervention, you need to find out if your plan is working. You need to collect data. In this section we examine why it is important to collect data, how to evaluate intervention, the types of data that you can collect, and what data can tell you about the efficacy of your intervention with a child.

■ Why do I have to collect data?

The evaluation of intervention is one of the most important yet often neglected aspects of clinical practice. Too often, student SLPs respond with a sense of urgency to start intervention, without giving much thought to how they are going to evaluate their efforts. Certainly experienced SLPs can know intuitively whether or not a child is responding to a particular type of teaching cue—the child's response in fact determines the clinician's subsequent utterance. A parent observing his or her child during an intervention session may also have a sense of whether or not his or her child is doing well. However, if informed decisions about the effectiveness of intervention are going to be made, then intuition is not enough. You need to collect data. Data help you answer fundamental questions about the impact of intervention on a child and his or her family, such as "Is the client responding to the treatment program?" (Olswang & Bain, 1994, p. 56). The data that you collect also help you to be accountable for your service—accountable to the children and families you work with, accountable to your employer, and accountable to third-party payers.

> **COMMENT:** *Fun-ology is important, but don't let it detract from learning*
>
> Session activities can be fun—every session needs an element of fun-ology (Bernhardt et al., 2010). Activities are the means by which you work on specific goals with children. As a beginning clinician it can be tempting to spend time creating fun and engaging activities for children. However, a good session is not necessarily measured by a child's degree of fun (although fun is important). It is measured by the degree to which a child has the opportunity to learn and engage in practice. If you spend more time setting up or playing an activity than focusing on the purpose of session, rethink your activities. By contrast, if your sessions are devoid of fun and children are distracted or not motivated, rethink your session activities. As Bernhardt et al. (2010) suggest, inject some fun into your sessions through "creative activities that fit the child and target, using props, costumes, wands, and a warped sense of fun-ology" (p. 326).

▬ ░▬ ░▬ ░▬ ░▬ ░▬ ░▬ ░▬ ░▬ ░▬ ░▬ ░▬ ░▬ ░▬ ░▬ ░▬ ░▬ ░▬ ░▬

 APPLICATION: *Questions parents ask about intervention: "Is Luke's speech getting better?"*

Once you begin intervention with a child, parents often want to know if their child's speech is improving. Luke (4;3 years) has a severe phonological impairment. You have completed an analysis of Luke's speech and identified goals. How could you answer the following questions from Luke's mother about intervention?

- "Is the intervention working?"
- "Is Luke's speech getting better?"
- "Do you think Luke's speech is good enough now to stop coming to therapy?"
- "Do you think regular intervention and homework is actually causing the improvement in Luke's speech?"

Revisit your answers once you have finished reading this section on intervention evaluation, and again once you have selected a suitable intervention approach for Luke, based on the approaches covered in Chapter 13.

Read more about Luke (4;3 years), a boy with a phonological impairment, in Chapter 16 (Case 1).

▦ How do you evaluate intervention?

Intervention evaluation requires a plan. You need to know what you want to evaluate, who will collect data, when, where, and why. A helpful starting point can be to think about how you would answer the following questions:

- ▦ Is there a problem that needs intervention?
- ▦ Is the problem improving, deteriorating, or remaining the same?
- ▦ Is the child responding positively to the teaching and learning moments?
- ▦ Is improvement evident in short- and long-term goals?
- ▦ Can the child be dismissed?
- ▦ Is the intervention responsible for improvement in the child's speech? (Baker & McLeod, 2004; Olswang & Bain, 1994).

Types of data

Five different types of data are useful for evaluating intervention and answering questions about the efficacy of intervention (see Figure 12-1). Based on Olswang and Bain (1994), they include:

- ▦ **Assessment data:** information from an initial screening or assessment session (e.g., standard score or percentile rank from a standardized test, single-word speech sample, conversational speech sample, case history questionnaire) that helps you work out whether there is a problem requiring intervention. Assessment data answer the question: "Is there a problem that needs intervention?" Assessment data are collected during an assessment.
- ▦ **Baseline data:** information about a particular skill (identified as a problem during an assessment) that is collected *before* intervention is started. Baseline data answer the question: "Is the problem improving, deteriorating, or remaining the same?" Baseline data serve as a reference point for comparison with treatment data, generalization probe data, and control data. You analyzed Susie's baseline data when you completed a SODA analysis of her production of 24 words containing /s, z/ (see Chapter 9). Analysis of these data revealed 100% (15/15) lateralization of /s, z/ in singleton contexts, in initial, within word, and word-final positions, and 100% (9/9) lateralization of /s/ in consonant cluster contexts. If Susie completed this same baseline task three times (e.g., twice during an assessment session and then again at the beginning of the first intervention session) and her performance was identical or

Read more about Susie (7;4 years), a girl with an articulation impairment (lateral lisp), in Chapter 16 (Case 2).

very similar each time, then we have evidence that her problem with /s, z/ is stable and not improving. Usually three stable baseline measures are needed before starting intervention.

■ **Treatment data:** information collected during an intervention session that provides a measure of a child's response to teaching procedures (Olswang & Bain, 1994). Treatment data are the data specified in your session goals. Treatment data answer the question: "Is the child responding positively to teaching and learning moments?" For Susie, treatment data could consist of the number of accurate productions of /s/ out of the total number of opportunities she had to produce /s/ (e.g., 45/50) during the pre-practice phase of her first intervention session using Skelton's (2004a) concurrent intervention approach (see Chapter 14).

■ **Generalization data:** information that is gathered once intervention has started but is outside of intervention conditions. Outside does not mean outside the clinic room, it merely means at a time when teaching procedures are not being used. This could occur at the beginning of a clinic session rather than the end, so that your data are not influenced by the session's practice or at another time in another location (e.g., home). Generalization data are the data specified in your short- and long-term goals. They provide a measure of one or more skills thought to be related to the behaviors targeted in intervention sessions. Generalization data answer two important questions: "Is improvement evident in short- and long-term goals?" and "Can the child be dismissed?" The type of generalization data gathered depends on a number of factors, including:

■ type of SSD,
■ intervention target being worked on during a session, and
■ intervention approach.

FIGURE 12-1 Types of data collected when managing SSD in children: Assessment, baseline, treatment, generalization, and control data

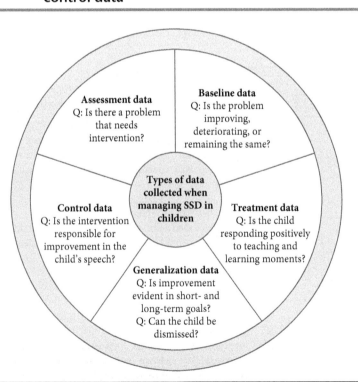

COMMENT: *Treatment data collection gets in the way of intervention*

SLPs sometimes find that quantitative treatment data collection can become intrusive during a teaching and learning moment, as it can break the conversational momentum between you and the child. It can also seem like a juggling act when running a small group. However, this does not mean that data collection should fall by the wayside. Rather, with a little planning prior to the session, alternate strategies can be used. For instance, you could collect treatment data using a qualitative rating scale (1 = consistently incorrect, 2 = mostly incorrect, 3 = sometimes correct, 4 = often correct, and 5 = consistently correct). You could note down your rating of a child's performance at the end of each activity in a session. Alternatively, you could put the picture cards into one of two piles as they are used during an activity—one pile for correct productions and another pile for incorrect productions. At the end of the activity, tally the cards in each pile. This usually requires multiple copies of the picture cards so that they are used once during an activity for counting purposes. Multiple copies of cards during an activity also helps you control and measure dose during a drill-play activity (e.g., five copies of the five words you are targeting during the session per activity equates to 25 trials per activity, with four activities reaching a dose of 100 trials in the session).

COMMENT: *How do I know if intervention is really working?*

Treatment data, generalization data, and control data all help you determine if intervention is really working. Of these three types of data, the most important is generalization data. The following two studies provide a helpful illustration. Baker and McLeod (2004) described the effect of minimal pairs intervention for two boys with phonological impairment. One boy (Cody) responded to the intervention—treatment data and generalization data showed an improvement, while the control behavior did not change. The other boy (James) showed an improvement in treatment data (e.g., he achieved 100% correct production of the target consonant clusters in trained words at sentence level without a model or feedback by the 11th intervention session). However, his generalization data indicated that significant and important change was not occurring (Baker & McLeod, 2004). Consequently, changes were made to James' intervention in an effort to facilitate his progress (Baker & Bernhardt, 2004). In another study, Ballard et al. (2010) reported that although response generalization occurred for three children (who had CAS and received Rapid Syllable Transition Treatment [ReST] targeting three syllable nonwords with varying lexical stress), generalization was only evident on untreated nonword stimuli, not real words. In both these studies, generalization data (not treatment data) were used to understand the effect of intervention and inform clinical decisions.

As discussed in Chapter 10 (goal setting), you would gather both stimulus and response generalization (e.g., stimulus: improved speech with other people in other settings; response: generalization to non-treatment words, across word positions, within sound classes, across sound classes and conversational speech). For Susie, generalization data could consist of:

- baseline probe of 24 words administered at the beginning of every third intervention session,
- 10-minute conversational speech sample in the clinic with the clinician, and
- 10-minute conversational speech sample at home with another family member—the behaviors noted in Susie's short-term goals in Chapter 10.

The actual words or stimulus that make up baseline and generalization data can be identical—the only difference between the two types of data is when the data are gathered. Baseline data are gathered before intervention starts. Generalization data are gathered regularly once intervention has started (e.g., at the beginning of every third session).

Control data: information gathered outside treatment conditions on a behavior that is unrelated to the behavior(s) being targeted in intervention. According to Olswang and Bain (1994), "These data reflect behaviors that could change as a result of other 'cosmic occurrences,' but their change would not be considered directly tied to treatment effects" (p. 57).

COMMENT: *Help! What can I use as a control behavior?*

A control behavior can sometimes be challenging to identify if a child only has one area of difficulty (e.g., Susie's only difficulty was lateralization of /s, z/), or if the intervention that you plan to use could induce widespread implicationally related change in a child's phonological system. In such instances, you could consider an alternative method for evaluating the effect of intervention. For instance, you could plot three baseline points (condition A) and the generalization probe data (condition B) and visually inspect the two conditions with respect to the **magnitude of change** (i.e., mean and level of performance) and **the rate of change** (i.e., trend and latency of change) (Kazdin, 1982). Figure 12-2 displays graphs for two preschoolers who received minimal pairs intervention targeting /s/ clusters. The data show the percent occurrence of cluster reduction in a single-word probe. During baseline, both children exhibited 100% cluster reduction. Once intervention started, Wayne showed a relatively steep and immediate decline in his percent occurrence of cluster reduction, dropping to 5% by the sixth probe. The mean of condition A was 100% while the mean of condition B was 34%. By contrast, Ben showed relatively little change in his percentage occurrence of cluster reduction between condition A and condition B, with the means being 100% and 80% respectively. The data for Ben guided the clinical decision to change his intervention target, approach, and intensity in an effort to facilitate achievement of his short- and long-term goals.

FIGURE 12-2   **Baseline and generalization probe data for two children who received twice weekly minimal pairs intervention targeting word-initial /s/ consonant cluster reduction**

Wayne's generalization data show improvement while Ben's data show minimal progress.

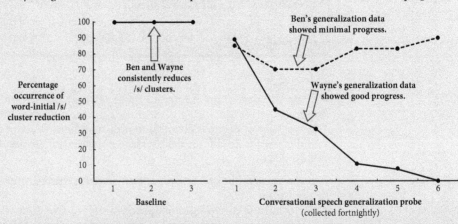

The behaviors that you select for control data need to be related developmentally but not phonologically and/or motorically. For example, if you used a developmental approach to target selection and prioritized Luke's stopping of early fricatives, it would be unlikely to see an improvement in Luke's production of affricates or consonant clusters, as early fricatives do not imply affricates or true consonant clusters (Gierut, 2007).

Data collection plans

A data collection plan outlines the types of data that will be collected, by who, where and when. It is important to develop a data collection plan before you start intervention, so that you know what type(s) of data will be gathered during an intervention session, and what types of data you need other people to collect. Table 12-2 provides examples of the types of data that could be collected as part of an evaluation plan. The information in this table is incorporated in the SSD Management Plan Template in Appendix 11-1.

TABLE 12-2 Data evaluation plans for children with SSD

Data to be collected	Who will collect the data?	Where will the data be collected?	When will the data be collected?
Treatment data: ■ Quantitative measure of percentage correct production of a targeted skill.	Clinician	Clinic	Every session
Treatment data: ■ Qualitative rating of the children's learning and enjoyment during clinic intervention sessions and homework sessions with parent/caregiver to consider changes in children's feelings about their speech (e.g., ☺☺☹).	Clinician Parent/caregiver	Clinic Home	Every clinic session Every homework session
Response generalization data: ■ Quantitative measure of non-treatment words containing the intervention target, and non-treatment words containing implicationally related targets, in a single-word probe and in a 5-minute sample of conversational speech.	Clinician	Clinic	At the beginning of every fourth intervention session
Stimulus (and response) generalization data: ■ Qualitative ratings by parent/caregiver of the child's intelligibility using the Intelligibility in Context Scale (McLeod et al., 2012a); child completing the Speech Participation and Activity Assessment of Children (SPAA-C) (McLeod, 2004) plus a drawing of themselves talking.	Parent/caregiver and child	Home	Once every three months
■ Quantitative measure of non-treatment words containing the intervention target and non-treatment words containing implicationally related targets in a 5-minute sample of conversational speech.	The parent/caregiver could record the sample and give it to the clinician for determining percentage correct production of selected behaviors.	Home	Once every three months
Control data: ■ Quantitative measure of the child's percentage accuracy of a behavior unrelated to the intervention target.	Clinician	Clinic	At the beginning of every fifth treatment session

Sources: Based on Baker & McLeod (2004); Olswang & Bain (1994).

■ ■

 APPLICATION: *Evaluation plan for Luke (4;3 years)*

Luke (4;3 years) has a severe phonological impairment. As discussed in Chapter 9, a few different target selection options are possible for him. Each option requires a unique evaluation plan. Using Table 12-2 as a guide, develop data collection plans for intervention targeting:

- one of Luke's earlier developing phonological processes (e.g., stopping of early developing fricatives starting with word-final position or velar fronting in word-initial position);

- Luke's largest word-initial collapse of contrast based on Williams' (2003) systemic approach; and

- complexity-based goals targeting true consonant clusters with small sonority differences based on Gierut (1999).

As part of your plan, generate word lists for measuring quantitative response generalization data. For instance, if you are targeting the phonological process of early stopping focusing on /f, s/ in word-final position, then you would sample non-treatment words containing /f/ and /s/ across word-initial, within word, and word-final positions. You could also sample Luke's production of other fricatives that may change (e.g., /h, ʃ, z, v/). If you target a complex cluster such as /sl/, your generalization probe should contain non-treatment real words starting with /sl/, and words containing other consonant clusters with similar and larger sonority difference scores. You would also include implicationally related fricatives and affricates across word positions (e.g., /s, ʧ/), as the evidence suggests that these targets might also change (e.g., Gierut, 2007). If you target four consonants (including one consonant cluster) from Luke's largest collapse of contrast, then your generalization probe should contain non-treatment words that sample the four targets in addition to words containing the other singleton consonants and consonant clusters within that collapse.

Read more about
Luke (4;3 years),
a boy with a phonological
impairment,
in Chapter 16 (Case 1).

 COMMENT: *Single-case experimental designs (SCED) and SSD intervention*

Just because you are collecting data does not mean that you are conducting experimental research. Routine data collection is a part of everyday clinical practice—you need to collect data to know if what you are doing (or have suggested that someone else do) is having the desired effect. You use interventions supported by evidence generated by researchers. This evidence typically comes from experimental group research (e.g., randomized and non-randomized controlled trials) and research involving single-case experimental designs (SCED).

There are many different types of SCED designs, such as simple withdrawal designs, multiple baseline designs (across subjects and/or behaviors), changing criterion designs, interactive additive designs, and alternating treatments designs (Kazdin, 1982). SCED designs have been used by researchers to study the effect of SSD interventions. For example, Koegel, Koegel, and Ingham (1986) used a multiple baseline design across subjects and behaviors to study the effect of self-monitoring on generalization. Gierut (1992) used an alternating treatments design combined with a staggered multiple baseline design across subjects to study the effect of target selection on phonological generalization. In each study, the research was experimental (rather than from routine clinical practice) because there were elements of control about the way children received intervention (e.g., some children remained in a baseline condition and did not receive intervention while other children received intervention), and the researchers were testing out an idea or theoretical prediction. Ethical approval was also sought to conduct the research.

While the majority of children who need intervention can be managed through routine data collection, there will be times when you have "substantial uncertainty about a treatment decision for a particular patient" (Dollaghan, 2007, p. 122). In such situations, it can be helpful to identify a SCED design that will answer the question raised by your uncertainty. For instance, you could use a multiple baseline design across behaviors to clearly determine whether your intervention is causing any improvement in a child's speech. To do this, you need to have identified two or more unrelated goals requiring intervention. Before beginning intervention, you would gather baseline data relevant to both goals. Three baseline points is usually considered adequate. You then provide intervention on the first goal. Regular probes of the child's performance on the first goal become your generalization data. Regular probes of the second goal that you plan to treat (once the first goal reaches a predetermined criterion) become your control data. You would then compare generalization data (for the first goal) with control data (for the second goal) to address your uncertainty about whether intervention is causing an improvement in the first goal. It can be helpful to visually inspect graphs of the data for change in mean, level, and slope of performance between the baseline, generalization, and control data (Morgan & Morgan, 2009). See Dollaghan (2007) for further ideas about using SCED designs to address clinical uncertainty.

A FRAMEWORK FOR PROBLEM-SOLVING SLOW PROGRESS

Children are individuals. Even though two children can present with similar clinical presentations, one child may progress more quickly than the other (Baker & McLeod, 2004). Baker and Bernhardt (2004) provided a helpful framework for problem-solving slow progress. Table 12-3 outlines a framework for problem-solving slow progress when working with children with SSD. Use the table as a guide to systematically think through and identify issues that could be hampering progress, and then generate possible solutions.

TABLE 12-3 A framework for problem-solving slow progress in children with SSD

Area	Skills or issues to consider
Child	
Speech production skills[a]	■ **Diagnosis:** Do you need to revisit and/or collect additional assessment data to reexamine your initial diagnosis of the child's SSD?
	■ **Delay versus disorder:** Does the child present with disordered rather than delayed patterns of acquisition?
	■ **Sampling and analysis:** Have you completed an adequate analysis of the child's phonological skills to identify specific skills requiring intervention?
	■ **Consistency:** Have you considered the consistency of the child's speech production skills?
	■ **Prosody:** Do the child's prosodic abilities require further investigation (e.g., juncture, lexical and phrasal stress, ability to produce polysyllables)?

(Continued)

Area	Skills or issues to consider
Body functions relevant to speech[b]	Do the following areas require further investigation and/or consideration? ■ **Mental functions** such as intellectual ability, energy and drive, sleep, attention, memory, auditory perception, visual perception, higher-level cognition functions (e.g., executive function and problem solving), phonological processing skills (including phonological working memory, phonological retrieval, and phonological awareness), receptive and/or expressive language ■ **Sensory functions** such as vision, hearing, or proprioceptive function ■ **Voice and speech functions** such as voice quality, fluency, or oromotor abilities and stimulability ■ **Functions of the respiratory system** ■ **Neuromusculoskeletal and movement-related functions** such as muscle power, tone, endurance, reflexes, and sensation (particularly for children with dysarthria)
Body functions relevant to attendance at or conduct during intervention or homework sessions[b]	Do the following areas require further consideration or call for adjustments to the intervention plan? ■ **Disposition and intra-personal functions** (b125) (WHO, 2007) such as: 　■ **Adaptability** (e.g., Is the child accepting or resistant to new experiences such as parent/caregiver conducting intervention at home?) 　■ **Responsivity** (e.g., Does the child react in a positive or negative way to practice?) 　■ **Activity level** (e.g., Is the child active with energy or tired and lethargic?) 　■ **Predictability** (e.g., Are the child's reactions to session activities predictable and stable, or unpredictable, making it difficult to plan tasks that would be interesting and engaging?) 　■ **Persistence** (e.g., Does the child sustain effort on a task or give up quickly when a task seems too challenging?) 　■ **Approachability** (e.g., Does the child initiate or withdraw from interactions with others in small group sessions? Does the child approach or withdraw from working with a new speech-language pathologist or other intervention agent?) ■ **Temperament and personality functions** (b126) (WHO, 2007) such as: 　■ **Extraversion** (e.g., Is the child outgoing and sociable or overly shy or inhibited during intervention sessions, resulting in considerable time coaxing the child to participate?) 　■ **Agreeableness** (e.g., Is the child cooperative, amicable, and accommodating or oppositional and defiant during sessions, reducing opportunities for practice or hindering opportunities for others to practice in a group session?) 　■ **Conscientiousness** (e.g., Is the child hard-working and methodical or does the child seem uninterested, not bothering to practice or seeing the point of practice between sessions?) 　■ **Stability** (e.g., Is the child calm, even-tempered, and composed, or often worried about his or her speech intelligibility to the point he or she will not communicate with others or practice during intervention sessions?) 　■ **Openness to experience** (e.g., Is the child curious and imaginative, or inattentive and inexpressive in activities during intervention sessions? Does the child understand why he or she attends speech-language pathology?) 　■ **Optimism** (e.g., Is the child cheerful, hopeful, and buoyant, or is the child's reaction to intervention negative and gloomy, responding such that the child cannot or will not say targeted words or utterances?) 　■ **Confidence** (e.g., Is the child assertive, self-assured, and bold, or does the child self-doubt his or her ability to communicate with others? Does the child doubt that practice and/or attending speech-language pathology could improve his or her communication skills?)

| TABLE 12-3 | *(Continued)* |

Area	Skills or issues to consider
Body structures relevant to speech[b]	Are there particular body structures that require further investigation and/or consideration? ■ **Structures of the nervous system** ■ **Structures of the eye, ear, nose, mouth, hard and/or soft palate, tongue, pharynx, larynx** ■ **Structure related to the respiratory system** (particularly for children with childhood dysarthria)
Family[c]	Does one or more of the following issues require further investigation or consideration? ■ **Knowledge and belief about SSD,** the consequence of SSD, and the value of speech-language pathology intervention ■ **Parent/caregiver training** (including confidence and knowledge) to implement intervention and/or home activities ■ **Family involvement** in intervention ■ **Family circumstances** and home environment

Intervention Plan

Intervention goals	■ Modify your target selection strategy. ■ Change your goal attack strategy. ■ Change and/or expand the intervention goals.
Intervention approach	■ Modify or change the intervention approach in keeping with revised analysis and/or the child's response to intervention.
Service delivery	■ Consider modifying the intervention agent and/or setting. ■ Modify the session duration, frequency, and/or dose.
Instructional cues	■ Examine the range of cues that have been used in intervention and identify other auditory and/or production cues that could be useful.
Intervention stimuli and activities	■ Increase the number of words used in intervention. ■ Reconsider the words according to their lexical and/or sublexical characteristics (e.g., real versus nonwords, high- versus low-frequency words, high versus low neighborhood density). ■ Reconsider the communicative potency of the words, particularly for young children or children with severe SSD. Consider activities in line with the child's interests.

Clinician

Knowledge[d]	■ Learn more about a particular type of SSD, assessment tool, analysis method, target selection strategy, or intervention approach.
Procedural and problem-solving skills[d]	■ Learn how to administer a new assessment, counselling technique, or intervention procedure. ■ Ask an expert clinician to observe you or observe an expert clinician to identify skills that you need to learn or refine.
Interpersonal skills attitude[d]	Reflect on your: ■ **Attitude** towards and rapport with the children and families you work with. ■ **Confidence** to work with children with SSD. ■ **Adaptability;** that is, your ability to readily modify your teaching procedures, session activities, or behavioral strategies when a child disengages or does not want to respond during an intervention session. ■ **Motivation** to deliver the best service possible within the constraints of your workplace setting.

Sources: [a]Based on Baker and Bernhardt (2004) and Powell (2002). [b]Based on the International Classification of Functioning, Disability and Health – Children and Youth (ICF-CY) (World Health Organization, 2007). [c]Based on Baker and Bernhardt (2004) and Watts Pappas, (2010). [d]Based on Baker and Bernhardt (2004) and Kamhi (1995).

COMMENT: *Help! Carryover is not happening!*

Carryover occurs when a child shows habitual use of a targeted speech skill in everyday conversational speech in a variety of speaking contexts (Gordon-Brannan & Weiss, 2007). For some children, carryover occurs automatically with little effort. For others, carryover needs explicit attention and effort from the SLP and the child. Ertmer and Ertmer (1998) describe a **constructivist approach** for helping children achieve carryover. Their approach involves the clinician understanding that given the right opportunity and support, children can figure out what it is they need to do to achieve carryover, through increasing motivation, metacognitive knowledge, and metacognitive control (Ertmer & Ertmer, 1998).

- **Metacognitive knowledge** refers to a child's awareness of the task and resources needed to achieve carryover (Ertmer & Ertmer, 1998).

- **Metacognitive control** refers to three interconnected processes, including (1) developing a plan of action, (2) self-monitoring progress and performance, and (3) engaging in self-evaluation of one's own performance and the success of the plan itself (Ertmer & Ertmer, 1998).

Ertmer and Ertmer (1998) offer a helpful sequence of seven goals when targeting carryover, including:

1. Increase motivation for carryover.
2. Increase knowledge of barriers to carryover.
3. Increase awareness of personal resources for carryover.
4. Plan strategies for carryover during performances.
5. Increase self-monitoring during rehearsals and performances.
6. Increase self-evaluations of performance and plan.
7. Revisit previous goals as needed.

You will need to help children develop their plan for carryover; however, if the plan is going to work, the ideas for the plan needed to be generated by the children. Marshalla (2010) offers practical suggestions and ideas for facilitating carryover, such as practicing a new speech skill during grocery shopping. As part of this activity, the child and parent work together to generate a shopping list, paying particular attention to words containing the child's target sound. The child then practices the target words to and from the grocery store. During the actual shopping experience, the child is given the opportunity to use the target sound in everyday conversational speech. As an incentive, the child could be offered a reward for the number of times the target sound is produced correctly during the shopping experience.

Chapter summary

In this chapter you learned about intervention procedures and evaluation. You learned that intervention procedures comprise teaching cues, stimuli, resources, materials, and activities and that the crux of intervention is the teaching and learning moment—the moment in time when teaching cues are used to address a particular goal using carefully selected stimuli (e.g., words) with corresponding resources (e.g., pictures) in an activity (e.g., bowling, posting letters, playing a fishing game). You also learned about the importance of evaluating intervention through the collection of data. A framework for problem-solving slow progress was also outlined. The knowledge you have gained from this chapter serves as a foundation for the following two chapters: intervention approaches for phonological impairment (Chapter 13) and intervention approaches for motor speech difficulties (Chapter 14).

Suggested reading

Teaching and learning moment

■ McLeod, S., & Singh, S. (2009b). *Seeing speech: A quick guide to speech sounds.* San Diego, CA: Plural Publishing.

■ Secord, W., Boyce, S. E., Donohue, J. S., Fox, F. A., & Shine, S. E. (2007). *Eliciting sounds: Techniques and strategies for clinicians* (2nd ed.). Clifton Park, NY: Thomson Delmar Learning.

Evaluation of intervention

■ Baker, E., & Bernhardt, B. H. (2004). From hindsight to foresight: Working around barriers to success in phonological intervention. *Child Language Teaching and Therapy, 20*(3), 287–318.

■ Baker, E., & McLeod, S. (2004). Evidence-based management of phonological impairment in children. *Child Language Teaching and Therapy, 20*(3), 261–285.

■ Olswang, L., & Bain, B. (1994). Data collection: Monitoring children's treatment progress. *American Journal of Speech-Language Pathology, 3,* 55–66.

Application of knowledge from Chapter 12

1. Review the auditory and production cues mentioned in this chapter. With a peer, demonstrate teaching and learning moments comprising one or more cues. Ask your peer to identify the cue(s) in your demonstration.
2. Observe a clinician conducting intervention with a child with SSD. Identify the types of cues comprising the clinician's teaching and learning moments. Note down what the clinician says, does, and uses (e.g., pictures, objects, books, mirror, instrumentation) within a teaching and learning moment. Observe the child's response for each teaching and learning moment.
3. Assume you will be conducting intervention with Susie (7;4 years) focused on /s, z/. Develop a resource to collect a baseline measure of Susie's production of /s, z/.
4. Outline the types of generalization data would you need to collect to identify progress on the short- and long-term goals you developed for Susie in Chapter 10.
5. Assume that Susie is making slow progress—carryover to everyday conversational speech (as measured by your stimulus and response generalization probes) is not happening, despite treatment data showing that Susie can produce /s, z/ clearly, without lateralization, during intervention sessions. Develop a plan for Susie to facilitate carryover of /s, z/ into everyday conversational speech.

13

Phonological Intervention Approaches

KEY WORDS

Interventions for phonological impairment: minimal pair approach, maximal oppositions and treatment of the empty set, multiple oppositions, Metaphon, cycles approach, Parents and Children Together (PACT), intervention targeting complex onsets, speech perception intervention, intervention for concomitant phonology and morphosyntax difficulties, stimulability intervention

Intervention for inconsistent speech disorder: core vocabulary intervention

Intervention: for children who are late talkers, multilingual children

Emergent literacy intervention

OVERVIEW

This chapter is about intervention for children with phonological difficulties, including phonological impairment and inconsistent speech (phonological) disorder. You will become familiar with different phonological intervention approaches including the history of each approach, theoretical background, procedure, evidence base, and resources. You will also learn strategies for promoting babbling in infants, and toddlers' speech sound acquisition, strategies for managing multilingual phonological impairment, and the important role of emergent literacy intervention for children with phonological difficulties. Figure 13-1 provides a schematic timeline of phonological intervention approaches, including who developed the approaches and when they first emerged. Use this figure to orientate your reading of the chapter. Notice how the approaches above the timeline are classified as contrastive approaches, while approaches below the line are non-contrastive. In this chapter, the **contrastive approaches** (approaches that use minimal pair words) are presented first, followed by **non-contrastive approaches** (approaches in which minimal pair words are an optional component). More space is devoted to the minimal pair approach simply because this approach was one of the first to be developed and is assumed understanding for a number of other approaches. Given that the main focus of this chapter is on phonological interventions, we use the term **phonological impairment** rather than the broader term SSD, to specify the type of SSD suited to the majority of intervention approaches described in this chapter. We use the term **inconsistent speech disorder** when referring to the specific intervention approach suited to that disorder—core vocabulary therapy. Interventions for other types of SSD (e.g., lateral lisp, CAS, childhood dysarthria) are addressed in Chapter 14.

FIGURE 13-1 Schematic timeline of phonological intervention approaches highlighting who developed the different approaches and when they first emerged

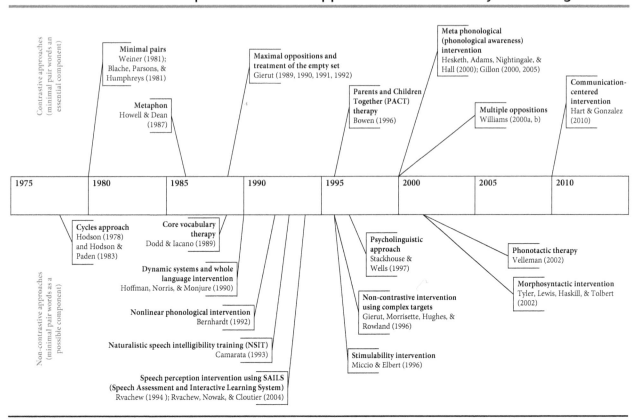

PRINCIPLES OF PHONOLOGICAL INTERVENTION IN PRACTICE

Phonological intervention is based on the premise that children who have a phonological impairment have a linguistic difficulty rather than an articulation or motor speech difficulty (Gierut, 2005; Grunwell, 1987). Change needs to occur primarily in a child's mind rather than his or her mouth (Grunwell, 1983). This can be a difficult concept to grasp. Intuitively, it makes sense to focus exclusively on children's production of speech sounds if their speech is unintelligible. However, consider the following cases where children can produce the consonant, but not in the required contexts:

- James (5;4 years) says *sing* as [θɪŋ] but *thing* as [fɪŋ]
- John (4;11 years) says *she* as [si] but says /ʃ/ when gesturing to his younger sister to be quiet

In each case, the problem is not limited to the child's ability to articulate speech sounds. You can see that James can articulate /θ/ and John can articulate /ʃ/, but not in the appropriate context. That is, the problem is associated with each child's ability to use the appropriate speech sounds for meaning in accordance with the phonological rules of the language they are learning. Recall the five phonological principles of intervention covered in Chapter 11:

1. Intervention should focus on children learning phonological systems rather than just the articulation of individual phonemes (Stoel-Gammon & Dunn, 1985).
2. Intervention targets can be carefully selected to facilitate generalization or widespread change in children's phonological systems (Gierut, 2001, 2005, 2007; Stoel-Gammon & Dunn, 1985).
3. Intervention should help children discover and learn the rules (Lowe, 1994).
4. Intervention procedures should be meaning-based (Lowe, 1994; Weiner, 1981).
5. Intervention can include conversational repair sequences (e.g., listener requests for clarification) to facilitate improved speech intelligibility (Weiner, 1981).

In practice, principles 1 and 2 direct what is targeted and what data are monitored during intervention. Principles 3 through 5 direct the types of procedures and teaching cues used in intervention, notably, pragmatic cues and metaphonological cues.

As you will learn, different intervention developers have applied the five phonological principles of intervention in different ways. Some approaches also use other auditory-perceptual, cognitive, motor, behavioral, or neurological principles to guide intervention procedures. The different combination of principles and procedures is what makes each of the phonological intervention approaches unique.

> **COMMENT:** *Why cover so many phonological intervention approaches?*
>
> The answer to this question reflects the state of the literature. No single phonological intervention approach has proven to be THE most effective and efficient approach for all children with phonological impairment. Rather, it would seem that different approaches are better suited to different children. If you are a novice SLP, we recommend that you start out small. Learn one approach at a time, and learn it well. Become familiar with the literature on the approach and the resources available to apply the approach to clinical practice. The first few children you see may dictate the order in which you become familiar with the approaches. Over time, you will find that it can be helpful to have knowledge of and experience with a range of approaches. What may work with one child may not work with another. You need to have evidence-based intervention options. You may also need to trial a different approach if a child's intervention progress is relatively slow. Knowledge of a broad range of approaches not only provides you with a broad range of expertise from which you can draw upon, but helps to keep your mind open to new research and adopting new methods of practice.

MINIMAL PAIR APPROACH

Minimal pairs are word pairs that differ or contrast by one phoneme; a change in one phoneme results in a change in word meaning (Barlow & Gierut, 2002). The contrasting phonemes can have **minimally opposing features** (e.g., *key* and *tea*, due to the one difference in place of articulation, with /k/ being velar and /t/ being alveolar), **maximally opposing features** (e.g., *key* and *me*, due to the multiple feature differences, with /k/ being an obstruent, voiceless, velar, and plosive, and /m/ being a sonorant, voiced, bilabial, and nasal), or they can be **near minimal pairs** (e.g., *ski* and *key*, due to the presence and absence of the phoneme /s/ to create a consonant cluster). The minimal pair approach uses minimal pair word pairs that a child produces as homonyms—they usually have minimally opposing features or are near minimal pair words. For example, if a child's speech shows the phonological process of stopping of fricatives (e.g., says *shoe* /ʃu/ as [tu]), then rhyming word pairs that start with /ʃ/ and /t/ form the minimal pair words to be used in minimal pair intervention (e.g., *shoe* and *two*; *shape* and *tape*; *shy* and *tie*; *shell* and *tell*; *ship* and *tip*).

Historical background

The minimal pair approach is one of the oldest, most well-known and widely used contrastive approaches for phonological intervention (Baker, 2010b). As one of the oldest approaches, it has served as the basis from which a number of other contrastive approaches have developed, such as **maximal oppositions** (Gierut, 1990), **treatment of the empty set** (Gierut, 1992), and **multiple oppositions** (Williams, 2000a, b, 2005a, 2010). Minimal pair words are also used in other approaches such as **Metaphon** (Howell & Dean, 1994) and **Parents and Children Together (PACT)** intervention (Bowen, 2015; Bowen & Cupples, 2006). The inclusion of minimal pair words within these approaches does not make them modified versions of the minimal pair approach per se, but rather phonological intervention approaches that use minimal pairs (Baker, 2010b).

Theoretical background

According to Weiner (1984), the minimal pair approach is based on two basic tenets: (1) Stampe's (1979) theory of natural phonology and (2) Greenfield and Smith's (1976) pragmatic principle of informativeness. Stampe's theory of natural phonology guides *what* to target and monitor over a course of intervention: phonological patterns rather than individual speech sounds. Greenfield and Smith's pragmatic principle of informativeness guides *how* targets might be worked on and changed during intervention sessions: through the phenomenon of speakers accommodating to their listeners' needs by repairing their speech when a breakdown in communication has occurred. In Weiner's (1981) classic study, the phonological processes of final consonant deletion, stopping of fricatives, and fronting of velars were selected as intervention targets, and the children were confronted with the homonymy in their speech within the context of a communication breakdown, and given instruction on how to repair the breakdown (e.g., "You keep saying *bow*. If you want me to pick up the *boat* pictures, you must say the /t/ sound at the end. Listen, *boat, boat, boat*. You try it. Okay. Let's begin again," Weiner, 1981, p. 98).

Procedure

The minimal pair approach has been implemented by different researchers in different ways (see Baker, 2010b). If you compare and contrast the teaching procedures across the evidence base, there are basically two different ways in which the approach can be implemented: (1) meaningful minimal pair intervention and (2) perception-production minimal pair approach. The main difference is when minimal pair words are introduced to a child (Baker, 2010b). A brief procedural description for each approach follows.

Meaningful minimal pair intervention (adapted from Baker, 2010b)

The meaningful minimal pair approach is based on the early works of Blache, Parsons, and Humphreys (1981) and Weiner (1981). Pragmatic cues typify the approach, as you confront the child with the impact of the homonymy in his or her speech via a request for clarification. For example, if you showed pictures of a superhero *cape* and adhesive *tape* to a child who had velar fronting, the child would probably say [tep] when asked to tell you which picture you should pick up. Regardless of the child's intent, you would pick up the [tep], as that is what you understood. This creates a breakdown in communication if the child meant *cape*. The child might try to clarify the request (e.g., "No, not the [tep], the [tep]"). You then offer the child a solution to the conversational confusion in the form of a request for clarification containing the child's production and the target contrast (e.g., "Do you mean *tape* or *cape*?"). If the child's attempted repair does not make the contrast, you provide the child with additional cues (e.g., phonetic cues, successive approximation/shaping) about how to make the contrast. Three steps make up the meaningful minimal pair approach:

1. Familiarization
2. Listen and pick up
3. Production

The first two steps are completed within the first session. The third step commences during the first session and continues in subsequent sessions until predetermined phonological generalization performance criteria are met. During the intervention sessions, pictures, real objects, toys, or the actions representing the words may be used. Typically, only three to five word pairs (that is, 6 to 10 pictures or objects) are necessary to facilitate generalization for the majority of children, although some children may need more word pairs (Elbert, Powell & Swartzlander, 1991).

■ **Step one: Familiarization.** You sit facing the child at a small table. You show the child the picture for each word, saying, "This is a *cape*. It starts with the /k/ sound. You can wear a *cape*. Superheroes like to wear capes when they fly! This is a picture of *tape*. You can use *tape* to stick paper together. *Tape* starts with the /t/ sound." Assuming five word pairs are being used (e.g., *cape-tape; key-tea; call-tall; corn-torn; kick-tick*), this step continues until you have shown the child all 10 pictures.

■ **Step two: Listen and pick up.** Once the child is familiarized with the pictures, you spread out one picture for each word on the table and ask the child to listen and pick up one picture at a time (e.g., "Pick up *cape*"). This process continues until all 10 pictures have been picked up by the child. You provide praise for a correct response (e.g., "Great listening, that's the *cape*") and instructional feedback, in the form of a metaphonological cue, following an incorrect response (e.g., "The *tape*? The word I said sounds a bit like *tape*, but it's different. Listen again: pick up the *cape*.")

■ **Step three: Production of minimal pair words.** During the third and final step, the child is given a turn to be the teacher. The child is instructed to tell you which word to pick up. It is during this step that the child is likely to experience communication failure or semantic confusion and is challenged to produce a phonemic contrast between the word pairs in order to be understood. You provide praise for a correct response (e.g., "The *cape*, I know what you mean!") and a pragmatic cue if semantic confusion occurs (e.g., "I'm not sure what you mean. Do you mean *tape* or *cape*? Tell me again"). If on a second attempt the child does not make a contrast between the word pairs, you provide additional cues as necessary (e.g., auditory model for immediate or delayed imitation, visual-phonetic cues, verbal-phonetic cues, manual guidance, successive approximation/shaping, orthographic cues, metaphor, pragmatic cue) regarding the articulation of the target word. The moment the child accurately produces or approximates the target word, you provide meaning-based praise (e.g., "Oh, I can understand you now! You meant the *cape*, not the *tape*, the *cape* with the /k/ sound"). Step three of the meaningful minimal pair approach continues at word level until a performance-based phonological generalization criterion has been met. Following the first session, subsequent sessions usually consist of 20 trials of each of the five target words (with or without the pictures or objects for the minimal pair cognates, as the instructional feedback already contains the minimal pair cognate), totaling 100 trials. Production practice activities could include a few games, each lasting approximately 10 minutes, in which multiple opportunities are provided for the child to produce the target words within a meaningful context.

Perception-production minimal pair intervention (adapted from Baker, 2010b)

The perception-production minimal pair approach is based on the work of Crosbie et al. (2005), Elbert et al. (1990, 1991), and Tyler et al. (1987, 1990). Within a perception-production approach, a child is taught how to produce the target words via imitation activities and becomes relatively proficient at production before he or she is introduced to the minimal pair words. This is done to ensure the child has a greater chance of successfully repairing a communication breakdown given a request for clarification. The repeated opportunities to learn the target word are also thought to minimize the possibility of a child becoming frustrated. This contrasts with the meaningful minimal pair approach, in which the semantic confusion or frustration is thought to help raise a child's awareness of the need change his or her speech. There are four steps within a perception-production minimal pair approach. The first step combines steps 1 and 2 in the meaningful minimal pair approach.

- **Step one: Familiarization and perception training.** Sit at a small table, facing the child. You show the child the minimal pair pictures (e.g., "This is *cape*, and this is *tape*"). Assuming that pictures of five word pairs are being used, the 10 pictures would be spread out on the table, and the child would be asked to pick up the word you say. The child moves on to step two once he or she identifies the picture corresponding to each treatment word with 90% accuracy. Crosbie et al. (2005) include a sorting activity at this step, whereby the child is expected to listen to and sort the word pairs into their respective categories (e.g., compiling /k/ pictures versus /t/ pictures). You offer praise for correct responses (e.g., "Great listening, yes, that's the *cape*") and instructional feedback and cues for incorrectly identified or sorted pictures (e.g., "Uh oh, that's the *tape* that starts with the /t/ sound. Listen again and find the *cape* that starts with the /k/ sound.").

- **Step two: Production involving word imitation.** Of the five minimal pairs (five target words and five cognate pairs), the child is to imitate each of the five target words given auditory and production cues, as necessary (see Chapter 12). Praise regarding the articulatory accuracy of the word is provided for correct responses (e.g., "Great /k/ sound when you said *cape*") and instructional feedback for incorrect responses (e.g., "Try again. Watch me and listen, *cape*, remember to use the /k/ sound when you say *cape*"). This step continues until the child can imitate the target words with 90% accuracy in at least 50 trials.

- **Step three: Production involving independent naming.** Using the five target words, you then ask the child to name each picture without a model. You provide praise and instructional feedback, similar to step two, as necessary. This step continues until the child independently produces the target words with 50% accuracy in at least 50 trials.

- **Step four: Production of minimal pair words.** This step is identical to step three of the meaningful minimal pair approach, in which you give the child the opportunity to request either a target word or a minimal cognate pair of the 10 words. Pragmatic feedback is provided in conjunction with other cues, as necessary. According to Tyler et al. (1987), the inclusion of imitation and independent naming of the target words prior to the child naming the minimal pairs in this final step helps facilitate success, and avoids potential frustration resulting from the semantic confusion that can arise when children are confronted with the homonymy in their speech.

Evidence

The minimal pair approach has a relatively large evidence base, primarily because it has been around since the early 1980s. In the Baker and McLeod (2011a) narrative review of 134 published peer-reviewed studies of phonological intervention, there were 43 studies on the minimal pair approach, including two **randomized controlled trials** (Dodd et al., 2008; Ruscello, Cartwright, Haines, & Shuster, 1993), six studies using a **within-group design**, 20 **single-case experimental design studies**, and 15 **case studies**. The appendix of Baker and McLeod (2011a) provides details regarding the research designs, participant numbers and ages, service delivery, study duration, and level of evidence (based on ASHA, 2004a). The repeated outcome across the evidence was that the minimal pair approach was effective. However, in a few studies using single-case experimental designs, the approach was less efficient for children with more severe phonological impairment compared to maximal oppositions intervention (Gierut, 1990) and the multiple oppositions approach (Williams, 2005a).

■ Children suited to the minimal pair approach

The minimal pair approach has been used with children who have a mild through to severe phonological impairment. Although the approach was originally developed for children with unintelligible speech (Weiner, 1984), Williams (2000a) suggests the minimal pair approach may be more appropriate for children who have mild-to-moderate phonological impairment. Basically, you need to make sure that a child's speech production error is consistent (e.g., *cape* consistently said as *tape* rather than variable or inconsistent productions such as *tape, gape, ape,* and *kay* during an assessment). You also need to make sure that the errors are phonological rather than articulatory. Word pairs need to show a loss of contrast.

■ Resources for conducting minimal pair intervention

There are a variety of commercially available minimal pair resources (see Table 13-1) for English-speaking children. The Internet, including Caroline Bowen's speech-language-therapy website, is also an invaluable resource for SLPs in search of minimal pair stimuli. It is important to note the country of origin of minimal pair stimuli or commercially available resources, as dialect differences can influence whether word pairs are in fact minimally contrastive (Baker, 2010b). For example, in General American English, the words *new* /nu/ and *do* /du/ are minimal pairs, while in British, Australian, and New Zealand English they are not, because *new* is said as /nju/ while *do* is /du/. Your colleagues are also invaluable for ideas about games to play during intervention to keep children motivated and to help ensure that intervention sessions are fun. Remember—your games and activities are a means to an end for creating multiple opportunities for production practice. They should not be complicated to set up or play, and they should not detract from your valuable session time.

■ Minimal pairs for children who speak languages other than English

Minimal pair intervention may be used in languages other than English. For instance, minimal pair words were included in intervention for monolingual children learning Swedish (Palle, Berntsson, Miniscalco, & Persson, 2014). Gildersleeve-Neumann and Goldstein (2015) used a minimal pair approach as part of their intervention with multilingual

---

TABLE 13-1   Examples of commercially available phonological intervention resources

- *Scissors, glue, and phonological processes, too!* (Daly, 1999)
- *Contrasts: The use of minimal pairs in articulation training* (Elbert, Rockman, & Saltzman, 1980)
- *Just for kids: Phonological processing* (Flahive & Lanza, 1998)
- *Webber Spanish phonology cards* (Frederick, 2005)
- *Have you ever …? Eight interactive books for phonological processes* (Hall, 2006)
- *Minimal contrast stories* (Krupa, 1995)
- *Preschool phonology cards* (LinguiSystems, 2007)
- *Webber photo phonology minimal pair cards* (Webber, 2005)
- *SCIP—Sound contrasts in phonology: Evidence-based treatment program* (Williams, 2006) [computer program]
- *Phoneme Factory Sound Sorter* (Wren & Roulstone, 2006, 2013) [computer program]

children learning English and Spanish. It is important to note that some languages (e.g., Icelandic) have very few minimal pairs. You therefore need to determine whether minimal pairs intervention is suitable for the language(s) spoken by the children you are working with. In tonal languages, such as Cantonese, Mandarin, and Vietnamese, you need to think about the role of tone in selecting minimal pair words. If you are targeting a consonant phoneme, then the tone should be the same for each word that is part of the minimal pair. If tone is being targeted, then all other phonological characteristics need to remain the same. Table 13-2 provides some examples of words to use in Spanish, Cantonese, and Vietnamese.

TABLE 13-2 Minimal pair words for fronting and stopping in Spanish, Cantonese, and Vietnamese

Process	Language	Pair of words	Transcription using the International Phonetic Alphabet	Word position	English translation
Fronting	Spanish	casa – masa	/kasa/ – /masa/	initial	house – corn meal
		gata – rata	/gata/ – /rata/	initial	cat – rat (feminine)
		caro – paro	/kaɾo/ – /paɾo/	initial	expensive – arrest
		capa – mapa	/kapa/ – /mapa/	initial	cape – map
		casa – raza	/kasa/ – /rasa/	initial	house – race (group of people)
		cama – rama	/kama/ – /rama/	initial	bed – branch
		carro – raro	/karo/ – /raro/	initial	car (Mexican Spanish) – strange
		cara – para	/kaɾa/ – /paɾa/	initial	face – for
		gallo – rayo	/gajo/ – /rajo/	initial	rooster – ray
		gancho – rancho	/gantʃo/ – /rantʃo/	initial	hook – ranch
	Cantonese	高 – 刀	/kou₁/ – /tou₁/	initial	tall – knife
		狗 – 豆	/kɐu₂/ – /tɐu₂/	initial	dog – pea
		雞 – 低	/kɐi₁/ – /tɐi₁/	initial	chicken – low
		橋 – 條	/kʰiu₄/ – /tʰiu₄/	initial	bridge – classifier
		鯨 – 停	/kʰɪŋ₄/ – /tʰɪŋ₄/	initial	whale – stop
	Vietnamese	cáo – táo	/kɑw⁵/ – /tɑw⁵/	initial	fox – apple
		cay – tay	/kăj¹/ – /tăj¹/	initial	hot (chilli) – hand
		cóc – tóc	/kɔ̆kᵖ⁵/ – /tɔ̆kᵖ⁵/	initial	toad – hair
		cáo – cháo	/kɑw⁵/ – /cɑw⁵/	initial	fox – congee
		kim – chim	/kim¹/ – /cim¹/	initial	needle – bird
		ngà – nhà	/ŋɑ²/ – /ɲɑ²/	initial	ivory – house
		ngồi – nhồi	/ŋoj²/ – /ɲoj²/	initial	sit – knead flour
		mặc – mặt	/măk⁶/ – /măt⁶/	final	put on (clothes) – face
		ước – ướt	/ɯɤk⁵/ – /ɯɤt⁵/	final	wish – wet
		thang – than	/t̪ʰɑŋ¹/ – /t̪ʰɑn¹/	final	ladder – coal
		chuồn – chuồng	/cuon²/ – /cuoŋ²/	final	dragonfly – cage

Stopping	Spanish	sala – pala	/sala/ – /pala/	initial	room – stick
		fama – dama	/fama/ – /dama/	initial	fame – lady
		fe – de	/fe/ – /de/	initial	faith – from
		sé – de	/se/ – /de/	initial	I know – from
		soy – doy	/soi/ – /doi/	initial	I am – I give
		saca – vaca	/saka/ – /baka/	initial	He/she/it takes – cow
		sala – bala	/sala/ – /bala/	initial	room – bullet
		saga – paga	/saɣa/ – /paɣa/	initial	saga – he/she/it pays
		salón – balón	/salon/ – /balon/	initial	room – large ball
	Cantonese	花 – 爸	/fa₁/ – /pa₁/	initial	flower – dad
		快 – 拜	/fai₃/ – /pai₃/	initial	fast – worship
		方 – 幫	/fɔŋ₁/ – /pɔŋ₁/	initial	square – help
		灰 – 杯	/fui₁/ – /pui₁/	initial	gray – cup
		手 – 豆	/sɐu₂/ – /tɐu₂/	initial	hand – pea
		瘦 – 鬥	/sɐu₃/ – /tɐu₃/	initial	thin – compete
		粥 – 篤	/tsʊk₁/ – /tʊk₁/	initial	congee – poke
	Vietnamese	khô – cô	/xo¹/ – /ko¹/	initial	dry – teacher
		khâu – câu	/xɤ̆w¹/ – /kɤ̆w¹/	initial	sewing – fishing
		khát – cát	/xɑt⁵/ – /kɑt⁵/	initial	thirsty – sand

Note: Lexical items and pronunciation may differ across dialects. The numbers within the transcription columns for Cantonese and Vietnamese correspond to the tone value.

Sources: The Spanish minimal pairs were created by Dr. Leah Fabiano-Smith, University of Arizona (2014). Used by permission; The Cantonese minimal pairs were created by Dr. Carol Kit Sum To, University of Hong Kong, SAR China (2014). Used by permission; The Vietnamese minimal pairs were created by Lê Thị Thanh Xuân, Ho Chi Minh City, Vietnam (2014). The transcription of the Vietnamese words was undertaken by Lê Thị Thanh Xuân and Ben Phạm, Charles Sturt University, Australia and Ha Noi National University of Education, Vietnam using the Vietnamese transcription conventions described in Phạm and McLeod (2016). Used with permission.

> ### MULTILINGUAL INSIGHTS: *Minimal pairs for tonal languages*
>
> When selecting minimal pairs for tonal languages such as Cantonese and Vietnamese, you need to match the consonants, vowels, *and* tones.
>
> ### Cantonese
> To contrast alveolar and velar consonants (fronting or backing) in Cantonese, the following word pairs can be selected, since they contrast the consonants /t/ and /k/ but use the same vowels and tones:
>
> - 豆 'pea' /tɐu₂/ – 狗 'dog' /kɐu₂/
> - 刀 'knife' /tou₁/ – 高 'tall' /kou₁/
>
> It would not be appropriate to contrast alveolar and velar consonants using the words 雞 'chicken' /kɐi₁/ – 弟 'little brother' /tɐi₆/, because 雞 uses tone 1 and 弟 uses tone 6; thus, 雞 and 弟 contain two contrasts: the initial consonant and the tone. In Cantonese, a minimal pair to target differences between tones 1 and 6 would be
>
> - 書 'book' /syu₁/ – 樹 'tree' /syu₆/

The consonants and vowels are the same, /syu/, the tones are the only difference: tone 1 versus tone 6.

Vietnamese

To contrast stops and fricatives (stopping) in Vietnamese, the following word pairs can be used, since they use the same tones within each word pair:

- bê 'a calf' /be¹/ – dê 'a goat' /ze¹/

To contrast alveolar and velar consonants (fronting or backing) in Vietnamese, the following word pairs can be used, since they use the same tones within each word pair:

- thỏ 'a rabbit' /tʰɔ⁴/ – cỏ 'grasses' /kɔ⁴/

To contrast nasalized and non-nasal consonants in Vietnamese, the following word pairs use the same tones within each word pair: *một – bột, na – đa, ngon – con, ngô – cô.* It would not be appropriate to contrast nasalization using the words bé 'baby' /bɛ⁵/ – mẹ 'mother' /mɛ⁶/, because bé uses tone 5 and mẹ uses tone 6; thus, bé and mẹ contain two contrasts: the initial consonant and the tone.

A Vietnamese minimal pair to target differences between tones 1 and 5 would be

- ca 'glass of water' /kɑ¹/ – cá 'fish' /kɑ⁵/

The consonants and vowels are the same, /kɑ/, the tones are the only difference: tone 1 versus tone 5.

APPLICATION: *Compare David and Peter*

Consider the following two cases. David (4;11 years) consistently says *see* /si/ and *she* /ʃi/ as *see* [si] and does not produce a contrast between the word pairs. Peter (4;3 years) consistently says *see* /si/ as [ɬi] but *she* /ʃi/ as *she* [ʃi] and does produce a contrast between the word pairs.

1. Who is suited to the minimal pair approach and why?
2. Write five suitable minimal pair words for contrasting /s/ from /ʃ/.

Answers:

1. David, because he does not have a phonemic contrast between /s/ and /ʃ/.
2. *shell, sell; she, see; ship, sip; show, sew; shower, sour.*

APPLICATION: *Minimal pair management plan and session plan for Kevin*

Kevin (4;11 years) has a mild phonological impairment. His interests include bugs, superheroes, and craft. You will be seeing him for individual 30-minute sessions twice per week at preschool, using the minimal pair approach. You have completed a CHIRPA analysis and identified one phonological process in word-initial position requiring intervention: velar fronting of /k, g/ to [t, d] respectively. Briefly, the long-term goal will be for Kevin to improve his everyday speech intelligibility and accuracy, so that it is equivalent to his same-age peers. The short-term goal will be to eliminate velar fronting in conversational speech. Using the templates for the SSD management plan (Appendix 11-1, in Chapter 11) and SSD session plan (Appendix 11-2, in Chapter 11), prepare for your first intervention session with Kevin. As you complete the management plan and session plan, integrate what you have learned in Chapter 10 (on goals), Chapter 11 (on principles and plans), and Chapter 12 (on procedures) with what you have learned in this chapter about the minimal pair approach. Compare your management plan and session plan with a peer.

Maximal oppositions (Gierut, 1990) and treatment of the empty set (Gierut, 1992) are two contrastive approaches to intervention grounded in the principles of language learnability and complexity.

■ Historical background

Maximal oppositions and treatment of the empty set approaches were developed by Judith Gierut (Gierut, 1989, 1990, 1991, 1992) and emerged out of a series of studies during the 1980s and early 1990s investigating the role of children's pre-treatment phonological knowledge and feature distinctions on target selection and generalization learning.

■ Theoretical background

Although maximal oppositions and treatment of the empty set use minimal pair words, they are each theoretically and practically different from conventional minimal pair intervention. Let's consider the theoretical differences first. According to Gierut (1992), contrasting word pairs such as *sock* and *lock* can differ theoretically in three ways:

1. the **number** of distinctive feature differences (i.e., /s/ and /l/ differ by four features, with /s/ being + obstruent and + strident, and /l/ being + lateral and + voice).
2. the **nature** of those feature differences (i.e., /l/ and /s/ differ according to the major class distinction of obstruent and sonorant, with /s/ an obstruent and /l/ a sonorant).
3. the **relationship** of the targeted phonemes to a child's pre-treatment grammar (i.e., whether the child has phonological knowledge of /l/ and/or /s/).

The greater the **number**, **nature**, and **relationship** differences between the consonants in a word pair, the greater the potential system-wide change in children's phonological systems following intervention (e.g., Gierut, 1992; Topbaş & Ünal, 2010).

In practice, the word pairs do not result in **homonymy**. You might be thinking that this seems to contradict one of the principles of phonological intervention (that intervention should include conversational repair sequences to facilitate improved speech intelligibility). However, Gierut's (1991) point is this—the underlying theoretical feature differences between sounds is thought to be more important for promoting the change in children's phonological systems than the explicit, functional confrontation of the homonymy, as is done in meaningful minimal pair intervention.

■ Procedure

The procedures for implementing **maximal oppositions** and treatment of the **empty set** are the same. The only difference between them is whether one or two sounds unknown to a child are paired, in non-homonymous contrasts. Suppose a child's consonant phonetic inventory consists of [m, n, t, d, p, b, w, j, h]. **Maximal oppositions** pairs one sound that is known (i.e., used) by the child (e.g., /m/) with one sound that is unknown (i.e., not used) by the child (e.g., /ʧ/); whereas treatment of the **empty set** pairs two sounds that are unknown (i.e., not used) by the child (e.g., /l/ versus /ʧ/). Both pairs still reflect major class distinctions (**sonorant** versus **obstruent**) and have maximal or many feature differences. For example, /l/ and /ʧ/ differ in place (**alveolar** versus **postalveolar**), manner (**approximant** versus **affricate**), and voicing (**voiced** versus **voiceless**). Having identified the sounds to be paired, eight novel word pairs are developed in accordance with individual children's phonological needs and abilities. A **novel word** is simply a new word unknown to the child. Through the literature the terms *novel*, *nonce*, *nonsense*, and *nonword* are used interchangeably. Typically, novel words are newly created words assigned a newly created meaning. According to Gierut (2008), the eight novel word pairs may consist of varying phonotactically permissible syllables with the target phoneme(s) in syllable-initial word-initial position. A variety of vowels can also be used. For example, assuming that /tʃ/ and /l/ are to be paired in treatment of the empty set, novel words could be:

- [tʃi] [li]
- [tʃimu] [limu]
- [tʃɛp] [lɛp]
- [tʃun] [lun]

- [tʃɔt] [lɔt]
- [tʃæn] [læn]
- [tʃæbi] [læbi]
- [tʃʊtə] [lʊtə]

The novel stimuli are assigned lexical meaning via stories in order to familiarize a child with the words. According to Gierut (2008), the novel words are associated with names for characters, unusual objects, or actions via stories. Having familiarized a child with the words, you conduct intervention in two phases: imitation followed by spontaneous production.

During the imitation phase, you prompt the child to repeat your model of each word. A continuous positive verbal feedback schedule follows correct responses, while instructional feedback regarding the accuracy of the child's production follows inaccurate responses. You would provide cues as needed (e.g., auditory model for imitation, visual-phonetic cues, verbal-phonetic cues about place or manner of articulation, manual guidance, successive approximation/shaping, orthographic cues, metaphor, pragmatic cues) to elicit the target sound(s). Intervention continues at this phase until a child maintains 75% accurate imitated productions over two consecutive sessions or until seven sessions have been completed (Gierut, 1992). Intervention then shifts to the spontaneous phase.

During the spontaneous phase, you encourage the child to produce the target words without your model. Intervention continues at this phase until the child achieves 90% accuracy in production over three consecutive sessions or until a further 12 intervention sessions have been completed (Gierut, 2008). During the spontaneous phase, you provide verbal praise on an intermittent schedule.

According to Gierut (1992), activities during the imitation and spontaneous production practice phases may include various conceptual activities such as sorting and matching of word pairs, informal storytelling, and "disambiguation of word pairs" (p. 1053). To achieve a relatively high response rate (e.g., approximately 100 responses per session), Gierut (1999) suggests the use of a drill-play format (Shriberg & Kwiatkowski, 1982b) to maintain a child's interest and motivation. Production practice between sessions is also encouraged through caregivers helping their child complete individualized homework sheets, coloring books, and the child listening to audio recordings of the target words. Having achieved the criterion to finish the spontaneous phase, you need to evaluate a child's performance on a phonological generalization probe. Ideally, a child would need to achieve approximately 70% accuracy in conversational speech on a probe of the targeted speech sound(s) in non-treatment words before stopping intervention on that target and starting intervention on a new target or discontinuing intervention altogether. The criterion of 70% is a guide, based on Tyler (1995), Tyler, Figurski, and Lansdale, (1993), and Williams (1991). You would also regularly probe any other implicationally related phonemes that may improve as a result of intervention on the target sound(s), in order to monitor changes to the child's phonological system.

■ Evidence

Judith Gierut and colleagues from the University of Indiana are the main proponents of maximal oppositions and treatment of the empty set. The evidence for each approach could be described as emerging, with a between-group study (Mota, Keske-Soares, Bagetti, Ceron, & Melo Filha, 2007), four single-case experimental studies (e.g., Gierut, 1989, 1992; Topbaş & Ünal, 2010), and case studies (Donicht, Pagliarin, Mota, & Keske-Soares, 2011; Mota, Bagetti, Keske-Soares, & Pereira, 2005) published on maximal oppositions. Regarding treatment of the empty set, a between-group study (Pagliarin, Mota, & Keske-Soares, 2009), three single-case experimental studies (Gierut, 1991, 1992; Gierut & Neumann, 1992), and

> **MULTILINGUAL INSIGHTS:** *Minimal pairs versus maximal pairs in Turkish*
>
> Topbaş and Ünal (2010) compared the effect of minimal pairs versus maximal oppositions for two 6-year-old monolingual Turkish-speaking twins. For each approach, a known phoneme was paired with an unknown phoneme. For minimal pairs, an unknown phoneme was paired with the child's minimally opposing substitute (e.g., /s/ versus /t/—both voiceless obstruents). For maximal pairs, an unknown phoneme was paired with a known phoneme reflecting a major class distinction (e.g., obstruent /s/ versus sonorant /m/). Topbaş and Ünal (2010) reported greater change for the maximal opposition condition. Singleton consonants (rather than consonant clusters) were the focus of this investigation on complex target selection, as Turkish does not have word-initial consonant clusters (Topbaş & Ünal, 2010).

case studies (Mota et al., 2005) have been published on the approach. The repeated finding across this research has been that complex targets facilitate more widespread change in children's phonological systems relative to less complex targets. Other researchers have reported on the benefit of *modified* versions of maximal oppositions, including Dodd et al. (2008) and Williams (1993). Given the differences in the way intervention was delivered, how targets were selected, and the duration of intervention, it is difficult to make meaningful comparisons between the studies of the modified approaches and the original approaches. Dodd et al. (2008) reported no difference between groups given minimal pairs intervention versus modified maximal oppositions.

■ Children suited to maximal oppositions and treatment of the empty set approaches

According to Gierut (1989, 2008), children suited to maximal oppositions or treatment of the empty set typically have a functional phonological impairment characterized by the exclusion of at least six or more speech sounds from their phonetic and phonemic inventories. Research by Helena Mota and colleagues from the Universidade Federal de Santa Maria (UFSM) in Brazil (Mota et al., 2005) supports the use of maximal oppositions with children who have a mild-moderate phonological impairment, based on a PCC score.

■■ ■■ ■ ■■ ■ ■ ■ ■ ■ ■■ ■ ■ ■ ■■ ■ ■ ■ ■ ■ ■ ■■ ■ ■ ■ ■ ■ ■ ■ ■■

 APPLICATION: *Intervention for Dylan*

Dylan (4;2 years) does not have the following sounds in his phonetic or phonemic inventories: /l, ɹ, ʃ, ʒ, ʧ, ʤ, ð, θ, s, z, v/.

1. Select one of Dylan's unknown sounds and pair it with one of the following known sounds /m, n, t, d/ to create a maximal opposition word pair reflecting major class distinctions (i.e., obstruent and sonorant), and write down five suitable maximal opposition novel pairs.
2. Select two of Dylan's unknown sounds to be used in word pairs for treatment of the empty set, and write down five suitable novel pairs to be used in intervention.

Suggested answers:

1. Pair /m/ with /ʧ/. Possible word pairs include [mɔt] [ʧɔt]; [mɪdi] [ʧɪdi]; [mætu] [ʧætu]; [mʊp] [ʧʊp]; [mɔɪ] [ʧɔɪ].
2. Pair /l/ with /ʧ/. Possible words pairs include: [lɔt] [ʧɔt]; [lɪdi] [ʧɪdi]; [lætu] [ʧætu]; [lʊp] [ʧʊp]; [lɔɪ] [ʧɔɪ].

MULTIPLE OPPOSITIONS

The multiple oppositions approach is another type of contrastive phonological intervention approach. Unlike other contrastive approaches such as the minimal pair approach (Weiner, 1981), maximal oppositions (Gierut, 1990), and treatment of the empty set (Gierut, 1992), multiple oppositions targets *several* error sounds that are part of a phoneme collapse in a child's phonological system (Williams, 2000b).

■ Historical background

The multiple oppositions approach was developed by A. Lynn Williams during the 1990s and 2000s (Williams, 1991, 2000a, b, 2005a, b, c, 2006). The approach emerged out of Williams' work with Michelle (3;5 years), a young child with SSD who had an unusual pattern of using [l] for /w/, /s/, and /ʃ/ word-initially (Williams, 2005c). Following a 5-week period of relatively little progress with conventional minimal pair intervention, Williams reanalyzed Michelle's speech and noticed "that rather than the child exhibiting three separate, idiosyncratic errors involving target /w/, /s/ and 'sh,' all of the errors were related to a single rule in which the child collapsed all of these continuants to [l], which was also a continuant" (Williams, 2005c, pp. 189–190). In the subsequent session, Williams provided Michelle with multiple rather than minimal pairs (e.g., *lee, we, see, she; lock, wok, sock, shock; lamb, wham, Sam, sham*). Given another two sessions, phonological generalization was evident in untreated words containing trained sounds and a selection of untrained sounds (Williams, 2005c).

■ Theoretical background

Williams' (2000a, b) multiple oppositions approach is based on the systematic nature of phonology, with respect to the **structure** and **function** of phonemes (singletons and consonant clusters) within a language. A child's phonemic system is analyzed using Williams' (2003) Systemic Phonological Analysis of Child Speech (SPACS), and multiple collapses of contrast are identified. Through targeting several strategically selected sounds from a collapsed contrast at one point in time, Williams (2005c) believes that the task of learning the phonological system is made easier, because the child is made aware of the system as a whole rather than simply isolated parts of the system—an idea reminiscent of Aristotle's belief that a whole is more than the sum of its parts. (See Chapter 10 for further information about the systemic approach to target selection that it used with multiple oppositions.)

Williams (2010) also believes that the difficulties underlying a child's collapses of contrast are not solely phonemic or phonetic but a combination of both skills along a continuum. Although most children with SSD may be considered to primarily have a phonemic (phonological) difficulty, it is possible for phonetic or articulatory difficulties to be present. Consequently, Williams (2005c) proposes that multiple oppositions address both skills through the following four goals:

1. Providing children with opportunities to discover the rule(s) being targeted.
2. Ensuring opportunities for focused practice, so that new targets become automatic.
3. Including communicative feedback about the semantic meaning of children's productions.
4. Providing children with opportunities to use the targets they are learning in everyday play activities.

■ Procedure

The multiple oppositions approach, as developed by Williams (2000a, b, 2003, 2005c) consists of four phases:

1. Familiarization and production of contrasts.
2. Contrasts and interactive play (including imitation followed by spontaneous production)
3. Contrasts within communicative contexts.
4. Conversational recasts.

During Phase 1, the familiarization and production of contrasts phase, there are three steps. Children are (i) familiarized with the contrasts they need to learn (e.g., if the targets are [d] contrasted with /k, ʃ, ʤ, sl/, conceptual contrasts could include short sound /d/, long quiet sound /ʃ/, front sound /k/, jeep sound /ʤ/, and friendly sounds /sl/); (ii) familiarized with the vocabulary and stimuli; and (iii) given the opportunity to imitate the contrasts given the SLP's model (Williams, 2010). Williams (2003) suggests that the first step of Phase 1 takes about 10 to 15 minutes of the first session. In the second step, children are also exposed to the vocabulary and the stimuli (usually picture stimuli). Williams (2003) suggests telling the child a story about each word. This story might define the word, providing a description of features and function. The child could also be given an opportunity to identify named items. This provides an opportunity to see how familiar a child is with the words in a set. Ideally, the selected words need to be familiar and frequently occurring. However, some words may be less familiar to children and so require extra learning opportunities. The third and final step of Phase 1 involves the production of the contrast. According to Williams (2003), children should begin by imitating the SLP's model of each of the word pairs. This model is be accompanied by metaphonological cues, metaphor, and metaphoric gesture for each target in the collapse (e.g., telling a child that a depicted word *sheep* begins with the long quiet sound /ʃ/ while performing a gesture of a long arm movement, in contrast with the depicted word *deep* that begins with the short sound /d/ while performing a gesture of a short arm movement). Other types of cues can be used if a child has difficulty articulating a specific target (e.g., visual-phonetic cues, verbal-phonetic cues about place or manner, manual guidance, successive approximation/shaping, orthographic cues). Pragmatic cues can also be provided in response to each attempt, focusing a child's attention on the meaning of his or her production (Williams, 2003). Phase 1 typically lasts about one to two sessions and is primarily dependent on the child's familiarization with the training stimuli rather than production performance.

Phase 2 of the multiple oppositions approach involves contrasts and interactive play. There are two steps: imitation followed by spontaneous production practice of the contrasts. During the first step of Phase 2, imitation practice is believed to help children learn the articulatory requirements of the contrasts, while the spontaneous productions in the second step help children learn the phonological rule (Williams, 2003). A child is required to achieve 70% correct production across two consecutive treatment sets at the first step (imitation) before progressing to the second step (spontaneous production). One treatment set comprises 20 to 40 responses, depending on the number of contrasts being targeted (Williams, 2006). For instance, if [d] is contrasted with /k, ʃ, ʤ, sl/ for Luke (4;3 years, Chapter 16), then five word sets (e.g., *door, core, shore, jaw, slaw; dough, Koh, show, Joe, slow; day, K, Shay, J, sleigh; deep, keep, sheep, jeep, sleep; dam, Cam, sham, jam, slam*) would constitute a set of 20 responses of the targets /k, ʃ, ʤ, sl/. If the words are repeated, you would have a treatment set of 40 responses. The cues used in Phase 2 are similar to the cues used during the third step of Phase 1. Once a child achieves 90% correct production across two consecutive treatment sets in the second step of Phase 2, he or she can progress to Phase 3. A brief period of naturalistic interactive play is also encouraged at the end of each session in Phase 2 (e.g., craft activity, playing with farm animals, tea party) (Williams, 2006, 2010). The period of naturalistic play provides opportunities for children to use their intervention targets in a meaningful context, in a variety words in a play activity (Williams, 2006).

During Phase 3, the contrasts are used spontaneously within communicative contexts. For example, a child and the SLP may play a game of Concentration or What's Missing? (Williams, 2003). Pragmatic cues characterize Phase 3, given the focus on communication. Intervention continues at this phase until a child achieves 90% accuracy in communicative activities using the treatment words. A generalization probe is administered, ideally every third session, to determine whether intervention needs to continue. The generalization criterion is defined as 90% accuracy of a target sound in untrained words. If this criterion has been met, then the child's production of the target sound in conversational speech is evaluated. If the child is showing > 50% accuracy of that targeted sound during conversational speech, then intervention on that target discontinues. In the event that a child has met the Phase 3 training criterion (90% accuracy in communicative activities using target words) but shows difficulty meeting the generalizing criterion (generalization to untrained words) and/or the dismissal criterion, then Phase 4 is commenced (Williams, 2006). Phase 4 is essentially another intervention approach—naturalistic intervention for speech intelligibility and speech accuracy developed by Camarata (1993, 1995, 2010). This approach involves the SLP using conversational recasts during naturalistic play activities. The recasts provide children with opportunities to self-correct their speech, without imitative prompts.

■ Evidence

Williams has published a series of papers on the positive effect of multiple oppositions, comprising case studies and research using single-case experimental designs (see Williams, 2000a, b, 2005a, 2012). Ceron and Keske-Soares (2012) reported five case studies for Brazilian Portuguese-speaking children. In a large randomized controlled trial involving 54 children, Allen (2013) reported the effect of session frequency (three times per week for 8 weeks; weekly for 24 weeks) using multiple oppositions intervention. A control group of children received storybook intervention weekly for 8 weeks. The children who received more frequent sessions significantly outperformed the children who received weekly multiple oppositions intervention and the children in the control condition (Allen, 2013). Allen's findings highlight the importance of intervention intensity. You need to administer intervention, in this case multiple oppositions, at the recommended intensity to achieve optimal outcomes. Regarding dose, Williams (2012) reported that a *minimum* dose of 50 trials for a child with moderate phonological impairment and 70 trials for children with more severe impairment was needed in 30-minute intervention sessions for intervention to be effective. With regards to total intervention duration, Williams (2000a) provides helpful case study accounts of 10 children's therapy journey from the point of referral to discharge. On average, the number of sessions required to become intelligible using multiple oppositions with 10 children was 60.3 (range = 26–105), which was equivalent to approximately 30 SLP intervention hours (range = 13–52.5).

■ Children suited to the multiple oppositions approach

Children best suited to the multiple oppositions approach have a severe or profound phonological impairment characterized by multiple collapses of contrast (Williams, 2010). We would add that children with a severe or profound phonological impairment dominated by syllable structure or prosodic difficulties (e.g., *helicopter* /hɛlikɒptɚ/ as [kɒtɚ]; *caterpillar* /kætəpɪlɚ/ as [kæ.tɜ.pɪ.wɑ]) would be not appropriate.

■ Resources for conducting multiple oppositions intervention

Williams (2006) published a computer program called Sound Contrasts in Phonology (SCIP). This program is an automated database of over 8,000 illustrated intervention targets (real and nonsense), developed primarily for constructing word sets for contrastive approaches to intervention, including the minimal pair approach, maximal oppositions, treatment of the empty set, and multiple oppositions (Williams, 2006). You can use the program with a computer, or you can print out individualized word sets. The program also enables you to enter treatment data (online or offline) to help monitor a child's progress. SLPs could also develop their own word sets using their own picture database or sources on the Internet.

 APPLICATION: *Multiple oppositions intervention for Luke (4;3)*

Read more about Luke (4;3 years), a boy with a phonological impairment, in Chapter 16 (Case 1).

Using your analysis of the phonological patterns in Luke's speech (from your CHIRPA analysis in Chapter 9) and the phoneme collapses identified as short-term goals (from Chapter 9), prepare a speech sound disorder management plan (Appendix 11-1) and a speech sound disorder intervention session plan (Appendix 11-2) for Luke, based on the multiple oppositions approach. Ensure that your activities are fun and motivating and account for Luke's interests (see Chapter 16).

■■■

 APPLICATION: *Multiple oppositions intervention for Kathy*

Kathy (4;8 years) has a severe phonological impairment. She enjoys learning about animals, doing crafts, and engaging in pretend play. The following consonants are absent from her phonetic inventory: /f, h, v, s, z, ʃ, ʒ, ʧ, ʤ, l, ɹ, θ, ð/ as well as all consonant clusters. She can produce a relatively wide range of nasals, plosives, and the glides /w, j/. Velars have a positional constraint, only evident in within word and word-final positions. The largest collapse of contrast in word-initial position in her speech is [t] for: /s, ʃ, ʧ, tw, tɹ, st, sl, sk, k, ʃɹ, stɹ, skɹ, skw, kɹ, kw, kl, tɹ, tw/. Kathy can imitate the following phonemes absent from her inventory, in isolation, given an auditory model from the SLP: /f, h, v, s, z, θ, ð/.

1. Which four targets could you select to contrast with [t] as part of the multiple oppositions approach, and why? (Review the systemic approach in Chapter 10 to answer this question.)
2. What are three word sets that you could use in intervention to work on your targeted sounds?
3. Prepare for your first multiple oppositions session with Kathy by completing a speech sound disorder intervention session plan (see Appendix 11-2). Assume that you will see Kathy for individual 30-minute sessions twice weekly at preschool.

Metaphon

Metaphon, as the name suggests, is an intervention approach that uses children's metalinguistic abilities to improve their phonological system (Howell & Dean, 1994). The defining feature of this approach is metalinguistic talk during intervention.

■ Historical background

Metaphon was developed in the United Kingdom by two SLPs, Janet Howell and Elizabeth Dean, during the mid-to late 1980s. Howell and Dean wanted to develop an approach that targeted children's phonological systems rather than simply their articulation of individual speech sounds. They also wanted to encourage children to take an active role in intervention through discovering that communicative success depends on speakers being understood by listener(s) (Howell & Dean, 1994).

■ Theoretical background

The Metaphon approach is grounded in the idea that change or improvement in children's phonological systems occurs when the following three conditions are met:

1. Children understand that change is required.
2. Children learn that change can be made.
3. Children acquire information about how change might be achieved (Howell & Dean, 1994).

The approach integrates principles of phonology with principles of cognition and metacognition, with particular focus on children's metaphonological and metacommunicative abilities. **Metaphonology** refers to children's abilities to attend to and reflect on phonology (e.g., words can start with long or short sounds), while **metacommunication** is about knowing that communicative success depends on speakers being understood by listeners and that breakdowns in communication can be repaired through speakers revising their speech (Howell & Dean, 1994). Further information about the theoretical basis for Metaphon can be found in Chapters 4 and 5 of Howell and Dean (1994).

Procedure

The following description of the Metaphon procedure is based on Howell and Dean (1994). Metaphon is divided into two phases, with levels within each phase. Phase 1 focuses on developing children's metaphonological abilities, while Phase 2 targets children's metaphonological and metacommunication abilities. Relative to other interventions focused on production practice, Metaphon dialogue spends more time on metaphonological and metacommunication awareness (Hulterstam & Nettelbladt, 2002).

Phase 1: Listening and developing metaphonological awareness

- **Concept level** (for systemic and structural phonological processes): A child is introduced to and learns vocabulary concepts for the contrastive characteristic of a targeted phonological process. For example, if targeting the systemic phonological process of stopping of fricatives, a child could be familiarized with the concepts of *long* and *short*. Activities could be played where a child identifies and categorizes objects according to their contrastive feature (e.g., sorting long from short socks; cutting long versus short strips of paper). For intervention targeting a structural phonological process such as final consonant deletion, the child could be familiarized with the concept of animals with and without tails (Howell & Dean, 1994). Activities could include identifying animals that do and do not have tails and matching pictures of animals to their tails. Once a child understands the concept, he or she progresses to sound and then phoneme level (for systemic phonological processes) or syllable level (for structural phonological processes).
- **Sound level** (for systemic phonological processes only): The metaphonological concepts are applied to sounds. For example, the child could be given a drum or similar musical instrument and asked to identify or produce *long* versus *short* sounds.
- **Phoneme level** (for systemic phonological processes only): The metaphonological concept is applied to speech sounds. For example, a child could be asked to label a speech sound produced by an SLP as a long (e.g., /f, v, s, z, ʃ, ʒ/) or short sound (e.g., /p, b, t, d/). A visual referent or picture showing a mnemonic of the sound property could be used to facilitate a child's understanding of the concept at phoneme level (Howell & Dean, 1994).
- **Syllable level** (for structural phonological processes only): Structural phonological processes (e.g., final consonant deletion, cluster reduction) are somewhat different to systemic processes, in that the concept is not applied to a specific sound or group of sounds, but a particular speech structure such as final consonants, clusters, or weak syllables. For example, for final consonant deletion, the child could be asked to indicate whether a series of silly words have a tail sound or no tail sound (e.g., /ɪ/ versus /ɪp/). For cluster reduction, the child could be asked to identify silly words as either friendly (e.g., /spʌ/) or lonely (e.g., /pʌ/). As with phoneme level, a visual referent could be used to illustrate the concept.
- **Word level** (for systemic and structural phonological processes): Children are introduced to minimal pair words containing the phonological contrast and apply their metaphonological knowledge in listening activities. For example, a child could be asked to identify and sort pictures representing minimal pair words into one of two piles, as they are spoken by the SLP (e.g., "That word has a long sound"; "That word has a tail sound").

Phase 2: Speech production and developing metaphonological awareness and metacommunication

- **Word level:** Using minimal pair words, children apply their metaphonological knowledge to communication-centered speech production activities. Children are encouraged to use their metaphonological skills to talk about, reflect on, and where necessary repair their speech. One of the main goals of Phase 2 is that children explore the sound system via developing their metaphonological and metacommunicative awareness. This occurs within word-level speech production activities akin to those used in meaningful minimal pair intervention. During these activities children are confronted with the consequence of a breakdown in communication when they fail to produce a contrast between minimal pair words. Feedback and praise primarily focuses on the targeted phonological property using pragmatic (metacommunication) cues and metaphonological cues, such as "I heard you say a lonely word. Should it have been a friendly word?"; "I heard a long sound on that word. What are some other words with long sounds?"

■ **Sentence level:** Practice at sentence level using communication-centered activities can be introduced for children not showing generalized change in their phonological system in response to intervention at word level. Howell and Dean (1994) recommended that target phrases and sentences are kept constant for both minimal pair words, that the meaning is still conveyed by the single distinction between the minimal pair words. For example, while playing a treasure hunt game, the child could be instructed to say, "I found ... *key*" or "I found ... *tea.*"

Children suited to the Metaphon approach

The Metaphon approach was designed for children who have a phonological impairment. Children involved in Metaphon research have typically been of preschool age onwards (e.g., Dean et al., 1995; Dodd & Bradford, 2000; Harbers, Paden & Halle, 1999; Howell & Dean, 1994; Jarvis, 1989). Given the reliance of the approach on children's metalinguistic abilities, it may not be suitable for younger children. Howell and Dean (1994) suggest that the approach could be modified to meet the needs of children who have SSD characterized by both phonological and speech motor difficulties, speech difficulties resulting from cleft lip, and hearing impairment (Howell & Dean, 1994).

Evidence

Research on the Metaphon approach includes quasi-experimental group research (Dean, Howell, Reid, Grieve, & Donaldson, 1996; Dodd & Bradford, 2000), case studies (Dean, Howell, Waters, & Reid, 1995; Jarvis, 1989), and a book chapter (Howell & Dean, 1994). A modified version of the approach involving cycles and Metaphon was reported by Harbers, Paden, and Halle (1999). Across this research, improved speech accuracy has been reported for children with consistent developmental or nondevelopmental phonological errors.

Gillon (2005) compared retrospective data from a group of children—some of whom had received Metaphon or cycles intervention—with prospective data from a group of children who had received cycles intervention in addition to integrated phonological awareness intervention. Although improvements in speech accuracy were similar for both groups, the children in the prospective group show significantly better performance on early literacy measures. These results suggest that although Metaphon may help improve children's speech production skills, the metaphonological focus of Metaphon (i.e., focusing children's attention on features of the phonological system such as long/short), it does not necessarily address children's phonological awareness (i.e., ability to reflect upon and manipulate speech sounds in words, such as identifying the first sound in *mat* and replacing it with /k/ to create *cat*). Jarvis (1989) reported that a boy, Luke (4;9 years), was dismissed from intervention following approximately 1 academic year of Metaphon intervention. Dodd and Bradford (2000) reported that the approach was not appropriate for children with inconsistent speech errors.

Resources for conducting Metaphon intervention

The Metaphon Resource Pack (Dean, Howell, Hill, & Waters, 1990) was developed by Elizabeth Dean, Janet Howell, and colleagues to guide SLPs' conduct of Metaphon. The Metaphon Resource Pack includes screening assessment, process-specific evaluation or probe, resources for monitoring progress, and black-and-white line drawings of minimal pair pictures for nine common phonological processes. SLPs could also use commercial or freely available minimal pair resources in their conduct of Metaphon.

CYCLES

The Cycles Phonological Remediation Approach (Hodson, 1978; Hodson & Paden, 1983, 1991), known as the cycles approach, targets phonological patterns over designated periods of time, or cycles.

■ Historical background

The cycles approach was developed by Barbara Hodson and Elaine Pagel Paden in the mid-1970s at a communication disorders research clinic at the University of Illinois in Champaign-Urbana (Paden, 2007). Since that time, the approach has been developed and modified. Hodson and Paden's classic text on the approach was published in 1983, titled *Targeting Intelligible Speech*. A revised version of this text was published in 1991. A series of landmark papers and book chapters have been published along the way (e.g., Hodson, 1982, 1989, 1992, 1994, 1997, 1998, 2006; Hodson & Scudder, 1990; Prezas & Hodson, 2010), including Hodson's (2007) text *Evaluating and Enhancing Children's Phonological Systems: Research and Theory to Practice*. Modified applications of the approach have also been reported (e.g., Almost & Rosenbaum, 1998; Gillon, 2005).

■ Theoretical background

To facilitate efficient change in children's phonological systems, the cycles approach targets phonological patterns rather than individual phonemes. Seven important concepts or principles underlie the cycles approach to targeting patterns (Prezas & Hodson, 2010).

First, phonological acquisition is considered to be gradual. One carefully selected pattern after another is given intervention for a period of time, until a child's performance is reviewed. It is on this basis that the concept of a cycle or period of time for targeting deficient patterns is based. Second, children learn speech through listening (Van Riper, 1939). This is why the approach incorporates slightly amplified auditory stimulation, as it is thought to help children become more aware of the speech sounds they need to learn (Hodson, 2007). Third, children develop kinesthetic and auditory associations for the speech sounds and syllables as they learn to produce them. Consequently, errorless (rather than errorful) practice of stimulable targets is emphasized. Fourth, the phonetic environments can help (or hinder) children's productions of new speech sounds (Hodson, 2007). This means that the words selected for production practice must reflect the most conducive phonetic environment for successful production. Fifth, children should be actively involved in phonological acquisition, as they learn better when they are mentally and physically engaged. This translates as including fun, drill-play activities during production practice (Prezas & Hodson, 2010). Sixth, intervention needs to target a select group of speech sounds or syllable shapes representative of phonological patterns to facilitate phonological generalization in children's phonological systems. The seventh and final concept aligns with Vygotsky's (1978) idea of children having a zone of proximal development, and that tasks children cannot yet handle alone may be handled with the help of a more skilled partner (Berk, 2007). In practice this means finding out what a child is phonologically capable of and what he or she finds challenging, and focusing intervention at a point just beyond the child's current capabilities (Hodson, 2007).

■ Procedure

The cycles approach involves the careful selection, targeting, and cycling of deficit patterns for a predetermined period of time, in addition to using a prescribed sequence of session activities and procedures (Hodson, 2011). Target patterns are identified following a comprehensive analysis of a child's speech production skills. Patterns occurring 40% or more of the time (typically based on results from the Hodson Assessment of Phonological Patterns, HAPP-3, Hodson, 2004) are prioritized for intervention (Hodson & Paden, 1991). Those patterns occurring less than 40% of the time are monitored. Patterns occurring more than 40% of the time are then grouped into **primary**, **secondary**, and **advanced target patterns** (see Chapter 10).

Having identified and grouped an individual child's patterns into primary, secondary, and advanced, the child's first cycle is planned. A cycle constitutes the period of time in which all of the phonological patterns (initially, all primary patterns only) are targeted. According to Hodson (2007), each pattern is targeted for approximately 2 to 6 hours per cycle, depending on the number of target phonemes within a pattern that are stimulable, with each stimulable phoneme or consonant cluster within a pattern being targeted for 1 hour. A cycle may last for approximately 5 to 6 weeks or may be as long as 15 or 16 weeks, with there being 1 SLP contact hour per week (Hodson, 2007). At the conclusion of a cycle, children's phonological skills are reexamined and phonological patterns are recycled, until they begin to emerge in conversational speech. Secondary patterns are not included in a cycle until certain primary patterns have become established, including syllableness (production of at least two-syllable compound words and three-syllable word combinations); basic word structure (i.e., no omissions of singleton consonants); anterior-posterior contrasts (although some assimilations are still acceptable); the emergence of stridency; and the suppression of the glide substitution/insertion for production practice words that contain liquids (Hodson, 2007).

Based on the work of Prezas and Hodson (2010), cycles sessions comprise eight components:

1. Review of the previous session's production practice words. (If it is the first session, this step is not necessary.)
2. Amplified auditory stimulation of a list of approximately 20 words containing the session's intervention target. The list of words is read for approximately 30 seconds (Hodson, 2011).
3. Selection of words with facilitating phonetic contexts. Four or five strategically selected words are depicted and written on a large card. During this activity the child could draw and/or color the picture on each card. Depending on the child's age and abilities, the child could write the word, or part thereof, on the card.
4. Production practice activities of the selected words using drill play. Typically, five or six activities may be used during a 1-hour session, while two or three activities may be used during a half hour session (Hodson & Paden, 1991). Instructional cues (e.g., auditory, visual, verbal, tactile) are used as needed.
5. Stimulability testing to determine which phoneme from a pattern or which pattern will be targeted in the following session.
6. Emergent literacy activity focused on phonological awareness. (See the section on emergent literacy intervention later in this chapter for further information.)
7. Repetition of the amplified auditory stimulation.
8. Review of homework (auditory stimulation using the word list from the session, the child naming the production practice words, and a brief emergent literacy activity).

■ Children suited to the cycles approach

The cycles approach was developed to address the needs of children with highly unintelligible speech, characterized by multiple phonological patterns (including segmental and syllable structure difficulties). Hodson (2011) suggests that the approach can be modified for toddlers by focusing on auditory stimulation of primary patterns.

■ Evidence

Research evidence on the cycles approach first emerged from a phonological intervention clinic at the University of Illinois in 1975 (Hodson, 1997). Research clinics were also established at San Diego State University in 1981 and Wichita State University in 1989 (Hodson, 1997). In 1991, Hodson and Paden reported that over 200 children had been involved in their ongoing efforts to research and develop the approach. According to Hodson (2007), children with a severe phonological impairment have become intelligible in less than a year given three to four cycles (equivalent to approximately 30 to 40 hours of an SLP's time). The evidence base for the cycles approach includes a series of experimental group studies of the cycles approach or modified versions of the approach (e.g., Almost & Rosenbaum, 1998; Conture, Louko, & Edwards, 1993; Gillon, 2005; Mota, et al., 2007; Rvachew, Nowak, & Cloutier, 2004; Tyler & Watterson, 1991), single-case experimental design research (e.g., Harbers, Paden, & Halle, 1999; Rvachew, Rafaat, & Martin, 1999; Tyler, Edwards, & Saxman, 1987),

APPLICATION: *Cycles approach to intervention for Luke (4;3)*

Using your analysis of the phonological patterns in Luke's speech (from your CHIRPA analysis in Chapter 9) and the cycles-based goals that would be suitable for Luke (from Chapter 10), prepare a speech sound disorder management plan (Appendix 11-1), and a speech sound disorder intervention session plan (Appendix 11-2) for Luke. Use the information about Luke's case in Chapter 16 to guide your ideas about the types of activities that Luke would find interesting and motivating in his first session with you.

Read more about
Luke (4;3 years),
a boy with a phonological
impairment,
in Chapter 16 (Case 1).

 COMMENT: *PACT intervention (Bowen, 2015)*

Caroline Bowen developed and tested a phonological intervention approach called PACT (Parents and Children Together) (Bowen, 2010). According to Bowen (2015), this approach includes five components: parent education and involvement; metalinguistic training (i.e., using metaphonological cues and teaching children to use language to talk about speech sounds); phonetic production training (i.e., learning to hear and produce word structures or speech sounds in syllables and words via auditory discrimination activities and various speech production cues); multiple exemplar training (i.e., practicing targeted speech skills via auditory input tasks and through the use of minimal pair words reflecting minimal oppositions, maximal pairs, or multiple oppositions); and homework. PACT contains elements of intervention in other approaches, such as Metaphon (Howell & Dean, 1994), cycles (Hodson, 2007), and the contrastive interventions (e.g., Baker, 2010b; Gierut, 1992; Williams, 2010). Intervention targets may be developmental or complex, depending on a child's needs and the SLP's informed opinion (Bowen, 2015). The deliberate focus on educating and involving parents is the defining feature of PACT intervention.

and non-experimental case reports (e.g., Culatta, Setzer, & Horn, 2005; Glaspey & MacLeod, 2010; Glaspey & Stoel-Gammon, 2005, 2007; Gordon-Brannan, Hodson, & Wynne, 1992; Hodson, Chin, Redmond, & Simpson, 1983; Hodson, Nonomura, & Zappia, 1989; Hodson & Paden, 1983; MacLeod & Glaspey, 2014; Montgomery & Bonderman, 1989). The repeated finding across the evidence base has been that the cycles approach (and modified versions of the cycles approach) improves children's speech intelligibility. Almost and Rosenbaum's (1998) experimental study reported that children who received modified cycles had significantly improved speech intelligibility relative to a control group of children who were waiting for intervention. Relative to other approaches, Mota et al. (2007) found no difference in outcomes between the cycles approach, maximal oppositions, and an approach described as ABAB withdrawal and multiple probes that prioritized complex targets.

■ Resources for conducting the cycles approach

The cycles approach to intervention requires a few different resources, including:

1. Word lists to provide the amplified auditory stimulation: Word lists are available in commercial intervention resources (e.g., Foster & Gold, 2002), with some freely available on the Internet.[1]
2. Small amplifier and microphone: You could purchase a small amplifier and microphone, or connect a microphone to your computer to play back live voice, using relevant software.

---

[1]For example, Peter Flipsen Jr.'s list: http://speech-language-therapy.com/pdf/listeninglists2010pf.pdf.

3. 5 × 8 inch blank card stock, and/or pictures representing real-word stimuli: You could source the minimal pair stimuli available on the Internet, or invest in a commercially available resource suited to the cycles approach (e.g., Foster & Gold, 2002).
4. Phonological-awareness resources suitable for children with SSD (discussed later in this chapter).
5. Equipment/toys for use during production practice games. Appendix E of Hodson and Paden (1991) and Appendix C of Hodson (2007) provide a list of fun and easy production practice games to play with children.

 APPLICATION: Which intervention approach for Jonathon?

Jonathon (4;4 years) has a percentage of consonants correct (PCC) of 42% and is highly unintelligible. His speech production errors are consistent and characterized by early developing error patterns. Jonathon also has a history of repeated middle ear infections.

1. Which of the following three intervention approaches would you select for Jonathon?
   ■ Hodson's (2007) cycles approach
   ■ Bowen's (2015) PACT intervention approach
   ■ Howell and Dean's (1994) Metaphon approach

2. Justify your decision based on research evidence and client factors.

Answer: You could select any of the three approaches for Jonathon. All three approaches have peer-reviewed published evidence of cases similar to Jonathon's with respect to age and severity and nature of impairment. The approach that a practicing SLP selects may be based on knowledge, resources, and experience with the approach. You would, however, supplement your selected intervention with emergent literacy intervention focusing on phoneme awareness and letter knowledge (e.g., Gillon, 2005) to address Jonathon's risk of literacy difficulties. You would also assess Jonathon's speech perception skills and provide speech perception training, if needed.

SPEECH PERCEPTION INTERVENTION

Speech perception intervention was designed to help children with phonological impairment develop better underlying phonological representations for speech and literacy. It is an input-based intervention that can supplement a production-based intervention approach.

■ Historical background

The role of speech perception training in intervention for children with SSD has a long history (see Rvachew & Brosseau-Lapré, 2012). Since the 1930s, some researchers have included direct speech perception training as a component of intervention (e.g., Howell & Dean, 1994; Rvachew, 1994; Van Riper, 1939) while others have not (e.g., Gierut, 1992; McCabe & Bradley, 1975). In 1980, John Locke suggested that

> speech perception deserves clinical interest to the extent that production difficulties are linked to problems of perceptual processing, and that the elicitation of perceptual responses is one of the few good ways of inferring what a child knows about the phonological structure of language. (Locke, 1980b, p. 445)

Although speech perception training (in various forms) has been included within some phonological intervention approaches, Susan Rvachew's work on the role and benefit of speech perception training that incorporates multiple speakers and lexical judgment tasks has confirmed Locke's (1980b) suggestion.

> **COMMENT:** *What about intervention targeting complex onsets?*
>
> Complex onsets are word-initial two- and three-element consonant clusters. Research by Judith Gierut and colleagues has suggested that intervention targeting word-initial two-element consonant clusters with small sonority difference score facilitates more widespread change in children's phonological systems compared to intervention targeting consonant clusters with large sonority difference scores (Gierut, 1999). Word-initial three-element consonant clusters can also be targeted. (See Chapter 10 for further information about the complexity approach to target selection and when you might prioritize two- versus three-element word-initial consonant clusters.)
>
> Drawing on the work of Gierut and colleagues, one approach for targeting complex onsets could be to use similar procedures as maximal oppositions and treatment of the empty set. Up to 15 novel words containing strategically selected word-initial consonant clusters could serve as the word stimuli. The novel words would need to be phonotactically permissible and ideally balanced for canonical structure, phonetic environment, and syntactic category (a mix of nouns and verbs) (Gierut, 2008). Various word shapes and lengths could be used, including monosyllables (e.g., [flim]), disyllables (e.g., [flupi]), and polysyllables (e.g., [flɛdupɪk]). The appendix of Gierut and Champion (2001) provides helpful suggestions for constructing suitable novel word stimuli for three-element consonant clusters. Examples of words from their 2001 study targeting the cluster /spɹ/ include: [spɹin], [spɹɪb], [spɹeb], [spɹɛm], [spɹæd], [spɹidɛb] and [spɹudəm]. Using a procedure similar to maximal oppositions, the novel words could be assigned lexical meaning in a story. Two phases may be used: imitation followed by spontaneous production. The criterion for progressing from one phase to the next could be identical to the criteria outlined in the maximal oppositions/empty set procedure. The children involved in the research by Gierut (1998, 1999) and Gierut and Champion (2001) were of preschool age (the youngest across the research was 3;2 years), and all had a phonological impairment, characterized by the exclusion of six or seven consonants from their phonemic inventories.
>
> Alternatively, you could target word-initial two-element consonant clusters with small sonority difference scores using the minimal pair approach. For example, for Luke (4;3 years) a complex onset target could be /sl/. You could then pair /sl/ with /d/ in near minimal pair words (e.g., *sleep* versus *deep*; *slow* versus *dough*), because he uses [d] for /s/. You would then monitor Luke's phonological system for generalization.

▪ Theoretical background

Speech perception intervention is based on an understanding that as children learn to talk they develop and refine multiple underlying representations for words, including **acoustic-phonetic**, **articulatory-phonetic**, and **lexical representations** (Rvachew & Brosseau-Lapré, 2010). Children's underlying acoustic-phonetic representations are believed to become increasingly refined in infancy as children learn to understand the words spoken by different speakers, of different ages and genders, in different environmental or speaking conditions. Children then use their underlying acoustic-phonetic representations of words to create and refine their articulatory-phonetic representations of those words (Rvachew & Brosseau-Lapré, 2012).

The importance of the link between perception and production is evident in the relationship between children's speech perception skills and their expressive vocabulary—the better the speech perception as an infant, the larger the vocabulary as a toddler (Tsao, Liu, & Kuhl, 2004). Speech perception skills also have been shown to predict growth in children's speech production skills—the better the speech perception, the better the growth in children's speech production (Rvachew & Brosseau-Lapré, 2012).

Children with phonological impairment are thought to struggle with the creation and refinement of acoustic-phonetic representations and the subsequent creation and refinement of articulatory-phonetic representations. This idea is based on evidence that these children perform significantly more poorly on tests of speech perception and phonological processing relative to their typically developing peers (e.g., Munson, Baylis, Krause, & Yim, 2010; Rvachew, 1994). Rvachew and Brosseau-Lapré (2010) suggest that children with phonological impairment have acoustic-phonetic representations that are not like adults; their perceptual categories are too broad, including both correct and incorrect productions of specific phonemes. This is why children with phonological impairment are thought to benefit from intervention targeting their speech perception ability.

■ Procedure

In this section we describe speech perception intervention based on the Speech Assessment and Interactive Learning System (SAILS) (Rvachew, 2009) developed by Susan Rvachew. This program was designed to help children develop stable, detailed underlying acoustic-phonetic representations of words through completing lexical judgment and mispronunciation detection tasks using speech samples from multiple speakers. During intervention, children are instructed to listen to carefully selected and strategically designed samples of spoken words and decide whether the words heard are consistent with a predetermined target word (Rvachew & Brosseau-Lapré, 2010). The words include pronunciations of the same word spoken by different speakers (children and adults, male and female speakers) in addition to error productions of the target word. Children listen to the words via headphones and indicate whether the word they hear is their target word or a different word (i.e., make a lexical judgment about which word they hear) or detect whether the word they hear is an accurate way of pronouncing the target sound (i.e., mispronunciation detection). The child's SLP would typically sit with the child as they use the SAILS program to provide the child with relevant feedback. Correctly identified pictures would be followed by positive metaphonological feedback (e.g., "Great, you heard the /k/ in *kick*"). Incorrect responses would be followed by instructional feedback (e.g., "I heard /k/ in *kick*. Listen and try again"). Speech perception intervention can be provided prior to or alongside production-based intervention. From the research evidence, the production component has included the cycles approach (e.g., Rvachew, Rafaat, & Martin, 1999), traditional articulation intervention (e.g., Rvachew, 1994), and a speech production approach considered appropriate by a child's SLP (e.g., Rvachew, Nowak, & Cloutier, 2004).

■ Children suited to speech perception intervention

According to Rvachew and Brosseau-Lapré (2010), most children who have a phonological impairment have difficulty with the perception of at least some of the phonemes in error in their speech, and are therefore suited to speech perception intervention. Children who have SSD second to cleft palate or Down syndrome, and second language learners, may also benefit from speech perception intervention. According to Rvachew and Brosseau-Lapré (2010), children younger than 4 years may find the SAILS tasks somewhat difficult. In such situations, you could apply the principles underlying SAILS of listening to multiple speakers, making lexical judgments, and detecting mispronunciations. Research is needed to determine how this might best be done. Jamieson and Rvachew (1992) noted that speech perception intervention is unlikely to improve a child's speech production if the child does not have difficulty with speech perception.

■ Evidence

Most of the evidence base associated with SAILS has been published by Rvachew and colleagues. Randomized controlled trials and one non-randomized controlled trial have been conducted on the approach (Rvachew, 1994; Rvachew, Nowak, & Cloutier, 2004; Rvachew, Rafaat, & Martin, 1999; Wolfe, Presley, & Mesaris, 2003), in addition to case studies (Jamieson & Rvachew, 1992). The repeated finding from this research is that it is beneficial (with respect to intervention efficiency and effectiveness) to provide speech perception intervention prior to or alongside a production-based approach for children who have speech perception and production difficulties.

■ ■

 APPLICATION: *Speech perception intervention for Courtney*

Courtney (5;2 years) has persistent velar fronting for all velars across all word positions (e.g., /k/→ [t]). Assessment using SAILS (Rvachew, 2009) identified that she is having difficulty perceiving velars—Courtney accepts both correct and incorrect productions as correct. Prepare an SSD management plan and SSD session plan for Courtney, addressing her difficulty with perception using Rvachew's (2009) SAILS approach.

■ Resources for speech perception intervention

The Speech Assessment and Interactive Learning System (SAILS) (Rvachew, 2009) could be used by SLPs working with children learning to speak American English or Canadian English. If you do not have access to SAILS or work with children who speak another dialect of English or another language, you could apply Locke's (1980b) idea and use pictures of minimal pair words relevant to a child's particular speech production error with a speech perception task. For example, suppose a child does not produce a contrast between /k/ and /t/ and says *key* and *tea* as [ti]. To determine whether the child hears the contrast between the word pairs, you could play the child recordings of different speakers saying minimal pair words containing the child's target sound /k/, the child's substitute sound, and an unrelated sound (e.g., *key, tea, me*). The different speakers could include males and females of various ages, including children (with and without SSD). Given a picture of a word containing the target sound (e.g., *key*), you would play the child the various renditions of the words that you have recorded, and the child would decide whether the word is the target word (i.e., *key*) or another word (i.e., *tea* or *me*). The variety of speakers could provide the child with opportunities to better refine their underlying representation of /k/. Speech perception instructions and feedback would be in keeping with the procedures described in this chapter. Evidence in support of this more informal approach to speech perception training based on SAILS has not been established, so, as with any adaptation to an evidence-based approach, you would need to gather your own internal clinical evidence to determine if it is helping a child.

INTERVENTION FOR CONCOMITANT PHONOLOGY AND MORPHOSYNTAX DIFFICULTIES

Children who have phonological impairment can have concomitant language impairment (Shriberg & Kwiatkowski, 1994; Tyler & Haskill, 2010). A particular skill that can be problematic is the production of finite morphemes (Tyler, Gillon, Macrae, & Johnson, 2011). Finite morphemes include:

1. third-person singular regular (e.g., -s as in *eats, drinks, looks, finds, puts, wants, makes*).
2. regular past tense (e.g., -ed as in *jumped, skipped, hopped, looked*).
3. irregular past tense (e.g., *ran, fell, ate, found, drank*).
4. copula and uncontractible and contractile auxiliary BE verbs (e.g., *is, are, am, was, were*).

The morphosyntactic approach was developed specifically for children who have concomitant phonology and morphosyntax difficulties.

■ Historical background

Ann Tyler and colleagues developed the morphosyntactic approach to directly target children's acquisition of finite morphemes (e.g., Tyler, 2002, 2008; Tyler et al., 2011; Tyler, Lewis, Haskill, & Tolbert, 2002, 2003; Tyler, Lewis, & Welch, 2003).

■ Theoretical background

Tyler and colleagues' approach to targeting morphosyntactic difficulties in children is based on two theoretical rationales. Firstly, children with language impairment often need intervention targeting difficulty with their use of finite morphemes. Why these particular morphemes can be challenging is not well understood. It is thought that children either have a linguistic problem learning grammatical rules, or a broader cognitive-linguistic problem (characterized by either a generalized slower processing system or phonological working memory limitations) (Tyler & Haskill, 2010). Either way, finite morphemes are important in children's development of syntax (sentence structure) (Haskill & Tyler, 2007; Rice & Wexler, 1996).

The second rationale underlying Tyler and colleagues' intervention approach is the notion of cross-linguistic generalization, that is, intervention targeting one domain can (but not always will) indirectly benefit another domain. Consider the phonological structure of some finite morphemes. Third-person present singular (e.g., *runs, eats, hops*) is typically realized via the production of final consonant clusters (e.g., /nz, ts, ps/). Given that children with phonological impairment often present with cluster reduction, Tyler and Haskill (2010) suggest that morphosyntax intervention might indirectly improve these children's phonological abilities through the production of complex morphophonemic markers such as /nz/ in *runs*, /ts/ in *eats*, and /ps/ in *hops*.

■ Procedure

Morphosyntax intervention is usually provided alongside another approach targeting children's speech production. Evidence from Tyler, Lewis, Haskill, and Tolbert (2003) suggests that optimal morphosyntax outcomes are achieved when an alternating goal attack strategy is used. This involves directly targeting children's phonological abilities one week (e.g., odd weeks 1, 3, 5, 7, 9, 11 of a 12-week block) and production of finite morphemes on alternate weeks (e.g., even weeks 2, 4, 6, 8, 10, 12). In keeping with the evidence, sessions could be conducted twice weekly in a cycles format (e.g., 4 weeks × 3 cycles), with one session per week being a 30-minute individual session and the other a small group session (comprising two to four children) for 45 minutes (Tyler, Lewis, Haskill, & Tolbert, 2003). Having considered the service delivery format, let's now turn our attention to Tyler and colleagues' morphosyntax intervention procedure.

Morphosyntax intervention is provided within a cycles format, targeting a different finite morpheme each week (Tyler & Haskill, 2010). A session typically begins with a series of focus stimulation activities followed by an elicited production activity in keeping with a particular theme such as water, animals, or food (Haskill, Tyler, & Tolbert, 2001).

- **Focus stimulation** activities typically involve the SLP providing a child with at least 40 correct productions of the target finite morpheme within a literacy, narrative, or singing activity (Haskill et al., 2001). For example, when recounting a picture book about a father bathing his baby, the script could be: "Dad *washes* baby's hair. Dad *cleans* baby's face. Dad *blows* the bubbles. Dad *pops* the bubbles in the bath. Dad *sings* to the baby. The baby *looks* at Dad. The baby *smiles* at Dad. Dad *smiles* at the baby."
- **Elicited production activities** occur within the context of play, craft, or a story recount in keeping with the theme introduced during the focused stimulation. The target morpheme is elicited via the SLP's dialogue. Specifically, Tyler and Haskill (2010) recommend that the SLP elicit the target morpheme initially via a simple forced choice question, progressing to a cloze task followed by a preparatory set:

  1. **Forced choice:** The SLP provides the child with an opportunity to attempt a production of the target morpheme given a choice of two options, both of which provide an opportunity for the child to produce the marker, such as: "Tell me how Dad gives his baby a bath. He *washes* the hair or *brushes* the hair?"
  2. **Cloze task:** The SLP gives the child an opportunity to complete a sentence, such as: "Look at what Dad does to the bubbles, he ..."

3. **Preparatory set:** The SLP models a type of utterance for a child, and then provides a prompt for the child to generate his or her own utterance containing the target morpheme, such as: "The baby *looks* at Dad, and the baby *smiles* at Dad. You tell me what Dad does."

With regards to the type of feedback that you would give the child, Tyler and Haskill (2010) provide some helpful suggestions. If the child says the target morpheme correctly, a positive, encouraging response reiterating the correct production could be provided (e.g., SLP: "Yes, Dad *pops* the bubbles"). In the event that the child does not produce the target morpheme, the SLP could provide either a relatively simple expansion recast (e.g., SLP: "Dad *pops* the bubbles"), or a growth recast (Nelson, 1989) by rewording the child's utterance and adding further information (e.g., SLP: "Dad *pops* all the bubbles in the air").

◼ Children suited to the intervention for concomitant phonology and morphosyntax

Children with concomitant phonological and language impairment are suited to morphosyntax intervention when the child's language difficulties are characterized by a problem with marking finite morphemes (Tyler & Haskill, 2010).

◼ Evidence

Tyler and colleagues' morphosyntax intervention approach has been tested empirically via a number of randomized controlled trials (Tyler, Lewis, Haskill, & Tolbert, 2003; Tyler, Lewis, & Welch, 2003; Tyler, Gillon, Macrae, & Johnson, 2011), non-randomized controlled trials (Tyler et al., 2002; Tyler & Watterson, 1991), quasi-experimental group studies (Tyler & Lewis, 2005; Tyler, Williams, & Lewis, 2006), and a case study (Tyler, 2002). The morphosyntax outcomes were measured via the analysis of a 200-word language sample and subsequent calculation of a finite morpheme composite (FMC). The FMC was calculated by determining the percentage correct usage of finite morphemes in the sample (Tyler, Lewis, Haskill, & Tolbert, 2003). The phonology outcomes were measured via computerized analysis of a single-word speech sample and subsequent calculation of the PCC for the target and generalization sounds relevant to each individual child.

The main findings from this body of research are interesting, yet somewhat complicated. First, Tyler et al. (2002) examined the benefit of two 12-week blocks of intervention. Participants ($n = 20$) were randomly assigned to begin with a block of phonology or morphosyntax intervention. Relative to a non-randomized controlled group, children receiving a block of either phonology or morphosyntax intervention showed a statistically significant improvement in their respective targets after the first 12-week block (Tyler et al., 2002). Cross-domain generalization, in the form of changes in the children's phonological systems, was evident for the children receiving the morphosyntax intervention. Such cross-domain effects were not evident with the phonology intervention. Tyler et al. (2002) recommended "targeting morphosyntax intervention first, followed by phonology, if using a block intervention sequence for children with concomitant morphosyntactic and phonology impairments" (p. 52). In an extension of this work, Tyler et al. (2003) examined the relative benefits of three different goal attack strategies: simultaneous (both interventions provided within same session), block (12 weeks of morphosyntax or phonology), and weekly alternating (odd weeks = phonology, even weeks = morphosyntax). Tyler et al. (2003) reported that "morphosyntactic change was greatest for children receiving the alternating strategy after 24 weeks of intervention" and that "no single goal attack strategy was superior in facilitating gains in phonological performance" (p. 1077). The children showed similarly significant improvements in their phonological abilities. The main clinical recommendation from this study was that a weekly alternating intervention strategy may be preferable for children with concomitant morphosyntactic and phonology difficulties. It is important to note that the morphosyntax intervention targeted finite morpheme targets realized by the production of final consonant clusters.

In a comparison study, an alternating sequence of phonology and morphosyntax intervention was compared with a block of integrated phonological awareness intervention that included production practice for targeted phonological processes

(Tyler et al., 2011). The participants in both groups improved their speech, with more marked improvements in phonological awareness evident for the children who received phonological awareness intervention, and more marked improvements in morphosyntax for the children receiving morphosyntax intervention. These findings suggested that children's speech can be indirectly improved via phonological awareness and morphosyntax intervention, but that marked improvements in phonological awareness and morphosyntax tend to occur with intervention directly targeting these skills.

■ Resources for conducting intervention for concomitant phonology and morphosyntax difficulties

The morphosyntax intervention approach described in Tyler and colleagues' research was developed into an intervention resource titled *Months of Morphemes* (Haskill et al., 2001). If you cannot access this resource, then locate a series of children's books that contain multiple occurrences of the target finite morphemes, or create your own stories comprising finite morphemes. A variety of craft resources (e.g., scissors, paper, glue) may be required for the elicited production activities.

STIMULABILITY INTERVENTION

Stimulability refers to a child's ability to "immediately modify a speech production error when presented with an auditory and visual model" (Miccio, 2009, p. 97). Stimulability intervention was designed to enhance young children's speech sound stimulability so that they could more readily participate and benefit from a production-based approach, such as minimal pairs or multiple oppositions.

■ Historical background

Stimulability intervention was developed by Adele Miccio and Mary Elbert (Miccio & Elbert, 1996; Miccio, 2005, 2009). The main aim of the approach is to facilitate young children's speech sound stimulability.

■ Theoretical background

Stimulability intervention targets all consonants at once during a session (stimulable and non-stimulable, whether present or absent from a child's phonetic inventory) through the use of auditory, verbal, visual, and gestural cues (Miccio, 2015). The approach is grounded in three ideas: the role of stimulability in speech sound learning, the basic principles of complexity (what to target), and an understanding about the types of teaching cues that best help children learn (how to target).

First, regarding the role of stimulability speech sound learning, the ability to perceive speech and produce speech are independent but related abilities. This connection between perception and production is evident in the DIVA model (Guenther, 1995) mentioned in Chapter 5. Researchers have suggested that when children engage in speech perception training for sounds in error in speech production, their stimulability can improve (Rvachew, 1994). Second, the complexity approach to target selection promotes targeting non-stimulable over stimulable sounds, as stimulable sounds are more likely to be learned without direct instruction compared to non-stimulable sounds (e.g., Powell et al., 1991). However, SLPs have been reluctant to target non-stimulable sounds because of a potential for children to be frustrated by the intervention experience, and because of a lack of certainty about how best to target non-stimulable sounds (McLeod & Baker, 2014; Miccio & Williams, 2010). Miccio and Elbert (1996) developed stimulability intervention in an effort to meet the need for an approach targeting stimulability in younger children. Third, it is thought that multimodal cues including auditory, verbal, visual, and gestural cues can help children learn to talk. For instance, being able to gesture while speaking has been associated with better word retrieval (Rauscher, Krauss, & Chen, 1996). The use of gesture can also help ensure successful communication (Miccio, 2005). Stimulability intervention uses multimodal cues by including alliterative names for characters associated with each consonant (e.g., Munchie Mouse, Zippy Zebra) in addition to speech sounds, pictures, and hand/body gestures specific to each character.

Procedure

Stimulability intervention targets 21 consonants within a session (that is, all consonants in English with the exceptions of [ʒ], [ŋ], and [ð]) at the level of isolation for fricatives, affricates, and nasals (e.g., /z::::/), and in consonant-vowel (CV) contexts for plosives and glides, with /h/ classified as a glide rather than a fricative (e.g., /hə/). During a session children are taught the names of 21 alliterative characters, their corresponding gesture, picture, and speech sound (e.g., Zippy Zebra is associated with the speech sound /z::::/ and the action of zipping a jacket). Miccio and Williams (2010) describe a typical session as follows:

1. Elicit of one third of a stimulability probe (5 minutes): This task examines a child's ability to produce each of the 24 English consonants in isolation and in one of three vowel contexts (/i/, /ʌ/, /u/), depending on whether or not a sound occurs in that position (e.g., /ŋ/ is not assessed in syllable-initial position). During subsequent sessions another third of the stimulability probe is administered, so that by the end of every third session the entire stimulability probe has been administered. For example:
   - Session 1: consonants with /i/ e.g., /z::/, /zi/, /izi/, /iz/
   - Session 2: consonants with /ʌ/ e.g., /z::/, /zɒ/, /ɒzɒ/, /ɒz/
   - Session 3: consonants with /u/ e.g., /z::/, /zu/, /uzu/, /uz/
2. Review of alliterative characters (5 minutes): Using focused joint attention, the SLP reviews the names for the 21 alliterative characters and their associated pictures, speech sounds, and gestures. Children are encouraged but not required to articulate the speech sound associated with each alliterative character (Miccio & Williams, 2010).
3. Play-based stimulability activities (30 minutes): Play-based activities constitute the majority of a stimulability intervention session. Play-based activities typically involve turn-taking activities (e.g., Go Fish, Lotto boards) using the picture cards depicting the alliterative characters (Miccio & Williams, 2010). During the SLP's turn, the name of the character, speech sound, and gesture are produced by the SLP. During the child's turn, the child is encouraged to name the character and use the gesture, but only to attempt to imitate the target speech sound. Imitation of the child's non-stimulable speech sounds is not essential for a child to complete his or her turn. Phonetic cues, in addition to successive approximation/shaping, can be used to shape a child's production, if the child is amenable to such instruction. Through play-based activities, children are provided with multiple opportunities to listen to and attempt the 21 target consonants.
4. Palindrome generalization probe (5–8 minutes): A brief single-word imitation task comprising palindromes (e.g., *pop, bub, Dad, Nan*) is administered to monitor response generalization to simple CVC words.

Stimulability intervention typically lasts around 12 sessions over 6 weeks, given that 45-minute sessions are scheduled twice weekly; however, intervention could last as long as 12 weeks (Miccio, 2015; Miccio & Williams, 2010). The approach could be used as a precursor to a contrastive approach (e.g., Miccio's case study of a girl called Fiona) (Miccio, 2015).

Children suited to the stimulability approach

The stimulability approach is suitable for 2- to 4-year-old children who have small phonetic inventories and are not stimulable for the phones absent from their inventories (Miccio & Williams, 2010).

Evidence

Stimulability intervention has a relatively small evidence base, limited to published peer-reviewed case study reports (Miccio & Elbert, 1996; Powell, 1996) and case descriptions in book chapters (Miccio, 2009; Miccio & Williams, 2010). Across this evidence, the outcomes have been positive, with children who were non-stimulable for a range of speech sounds becoming more stimulable. It is important to add that this approach is not designed to improve children's overall speech intelligibility but simply their speech sound stimulability. Consequently, based on the case study evidence available, the approach is recommended as a first stage of intervention, making way for a contrastive phonological intervention approach such as minimal pairs, maximal oppositions, treatment of the empty set, or multiple oppositions, or, a non-contrastive intervention.

■ Resources for conducting stimulability intervention

To conduct stimulability intervention you will need pictures of alliterative characters. You will also need to have gestures that correspond with the alliterative characters. Given that much of a stimulability intervention session is comprised of play-based stimulability activities using the picture cards, it would be helpful to laminate multiple copies of the pictures for use during activities. Additional materials would be required depending on the activities to be conducted during the session (e.g., magnetic fishing rod and paper clips attached to each picture card to conduct a fishing game; Lotto boards depicting the alliterative characters; envelopes to put the cards in during a pretend mailbox activity).

INTERVENTION FOR INCONSISTENT SPEECH DISORDER

There is currently only one intervention approach specifically designed to target lexical inconsistency: core vocabulary intervention (Dodd et al., 2010). This approach is designed to help these children with phonological planning.

■ Core vocabulary: Intervention for inconsistent speech disorder

Core vocabulary intervention is for children with inconsistent speech disorder—children who have lexical inconsistency and tend to say the same word in different ways.

Historical background

Core vocabulary was developed by Barbara Dodd and colleagues during the late 1980s and 1990s (e.g., Dodd & Iacano, 1989; Bradford & Dodd, 1997; Bradford-Heit & Dodd, 1998). It was developed in response to a need for an intervention for a child with inconsistent productions of the same lexical item (Dodd & Iacano, 1989). The child was a participant in an 8-month phonological intervention study involving seven children. Six of the seven children showed an improvement in their speech. The child who did not improve needed another approach. He needed to learn to produce the same word in the same way each time he said it. Given 2 months of weekly intervention targeting consistent (although not necessarily accurate) production of a group of highly functional words, he showed generalization of consistency in his phonological system (Dodd et al., 2010). The words used in intervention were highly functional and relevant to the child, hence the name core vocabulary intervention.

Theoretical background

Core vocabulary is based on a theoretical understanding that "children whose speech is characterized by inconsistent errors may have difficulty selecting and sequencing phonemes (i.e., in assembling a phonological template or plan for production of an utterance)" (Dodd et al., 2010, p. 122). This idea has been supported through research examining children's responses to different types of interventions. For instance, when children with inconsistent speech disorder received phonological contrast intervention, they made little progress (Crosbie, Holm, & Dodd, 2005; Dodd & Bradford, 2000). When they were given PROMPT intervention (targeting articulatory gestures), they also made little progress (Dodd & Bradford, 2000). However, when they were given core vocabulary intervention targeting lexical consistency, their speech intelligibility improved (e.g., Crosbie et al., 2005; Holm, Crosbie, & Dodd, 2013; McIntosh & Dodd, 2008).

Procedure

Core vocabulary differs from other approaches to intervention because it targets lexical consistency. The types of words selected and the way in which they are taught and then practiced is what makes this approach unique. An overview of the core vocabulary approach as described by Dodd et al. (2010) and Holm et al. (2013) follows.

Selection of a core vocabulary

Core vocabulary intervention begins with parents/caregivers, the child, and the child's teacher generating a list of 50 to 70 functionally powerful words relevant to a child that the child has the opportunity to produce in day-to-day interactions (Holm et al., 2013). The words are selected based on their relevance rather than their phonological content. The words can include names (people and pets), places, functional words (e.g., *please, thank you, sorry*), foods, and favorite things (Dodd et al., 2010). At least 50 words are selected and practiced over a period of time, due to evidence suggesting that lexical consistency only generalizes once around 50 words have been targeted (Holm et al., 2013). Appendix 13-1 provides a list of core vocabulary words in Cantonese, Appendix 13-2 provides a list of core vocabulary words in Vietnamese, and Appendix 13-3 provides a list of core vocabulary words in Spanish that may be a starting point when discussing functional words with multilingual families.

Once you have the list of words, you (and/or the child's family) will need to generate pictures of the target words, with the name written beneath each picture. You will also need a box or bag for storing and selecting words for practice from session to session. The number of words practiced in a session can vary from a few up to as many as 10 (Holm et al., 2013).

Service delivery for core vocabulary

It is recommended that core vocabulary intervention be scheduled in twice weekly in 30-minute individual sessions, with home practice between sessions, for a total intervention duration of approximately 6 to 8 weeks (Dodd et al., 2010). During the first session in a week, the child's best production of a selected subset of words is established. During the second session for the week, the child engages in massed practice of those words, with feedback focusing on consistency rather than accuracy (Holm et al., 2013). Although SLPs are recommended to be the primary agents of intervention, parents and teachers have an important role to play. They need to monitor the child's speech and encourage the child to use his or her best production in the home and school environments (Holm et al., 2013).

Establish best production

A child's best production of a word (during the first of the two sessions in a week) is achieved through the use of multiple production cues as necessary, including an auditory model for immediate or delayed imitation, visual-phonetic cues, verbal-phonetic cues, manual guidance, prosodic cues, successive approximation/shaping, orthographic cues, metaphor, metaphonological information (e.g., information about phonological properties of sounds such as a fricative being a long sound), and phonological awareness instruction (e.g., information about the syllables and phonemes that comprise words and how syllables and phonemes can be segmented and/or blended to form spoken words). Of these cues, the dialogue during the antecedent event focuses primarily on the child's phonological awareness, to help the child learn how to phonologically plan words. For example:

> to teach *Joseph*, the clinician would explain that Joseph has two syllables—[ʤoʊ] and [sɛf]. The first syllable [ʤoʊ] has two sounds—/ʤ/ and /oʊ/—and the second syllable [sɛf] has three sounds—/s/, /ɛ/ and /f/. The child attempts the first syllable—[ʤoʊ]—receives feedback and makes further attempts after being given models and receiving feedback about each attempt. When the child's best production of the first syllable has been established, the second—[sɛf]—is targeted, and then the two syllables are combined—[ʤoʊ-sɛf]. (Holm et al., 2013, pp. 191–192)

If it proves difficult to establish an accurate production, then a child's best production may include an acceptable developmental error (Holm et al., 2013), given that the main focus of this intervention is on consistency, not necessarily accuracy. In such instances, accuracy can be targeted using another suitable intervention approach following a discrete period of core vocabulary intervention.

Practicing consistent production

Once you have established the child's best production of the 10 words to be practiced for the week, the second session focuses on massed practice. The aim of this session is for the child to learn how to phonologically plan production of the target words. The child needs to learn to say the word the same way each time it is said (Dodd et al., 2010). While some of the cues used during the first session can be used during the second session (e.g., metaphor, phonological awareness instruction), opportunities to imitate should be kept to a minimum. This is because an auditory model is thought to provide a child with a phonological plan (Holm et al., 2013). This is akin to giving a child an answer to a question that you asked the child to figure out. The child needs to learn how to phonologically plan and retrieve words in a consistent way. The amount of practice completed during motivating activities or games during the session needs to be quite high, such as 150 to 170 responses in 30 minutes (Dodd et al., 2010). Towards the end of the second session, the target words are tested by examining their consistency across three repetitions. Any words produced consistently are subsequently removed from the list, while any inconsistent words are retained on the list for further intervention.

Monitoring and generalization

A response generalization probe evaluating production consistency is examined once a fortnight, using a set of 10 untreated words (Dodd et al., 2010). Once the untreated words become consistent, Dodd et al. (2010) recommend that the Inconsistency subtest of the Diagnostic Evaluation of Articulation and Phonology (DEAP) (Dodd, Hua, et al., 2002, 2006) is administered to confirm whether generalization (in the form of lexical consistency) has occurred.

Evidence

Core vocabulary intervention has been examined in intervention research by Dodd and colleagues in a randomized controlled trial (Broomfield and Dodd, 2011), a between-group study (Crosbie, Holm, & Dodd, 2005), single-case experimental studies (e.g., Dodd & Bradford, 2000), and case studies (e.g., Crosbie, Pine, Holm, & Dodd, 2006; Holm & Dodd, 1999; McIntosh & Dodd, 2008). The case study by Holm and Dodd (1999) reported cross-linguistic generalization from English to Punjabi in a bilingual Punjabi–English-speaking boy (4;6 years) whose speech was inconsistent in both languages (Holm & Dodd, 1999). Studies by other researchers are needed. Dodd (2014) notes that some children may need a period of contrastive phonological intervention (e.g., minimal pairs) once their speech is more consistent.

Children suited to core vocabulary intervention

Core vocabulary intervention is suitable for children with inconsistent speech disorder—children who show at least 40% variability on a single-word sample (Dodd et al., 2010). Inconsistent errors are characterized by different versions of the same lexical item. For further information, refer back to Chapters 7, 8, and 9 on assessment, analysis, and differential diagnosis.

Resources for conducting core vocabulary

Dodd, Crosbie, and Holm developed a resource for implementing core vocabulary—the Core Vocabulary Therapy CD available from Grow Words. You can implement the approach without the CD. You would need to source pictures relevant to a child's core vocabulary word list and materials such as a bag for storing and selecting the picture, record forms, a generalization word list with corresponding pictures, and motivating drill-play toys and games.

APPLICATION: *Intervention approaches suitable for Jarrod*

Jarrod (7;0) has inconsistent speech disorder (Chapter 16). What intervention approach might be suitable for Jarrod?

Read more about
Jarrod (7;0 years),
a boy with inconsistent
speech disorder,
in Chapter 16 (Case 3).

Answer: You could start with a period of core vocabulary intervention (Dodd et al., 2010). Once generalization data indicate that Jarrod's speech is consistent, you would select a suitable phonological intervention approach to address any remaining error patterns in his speech. Crosbie et al. (2006) report on Jarrod's progress given one block of core vocabulary intervention.

BRIEF OVERVIEW OF OTHER APPROACHES FOR MANAGING PHONOLOGICAL IMPAIRMENT IN CHILDREN

In this chapter we have reviewed a range of different intervention approaches, with varying levels of empirical support, for children who have a phonological impairment or inconsistent speech disorder. The range we have presented in this text is not exhaustive. In a narrative review of 134 intervention studies designed to address phonological impairment in children, Baker and McLeod (2011a) identified 46 different approaches. This number halved when approaches were limited to those that had more than one research paper providing evidence for the approach (*n* = 23). As a beginning SLP, it is important that you are familiar with a range of approaches. In this chapter we have reviewed approaches that would address the needs of the majority of children with phonological impairment on your caseloads. As you gain experience and knowledge, you are encouraged to add more breadth and depth to your intervention knowledge base. Other approaches you might like to learn about include:

- **Naturalistic intervention for speech intelligibility and speech accuracy**, developed by Stephen Camarata for children with severe SSD who do not respond readily to imitation and drill-based approaches to intervention (Camarata, 2010) in addition to children who have more complex communication needs, such as autism or Down syndrome. The primary goal of this approach is to improve children's speech intelligibility in naturalistic, child-directed, play-based contexts in which children's verbal initiations are followed by conversational recasts comprising words with the target speech sound(s). Suggested reading: Camarata (2010).

- **Constraint-based nonlinear phonology intervention**, developed by May Bernhardt and Joe Stemberger (2000). Unlike some other approaches to phonological intervention, nonlinear intervention is not a series of predetermined phases and stages with criteria for progression. Rather, nonlinear intervention could be described as a series of theoretically motivated techniques for addressing carefully identified goals targeting the segmental and prosodic tiers. Often these techniques rely on using the strengths of one tier to support the development of another tier. For instance, building new structures using established structures and segments (e.g., building the disyllable word *window* from *win-dough*), transferring codas in a rhyme to an onset (e.g., repeating [ɪk ɪk ɪk ɪk ɪk] to create *kick* /kɪk/) or establishing lab-cor sequences for a child limited to cor-cor sequences using rebuses or pictures representing each syllable (e.g., adding *baa, ma,* or *bee* to the word *knee* /ni/ to create *bunny, money,* and *beanie*) (Bernhardt, 1994). Suggested readings: Bernhardt (1994) and Bernhardt and Stemberger (2000).[2]

- **Psycholinguistic approach for managing SSD in children**, developed by Joy Stackhouse and Bill Wells (1997). This approach uses psycholinguistic principles to guide SLPs' assessment, goal identification, and intervention with children who have SSD and/or literacy difficulties. Like constraint-based nonlinear phonology, it is not a specific intervention approach per se, but a collection of ideas and strategies that could be used with children who have SSD. Suggested readings: Stackhouse and Wells (1997, 2001), Pascoe, Stackhouse, and Wells (2006), and Stackhouse, Vance, Pascoe, and Wells (2007).

---

[2]See also phonodevelopment.sites.olt.ubc.ca.

- **Dynamic systems and whole-language intervention**, developed by Paul Hoffman and Janet Norris (2010). This approach was designed to be used during interactive storybook reading with preschoolers who have concomitant speech and language (syntactic and/or morphological and/or semantic) difficulties. The approach is based on the premise that phonology is part of the linguistic system, and that as a linguistic difficulty it can be remediated through sequences of communication failure and repair rather than drill-type activities. The approach is considered to be more of a philosophy about learning rather than a prescriptive approach (Hoffman, Norris, & Monjure, 1990). Suggested reading: Hoffman and Norris (2010).
- **Mnemonic method for teaching disyllabic and polysyllabic words**, developed by Edna Carter Young (1987, 1995). This approach applies the concept of mnemonics to syllable-based speech production problems. A mnemonic is simply a memory stimulator that prompts learning (Young, 1995). The approach begins with stress equalization of syllables, and the replacement of syllables with sound-referenced rebuses that serve as visual guides to aid in production. Using the word *mosquito*, you could have three pictures: *moss, key, toe*. Together, the individual words make the word *mosquito*. As children learn to articulate each syllable, they are encouraged to produce the words with fewer prompts and models, and increasing speech naturalness. This approach would not be suitable for children with CAS, as they are likely to have stress equalization of syllables. Suggested reading: Young (1995).
- **Phonotactic therapy**, as described by Shelley Velleman (2002). Velleman describes a series of theoretically motivated therapy techniques designed to help children develop specific phonotactic structures, such as final consonants, consonant clusters, and weak syllables. For instance, Velleman (2002) suggests that to help children with word-initial weak syllable deletion (e.g., *potato* /pəteto/ → [teto]), it can be helpful to begin at phrase level. Specifically, embed two- and three-syllable iambic words (i.e., words starting with weak stress) in a two-word phrase so that words with iambic stress are second (e.g., big potato). The stress pattern of the phrase (e.g., SwSs) provides a scaffolding structure for the child to learn the stress pattern of the word (e.g., wSs). This would be a helpful strategy for children with CAS to learn how to produce polysyllables with natural stress. Suggested reading: Velleman (2002).

ALIGNING PHONOLOGICAL TARGET SELECTION APPROACHES WITH PHONOLOGICAL INTERVENTION APPROACHES

The task of selecting intervention approaches for children with phonological impairment can seem daunting, given the range of empirically supported choice in the literature. As we discuss in more detail in Chapter 15, evidence-based decisions for children with SSD are made by integrating research findings with internal evidence from clinical practice and client factors, values, and preferences (Baker & McLeod, 2011b). While you do have choices (and therefore decisions to be made), the phonological intervention approach you select will, in part, be influenced by the findings from your assessment and in particular the goals you identify from your phonological analysis of a child's speech sample. Figure 13-2 shows which target selection approaches align with the various intervention approaches addressed in this chapter. You will notice on Figure 13-2

APPLICATION: *Which phonological intervention approach(es) would you select for Luke?*

Read more about Luke (4;3 years), a boy with a phonological impairment, in Chapter 16 (Case 1).

Consider the case study of Luke in Chapter 16. Using the results of your analysis of Luke's speech sample from Chapter 9 and the goals you identified for him from Chapter 10, which phonological intervention approach(es) might be suitable for Luke? Which phonological intervention approach would you select, and why? Discuss your answers with a peer.

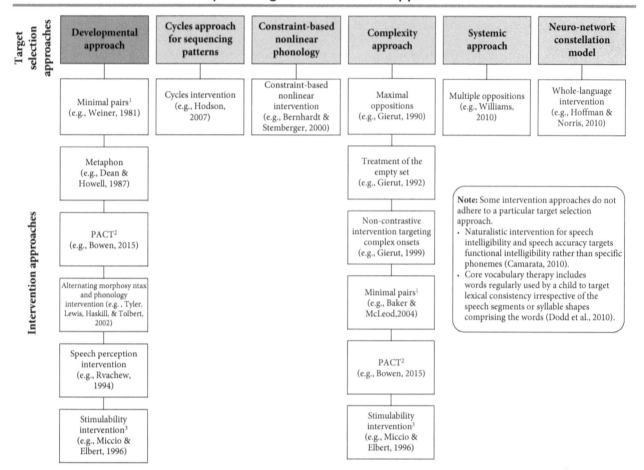

FIGURE 13-2 Recommendations for aligning target selection approaches (shaded boxes) with selected phonological intervention approaches.

[1]Minimal pairs intervention has been studied with developmental targets (e.g., Weiner, 1981) and complex targets (e.g., Baker & McLeod, 2004; Miccio & Ingrisano, 2000). [2]PACT intervention has a flexible approach to target selection, either developmental and/or complex targets (e.g., Bowen, 2015). [3]Stimulability intervention includes both developmental and complex targets (Miccio & Williams, 2010).

that some intervention approaches have a flexible approach to target selection. For example, minimal pairs and PACT intervention can be used with developmental or complexity targets. Stimulability intervention uses both development and complex targets, as all consonants (stimulable and non-stimulable) are selected. Other interventions have a prescribed approach to target selection. For example, Williams' (2000a, b) multiple oppositions approach aligns with the systemic approach to target selection, and Hodson's (2007) cycles approach aligns with Hodson's (2007) sequence of primary, secondary, and advanced phonological patterns.

PHONOLOGICAL INTERVENTION FOR CHILDREN WHO ARE LATE TALKERS

Children who are late to talk pose an interesting challenge for SLPs. Late talkers typically have smaller expressive vocabularies of no more than 50 words and no word combinations by the age of 2 years or are not performing within the normal range on standardized test (Stokes & Klee, 2009). Children who are late to talk can also have limited phonetic inventories, PCC lower than expected, atypical error patterns, greater speech sound variability, and a slow rate of resolution of their reduced speech intelligibility (Williams & Elbert, 2003). The dilemma for SLPs is how to best address their speech and language needs. For example, late-talking toddlers not only need to expand their expressive vocabulary and use two-word utterances, but also to increase their repertoire of consonant sounds and syllable shapes in order to improve their speech intelligibility. While there is much evidence about strategies for facilitating language acquisition in late-talking toddlers (e.g., Girolametto, Pearse, & Weitzman, 1997), there is relatively little robust experimental evidence on intervention approaches suitable for targeting the emerging phonological abilities of infants showing signs of the late onset of canonical babbling, and toddlers who are late to talk. Therefore, this section outlines potential goals for infants and toddlers, and evidence-based strategies (as opposed to descriptions of evidence-based intervention approaches) that might facilitate their phonological and lexical acquisition.

■ Goals and intervention strategies to use with infants and toddlers at risk of or showing early signs of SSD

According to Stoel-Gammon (2011), phonological and lexical acquisition interact in a bidirectional manner. Caregiver input and responsiveness also have an important role to play in facilitating children's early speech and language acquisition. Intervention therefore needs to target all three issues: phonological acquisition, word learning, and caregiver input. Table 13-3 outlines a series of goals that may be suitable for infants and toddlers who are at risk of or showing early signs of SSD. Table 13-4 provides a series of evidence-based suggestions designed to justify and address the goals in Table 13-3. The suggestions are based not on direct evidence from an established intervention approach, but rather evidence about factors known to influence infant and toddlers' phonological and lexical learning. Read Stoel-Gammon (2011) for a helpful review of this literature. For late-talking toddlers who are not readily imitating, DeThorne, Johnson, Walder, and Mahurin-Smith (2009) offer six evidence-based suggestions for facilitating early speech development:

1. Provide a child with access to augmentative and alternative communication (AAC).
2. Minimize pressure on the child to speak.
3. Imitate the child, and in doing so model the skill of imitation to the child.
4. Use a slower tempo and exaggerated intonation when talking with the child.
5. Augment auditory, visual, tactile, and proprioceptive feedback to enhance the child's sensory experience when attempting to speak.
6. Avoid emphasis on non-speech-like movements of the articulators and focus on function.

For late-talking toddlers approaching their third birthday (who are talking in short yet unintelligible sentences due to a limited phonetic inventory and limited speech sound stimulability), Miccio and Elbert's (1996) stimulability approach would be a suitable intervention option. As the child's phonetic repertoire expands and the type of SSD is more readily apparent, then another intervention approach would be selected.

TABLE 13-3 Goals for infants and toddlers at risk of or showing early signs of SSD	
Goals for infants at risk of SSD due to delayed onset of canonical babbling[a]	**Goals for late-talking toddlers showing early characteristics of SSD**[a,b]
Increase the amount of vocalization.	Expand the consonant inventory.
Increase the quality of vocalizations—specifically, canonical babbling characterized by varied vowel-like and consonant-like vocalizations in CV syllable strings.	Expand the syllable-shape inventory.
	Increase vocabulary size, including words from a variety of grammatical classes.
Develop the ability to imitate, initially in non-speech (e.g., imitating raspberries) and then speech contexts (e.g., imitating vowel- and consonant-like sounds) during vocal play.	Encourage the development of two-word utterances as the expressive vocabulary increases.
Encourage caregiver responsiveness.	Encourage caregiver responsiveness.

[a]Adapted from Stoel-Gammon (2011). [b]Adapted from Bauman-Waengler (2014).

TABLE 13-4 Evidence-based strategies for facilitating the emergence of babbling in infants and first words in late-talking toddlers

Evidence-based statement*	Clinical implication	Example
1. The sounds in an infant's babble underlie the speech sounds evident in a child's first words (e.g., Bernhardt & Stoel-Gammon, 1996; Stoel-Gammon, 2011; Stoel-Gammon & Cooper, 1984).	Encourage first words containing sounds in an infant's babbling repertoire.	The infant uses /b/ in babbling, therefore target /b/ initial in CV and CVCV words, such as *boo, bee, baby*.
2. Babbling creates opportunities for motor practice of the spoken form of early words and the creation of an auditory-articulatory loop (Stoel-Gammon, 2011).	Facilitate babbling in infants at risk for SSD (e.g., infants with Down syndrome) in terms of: ■ *quantity* (i.e., the amount of babbling an infant engages in), and ■ *quality* (i.e., varied babbling with respect to consonant and vowel-like sounds, and variety in canonical sequences).	Engage in vocal play following each diaper change, each day.
3. Adult–child vocal interactions can influence infant babble and help early lexical development, specifically: ■ adult imitation of infants' CV babble (as opposed to infant vowel-like vocalizations) has been associated with increased production of CV babble; ■ greater caregiver responsiveness to infant's vocalization (in the form of imitation and expansion of an infant's babble) has been associated with lexical development (Stoel-Gammon, 2011).	Encourage caregivers to be responsive to the infant's babbling so that they imitate and expand upon their infant's babble.	An infant vocalizes [ba]. In response, the caregiver makes eye contact with the infant and says [bababa]. Subsequent conversational exchanges would involve the adult modelling expanded babbling sequences with respect to length and variety of consonants and vowels (e.g., [ba ma ba ma], [ba bu ba bu]).
4. Toddlers can have selection-avoidance strategies whereby new words are more likely to be acquired if those words contain the toddler's IN sounds (i.e., specific sounds or sound classes already used in words or babble) (e.g., Schwartz & Leonard, 1982). Toddlers can also have whole-word strategies for learning words, such that words might be learned if they have a whole-word pattern common to the toddler's known or IN words (e.g., Leonard & McGregor, 1991; Stoel-Gammon, 2011)	As part of a comprehensive assessment of toddlers' emerging language, it would be important to analyze the phonological characteristics of toddlers' words to determine whether toddlers have individualized selection-avoidance strategies with respect to speech sounds and/or whole-word patterns to acquire new words. Having identified toddlers' strategies, encourage the acquisition of new words containing the phonological characteristics of known words.	A toddler may have three words containing /m/, *more* [mɔ], *milk* [mɪ], and *mom* [ma], and two words containing /b/, *ball* [bɔ] and *bye* [baɪ]. New words to be included in a language stimulation session could include words containing /b/ and /m/, in simple syllable shapes CV and CVCV, such as: *me, moo, bee, baby*.
5. A toddler's productions of words beyond the 50-word period tend to consist of CVCV and CVC syllable shapes; disyllables tend to have strong stress on the first syllable; and words often begin with stops, particularly /b/ (e.g., Stoel-Gammon & Peter, 2008).	Consider the phonological characteristics of words to be included in an intervention program targeting the expansion of a toddler's lexicon. Select words characterized by CVCV, CV, and CVC syllable shapes, words beginning with stops (e.g., /b/), and disyllabic words beginning with a stressed onset (e.g., *baby*) rather than weak onsets (e.g., *guitar*).	A late-talking toddler has an expressive vocabulary of approximately 50 words. New words to be introduced into the child's lexicon could have CV, CVCV, and CVC syllables and begin with stops, particularly /b/ (e.g., *bee, bunny, bang!*). Disyllables would have strong stress on the first syllable.

*Adapted from Stoel-Gammon (2011).

PHONOLOGICAL INTERVENTION FOR MULTILINGUAL CHILDREN

It has been suggested that the majority of children in the world speak more than one language (Tucker, 1998). Recall from Chapters 7 through 9 that your comprehensive assessment and analysis needs to determine whether a child's reduced speech intelligibility is due to SSD or cross-linguistic transfer during **multilingual** speech acquisition. If you establish that SSD exists, you need to provide intervention in accordance with individual children's needs. Do you work with a multilingual child in the same way as you would a **monolingual** child? According to Gildersleeve-Neumann and Goldstein (2012), the answer is both yes and no. Yes, because the intervention approaches you would use with a monolingual child are equally suitable for a multilingual child. Table 13-5 provides an overview of languages other than English in which various phonological intervention approaches have been reported to be used. However, the answer regarding whether you

TABLE 13-5 **Languages other than English in which phonological intervention approaches have been reported to be used**

Approach	Languages in which the approach has been used by SLPs
Minimal pairs	Finnish (Kunnari & Savinainen-Makkonen, 2007), German (Fox, 2007), Greek (Mennen & Okalidou, 2007), Israeli Hebrew (Ben-David & Berman, 2007), Japanese (Ota & Ueda, 2007), Korean (Kim & Pae, 2007), Maltese (Grech, 2007), Turkish (Topbaş, 2007)
Complexity-based approaches (maximal oppositions, treatment of the empty set, intervention targeting complex onsets)	Brazilian Portuguese (Donicht, Pagliarin, Mota, & Keske-Soares, 2011; Mota et al., 2007; Yavaş & Mota, 2007), Turkish (Topbaş and Ünal, 2010)
Multiple oppositions	Brazilian Portuguese (Mota et al., 2007; Pagliarin et al., 2009; Ceron & Keske-Soares, 2012)
Cycles	Jordanian Arabic (Dyson & Amayreh, 2007), Cantonese (So, 2007), Dutch (Mennen, Levelt, & Gerrits, 2007), German (Fox, 2007), Korean (Kim & Pae, 2007), Spanish (Goldstein, 2007)
Metaphonological approaches (including Metaphon)	Dutch (Mennen, Levelt, & Gerrits, 2007), German (Fox, 2007), Korean (Kim & Pae, 2007), Norwegian (Kristoffersen, 2007), Brazilian Portuguese (Yavaş & Mota, 2007), Turkish (Topbaş, 2007), Welsh (Munro, Ball, & Müller, 2007)
Integrated phonological awareness intervention	Portuguese (Lousada et al., 2013; Lousada, Jesus, Hall, & Joffe, 2014)
PACT intervention	Afrikaans, Bahasa Melayu, Cantonese, Egyptian Arabic, French, Portuguese, Spanish, and Tamil (Bowen, 2010)
Stimulability intervention	–
Speech perception intervention	A version of SAILS is being developed for French and American Spanish (Rvachew & Brosseau-Lapré, 2010)
Core vocabulary	Cantonese (So, 2007), Greek (Mennen & Okalidou, 2007), Punjabi-English (Holm & Dodd, 1999)
Morphosyntax intervention	–
Constraint-based nonlinear phonological intervention	Cantonese (So, 2007), German (Ullrich, Stemberger, & Bernhardt, 2008), Kuwaiti Arabic (Ayyad & Bernhardt, 2007)
Auditory discrimination	Cantonese (So, 2007), Welsh (Munro, Ball, & Müller, 2007)
Psycholinguistic approaches	French (Rose & Wauquier-Gravelines, 2007), German (Fox, 2007), Turkish (Topbaş, 2007)
Phonological Intervention Approach to Articulation Disorders	Israeli Hebrew (Ben-David & Berman, 2007)
Other phonological intervention (unspecified)	Hungarian (Zadjó, 2007), Spanish (Goldstein, 2007), Thai (Lorwatanapongsa & Maroonroge, 2007), Turkish (Topbaş, 2007)

work with a multilingual child with SSD in the same way as you would a monolingual child is also no, because you need to consider which language(s) should be the target of intervention, whether the approach is suitable for all languages (e.g., Icelandic has few minimal pairs), what are the most appropriate goals of intervention, in what order should both languages be treated (if both are to be treated), and who will provide the intervention.

SLPs tend to provide intervention to multilingual children in the language spoken by the SLP rather than the languages spoken by the child (Gildersleeve-Neumann & Goldstein, 2012; Jordaan, 2008; Williams & McLeod, 2012). Is this OK? Let's take a look at what the evidence suggests. Researchers suggest that instruction in the child's first language (i.e., language learned at home) helps (and does not hinder) the acquisition of English (Gildersleeve-Neumann & Goldstein, 2012; Kohnert, 2013). The research on intervention for multilingual children with phonological impairment is limited. Essentially, the evidence is confined to a small number of peer-reviewed published pre-post case studies in which English-speaking SLPs have provided intervention in English to bilingual or multilingual children. The question of interest across the peer-reviewed published research has been whether intervention in English facilitates generalized phonological improvement across the languages spoken by the child. The findings have been mixed. Ray (2002) reported using the minimal pair approach in English with a child learning to speak English, Hindi, and Gujarati and noted cross-linguistic generalization from English to the other two languages over a period of 40 intervention sessions. Holm, Dodd, and Ozanne (1997) reported using the minimal pairs approach and traditional articulation intervention in English with a Cantonese–English-speaking boy of 5;2 years who had phonological and articulatory errors in both English and Cantonese. Articulation therapy targeted his distorted [s], with generalized improvement noted across English and Cantonese. By contrast, generalized improvement was not seen in the child's phonological errors (cluster reduction[3] and gliding of /ɹ/ and /l/). Improvements were limited to English, which was the language targeted in intervention. In another study using a multiple baseline design across behaviors, Gildersleeve-Neumann and Goldstein (2015) reported that bilingual intervention for SSD (in English and Spanish) was associated with improvements in both languages.

Based on this small amount of evidence, there is a need to better understand when and how cross-language generalization does and does not occur, and whether it is necessary to provide intervention in one or more languages. Until that research is undertaken, it would seem that cross-generalization is possible for phonetic errors such as a lisp but perhaps not for phonological impairment. This makes sense, because children can exhibit different types of errors between the languages that they are learning. For example, in the case study by Holm et al. (1997), although the boy had cluster reduction in both languages, some processes were only evident in English (e.g., gliding, fronting, final consonant deletion, voicing, stopping of affricates, deaffrication), while others were only evident in Cantonese (e.g., consonant harmony, backing, affrication, nasalization, blending of two words). Interestingly, he had deaffrication in English and affrication in Cantonese. What, then, is the best way to help children with phonological impairment?

Gildersleeve-Neumann and Goldstein (2012) offer some helpful guidelines. You need to think about each child's individual goals and how to best to work on them in accordance with each child's needs and circumstances. Consider the case of Antonio, a Spanish–English-speaking boy who had SSD diagnosed at 2;3 years (Gildersleeve-Neumann & Goldstein, 2012). Antonio's parents spoke only Spanish with him, as did his younger sister and extended family. As a preschooler, Antonio was enrolled in a Spanish-only Head Start Program in the United States. Spanish was Antonio's main language before he started school. Antonio was exposed to English via his English-speaking SLP. When Antonio received SLP intervention in English as a preschooler, there was little or no improvement in his speech production skills. When intervention was provided in Spanish, improvements were noted. Once Antonio started school, the need for English proficiency became greater. Although Antonio's speech intelligibility had improved, intervention was still required to target later developing phonemes. Using a horizontal goal attack strategy, Antonio's school-based SLP provided intervention targeting /ɹ/ in English, while his local university clinic provided intervention in Spanish, targeting his production of the trill /r/. In summary, as Antonio's case illustrates, you need to consider the phonological characteristics of the languages a child is learning, the child's past and present language learning experiences, the findings from your phonological analysis of speech samples for each of

---

[3]Zee (1999) indicates Cantonese does not contain consonant clusters; instead /kw/ and /kwh/ are labialized consonants /kʷ/, /kwʰ/.

the languages being learned by a child, suitable goal attack strategies, your service delivery options, and, of course, the preferences of the child and his or her family. Plans need to be revised in accordance with each individual child's needs and circumstances. Table 13-6 provides an overview of each of these issues and recommendations to guide your intervention decisions with multilingual children who have SSD.

TABLE 13-6   Factors to consider when developing an intervention plan for a multilingual child who has SSD

Phonological characteristics of the languages the child is learning and recommended priorities for intervention targets	Child and family factors	Intervention approach
Investigate ■ Consonants, vowels, tones[a], syllable shapes, word lengths, and stress patterns shared by the child's languages ■ Consonants, vowels, tones[a], syllable shapes, word lengths, and stress patterns unique to each individual language ■ Common phonological processes shared by the child's languages ■ Common phonological processes unique to each individual language **Action (in order of priority)** ■ Prioritize error patterns and/or phonemes common to the child's languages with similar error rates. ■ Target error patterns and/or phonemes common to both languages but occurring with different frequencies and having different importance between the languages. ■ Target error patterns and/or phonemes that only exist in one language and/or are only in error in one language.	**Investigate** ■ When and how did the child learn the languages that he or she is learning? ■ Who is in the child's life, and what languages do they speak? ■ Who in the child's life is willing to be trained and assist with providing intervention? ■ What is the family's preference regarding the language of intervention? **Action** ■ Account for child and family factors with respect to service delivery and language of intervention, knowing that if one language is to be targeted rather than all the child's languages, then preference is given to the child's stronger, more dominant language. ■ Review clinical decisions as the child and family life and language circumstances change.	**Investigate** ■ Are the child's errors consistent or inconsistent? ■ Are the child's errors phonetic or phonological? ■ Does the child have speech perception plus production difficulties? ■ Does the child have morphosyntactic errors? **Action** ■ Core vocabulary if errors are inconsistent ■ Phonetic approach if errors are phonetic, and phonological approach if errors are phonological ■ Include speech perception training, if speech perception is problematic. ■ Target morphosyntax using an alternating or block strategy, if concomitant phonology and morphosyntax difficulties are present.

Source: Adapted from Gildersleeve-Neumann and Goldstein (2012).
[a]If appropriate for the language.

FIGURE 13-3   Transcription conversion chart for English-speaking SLPs' transcription of Cantonese. Shaded sections show matches between Cantonese and English-speaking SLPs' transcription

Word-initial consonants

Cantonese	p^h	p	t^h	t	k^h	k	k^{wh}	k^w	m	n	ŋ	f	s	h	ts^h	ts	j	w	l
English	p	b	t	d	k	g	kw	kw, gw	m	n	m, n	f	s	h	tʃ, t	dʒ, t	j	w	l

Word-final consonants

Cantonese	p	t	k		m	n	ŋ
English	p	t	omitted		m	n	ŋ, omitted

Source: Lockart & McLeod (2013), Figure 1, p. 529. Used by permission from American Speech-Language-Hearing Association (ASHA).

COMMENT: *What if I do not speak the language(s) spoken by children on my caseload?*

When selecting the language to work on with a multilingual child who has a phonological impairment, you need to think about (1) the child, (2) the child's community, (3) yourself, and (4) your workplace resources. It is important that you think about these four issues in that order. Consider the needs of the child first, then the resources available within the family and community, what skills you have, and finally the workplace resources you have available to meet the child's needs. This does not mean that you work on goals in English, when English is not a child's primary language, simply because English is the language that you are competent in. You need to think about the nature of the child's SSD; the child's past and present language learning experiences; the child's current language-learning support at home, preschool, or school; the languages spoken by the child's family members and friends; and how much time in a typical day a child spends conversing in the languages he or she is learning (Gildersleeve-Neumann & Goldstein, 2012; International Expert Panel on Multilingual Children's Speech, 2012; Peña-Brooks & Hegde, 2007). If you are not familiar with the child's language(s), then consider who you know who is, and learn about the child's language(s) and culture(s). Become equipped to work with the culturally and linguistically diverse families on your caseload. Consider the following ideas:

- Create a database of languages spoken by your colleagues, whether they be health or education professionals, SLP assistants, itinerant SLPs, SLP students, teaching assistants, administrative assistants, or trained volunteers.

- Find out who in a child's life speaks the child's languages, and consider who could be available and willing to receive training and supervision to provide appropriate intervention.

- Look for information created by SLPs in the countries that speak the languages of your clients (e.g., McLeod, 2007a; Multilingual Children's Speech website[1]).

- Look at the modules in the Training to Enhance Services for English Language Learners website.[2]

- Create a conversion chart between English and the other language (see Figure 13-3 and Lockart & McLeod, 2013).

- Have information and intervention resources about SSD in children translated into the languages spoken by the children and their families who live in your service area.

- Read the American Speech-Language-Hearing Association guidelines (2004b) regarding the knowledge and skills needed by SLPs to provide culturally and linguistically appropriate services.

- Consider the six Principles of Culturally Competent Practice (Verdon, 2015; Verdon, McLeod, & Wong, 2015): "(1) identification of culturally appropriate and mutually motivating therapy goals, (2) knowledge of languages and culture, (3) use of culturally appropriate resources, (4) consideration of the cultural, social and political context, (5) consultation with families and communities, and (6) collaboration between professionals" (Verdon et al., 2015, p. 74).

The ASHA (2004b) guidelines state that SLPs have an ethical obligation to "continue in lifelong learning to develop those knowledge and skills required to provide culturally and linguistically appropriate services" (p. 2). Chabon (cited in Gildersleeve-Neumann & Goldstein, 2012) takes this further by suggesting that if you accept employment with a service in which many of the children and their families on your caseload have a shared linguistic background dissimilar to yours, then you have an ethical obligation to at least learn the language well enough to communicate with these children and their families.

[1]http://www.csu.edu.au/research/multilingual-speech
[2]http://www.tesell.org/

ADDRESSING THE RISK OF LITERACY DIFFICULTIES IN PRESCHOOLERS WITH PHONOLOGICAL IMPAIRMENT

Young children with phonological impairment are at risk of future literacy difficulties. We know this because 30% to 77% of children with SSDs struggle with reading (Anthony et al., 2011). Can this risk of literacy difficulties be addressed? Research by Gillon (2005) and Kirk and Gillon (2007) suggests so. The key seems to lie in the provision of an emergent literacy program that helps children develop an awareness of the sound structure of words and the ability to manipulate that structure (i.e., phonological awareness) and letter knowledge (name and sound) during the years before children start school.

The aim of emergent literacy intervention is not to treat a presenting problem but to avert a problem from emerging (Justice, 2006). In contrast to many of the intervention approaches described in this chapter, emergent literacy intervention is a **primary prevention approach** rather than **secondary** or **tertiary intervention**. In this section we describe how you can target young children's emergent literacy alongside or while working on their speech intelligibility.

Gillon (2005) reported a study in which 12 preschool children (3;0–3;11 years) with a moderate or severe phonological impairment received regular phonological intervention—in the form of Hodson and Paden's (1991) cycles approach—in conjunction with activities targeting **phonemic awareness** and **letter-sound knowledge**. Gillon's (2005) **phoneme awareness** tasks included:

- phoneme detection (e.g., "Does *dog* start with the /s/ sound?" "No!" "Let's go on a treasure hunt and find a word that starts with the /s/ sound.");
- phoneme categorization (e.g., "Let's find all the toys in the box that start with the /s/ sound.");
- initial phoneme matching (e.g., "*Sun* starts with /s/. Let's find more pictures that start with /s/. Which one of these two starts with /s/, *sea* or *ball*?");
- phoneme isolation (e.g., "What sound does *sun* start with?"); and
- segmentation and blending at the level of onset-rime (e.g., "*s-un*") and the level of the phoneme (e.g., "*s-u-n*") of common CVC words, as children approach school age.

Letter-sound knowledge activities involved simple recognition tasks, whereby the children were made aware of the relationship between phonemes and graphemes in word-initial position. In Gillon's (2005) study, phoneme awareness and letter knowledge activities were interspersed in the activities targeting the children's speech intelligibility.

Intervention was conducted twice weekly in the form of one individual session and one small group session. Each session was 45 minutes in duration. On average, the children received 25.5 sessions (range 16 to 34) (Gillon, 2005). The children's speech, phonological awareness, and early literacy skills were monitored over a 3-year period. Gillon compared the children's speech, phonological awareness, and early literacy performance with a retrospective matched control group who received similar phonological intervention (either cycles or Metaphon) but no activities explicitly targeting phonemic awareness or letter-sound knowledge. Gillon reported that the children in the experimental group performed similarly to the retrospective control group on measures of speech production and letter-sound knowledge. However, the experimental group performed significantly better than the controls on a combined measure of phonological awareness in addition to word recognition, nonword reading, and spelling. Gillon (2005) noted that

> Despite a history of moderate or severe speech impairment and a known risk factor of commencing literacy instruction with persistent speech impairment, the children in the experimental group demonstrated average or well above average reading performance in their first or second year at school. (p. 322)

Follow-up assessment of these children's literacy, morphological awareness, and spelling skills during the school years (age 7;6–9;5 years) found that the children who received phonological intervention in addition to emergent literacy intervention (focusing on phoneme awareness and letter-sound knowledge) were continuing to do well (Kirk & Gillon, 2007). The findings from Gillon's research are encouraging, because the results suggest that preschoolers' risk of literacy difficulties might be reduced given the right kind of intervention at an early age.

■ Resources for emergent literacy intervention with children with phonological impairment

According to Cabell, Justice, Kaderavek, Pence Turnbull, and Breit-Smith (2009), emergent literacy programs target those skills identified as strong predictors of later reading and spelling achievement, which typically include:

- phonological awareness (particularly at a phonemic level);
- print awareness (including print conventions, function, and form);
- alphabet knowledge (including knowledge of letter shapes, names, and sounds);
- emergent writing; and
- oral language (inferential language and vocabulary).

There are many commercially available resources, journal articles, books, and websites that describe how you could target one or more of the above emergent literacy skills (e.g., Cabell et al., 2009). The resources used to conduct the emergent literacy intervention in Gillon's (2005) research are available at Gail Gillon's website at the University of Canterbury, New Zealand. Whatever program or resource you use, it is important to remember that the results from Gillon's (2005) research were based on an emergent literacy program that specifically targeted alphabet knowledge in the form of letter-sound knowledge activities and phonological awareness at the phonemic level via play-based activities for children in New Zealand. It is also important to remember that the long-term benefit of such a program on children's literacy skills during the teenage and early adult years remains to be established. Given the early signs of the benefits of such intervention, however, phonemic awareness and letter knowledge activities would seem to be a valuable adjunct to a comprehensive intervention plan designed to improve preschool children's speech intelligibility. Further information about this approach and accompanying evidence for children with CAS is provided in Chapter 14.

Chapter summary

In this chapter you learned about approaches for managing phonological impairment in children, such as minimal pairs, maximal oppositions, treatment of the empty set, multiple oppositions, Metaphon, cycles, PACT intervention, intervention targeting complex onsets, speech perception intervention, morphosyntax intervention, and stimulability intervention. You also learned about core vocabulary—an intervention suited to children with inconsistent speech disorder. You learned about strategies for working with infants and toddlers, multilingual children, and methods for reducing children's risk of literacy difficulties.

As a beginning SLP armed with knowledge about intervention approaches, your job is to learn how to put the approaches into practice. As your practical skills develop, remember that peer-reviewed published intervention research evidence is like an ever-expanding universe. There is no end point. Make a concerted effort to keep up to date with the evidence associated with each intervention approach so that your application is in keeping with the latest evidence-based recommendations.

Suggested reading

Phonological intervention approaches

■ Williams, A. L., McLeod, S., & McCauley, R. J. (Eds.). (2010). *Interventions for speech sound disorders in children*. Baltimore, MD: Paul H. Brookes.

Phonological and lexical learning in late talkers

■ Stoel-Gammon, C. (2011). Relationships between lexical and phonological development in young children. *Journal of Child Language, 38*(1), 1–34.

Phonological intervention with multilingual children

■ Gildersleeve-Neumann, C., & Goldstein, B. (2012). Intervention for multilingual children with speech sound disorder. In S. McLeod & B. Goldstein (Eds.), *Multilingual aspects of speech sound disorder in children* (pp. 214–227). Clevedon, UK: Multilingual Matters.

Emergent literacy intervention for children at risk of literacy difficulties

■ Gillon, G. T. (2005). Facilitating phoneme awareness development in 3- and 4-year-old children with speech impairment. *Language, Speech, and Hearing Services in Schools, 36*, 308–324.

Application of knowledge from Chapter 13

The ability to conduct phonological intervention requires knowledge, practice, feedback, and self-reflection. Apply and extend your knowledge about phonological intervention by completing one or more of the following tasks.

1. Prepare a parent-friendly handout summarizing the history, general procedure, and evidence base for one or more of the phonological intervention approaches described in this chapter.
2. Select two phonological intervention approaches: compare and contrast the approaches with respect to history, theoretical background, procedure (including cues that typify a teaching moment), and their evidence base.
3. With a partner, demonstrate a phonological intervention session to a small group of your peers—

they are the observers. Do not tell your observers what intervention approach you are demonstrating. Rather, ask your observers to figure out what approach you are using, through observing your teaching moment dialogue and stimuli.

4. Observe an expert clinician conduct a phonological intervention session.
5. Compile a resource folder (or box) with resources suitable for each intervention approach discussed in this chapter. For example, print and laminate the character cards for the stimulability approach (Miccio & Elbert, 1996); prepare stimulus words, picture cards, and activities for a minimal pairs session targeting velar fronting in word-initial position.

Appendix 13-1. Core Vocabulary Words That May Be Relevant for Working with Children Who Speak Cantonese

Here are some words commonly used by Cantonese-speaking children in Hong Kong that may be relevant to use in core vocabulary intervention.

Cantonese word	Transcription using the International Phonetic Alphabet	English translation
書	/sy$_1$/	book
包	/pau$_1$/	bread
飲	/jɐm$_2$/	drink
食	/sɪk$_6$/	eat
肚餓	/t^{h}ou$_5$ ɔ$_6$/	hungry
幫	/pɔŋ$_1$/	help
無	/mou$_5$/	none
買	/mai$_5$/	buy
聽	/t^{h}ɛŋ$_1$/	listen
廁所	/ts^{h}i$_3$ sɔ$_2$/	toilet
碗	/wun$_2$/	bowl
羹	/kɐŋ$_1$/	spoon
車	/ts^{h}ɛ$_1$/	car
水	/sɵy$_2$/	water
汁	/tsɐp$_1$/	juice
衫	/sam$_1$/	clothes
凍	/tʊŋ$_3$/	cold
痛	/t^{h}ʊŋ$_3$/	painful
開	/hɔi$_1$/	open
天	/t^{h}in$_1$/	sky
蛋	/tan$_2$/	egg
麵	/min$_6$/	noodle
飯	/fan$_6$/	rice
凳	/tɐŋ$_3$/	chair
紙巾	/tsi$_2$ kɐn$_1$/	tissue

Note: Lexical items and pronunciation may differ across dialects. The numbers within the transcription column correspond to the tone value. The list was created and transcribed by Dr. Carol Kit Sum To, University of Hong Kong, SAR China. Used with permission.

Appendix 13-2. Core Vocabulary Words That May Be Relevant for Working with Children Who Speak Vietnamese

Here are some words commonly used by Vietnamese-speaking children in Ho Chi Minh City (Saigon), Vietnam, that may be relevant to use in core vocabulary intervention.

Vietnamese word	Transcription using the International Phonetic Alphabet	English translation
bái bai	/bɑj⁵ bɑj¹/	bye bye
bạn	/ban⁶/	friend
bò	/bɔ²/	cow
bố mẹ	/bo⁵ mɛ⁶/	parents
bún bò	/bun⁵ bɔ²/	Hue beef noodle
cam	/kɑm¹/	orange
cảm ơn	/kɑm⁴ ɤn¹/	thank you
cặp	/kăp⁶ /	school bag
chân	/cɤ̆n¹/	leg
cháo	/cɑw⁵/	congee (food)
cho	/cɔ¹/	give
chó	/cɔ⁵/	dog
chơi	/cɤj¹/	play
cơm	/kɤm¹/	cooked rice
công viên	/koŋᵐ¹ vien¹/	park
đau	/dăw¹/	pain
dép	/zɛp⁵/	slipper
dưa hấu	/zɯɤ¹ hɤ̆w⁵ /	watermelon
gà	/ɣɑ² /	chicken
hổ	/ho⁴/	tiger
hỏi	/hɔj⁴/	ask
ipad	/ipɑt⁵/	iPad
kem	/kɛm¹/	ice cream
kẹo	/kɛw⁶/	candy
KFC	/kɑ¹ ɛp⁵ se¹/	KFC (fast food)
mắt	/măt⁵/	eye

mèo	/mɛw²/	cat
miệng	/mieŋ⁶ /	mouth
mũ bảo hiểm	/mu³ ɓɑw⁴ hiem⁴/	helmet
mũi	/muj³/	nose
ngồi bô	/ŋoj² ɓo¹/	potty
nho	/ɲɔ¹/	grapes
nóng	/nɔ̌ŋᵐ⁵/	hot
nước	/nɯɤk⁵/	water
phở	/fɤ⁴/	beef (chicken) noodle
quần áo	/kwɤ̌n² ɑw⁵/	clothes
sư tử	/ʂɯ¹ tɯ⁴/	lion
sữa	/ʂɯɤ³/	milk
tắm	/tăm⁵/	bathe
táo	/tɑw⁵/	apple
tay	/tăj1/	hand
trò chơi	/ʈɔ² cɤj¹/	game
uống	/uoŋ⁵ /	drink
xe máy	/sɛ¹ măj⁵/	bike
xin	/sin¹/	ask for
xin chào	/sin¹ cɑw²/	hello

Note: Lexical items and pronunciation may differ across dialects. The numbers within the transcription column correspond to the tone value. Students from Pham Ngoc Thach Medical University in Ho Chi Minh City, Vietnam, worked with Sharynne McLeod to generate words in Vietnamese that may be relevant to use for children who lived in their city. The word list was transcribed by Lê Thị Thanh Xuân, Ho Chi Minh City, Vietnam and Ben Phạm, Charles Sturt University, Australia and Ha Noi National University of Education, Vietnam using the Vietnamese transcription conventions described in Phạm and McLeod (2016). Used with permission.

Appendix 13-3. Core Vocabulary Words That May Be Relevant for Working with Children Who Speak Spanish

Here are some words commonly used by Spanish-speaking children in the United States that may be relevant to use in core vocabulary intervention.

Spanish word	Transcription using the International Phonetic Alphabet	English translation
yo	/jo/	me
mamá	/mama/	mommy
papá	/papa/	daddy
perro	/pero/	dog
casa	/kasa/	house
pelota	/peolota/	ball
juguete	/xugete/	toy
hambre	/ambre/	hunger
sed	/sed/	thirst
pañal	/paɲal/	diaper
nariz	/naɾis/	nose
ojo	/oxo/	eye
boca	/boka/	mouth
mano	/mano/	hand
peluche	/pelutʃe/	stuffed animal
jugo	/xugo/	juice
leche	/letʃe/	milk
pan	/pan/	bread
gato	/gato/	cat
osito	/osito/	teddy bear
parque	/paɾke/	park
afuera	/afuera/	outside
cama	/kama/	bed
manta	/manta/	blanket
comida	/komida/	food

Note: Lexical items and pronunciation may differ across dialects.
Source: This list was created by Dr. Leah Fabiano-Smith, University of Arizona, 2014, and transcribed by Dr. Brian Goldstein, La Salle University, 2015. Used with permission.

14

Articulatory and Motor Speech Intervention Approaches

KEY WORDS

Historical perspectives

Intervention for articulation impairment: traditional articulation intervention, concurrent treatment (articulation intervention based on principles of motor learning), articulation intervention using instrumental feedback (electropalatography, ultrasound, spectrography)

Intervention for childhood apraxia of speech (CAS): Dynamic Temporal and Tactile Cueing (DTTC), Rapid Syllable Transition Treatment (ReST), Prompts for Restructuring Oral Muscular Phonetic Targets (PROMPT), integrated phonological awareness intervention

Intervention for childhood dysarthria: systems approach

Augmentative and Alternative Communication (AAC)

LEARNING OBJECTIVES

1 Align the different types of motor speech difficulties and disorders (including articulation impairment, CAS, and childhood dysarthria) with suitable intervention approaches.

2 Describe, compare, and contrast traditional articulation intervention with concurrent treatment for articulation impairment.

3 Demonstrate teaching cues suitable for eliciting /s/ and /ɹ/ with children.

4 Describe and appraise interventions for childhood motor speech disorders: CAS and childhood dysarthria.

5 Compare and contrast teaching moments for different types of interventions for motor speech difficulties and disorders in children.

6 Consider the scientific rigor of the evidence base associated with motor speech interventions.

7 Create an intervention session plan for a child with motor speech difficulties and disorders.

OVERVIEW

In this chapter we provide an overview of intervention approaches suitable for motor speech difficulties and disorders in children, including interventions for articulation impairments involving sibilants and rhotics, CAS, and childhood dysarthria (see Figure 14-1 for a list of the approaches mentioned in this chapter). The structure of this chapter is similar to Chapter 13. For each intervention approach we provide a brief overview of the historical and theoretical background, general procedure, the evidence base, and suggested resources. We suggest that you learn about one approach at a time. Add depth to your understanding about an approach by reading associated references. Remember—the greater your knowledge, the better equipped you will be to implement intervention approaches in accordance with developers' intentions.

FIGURE 14-1   **Intervention approaches for different types of motor speech difficulties and disorders in children**

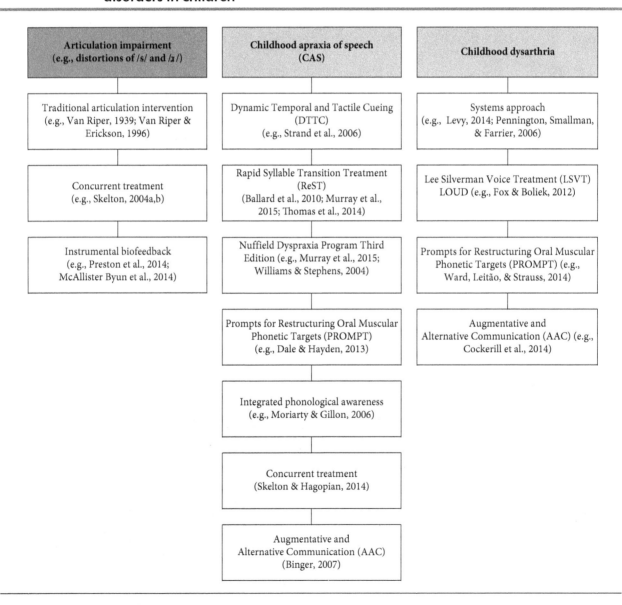

HISTORICAL PERSPECTIVES ON ARTICULATION AND MOTOR SPEECH INTERVENTIONS

Interventions focused on the physical articulation of speech have a long history in speech-language pathology. Unlike phonological interventions (which emerged in the mid to late 20th century), interventions targeting children's physical production of speech emerged in the early 20th century, when university programs began to offer speech-language pathology courses (Paden, 1970). See Figure 14-2 for a timeline depicting when various approaches targeting speech perception and/or production emerged.

As shown on the timeline, one of the earliest books about intervention for SSD in children was May Scripture and Eugene Jackson's (1919) book *A Manual of Exercises for the Correction of Speech Disorders.* The book included information about articulation placement for English consonants, drawings of the mouth during articulation (including coronal and sagittal images), and production practice exercises for consonants and vowels (e.g., drills of the sound in isolation, syllable chants, saying words with rising intonation, practicing everyday expressions and proverbs, rhythmic reading, reciting poems, rehearsing scripted dialogue, picture description, and storytelling). Scripture and Jackson (1919) also advocated breathing and relaxation exercises, lengthening and strengthening of vowels, mouth gymnastics, the use of mirrors, and exercises with a variety of tools such as a pipe for making soap bubbles (during breathing exercises), metronomes, and megaphones. Their approaches were based on experience.

FIGURE 14-2 Timeline of intervention approaches for different types of motor speech difficulties and disorders in children

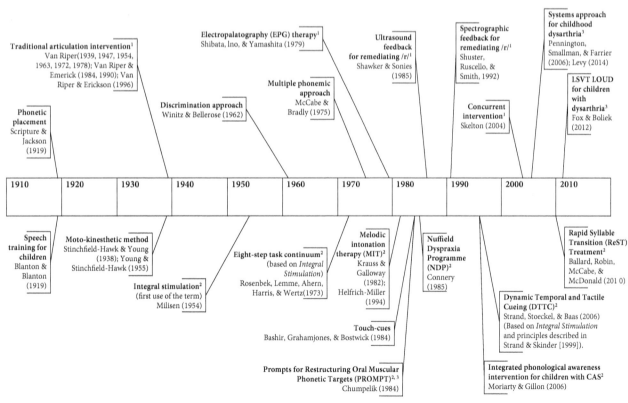

[1]Intervention suitable for simple articulation errors (e.g., /s/ distortion).
[2]Intervention suitable for CAS.
[3]Intervention suitable for childhood dysarthria

Although Scripture and Jackson's (1919) approach may have improved children's speech, it is difficult to know what elements in their approach worked and whether their approach was efficient. As you will learn, some of the empirically supported approaches used by SLPs in the 21st century include procedures similar to Scripture and Jackson's approach, such as practicing speech sounds in a variety of linguistic contexts (e.g., Skelton, 2004a). You will also learn that some procedures are no longer used and/or are considered ineffective or inefficient.

INTERVENTION FOR ARTICULATION IMPAIRMENT

In this section we describe three different options for managing articulation impairment in children. We describe one of the oldest approaches still used by SLPs today, a recent approach based on principles of motor learning, and intervention based on visual biofeedback.

■ Traditional articulation intervention for articulation impairment

Traditional articulation intervention is suitable for children with articulation difficulties, typically distortion errors involving sibilants and rhotics. Elements of the approach are common to other interventions for children with SSD.

Historical background

Traditional articulation intervention was developed by one of the pioneers of speech-language pathology, Charles van Riper (1939). His approach is considered to be one of the first organized methods for treating SSD in children (Secord, 1989). Van Riper's text *Speech Correction: Principles and Methods* was a classic for SLPs throughout the 20th century, with nine editions being published from 1939 through to 1996. Even though traditional articulation intervention is one of the oldest approaches (and therefore might seem outdated), we have included in this book because:

- it continues to be the approach of choice for many SLPs working with children who have SSD (Brumbaugh & Smit, 2013; McLeod & Baker, 2014),
- many of the elements of traditional articulation intervention form the basis of other approaches described in this chapter, and
- it is often assumed knowledge when reading intervention research from the late 20th and early 21st centuries.

Theoretical background

Traditional articulation intervention was based on the assumption that speech errors were due to defective speech sounds. Defective sounds were presumed to spoil syllables, which in turn were thought to spoil words and sentences (Van Riper, 1963). This focus on individual speech sounds informed ideas that:

- "the client's articulation errors have become so fixed, reinforced, and automatized by the time he comes for help that not only does he not recognize them but also that he does not know how to produce the correct phonemes" (Van Riper & Erickson, 1996, p. 238);
- a child needs to learn how to listen to the target sound, because the sound is buried with the flow of every day (Van Riper, 1963);
- it is better to initially teach a new sound in isolation or in nonsense syllables than in words;
- once a child is able to produce a targeted sound correctly, that is weak and needs to be strengthened "to win the competition with an error that has had a long history of usage" (Van Riper & Erickson, 1996, p. 238); and
- it is preferable to target only one or two sounds at a time (Van Riper & Erickson, 1996).

Procedure

The hallmark of traditional articulation intervention is

> its sequencing of activities for (1) sensory-perceptual training, which concentrates on iden-
> tifying the standard sound and discriminating it from its error through scanning and com-
> paring; (2) varying and correcting the various productions of the sound until it is produced
> correct; (3) strengthening and stabilizing the correct production; and finally, (4) transferring
> the new speech skill to everyday communication situations [and that] this process is usually
> carried out first for the standard sound in isolation, then in the syllable, then in a word, and
> finally in sentences. (Van Riper & Erickson, 1996, p. 237)

If you access one of Van Riper's texts you will find this idea of the gradual mastery of a
speech sound from easier through to more challenging contexts depicted as a staircase
(e.g., Van Riper & Erickson, 1996). The staircase includes four successive levels (isolation,
syllables, words, sentences) with a sequence of four activities to be completed at each level
(sensory-perceptual training, learning how to produce the target, stabilizing [practicing]
the target, and transferring the target). Van Riper and Erickson (1996) also advocated a
period of ear training prior to starting production training. Transfer/carryover activities
and maintenance were recommended once a child reached the top of the staircase (e.g.,
Secord, 1989; Van Riper & Erickson, 1996).

If you were to ask practicing SLPs to describe traditional articulation intervention,
they would probably say it involves listening to and then practicing a targeted speech sound
in isolation, syllables, words, phrases, sentences, and then conversation. Practice would
begin with imitation and then progress to spontaneous speech in drill or drill-play contexts.
Production cues such as auditory models for imitation, visual- and verbal-phonetic cues,
and successive approximation and shaping would be used. When you read contemporary
researchers' experimental accounts of traditional articulation intervention, similar descriptions are evident—they focus on incremental levels of production training (e.g., Hesketh,
Adams, Nightingale, & Hall, 2000; Klein, 1996b; Lipetz & Bernhardt, 2013; Powell, Elbert,
Miccio, Strike-Roussos, & Brasseur, 1998). Compared with Van Riper's original 1939 text,
traditional articulation intervention has evolved. Our rendition of traditional articulation
intervention therefore reflects a combination of Van Riper and Erickson's (1996) enduring ideas in addition to contemporary descriptions from empirical research (e.g., Hesketh
et al., 2000; Klein, 1996b; Lipetz & Bernhardt, 2013; Powell et al., 1998). We depict traditional articulation intervention as a pyramid (see Figure 14-3). **Sensory-perceptual (ear)
training** forms the base of the pyramid. We refer to Van Riper and Erickson's (1996) concept of producing activities (i.e., when children are acquiring the knowledge and ability
to articulate a new speech sound) as **pre-practice instruction**, and stabilizing activities
(i.e., when children are practicing a targeted skill in increments or steps) as **incremental
production practice**. A description of each component of the pyramid follows.

Sensory-perceptual (ear) training

Traditional articulation intervention begins with sensory-perceptual training (or ear
training). Sensory-perceptual training includes four tasks: **identifying**, **locating**, **stimulation**, and **discrimination**. A child progresses from one task to the next based on performance. A description of each type of training follows.

- **Identifying:** listening to and learning about the auditory, visual, and movement features of a target sound in an isolation context (Van Riper & Erickson, 1996). Metaphor
can be used to talk about the target sound (e.g., "Listen to the snake sounds /s/"). Auditory cues (including auditory detection phonetic cues of a target sound—see Chapter 12)
can be used to help the child identify the sound (e.g., "I'm going to say some different
speech sounds. Raise your hand when you hear the snake sound"). Treatment data
would capture the percentage of times the child correctly identifies the target sound.
- **Locating:** detecting the target sound in a variety of linguistic contexts (e.g., words,
phrases, oral reading, and conversation). You would encourage the child to signal
when he or she hears the target sound spoken by the clinician. For example, "Put on
your listening ears now. I am going to name some pictures—some have our sound
/s/ and some don't. When you hear the /s/ sound, put a bean in this jar, Ready? First
word, '*sun*'" (Van Riper & Emerick, 1990, p. 209). Treatment data would be the percentage of times the child correctly correct detects the target sound.

FIGURE 14-3 **Traditional articulation intervention**

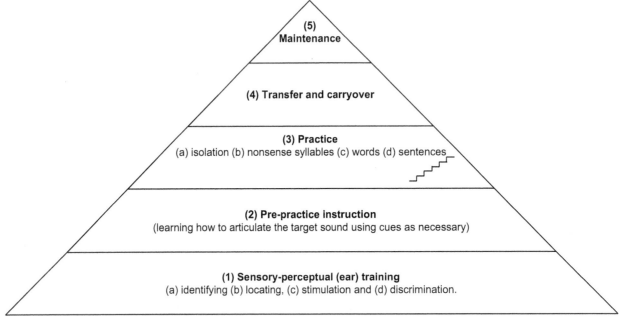

Sources: Based on Van Riper and Erickson (1996) and Secord (1989).

■ **Stimulation:** listening to multiple productions of the target sound, akin to focused stimulation. In 1963, Van Riper also suggested that children listen to the sound spoken by a variety of people—consistent with the concept of speaker variance (discussed in Chapter 5) and the speech perception principle that intervention should exploit varied speakers. In contrast with the other three tasks, progression towards discrimination activities is based on the child receiving a predetermined dose of stimulation rather than a particular level of performance as measured by treatment data.

■ **Discrimination:** differentiating the target sound from other speech sounds (including the child's error of the target sound). Using information about auditory cues in Chapter 12, this could involve auditory discrimination and judgment of correctness tasks in others' speech (inter-auditory comparison) (Secord, 1989). Van Riper and Erickson (1996) also recommend error correction, that is, the child detecting then correcting an error in a speaker's utterance (e.g., "Your tongue poked out between your teeth"). Such tasks can help children develop their ability to detect and self-correct their own errors once they start production practice (Secord, 1989). Van Riper and Erickson (1996) also suggest that it is helpful for children to learn this skill not only by **recalling** a sound they have just heard but **perceiving** errors as they occur and **predicting** the possible occurrence of an error. The treatment data that you collect would depend on the type of task (e.g., percentage of correct discrimination, percentage of correct judgment of correctness, percentage of correct error correction).

Van Riper and Erickson (1996) suggest that you can work on all four tasks during a session. Once treatment data indicate that a child can identify, locate, and discriminate the target sound, pre-practice instruction begins.

Pre-practice instruction
Pre-practice instruction involves teaching a child to articulate a targeted speech sound with cues as necessary. This could involve auditory cues, such as auditory detection of a target sound, in addition to one or more production cues (see Chapter 12 for further information about cues). For instance, to elicit a clear /s/ you could provide an auditory model

COMMENT: *Cues for eliciting /s/*

How do you teach a child who has a lateral or interdental lisp to articulate a clear /s/? Several authors provide helpful cues (e.g., Bleile, 2014; Marshalla, 2007; Secord et al., 2007; Shine, 2007). What follows is a brief summary of common ideas across this literature:

- Shape /s/ from a long (aspirated) [tʰ] or a rapid succession of [t], turning the last one into [s] (Secord et al., 2007).

- Shape /s/ from a long [t] then in the cluster [ts], followed by production practice in VC syllables—a method known as the Long T Method (Marshalla, 2007). As the child learns to produce [ts], Marshalla suggests that it is better for the child to focus on learning a new sound, rather than teaching him or her to think about correcting /s/. Marshalla also recommends beginning intervention with [ts] consonant clusters in word-final position at syllable level.

- Provide verbal-, visual- and tactile-phonetic instruction about the place and manner of the articulators when producing /s/ (including the need for lateral bracing). You could use an EPG image to help a child understand the need for lateral bracing of the tongue (e.g., Dagenais, Critz-Crosby, & Adams, 1994; McAuliffe & Cornwell, 2008). See Chapter 4 for EPG images of /s/.

- Use butterfly imagery to guide phonetic placement—the lateral tongue edges are the wings pressed against the top molars to prevent lateral air from escaping and the midline of the tongue is grooved (i.e., the butterfly body) (Bleile, 2014).

- Use the straw technique (Usdan, 1978). This approach requires a thin straw, half a cup of water, and a mirror. The child is initially instructed to hold the straw between the tongue tip and alveolar ridge while keeping the teeth apart; that is, holding the straw into position with the tongue. Next, the child is instructed to blow bubbles in the half cup of water. Initially air may escape laterally. With practice, the child learns to direct airflow through the straw to create bubbles. Next, the child is asked to remove the straw from the water but to keep blowing and directing air through the straw. The straw is gradually cut into smaller and smaller lengths and eventually removed from the child's mouth while the child is blowing. In a study of 18 children who had a lateral lisp, it was reported that "when the straw was withdrawn their blowing approximated a 'loose /s/ sound with no lateral emission'" (Usdan, 1978, p. 7). Van Riper's incremental articulation hierarchy was then used to practice /s/.

for imitation, phonetic placement instruction (including visual-, verbal-, tactile-phonetic cues and manual guidance), orthographic cues, shaping, a facilitating phonetic context, and metaphor. An overview of teaching cues for eliciting sibilants and rhotics is provided in the comment boxes on cues for eliciting /s/ and cues for /ɹ, ɚ, ɝ/.

Practice

Once a child is stimulable for the target sound, it needs to be practiced or stabilized (Van Riper & Erickson, 1996). In traditional articulation intervention, practice progresses incrementally: isolation, syllables, words, sentences (as shown in Figure 14-3). Additional levels (e.g., short phrases, conversation) could be added, if needed.

- **Isolation:** Children practice continuant sounds in true isolation while plosives are practiced with the schwa. For school-age children, simultaneous talking and writing (i.e., saying the sound while writing the sound) can be helpful (Van Riper & Erickson, 1996).
- **Nonsense syllables:** Practice the target sound in a variety of syllable shapes (e.g., CV, VC, CVC, VCV) with a variety of vowels (e.g., /sɑ, is, sɔp, usu/). Recall from Chapter 12 that some vowels facilitate accurate production more than others. When dealing with phonetic errors involving /ɹ/ or /s/, the high front vowel /i/ can serve as a facilitating phonetic context (Bleile, 2014).

COMMENT: *Cues for eliciting /ɹ, ɚ, ɝ/*

When starting intervention targeting consonantal /ɹ/ (and the rhotic vowels /ɚ, ɝ/ for those children learning to speak a rhotic dialect of English), you need to consider three questions.

1. What is the child's dialect? If the child speaks a rhotic dialect, you will need to decide whether you need to focus on one allophonic variant for a child (the consonantal /ɹ/, the stressed /ɝ/, or the weak /ɚ/ rhotic vowel), or whether you focus on all variants. Evidence is divided regarding allophonic generalization from one variant to another (e.g., Elbert & McReynolds, 1975; Hoffman, 1983; Preston et al., 2014). It would seem that generalization occurs, but not in a uniform way for all children. We suggest that you start with the most stimulable variant in a child's dialect and closely monitor the other variants.

2. Can the child accurately perceive correct and incorrect or distorted productions of /ɹ/ in others' speech and their own speech? Researchers who have studied children and adults who have difficulty producing /ɹ/ have suggested that these speakers might also have difficulty perceiving /ɹ/, especially their own incorrect productions—accepting incorrect productions as correct (Shuster, 1998). Children can also have difficulty accepting that their correct productions are indeed correct. They comment that productions identified by others as correct do not sound right (Shuster, Ruscello, & Toth, 1995). These findings have implications for intervention. When you begin intervention targeting /ɹ/ distortion, you need to consider the role of the child's speech perception skills. If speech perception skills are poor, visual biofeedback can help guide production, as children can learn to rely on the visual (rather than auditory) feedback to improve their articulation (Shuster et al., 1995).

3. Which articulatory gestures you will use to elicit /ɹ/? There are actually many different ways to shape the tongue (including the tongue root, tip, blade, and dorsum) to produce the [ɹ] sound (Secord et al., 2007). Across the intervention literature, recommendations focus on two broad types—the bunched (molar) production and the retroflex (apical) production (Ball, Müller, & Granese, 2013). Some authors recommend starting with the bunched gesture (e.g., Bleile, 2014) while others recommend starting with the retroflex gesture (e.g., Ball et al., 2013). We suggest that you select suitable gestures on a case-by-case basis. Use what works for the child. Review Chapter 4 for further information about the articulation of /ɹ, ɚ, ɝ/.

Some suggestions for eliciting consonantal /ɹ/:

■ Provide an auditory model for imitation. If a child can imitate you correctly, further cued instruction would be unnecessary, as you (and the child) may not actually know how they articulated the sound correctly, just that it was correct.

■ Provide instrumental visual-phonetic cues, such as a spectrogram or ultrasound image (e.g., Lawson, Scobbie, & Stuart-Smith, 2013; McAllister Byun & Hitchcock, 2012; Preston et al., 2014).

■ Provide verbal-phonetic cue about the place and manner of the articulation. For example, to produce a bunched /ɹ/, Bleile (2014) suggested that you "ask the student to place the tongue tip behind the lower front teeth and to raise the body of the tongue toward the mouth roof" (p. 214). To produce a retroflex /ɹ/, Bleile (2014) suggests that you first "ask the student to place the tongue tip behind the upper front teeth" and then "ask the student to curl the tongue backward without touching the roof of the mouth until it cannot go back farther" (p. 215).

(continued)

- Trial successive approximation/shaping of /ɹ/ from [l]. For example, Shriberg (1975) suggests that you say to the child, "Say a long /l/ but this time as you're saying it, drag the tip of your tongue slowly back along the roof of your mouth—so far back that you have to drop it" (p. 105). Shriberg (1975) also suggests that the clinician also use a hand gesture of the palm up and the fingertips slowly moving back.
- Elicit /ɹ/ before a high front vowel [i], between vowels, or in a syllable-initial velar plosive cluster /kɹ, gɹ / (for bunched /ɹ/) or alveolar plosive cluster /tɹ, dɹ / (for retroflex /ɹ/) (Bleile, 2014).
- Ask the child to produce the /ɑ/ sound, then ask the child to "move the tongue dorsum up toward the palate while continuing to produce /ɑ/" (Secord et al., 2007, p. 146).
- "Sometimes, merely telling the client [child] to tighten tongue muscles in the pharynx is enough to produce the /r/ quality" (Secord et al., 2007, p. 147).*
- "A good [r] is often more easily achieved if the student is encouraged to say the sound while keeping the sides of the tongue touching the insides of the teeth" (Bleile, 2014, p. 215).*
- Shape the consonantal /ɹ/ from the vocalic /ɹ/ by asking a child to say the vocalic /ɹ/ before starting words with the consonantal /ɹ/ (Bleile, 2014).

*Note, in these quotes r = ɹ.

- **Words:** Practice the target sound in a variety of positions in words. Van Riper and Erickson (1996) recommended starting with the target sound in monosyllables in prevocalic position (e.g., *sea, saw, sock, soap, sing*) followed by monosyllables in postvocalic position (e.g., *bus, kiss, moose, rice, mess*) and then consonant clusters in pre- and postvocalic contexts (e.g., *stop, star, spot, skip, sleep, smell, snow, bats, cats, oats, mitts, dots*). Move on to words containing two or more syllables with increasing complexity across positions (e.g., *dinosaur, octopus, castle, ice cream, sausage, sunglasses, principal, stethoscope,* and *rhinoceros*). It can be helpful to select words that are highly meaningful to a child, such as family names, pet's names, and the names of favorite toys, superheroes, and television and movie characters.
- **Sentences:** Once a child can produce the target sound in words to a predetermined performance criterion (e.g., 90% correct without a model) and displays evidence of self-correction, sentence level begins. Meaningful sentences varying in purpose are recommended—for instance, statements (e.g., "I like *sausages*"), questions (e.g., "Do you like *sausages*?"), and commands (e.g., "Don't eat that *sausage!*").

Transfer and carryover
Use of the targeted speech sound in spontaneous speech in everyday situations is needed for children to achieve the long-term goal. If stimulus and response generalization data suggest that carryover is not occurring, you may need to facilitate a child's motivation, metacognitive knowledge, and metacognitive control. (See Chapter 12 for further information about carryover.) You could also apply principles of motor learning, including (1) random variable practice and (2) reduced feedback with a delay reflecting knowledge of results only, to better facilitate transfer and carryover.

Maintenance
Once a child has achieved the long-term goal, such as use of the targeted sound in everyday conversational speech with a variety of conversational partners, periodic review assessments (e.g., 1, 3, then 6 months following the cessation of intervention) may be conducted to ensure sustained achievement of the goal (Secord, 1989).

■ ■■ ■ ■■ ■ ■■ ■ ■■ ■ ■■ ■ ■■ ■ ■■ ■ ■■ ■ ■■ ■ ■■ ■ ■■ ■ ■■ ■ ■■ ■ ■ ■■ ■ ■■ ■ ■■ ■

✓ **APPLICATION: Traditional articulation intervention and the principles**
of motor learning

As you read through the information about traditional articulation intervention, you may have wondered how the approach aligns (and in some respects does not align) with the principles of motor learning. This is certainly what some clinicians and researchers have been thinking about in the 21st century (e.g., Hageman, 2014; Skelton, 2004a, Skelton & Funk, 2004; Taps, 2006). Consider the following questions.

1. What are the similarities and differences between the structure of traditional articulation intervention and the principles of motor learning (particularly the conditions and structure of practice)?
2. Why might a child struggle to generalize /s/ to everyday conversational speech using the traditional approach to articulation intervention?

Suggested answers:

1. Although a period of pre-practice followed by production practice aligns with Fitts' (1964) idea that motor learning can be divided into phases, the incremental levels of production practice seem at odds with recommended randomized variable practice conditions and practice task complexity. Research is needed to compare outcomes of intervention using traditional articulation intervention and articulation intervention guided by principles of motor learning.
2. A child might struggle with generalization because the conditions of practice and the type, frequency, and timing of feedback during practice may not follow principles of motor learning.

Evidence

The evidence associated with traditional articulation intervention is complicated to navigate. This is because it has been examined over decades by various researchers with children with different types of SSD (including phonological and articulation impairment) for various reasons (e.g., Arndt, Elbert, & Shelton, 1971; Carrier, 1970; Galloway & Blue, 1975; Gray, 1974; Klein, 1996b; Pamplona, Ysunza, & Espinosa, 1999; Sommers et al., 1966; Sommers et al., 1970; Weston & Harber, 1975). The procedures have not consistently mirrored Van Riper's rendition of traditional articulation intervention (particularly the inclusion of ear training). Intervention intensity and service delivery have also varied. What the research does have in common is consideration of an incremental hierarchy for practicing a targeted speech sound. Given that we have focused on articulation impairments involving sibilants and/or rhotics (typically /s, z, ɹ/), we provide an overview of a selection of the evidence limited to these phonetic errors in Table 14-1. Note that this table does not include articulation intervention studies that have used visual biofeedback. These studies are addressed later in the chapter.

Children suited to traditional articulation intervention

Traditional articulation intervention has been used with children who have articulation impairments and children who have phonological impairments (e.g., Klein, 1996b; Pamplona et al., 1999). The evidence suggests that phonological intervention is better suited to children with phonological impairment, while traditional articulation intervention is better suited to articulation impairment involving residual speech sound errors (e.g., Klein, 1996b). Further research is needed to compare outcomes between traditional articulation intervention and contemporary renditions of articulation intervention based on principles of motor learning and interventions that incorporate instrumental feedback (e.g., ultrasound, electropalatogram, spectrogram).

TABLE 14-1 **Selected studies of traditional articulation intervention targeting phonetic errors involving sibilants or rhotics**

Error type	Reference	Focus	Nature of the evidence
Interdental lisp	Costello & Schoen (1978)	Delivery of Mower's (1968) S-Pack by SLPs versus paraprofessionals	RCT involving 15 children
	Engel & Groth (1976)	Carryover	Six case studies
	Masterson & Daniels (1991)	Benefit of contrastive (phonology-based) intervention versus articulation intervention for errors involving /ɹ/ and /s/	Case study
	Ruscello (1975)	The role of word position in generalization	Six case studies
Nasal lisp	Hall & Tomblin (1975)	Shaping of nasal lisp using [ts] cluster	Single case study
Errors on /s/ or /ɹ/	Gray & Shelton (1992)	Self-monitoring and carryover	Multiple baseline design across eight participants
	Koegel, Koegel, & Ingham (1986)	Self-monitoring in carryover	Multiple baseline design across behaviors and across 13 participants
	Koegel, Koegel, Ingham, & Van Voy (1988)	Self-monitoring in carryover	Multiple baseline design across seven participants
Distortion of /ɹ, ɝ, ɚ/	Hoffman (1983)	Interallophonic generalization between /ɹ, ɝ, ɚ/	Non-RCT involving 12 children
	Shriberg (1975)	The /ɝ/ evoke program	Case study from 65 children, across 19 clinicians

Note: RCT = randomized controlled trial

Resources for conducting traditional articulation intervention

If you type the words "articulation therapy" and "resources" into your Internet browser, you will find a wealth of pictures in addition to activities, ideas for games, worksheets, and forms for conducting traditional articulation intervention with children. Commercial resources (e.g., activity books, picture cards, computer- and tablet-based activities) are available from companies that publish in the area of speech-language pathology.

◼ Concurrent treatment: Articulation intervention based on principles of motor learning

Concurrent treatment is another intervention option for children with articulation impairment. Grounded in principles of motor learning, concurrent treatment differs from traditional articulation intervention in the way that treatment exemplars are practiced.

Historical background

Concurrent treatment was developed by Steve Skelton (Skelton, 2004a, b). He developed the approach in light of questions about the necessity of the incremental practice sequence in traditional articulation intervention (i.e., isolation, syllables, words, sentences, then transfer and carryover to conversational speech). Skelton (2004a) was particularly interested the effect of randomized variable practice on children's generalized learning of targeted speech sounds. As shown in Figure 14-2, concurrent treatment is a relatively recent addition to approaches suitable for treating children with SSD.

Theoretical background

The concurrent approach is based on theoretical principles of motor learning. Recall from Chapter 11, practice conditions include practice amount (large versus small), distribution of practice (massed versus distributed), practice variability (constant versus variable), and practice schedule (blocked versus random). Generalized learning is thought to be best when the practice is large, distributed, variable, and random (Maas et al., 2008). The incremental or easy-to-hard sequence used in traditional articulation intervention reflects blocked constant practice. Concurrent treatment uses a randomized variable practice schedule, with the aim of facilitating better generalized learning.

Procedure

Concurrent treatment is similar to traditional articulation intervention in that it focuses on production practice of individual speech sounds, in a variety of linguistic contexts or exemplar types. What makes it different is the use of a randomized variable practice schedule or intermixing of the easy and harder exemplars that make up the incremental hierarchy in traditional articulation intervention (Skelton, 2004a). Concurrent treatment begins with a period of orientation training (i.e., instruction about the different types of exemplars to be used during practice), pre-practice, and then randomized variable practice.

Orientation training

Concurrent treatment uses multiple exemplars—that is, different ways or linguistic contexts for practicing speech sounds. Skelton (2004a) reported using 29 different exemplars involving syllables, words, two- to four-word phrases, and sentences in word-initial singleton, word-initial consonant cluster, word-final singleton, and intervocalic contexts. The words, phrases, and sentences were elicited in both an imitative and evoked (spontaneous) context. The syllables were elicited via imitation. A brief portion of conversational speech (in the form of a short story) was elicited in an evoked context. This created 29 different exemplars. During orientation training children learn about each exemplar type and the expected length and mode of response, using a consonant that does not requiring training (Skelton, 2004a). Table 14-2 provides an example of stimuli that could be used during orientation training (using a consonant /p/ already produced accurately by a child) and production practice during intervention targeting /s/.

Pre-practice instruction

During pre-practice instruction, cues are used to help children articulate the target sound in a limited number of contexts (e.g., isolation, CV and VC syllables, and/or three or four words) (Skelton, 2004a; Skelton & Taps, 2008). The auditory and production cues used would be similar to those used in traditional articulation intervention; the approach differs in the randomized variable practice schedule. Additive segmentation rather than fractionation could also be used to teach a child how to articulate the target sound in words (Skelton & Taps, 2008). The purpose of pre-practice is to ensure that the child is stimulable for the target in a blocked constant format, in preparation for randomized variable practice of the different exemplar types (Skelton, 2004a). Pre-practice instruction continues until performance criterion is met. Skelton (2004a) reported using a criterion of 8 out of 10 correct consecutive attempts (Skelton, 2004a).

Practice

Once a child is able to perform the task in limited contexts, practice is needed to facilitate learning—that is, generalization of the target sound to everyday speech. During practice a random-variable practice structure is used, mixing the full range of exemplar types. A relatively high dose is recommended (at least 150 production practice trials per session), with 30-minute sessions distributed twice weekly (Taps, 2006).

You could implement randomized variable practice in a few different ways. You could begin the practice session with predetermined randomized variable lists of the different exemplar types and work through the randomized lists to yield the recommended dose (Skelton, 2004a). You could use a spinner with eight different exemplar types noted as options for random selection: imitated syllable, imitated and evoked words, imitated and evoked phrases, imitated and evoked sentences, and evoked conversation/story (Skelton & Taps, 2008).

| TABLE 14-2 | Exemplar types used during Skelton's concurrent treatment: Orientation and production practice examples |

	Imitated production	Imitated and evoked (spontaneous) production			Evoked production
	Syllable	Word	Two- to four-word phrase	Sentence	Conversation topic
Word-initial singleton: *orientation*	/pɑ/	pen	chicken pasta	She is eating a pancake.	*Orientation training*: Tell me a short story about a pool party.
Word-initial singleton: *production practice*	/sɑ/	sun	chicken noodle soup	She put sauce on her hotdog.	
Word-initial consonant cluster: *orientation*	/pli/	play	red plate	She is watering the plant.	*Production practice*: Tell me a short story about a stick insect.
Word-initial consonant cluster: *production practice*	/sni/	snow	brown snail	The snake is curled up on the rock.	
Word-final singleton: *orientation*	/ip/	cup	the big blue cup	He is washing his hands with soap.	*Note*: The short story should contain at least four sentences and exemplars across different word positions.
Word-final singleton: *production practice*	/is/	bus	the big blue house	The mouse is hiding under the table.	
Intervocalic context: *orientation*	/upu/	happy	happy dog	She is hopping on one foot.	
Intervocalic context: *production practice*	/usu/	messy	green grasshopper	Her pet rabbit escaped.	

Source: Skelton (2004a).

These options require you to have your stimuli for the different exemplar types sorted into piles (e.g., a pile of word-initial pictures, word-final pictures, written sentences targeting word-initial clusters, story topics). Alternatively, you could have your stimuli for the different exemplar types shuffled into one pile and have the child work through the pile. The number of times a child works through the pile to achieve the recommended dose depends on the number of stimuli in the pile. You would include age-appropriate activities and positive verbal and tangible reinforcement throughout practice to ensure that the child was engaged and motivated to practice. Skelton (2004a) provided token reinforcement initially using a continuous reinforcement schedule and then changed to a fixed ratio as a child improved. You would monitor progress over time using response generalization probes of non-treatment words for the different exemplar types, in addition to a sample of conversational speech. Skelton (2004a) used a generalization (maintenance) criterion of 80% correct.

Evidence

Concurrent treatment is a relatively new approach for treating SSD in children, and so has limited evidence. Using a multiple baseline design across participants, Skelton (2004a) reported that it was successful with four 7-year-old children who had an interdental lisp. Using an AB design replicated across three younger children (4;8 to 5;11 years), Skelton and Funk (2004) reported that "once placement position has been taught in a limited context, the target speech sounds were successfully acquired using a randomized, variable sequence of presumed easy to hard tasks" (p. 603) and that modest within-clinic generalization to conversational speech occurred. Using a multiple baseline design across participants, Skelton and Hagopian (2014) tested the approach with three children with CAS and reported generalized acquisition of targeted sounds in untreated words and phrases. Using practice-based evidence from San Diego Unified School District (the eighth-largest school district in United States), Taps (2006, 2008) reported that most children with mild articulation difficulties completed intervention characterized by randomized variable practice in

17 to 20 SLP hours (equivalent to approximately forty 30-minute sessions) plus home practice. Further research is needed to compare concurrent treatment with other intervention approaches suitable for children with SSD and to examine the effect of adding randomized variable practice to other existing intervention approaches.

Children suited to concurrent treatment

Concurrent treatment has been examined with children who have relatively mild articulation impairment (e.g., Skelton, 2004a; Skelton & Taps, 2008; Taps, 2006), children with phonological impairment (e.g., Skelton & Kerber, 2005; Skelton & Resciniti, 2009), and children with CAS (Skelton & Hagopian, 2014). Of this relatively small body of research, it would seem that randomized variable practice can be helpful for children when learning to produce targeted consonants. Of the clinical cases described in Chapter 16, it would seem that randomized variable practice might be beneficial for Luke, Susie, and Michael.

Resources for conducting concurrent treatment

Resources suitable for traditional articulation intervention are also suitable for concurrent treatment. However, your preparation and use of the resources will differ. Rather than completing activities in an incremental manner, you would prepare and implement activities using a randomized variable sequence. You could create a picture card resource for the different types of exemplars. You could also create materials such as a spinner with the various practice options to create a random practice schedule (e.g., Skelton & Taps, 2008).

■ Articulation intervention using instrumental feedback: Ultrasound, electropalatography, and spectrography

Articulation intervention can be facilitated using visual biofeedback from a range of tools, including ultrasound, the electropalatograph (EPG), and the spectrograph. Ultrasound and EPG are useful for providing feedback on tongue placement, shapes, and movement (Lipetz & Bernhardt, 2013; McAuliffe & Cornwell, 2008). Intervention using EPG requires relatively expensive medical equipment, so it is more frequently used in university clinics and medical centers with children who have protracted difficulties who have not responded to traditional intervention. Traditionally, access to spectrographic feedback or ultrasound images required expensive equipment. Spectrographic feedback is now more readily available via computerized shareware (e.g., Praat: Boersma & Weenink, 2013; see Chapter 9 for a list of available programs). You can also turn a computer into an ultrasound machine, by using an ultrasound imaging probe and accompanying software that connects to your computer via a USB port (e.g., SeeMore Ultrasound Imaging Probes; ClearProbe Ultrasound).

Historical background

While ultrasound and spectrography have more recently been applied to speech intervention, EPG was one of the earliest instruments to assist with articulation intervention.

Ultrasound

The earliest accounts of using ultrasound in speech intervention describe work on vowel production with children with hearing loss across a range of countries including the United States, Germany, and Poland (Foss, Whitehead, Paterson, & Whitehead, 1990; Klajman, Huber, Neumann, Wein, & Bockler, 1988; Shawker & Sonies, 1985; Wein, Böckler, Klajman, & Obrebowski, 1991). Since this time, researchers in Canada, Scotland, and the United States have conducted research using ultrasound for speech intervention. Researchers from Canada predominantly have targeted /ɹ/ during intervention (although some of their studies have targeted vowels and fricatives) for children, adolescents, and adults with residual speech sound errors (Adler-Bock, Bernhardt, Gick, & Bacsfalvi, 2007; Bernhardt et al., 2008), hearing loss (Bernhardt, Gick, Bacsfalvi, & Ashdown, 2003; Bernhardt, Gick, Bacsfalvi, & Adler-Bock, 2005), and Down syndrome (Fawcett, Bacsfalvi, & Bernhardt, 2008). They have demonstrated long-term outcomes of intervention (Bacsfalvi & Bernhardt, 2011). Researchers from Scotland have used ultrasound to target either /ɹ/, /ʃ/, /t/ or velars with children with persistent SSD (Cleland, Scobbie, & Wrench, 2015). In the

United States, Preston and colleagues have successfully used ultrasound to target a range of consonants for children with CAS (Preston, Brick, & Landi, 2013) and residual speech sound errors (Preston et al., 2014). McAllister Byun and colleagues have used ultrasound as part of an intervention to treat persistent /ɹ/ distortion (e.g., Hitchcock & McAllister Byun, 2015; McAllister Byun & Hitchcock, 2012; McAllister Byun, Hitchcock, & Swartz, 2014).

Electropalatography

In the early 1800s and 1900s, tin foil, chalk, and ink were used to create static images of contact between the tongue and the hard palate (Darwin, 1803; Moses, 1939; Shohara & Hanson, 1941). Then, in the early 1900s, tongue markers (Stetson, 1928) were used to document the position and timing of the articulators. These technologies led the way to the development of the EPG (see Chapter 4 for EPG images and Chapter 9 for information about the use of EPG in speech analysis). In the mid-1900s, different versions of EPGs were created in Japan (Rion: Shibata, 1968), the United Kingdom (Reading/WinEPG: Hardcastle, 1972), and the United States (Kay Palatometer: Fletcher, McCutcheon, & Wolf, 1975). Currently, two EPG systems are available for use in assessment and intervention: Articulate Instruments[1] (UK, Wrench, 2007) and CompleteSpeech[2] (US). One of the earliest accounts of using EPG for intervention was by Japanese researchers Shibata, Ino, and Yamashita (1979). Since this time, the majority of EPG intervention research has been undertaken using the Reading/WinEPG. Researchers across the world have used the Reading/WinEPG for speech intervention (e.g., Canada, England, Hong Kong, Japan, New Zealand, Scotland, Sweden, United States) and have consistently documented improvements in the articulation of lingual consonants by children and adolescents with SSD (e.g., Dagenais, 1995; Gibbon & Hardcastle, 1987; McAuliffe & Cornwell, 2008), dysarthria as a result of cerebral palsy (e.g., Gibbon & Wood, 2003; Nordberg, Carlsson, & Lohmander, 2011), hearing loss (e.g., Bernhardt, Gick, Bacsfalvi, & Ashdown, 2003; Martin, Hirson, Herman, Thomas, & Pring, 2007), and cleft palate (e.g., Fujiwara, 2007; Stokes, Whitehill, Tsui, & Yuen, 1996).

Spectrography

Spectrographic images primarily have been used as a speech analysis tool rather than a speech intervention tool. In the 1980s, researchers in the United States used the Kay Elemetrics Sonograph to facilitate intervention for the production of /ɹ/ (Shuster, Ruscello, & Smith, 1992; Shuster, Ruscello & Toth, 1995). More recently, the Kay-Pentax CSL SonaMatch has been used to remediate /ɹ/ production in children with SSD who previously had limited success with traditional articulation intervention (McAllister Byun & Hitchcock, 2012). Spectrography also has been used in conjunction with ultrasound intervention to remediate a persistent frontal lisp in an adolescent (Lipetz & Bernhardt, 2013).

Theoretical background

Most interventions for children with SSD rely on auditory input, where children listen to the productions of themselves and others to monitor their output; however, some children have difficulties changing their speech production using perceptual cues. Additionally, children with motor speech difficulties traditionally receive auditory directions from the SLP regarding how to move their articulators (e.g., move your tongue to the back of your mouth to produce /k/, make a central groove along your tongue to produce /s/). These directions can be difficult for children to imagine, since the articulators are largely invisible during speech. Visual biofeedback using technology such as ultrasound, EPG, and the spectrograph provides a mirror to previously invisible movements. As discussed in Chapter 11, knowledge of performance (KP) helps shape incorrect responses towards accurate responses. Recently researchers have suggested that mirror neurons facilitate this learning by coding representations of actions that can be replicated (Buccino, Binkofski, & Riggio, 2004). It has been suggested that the synaptic connection becomes stronger the more frequently it is activated with frequent practice. However, there is dissent regarding the link between mirror neurons and speech perception and production (Hickok, 2010), with some authors indicating that mirror neurons are too simplistic to explain the link between speech perception and motor learning (Lotto, Hickok, & Holt, 2009).

---

[1]http://www.articulateinstruments.com
[2]http://www.completespeech.com/

Procedure

To use **ultrasound** during intervention, an ultrasound probe is held beneath the chin and the ultrasound waves are directed through the muscle tissue into the oral cavity. The air shadow of the tongue is seen as a white line on the monitor, and the tongue's movement can be followed in real time along the sagittal plane (see Chapter 4 for examples). Ultrasound can provide visual biofeedback during intervention for consonants and vowels where the adult target has a different tongue shape and placement to the child's typical production (e.g., /k/ → [t], /ɹ/ → [w]). It can also be useful for identifying the type of tongue shape (either bunched or reflex) that best suits individual children needing to improve persistent rhotic distortions (McAllister Byun et al., 2014).

To use **EPG** during intervention, children need to visit a dentist to have a cast made of their teeth and mouth, which is sent to a company to create a custom-made EPG palate. The EPG palate is worn during intervention, and real-time coronal (transverse) images can be compared with images either provided on paper (cf. Chapter 4) or created by the SLP, who also wears an EPG palate. Electropalatography is also useful for providing biofeedback during intervention for lingual consonants, particularly when the target tongue/palate contact is different from the child's typical tongue placement (e.g., /k/ → [t], /s/ → [ɬ], lateral and interdental lisps).

To use **spectrography** during intervention, the child produces speech into a microphone that is linked to an acoustic display set at approximately 2 seconds per screen (Shuster et al., 1995). The child is directed to consider the number of lines (formants) on the screen, and attempts to match the spectrogram produced by the SLP. Spectrography has primarily been used to remediate distortions of consonantal /ɹ/, vocalic /ɝ, ɚ/ and /s/ → [θ] (e.g., Lipetz & Bernhardt, 2013; McAllister Byun & Hitchcock, 2012). Teaching moments would focus on visual-phonetic cues (see Chapter 12); however, other auditory and production cues could be used as needed.

Evidence

To date, the evidence regarding the outcomes of articulation intervention using visual biofeedback via ultrasound, EPG, and spectrograph is primarily limited to case studies (e.g., Gibbon & Wood, 2003; Hitchcock & McAllister Byun, 2015; McAuliffe & Cornwell, 2008; Modha, Bernhardt, Church, & Bacsfalvi, 2008), single-case experimental designs (e.g., Preston et al., 2014), and a non-experimental within-group study (McAllister Byun & Hitchcock, 2012). Gibbon (2003) indicated that over half the 150 research papers on clinical applications of EPG have described children with SSD or cleft palate. Overall, children have demonstrated positive outcomes from visual biofeedback intervention, particularly since many of these children were working on targets that had not been remediated using traditional articulation intervention. Some examples will be described. First, Preston, Brick, and Landi (2013) found significant improvements using **ultrasound** for 23 of 31 "treated sequences" (p. 627) for six children over an average of five sessions. Similarly, Cleland et al. (2015) reported significant improvements over a 12-week block of intervention using **ultrasound** for six of the seven children with persistent SSD targeting a range of errors (e.g., idiosyncratic backing, errors on /ɹ/ and velars). McAuliffe and Cornwell (2008) worked with an 11-year-old girl with persistent lateral /s/ using **EPG** during 12 sessions across 4 weeks plus 6 weeks of home practice. Improvements in her production of /s/ were verified using perceptual and acoustic analysis. Finally, McAllister Byun and Hitchcock (2012) found significant improvements in the production of /ɹ/ over 10 weeks of intervention (traditional articulation + visual biofeedback using **spectrography**) for eight of the 11 children who produced /ɹ/ in isolation and four of the 11 children who produced /ɹ/ in untreated words.

Children suited to articulation intervention using instrumental feedback

Intervention using visual biofeedback is often used with children who have not benefitted from traditional articulation intervention. **Ultrasound** has been used in intervention studies with children and adolescents with persistent SSD typically involving rhotics and sibilants (Adler-Bock et al., 2007; Bernhardt et al., 2008; Cleland et al., 2015; Lipetz & Bernhardt, 2013; McAllister Byun, Hitchcock & Swartz, 2014; Preston et al., 2014), CAS (Preston et al., 2013), hearing loss (Bernhardt et al., 2003; Bernhardt Gick, Bacsfalvi, & Adler-Bock,

2005), in addition to children with cochlear implants (Bacsfalvi, 2010) and adults with Down syndrome (Fawcett et al., 2008). While the primary target has been /ɹ/, other targets have included vowels, velars, and fricatives. **EPG** has been used for speech sound intervention for children and adolescents with SSD, CAS, dysarthria, cleft palate, and hearing loss. Intervention targets have included lateral /s/ (Dagenais, Critz-Crosby, & Adams, 1994; Gibbon & Hardcastle, 1987), velars (Friel, 1998; Gibbon, Dent, & Hardcastle, 1993), and reduction of the use of undifferentiated lingual gestures (i.e., tongue contact across the entire palate) (Gibbon, 1999). To date, **spectrography** primarily has been used to remediate /ɹ/ and a frontal lisp; but it has potential for providing visual feedback regarding the production of other speech targets including fricatives and approximants (McLeod & Isaac, 1995).

Resources for conducting articulation intervention using instrumental feedback

Resources for using EPG are available from Articulate Instruments[3] and CompleteSpeech.[4] Portable ultrasound devices that connect to a computer via a USB port are available from Interson (e.g., SeeMore Ultrasound Imaging Probes[5]) and GlobalMed (e.g., ClearProbe Ultrasound[6]). See Chapter 9 for a list of spectrographic software programs.

COMMENT: *Why are some outdated therapies and procedures still used by SLPs?*

Surveys of SLPs' methods of practice suggest that some outdated therapies and procedures are still used by SLPs (McLeod & Baker, 2014). Why? Sometimes the answer is as simple as SLPs use what other SLPs use. Sometimes the answer is more complicated—because there are attractively marketed (untested) tools and resources steeped in folklore being used and recommended by clinicians (Lof, 2011). An example is the use of nonspeech oral motor exercises (NSOMEs) for children with articulation and phonological impairments. Although they are still used by some SLPs, Forrest and Iuzzini (2008) state, "Strong evidence for the efficacy of NSOMEs should be demonstrated before the inclusion of such exercises" (p. 310). See Forrest (2002) and Lof (2003) for further information about this controversial practice. Remember, although it is helpful to understand and appreciate professional ancestry and history (see Duchan, 2010), question the evidence for your clinical practice. As evidence-based SLPs, do not let heritage cloud clinical decisions.

■ ▪ ■ ▪▪ ■ ▪ ■ ▪ ■ ▪▪ ■ ▪ ■ ▪ ■ ▪▪ ■ ▪ ■ ▪ ■ ▪▪ ■ ▪ ■ ▪ ■ ▪▪ ■ ▪ ■ ▪ ■ ▪▪ ■ ▪ ■ ▪ ■ ▪▪ ■ ▪ ■

 APPLICATION: *Intervention approaches suitable for Susie*

Susie has a lateral lisp. What intervention approaches might be suitable for Susie?

Answer: You could trial articulation intervention (based on Van Riper & Erickson, 1996) or concurrent treatment (Skelton, 2004a). If you have the technology available, you could also include visual biofeedback (e.g., EPG, ultrasound), particularly during the pre-practice phase of intervention, to help Susie learn how to articulate a clear /s/.

Read more about Susie (7;4 years), a girl with an articulation impairment (lateral lisp), in Chapter 16 (Case 2).

---

[3]http://www.articulateinstruments.com
[4]http://www.completespeech.com/
[5]http://www.interson.com/products/seemore-153-usb-probes
[6]http://www.ivci.com/product/globalmed-clearprobe-ultrasound/

INTERVENTION FOR CHILDHOOD APRAXIA OF SPEECH (CAS)

A range of intervention options exists for CAS, such as:

- Dynamic Temporal and Tactile Cueing (DTTC) (e.g., Strand et al., 2006);
- Rapid Syllable Transition Treatment (ReST) (Ballard et al., 2010; Thomas, McCabe & Ballard, 2014);
- Prompts for Restructuring Oral Muscular Phonetic Targets (PROMPT) (e.g., Dale & Hayden, 2013);
- Integrated phonological awareness intervention (e.g., Moriarty & Gillon, 2006);
- Nuffield Centre Dyspraxia Programme-3 (NDP-3) (Williams & Stephens, 2004);
- Melodic intonation therapy (e.g., Helfrich-Miller, 1994);
- Touch-cue method (e.g., Bashir, Grahamjones, & Bostwick, 1984);
- Combined melodic intonation therapy and touch-cue intervention (Martikainen & Korpilahti, 2011);
- Combined stimulability and core vocabulary (Iuzzini & Forrest, 2010);
- Rate control therapy (Rosenthal, 1984);
- Biofeedback (e.g., Lundeborg & McAllister, 2007; Preston, Brick, & Landi, 2013); and
- Alternative and augmentative communication (AAC) (e.g., Binger, 2007).

In this section we provide a summary of four approaches (DTTC, ReST, PROMPT, and integrated phonological awareness intervention) that have supporting peer-reviewed published evidence. These four approaches also cover different age groups and severities of impairment. Our focus on four approaches does not mean that other approaches such as the Nuffield Centre Dyspraxia Programme-3 (NDP-3) (Williams & Stephens, 2004), melodic intonation therapy (Helfrich-Miller, 1994), and the touch-cue method (Bashir et al., 1984; Martikainen & Korpilahti, 2011) are ineffective. It simply means that more experimental evidence is needed on these approaches for clinicians to make informed clinical decisions guided by empirical research. Refer to Murray, McCabe, and Ballard (2014) for a systematic review of intervention outcomes for children with CAS.

■ Dynamic Temporal and Tactile Cueing (DTTC): Intervention for CAS

Dynamic Temporal and Tactile Cueing (DTTC) is an approach for children with severe CAS. As the name implies, DTTC is characterized by dynamic teaching and learning moments—carefully selected cues that change from one teaching moment to the next depending on a child's response.

Historical background

Dynamic Temporal and Tactile Cueing (DTTC) is an intervention based on principles of motor learning (Strand, Stoeckel, & Baas, 2006). It was developed and refined by Edythe Strand over a number of years, with early publications of the approach referring to it as a form of integral stimulation (e.g., Strand & Skinder, 1999; Strand & Debertine, 2000). It was designated as DTTC by Strand, Stoeckel, and Baas (2006).

Theoretical background

DTTC is based on the understanding that CAS is a problem with motor planning and programming. This translates into a focus on **movement sequences**, rather than individual phonemes (Strand, 1998). Children with CAS therefore need to learn the movement parameters needed to produce particular articulatory configurations and the transitions into and out of these configurations (Strand, 2012). The approach uses various types of imitation, multiple cues, and a slowed speech rate to shape movement sequences and practice of those sequences in speech (Strand et al., 2006). Imitation and cues are used to support and encourage the child's motor planning and programming skills. Refer to Chapter 5 for further information about motor planning and programming, and Chapter 11 for further information about the principles of motor learning.

Procedures

Unlike other approaches to intervention that are programmed and follow a sequence of phases (e.g., multiple oppositions), DTTC is based on principles of motor learning and guidelines about how those principles can be implemented with children with CAS. In this section we outline procedures, including different types of cues (and the timing of those cues), that characterize DTTC.

General overview of DTTC

DTTC is typified by a dynamic response to children's efforts to produce speech from one teaching moment to the next. To appreciate the dynamic nature of this teaching moment, it is important to understand the similarities and differences between conventional descriptions of integral stimulation (e.g., Rosenbek et al., 1973) and DTTC. Integral stimulation involves imitation supported by the gradual withdrawal of multiple cues, notably auditory and visual models (Jakielski, 2011). One of the earliest and best examples of integral stimulation is the Eight-Step Continuum—an approach originally developed for adults with acquired apraxia (Rosenbek et al., 1973). This approach begins with maximally supportive cues that slowly fade in a hierarchical manner from mimed imitation to immediate imitation, followed by successive repetition and then delayed imitation, culminating with spontaneous production "as the speaker is able to take increasing responsibility for the assembly, retrieval, and execution of the motor plan" (Yorkston et al., 2010, p. 400). Refer to Chapter 12 for descriptions of these different types of imitation.

DTTC is similar to conventional descriptions of integral stimulation, in that it is characterized by different types of imitation and multiple supporting cues. However, it differs in its **dynamic** or "back-and-forth, adding and fading of cues" from one teaching moment to the next (Yorkston et al., 2010, p. 417). The term **temporal** reflects the process of "varying the amount of time between the clinician's stimulus and the child's imitative response" (p. 417). The term **tactile** refers to the use of tactile-phonetic cues, manual guidance (motokinesthetic cues), and gestural cues to help a child achieve initial articulatory configurations and, if needed, guidance through the movement sequence.

Unlike integral stimulation proposed by Rosenbek et al. (1973), there is no strict incremental hierarchy or predetermined set of criteria that a child must work through when using DTTC. Rather, DTTC uses intervention procedures guided by principles of motor learning, providing cues based on individual children's ages, ability, and difficulties, and most importantly, their moment-to-moment response to intervention. You still strive towards a goal, progressing from easier to more challenging stimuli with fewer cues or supports. However, the journey taken to get there is dynamic and gradual in nature—supporting children as they need support and withdrawing support as they develop their motor planning and programming abilities. Essentially, you focus your teaching moments on the child's challenge point—the point at which the child is learning without being overwhelmed and unable to produce the desired response (Guadagnoli & Lee, 2004). What follows is an overview of teaching procedures that characterize DTTC, based on Strand (2012) and Yorkston et al. (2010).

Provide auditory and visual models

Establish the minimal conditions required to elicit a targeted response from a child. Begin with an auditory and visual model of a target word or functional phrase and request that the child imitate your model. You could start with immediate repetition. If that is too challenging for the child, step down and try simultaneous or mimed imitation. If the child's imitation response is generally correct, continue with repeated practice of that word or phrase, to ensure that the child's production is segmentally accurate and natural with respect to rate and prosody (Yorkston et al., 2010). Work towards delayed imitation (providing a delay between your model and the child's opportunity to imitate you) and spontaneous productions.

Provide supporting cues as needed

If a child has difficulty imitating you (i.e., using only auditory and visual cues), then provide additional supporting cues as needed. The types of cues that you will use will depend on the child's age and area of difficulty. You could use manual guidance (i.e.,

COMMENT: *"Let's say it together!"*

Imitation is an important element of DTTC. However, not all children with CAS will simply repeat back what you say. Rosenbek et al. (1973) proposed a useful verbal imitation hierarchy. We illustrate it below using the word *bye*:

■ **Simultaneous imitation:** "Let's say it slowly together, *bye*."

■ **Mimed production:** "Let's say it together. I will pretend to say it while you say it out loud, *bye*."

■ **Immediate repetition:** "You say it straight after me, ready, look and listen, *bye*."

■ **Successive repetition:** "You say it straight after me five times, ready, look and listen, *bye*."

■ **Delayed repetition:** "You say it after me, but only when I point to you. You have to wait, ready, *bye*." (The clinician counts from 1 to 5 seconds and then points to the child indicating that it is his or her turn.)

During an imitation attempt, the child is encouraged to intently watch the clinician's face and listen to the clinician's speech as speech movements are made. Strand and Skinder (1999) suggest that young children's visual attention to a person's face and general imitation skills can be encouraged through behavioral principles, particularly positive reinforcement.

motokinesthetic cues) in addition to visual-, verbal-, and tactile-phonetic cues, and/or prosodic cues, orthographic cues, sound-referenced rebuses, shaping, a key phonetic environment, a gestural cue, and/or metaphonological instruction to help a child achieve initial articulatory configurations and the ensuing movement sequence. For instance, to help a child say *bye* you could physically assist the child to achieve the correct jaw and lip position, then say the rest of the word together, slowly. Yorkston et al. (2010) recommend that you encourage children to stay in an initial articulatory configuration "for a few moments, to maximize proprioceptive processing" before articulating the rest of the word (p. 417). If a child finds this task challenging, you could simplify it even further by temporarily removing the voicing component of a spoken word and focusing the child's attention on production of a smooth, continuous movement (Strand, 2012). Once the child is able to make the speech-related mouth movement, reinsert the voicing characteristic.

Movement sequences

Avoid pausing during a syllable and segregating the movement, as the child will miss out on the opportunity to practice movement sequences—the very problem the child needs to work on (Strand, 2012). For instance, if the target word is *bye*, do not insert a breath between the [b] and the vowel. If you need to help a child sequence syllables (e.g., *butterfly*), you can start with part practice, but only if it involves simplification or additive segmentation (i.e., the progressive parts method), not fractionation (Skelton, 2004b). Refer to Chapter 11 for further information about the practice fraction principle of motor learning.

Speech rate

Use a slowed speech rate when a child is first acquiring a new speech production skill (Yorkston et al., 2010). As the child's production of a word or phrase improves, reduce the amount of additional support provided and increase the child's rate until it is natural.

Encourage conscious attention

Encourage a child to think about or consciously attend to the speech movements being produced, rather than mindlessly imitating you, in an effort to help the child refine and improve subsequent attempts at the movement (Strand, 2012). It would be important that this focus occurs during the pre-practice phase of intervention, when the child is first acquiring a

> **COMMENT:** *What type and amount of stimuli are used in DTTC?*
>
> The type and amount of stimuli that you target during a DTTC session depends on the severity of a child's problem and the findings from your analysis. For a child with limited, highly unintelligible speech, you could start with simple syllables (CV, VC) comprising early developing stimulable consonants (e.g., [h], glides, nasals) and vowels in meaningful words (e.g., *hi, me, more, no, wow!*) (Strand & Skinder, 1999). It is important that you start with syllables (rather than speech sounds in isolation), because you are addressing a movement problem that includes difficulty making smooth articulatory transitions from one sound to the next (Strand & Skinder, 1999). The inclusion of some two- or three-word functional phrases comprising simple syllable structures for young children (e.g., *hi Dad; me too!*) is also recommended with young children to encourage intelligible and functional communication. As the child improves, you would increase the syllabic and segmental complexity of the stimuli. By contrast, for an older school-age child with mild or moderate difficulties, your stimuli might focus on multisyllabic real words or nonwords representing various types of lexical stress (e.g., Sws, wSs) (e.g., Ballard et al., 2010; Maas & Farinella, 2012).

particular skill. Once the child is engaged in intensive practice, external (rather than internal) attentional focus may help facilitate generalization (Lisman & Sadagopan, 2013).

Encourage intense production practice

Incorporate opportunities for production practice—ideally, frequent sessions involving massed blocked and random practice. Strand (2012) recommends five 20- or 30-minute sessions per week comprising a high dose. Edeal and Gildersleeve-Neumann (2011) found that a dose of 100 to 150 productions in a 15-minute period was better than 30 to 40 productions during the same period. This equated to two 15-minute blocks (i.e., 200 to 300 trials) per 30-minute session. Regarding blocked and random practice, Maas and Farinella (2012) suggest that blocked practice might be useful to establish basic motor patterns early on in DTTC intervention for CAS, with random practice being introduced at a later point to facilitate generalization. Edeal and Gildersleeve-Neumann (2011) used a combination of blocked and random. They began with blocked practice until the child was able to produce the targeted speech skill with 80% accuracy over two sessions. Once achieved, random practice was employed until an error occurred. Blocked practice was re-implemented until the target was reestablished in 5 to 10 correct productions. In this way, practice was dynamic and in keeping with the child's response to during teaching moments. Use these empirically based suggestions to guide your schedule of blocked and random practice for the children you work with.

Encourage attention and motivation

Ensure that children are attentive and motivated during drill-play activities. Strand and Skinder (1999) offer some helpful suggestions:

- Change the position of the child and the therapist every 10 to 20 trials (e.g., stand up, sit under the table, sit backward on the floor, put one hand in the air, and put both hands in the air).
- Change the inflection of the target utterance once the child has accurate movement and rate. (e.g., say the utterance with a high pitch followed by low pitch, sing the utterance, say the utterance with different feelings, say the utterance varying the intensity—loud and quiet). This encourages varied (rather than constant) practice, and as such helps facilitate generalization.
- Use reinforcers that do not take too much time during the session and, ideally, keep the child's attention on the clinician's face (refer to Chapter 11 for further ideas).

COMMENT: *How do you collect treatment data during dynamic teaching and learning moments?*

Data collection during the implementation of DTTC can seem challenging because you are not providing a child with opportunities to practice a particular intervention target with one type of support for a prescribed dose (e.g., 100 trials without a model). The support you provide can change from one teaching moment to the next. How then do you evaluate the efficacy of your intervention, particularly the collection of quantitative treatment data? As discussed in Chapter 12, there are different types of data. You can still plan for and collect quantitative and qualitative generalization and control data when implementing DTTC. Treatment data, however, may need to be qualitative— collecting ratings of the child's overall level of support (both frequency and type) per set of trials or per activity. For instance, using a rating scale you would write down your numeric rating of the child's response to intervention at the end of every 20 trials. The ratings could include:

1 = constant maximal cues (e.g., simultaneous model, manual guidance, slow speech rate)

2 = frequent maximal cues (e.g., mimed imitation and slowed speech rate)

3 = occasional fading cues (e.g., immediate or successive imitation)

4 = few cues fading (e.g., successive or delayed imitation)

5 = no cues needed

Evidence

In a systematic review of treatment outcomes for children with CAS, DTTC was identified as one of three approaches with preponderant evidence (Murray et al., 2014). Most of the evidence for DTTC has used single-case experimental designs (e.g., Baas, Strand, Elmer, & Barbaresi, 2008; Edeal & Gildersleeve-Neumann, 2011; Maas, Butalla, & Farinella, 2012; Maas, & Farinella, 2012; Strand & Debertine, 2000; Strand, Stoeckel, & Baas, 2006). The approach has been replicated by researchers other than the developer.

Children suited to DTTC

DTTC is suitable for young as well as older children with CAS. It is recommended for children with more severe CAS, with other approaches considered more suitable for children with primarily prosodic difficulties or mild-moderate impairment (Murray et al., 2014).

Resources for conducting DTTC intervention

The resources needed to implement this approach will depend on the child's age, severity, attention, and intervention targets. You will need basic resources such as picture stimuli or objects in addition to materials such as motivating yet simple reinforcers and activities that do not take time and distract a child from production practice. A helpful overview of the approach is available on DVD (Strand, 2010). As a beginning clinician, talk with and observe an experienced clinician conducting DTTC. Like other intervention approaches for managing SSD, implementation of DTTC requires practice and good observation skills. Some of the commercially available intervention programs (e.g., Czarnik, 2010; Williams & Stephens, 2004) include resources that could be adapted to suit DTTC intervention.

■ Commercial intervention programs for CAS

There are a number of commercial intervention programs suitable for children with CAS that have been developed by and are used by SLPs. Most of these programs are based on one or more principles of motor learning (see Chapter 11) and advocate a developmental approach to target selection, moving from easier to more challenging speech production tasks. Table 14-3 provides a summary of a selection of these programs, including comments on the amount and type of peer-reviewed published evidence. As a beginning clinician, it can be appealing to use ready-made programs such as these, as they provide you with a detailed program, descriptions of teaching procedures, record forms, and resources for the stimuli to be targeted in intervention. As an evidence-based clinician, we encourage you to consider the underlying theory motivating the programs and their evidence base (including peer-reviewed published experimental evidence and your own practice-based evidence).

TABLE 14-3　**Commercial intervention programs for CAS**

Program	Description	Evidence
Nuffield Centre Dyspraxia Programme-3 (NDP-3) (Williams & Stephens, 2004)	■ Based on the psycholinguistic model by Stackhouse and Wells (1997) (see Chapter 5). ■ Contains an assessment, therapy manual, and extensive picture resource. ■ The picture stimuli are divided into three sections: (i) single sounds, (ii) words of different phonotactic structures, and (iii) combinations of words in phrases, clauses, and sentences (Williams & Stephens, 2010). ■ Available in paper and electronic versions.	■ Murray, McCabe, and Ballard (2015) presented results of an RCT comparing NDP-3 with ReST (Ballard et al., 2010). Study protocol was reported in Murray et al. (2012). ■ Williams and Stephens (2004): six case studies in the NDP-3 manual. ■ Belton (2006) and Teal (2005): unpublished master's dissertations.
Kaufman Speech to Language Protocol (K-SLP) (Kaufman, 1998)	■ Targets simple syllable shapes and words through to more complex two- and three-syllable words. ■ Various materials have been produced by the developer (e.g., instructional DVD; Kaufman K-SLP Treatment Kit: Basic Level; Kaufman K-SLP Treatment Kit: Advanced Level)	■ Unpublished case study data, available from the Kaufman Children's Center website.
Treatment Program for Childhood Apraxia of Speech (Czarnik, 2010)	■ Based on principles of motor learning, emphasizing movement sequences (Czarnik, 2010). ■ The program includes an instruction manual, stimulus cards, and tactile-kinesthetic cue cards.	■ Expert opinion
Speech-EZ Apraxia Program (Carahaly, 2010)	■ The main focus of the program is on motor planning; however, it does cover other areas such as phonological awareness, auditory perception, and auditory working memory. ■ Multiple cues are used (e.g., visual, auditory, proprioceptive, gestural, and tactile), including symbolic hand cues. ■ The program emphasizes the importance of regular home practice and includes a parent manual. ■ Paper-based and electronic resources are available.	■ Expert opinion

> **COMMENT:** *A rare case of obstructive sleep apnea and CAS*
>
> Caspari, Strand, Kotagal, and Bergqvist (2008) report an interesting case of a child (6 years old) with obstructive sleep apnea, seizures, and CAS. The child was essentially nonverbal, having made no functional gains in his speech productions despite receiving intervention for many years. Following tonsillectomy for obstructive sleep apnea "he experienced a reduction in seizures and rapid growth in speech production" (Caspari et al., 2008, p. 422). At age 6;2 years, he had four intelligible words. Nine months after the tonsillectomy he had at least 100 intelligible words. This rare case highlights the importance of thorough clinical investigation and collaboration with health professionals.

■ Rapid Syllable Transition Treatment (ReST): Intervention for dysprosody in CAS

Rapid Syllable Transition Treatment (ReST) is an intervention that targets lexical stress. You would consider this approach for children with CAS whose speech sounds robotic. Robotic speech can be a symptom of a syllable sequencing difficulty, whereby strong and weak syllables in words all sound strong.

Historical background

ReST was designed to address one of the three key characteristics of CAS: "inappropriate prosody, especially in the realization of lexical or phrasal stress" (ASHA, 2007b, p. 2). It was conceived by Donald A. Robin, with the first experimental rendition for children reported by Ballard et al. (2010). The approach emerged out of an interest in the therapeutic application of the principles of motor learning for motor speech disorders.

Theoretical background

ReST is influenced by Schmidt's (1975) schema theory of motor control and learning (see Chapter 5), and the principles of motor learning (see Chapter 11). These principles guide the initial acquisition and then generalized learning of a motor skill through recommendations about the structure and conditions of practice; the type, frequency, and timing of feedback; and attentional focus. As you read through the procedures for conducting ReST, reflect on the theoretical principles that underlie the approach.

ReST intervention is also influenced by knowledge and theories about children's acquisition of lexical stress, how stress is marked in words, and the challenges for children with CAS in assigning stress. Lexical stress is usually realized through changes in vowel duration, vocal pitch, and vocal intensity. Words with a trochaic stress pattern (i.e., Sw stress) begin with stressed syllables that have longer vowel durations, higher peak intensity, and higher pitch (Ballard et al., 2010). Words with iambic stress (i.e., wS stress) can be more challenging for children, as they begin with syllables that are shorter, softer, and lower in pitch (McCabe, Macdonald-D'Silva, Van Rees, Ballard, & Arciuli, 2014). Polysyllabic words can be particularly challenging because they require children to vary their realization of stress from one syllable to the next. For example, correct realization of lexical stress in *computer* /kəmpjutɚ/ requires that you start with a weak syllable, transition to a strong syllable, and then finish with a weak syllable. Children with CAS can present with excessive, equal, or misplaced stressed in words and inconsistencies in the way they mark stress (e.g., Ballard et al., 2010; Munson, Bjorum, & Windsor, 2003; Peter & Stoel-Gammon, 2005; Shriberg, Aram, & Kwiatkowski, 1997). Authors differ on the underlying nature of this difficulty, with some viewing it as primarily a speech-related difficulty (e.g., Shriberg, Aram, & Kwiatkowski, 1997) and others suggesting that it reflects a broad problem with internal timing mechanisms: the Internal Metronome Hypothesis (Peter & Stoel-Gammon, 2005). The developers of ReST ascribe to the understanding that CAS "is a speech motor disorder that, in part, affects control of temporal parameters of speech movements that underlie production of prosodic features at the syllable level" (Ballard et al., 2010, p. 1228).

Procedure

ReST intervention involves intensive practice of multisyllabic pseudo-words (Murray, McCabe, & Ballard, 2012). Although the main focus of the intervention is lexical stress, the approach also targets difficulties with transitions from sound to sound or syllable to syllable, and articulation accuracy (McCabe & Ballard, 2015). An overview of ReST intervention follows.

Prepare pseudo-word stimuli

You will need to prepare a list of multisyllabic pseudo-words comprising two or three syllables in length. The words need to have a variety of stress patterns, beginning with weak and strong onsets (e.g., wS, Sw, wSs, Sws). The words should adhere to the phonotactic rules of the child's ambient language and should contain consonants and vowels that a child is capable of producing accurately (McCabe & Ballard, 2015). The words can be presented as a written stimulus (rather than assigned to a referent and given meaning) with the spelling orthographically biased so some words begin with weak onsets while others begin with strong onsets (McCabe et al., 2014). For example, be**doon** (wS), and **far**begee (Sws). In Ballard et al. (2010), strong syllables were depicted in bold font to contrast with the weak syllables—for example, **baa**teegoo (Sws) versus baateegoo (wSs). Ballard et al. (2010) provide an example of the words used in an intervention study with children aged 7 to 10 years. If a child does not have adequate literacy to read the novel stimuli, then the clinician can provide an auditory model for direct imitation (McCabe et al., 2014). Across published research on ReST intervention, the words have comprised the consonants [t, m, n, f, b, g], the vowels [ɑ, i, u, ə], and the syllable shapes CVCV and CVCVCV (e.g., Ballard et al., 2010; McCabe et al., 2014; Murray et al., 2012; Thomas et al., 2014). McCabe and Ballard (2015) suggest that the starting point in intervention should be CVCVCV words. If a child struggles at this level, two-syllable words would be used. As a child improves, more complex word shapes and segments (including clusters) can be practiced. The words can also be practiced in short sentences such as "Can you find my ___" (Ballard et al., 2010, p. 1232). Once you have your list of words, divide it into words for treatment and words to be monitored for change in a generalization probe.

Instructions and feedback

ReST focuses on three skills: lexical stress, smooth articulatory transitions, and articulation accuracy. The instruction and feedback that you use needs to facilitate children's understanding of these three skills, in addition to their ability to self-monitor. You could begin by talking about how:

- words are made up of speech sounds and syllables,
- some syllables have long strong beats and some have short quiet beats, and
- syllables in words glide from one to another without stops in between.

You could supplement your verbal description with auditory models in addition to prosodic, gestural, and metaphoric cues as needed. To ensure that a child has understood the concepts, you could also include opportunities for auditory detection of prosodic characteristics (see Chapter 11). In a study with three children aged 7 to 10 years, Ballard et al. (2010) used the terms **emphasis**, **fluency**, and **loudness** to address problems with lexical stress and articulatory transition. The word "emphasis referred to getting the durational contrast; fluency to speaking at a habitual rate without pauses, hesitations, or repetitions; and loudness to overall intensity level for the sentence" (Ballard et al., 2010, p. 1232). These

COMMENT: *Why pseudo-words in ReST?*

McCabe and Ballard (2015) suggest that pseudo-words (as opposed to real words) are useful for practicing rapid, fluent, and natural-sounding multisyllabic sequences without the interference of ingrained errors from real words in a child's linguistic/semantic system. They also suggest that rearranging the syllables in a pseudo-word to create other pseudo-words encourages a child work on the underlying problem of motor planning and programming.

terms translated into knowledge of performance feedback, such as "emphasis and fluency were spot on, but your voice was too loud" (Ballard et al., 2010, p. 1232).

One of the participants in the study by Ballard and colleagues also required rhythmic tapping and metaphoric visual aids (long and short blocks arranged on a table) to encourage appropriate syllable durations at a natural speech rate. For younger children, McCabe and Ballard (2015) recommend using simpler terms such as beats for syllable stress and smoothness for articulatory transitions. Your feedback about articulation accuracy may be minimal (e.g., correct or incorrect) because consonants and vowels are selected that the child can already produce accurately (McCabe et al., 2014). However, if a child's articulation is inaccurate during an attempt at one of the pseudo-words, you could provide relevant phonetic cues to encourage articulation accuracy. A production is considered correct if all three characteristics are accurate (McCabe & Ballard, 2015).

Pre-practice

An intervention session begins with a period of pre-practice. This is an opportunity for the child to acquire knowledge and the ability to produce the targeted skill. A child's knowledge could initially be developed through an auditory detection activity, that is, identifying whether words have a long-short (Sw) or short-long (wS) stress pattern (McCabe et al., 2014). You could then use production cues (see Chapter 12) and feedback (including knowledge of results and knowledge of performance) to help a child produce the target words. During the first few sessions, pre-practice may last as long as 20 minutes in a 50- to 60-minute session. As a child's understanding of the response requirement and skill improves, the pre-practice phase of a session can be shorter (e.g., 10 minutes) (Thomas et al., 2014). The pre-practice phase of a session finishes when a child produces five consecutive trials of a random selection words (including Sw and wS onsets) correctly (McCabe et al., 2014).

Practice

The practice phase of a session involves drill-style practice—at least 100 productions—divided randomly into sets of 20 to 25 trials with a brief 2-minute rewarding activity between sets (McCabe & Ballard, 2015). Children who can read the pseudo-words do so, while younger children (or children who struggle to read the words accurately) can repeat the word after the clinician (McCabe et al., 2014). In contrast with pre-practice, feedback during practice is limited to knowledge of results (KR) (i.e., letting a child know if the response was right or wrong), delayed by a few seconds following each attempt, and reduced from high to low frequency across the total number of trials in a session (Murray, McCabe, & Ballard, 2015). For example, Ballard et al. (2010) and Murray, McCabe, and Ballard (2015) provided knowledge of results on 50% of responses on a sliding scale, with 100% on the first 10 trials through to 10% on the last 10 trials. You will need to let the children know the difference between pre-practice and practice (i.e., delayed and limited feedback) and encourage them to listen to and self-evaluate each production attempt (Ballard et al., 2010).

Generalization probes

It is important to include response generalization probes over the course of this intervention, because the research on this approach suggests that the use of pseudo-words does not necessarily guarantee an improvement in real words and/or connected speech (e.g., Ballard et al., 2010; McCabe et al., 2014).

Service delivery

ReST should be delivered intensely, such as four times a week in 50- or 60-minute sessions (McCabe & Ballard, 2015). It can be delivered less frequently (e.g., twice weekly), although the effect of intervention (particularly on maintenance and generalization to real words) may be diminished (Thomas et al., 2014).

Evidence

ReST is a relatively new intervention option for managing dysprosody in children with CAS. To date the approach has been investigated by Ballard and colleagues. This evidence includes a randomized controlled trial comparing ReST with the Nuffield Centre Dyspraxia Programme (Murray, McCabe, & Ballard, 2015) and three studies using single-case experimental designs (Ballard et al., 2010; McCabe et al., 2014; Thomas et al., 2014). Across the evidence, ReST can improve children's production of treated and untreated pseudo-word stimuli. More frequent sessions and performance criterion of at least 80% correct during intervention seemed to be important for generalization (Thomas et al., 2014). Generalization to real words and conversational speech has varied across participants, with some showing minimal change and others showing improved production. We encourage you to read further research on this approach as it is published, as researchers refine the procedure and identify strategies for ensuring functional generalization.

Children suited to ReST

ReST is suited to children with mild or moderate CAS characterized by dysprosody, particularly poor lexical stress (Murray et al., 2014). Children who cannot produce words comprising two or more syllables with differing consonants and vowels such as *bedoon* (regardless of stress accuracy) are not suitable (McCabe & Ballard, 2015). Based on previous research, it would be suitable for children from 4 years; however, more of the participants involved in the research have been of school age. Children would need to have relatively good comprehension and metalinguistic abilities to understand the prosodic feedback, such as "Emphasis and fluency were spot on, but your voice was too loud" (Ballard et al., 2010, p. 1232).

Resources for conducting ReST intervention

You need to compile stimuli comprising pseudo-words with varying stress patterns, ideally two and three syllables in length. For resources, Ballard et al. (2010) presented their written words such as **baa**teegoo (Sws) and baa**tee**goo (wSs) in 24-point Times New Roman font on individual cards, with the stressed syllables in bold font. You would also need a rewarding activity that can be played for a few minutes between practice sets. For some children you may need short and long building blocks as visual aids to symbolize the relative durations of the strong and weak syllables (Ballard et al., 2010).

■ Prompts for Restructuring Oral Muscular Phonetic Targets (PROMPT): Intervention for motor speech disorders

The Prompts for Restructuring Oral Muscular Phonetic Targets (PROMPT) program "uses tactile cues to support and shape movements of the oral articulators in order to improve the production of individual sounds, syllables, words, and eventually connected speech" (Grigos, Hayden, & Eigen, 2010, p. 46).

Historical background

PROMPT was developed by Deborah Hayden in the 1980s (e.g., Chumpelik, 1984) as a tactile-kinesthetic method for assessing and treating motor speech disorders in children and adults (Dale & Hayden, 2013). The PROMPT program's focus on tactile cues or physically assisted articulation echoes aspects of moto-kinesthetic therapy developed by Stinchfield-Hawk and Young (1938). You need to be trained as a PROMPT-certified SLP to use the approach. This certification involves post-qualification training over 1½ to 2 years and includes "two courses and two self-study projects" (Hayden, Eigen, Walker, & Olsen, 2010, p. 464). Given that specialist knowledge and skill is required to implement this approach, we provide only a brief overview. If you are interested in learning more about PROMPT, visit the PROMPT Institute website, and review peer-reviewed published evidence on the approach.

Theoretical background

PROMPT is influenced by a number of different theories that focus on the role of somatosensory input in speech development, including dynamic systems theory (Thelen & Smith, 1994), neuronal group selection theory (Edelman, 1987), and motor learning theories (e.g., Schmidt, 1975). Drawing on these theories, PROMPT is based on the understanding that "tactile input is used to effect somatosensory change and promote motor speech accuracy while the motor skill is simultaneously linked to cognition and socially relevant communication content" (Hayden et al., 2010, p. 459). Although verbal-tactile cues and hands-on manual guidance (i.e., physical prompts) are characteristic of the approach, PROMPT is not limited to these cues. As Hayden (2006) emphasizes, PROMPT is a broad-based approach capitalizing on "the entire act of communication, including how the physical-sensory, cognitive-linguistic and emotional-social domains develop and interact in normally developing humans" (Hayden, 2006, p. 265). Refer to Hayden et al. (2010) for further information about the theoretical background.

Procedure

PROMPT begins with a comprehensive assessment of a child across the three domains: physical-sensory, cognitive-linguistic, and emotional-social. Assessment findings are then used to form a Global Domain Profile, which is a profile of the child's areas of strength and weakness (Hayden, 2006). A detailed assessment of a child's speech subsystems is also conducted, with results interpreted against a motor speech hierarchy (MSH) (Hayden, 2006). This hierarchy is divided into seven stages of motor speech development and control, including: "Stage I: tone, Stage II: phonatory control, Stage III: mandibular control, Stage IV: labial–facial control, Stage V: lingual control, Stage VI: sequenced movements, and Stage VII: prosody" (Dale & Hayden, 2013, p. 646). Intervention then targets a child's identified areas of difficulty through relevant "dynamic TKP [tactual-kinesthetic-proprioceptive] cues that physically guide the child's speech movements with concurrent auditory and visual input," with cues being "faded as speech movement patterns improve" (Dale & Hayden, 2013, p. 646).

Four different types of PROMPT cues can be used in intervention: **parameter**, **syllable**, **complex**, and **surface** prompts (Hayden, 2006). Parameter prompts provide maximal support and stability for one parameter (the face or the jaw); surface prompts provide tactile information about the place, timing, or transition of an articulator; syllable prompts are a combination of parameter and surface prompts that shape CV and VC syllables, and complex prompts provide information about the production of a specific phoneme (Dale & Hayden, 2013). This is a brief overview PROMPT. As we have mentioned, correct implementation of PROMPT requires training from a certified PROMPT instructor.

Evidence

Peer-reviewed published evidence on PROMPT has been based on pre-post within-group studies (Kadis et al., 2014; Namasivayam et al., 2015), single-case experimental research (Dale & Hayden, 2013; Square, Namasivayam, Bose, Goshulak, & Hayden, 2014; Ward, Leitão, & Strauss, 2014; Ward, Strauss, & Leitão, 2013), and case study data (Grigos, Hayden, & Eigen, 2010). Across this research, positive reports about the effect of PROMPT intervention have been noted. Dodd and Bradford (2000) reported that the approach was not effective for three children with phonological impairment. The approach has been replicated by researchers other than the developer.

Children suited to PROMPT

PROMPT is suitable for children with mild-to-severe motor-speech-based SSD such as CAS (e.g., Kadis et al., 2014), and childhood dysarthria (e.g., Ward et al., 2014). Hayden et al. (2010) also suggest that it is suitable for children with SSD accompanied by hearing impairment, Down syndrome, attention deficit disorder (ADD), attention-deficit/hyperactivity disorder (ADHD), pervasive developmental disorders, or autism spectrum disorder. Dodd and Bradford (2000) indicated it is not suitable for children with phonologically based SSD. Hayden et al. (2010) suggest that children as young as 18 months may be suitable for PROMPT; however, "it is generally recommended for use with children from 2 years or older" (p. 454).

Resources for conducting PROMPT intervention

You need to complete post-qualification training with a certified PROMPT trainer associated with the PROMPT Institute to conduct this approach. Refer to the PROMPT Institute website for further information.

■ Integrated phonological awareness intervention for CAS

Integrated phonological awareness intervention targets speech production, phonological phoneme awareness, and letter knowledge in children with SSD. In Chapter 13, we provided an overview of this approach for preschoolers with phonological impairment. In this section, we provide an overview of the approach as it has been applied to children with CAS.

Historical background

Integrated phonological awareness intervention was developed by Gail Gillon. Gillon (2000) reported that the approach improved the speech production and phonological awareness abilities of 5- to 7-year-old children diagnosed with phonological impairment (and in some cases concomitant semantic or syntactic difficulties). Gillon (2005) applied a similar version of this approach to preschoolers with phonological impairment (see Chapter 13). Moriarty and Gillon (2006) applied the approach to children with CAS, targeting speech production, phoneme awareness, and letter knowledge.

Theoretical background

Integrated phonological awareness intervention is built on two understandings: (1) children with CAS have difficulty with motor speech processes and the establishment of detailed underlying phonological representations of words (Moriarty & Gillon, 2006), and (2) young children with CAS are at risk of future literacy difficulties (Stackhouse & Snowling, 1992a). It is thought that "traditional approaches used to target articulation in CAS may do little to develop skills that are critical to early literacy acquisition" (Gillon & Moriarty, 2007, p. 48). If these children's risk of literacy difficulties is to be addressed, then they need intervention that integrates speech production, phonological awareness, and letter knowledge (McNeill, Gillon, & Dodd, 2009a). Integrated intervention is thought to facilitate more detailed underlying phonological representations and more stable motor programs, improved speech production, phoneme awareness, letter knowledge, word decoding, and spelling (McNeill et al., 2009a).

Procedure

Integrated phonological awareness intervention includes speech production practice with phonological awareness and letter knowledge activities (McNeill et al., 2009a). The phonological awareness activities focus on the phonemic level. Letter knowledge activities focus on letter names and sounds, targeting explicit links between phonemes and graphemes. An overview of the approach follows, including targets and stimuli, phoneme awareness, and letter knowledge tasks, and how speech production practice is integrated in phoneme awareness tasks.

Intervention targets and stimuli
Intervention targets include phonemic awareness, letter knowledge (names and sounds), and phonological error patterns in a child's speech. McNeill et al. (2009a) targeted substitution (e.g., velar fronting) and structural phonological processes (e.g., final consonant deletion, cluster reduction) in 12 children with CAS, using real-word stimuli.

Phonemic awareness and letter knowledge tasks
Intervention sessions include phonological awareness tasks focused on phoneme (rather than syllable or rhyme) awareness and include phoneme identification, blending, segmentation, and manipulation (Moriarty & Gillon, 2006). Letter name and sound knowledge tasks (using written letters and written words beneath picture stimuli) are incorporated during the phoneme awareness tasks. These tasks focus on developing children's knowledge of letter names and their corresponding sounds, with an emphasis on recognition. Table 14-4 provides an overview of the types of tasks that have been used in research on this approach with children with CAS.

Integration of speech production practice during phoneme awareness tasks
Children's speech production skills are targeted through metalinguistic talk and production practice during phoneme awareness activities. For example, "if the child was working

TABLE 14-4   Integrated phonological awareness intervention: Example phoneme awareness and letter knowledge tasks

Task	Description and example
Phoneme identification	Identify, categorize, and sort phonemes at the beginning, middle, and end of words. For example, find all the toys/pictures starting with the same sound as a target word; group pictures according to their first sound or last sound; memory games matching words that have the same first or last sound; generate words that begin with the same sound as a target word.
Blending	Combine phonemes to form spoken syllables and words. For example, blending onsets with rimes (e.g., "d-og"), blending single-syllable words without clusters (e.g., "d-o-g"), blending phonemes in single-syllable words with clusters (e.g., "s-t-o-p").
Segmentation	Separate the phonemes that make up a word. For example, "segmenting single-syllable words into phonemes using colored blocks to represent different phonemes" (Gillon, 2004, p. 166). For younger children, Moriarty and Gillon (2006) suggest an activity where a child teaches a puppet to talk, by saying the words slowly, eventually separating out all the sounds.
Manipulation	Removing and replacing phonemes in words to make new words. For example, erasing the first consonant of a written word and replacing it with another consonant to make a new word
Letter-sound knowledge activities	Develop children's knowledge of letter names and their corresponding sounds. In a study with 3- and 4-year-old children, Gillon (2005) targeted letter-sound knowledge using recognition (rather than recall) activities, beginning with letters with a wide visual contrast. Letters can be incorporated into phoneme awareness activities such as bingo (e.g., "Do you have a word that starts with the letter s that makes an /s/ sound?" Gillon, 2005, p. 315).

Sources: Adapted from Gillon (2004, 2005); McNeill, Gillon, and Dodd (2009); and Moriarty and Gillon (2006).

on suppressing the s-cluster reduction error pattern, he or she would be required to segment words that contained an s-cluster" (McNeill et al., 2009a, p. 351). If a child's production of a target word is incorrect, phonological awareness cues would be used to facilitate correct production. For example, if the target word is *step* /step/ and a child says [tep], the clinician could say, "Nice try. I heard you say three sounds. Step has four sounds (pointing to the blocks). There's a /s/ sound at the start (pointing to the first block). Try and say step again with a /s/ sound at the start" (Moriarty & Gillon, 2006, p. 734). This focus on metalinguistic talk is a unique aspect of this approach. Rather than imitating an auditory model only, children are expected to use the phonological awareness cues from a clinician to create motor plans. The cues for this teaching moment are based on research by Bradford-Heit and Dodd (1998), who reported that "imitation on its own was not at all useful in improving production accuracy" (p. 173) for children with CAS. Rather, the children benefitted from imitation combined with phonological awareness cues to facilitate phonological planning. For example, if the target word is *cat*, the clinician could say, "Good try. It sounds like the word *bat* but starts with /k/. Try again, *cat*." This is slightly different to Gillon's (2005) application of the approach for children with phonological impairment, as those children received phonological intervention (specifically the cycles approach) concurrent with activities targeting phonemic awareness and letter knowledge.

Service delivery

The approach has been administered two and three times weekly, in 45-minute sessions with an SLP (McNeill et al., 2009a, b; Moriarty & Gillon, 2006). Research is needed on the recommended dose and total intervention duration, in addition to the value of follow-up home practice.

Evidence

Evidence on integrated phonological awareness intervention for children with CAS has been reported in studies involving single-case experimental designs (McNeill et al., 2009a; Moriarty & Gillon, 2006) and a longitudinal case study (McNeill et al., 2009b).

APPLICATION: *Intervention approaches suitable for Michael*

Michael (4;2 years) has CAS, characterized by dysprosody (e.g., *caterpillars* /kætə-pɪlə-z/ was pronounced as [kæʔ.pɪʔ.wəs]). Assessment indicated that he tended to produce words with two or more syllables with equal stress. There was also evidence of syllable segregation. What intervention approaches might be suitable for Michael?

Answer: ReST (McCabe & Ballard, 2015) would be suitable for Michael, as it was designed to specifically address dysprosody. It would be important to collected response generalization data to monitor generalization to non-treatment words and everyday conversational speech. Given Michael's age, he would also benefit from integrated phonological awareness intervention (McNeill et al., 2009a) to mitigate his increased risk of future literacy difficulties.

Read more about
Michael (4;2 years),
a boy with childhood
apraxia of speech (CAS),
in Chapter 16 (Case 4).

The approach has also been reported in a retrospective control study (with two groups) involving children with phonological impairment (Gillon, 2005), and in a two-group randomized experimental design involving children with concomitant morphosyntax and phonological impairment (Tyler et al., 2011). Kirk and Gillon (2007) reported that children with phonological impairment who received integrated phonological awareness intervention during the years before school became proficient readers. By contrast, McNeill, Gillon, and Dodd (2010) found that children with CAS who received a similar intervention would require additional support to develop their written language skills.

Children suited to integrated phonological awareness intervention

Integrated phonological awareness intervention is suitable for children with CAS (e.g., Moriarty & Gillon, 2006), phonological impairment (Gillon, 2005), and Down syndrome (e.g., Van Bysterveldt, Gillon, & Foster-Cohen, 2010).

Resources for conducting integrated phonological awareness intervention

You will need a variety of resources such as pictures that include the written word and large cards displaying lowercase letters. The materials that you need would depend on the activities played during intervention sessions. An instruction manual including word list stimuli, pictures, and letter resources (Gillon & McNeill, 2007) is freely available on Gail Gillon's website at the University of Canterbury, New Zealand.

INTERVENTION FOR CHILDHOOD DYSARTHRIA

Intervention for childhood dysarthria depends on the type and severity of the problem. Just as no two children are the same, no two interventions for children with childhood dysarthria will be the same. It will depend on the type and severity of the dysarthria and range of speech subsystems affected.

■ Systems approach: Intervention for childhood dysarthria

The systems approach is a broad-based method for addressing multiple areas or speech subsystems. Interventions that target a particular subsystem (e.g., laryngeal, respiratory) are embedded within the systems approach.

Historical background

A systems approach for managing childhood dysarthria has a long history in speech-language pathology (e.g., Froeschels, 1952; Hodge & Wellman, 1999; Levy, 2014; Love, 1992,

2000; Pennington, Miller, Robson, & Steen, 2010). During the 1950s and 1960s it was recognized that speech subsystems—respiratory, laryngeal (phonation), velopharyngeal (resonance), and articulatory systems—could be negatively impacted when a neurological impairment affects muscles needed to produce clear, intelligible speech (Love, 2000). Over time, various researchers have used the generic label, a systems approach (e.g., Pennington et al., 2010), when referring to methods for improving speech intelligibility through targeting subsystems. Levy (2014) designated it as Speech Systems Intelligibility Treatment (SSIT).

Theoretical background

A systems approach to intervention is based on an understanding that impairments in speech subsystems (respiratory, laryngeal, velopharyngeal, and articulatory) can have a negative impact on a child's speech intelligibility (Love, 2000). Depending on the severity of impairment, this impact could be minor or profound. If an assessment reveals that it is abundantly clear that intelligible speech is unlikely, then augmentative and alternative forms of communication (AAC) would be investigated (Love, 2000). However, if an assessment indicates that a child has the potential to use speech, a systems approach could be used to ensure that the child's potential is realized. This section is about management strategies for those children. The role of AAC when working with children with motor speech disorders is addressed later in this chapter. Across the evidence on a systems approach to intervention, procedures involving practice of a particular motor skill are usually based on principles of motor learning (e.g., Levy, 2014; Pennington et al., 2010; Pennington et al., 2013).

Procedure

A systems approach is characterized by procedures and strategies designed to improve a child's speech intelligibility. The procedures focus on one or more subsystem (e.g., adequate seating for speech respiration) and/or speech characteristics (e.g., loudness). An overview of selected strategies and procedures designed to improve a child's speech intelligibility follows.

Encourage respiratory support and breath control for speech

Trying holding your breath and talking at the same time, it is not possible. Although you can move your articulators, your words will be inaudible. Audible speech requires breath. That breath needs to be controlled, so that phonation can be sustained over an utterance. Speech breathing, as opposed to tidal breathing, involves quicker inhalation of larger volumes of air and slower exhalation in accordance with the needs of an utterance (Parham, 2013). For children with cerebral palsy, such breathing can be challenging. Pennington and colleagues developed and tested a program to help with this difficulty (Pennington, Smallman, & Farrier, 2006; Pennington et al., 2010; Pennington et al., 2013). In summary, their program focuses on:

- increasing children's awareness about breathing and its importance for speech;
- discussion about the importance of correct seating and posture;
- speech production exercises focused on speaking at the beginning of exhalation—beginning with sustained vowels followed by phrases;
- practice "speaking slowly and maintaining breath supply across a phrase, taking a new breath at syntactically appropriate places" (Pennington et al., 2010, p. 339);
- production practice adhering to a hierarchy and performance criteria for advancing from one level to the next. The hierarchy includes: (1) 10 frequently used phrases, (2) novel phrases comprising single words, (3) sentences, then (4) conversation (Pennington et al., 2010); and
- exercises to practice breath control during phrases to ensure adequate intensity and stress (Pennington et al., 2006).

Throughout production practice, principles of motor learning are applied, including "high-intensity practice, random practice of target behaviors within each exercise and then between exercises once the criterion was reached, frequent feedback initially to aid skill acquisition, and then fading feedback to promote skill retention, knowledge of results and knowledge of performance" (Pennington et al., 2010, p. 339). In an effort to promote generalization, a stimulus or cue phrase that conversational partners could use with the children can be included to encourage and provide opportunities for practice. Pennington et al. (2006) reported that their participants' speech intelligibility improved at word level only. Their intervention was provided 5 days per week, in 20- to 30-minute sessions, for 5 weeks. Pennington et al. (2010) reported that 30- to 45-minute intervention sessions 3 times per week for 6 weeks resulted in improvements in both word level and conversational speech intelligibility in children aged 12 to 18 years. A similar finding was reported for younger children aged 5 to 11 years (Pennington et al., 2013).

Reduce hypernasality

Hypernasality is a common problem for children with childhood dysarthria. A range of procedures and strategies have been reported in the literature, with success often dependent on a child's broader characteristics. For example, Davison, Razzell, and Watson (1990) reported that pharyngoplasty (a surgical technique designed to reduce nasal air escape) in conjunction with speech-language pathology intervention improved the speech intelligibility in 11 out of 16 children. Davison et al. (1990) suggested that good lip posture and tongue function were important presurgical characteristics for a good outcome. Other options have included the use of a palatal lift (e.g., Holley, Hamby, & Taylor, 1973; Shaughnessy, Netsell, & Farrage, 1983). The behavioral strategy of encouraging a reduced speaking rate (in an effort to reduce nasal air emission and hypernasality) might be helpful for some children; however, as Yorkston et al. (2010) point out, behavior-based strategies may only be suitable in very mild cases of velopharyngeal dysfunction.

Improve speech intelligibility through targeting articulation

A common feature of childhood dysarthria is imprecise articulation. A variety of strategies can be trialed to address this imprecision and improve speech intelligibility. Ward et al. (2014) reported that PROMPT intervention was associated with an improvement in the speech production accuracy in six children with cerebral palsy. Significant changes were also detected in "specific movement characteristics of the jaw and lips" (Ward et al., 2013, p. 136). Hustad (2010) suggests that "for those children who do not have respiratory, phonatory, or velopharyngeal impairments that make significant contributions to intelligibility deficits, traditional articulation therapy may be useful"; however, she emphasizes that mastery of speech targets (i.e., adultlike production) "is almost never a realistic goal because of underlying neurological impairment" (p. 374). Phonological interventions such as minimal pairs intervention (see Chapter 13) could also be a useful option, particularly if a child has existing error patterns or a difficulty contrasting phonemes (Hustad, 2010). Another option is to target another speech subsystem. Pennington (2012) suggests that more precise articulation and improved intelligibility can be achieved "through developing control of breathing for speech, increasing background effort and slowing speech rate" (p. 172).

Interventions involving instrumental biofeedback have also shown promise at improving the articulation of children with childhood dysarthria. Marchant, McAuliffe, and Huckabee (2008) trialed phonetic (articulation) placement intervention combined with surface electromyography (sEMG) facilitated biofeedback relaxation intervention with a 13-year-old girl with severe spastic dysarthria. Improvements were reported in single-word articulation but not overall speech intelligibility. Nordberg, Carlsson, and Lohmander (2011) reported that EPG feedback for alveolar consonants [t, d, n, s] resulted in improved patterns of articulatory contact in five children with cerebral palsy. Nordberg et al. (2011) also noted that EPG was a useful tool for detecting abnormal tongue-palate contact patterns associated with dental and alveolar consonants in children with dysarthria and cerebral palsy. Morgan, Liégeois, and Occomore (2007) reported that EPG may help improve speech accuracy in adolescents with dysarthria following traumatic brain injury.

Increase healthy loudness

Speech intelligibility in children with childhood dysarthria can be compromised because of reduced volume. Several researchers have reported that LSVT LOUD (Lee Silverman Voice Treatment)—an intensive intervention designed to increase sound pressure level (loudness), intelligibility, and vowel space in adults with Parkinson's disease—can improve speech function in children with cerebral palsy (Boliek & Fox, 2014; Fox & Boliek, 2012; Fox et al., 2008; Levy, 2014; Levy, Ramig, & Camarata, 2012). To implement LSVT LOUD, you need to be certified through post-qualification training with LSVT Global.[7] The LSVT LOUD program is conducted in an intensive format, such as 1-hour sessions scheduled four times a week for 4 weeks in conjunction with structured daily home practice (Levy, 2014). Each session is divided in half. During the first half, the focus is on "sustained vowel phonation, maximal pitch range (rising and falling), and functional phrases" (Levy, 2014, p. 346). During the second half, the session focuses on hierarchically based speech production tasks that change from week to week (e.g., words or phrases followed by sentences, reading, and conversational speech). Given the intensity of the intervention, motivating activities are used as part of the practice. See Levy (2014) for a helpful example of how motivating activities were used as part of a 7-year-old boy's intervention involving LSVT LOUD.

Evidence

The evidence for a systems approach to intervention covers all speech subsystems, albeit in a limited manner for some subsystems (e.g., resonance) and with mostly low levels of evidence. Most of the research has included single-case experimental designs (e.g., Dale & Hayden, 2013; Fox & Boliek, 2012; Morgan et al., 2007) and case studies (e.g., Boliek & Fox, 2014; Levy et al., 2012; Pennington et al., 2006; Shaughnessy et al., 1983), with a limited number of group studies (e.g., Pennington et al., 2010).

Children suited to the systems approach

Children with childhood dysarthria who have been assessed as having the potential to use speech are suitable for intervention based on the systems approach. The type of intervention that a child receives depends on the speech subsystem that most impacts a child's speech intelligibility.

Resources for conducting the systems approach

The resources needed to implement a systems approach to intervention depend on the speech subsystem of focus. Intervention targeting respiration and phonation would include stimuli relevant to an individual child (e.g., functional words and phrases) and corresponding resources (e.g., pictures of functional words and phrases). Intervention using a specific program such as PROMPT or LSVT LOUD requires post-qualification training and certification.

■ Using Augmentative and Alternative Communication (AAC) to improve speech and/or enhance activity and participation for children with severe motor speech disorders

Children with motor speech disorders, particularly children with severe CAS or childhood dysarthria, may benefit from using augmentative or alternative communication (AAC). AAC refers to "some form of communication intended to supplement or replace typical communication skills when an individual has difficulty communicating" (Oommen & McCarthy, 2014, p. 118). There are two broad types: unaided and aided communication. Unaided communication does not need an additional device, such as using the hands for sign language, the face to communicate facial expression, and the voice to communicate non-symbolic vocalization (Hourcade, Everhart Pilotte, West, & Parette, 2004). Aided communication uses external equipment for communication, such as an alphabet supplementation board, theme-specific communication boards, communication books, and dictionaries in addition to speech-generating devices (Binger, 2007).

Questions SLPs might consider when working with a child with a severe motor speech disorder include: does the child need AAC, is the child and/or family open to using AAC, when should AAC be introduced, what type of AAC should be recommended, and does the child have the prerequisite skills (e.g., fine motor skill, reading ability, cognition) needed to use a particular type of AAC? Your answers will depend on each child's situation. For some children you might recommend augmenting their spoken language with

---

[7]http://www.lsvtglobal.com

sign language or an alphabet supplementation board (pointing to the first letter of each word while speaking), so that they use multimodal forms of communication (Binger, 2007; Hanson, 2014). Dowden (1997) provides a helpful overview of speech supplementation strategies for children with motor speech disorders. For other children, with highly unintelligible speech even with familiar listeners, you might recommend alternative forms of communication. Detailed discussion of the issues regarding the use, timing, type, and training of AAC for children with motor speech disorders is beyond the scope of this book.

APPLICATION: *Alphabet supplementation board: Make sure communication partners know how to use them*

Children with severe motor speech disorders need to have "spelling skills that are sufficient to correctly identify initial letters of words" (Yorkston et al., 2010, p. 347) if they are to successfully use an alphabet supplementation board. It is also important that communication partners know how to communicate with children (or adults, for that matter) who use a board. How could you do this?

Answer: Yorkston et al. (2010) suggest that you include instructions for communication partners, such as: "To help you understand me, I will point to the first letter of each word as I speak. Please say each word after me. I'll let you know if you are wrong. If you don't understand a word, let me know and I will repeat it or spell it for you. Please don't finish the sentences for me unless I ask you to do so. Thank you for your patience" (p. 338).

APPLICATION: *Will AAC discourage my child from using speech?*

Imagine you are working with a 3-year-old child with highly unintelligible dysarthric speech. The child is frustrated and unable to communicate his basic needs and wants. During a discussion with the child's family, you recommend that AAC be trialed. The family asks you, "Will AAC discourage my child from using speech?" As an evidence-based clinician, what would your answer be?

Answer: You would reassure the family that AAC is a viable option for children with highly unintelligible speech, because it offers children a means of developing functional communication. Using supporting evidence (e.g., Silverman, 1995), you would also explain that AAC strategies can actually encourage (as opposed to discourage) children to use speech.

COMMENT: *Intervention is more than speech; it is about activities and participation*

When you work with children with childhood dysarthria, particularly associated with cerebral palsy, you will be a member of a multidisciplinary team. This team could include a neurologist, physiatrist, ophthalmologist, pediatrician, psychologist, SLP, physical therapist, occupational therapist, educator, and expert in computer-assistive technology (Trabacca et al., 2012). You work together with the child and his or her family to enhance the child's activity and participation in society. Trabacca et al. (2012) describe a helpful ICF-CY-based neurorehabilitation program for a 12-year-old boy with cerebral palsy. The case study highlights the importance of tailoring intervention to an individual child's needs.

■■■■■■■■■■■■■■■■■■■■■■■■■■■■■■■■■■■■■■■

 APPLICATION: Intervention options for Lian

Lian has spastic dysarthria. In light of her assessment results (see Chapter 16) and goals (see Chapter 10), what intervention approaches would be suitable for Lian?

Answer: Lian was motivated to improve her contrast between the consonants /ʃ, ʧ, ʤ/. Lian's speech intelligibility was also negatively influenced by other factors such as reduced loudness, mild hypernasality, and difficulty with breath control. A systems approach would be suitable for Lian, addressing respiration/phonation, loudness, resonance, and articulation. Within this broad-based approach, a number of options are possible. In light of Lian's motivation and own goals, minimal pairs intervention could be trialed to improve her contrast between the phonemes /ʃ, ʧ, ʤ/ in English. Regarding respiration/phonation, the approach described by Pennington et al. (2010) could be trialed to improve Lian's speech breathing and breath control. Her hypernasality may improve as a result of learning how to better manage speech breathing for intelligibility. Another option could be to trial an intensive period of LSVT LOUD (Levy, 2014).

Read more about Lian (14;2 years), a girl with childhood dysarthria, in Chapter 16 (Case 5).

Chapter summary

In this chapter you learned about motor speech interventions for children with articulation impairment characterized by residual errors, CAS, and childhood dysarthria. You learned about the history and theory underlying various approaches. You also learned about the procedures and resources needed to implement the approaches, and the evidence underscoring them.

Suggested reading

You can learn more about motor speech interventions for children in Caruso and Strand (1999) and Yorkston et al. (2010). Yorkston et al. include a DVD of three children with CAS and two children with childhood dysarthria. Other helpful texts for beginning clinicians include Fish (2011) and Velleman (2003). The following readings relate to each of the intervention approaches:

Traditional articulation intervention

■ Secord, W. A. (1989). The traditional approach to treatment. In N. Creaghead, P. W. Newman, & W. A. Secord (Eds.), *Assessment and remediation of articulatory and phonological disorders* (pp. 129–158). New York, NY: Macmillan.

■ Van Riper, C., & Erickson, R. L. (1996). *Speech correction: An introduction to speech pathology and audiology* (9th ed.). Needham Heights, MA: Allyn & Bacon.

Concurrent treatment

■ Skelton, S. L. (2004a). Concurrent task sequencing in single-phoneme phonologic treatment and generalization. *Journal of Communication Disorders, 37*(2), 131–155.

■ Skelton, S. L., & Hagopian, A. L. (2014). Using randomized variable practice in the treatment of childhood apraxia of speech. *American Journal of Speech-Language Pathology, 23*(4), 599–611.

Articulation intervention using instrumental feedback

■ Bernhardt, B. M., Stemberger, J., & Bacsfalvi, P. (2010). Vowel intervention. In A. L. Williams, S. McLeod, & R. McCauley (Eds.), *Interventions for speech sound disorders in children* (pp. 537–555). Baltimore, MD: Paul H. Brookes.

■ Gibbon, F., & Wood, S. (2010). Visual feedback therapy with electropalatography. In A. L. Williams, S. McLeod, & R. McCauley (Eds.), *Interventions for speech sound disorders in children* (pp. 509–536). Baltimore, MD: Paul H. Brookes.

■ McAllister Byun, T., & Hitchcock, E. R. (2012). Investigating the use of traditional and spectral biofeedback approaches to intervention for /r/ misarticulation. *International Journal of Speech-Language Pathology, 21*(3), 207–221.

Dynamic Temporal and Tactile Cueing (DTTC)

- Maas, E., & Farinella, K. A. (2012). Random versus blocked practice in treatment for childhood apraxia of speech. *Journal of Speech, Language, and Hearing Research, 55*(2), 561–578.

- Strand, E. A., & Skinder, A. (1999). Treatment of developmental apraxia of speech: Integral stimulation methods. In A. Caruso & E. A. Strand (Eds.), *Clinical management of motor speech disorders in children* (pp. 109–148). New York, NY: Thieme.

Rapid Syllable Transition Treatment (ReST)

- Ballard, K. J., Robin, D. A., McCabe, P., & McDonald, J. (2010). A treatment for dysprosody in childhood apraxia of speech. *Journal of Speech, Language, and Hearing Research, 53*(5), 1227–1245.

- McCabe, P., & Ballard, K. (2015). ReST program. In C. Bowen (Ed.), *Children's speech sound disorders* (2nd ed.). Oxford, UK: Wiley-Blackwell.

Prompts for Restructuring Oral Muscular Phonetic Targets (PROMPT)

- Hayden, D., Eigen, J., Walker, A., & Olsen, L. (2010). PROMPT: A tactually grounded model for the treatment of childhood speech production disorders. In A. L. Williams, S. McLeod, & R. J. McCauley (Eds.), *Interventions for speech sound disorders in children* (pp. 453–474). Baltimore, MD: Paul H. Brookes.

Integrated phonological awareness intervention

- McNeill, B. C., Gillon, G. T., & Dodd, B. (2009a). Effectiveness of an integrated phonological awareness approach for children with childhood apraxia of speech (CAS). *Child Language Teaching and Therapy, 25*(3), 341–366.

Systems approach

- Hodge, M., & Wellman, L. (1999). Management of children with dysarthria. In A. Caruso & E. A. Strand (Eds.), *Clinical management of motor speech disorders in children* (pp. 209–280.). New York, NY: Thieme.

- Levy, E. S. (2014). Implementing two treatment approaches to childhood dysarthria. *International Journal of Speech-Language Pathology, 16*(4), 344–354.

Augmentative and Alternative Communication (AAC)

- Hanson, E. K. (2014). My client talks! Do I still need to consider AAC in my treatment planning? Speech supplementation strategies: AAC for clients who talk! *Perspectives on Augmentative and Alternative Communication, 23*(3), 124–131.

- King, A. M., Hengst, J. A., & DeThorne, L. S. (2013). Severe speech sound disorders: An integrated multimodal intervention. *Language, Speech, and Hearing Services in Schools, 44*(2), 195–210.

- Oommen, E. R., & McCarthy, J. W. (2014). Natural speech and AAC intervention in childhood motor speech disorders: Not an either/or situation. *Perspectives on Augmentative and Alternative Communication, 23*(3), 117–123.

Application of knowledge from Chapter 14

1. Select one of the cases of children with a motor speech disorder from Chapter 16 (Michael or Lian) and prepare a session plan. Target a short-term goal (based on what you learned in Chapter 10), using one of the suitable approaches described in this chapter. Compare and contrast your session plan with that of a peer.

2. At the end of Chapter 11, you were asked to draft a management plan and session plan for Susie. Now that you are familiar with intervention approaches suited to articulation impairments, complete your management plan and session plan for Susie.

3. Create stimuli for conducting Skelton's (2004a) concurrent treatment approach with Susie. The stimuli should address all relevant exemplar types including /s/ in word-initial singleton, word-initial consonant cluster, within word, and word-final contexts in syllables, words, and two- to four-word phrases and sentences, in addition to a conversation topic strategically designed to elicit /s/. Use the examples in Table 14-2 as a guide. Create a suitable resource (e.g., paper-based picture cards, electronic picture resource) to elicit the stimuli with Susie in a randomized order.

4. Assume you are going to use the ReST approach with Michael (4;2 years) to address his difficulty with lexical stress, associated with CAS. Prepare a list of 40 multisyllabic pseudo-words comprising two or three syllables in length to use with Michael, dividing them evenly between wS, Sw, wSs, Sws stress patterns. Make sure that the words contain consonants and vowels that Michael is capable of producing accurately (see Chapter 16 for Michael's speech assessment results) (McCabe & Ballard, 2015). Your list could be written so that strong syllables are depicted in bold font.

15

Evidence-Based Practice in Practice

LEARNING OBJECTIVES

1 Describe the seven-step process for engaging in evidence-based practice.

2 Compare and contrast the terms *evidence-based practice, empirically supported practice,* and *practice-based evidence.*

3 Appraise the scientific rigor of assessment, diagnostic, and intervention evidence for working with children with SSD.

4 Explain how ethical guidelines direct clinical practice with children with SSD.

5 Compare and contrast international policies relevant to the management of SSD in children.

KEY WORDS

Evidence-based practice: PICO questions, external published evidence, clinical practice, client factors, values, and preferences

Ethics: respect for autonomy, nonmaleficence, beneficence, justice

Policies, conventions, and laws: international, national, speech-language pathology professional associations

OVERVIEW

Good clinical decisions are grounded in knowledge and motivated by expertise. In Chapter 1 of this book you learned about evidence-based practice (EBP)—a helpful framework for guiding your clinical decisions. In subsequent chapters of this text you learned about typical speech acquisition, assessment, analysis, goal setting, intervention, and how to monitor and evaluate children's progress over the course of intervention. Throughout the chapters you have applied your knowledge to cases of children with SSD to make clinical decisions. You now need to think about how you will integrate that knowledge in the context of everyday clinical practice with real children and their families. This chapter describes a seven-step process for making evidence-based decisions when working with children with SSD, using Dollaghan's (2007) E^3BP framework. You will learn how to use your clinical expertise to integrate published research evidence (external evidence) with two complementary sources of evidence from everyday clinical practice (internal clinic and client evidence). The better you understand these different sources of evidence, the better prepared you will be to work with children and their families. You will learn about a range of policies relevant to children with SSD, such as the United Nations Conventions on the Rights of the Child (UNCRC) and the No Child Left Behind (NCLB) Act. You will also become familiar with the ethical guidelines that direct your practice and the professional associations that support your practice.

WHAT IS EVIDENCE-BASED PRACTICE (EBP)?

EBP is a conceptual framework for guiding good clinical decisions. Recall from Chapter 1 that it refers to "the conscientious, explicit, and judicious integration of 1) best available *external* evidence from systematic research, 2) best available evidence *internal* to clinical practice, and 3) best available evidence concerning the preferences of a fully informed patient" (Dollaghan, 2007, p. 2). You use your clinical expertise to integrate the three sources of evidence to make decisions.

If it has been a while since you read Chapter 1, revisit the overview of EBP, E^3BP, and Figures 1-4 and 1-5 before reading any further. You need to understand Dollaghan's (2007) definition and the idea that there are three sources of evidence, to appreciate the steps involved in the conduct of EBP. You also need to have read the chapters on assessment and intervention to appreciate many of the examples in this chapter and to complete the clinical application tasks.

> **COMMENT:** *What's the difference between empirically supported practice and EBP?*
>
> Clinical practice based solely on good-quality peer-reviewed published research is empirically supported practice, not EBP. Although reasonable, clinical decisions are supported by only "one of the three components of evidence-based practice" (Schlosser & Sigafoos, 2008, p. 61). EBP is more encompassing. It is characterized by clinical decisions based on an integration of empirical evidence, evidence from clinical practice, and evidence on the characteristics, values, and preferences of children and their families, on a case-by-case basis.

Integrating External Published Evidence with the Reality of Clinical Practice and Client Factors, Values, and Preferences

Across literature on EBP, you will find a range in the number of steps involved in the conduct of EBP. Some literature outlines four steps (e.g., Brackenbury, Burroughs, & Hewitt, 2008; Justice, 2010), some outlines six steps (e.g., Johnson, 2006), and others up to seven steps (e.g., Baker & McLeod, 2011b; Gillam & Gillam, 2006). We adopt the seven-step process in this chapter, because it accounts for all three sources of evidence. Four-step frameworks do not tend to include steps for considering internal clinic and client evidence. The seven steps are outlined in Table 15-1.

■ Step 1: Generate a PICO clinical question

The first step in making a sound clinical decision requires the generation of a PICO clinical question. A PICO question should include four elements: Patient, Intervention, Comparison, Outcome (hence the acronym PICO) (Straus & Sackett, 1998). You can use a PICO question to consider the benefits and risks of using a particular intervention approach relative to another intervention approach (or no intervention) in achieving a specific outcome for a specific client population. You can also use a PICO question to evaluate the diagnostic value of one assessment tool or diagnostic marker compared to another for a specific client population. PICO questions typically emerge from preliminary thinking, questioning, discussion, and/or brief literature searching on a general topic. Examples of preliminary questions include: "What is the most reliable assessment tool for identifying CAS in children?" or "What evidence-based approaches exist for treating phonological impairment in children?" or "What intervention approaches are the most efficient for children diagnosed with CAS?" or "Is group therapy for children with phonological impairment effective?" or "Can the future risk of literacy difficulties associated with SSD be addressed before children start formal schooling?" or "Is my current approach to intervention as efficient as the new approach I just read about?"

Having thought through the general issue, it is important that a clearly defined, answerable PICO clinical question be generated. PICO questions may address an issue relevant to many of the children seen by an SLP in a particular clinical service, or they may focus on a specific clinical case that you have uncertainties about. Examples of diagnostic and intervention PICO questions that address specific aspects of clinical service include:

TABLE 15-1 **A seven-step decision-making process for engaging in EBP when working with children with SSD**

Step
1. Generate a PICO (Patient, Intervention, Comparison, Outcome) clinical question.
2. Find external evidence relevant to the question.
3. Critically evaluate the external evidence.
4. Evaluate the internal evidence from your clinical practice.
5. Evaluate the internal evidence with respect to child and family factors, values, and preferences.
6. Make a decision by integrating the evidence.
7. Evaluate the outcomes of the decision.

Sources: Adapted from Baker and McLeod (2011b), and Gillam and Gillam (2006).

- Diagnostic: Is the Diagnostic Evaluation of Articulation and Phonology (DEAP) (Dodd, Hua, et al., 2006) more accurate than the Hodson Assessment of Phonological Patterns: Third Edition (Hodson, 2004) for identifying 4-year-old children within my clinic with SSD?
- Intervention: Does the PACT approach (Bowen, 2010) lead to significantly greater gains in percent consonants correct (PCC) compared with the multiple oppositions approach (Williams, 2010) for children with severe phonological impairment and no other concomitant conditions?

PICO questions may also address the needs of a specific child or specific group of children on your caseload. For example:

- For Spanish-English bilingual children learning the Puerto Rican dialect of Spanish and General American English, is the Contextual Probes of Articulation Competence: Spanish (Goldstein & Iglesias, 2009) more reliable than the Hodson-Prezas Assessment of Spanish Phonological Patterns (Hodson & Prezas, 2010) for identifying SSD?
- For a child (4;5 years) with inconsistent speech errors, does the core vocabulary approach (Holm, Crosbie, & Dodd, 2013) lead to significantly improved consistency of speech production compared with traditional pairs intervention?
- For a 4-year-old child with CAS secondary to Russell-Silver syndrome, is three times weekly 30-minute SLP intervention sessions and daily home practice using the Nuffield Centre Dyspraxia Programme (NDP-3) (Williams & Stephens, 2004) associated with greater gains in speech intelligibility compared with once weekly 60-minute SLP sessions and daily home practice using the same intervention?

As the examples illustrate, each PICO component in a clinical question may be placed in any particular order, and may be specified to a greater or lesser degree, depending on the issue being considered (Dollaghan, 2007). It is important to add that formulating clinical questions to find evidence to support current practice is not EBP. As Kamhi (2011) states, "If evidence is sought solely to support one's prior beliefs, contradictory evidence will likely be ignored or discounted" (p. 59). This means that your clinical questions need to emerge from your uncertainty or curiosity about an issue and, more importantly, your genuine interest in what the answer might be (Dollaghan, 2007).

■ Step 2: Find external evidence relevant to the question

Having generated a PICO clinical question, you need to answer the question by searching for relevant external research evidence. Much has been written about how to conduct electronic searches for published research evidence (see Brackenbury et al., 2008; Dollaghan, 2007; Gillam & Gillam, 2006). It can be efficient to begin with freely available summaries or syntheses of external evidence generated by constituted evidence review groups and organizations that produce or compile evidence-based summaries and guidelines (Dollaghan, 2007), such as:

 APPLICATION: *Writing a PICO question*

Parent: "Do you know whether it would be better for Matthew (6;2 years with a lateral lisp) to stay in the group to improve his speech, or whether would it be better if he saw you one on one for therapy?"

1. Reword the parent's question into a PICO-style question.
2. How would you determine the answer to the parent's question?

- Agency for Healthcare Research and Quality (AHRQ) National Guideline Clearinghouse[1]
- American Speech-Language-Hearing Association's (ASHA) National Center for Evidence-Based Practice in Communication Disorders (N-CEP), which produces evidence-based systematic reviews (EBSRs)[2] and evidence maps[3]
- Cochrane Collaboration[4]
- Campbell Collaboration[5]
- U.S. Department of Education Institute of Education Sciences, What Works Clearinghouse (WWC)[6]

If you do not find a systematic review or clinical practice guideline addressing your particular clinical question, then consider searching one of the many available databases. A selection of databases relevant to SSD in children includes PubMed, Scopus, MEDLINE, Embase, speechBITE (Speech Best Interventions in Treatment Efficacy), CINAHL (Cumulative Index to Nursing and Allied Health Literature), PsycINFO, ERIC (Education Resources Information Center), ASSIA (Applied Social Science Index and Abstracts), and Web of Science. Some of these databases are open access (e.g., speechBITE), while others could be accessed through your university library website (e.g., Scopus), assuming your library has an annual subscription. If you are not familiar with one or more of these databases, set aside some time to speak with a librarian about databases relevant to speech-language pathology practice and develop your literature searching skills.

Journal review articles can also provide a helpful source of synthesized external evidence. Publications that have summarized intervention and/or assessment research specifically about SSD in children include:

- Baker and McLeod (2011a) offer a narrative review of 134 studies addressing phonological intervention or intervention for children with phonological impairment/delay or disorder spanning 30 years from 1979 through 2009.
- Law, Garrett, and Nye (2003) and Law, Garrett, Nye, and Dennis (2012) present a detailed, systematic review of speech and language interventions for children with speech and/or language impairment.
- Lee and Gibbon (2015) completed a systematic review of the evidence associated with non-speech oral motor treatment for children with developmental SSD.
- McCauley, Strand, Lof, Schooling, and Frymark (2009) offer a review of the evidence associated with non-speech oral motor exercises.
- Morgan and Vogel (2008b) review the evidence on intervention for dysarthria associated with acquired brain injury in children and adolescents.

■■

 APPLICATION: *Search the evidence*

The PICO question stated in step 1 said, "For a child (4;5 years) with inconsistent speech errors, does the core vocabulary approach (Holm, Crosbie, & Dodd, 2013) lead to significantly improved consistency of speech production compared with minimal pairs intervention?" Search for and read the following peer-reviewed published intervention study: Crosbie, S., Holm, A., & Dodd, B. (2005). Intervention for children with severe speech disorder: A comparison of two approaches. *International Journal of Language and Communication Disorders, 40* (4), 467–491. Using a database relevant to speech-language pathology practice and the references in Chapter 13 associated with core vocabulary intervention, search for at least one more recent peer-reviewed published study on the core vocabulary approach.

---

[1]http://guideline.gov

[2]http://www.asha.org/Members/ebp/EBSRs.htm

[3]http://www.ncepmaps.org/

[4]http://www.cochrane.org

[5]http://campbellcollaboration.org

[6]http://ies.ed.gov/ncee/wwc/

- Murray, McCabe, and Ballard (2014) provide a systematic review of intervention outcomes for children with CAS.
- Nelson, Nygren, Walker, and Panoscha (2006) provide a systematic review of interventions for speech and language impairment in the preschool population, including a review of screening resources for this same population.
- Pennington, Miller, and Robson (2009) provide a review on interventions for children with dysarthria acquired before three years of age.
- Tyler (2008) offers an expert summary of intervention for children with SSD, with a particular focus on children who have concomitant phonological and morphosyntax difficulties.

A search may stop at this point, particularly if the PICO question is relatively broad, as someone may have already conducted the review for you. For example, the Law et al. (2003) review answers the following question: "For children with a phonological impairment (patient), does phonological intervention (intervention) lead to improved speech production skills (outcome) as compared with no intervention (comparison)?" Of the 25 studies reviewed by Law et al. (2003), seven compared the effect of intervention versus no intervention using standardized measures of overall phonological development. Five of these seven studies were based on phonological principles, while two were based on principles of traditional articulation therapy. Meta-analysis of the results of the seven investigations indicated that:

> The overall effect estimate was statistically significant favoring the use of speech and language therapy when compared to no treatment ($n=264$; SMD=0.44, 95% CI: 0.01, 0.86). This estimate increased when parent administered treatments were removed ($n=214$; SMD=0.67, 95% CI: 0.19, 1.16), and when interventions lasting less than eight weeks were removed ($n=213$; SMD=0.74, 95% CI: 0.14, 1.33). (Law et al., 2003, p. 10)

Questions relevant to a specific type of intervention approach and/or specific type of clinical presentation usually require more extensive searching. The studies reviewed in Chapters 13 and 14 could serve as a useful starting point for gathering evidence about a specific intervention named in a clinical PICO question. Review the assessment tools described in Chapter 8 for diagnosing SSD in children. This would be a useful starting point for answering specific PICO questions relevant to diagnosis.

It is worth noting that you may need to modify each of the PICO components in a clinical question depending on the extent of evidence gathered on the topic. Very specific clinical questions focused on a unique or rare clinical presentation (e.g., a preschool child with Joubert syndrome learning to speak both General American English and Korean) may need to be rephrased if no literature is found. Likewise, clinical questions that yield an overwhelming disparate body of literature may benefit from being further specified.

■ Step 3: Critically evaluate the external evidence

Having identified external evidence, it is important that you consider the nature and credibility of the evidence. It would be irresponsible, if not unethical, for you to make a diagnosis without conducting a valid and reliable assessment or to administer intervention

---

 APPLICATION: *Talking with parents about advice found on the Internet*

Parent: "I found some interesting information on the Internet about how using whistles and bubble blowing can help children improve their speech. The website had lots of comments from parents about how satisfied they were with the mouth toys. I was thinking they might be good for Peter. Do you use these mouth toys, and how do they work?"

How would you as a clinician answer the parent?

Hint: Read the Lee and Gibbon (2015) and McCauley et al. (2009) reviews of evidence associated with non-speech oral motor exercises (NSOME).

based on scientifically untested ideas. What might seem like a good idea at the time could turn out to be a waste of time, or worse still, detrimental for the children and families you work with. Just as you trust your medical practitioner to prescribe medication proven to work (and not cause harm), so too do the children and families with whom you work trust you to offer the best available evidence-based management of SSD. They also rely on your expertise to critically evaluate the wealth of publically available information on working with children with SSD.

Let's now take a look at two parameters for evaluating published evidence: the nature of the evidence and the credibility of the evidence.

Nature of evidence

The **nature** of evidence relates to the type or phase of study. Using the Fey and Finestack (2009) 5-phase plan for studying the effectiveness of language intervention, you need to determine the phase a published investigation best represents (see Fey & Finestack, 2009; Williams et al., 2010, for further information). The five phases include:

- ■ **Pre-trial study:** Investigations at this phase are not clinical trials. They may be studies designed to test a particular theory or establish issues of reliability or validity and may be conducted with typically developing children.
- ■ **Feasibility study:** Investigations at this phase may be clinical in nature, but do not establish efficacy. Feasibility studies determine whether a clinical idea is feasible or doable, and as such, help to determine whether a more labor-intensive and costly efficacy trial would be worthwhile (Munro, Lee, & Baker, 2008).
- ■ **Early efficacy study:** Early efficacy studies may be quasi-experimental or experimental and are designed to answer the important question as to the cause-effect relationship between an intervention and targeted skill, using treatment and no-treatment groups. Early efficacy studies are typically conducted under carefully controlled conditions and have a surrogate or artificial end point (Fey & Finestack, 2009), such as an improvement in a specific speech production skill.
- ■ **Later efficacy study:** Investigations of later efficacy are experimental, establishing a cause-effect relationship between an intervention and targeted skill under more generalizable conditions with more meaningful, broader measures of improvement (Fey & Finestack, 2009). Ideally, efficacy studies compare a new intervention approach with current or standard clinical practice.
- ■ **Effectiveness study:** Effectiveness investigations are like large-scale community-based clinical trials. They are only conducted once efficacy has been experimentally established under controlled conditions. Effectiveness studies examine outcomes of particular intervention approaches under everyday clinical conditions, with different or heterogeneous populations, and with varying service delivery formats, intervention agents, and/or contexts.

Credibility of evidence

Credibility encompasses two dimensions: type of research design and scientific quality. Each is important for critically evaluating research evidence.

Type of research design

Not all research evidence is equally credible. Depending on the phase of investigation, available resources, and personnel, some studies for children with SSD are better designed and executed than others. In part, it is the task of journal editors and peer reviewers to act as gatekeepers so that only credible research is published. As a reader, you are also expected to critique research evidence and determine its hierarchical credibility, otherwise known as level of evidence (LOE). Most LOE frameworks (e.g., ASHA, 2004a) offer a hierarchy for sorting published research according to research design rigor (e.g., randomized controlled trial [RCT], single-case experimental design [SCED], case study). The freely available database of Best Interventions in Treatment Efficacy (speechBITE)[7] completes this task for clinicians,

---

[7]http://www.speechBITE.com

TABLE 15-2   **Levels of evidence**

Ia: Well-designed meta-analysis of > 1 randomized controlled trial

Ib: Well-designed randomized controlled study

IIa: Well-designed controlled study without randomization

IIb: Well-designed quasi-experimental study (including single-case experimental designs [SCED] such as multiple baseline design across participants or behaviors)

III: Well-designed non-experimental studies, i.e., correlational and case studies

IV: Expert committee report, consensus conference, clinical experience of respected authorities

---

Source: ASHA (2004a). Used by permission from American Speech-Language-Hearing Association (ASHA).

in part, by assigning an LOE to published research. If you are unfamiliar with the process of identifying and ranking research according to the LOE, it would be a helpful exercise to identify and critique published research associated with a particular intervention approach of interest, determine the LOE, and then check your ranking with the ranking suggested by speechBITE or the appendix from the narrative review by Baker and McLeod (2011a). Table 15-2 lists the LOE according to ASHA (2004a).

Evaluating scientific quality of intervention research

The second task you need to do when evaluating the credibility of research evidence is to consider the scientific quality of an investigation. As Brackenbury et al. (2008) point out, just because a study may have used a design associated with a high level of evidence (e.g., RCT), it does not negate consideration of the quality of the study, nor does it mean that a study has automatic credibility.

A variety of systems have been proposed for critically evaluating the quality of research evidence (e.g., Bhandari, Richards, Sprague, & Schemitsch, 2001; Dollaghan, 2007; Maher, Sherrington, Herbert, Mosley, & Elkins, 2003; Tate et al., 2008; Verhagen et al., 1998). Refer to Table 15-3 for an overview of frameworks useful for evaluating the quality of speech-language pathology research.

speechBITE uses two of the scales listed in Table 15-3 (PEDro and SCED) to rate the quality of published research, and as such provides a helpful starting point for busy SLPs wanting an independent evaluation of the quality of identified studies. Dollaghan's (2007) checklist forms (listed in Table 15-3) are also helpful for guiding your evaluation of the quality of external research evidence.

 APPLICATION: *Evaluating the quality of scientific evidence*

Review the quality of the paper by Crosbie et al. (2005). You would have searched for and read this paper when completing the previous application task in this chapter.

1. Describe the quality of the study using the SCED scale. See Tate et al. (2008), or the speechBITE website[1] for more information about the SCED scale.
2. Discuss your overview of the study quality with a peer.
3. Compare your quality review with the SCED rating offered by speechBITE. To do this, search for Crosbie et al. (2005) on the speechBITE website.[1] If you use the keyword "core vocabulary," you will find the review of the paper relatively quickly.

---

[1]http://www.speechBITE.com

| TABLE 15-3 | Frameworks for rating the methodological quality of published research |

Rating framework	Description
PEDro (Herbert, Moseley, & Sherrington, 1998/99)	The PEDro scale is an 11-item scale originally designed to assess the internal validity of RCTs archived in the Physiotherapy Evidence Database (PEDro: Herbert et al., 1998/99). It was intended to address issues such as whether participants were randomly allocated to intervention conditions and whether assessors were blind to the condition to which participants had been randomly allocated (see Maher et al., 2003). This scale is used in speechBITE to rate the quality of papers reporting outcomes from RCTs.
SCED (Tate et al., 2008)	The SCED scale can be used to assess the methodological quality of SCED research—addressing issues such as the definition of targeted behaviors, the type of design used, the reliability of the reported observations, and the independence of the assessors involved in evaluating the outcome of an intervention (see Tate et al., 2008). This scale is used in speechBITE to rate the quality of papers reporting outcomes from SCED research.
CADE, CATE, CASM (Dollaghan, 2007)	Dollaghan (2007) proposed a series of helpful templates for critiquing the quality of published diagnostic and intervention research: ■ CADE: Critical Appraisal of Diagnostic Evidence; ■ CATE: Critical Appraisal of Treatment Evidence; and ■ CASM: Critical Appraisal of Systematic Review of Meta-Analysis. Dollaghan (2007) also includes checklists for appraising internal evidence from clinical practice with the CAPE (Checklist for Appraising Patient/Practice Evidence) and internal evidence from the children and families we work with using the CAPP (Checklist for Appraising Evidence on Patient Preferences).

■ Step 4: Evaluate the internal evidence from your clinical practice

Having identified and appraised external evidence, you need to consider three issues before applying the empirical answer to the PICO question, to clinical practice. First, ask yourself whether the external evidence-based recommendations are consistent with your clinical practice (or, as a student, what an experienced SLP might recommend). Second, if the external evidence-based recommendations align with current clinical practice, you need to determine whether the procedures and outcomes are in fact the same. The application of research to clinical practice does not guarantee replication of published outcomes. The unique characteristics and constraints of individual clinical and educational workplaces combined with the unique knowledge and experiences of individual SLPs prevent procedures from being replicated in exactly the same way with every case as in published research (Dollaghan, 2007). You need to determine what is possible in your clinical practice. As Dollaghan (2007) points out, this is a challenging task because "our strong preferences for what we already believe to be true makes us poor judges of whether it is actually true" (p. 3). Third, if the recommendations contrast or even conflict with current clinical practice, you are faced with one of two options. You either disregard the research recommendations (not an appealing option if the evidence is compelling!) or you modify your clinical practice and align it with the external evidence. How do you make this decision? You need to gather and critically evaluate good-quality internal evidence from your own clinical practice. What is internal evidence?

There are two broad categories of internal evidence from clinical practice. Firstly, evidence from your own work with children and their families. We refer to this as **clinical**

case-based evidence. The second type is internal clinical evidence from a speech-language pathology service or a group of similar speech-language pathology services. We refer to this latter type of evidence as **practice-based evidence** (Dobinson & Wren, 2013; Evans, Connell, Barkham, Marshall, & Mellor-Clark, 2003). Let's consider each of these two different types of internal evidence from clinical practice.

Internal evidence from clinical practice: Clinical case-based evidence

Internal evidence about what is possible from your own clinical practice is best derived from the systematic and regular collection and analysis of data from the children and families that you work with. This idea is best understood in the context of two different clinical scenarios. Firstly, suppose a parent of a child who has a phonological impairment asks you how long it will take for you to treat his or her child using a particular intervention approach? As a beginning clinician, you could answer the parent based on recommendations from the external evidence and advice from an experienced SLP. As you gain experience you could complement your empirically supported answer with a summary of your own clinical case-based evidence. This internal evidence could take a number of forms. As described in Chapter 12, you could draw on your own de-identified qualitative and/ or quantitative treatment, generalization, and control data from similar cases. You could also use your own database of the children and families you work with, based on broad subtypes of SSD in children. Within each subtype, this database could include basic information such as age, gender, and severity in addition to other relevant characteristics such as speech perception and production skills; family history of speech, language, or literacy difficulties; history of OME; and receptive and expressive language abilities. It would be important that your database include information about intervention intensity (i.e., average dose, session duration, session frequency, total intervention duration) (Warren, Fey, & Yoder, 2007), given the empirical evidence suggesting that this is an important variable when working with children with SSD (Baker, 2012a, b; Williams, 2012). See Chapter 11 for further information about intensity.

Secondly, suppose you have been working with a child for a couple of months and you have concerns about the child's progress. You have doubts about the clinical decisions you made. In this context you could collect clinical case-based data using single-case experimental design (SCED) methodology (refer to Chapter 12 for further information). You would then use the data to inform your clinical decision about how to work with the child and his or her family. Bear in mind, evidence-based decisions are only as good as the quality of the evidence on which they are based. Dollaghan (2007) provides a checklist for evaluating this type of internal evidence from clinical practice. The issues for consideration are not that dissimilar from the issues to be addressed when conducting SCED research, such as the stability of baselines prior to starting intervention, the magnitude of a treatment effect, independent or blind assessment of behavioral outcomes, and evidence of stimulus and response generalization. Although it is not always feasible to use SCED designs in everyday clinical practice, the application of such designs may be particularly helpful when you need definitive evidence about the benefit (or lack thereof) of a particular intervention with a specific case, or when you are learning a new intervention approach. Refer to Chapter 12 for further discussion about how to evaluate the efficacy of your intervention.

Internal evidence from clinical practice: Practice-based evidence

The second broad type of internal evidence from clinical practice is practice-based evidence (PBE). This type of evidence is "derived from routine practice settings rather than from efficacy studies" (Evans et al., 2003, p. 375). It is typically based on a standard outcome measurement system. Unlike your own detailed clinical case-based evidence, practice-based evidence typically provides data about the functional outcomes associated with particular speech-language pathology service(s). The American Speech-Language-Hearing Association has one such system, known as the National Outcome Measurement System (NOMS). This system includes a series of seven-point functional communication measures (FCM) specific to each area of speech-language pathology practice. For children with SSD, the relevant FCM is Articulation/Intelligibility (American Speech-Language-Hearing Association, 2016). See Chapter 7 on assessment for more information about outcome measures that can be used for children with SSD. To enable meaningful interpretation of the evidence and meaningful comparison across speech-language pathology services, it is important that you understand how to use an outcome measurement system. Appropriate training will ensure that your practice-based measures are reliable. Remember, however, that practice-based evidence "does not provide strong causal attribution but it addresses generalizability and enables location of the activities and outcomes of a particular service within the range of data from other services" (Evans et al., 2003, p. 375). In other words, you cannot use practice-based evidence to claim that your intervention caused the improvement in a particular child's speech, because practice-based outcome measures are broad, non-experimental descriptive measures.

■ Step 5: Evaluate the internal evidence with respect to child and family factors, values, and preferences

The third element of EBP requires consideration of two issues: child and family factors and values known or believed to influence intervention outcomes, and the fully informed preferences of children and their families. Let's consider each of these two issues. Regarding child and family factors and values, there is relatively little published evidence about factors and values definitively known to facilitate or hinder intervention progress. Of the research that has been done, **motivation** has been identified as one important factor (Kwiatkowski & Shriberg, 1998). High motivation may be a positive factor contributing to intervention outcomes, while low motivation may hinder progress. Baker and Bernhardt (2004) described child-related factors thought to have negatively influenced one child's intervention progress such as the child's language abilities and limited communicative awareness. In a study on clinician-identified factors thought to influence the speech and language outcomes of children with early identified severe/profound hearing loss, Fulcher, Purcell, Baker, and Munro (2015) reported multiple child and family factors such as the age of identification of hearing loss, and families' distance to services.

Given the individuality of children and their families, many factors and values may have a positive or negative influence on intervention outcomes. How can you find out what they might be? You could ask the parents, caregivers, teachers, siblings, and the children themselves about what is important to them (Barr, McLeod, & Daniel, 2008; McCormack, McLeod, Harrison, & McAllister, 2010; McLeod, Daniel & Barr, 2013; Watts Pappas & McLeod, 2009). Children and their significant others can provide information about important (and difficult) activities they currently (or wish to) participate in for education, leisure, social, and religious purposes. Discussions about what is important to children and their families may also help you understand the cultural values and beliefs that shape family life. In general, cultures differ in the extent to which collectivism and individualism are emphasized (Berk, 2007). Children who are part of a collectivist family culture may have strong bonds with extended family. The influences, goals, and needs of these children may differ from those children who are part of an individualistic culture (McLeod, 2012a). Similarly, family beliefs

■■ ■■

☑ **APPLICATION:** Dealing with differences between empirically based recommendations and client preferences

Parent: "My mother is ashamed of Shu Xian's hearing loss. Whenever we go out or meet up with the family, she takes his hearing aids off. She does not like people to see that he has a problem. She thinks that he would be better if we went back home and saw a healer rather than come to speech-language pathology. What do you suggest I do?"

How would you answer the parent?

Hint: Read Fulcher et al. (2015), and the *Multilingual Children with Speech Sound Disorders: Position paper* (International Expert Panel on Multilingual Children's Speech, 2012).[1]

---

[1]http://www.csu.edu.au/research/multilingual-speech/position-paper

(including beliefs about SSD and the value of speech-language pathology services) may differ from one family to another. It is important to be aware of your own cultural values and beliefs and how they influence your perspective of SSD in children as you engage in EBP.

The second issue to consider when evaluating the internal evidence from children and their families is their informed preference for management of SSD. Consideration of an informed preference assumes that you have provided a child and his or her family with an unbiased appraisal of the relevant evidence in the first place. Exactly how you ensure (and measure) that families are fully informed is not well understood. Drawing on Dollaghan's (2007) work, suggestions for children with SSD and their families include:

- showing a video of a mock session for a particular intervention approach;
- compiling comments and feedback from previous children and their families about their experience with your speech-language pathology service; and
- providing an information sheet (including photos and drawings) about SSD and particular approaches to intervention.

Regardless of the strategies you use to fully inform the children and families you would work with, it is important that you be as honest as you can with what you know, the experience you have, and what is possible within the constraints of your clinical service. This is particularly important to remember if you are a beginning clinician, because undergraduate and graduate speech-language pathology students' first clients are often children with SSD (Flasher & Fogle, 2012). It is better to be honest about what you know (and do not know) and ask the experienced SLPs supervising you, rather than make a statement or recommendation without empirical support.

Step 6: Make a decision by integrating the evidence

Now that you have all the evidence, you need to make a clinical decision. You need to think about the pros and cons of the different options available. If a child's presenting clinical profile is similar to that of children involved in empirically robust intervention research associated with a particular approach, if the internal evidence from your clinical experience suggests that similar outcomes can be achieved within the constraints of the service in which you work, and if the family's preference aligns with this option, the decision may be straightforward. However, the literature on the barriers associated with engaging in EBP (e.g., O'Connor & Pettigrew, 2009) suggests that decision-making may not be that straightforward.

There does not seem to be one assessment tool, intervention approach, or target selection strategy that is superior to others (Baker & McLeod, 2011a). SLPs (including you) are in the unenviable position of having a wealth of external evidence to guide their decision-making. The task is further complicated by the fact that EBP requires integration of three sources of evidence. As a student, this may be frustrating to realize. There is no single gold-standard decision-making flow chart to guide you to the perfect decision with every case, every time. Similarly, as tempting as it may be, there is no single off-the-shelf assessment or intervention resource that you can prescribe as a cure-all for all children with SSD. So, how can the different sources of evidence be measured against each other? An inherent assumption across EBP literature is that higher-ranked external research carries more weight, and so it should direct clinical decisions. However, when other issues such as resource constraints or child factors preclude the application of the best available external evidence to practice, you need to use your clinical expertise. Clinical expertise is the centerpiece that integrates the three sources of evidence in the decision-making process (Dollaghan, 2007). But what exactly is it?

Clinical expertise

Clinical expertise is a difficult construct to define and measure. In a discussion on clinical expertise, Kamhi (1994, p. 117) suggested that it is "defined not only by technical, procedural, and knowledge-based (intellectual) qualities, but by interpersonal and attitudinal qualities as well." Examples of interpersonal and attitudinal qualities include your adaptability, enthusiasm and interest, your confidence as a clinician, and your ability to build rapport with young children and their families. Using the Dollaghan (2007) EBP framework, clinical expertise draws on your knowledge of the literature (i.e., external evidence), your technical and procedural experience applying that knowledge within the constraints of clinical practice (i.e., internal clinical evidence), and your interpersonal skills and attitudes to understand, connect, and relate with the children and families you work with (i.e., understanding of internal client-related evidence). In this context, evidence-based clinical decision-making is a delicate, evolving, and dynamic process that changes as expertise with all three sources of evidence develops and evolves (Baker & McLeod, 2011b). The dynamic nature of evidence-based clinical decision-making means your clinical decisions are open to change as evidence from different sources change. It also means that you need to reevaluate your clinical decisions regularly to ensure that the best possible outcomes for the individual children and families you work with are being achieved.

If you are a novice clinician, it may take you more time than you anticipate to familiarize yourself with the external evidence and to consider the factors, values, and preferences of individual children and their families. Qualified clinicians suggest that as experience grows, clinical decision-making becomes easier and more efficient (Kamhi, 1995). With experience, you will become more comfortable sharing your knowledge of the evidence with families, you will hone your technical skills, and you will develop your own "clinical style/approach that reflects a unique combination of knowledge, technical/problem-solving skills, and interpersonal abilities and attitudes" (Kamhi, 1995, p. 354). You will reach a point where there is no longer a divide between your clinical self and your personal self—you will be comfortable and confident with who you are as a clinician. Do not get too comfortable, though. As tempting as it may be to do as you have always done (because it is easier or seems more efficient), clinical decisions will no longer be evidence-based if you disconnect from the evidence. Later in this chapter we consider how you can stay up to date with the evidence by connecting with your professional association and remaining committed to continuing education opportunities.

■ Step 7: Evaluate the outcomes of the decision

Evaluations of clinical decisions typically require some forethought and planning. Goals need to be identified from the outset of intervention, and a plan or schedule for evaluating progress needs to be implemented. We addressed these issues in Chapter 10 (developing intervention goals) and Chapter 12 (developing a plan for evaluating intervention progress). In Chapter 12 you also learned about a framework for problem-solving slow progress. If your data suggest that progress is slowing down or indeed not occurring, it is important that you carefully think through possible reasons why. Think back over the decisions that you have made, beginning with the information you gathered at assessment. Reevaluate your initial diagnosis. Reflect on the possibility that client factors or values may be hindering progress, and consider how you could address them. If you are a novice clinician, it can be helpful to have a mentor to problem-solve difficult cases. You can draw on the mentor's expertise with similar cases as you consider evidence-based solutions.

■ Summarizing the importance of EBP

EBP provides a framework for considering integration of findings from published research with the complexities and constraints of everyday clinical practice to meet the needs of individual children with SSD and their families. The first element of EBP refers to the "best available external evidence from systematic research" (Dollaghan, 2007, p. 2). You can use findings from previously published reviews as an efficient initial step for searching for evidence associated with a specific clinical question. The second and third elements of EBP refer to the "2) best available evidence *internal* to clinical practice, and 3) best available evidence concerning the preferences of a fully informed patient" (Dollaghan, 2007, p. 2). This means collecting and contrasting your own outcomes from clinical practice with the external published evidence and the unique factors, values, and preferences of the individual children and families you work with. The seven-step process based on Baker and McLeod (2011b) and Gillam and Gillam (2006) serves as a guide for how this can be achieved.

ETHICAL GUIDELINES FOR CLINICAL PRACTICE

Ethics is "a process of deliberation about how best to act in the presence of others' lives" (Seedhouse, 1998, p. 47). Ethical practice relates to the way we work with children and their families, our colleagues, our employers, our profession, and the general public. According to Beauchamp and Childress (2012), there are four principles of ethical practice:

1. Respect for autonomy: respecting and supporting autonomous decisions.
2. Nonmaleficence: avoiding the causation of harm, or "don't make things worse" (Collicut McGrath, 2007, p. 85).
3. Beneficence: relieving, lessening, or preventing harm, and balancing benefits against risks and costs, or "the obligation to do good" (Body & McAllister, 2009, p. 17).
4. Justice: fairly distributing benefits, risks, and costs.

These four principles have been expanded within the Code of Ethics statements from many different speech-language pathology professional associations (see Table 15-4). Download the code of ethics for the professional association in the country you are working in, read it, and think about your professional practice for children with SSD. For example, the Principle of Ethics II from the American Speech-Language-Hearing Association Code of Ethics states: "Individuals shall honor their responsibility to achieve and maintain the highest level of professional competence and performance" (ASHA, 2010a). Reflect on your own practice and how this statement relates to undertaking EBP.

POLICIES AFFECTING CLINICAL PRACTICE

There are a number of national and international policies, frameworks, conventions, position papers, government inquiries, and laws that can guide SLPs' practice when working with children with SSD, or indeed with any children.

TABLE 15-4 Codes of ethics for SLPs practicing in different countries

Association	Title	Website
American Speech-Language-Hearing Association (ASHA)	Code of Ethics (2010)	http://www.asha.org/policy/ET2010-00309.htm
Hong Kong Association of Speech Therapists (HKAST)	Code of Ethics (1994)	https://speechtherapy.org.hk/uploads/doc/resources/Code%20of%20Ethics.pdf
New Zealand Speech-Language Therapists' Association (NZSTA)	Code of Ethics (2008)	http://www.speechtherapy.org.nz/about-nzsta/ethics
Royal College of Speech and Language Therapists (RCSLT)	Code of Ethics and Professional Conduct	http://www.rcslt.org/
South African Speech-Language-Hearing Association (SASLHA)	Code of Ethics (n.d.)	http://www.saslha.co.za/A_CodeOfEthics.asp
Speech-Language and Audiology Canada (SAC)	Code of Ethics (2005)	http://sac-oac.ca/professional-resources/resource-library/code-ethics
Speech Pathology Australia (SPA)	Code of Ethics (2010)	http://www.speechpathologyaustralia.org.au/library/Ethics/CodeofEthics.pdf

> **COMMENT:** *Children first*
>
> One everyday ethical issue is the way that we refer to those we work with. You will have noticed that throughout this book we use the person-first terminology "children with SSD." That is, we put the children center stage and recognize the separation between children and their areas of difficulty. Similarly, the main title of our book is *Children's Speech*. We purposefully chose the title of this book to profile children rather than the difficulties that they may have. There is a lot more to a child than his or her SSD. Think of the ways you refer to the children you work with.

■ International conventions and frameworks

International conventions and frameworks that can guide SLPs' professional practice include those by the United Nations and the World Health Organization.

United Nations conventions

The United Nations conventions are legally binding international documents that outline peoples' rights. There are two United Nations conventions that relate to children with communication disorders, including those with SSD: the United Nations Convention on the Rights of Children (UNCRC) (UNICEF, 1989) and the United Nations Convention on the Rights of Persons with Disability (CRPD) (United Nations, 2011). The UNCRC came into effect in September 1990 and has been ratified by 193 countries, with exceptions being the USA and Somalia (who are signatories). These documents state that children have the right to extra assistance (including speech-language pathology, although this is not explicitly stated) in order to fully participate in society.

Article 23 of the UNCRC states:

> Recognizing the special needs of a disabled child, assistance extended in accordance with paragraph 2 of the present article shall be provided free of charge, whenever possible, taking into account the financial resources of the parents or others caring for the child, and shall be designed to ensure that the disabled child has effective access to and receives education, training, health care services, rehabilitation services, preparation for employment and recreation opportunities in a manner conducive to the child's achieving the fullest possible social integration and individual development, including his or her cultural and spiritual development. (UNICEF, 1989)

Article 25 of the CRPD states:

> States Parties recognize that persons with disabilities have the right to the enjoyment of the highest attainable standard of health without discrimination on the basis of disability . . . Provide those health services needed by persons with disabilities specifically because of their disabilities, including early identification and intervention as appropriate, and services designed to minimize and prevent further disabilities, including among children and older persons. (United Nations, 2011)

Additionally, the UNCRC contains two articles that have been quoted extensively and have begun to influence speech-language pathology practice. These two articles have challenged adults (including SLPs) to listen to the views of children in matters that concern them:

> Article 12: Parties shall assure to the child who is capable of forming his or her own views the right to express those views freely in all matters affecting the child, the views of the child being given due weight in accordance with the age and maturity of the child.

> Article 13: The child shall have the right to freedom of expression; this right shall include freedom to seek, receive and impart information and ideas of all kinds, regardless of frontiers, either orally, in writing or in print, in the form of art, or through any other media of the child's choice. (UNICEF, 1989)

These conventions have provided the impetus for research that has aimed to listen to children's views about speech-language pathology (Merrick & Roulstone, 2011; Owen, Hayett, & Roulstone, 2004; Roulstone & McLeod, 2011) and SSD (e.g., McCormack, McLeod, McAllister, & Harrison, 2010; McLeod, Daniel, & Barr, 2013).

World Health Organization publications

In 1945, the World Health Organization defined health as ". . . a state of complete physical, mental and social well-being and not merely the absence of disease or infirmity." This definition is reflected in the International Classification of Functioning, Disability and Health – Children and Youth Version (ICF-CY) (WHO, 2007), an international classification system that can be used to guide a holistic view of children's lives. As demonstrated throughout this book, the ICF-CY describes children's body structures and functions, as well as factors such as their ability to perform daily activities, their ability to participate in society, personal factors, and the role the environment plays in their health and well-being. In 2011, the World Report on Disability (World Health Organization and the World Bank, 2011) was published, providing nine crosscutting recommendations:

1. "enable access to all mainstream systems and services" (p. 264)
2. "invest in specific programmes and services for people with disabilities" (p. 265)
3. "adopt a national disability strategy and plan of action" (p. 265)
4. "involve people with disabilities" (p. 265)
5. "improve human resource capacity" (p. 266)
6. "provide adequate funding and improve affordability" (p. 266)
7. "increase public awareness and understanding" (p. 267)
8. "improve disability data collection" (p. 267)
9. "strengthen and support research on disability" (p. 267)

The World Report on Disability included a recommendation to frame practice using the ICF and ICF-CY. A discussion of the application of the World Report on Disability to people with communication disorders was published in a special issue of the *International Journal of Speech-Language Pathology* (2013, volume 15, number 1), and a paper describing the application of the World Report on Disability to children's communication was written by McLeod, McAllister, McCormack, and Harrison (2014).

■ National policies and laws

The following acts that are relevant to the United States specifically name "speech and language impairment" in their definition of disability: Individuals with Disabilities Education Act (IDEA) and No Child Left Behind (NCLB) Act. IDEA explicitly identifies SLPs as professionals who assess and provide intervention for children with communication disorders as part of "special education" (Individuals with Disabilities Education Improvement Act, 2004, Section 300.39).

In the United Kingdom the government has focused on legislation, policies, and services for children with communication disorders. The overarching policy, Every Child Matters, was followed by the Children Act 2004, which established the role of a children's commissioner and provided a legal framework for considering children's well-being. The national government strategy, Every Child a Talker (Department for Children, Schools and Families, 2008), supported children's communicative abilities. Next, the government commissioned the Bercow Report of Services for Children with Speech, Language and Communication Needs (Bercow, 2008) to consider health and education services. In response to the report, the government published Better Communication: An Action Plan to Improve Services for Children and Young People with Speech, Language and Communication Needs, with one of the outcomes being that 2011 was the national year of communication (Dockrell, Lindsay, Roulstone, & Law, 2014).

In Australia children with speech, language, and communication needs were considered to be invisible within a review of state and national policies from the departments of education, health, and disability (McLeod, Press, & Phelan, 2010). The Australian government initiated an inquiry into the prevalence of speech, language, and communication disorders and speech pathology services in Australia (Commonwealth of Australia, 2014).

ASSOCIATIONS THAT SUPPORT SLPS' CLINICAL PRACTICE AND CONTINUING EDUCATION

Throughout the world there are many professional associations to support SLPs' clinical practice and continuing education when working with children with SSD. Some are directly related to speech-language pathology, and some are associated with phonetics, phonology, linguistics, and the study of children's language. The associations listed in Table 15-5 all publish journals that include papers that will be of interest to SLPs who work with children with SSD. The International Association of Logopedics and Phoniatrics (IALP) is the oldest international association, founded in 1924. IALP is auspiced by the World Health Organization and works from "a global perspective on scientific, educational and professional issues affecting persons with communication, language, voice, speech, hearing and swallowing disorders" (IALP, 2012). The American Speech-Language-Hearing Association is the largest association for SLPs in the world and provides extensive resources for SLPs, including their numerous journals. In addition to the associations and journals listed in Table 15-5, there are numerous associations and journals that are in countries where English is not spoken (Bleile, 2006). Some countries have community associations that provide support for children and their families (as well as professionals) (see Table 15-6).

COMMENT: *Finding speech-language pathology professional associations around the world*

The International Directory of Communicative Disorders[1] (Bleile, 2006) is a resource listing training programs and professional associations around the world.

[1]http://www.comdisinternational.com/agreement.html

| TABLE 15-5 | National and international professional associations that publish journals in English | | |

Country/ Region	Association	Website	Journals
Asia Pacific	Asia Pacific Society of Speech, Language and Hearing	http://www.apsslh.org	*Speech, Language and Hearing*
Australia	Speech Pathology Australia (SPA)	http://www.speechpathologyaustralia.org.au	*International Journal of Speech-Language Pathology, Journal of Clinical Practice in Speech-Language Pathology*
Canada	Speech-Language and Audiology Canada (SAC)	http://sac-oac.ca	*Canadian Journal of Speech-Language Pathology and Audiology/Revue canadienne d'orthophonie et d'audiologie*
International	International Association of Logopedics and Phoniatrics (IALP)	http://www.ialp.info	*Folia Phoniatrica et Logopaedica*
International	International Clinical Phonetics and Linguistics Association (ICPLA)	http://www.icpla.info	*Clinical Linguistics and Phonetics*
International	International Phonetic Association (IPA)	https://www.internationalphoneticassociation.org	*Journal of the International Phonetic Association*
Ireland	Irish Association of Speech and Language Therapists	http://www.iaslt.ie	*Journal of Clinical Speech and Language Studies*
New Zealand	New Zealand Speech-Language Therapists' Association (NZSTA)	http://www.speechtherapy.org.nz	*New Zealand Journal of Speech-Language Therapy*
South Africa	South African Speech-Language-Hearing Association (SASLHA)	http://www.saslha.co.za	*South African Journal of Communication Disorders, Die Suid-Afrikaanse Tydskrif vir Kommunikasie-afwykings*
United Kingdom	Royal College of Speech and Language Therapists (RCSLT)	http://www.rcslt.org	*International Journal of Language and Communication Disorders*
United States	American Speech-Language-Hearing Association (ASHA)	http://www.asha.org	*Journal of Speech, Language, and Hearing Research; American Journal of Speech-Language Pathology; Language, Speech, and Hearing Services in Schools; American Journal of Audiology; The ASHA Leader*

| TABLE 15-6 | Community associations that support children with SSD | |

Country	Association	Website
England	Afasic England	http://www.afasicengland.org.uk
Northern Ireland	Afasic Northern Ireland	http://www.afasicnorthernireland.org.uk
Scotland	Afasic Scotland	http://www.afasicscotland.org.uk
US	The Childhood Apraxia of Speech Association of North America (CASANA)	http://www.apraxia-kids.org
Wales	Afasic Cymru	http://www.afasiccymru.org.uk

■ Speech-language pathology position and policy papers

There are a few position papers that have been published by professional associations and international panels that directly or indirectly relate to working with children with SSD of known and unknown origins.

Position papers about working with children with SSD

The American Speech-Language-Hearing Association (2004c) Preferred Practice Patterns includes descriptions of the assessment and intervention for children with SSD:

> #15. Speech Sound Assessment. Assessment of articulation and phonology is provided to evaluate articulatory and phonological functioning (strengths and weaknesses in speech sound discrimination and production), including identification of impairments, associated activity and participation limitations, and context barriers and facilitators.

> #16. Speech Sound Intervention. Intervention in speech sound disorders addresses articulatory and phonological impairments, associated activity and participation limitations, and context barriers and facilitators by optimizing speech discrimination, speech sound production, and intelligibility in multiple communication contexts.

Each of these sections then addresses the following information: (1) individuals who provide the services, (2) expected outcome(s) based around the ICF (World Health Organization, 2001), (3) clinical indications, (4) clinical process, (5) setting, equipment specifications, safety, and health precautions, (6) documentation, (7) ASHA policy documents and selected references.

Position papers about working with children with childhood apraxia of speech

Two significant papers have been written about working with children with CAS. The American Speech-Language-Hearing Association (2007) published a position statement and comprehensive technical report that defined and summarized international literature about children with CAS. The Royal College of Speech and Language Therapists (RCSLT, 2011b) published a 60-page policy statement for SLPs working with children with CAS. The policy statement uses the term *developmental verbal dyspraxia*, in keeping with the UK convention. These are important international documents because they provide guidelines for identification, assessment, and intervention of this challenging and complex SSD in children.

Position papers about working with multilingual children

A number of position papers have been written about multilingual and multicultural considerations when working with children (and some also address working with adults).

- The International Expert Panel on Multilingual Children's Speech (2012) has written a position paper titled Multilingual Children with Speech Sound Disorders: Position Paper (see "Recommendations for Working With Multilingual Children With SSD" box).
- The American Speech-Language-Hearing Association (ASHA) has written three position papers, titled Bilingual Service Delivery (n.d.), Cultural Competence (2005), and Provision of Instruction in English as a Second Language by Speech-Language Pathologists in School Settings (1998).
- Speech-Language and Audiology Canada (previously the Canadian Association of Speech-Language Pathologists and Audiologists, CASLPA) has written the Position Paper on Speech-Language Pathology and Audiology in the Multicultural, Multilingual Context (1997).
- The International Association of Logopedics and Phoniatrics (IALP) has written Recommendations for Working with Bilingual Children.
- The Royal College of Speech and Language Therapists (RCSLT) has a document titled Communicating Quality that addresses multilingual and multicultural issues on pages 268–271.
- Speech Pathology Australia has written a position paper and clinical guidelines titled Working in a Culturally and Linguistically Diverse Society (Speech Pathology Australia, 2016a, b).

COMMENT: *Recommendations for working with multilingual children with SSD*

The International Expert Panel on Multilingual Children's Speech recommends that:

1. Children are supported to communicate effectively and intelligibly in the languages spoken within their families and communities, in the context of developing their cultural identities.
2. Children are entitled to professional speech and language assessment and intervention services that acknowledge and respect their existing competencies, cultural heritage, and histories. Such assessment and intervention should be based on the best available evidence.
3. SLPs aspire to be culturally competent and to work in culturally safe ways.
4. SLPs aspire to develop rich partnerships with families, communities, interpreters, and other health and education professionals to promote strong and supportive communicative environments.
5. SLPs generate and share knowledge, resources, and evidence nationally and internationally to facilitate the understanding of cultural and linguistic diversity that will support multilingual children's speech acquisition and communicative competency.
6. Governments, policy makers, and employers acknowledge and support the need for culturally competent and safe practices and equip SLPs with additional time, funding, and resources in order to provide equitable services for multilingual children. (International Expert Panel on Multilingual Children's Speech, 2012, p. 4)

 APPLICATION: *Evidence-based decisions with Luke*

Throughout this book there are a series of clinical tasks for Luke (4;3 years). If you have worked through these tasks, you would have completed an analysis of Luke's speech and identified possible intervention goals in addition to suitable intervention approaches. In light of what you have learned in this chapter, it is time to consider Luke's case within a clinical context. Discuss your answers for the following questions with a colleague.

1. Luke's mother asks you:
   a) "I'd like to read more about speech sound disorders in children. Can you recommend some helpful websites for parents?"
   b) "My mother suggested that Luke has a tongue-tie and that he should see an oral surgeon. What do you think?"
   c) "In your experience, how long it will take until Luke's speech is intelligible?"
   d) "How often should Luke attend therapy?"

Remember, even if a parent or caregiver asks you what you think, EBP means that your answers are based on what you know, from a combination of external and internal evidence.

2. Using a spreadsheet program, develop your own clinical case-based database template for children with an SSD, similar to Luke (4;3) (Chapter 16). You might like to include information such as age, gender, and severity in addition to other characteristics common across children with SSD. As part of your spreadsheet, make sure you include a series of columns about the intensity of your intervention plan for Luke (from Chapter 11) such as dose, session duration, session frequency, and total intervention duration in numbers of sessions and time.

3. Prepare a feedback form for Luke and his family to complete prior to Luke being discharged from speech-language pathology services. Think about the topics you would like Luke and his family to comment on. The information they provide could be used to inform future families on your caseload about your work with children with SSD.

Read more about Luke (4;3 years), a boy with a phonological impairment, in Chapter 16 (Case 1).

Chapter summary

In this chapter you learned about the steps involved in the conduct of EBP when working with children with SSD. You have been challenged to think about the different types of evidence that inform clinical decisions. You have also been challenged to think about clinical expertise—what it is and how it develops through knowledge and experience. You have also learned about ethical guidelines, national and international policies, position papers, professional associations, and journal publications that support and guide your work with children with SSD.

Remember—EBP is a process that you will continue to work at and refine over the course of your career. As Kent (2006) states, "EBP is very much a work in progress, not a polished perfection" (p. 268). Work through the process. Learn to ask clinical questions. Refine your literature search skills. Develop strategies for gathering and critiquing external evidence in addition to your own internal evidence from clinical practice. Continue to grow your knowledge as you gain experience, so that the decisions you make are the best possible for the children and families with whom you work.

Suggested reading

- Baker, E., & McLeod, S. (2011b). Evidence-based practice for children with speech sound disorders: Part 2 application to clinical practice. *Language, Speech, and Hearing Services in Schools, 42*(2), 140–151.

- Body, R., & McAllister, L. (Eds.). (2009). *Ethics in speech and language therapy.* Chichester, UK: Wiley-Blackwell.

- Dollaghan, C. A. (2007). *The handbook for evidence-based practice in communication disorders.* Baltimore, MD: Paul H. Brookes Publishing.

Application of knowledge from Chapter 15

1. In Chapters 13 and 14 you made a series of clinical decisions regarding your management of SSD for Luke, Susie, Jarrod, Michael, and Lian. Select one of those decisions (e.g., intervention approach, service delivery choice), and consider if alternate options are available. Complete steps 1 through 3 of the process of engaging in EBP as outlined in this chapter: create a PICO question, search for and then critique evidence relevant to your PICO question.

2. Gather policies at your workplace or clinical practicum site relevant to the conduct of clinical practice. Compare and contrast one of those policies with research evidence for managing SSD in children. Explain how the policy does (or does not) align with the research evidence.

3. List possible barriers to engaging in EBP with children with SSD. In a small group, discuss strategies for working around, reducing, or removing those barriers.

4. You are working as a school-based SLP. Your colleague (with more experience than you) is using an intervention approach for children with SSD that you are not familiar with. You are instructed by this colleague to use the same intervention approach. What do you do?

5. Create a plan (including time-bound actions) for keeping up to date with the evidence associated with the management of SSD in children. Ensure you include multiple strategies. For example, join your association, attend conventions, subscribe to and read journal articles, join an EBP network of clinicians who read and discuss research evidence, join and participate in a listserv or online discussion forum associated with SSD, attend topic-specific workshops, enlist the support of a mentor who can observe you engage in clinical practice, observe experienced SLPs conducting clinical practice, and look for or create opportunities to engage in clinical research.

16

Individual Children with Speech Sound Disorders: Case Studies

LEARNING OBJECTIVES

1. Write a case history summary for an individual child, using case-based data (e.g., developmental, medical, educational, and psychosocial history).

2. Generate a preliminary diagnosis about the nature of a child's SSD using case history information and assessment results.

3. Use the case history and assessment information to complete clinical exercises throughout this book.

KEY WORDS

Case 1: Luke (4;3 years): Phonological impairment

Case 2: Susie (7;4 years): Articulation impairment (lateral lisp)

Case 3: Jarrod (7;0 years): Inconsistent speech disorder

Case 4: Michael (4;2 years): Childhood apraxia of speech (CAS)

Case 5: Lian (14;2 years): Childhood dysarthria

OVERVIEW

In this chapter we provide case-based data for five children who have SSD. The cases cover the different types of SSD addressed in this book. The data include case history information and assessment results. Each case is either a composite based on the authors' own clinical experiences with a variety of children, or from colleagues with specialist experience, and published literature. Luke's case is the most comprehensive, because he presents with the most common type of SSD—phonological impairment. We hope that the cases promote your thinking and learning in ways that simulate clinical practice. We also hope that the cases remind you that you are not just learning about how to manage a phonological impairment, or [ɫ], or syllable segregation, but rather that you are learning how to work with families and their children who happen to have SSD. This chapter also contains a series of tables that summarize interesting case reports from peer-reviewed published literature. You may find these case reports helpful when you have a child on your caseload with an unusual or rare clinical presentation. As an evidence-based clinician, case study reports and detailed single-subject experimental reports can be a rich source of information for guiding clinical decisions (Crystal, 1987b; Vance & Clegg, 2012). Unlike previous chapters, this chapter is not meant to be read from beginning to end. Rather, you will read sections of this chapter as you come across clinical exercises in other chapters. If you started reading this book from the beginning, hopefully you are reading this chapter now because you just read the instruction in Chapter 1 to read this overview and Luke's case history.

LUKE (4;3 YEARS): PHONOLOGICAL IMPAIRMENT

Luke is a classic textbook case of a preschool child with SSD, who would be common in many speech-language pathology clinics throughout the world. He is described as a child who uses General American English; however, there are translations of Luke's speech assessment data into three other English dialects (African-American English, New England [Bostonian] English, and Spanish English). These translations will enable you to consider typical productions of the sampled words and Luke's likely production in those dialects. As discussed in Chapters 7 and 8, not all speech-language pathology assessments would include the breadth of information we have provided for Luke. We have used Luke's case to illustrate the range of information that could be gathered. Refer to Chapter 8 for further details about routine and strategic assessment, and developing individualized assessment plans.

■ Luke: Case history

Luke (4;3 years) was referred by his preschool teacher and mother for an assessment of his speech because he was difficult to understand. Luke is the younger of two boys. Luke's father was reported to be late to talk and to have struggled with reading at school. Luke's mother and father completed high school. Luke's mother works part-time as a receptionist. Luke's father works as a carpenter.

Luke's mother reported no problems during her pregnancy or birth with Luke. Luke was born naturally, at full term. There were no complications after birth. He was breast-fed for 10 months; however, Luke's mother did comment that feeding took a few weeks to get established. At the time of the initial speech-language pathology assessment, Luke was enjoying a varied diet without any dietary or allergy restrictions. Luke babbled a little around 10 months, and said his first word at 16 months. He started using short sentences by 2;6 years. Luke's motor milestones occurred at the expected ages; sitting without support by 6 months, crawling by 9 months and walking by 13 months. Luke was described as a generally healthy young boy, averaging about four head colds over the winter months. As a newborn, Luke passed his newborn hearing screening test. Audiometric evaluation at age 4;0 years confirmed that Luke's hearing was normal and adequate for speech acquisition. He did not wear glasses and did not use a hearing aid. He had no known additional medical diagnoses.

During a typical preschool day, Luke showed a preference for construction and gross motor play rather than pretend play. Luke's preschool teacher described him as a quiet yet friendly boy. On the case history questionnaire, Luke's mother commented that although

Luke had a couple of friends at preschool, he was not interested in playing with his friends outside of preschool time. At the time of the assessment, Luke was attending preschool three full days per week. Luke's interests included building with construction blocks, Play-Doh, and insects. He also enjoyed dressing up as a superhero, but did not engage in pretend play with other children.

Luke was described as social, moderately persistent, and moderately reactive on the Short Temperament Scale for Children (STSC) (Sanson, Prior, Garino, Oberklaid, & Sewell, 1987). Luke's parents indicated that Luke was usually in a happy mood, moderately active around him, somewhat slow to adjust to changes in his routine, and that he had a moderate attention span.

■ Luke: Assessment results

Luke's communication skills were assessed by a qualified SLP. A psychologist assessed Luke's cognition. Table 16-1 summarizes the results.

TABLE 16-1 | **Luke (4;3 years): Summary assessment results**

Skill area	Assessment	Measure and/or observation	Result
Receptive and expressive language	Clinical Evaluation of Language Fundamentals: Preschool-2 (CELF-P2) (Wiig, Secord, & Semel, 2004)	Receptive: 105 (SS) Expressive: 98 (SS)	✓
Receptive vocabulary	Peabody Picture Vocabulary Test-4 (PPVT-4) (Dunn & Dunn, 2007)	89 (SS)	✓ (low average)
Speech production: standardized single-word sample	Diagnostic Evaluation of Articulation and Phonology (DEAP): Phonology assessment (Dodd, Hua, et al., 2006)	PPC[1] = 56.7% PCC[1] = 38.6% PVC[1] = 89.6% (SS = 3; percentile rank = 1)	✗
Speech production: strategic single-word sample	Informal speech samples comprising simple CVC words, consonant clusters, and polysyllables (see Tables 16-3, 16-4, and 16-5)	Luke's inventory of consonant clusters was limited to nasal + plosive clusters in word final (e.g., [ŋk, mp, nt]) and [lt]. He could match most words with respect to length. He had no productive phonological knowledge of fricatives or affricates.	✗
Speech production: connected speech sample	Two samples of conversational speech were collected: one with a kitchen play set, Play-Doh, and pretend food, and one with toy transport items (e.g., cars, trucks, bus, boat, planes, helicopters) and a toy transport mat.	PPC[1] = 61.3% PCC[1] = 48.4% PVC[1] = 85.5%	✗
Speech production: stimulability	Informal assessment	Luke was stimulable for the following phones absent from his phonetic inventory [s, z, θ, ð, f, v, h] in isolation and simple CV and VC syllables, given cues. He was not stimulable for [ʃ, ʒ, ɹ, tʃ, dʒ].	✗
Speech production: intelligibility	Informal rating based on the Intelligibility in Context Scale (ICS) (McLeod, Harrison, & McCormack, 2012b), completed by Luke's mother.	Luke's mother usually understood Luke if the context of the conversation was known; otherwise she sometimes understood him. Luke's preschool teacher sometimes understood Luke. Strangers were reported to rarely understand Luke's speech. He achieved an average score of 3.2/5.	✗
Speech production: consistency	Visual inspection of data from single-word and conversational speech samples.	Luke's speech errors were generally consistent, so no further testing was conducted.	✓

(continued)

TABLE 16-1	*Continued*

Skill area	Assessment	Measure and/or observation	Result
Speech production: contextual testing	Observation of Luke's response to communication breakdown.	When Luke was not understood, he tended to simply repeat what he had said, in a louder voice, without changing his segments or syllable structure.	✗
	Visual inspection of Luke's speech across different sample contexts—single words and conversational speech.	There were no obvious differences between single-word and conversational speech samples, aside from there being a higher proportion of easier words (including repetitions of those words) in the conversational speech relative to the single-word task.	
Hearing function	Pure tone audiometric screening at 500, 1000, 2000, and 4000 Hz.	Luke responded to pure tone thresholds in his left and right ear, at 20 dB in a quiet room.	✓
	Tympanometry	Graph on tympanogram consistent with Type A, suggesting normal eardrum movement. No fluid was detected in Luke's middle ear cavity.	
Speech perception	Informal speech perception task, based on Locke (1980a, b).	Perception of /s, ʃ/ contrast was poor, typically responding to /ʃ/ as /s/. Other phonemes in error were adequately perceived.	✓✗
Assessment of phonological processing	Comprehensive Test of Phonological Processing 2 (CTOPP-2) (Wagner, Torgesen, Rashotte, & Pearson, 2013).	Composite scores: Phonological awareness = 90 Phonological memory = 92 Rapid symbolic naming = 94 Rapid non-symbolic naming = 92 Overall, low average performance.	✓[2]
	Distinctiveness of phonological representations was informally assessed based on the Articulation Judgment and Articulation Correction-Accuracy tasks by Anthony et al. (2010)	On the Articulation Judgment task Luke easily identified correctly produced words. Errors typically occurred when Luke judged incorrectly produced words (involving a vowel change) as correct. His responses to the Articulation Correction task showed improved syllable structure, albeit with his own segmental consonant singleton and cluster errors (e.g., he corrected *butterfly* /bʌflaɪ/ to [bʌtəbaɪ]).	
Emergent literacy skills	Pre-literacy rating scale of the Clinical Evaluation of Language Fundamentals: Preschool-2 (CELF-P2) (Wiig et al., 2004); informal assessment of letter name and sounds (based on Dodd & Carr, 2003)	Luke's book awareness was good. He could recognize common logos and a few printed numbers. He recognized and wrote two letters from his name, in capital form: L K. He knew the names of L and K. He did not know any letter sounds.	✓[2]
Oral structure and function	Oral and speech motor control protocol (Robbins & Klee, 1987)	Total structure score = 23/24. Total function score = 105/112. Luke had complete deciduous dentition. There was no evidence of tongue-tie. Some evidence of decay on his lower left first molar. Luke's structure and function scores were within the normal range for his age, based on normative data from Robbins and Klee (1987).	✓
	Diagnostic Evaluation of Articulation and Phonology (DEAP): Oral motor screen (Dodd, Hua, et al., 2006)	DDK (diadochokinetic) score = 5 (SS = 9) Isolated movements = 10 (SS = 10) Sequenced movements = 15 (SS = 11) Luke was able to complete all isolated and sequenced movements easily, except for tongue elevation outside his upper lip. He could elevate his tongue to the alveolar ridge.	

(continued)

TABLE 16-1	*Continued*

Skill area	Assessment	Measure and/or observation	Result
Pragmatics	Observation during conversational speech and completion of the Descriptive Pragmatics Profile from the Clinical Evaluation of Language Fundamentals: Preschool-2 (CELF-P2) (Wiig et al., 2004)	Descriptive Pragmatics Profile criterion score = 71, suggesting adequate communication abilities for his age. When Luke's speech could be understood, he displayed appropriate assertiveness and responsiveness with his conversation partners (SLP and mother). He initiated and responded to topics of conversation. When communication breakdowns occurred, Luke tried to repair the breakdown by repeating what he had said, or if it occurred with the SLP he would request that his mother interpret for him and tell the SLP what he had said. If this latter strategy was unsuccessful, the topic of conversation shifted.	✓
Fluency	Informal observation during conversational speech	Luke's fluency was informally assessed during conversational speech and found to be appropriate. He did not stutter.	✓
Voice	Informal observation during conversational speech	Luke's voice quality and pitch was perceived to be appropriate for age and gender.	✓
Activites and participation	Speech Participation and Activity Assessment of Children (SPAA-C) Version 2 (McLeod, 2004).	Luke indicated that he was ☺ happy to talk with his parents and brother. He circled ☹ when asked how he felt about people not understanding him. He shrugged his shoulders and circled "?" (don't know) in response to questions about talking with friends and teachers (see Figure 16-1).	✓✗
Environmental facilitators and barriers	Informal interview with Luke's parents	Luke's parents were both motivated to follow up and complete therapy activities at home; Luke's preschool teacher also reported that a teaching assistant could complete therapy activities given instruction.	✓
Cognition	Wechsler Preschool and Primary Scale of Intelligence-III (WPPSI-III) (Wechsler, 2002)	108 (SS)	✓

SS = standard score, ✓ = acceptable, ✗ = problematic.

[1]PPC = percentage of phonemes correct, PCC = percentage of vowels correct, PVC = percentage of vowels correct.

[2] Even though Luke's performance was adequate for his age, he is at risk for difficulties with phonological awareness and literacy given his phonological impairment. As discussed in Chapter 13, iIt is important to complement Luke's phonological intervention with emergent literacy intervention, particularly targeting phonemic awareness and letter name and sound knowledge.

Luke: Example single-word speech sample

The Diagnostic Evaluation of Articulation and Phonology (DEAP): Phonology Assessment (Dodd, Hua, et al., 2006) was used to elicit a 50-item single-word speech sample. Table 16-2 provides an example of Luke's responses for 3 of the 50 words from the DEAP: Phonology Assessment.

TABLE 16-2	Brief single-word speech sample for Luke (4;3 years)

Target word	Adult pronunciation	Luke's production
1. monkey	/mʌŋki/	[mʌŋki]
2. giraffe	/dʒəɹæf/	[dəwæp]
3. kitchen	/kɪtʃən/	[dɪtən]

Source: These three words are selected from the 50 words within the Phonology Assessment of the Diagnostic Evaluation of Articulation and Phonology (DEAP) (Dodd, Hua, et al. [2006]).

Luke: Conversational speech sample

Two samples of conversational speech were gathered. The clinician was the conversation partner for each sample. Each sample lasted approximately 10 minutes, yielding 262 word tokens and 169 word types. Six of Luke's utterances from one of these conversational speech samples follow. In this sample, Luke and the clinician are making shapes with Play-Doh.

LUKE   **Who made a star in there?**
Target (adult) production: /hu med ə staɹ ɪn ðɛɹ/
Luke's production: [u med ə dɑ ɪn dɛə]

SLP   Who? Oh, somebody else made a star in there.

LUKE   **A boy?**
Target (adult) production: /ə bɔɪ/
Luke's production: [ə bɔɪ]

SLP   No, it was a girl.

LUKE   **A girl, why?**
Target (adult) production: /ə gɝl waɪ/
Luke's production: [ə dʒʊ waɪ]

SLP   Because she liked making stars.

LUKE   **I like making stars ... little star little stars in the moon little stars in the moon.**
Target (adult) production: /aɪ laɪk mekɪn staɹz lɪtl staɹ lɪtl staɹz ɪn ðə mun lɪtl staɹz ɪn ðə mun/
Luke's production: [aɪ laɪk mekɪn dɑt lɪdʊ dɑ lɪdʊ dɑt ɪn ə mun lɪdʊ dɑt ɪn ə mun]

SLP   Little stars in the moon, is that a song?

LUKE   **Is this a star or not?**
Target (adult) production: /əz ðɪs ə staɹ ɔr nɑt /
Luke's production: [ə dɪt ə dɑ ɔ nɑt]

SLP   What do you think?

LUKE   **That looks like a man.**
Target (adult) production: /ðæt lʊks laɪk ə mæn/
Luke's production: [dæt lʊk laɪk ə mæn]

Luke: Strategic sampling of minimal pair words, consonant clusters, and polysyllabic words

Luke's responses during the DEAP: Phonology Assessment (Dodd, Hua, et al., 2006), and conversational speech suggested that further strategic sampling was needed, particularly of velars, fricatives, and affricates in minimal pair words, consonant clusters, and polysyllables. Tables 16-3, 16-4, and 16-5 provide a sample of Luke's responses across the strategically selected words. These samples were gathered to confirm and better understand the nature of Luke's difficulty across these different aspects of speech.

■ Adapting Luke's case study for different dialects

Luke's case study (presented above) is provided for a General American English-speaking boy. To help you appreciate the role of dialect in analysis, we have adapted Luke's speech sample (both the expected adult pronunciation and Luke's production) for three selected North American dialects (see Table 16-6). In each example of Luke's transcription, we have aimed to have a similar set of error patterns present (where appropriate) so that comparisons with the CHIRPA analyses in Chapter 9 may be possible. It is important to note that calculation of some measures (e.g., percentage of consonants correct, occurrence of cluster reduction) will differ across dialects, due to different acceptable adult pronunciations.

TABLE 16-3	Luke (4;3 years): Examples of monosyllabic words used to sample consonant singletons and identify phonemes in word-initial and word-final positions	
Target word	**Adult pronunciation**	**Luke's production**
1. sun	/sʌn/	[dʌn]
2. fan	/fæn/	[bæn]
3. light	/laɪt/	[laɪt]
4. fat	/fæt/	[bæt]
5. zip	/zɪp/	[dɪp]
6. meat	/mit/	[mit]
7. like	/laɪk/	[laɪk]
8. bite	/baɪt/	[baɪt]
9. seat	/sit/	[dit]
10. chip	/tʃɪp/	[dɪp]
11. ship	/ʃɪp/	[dɪp]
12. thin	/θɪn/	[dɪn]
13. feet	/fit/	[bit]
14. bike	/baɪk/	[baɪk]
15. that	/ðæt/	[dæt]
16. fun	/fʌn/	[bʌn]
17. cat	/kæt/	[dæt]
18. goo	/gu/	[du]
19. two	/tu/	[du]
20. neat	/nit/	[nit]
21. Pete	/pit/	[bit]
22. king	/kɪŋ/	[dɪŋ]
23. van	/væn/	[bæn]
24. hat	/hæt/	[æt]
25. read	/rid/	[wid]
26. weed	/wid/	[wid]
27. lead	/lid/	[lid]
28. chill	/tʃɪl/	[dɪl]
29. you	/ju/	[ju]
30. bag	/bæg/	[bæk]

■ Intervention studies of children who have phonological impairment

There are many helpful case studies of children (mostly of preschool age) who have a phonological impairment (Baker & McLeod, 2011a). Table 16-7 provides an overview of a selection of these cases.

TABLE 16-4	**Luke (4;3 years): Single-word sample of word-initial and word-final consonant clusters**	

Target word	Target (adult) production	Child's production
1. swim	/swɪn/	[dɪm]
2. square	/skwɛɹ/	[dɛə]
3. through	/θɹu/	[bu]
4. ant	/ænt/	[ænt]
5. jump	/ʤʌmp/	[dʌmp]
6. twin	/twɪn/	[dɪn]
7. blood	/blʌd/	[bʌd]
8. blue	/blu/	[bu]
9. clean	/klin/	[din]
10. clock	/klɑk/	[dɑk]
11. fly	/flaɪ/	[baɪ]
12. street	/stɹit/	[dit]
13. spring	/spɹɪŋ/	[bɪŋ]
14. playground	/pleɡɹaʊnd/	[bedaʊn]
15. sleep	/slip/	[dip]
16. drink	/dɹɪŋk/	[dɪŋk]
17. ski	/ski/	[di]
18. tree	/tɹi/	[di]
19. smell	/smɛl/	[mɛl]
20. snow	/sno/	[no]
21. space	/spes/	[bet]
22. splinter	/splɪntɚ/	[bɪntə]
23. scratch	/skɹæʧ/	[dæt]
24. throne	/θɹon/	[bon]
25. sleeve	/sliv/	[lip]
26. brush	/bɹʌʃ/	[bʌt]
27. story	/stɔɹi/	[dɔwi]
28. shrink	/ʃɹɪŋk/	[dɪŋk]
29. toast	/tost/	[tot]
30. green	/ɡrin/	[din]
31. pupil	/pjupəl/	[bupəl]
32. music	/mjuzɪk/	[mudɪk]
33. cute	/kjut/	[dut]
34. beautiful	/bjutɪfəl/	[butɪpəl]
35. pram	/pɹæm/	[bæm]

| TABLE 16-5 | Luke (4;3 years): Single-word sample of polysyllabic real words |

Target word[1]	Adult pronunciation	Child's production
1. spaghetti	/spəɡɛti/	[bədɛti]
2. caterpillar	/kætɚpɪlɚ/	[dætəbɪlə]
3. computer	/kəmpjutɚ/	[dəmbutə]
4. hippopotamus	/hɪpəpatəməs/	[ɪpəbatəmət]
5. animals	/ænɪməlz/	[ænɪməlt]
6. butterfly	/bʌtɚflaɪ/	[bʌtəbaɪ]
7. ambulance[2]	/æmbjələnts/	[æmbələnt]
8. caravan	/kæɹəvæn/	[dæəbæn]
9. vegetables	/vɛʤtəbəlz/	[bɛdəbʊt]
10. helicopter	/hɛlikaptɚ/	[ɛlidapə]

Source: [1]10 words from James (2006). Used with permission.

[2]*ambulance* may be pronounced with or without the /t/ in the final consonant cluster.

| FIGURE 16-1 | **(a) Luke's responses to the Speech Participation and Activity Assessment of Children (SPAA-C) and (b) Luke's drawing of himself talking to his mother.** |

Luke is on the left in the drawing. Notice Luke's rounded mouth and the closeness between the figures.

	Happy	In the middle	Sad	Another feeling	Don't know
1. How do you feel about the way you talk?	☺	⊝	☹	◐	?
2. How do you feel when you talk to your best friend?	☺	⊝	☹	◐	?
3. How do you feel when you talk to your [brothers and sisters]?	☺	⊝	☹	◐	?
4. How do you feel when you talk to your [mum and dad]?	☺	⊝	☹	◐	?
5. How do you feel when you talk to your [pre]school teachers?	☺	⊝	☹	◐	?
6. How do you feel when your teachers ask you a question?	☺	⊝	☹	◐	?
7. How do you feel when you talk to the whole class?	☺	⊝	☹	◐	?
8. How do you feel when you play with the children at [pre]school?	☺	⊝	☹	◐	?
9. How do you feel when you play on your own?	☺	⊝	☹	◐	?
10. How do you feel when people don't understand what you say?	☺	⊝	☹	◐	?

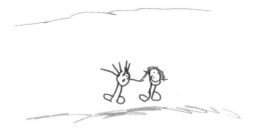

Source: Figure 16-1a. Sharynne McLeod (2004). Used by permission of Sharynne McLeod.
Source: Figure 16-1b. Copyright 2012 by S. McLeod, L. McAllister, J. McCormack & L. J. Harrison. Used by permission from Sharynne McLeod

TABLE 16-6   Single-word speech sample for Luke (4;3 years with phonological impairment) adapted for selected North American English dialects

Target word	General American English[2]		African-American English[3]		New England (Boston) English[4]		Spanish-influenced English[5]	
	Adult	Luke	Adult	Child	Adult	Child	Adult	Child
DEAP Phonology Assessment (Dodd, Hua, et al., 2006): Three words selected from the phonology assessment[1]								
1. monkey	/mʌŋki/	[mʌŋki]	/mʌŋki/	[mʌŋki]	/mʌŋki/	[mʌŋki]	/mʌŋki/	[mʌŋki]
2. giraffe	/dʒəɹæf/	[dəwæep]	/dʒəɹæf/	[dəwæep]	/dʒəɹæf/	[dəwæep]	/dʒəɹæf/	[dəwæep]
3. kitchen	/kɪtʃən/	[dɪtən]	/kɪtʃən/	[dɪtən]	/kɪtʃən/	[dɪtən]	/kɪtʃən/	[dɪtən]
Monosyllabic words used to sample consonant singletons and identify phonemes in word-initial and word-final positions								
1. sun	/sʌn/	[dʌn]	/sʌn/	[dʌn]	/sʌn/	[dʌn]	/sʌ̃/	[dʌ̃]
2. fan	/fæn/	[bæn]	/fæn/	[bæn]	/fæn/	[bæn]	/fæ̃/	[bæ̃]
3. light	/laɪt/	[laɪt]	/laɪt/	[laɪt]	/laɪt/	[laɪt]	/laɪt/	[laɪt]
4. fat	/fæt/	[bæt]	/fæt/	[bæt]	/fæt/	[bæt]	/fæt/	[bæt]
5. zip	/zɪp/	[dɪp]	/zɪp/	[dɪp]	/zɪp/	[dɪp]	/zɪp/	[dɪp]
6. meat	/mit/	[mit]	/mit/	[mit]	/mit/	[mit]	/mit/	[mit]
7. like	/laɪk/	[laɪk]	/laɪk/	[laɪk]	/laɪk/	[laɪk]	/laɪk/	[laɪk]
8. bite	/baɪt/	[baɪt]	/baɪt/	[baɪt]	/baɪt/	[baɪt]	/baɪt/	[baɪt]
9. seat	/sit/	[dit]	/sit/	[dit]	/sit/	[dit]	/sit/	[dit]
10. chip	/tʃɪp/	[dɪp]	/tʃɪp/	[dɪp]	/tʃɪp/	[dɪp]	/tʃɪp/	[dɪp]
11. ship	/ʃɪp/	[dɪp]	/ʃɪp/	[dɪp]	/ʃɪp/	[dɪp]	/ʃɪp/	[dɪp]
12. thin	/θɪn/	[dɪn]	/fɪn/	[dɪn]	/θɪn/	[dɪn]	/ti/	[dɪ]
13. feet	/fit/	[bit]	/fit/	[bit]	/fit/	[bit]	/fit/	[bit]
14. bike	/baɪk/	[baɪk]	/baɪk/	[baɪk]	/baɪk/	[baɪk]	/baɪk/	[baɪk]
15. that	/ðæt/	[dæt]	/dæt/	[dæt]	/ðæt/	[dæt]	/dæt/	[dæt]
16. fun	/fʌn/	[bʌn]	/fʌn/	[bʌn]	/fʌn/	[bʌn]	/fʌ̃/	[bʌ̃]
17. cat	/kæt/	[dæt]	/kæt/	[dæt]	/kæt/	[dæt]	/kæt/	[dæt]
18. goo!	/gu/	[du]	/gu/	[du]	/gu/	[du]	/gu/	[du]
19. two	/tu/	[du]	/tu/	[du]	/tu/	[du]	/tu/	[du]
20. neat	/nit/	[nit]	/nit/	[nit]	/nit/	[nit]	/nit/	[nit]
21. Pete	/pit/	[bit]	/pit/	[bit]	/pit/	[bit]	/pit/	[bit]
22. king	/kɪŋ/	[dɪŋ]	/kɪŋ/	[dɪŋ]	/kɪŋ/	[dɪŋ]	/kĩ/	[dĩ]
23. van	/væn/	[bæn]	/væn/	[bæn]	/væn/	[bæn]	/væ̃/	[bæ̃]
24. hat	/hæt/	[æt]	/hæt/	[æt]	/hæt/	[æt]	/xæt/	[æt]

(continued)

TABLE 16-6 *Continued*

Target word	General American English[2]	African-American English[3]	New England (Boston) English[4]	Spanish-influenced English[5]
25. read	/ɹid/ [wid̪]	/ɹit/ [wit]	/ɹid/ [wid]	/ɹid/ [wid̪]
26. weed	/wid/ [wid̪]	/wit/ [wit]	/wid/ [wid]	/wid/ [wid̪]
27. lead	/lid/ [lid]	/lit/ [lit]	/lid/ [lid]	/lid/ [lid̪]
28. chill	/tʃɪl/ [dɪl]	/tʃɪl/ [dɪl]	/tʃɪl/ [dɪl]	/tʃɪl/ [dɪl]
29. you	/ju/ [ju]	/ju/ [ju]	/ju/ [ju]	/ju/ [ju]
30. bag	/bæg/ [bæk]	/bæk/ [bæk]	/bæg/ [bæk]	/bæɣ/ [bæk]

Single-word sample of word-initial and word-final consonant clusters

Target word	General American English[2]	African-American English[3]	New England (Boston) English[4]	Spanish-influenced English[5]
1. swim	/swɪm/ [dɪm]	/swɪm/ [dɪm]	/swɪm/ [dɪm]	/swĩ/ [di]
2. square	/skwɛɹ/ [dɛə]	/skwæɚ/ [dæə]	/skwɛɚ/ [dɛə]	/skwɛɹ/ [dɛə]
3. through	/θɹu/ [bu]	/fɹu/ [bu]	/θɹu/ [bu]	/tru/ [bu]
4. ant	/ænt/ [ænt]	/æn/ [æn]	/ænt/ [ænt]	/ænt/ [ænt]
5. jump	/dʒʌmp/ [dʌmp]	/dʒʌm/ [dʌm]	/dʒʌmp/ [dʌmp]	/dʒʌmp/ [dʌmp]
6. twin	/twɪn/ [dɪn]	/twɪn/ [dɪn]	/twɪn/ [dɪn]	/twĩ/ [di]
7. blood	/blʌd/ [bʌd]	/blʌt/ [bʌt]	/blʌd/ [bʌd]	/blʌd̪/ [bʌd̪]
8. blue	/blu/ [bu]	/blu/ [bu]	/blu/ [bu]	/blu/ [bu]
9. clean	/klin/ [din]	/klin/ [din]	/klin/ [din]	/klĩ/ [di]
10. clock	/klɑk/ [dɑk]	/klɑk/ [dɑk]	/klɑk/ [dɑk]	/klɑk/ [dɑk]
11. fly	/flaɪ/ [baɪ]	/flaɪ/ [baɪ]	/flaɪ/ [baɪ]	/flaɪ/ [baɪ]
12. street	/stɹit/ [dit]	/stɹit/ [dit]	/stɹit/ [dit]	/strit/ [dit]
13. spring	/spɹɪŋ/ [bɪŋ]	/spɹɪn/ [bɪn]	/spɹɪŋ/ [bɪŋ]	/sprĩ/ [bi]
14. playground	/plegɹaʊnd/ [bedaʊn]	/plegɹaʊn/ [bedaʊn]	/plegɹaʊnd/ [bedaʊn]	/plegaʊ̃/ [bedaũ]
15. sleep	/slip/ [dip]	/slip/ [dip]	/slip/ [dip]	/eslip/ [edip]
16. drink	/dɹɪŋk/ [dɪŋk]	/dɹɪŋ/ [dɪŋ]	/dɹɪŋk/ [dɪŋk]	/dɹɪŋk/ [dɪŋk]
17. ski	/ski/ [di]	/ski/ [di]	/ski/ [di]	/eski/ [edi]
18. tree	/tɹi/ [di]	/tɹi/ [di]	/tɹi/ [di]	/tri/ [di]
19. smell	/smɛl/ [mɛl]	/smɛl/ [mɛl]	/smɛl/ [mɛl]	/esmɛl/ [mɛl]
20. snow	/snoʊ/ [no]	/snoʊ/ [no]	/snoʊ/ [no]	/esnoʊ/ [no]
21. space	/spes/ [bet]	/spes/ [bet]	/spes/ [bet]	/espes/ [bet]
22. splinter	/splɪntɚ/ [bɪmtə]	/splɪntə/ [bɪmtə]	/splɪntə/ [bɪmtə]	/esplɪntɚɹ/ [bɪmtə]
23. scratch	/skɹætʃ/ [dæt]	/skɹætʃ/ [dæt]	/skɹætʃ/ [dæt]	/eskɹætʃ/ [dæt]
24. throne	/θɹoʊn/ [bon]	/θɹon/ [bon]	/θɹoʊn/ [bon]	/tɹon/ [bon]
25. sleeve	/sliv/ [lip]	/slif/ [lip]	/sliv/ [lip]	/esliv/ [lip]
26. brush	/bɹʌʃ/ [bʌt]	/bɹʌʃ/ [bʌt]	/bɹʌʃ/ [bʌt]	/bɹʌʃ/ [bʌt]

(continued)

TABLE 16-6 Continued

Target word	General American English[2]		African-American English[3]		New England (Boston) English[4]		Spanish-influenced English[5]	
27. story	/stɔɹi/	[dɔwi]	/stɔɹi/	[dɔwi]	/stɔɹi/	[dɔwi]	/estɔɹi/	[dɔwi]
28. shrink	/ʃɹɪŋk/	[dɹɪŋk]	/ʃɹɪŋ/	[dɹɪŋ]	/ʃɹɪŋk/	[dɹɪŋk]	/ʃɹɪŋk/	[dɹɪŋk]
29. toast	/tost/	[tot]	/tost/	[tot]	/tost/	[tot]	/tost/	[tot]
30. green	/gɹin/	[din]	/gɹin/	[din]	/gɹin/	[din]	/gɾi/	[di]
31. pupil	/pjupəl/	[bupəl]	/pjupəl/	[bupəl]	/pjupəl/	[bupəl]	/pjupəl/	[bupəl]
32. music	/mjuzɪk/	[mudɪk]	/muzɪk/	[mudɪk]	/mjuzɪk/	[mudɪk]	/mjuzɪk/	[mudɪk]
33. cute	/kjut/	[dut]	/kut/	[kut]	/kjut/	[dut]	/kjut/	[dut]
34. beautiful	/bjutɪfəl/	[butɪpəl]	/buttfəl/	[butɪpəl]	/bjutɪfəl/	[butɪpəl]	/bjutɪfəl/	[butɪpəl]
35. pram	/pɹæm/	[bæm]	/pɹæm/	[bæm]	/pɹæm/	[bæm]	/pɹæ/	[bæ]

Single-word sample of polysyllabic real words[6]

Target word	General American English[2]		African-American English[3]		New England (Boston) English[4]		Spanish-influenced English[5]	
1. spaghetti	/spəgɛti/	[bədɛti]	/spəgɛti/	[bədɛti]	/spəgɛti/	[bədɛti]	/espæɣɛti/	[bædɛti]
2. caterpillar	/kætɚpɪlɚ/	[dætəbɪlə]	/kætɚpɪlɚ/	[dætəbɪlə]	/kætɚpɪlɚ/	[dætəbɪlə]	/kætɚpɪlɚɾ/	[dætəbɪlə]
3. computer	/kəmpjutɚ/	[dəmbutə]	/kəmputɚ/	[dəmbutə]	/kəmpjutɚ/	[dəmbutə]	/kəmpjutəɾ/	[dəmbutə]
4. hippopotamus	/hɪpəpɑtəməs/	[hɪpəbɑtəmət]	/hɪpəpɑtəməs/	[hɪpəbɑtəmət]	/hɪpəpɑtəməs/	[hɪpəbɑtəmət]	/hɪpəbɑtəməs/	[hɪpəbɑtəmət]
5. animals	/ænɪməlz/	[ænɪmɛlt]	/ænɪmɛlz/	[ænɪmɛlt]	/ænɪmɛlz/	[ænɪmɛlt]	/ænɪmɛls/	[ænɪmɛlt]
6. butterfly	/bʌtɚflaɪ/	[bʌtəbaɪ]	/bʌtɚflaɪ/	[bʌtəbaɪ]	/bʌtɚflaɪ/	[bʌtəbaɪ]	/bʌtɚflaɪ/	[bʌtɚflaɪ]
7. ambulance[7]	/æmbjələnts/	[æmbələn]	/æmbələn/	[æmbələn]	/æmbjələnts/	[æmbələn]	/æmbjulənts/	[æmbulənt]
8. caravan	/kæɹəvæn/	[dæəbæn]	/kæɹəvæn/	[dæəbæn]	/kæɹəvæn/	[dæəbæn]	/kaɾəvæ/	[dæəbæ]
9. vegetables	/vɛdʒtəbəlz/	[bɛdəbot]	/vɛdʒtəbəlz/	[bɛdəbot]	/vɛdʒtəbəlz/	[bɛdəbot]	/vɛdʒtəβɛlz/	[bɛdəβot]
10. helicopter	/hɛlɪkɑptɚ/	[elidɑpə]	/hɛlɪkɑptɚ/	[elidɑpə]	/hɛlɪkɑptɚ/	[elidɑpə]	/xɛlikɑptəɾ/	[elidɑpə]

[1]These three words are selected from the 50 words within the Phonology Assessment of the Diagnostic Evaluation of Articulation and Phonology (DEAP) (Dodd, Hua, et al., 2006).

[2]The first three target (adult) productions of General American English are adapted from the transcription from the DEAP (Dodd, Hua, et al., 2006), and the remainder is adapted from information from Smit (2007).

[3]The adult and child productions in the African-American English example were adapted from information from Stockman (2007). It is important to note that this presents one of many possible transcriptions; speakers of African-American English differ in the number, type, and frequency of dialectal features used in different contexts.

[4]The target (adult) productions in the New England (Boston) English example were adapted from Nagy and Roberts (2004).

[5]The adult and child productions in the Spanish-influenced English example were adapted from information from Goldstein (2007). It is important to note that this presents one of many possible transcriptions; speakers of Spanish-influenced English differ in the number, type, and frequency of dialectal features used in different contexts.

[6]Ten words adapted from James (2006). Used with permission.

[7]The word ambulance may be pronounced with or without the /t/ in the final consonant cluster.

TABLE 16-7				Intervention studies of children who have phonological impairment
Authors (year)	**Child(ren), gender, age, characteristics**	**Languages and/or dialects**	**Intervention approach**	**Why is this study interesting?**
Baker & Bernhardt (2004)	James: male (4;4 years)	Australian English	Minimal pairs	The study explores reasons underlying slow progress for a child with phonological impairment.
Bernhardt & Stemberger (2000)	Dylan: male (4;7 years)	Canadian English	Nonlinear phonology	The study provides detailed speech samples for Dylan (4;7 years) in addition to a step-by-step constraint-based nonlinear phonological analysis of his speech.
Bowen & Cupples (1998, 1999b)	Nina: female (4;4 years) Ceri: female (4;5 years)	Australian English	PACT therapy	Helpful overview of the management of moderate and severe phonological impairment from referral to discharge, using PACT therapy (Bowen, 2010).
Gierut & Champion (2000)	I.J.: male (4;5 years)	American English	Generic phonological intervention targeting ingressive substitution pattern	Interesting case of a child who used an ingressive fricative for sibilants /s, z, ʃ, ʧ, ʤ/.
Hodson & Paden (1991)	Annie: female (3;1 years) Brad: male (4;11 years)	American English	Cycles therapy	Practical case descriptions of two children with profound phonological impairment, who were managed using Hodson and Paden's (1991) cycles approach to phonological remediation.
Holm & Dodd (2001)	Michael: male (5;2 years)	Cantonese and English	Traditional articulation therapy and minimal pairs therapy	Interesting case of bilingual SSD (in Cantonese and English) characterized by both phonological (loss of phonemic contrast) and articulation impairment (interdental lisp).
Miccio & Elbert (1996)	Stacy: female (3;4 years)	American English	Stimulability intervention	Practical case description and application of stimulability intervention (Miccio & Elbert, 1996) for a young child with a small phonetic inventory, who was not stimulable for many speech sounds absent from her phonetic repertoire.
Miccio & Ingrisano (2000)	K: female (5;3 years)	American English	Minimal pairs	Overview of a complex case (child with bilateral recurrent otitis media with fluctuating conductive hearing loss; language, fine and gross motor delay) from assessment and analysis through to target selection and intervention.
Williams (2000a)	10 cases (4;6–5;6 years)	American English	Multiple oppositions	Overview of 10 cases of moderate, severe, and profound phonological impairment, from initial referral to discharge. The cases illustrate how children benefit from different types of intervention approaches over the course of intervention—beginning with multiple oppositions, progressing to minimal pairs therapy and, if needed, naturalistic speech intelligibility training.

SUSIE (7;4 YEARS): ARTICULATION IMPAIRMENT—LATERAL LISP

Susie (7;4 years) is described as a school-age girl with an articulation impairment involving the sibilants /s, z/. Susie is like many children throughout the world, with a relatively minor speech difficulty involving one or two speech sounds.

■ Susie: Case history

Susie is an above-average student, whose local dialect is General American English. Susie is an only child. She has no family history of SSD, language, or literacy difficulties. Birth and medical history were unremarkable. Susie's hearing was normal. Apart from a few head colds most winters, Susie was described as a healthy child. Major early developmental milestones (crawling, walking, talking) were all within the expected ranges.

Susie had lateralized production of /s, z/. Her parents first became concerned about the way Susie pronounced her /s/ in words when she was 4 years old. At that time, Susie's parents had decided to monitor her production of /s/ and simply remind her to say her /s/ more clearly. When Susie's upper central deciduous teeth fell out, her parents noticed that Susie's speech was less clear. They decided to seek the advice of an SLP when Susie's speech did not improve when her adult upper central front incisors grew.

During a case history interview with Susie and her family, Susie's parents described her as an outgoing and energetic child, when in the company of friends and family. In new situations or around new people, she was quiet and reluctant to join in conversation. Susie was aware that her pronunciation of /s, z/ was unclear. She was aware that her /s, z/ sounded different and was distressed by the fact that peers had commented on her "slushy" speech. Susie presented as highly motivated to work on her lisp and willing to complete follow-up practice at home. Up until 7;4 years, Susie had received no prior intervention. She enjoyed horse riding, reading, craft activities, and playing with her friends.

■ Susie: Assessment results

Susie saw an SLP for a routine speech and language assessment. Susie's receptive and expressive language tested as within normal limits on the Clinical Evaluation of Language Fundamentals (CELF-4) Screening Test (Wiig, Secord, & Semel, 2004). Susie passed a routine audiometric screening. Using the Robbins and Klee (1987) oral and speech motor control protocol, Susie's oral structures (lips, hard and soft palate, tongue, lingual frenulum, and teeth) and function were noted to be appropriate. Susie had mixed dentition characterized by mostly deciduous teeth with six adult teeth (four lower incisors and two upper central incisors). Her left upper lateral incisor was loose. Susie's fluency was normal. Her voice quality was appropriate for her age and gender. Susie was not stimulable for the production of /s/ or /z/ in isolation or in syllables, given an auditory model or phonetic placement cues.

Susie: Standardized and strategic speech assessment

The Goldman-Fristoe Test of Articulation-2 Sounds in Words subtest (Goldman & Fristoe, 2000) was used to assess Susie's articulation. Apart from /s, z/, all other consonants and vowels were perceived as correct. An informal single-word probe of Susie's production of /s, z/ in singleton and consonant cluster contexts, across initial, medial, and word-final positions was collected (see Table 16-8). A connected speech sample was gathered via a picture description task, strategically loaded to sample /s, z/. A 5-minute conversational speech sample was also gathered during the initial assessment session. Lateralized /s, z/ was evident in all sampling contexts.

■ Intervention studies of children who have an articulation impairment involving rhotics or sibilants

Case study reports of children who have an articulation impairment involving rhotics or sibilants either focus on the application of the principles of motor learning using conventional

TABLE 16-8	Susie's production of /s, z/ in single-words in singleton and consonant cluster contexts, in word-initial, -medial, and -final positions		
sun /sʌn/ → [ɬʌn]	*zip* /zɪp/ → [ʒɪp]	*lips* /lɪps/ → [lɪpɬ]	*missing* /mɪsɪŋ/ → [mɪɬɪŋ]
bus /bʌs/ → [bʌɬ]	*eats* /its/ → [itɬ]	*fuzzy* /fʌzi/ → [fʌʒi]	*hands* /hændz/ → [hændʒ]
has /hæz/ → [hæʒ]	*buzz* /bʌz/ → [bʌʒ]	*busy* /bɪzi/ → [bɪʒi]	*something* /sʌmθɪŋ/ → [ɬʌmθɪŋ]
skip /skɪp/ → [ɬkɪp]	*rats* /ɹæts/ → [ɹætɬ]	*handstand* /hændstænd/ → [hændɬtænd]	*zipper* /zɪpɚ/ → [ʒɪpɚ]
spaghetti /spəgɛti/ → [ɬpəgɛti]	*easy* /izi/ → [iʒi]	*hamster* /hæmstɚ/ → [hæmɬtɚ]	*kissed* /kɪst/ → [kɪɬt]
rice /ɹaɪs/ → [ɹaɪɬ]	*person* /pɝsən/ → [pɝɬən]	*stamp* /stæmp/ → [ɬtæmp]	*xylophone* /zaɪləfon/ → [ʒaɪləfon]

behavioral techniques (Skelton, 2004a) or describe innovative instrumental solutions where conventional methods have not been successful (e.g., McAllister Byun & Hitchcock, 2012). The children involved in this research have typically been school age (see Table 16-9).

Jarrod (7;0 Years): Inconsistent Speech Disorder

Jarrod is a 7-year-old boy who was diagnosed with inconsistent speech disorder. We selected Jarrod's case for this chapter because his case has been extensively documented and studied by different researchers (e.g., Bernhardt, Stemberger, & Major, 2006; Bowen & Cupples, 2006; Crosbie, Pine, Holm, & Dodd, 2006; Dodd, Holm, Crosbie, & McIntosh, 2006; Hodson, 2006; Hodson & Jardine, 2009; Holm & Crosbie, 2006; Stackhouse, Pascoe, & Gardner, 2006). You can also view a video sample of Jarrod's conversational speech within the supplementary material attached to the editorial at the Taylor & Francis Online website.[1] This video sample was part of a special issue about Jarrod's case in the *International Journal of Speech-Language Pathology*, volume 8(3). What follows is a brief history of Jarrod's case from that special issue, primarily drawing on the work of Holm and Crosbie (2006), Crosbie et al. (2006), and Dodd, Holm, et al. (2006).

▪ Jarrod: Case history

Jarrod is an Australian English-speaking boy who lives with his mother and older sister. He regularly sees his father and extended family. Jarrod has a positive family history of speech and literacy difficulties. At the time of the assessment, Jarrod's mother was a bookkeeper. His father was a builder. Jarrod was born full term. He was breastfed for 6 months. At 15 months Jarrod was diagnosed with asthma. At the time of the assessment, Jarrod's asthma was being managed with a nebulizer, Ventolin, and Flixotide. Jarrod has a history of otitis media. Pressure equalizer (PE) tubes (also known as grommets) were inserted at 2 and 4 years. A hearing test at 4;1 years indicated that his hearing was adequate for speech and language acquisition. Jarrod also had been diagnosed with attention-deficit/hyperactivity disorder (ADHD). At the time of the assessment, Jarrod had been taking Ritalin for 2 months. Although Jarrod's handwriting was considered good for his age, an assessment by an occupational therapist identified some fine motor difficulties (Holm & Crosbie, 2006).

▪ Jarrod: Assessment results

Jarrod started talking at around 30 months of age. It was suggested that he may have talked earlier than this, however his limited speech intelligibility meant that could not be understood

---

[1] http://www.tandfonline.com/doi/suppl/10.1080/14417040600861086#tabModule

(Holm & Crosbie, 2006). Jarrod's communication skills were first assessed by an SLP at 4;0 years. Over a 3-year period Jarrod was seen by four different SLPs (two in private practice and two school-based clinicians) for assessment and intervention. At 7;0 years Jarrod's speech was still mostly unintelligible. Table 16-10 provides a summary of the comprehensive assessment of Jarrod's language, speech, phonological processing (auditory discrimination, phonological working memory, phonological awareness), oromotor and nonverbal abilities at 7;0 years.

Jarrod: Single-word speech sample

A variety of formal and informal speech sampling tools were used to assess Jarrod's speech. The special issue of the *International Journal of Speech-Language Pathology* (volume 8, number 3)

TABLE 16-9 Intervention studies of children who have an articulation impairment involving sibilants or rhotics

Authors (year)	Child(ren), gender, age, characteristics	Languages and/or dialects	Intervention approach	Why is this case study interesting?
Adler-Bock, Bernhardt, Gick, & Bacsfalvi (2007)	VF: male (14 years) ML: male (12 years) with /ɹ/ distortion	Canadian English	Visual feedback using ultrasound	Valuable description of intervention using visual feedback from an ultrasound image to successfully treat persistent /ɹ/ distortion.
Dagenais, Critz-Crosby, & Adams (1994)	Child 1: female (8;8 years) Child 2: female (8;6 years) with lateral lisp	American English	Visual feedback using electropalatography (EPG)	Insight into how children with similar errors (lateral lisp) responded to intervention using EPG.
McAllister Byun & Hitchcock (2012)	11 children (6;0–11;9 years) with /ɹ/ distortion	American English	Visual feedback using linear predictive coding (LPC) spectrum of consonantal and vocalic /ɹ/	Overview of how linear predictive coding (LPC) spectrum showing F1, F2, and F3 formants can be a useful visual feedback device for helping children with persistent /ɹ/ distortion learn the motor skill required to produce (but not necessarily generalize) consonantal and vocalic /ɹ/.
McAuliffe & Cornwell (2008)	RB: female (11 years) with lateral lisp	Australian English	Visual feedback using electropalatography (EPG)	Description of how EPG can be used to provide visual feedback in conjunction with intervention based on the principles of motor learning (Maas et al., 2008) to treat persistent lateral /s/ lisp.
Shuster, Ruscello, & Toth (1995)	Jerry: male (10 years) and Tina: female (14 years) with /ɹ/ distortion	American English	Visual feedback using spectrogram	Interesting description of intervention targeting persistent /ɹ/ distortion in two children, who had not responded to other forms of intervention. Intervention involved visual feedback in the form of a real-time spectrogram.
Skelton (2004a)	Four children (7;5–7;10 years) with interdental lisp	American English	Concurrent treatment	Practical description about how traditional articulation therapy can be modified to align with the principles of motor learning by intermixing easy and more challenging exemplars when treating [θ] for /s/ substitution.

TABLE 16-10 Jarrod (7;0 years): Summary assessment results

Skill area	Assessment	Measure and/or observation	Result
Receptive and expressive language	Clinical Evaluation of Language Fundamentals-4 (CELF-4) (Semel, Wiig, & Secord, 2004)	Receptive language score: 103 (SS) Expressive language score: 112 (SS)	✓
Speech production	Diagnostic Evaluation of Articulation and Phonology (DEAP) (Dodd et al., 2002)	PPC = 44%; PCC = 29%; PVC = 70% Jarrod could produce all speech sounds except the affricates /tʃ, dʒ/ and the palatal fricative /ʒ/. He also produced some non-English sounds (e.g., /ɬ, y, x/) (Crosbie et al., 2006).	✗
Speech production	Hodson Assessment of Phonological Patterns-3 (HAPP-3) (Hodson, 2004)	Total occurrences of major phonological deviations = 157, consistent with profound severity rating.	✗
Speech inconsistency	Diagnostic Evaluation of Articulation and Phonology (DEAP): Inconsistency assessment (Dodd et al., 2002)	80% inconsistent	✗
Auditory discrimination	Auditory Discrimination Test involving real and nonwords (Bridgeman & Snowling, 1988)	Jarrod could perceive differences in simple CVC stimuli (in both real and nonword contexts), but had difficulty discriminating words with final consonant sequences (e.g., /st/ versus /ts/) in real and nonword contexts (Stackhouse et al., 2006).	✗
Lexical decision	Auditory Lexical Discrimination Tests (Locke, 1980a, b)	Given a task where Jarrod had to listen to and decide whether pictures of words (e.g., *brush*) were said correctly (e.g., *Is this a brush*) or incorrectly (e.g., *Is this a brish*), Jarrod did well, scoring at ceiling 46/48 (Stackhouse et al., 2006).	✓
Phonological working memory	Children's Nonword Repetition Test (CNRep) (Gathercole & Baddeley, 1996)	Below average.	✗
Phonological awareness and letter-sound knowledge	Preschool and Primary Inventory of Phonological Awareness (PIPA) (Dodd, Crosbie, McIntosh, Teitzel, & Ozanne, 2000)	Two subtests (Rhyme Awareness and Phoneme Isolation) significantly below average. Letter knowledge—borderline average.	✓
Cognition	Wechsler Intelligence Scale for Children—Fourth Edition (WISC-IV) (Wechsler, 2003)	Verbal Comprehension Index 81 (equivalent to 10th percentile). Perceptual Reasoning Index 111 (equivalent to 76th percentile).	✗ ✓
Oral structure and function	Verbal Motor Production Assessment for Children (VMPAC) (Hayden & Square 1999)	Based on Hayden (2006), Jarrod's performance was significantly below the 5th percentile for his age, in light of the following scores: ■ Global motor control 95% ■ Focal oromotor control 46% ■ Sequencing 57% ■ Connected speech and language control 53% ■ Speech characteristics 85%	✗
	Informal observation of oral structures	Jarrod had no obvious structural anomalies on informal observation. He had primary dentition only (McLeod, 2006b).	
Activity and participation	Speech Participation and Activity Assessment of Children (SPAA-C) (McLeod, 2004) and interview, including analysis using the ICF-CY (WHO, 2007)	Jarrod's mother reported that Jarrod "played with children in the neighbourhood and went to other children's birthday parties" (Holm & Crosbie, 2006, p. 168). By contrast, Jarrod's classroom teacher reported that Jarrod "did not have particularly good social interactions" (Holm & Crosbie, 2006, p. 168).	✗ ✓

SS = standard score, ✓ = acceptable, ✗ = problematic.

Sources: Adapted from Bernhardt et al. (2006); Crosbie et al. (2006); Dodd, Holm, et al. (2006); Hodson (2006); Holm and Crosbie (2006); McLeod (2006b); Stackhouse et al. (2006).

provides extensive single-word samples and analyses (see Bernhardt et al., 2006; Holm & Crosbie, 2006; Müller et al., 2006). Table 16-11 provides a brief sample of Jarrod's speech from the DEAP: Inconsistency test (Dodd et al., 2002) as reported by Dodd, Holm, et al. (2006) primarily for the purpose of illustrating the inconsistent nature of his single-word productions.

According to Dodd, Holm, et al. (2006), Jarrod's inconsistent production of identical lexical items and improved accuracy with imitation were symptomatic of inconsistent speech disorder. Jarrod's productions of intended consonants were mapped onto a substitution matrix (see Figure 16-2). This matrix shows all intended consonants as columns, and all realized consonants as rows. Consistent accurate speech would be depicted by a single diagonal line. Consistent errors are evident when one sound is always omitted or always substituted for another. Inconsistent errors are evident when a range of sounds is used for one sound. Jarrod's matrix of speech sound substitutions is shown in Figure 16-2. In this figure, the black squares reflect accurate productions. The gray squares show the range of substituted sounds for a target sound. For instance, although the consonant /l/ was correct on some occasions, it was also realized in 10 other ways (eight different consonants, including the glottal stop, and as an omission).

FIGURE 16-2   **Inconsistency matrix based on single-word samples collected for Jarrod (7;0 years)**

Note: The order of consonants depicted on the matrix is in keeping with the order of consonants on the IPA chart. The matrix in Dodd, Holm, et al. (2006) showed consonants in columns according to place of articulation from the front to back of the mouth.

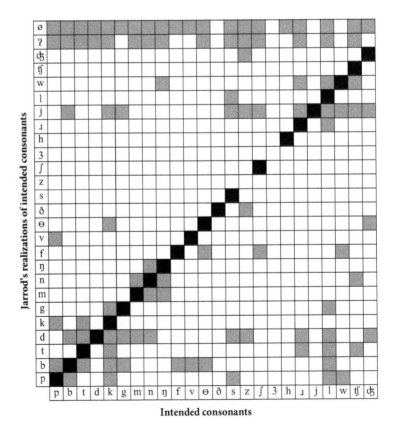

Source: Based on Dodd, Holm, et al. (2006).

| TABLE 16-11 | Brief single-word speech sample for Jarrod (7;0 years) showing inconsistent production of three words |

Target word[1]	Adult pronunciation	Jarrod's first production[2]	Jarrod's second production[2]	Jarrod's third production[2]
1. witch	/wɪtʃ/	[bwæːːtʃ]	[bwæ]	[bwɛʔt]
2. tongue	/tʌŋ/	[bʌns]	[dʌn]	[bʌʔm]
3. birthday cake	/bɜθdeɪ keɪk/	[bɜθdeɪkʰeɪʔk]	[bɜfdeːpʰeɪʔt]	[bɜθdæɪˌtʰʌʔt]

[1]These three words are selected from the 25 words within the Inconsistency Assessment of the Diagnostic Evaluation of Articulation and Phonology (DEAP) (Dodd, Hua, et al., 2002).
[2]Jarrod's productions as described in Dodd, Holm, et al. (2006).

| TABLE 16-12 | Intervention studies of children who have inconsistent speech disorder |

Authors (year)	Child(ren), gender, age, characteristics	Languages and/or dialects	Intervention approach	Why is this study interesting?
Crosbie, Holm, & Dodd (2005)	18 children including 10 diagnosed with inconsistent speech disorder	Australian English	Core vocabulary compared with minimal pairs therapy	This study illustrates how core vocabulary therapy was more effective than minimal pairs therapy for children with inconsistent speech disorder.
Holm & Dodd (1999)	Giuseppe: male (4;2 years)	Italian and English	N/A	Helpful discussion of the issues associated with the differential diagnosis of inconsistent speech disorder in children learning two languages.
Holm & Dodd (2001)	Hafis: male (4;8 years)	English and Punjabi	Core vocabulary	Helpful illustration of how a bilingual child with inconsistent speech disorder became consistent in both languages, given core vocabulary therapy in one language.
McIntosh & Dodd (2009)	Andrew: male (3;9 years) Benjamin: male (4;2 years) Cameron: male (4;3 years)	Australian English	Core vocabulary	Detailed case descriptions of three preschool English-speaking children with inconsistent speech disorder. The authors describe how they individualized core vocabulary therapy to meet the specific needs of each child.

■ Published intervention studies of children who have inconsistent speech disorder

According to Broomfield and Dodd (2004b), about 9.4% of all children with SSD have inconsistent speech disorder. Most of the research has been conducted by Barbara Dodd and colleagues. Table 16-12 provides an overview of a selection of the cases from this research.

MICHAEL (4;2 YEARS): CHILDHOOD APRAXIA OF SPEECH (CAS)

Michael has a motor speech disorder known as CAS. CAS occurs in approximately 1 to 2 children per thousand (Shriberg, Aram, & Kwiatkowski, 1997).

■ Michael: Case history

Michael is the youngest of two children. Michael is monolingual and learning General American English. Michael was referred for a speech-language pathology assessment by his parents and preschool teacher at 4;2 years. Although Michael's parents had been concerned about the naturalness of Michael's speech since he was a 2-year-old child, they acted on their concern on the advice of Michael's preschool teacher.

Michael was born full term with no complications during pregnancy or birth. Michael's mother reported that when Michael was awake and content, he was a quiet baby. Michael babbled somewhat less than his sister. First intelligible words appeared at around 18 months. Two and three-word utterances emerged at around 2 years. Michael's parents described Michael's speech as robotic and unnatural. With regards to other aspects of early development, gross motor milestones were as follows: unaided sitting (7 months), crawling (10 months) and walking (13 months). All other medical and developmental history was unremarkable. Although there was a positive family history of speech, language, or literacy difficulty in Michael's extended family, there were no prior cases of CAS.

■ Michael: Assessment results

Michael's communication skills were assessed using a range of standardized and informal, non-standardized assessment tools. Table 16-13 provides a summary of the results.

TABLE 16-13   Michael (4;2 years): Summary speech-language pathology assessment results

Skill area	Assessment	Measure and/or observation	Result
Receptive and expressive language	Clinical Evaluation of Language Fundamentals: Preschool-2 (CELF-P2) (Wiig, Secord, & Semel, 2004)	Receptive: 105 (SS) Expressive: 97 (SS)	Receptive ✓ Expressive ✓
Receptive vocabulary	Peabody Picture Vocabulary Test-4 (PPVT-4) (Dunn & Dunn, 2007)	Standard score = 98	✓
Speech production: standardized single-word sample	Goldman Fristoe Test of Articulation-2 (GFTA-2): Sounds in words subtest (Goldman & Fristoe, 2000)	GFTA-2 standard score = 12 (PPC = 73%; PCC = 70%; PVC = 78%)	✗
Speech production: strategic sampling	Nuffield Centre Dyspraxia Programme-3 (NDP-3) (Williams & Stephens, 2004)	Imitation of single consonants = 21/24. He did not imitate /θ, ð, ʒ/ accurately. Some imitated diphthongs were distorted or lengthened. Consonants in CV, VC, CVC, and CVCV words (with SS stress pattern) were correct except initial words containing /l, dʒ/. (The consonants /θ, ð, ʒ/ were not sampled in this task.) Articulation accuracy decreased in complex and multisyllabic words, with consonant omission, glottal insertion, imprecise voicing, cluster reduction, weak syllable deletion, stress equalization, and syllable segregation evident. Across the 20 consonant cluster words, 9 were correct. Michael's imitation of the 11 phrases and sentences were slow and deliberate. Equal stress, a level pitch, imprecise vowels, and difficulty with juncture were evident.	✗
Speech production: strategic sampling	Single-word test of polysyllables (Gozzard et al., 2004)	Polysyllabic words were particularly challenging for Michael. His words were either staccato-like (displaying syllable segregation and stress equalization) or reduced in length. Weak syllables in words with iambic (as opposed to trochaic) stress were particularly prone to omission.	✗

(continued)

TABLE 16-13 *Continued*

Skill area	Assessment	Measure and/or observation	Result
Speech production: conversational speech sample	Samples of connected speech were gathered during episodes of conversation during single-word testing, in addition to a 100-utterance conversational speech sample during play.	Due to Michael's reduced speech intelligibility, not all of Michael's utterances could be reliably glossed. His speech was noticeably dysprosodic.	✗
Speech production: speech inconsistency	Diagnostic Evaluation of Articulation and Phonology (DEAP): Inconsistency assessment (Dodd et al., 2002)	40% inconsistency	✗
Stimulability	Nuffield Centre Dyspraxia Programme-3 (NDP-3) (Williams & Stephens, 2004)	Michael was stimulable for all consonants except /θ, ð, ʒ/ in isolation and syllables.	✗
Verbal and nonverbal IQ	Primary Test of Nonverbal Intelligence (PTONI) (Ehrler & McGhee, 2008)	101 (SS)	✓
Oral structure and function	Nuffield Centre Dyspraxia Programme-3 (NDP-3) (Williams & Stephens, 2004)	Oral structures were normal. Muscle tone and facial symmetry were unremarkable. Michael had a complete set of deciduous dentition.	✗
		Oromotor (non-speech) skills: Michael's range of lip and tongue movement was good. Alternating mouth movements were adequate although slow. Voice quality was good during a sustained vowel. Volume was generally appropriate, although sometimes he spoke in a whisper. Pitch was generally flat; however, he was able to mark a rising intonation pattern on imitation. Connected speech was at times hypernasal.	
		DDK (diadochokinesis): Inconsistency was apparent on syllable and word sequencing tasks, especially those involving a change of consonant. Michael's attempts were slow and deliberate. Syllables were produced separately. He could not produce rapid alternating movements given trisyllabic sequences.	
Hearing function	Pure tone audiometric screening at 500, 1000, 2000, and 4000 Hz. Tympanometry	Michael responded to pure tone thresholds in his left and right ear, at 20 dB in a quiet room. Graph on tympanogram consistent with Type A, suggesting normal eardrum movement. No fluid was detected in Michael's middle ear cavity.	✓
Fluency	Informal observation during speech production assessment.	Although Michael did not present with obvious symptoms of stuttering (e.g., blocks, part-word repetitions), the staccato characteristic of his speech meant that he did not sound fluent.	✓ ✗
Voice	Informal observation during speech production assessment.	Michael's voice quality and pitch (based on a sustained vowel) was perceived to be appropriate for his age and gender. His conversational speech was somewhat monotone, and hypernasal at times.	✓

SS = standard score, ✓= acceptable, ✗ = problematic, PPC = percentage of phonemes correct, PCC = percentage of consonants correct, PVC = percentage of vowels correct.

Michael: Speech production skills

Michael is an interesting case. Although his case is similar to Luke's (e.g., both have normal receptive and expressive language, unremarkable medial and general developmental history, and SSD), Michael and Luke differ in a number of important ways. Michael's phonetic inventory was considerably more complete than Luke's. Based on single-word and connected speech samples, Michael's singleton consonant phonetic inventory included all consonants except /ɹ, ʒ, θ, ð/. He could imitate [r] and [ɝ] in isolation. This meant that all sound classes were present. Apart from [v] being present in word-final position only, there were no other singleton positional constraints. His consonant cluster inventory in word-initial position was limited to C + [w] and [s] + C clusters including word-initial [sp, sk, st, sn, sw, kw, gw] and the non-English clusters [pw, fw]. Michael produced a range of consonant clusters in word-final position including [mp, nt, ns, ps, nʤ, gz]. Three-element clusters were not sampled. His phonetic inventory of monophthong vowels included [i, ɪ, e, ɛ, æ, u, ʊ, o, ɔ, ɑ, ə, ʌ] but not [ɝ, ɚ]. With regards to diphthongs, he produced [aɪ, aʊ, ɔɪ, ɛə]. He did not produce rhotic diphthongs [ɪɹ, ɛɹ, ʊɹ, ɔɹ, ɑɹ]. He produced a range of syllable shapes including V, CV, VC, CVC, CCV(C+), (C+)VCC. He could produce words up to four syllables in length. Although he attempted words comprising Sw, Ssw, Sws, Swsw stress patterns, the weak syllables were perceived to be of a similar duration to the strong syllables. He tended to use loudness only to convey differences in syllable stress in words. Words comprising more than one syllable also contained brief pauses (i.e., syllable segregation) between the syllables. During conversational speech, Michael showed a preference for producing words with strong equally timed, segregated syllables. He did produce some words with weak onsets (i.e., iambic stress). Overall, the defining characteristic of Michael's speech was his dysprosody. Table 16-14 provides examples of the inconsistency in Michael's speech, while Table 16-15 illustrates his difficulty with polysyllables.

TABLE 16-14	Brief single-word speech sample for Michael (4;2 years) showing inconsistent production of three words			
Target word	Adult pronunciation	Michael's 1st production	Michael's 2nd production	Michael's 3rd production
1. witch	/wɪtʃ/	[wɜtʃ]	[ʰwɪtʃ]	[wʊtʃ]
2. tongue	/tʌŋ/	[tʌnd]	[tʌŋ]	[tʌŋ]
3. birthday cake	/bɜˑθde kek/	[bɜf.de.kek]	[bɜf.de.keʔ]	[bɜp.de.kek]

Source: These three words are selected from the 25 words within the Inconsistency Assessment of the Diagnostic Evaluation of Articulation and Phonology (DEAP) (Dodd, Hua, et al., 2006).

TABLE 16-15	Michael (4;2 years): Single-word sample of polysyllabic real words	
Target word	Adult pronunciation	Child's production
1. dinosaur	/daɪnəˑsɔɹ/	[daɪn.sɔ]
2. ambulance	/æmbjələnts/	[æm.bɜ.ʤəns]
3. medicine	/medɪsən/	[med.sən/
4. spaghetti	/spəgɛti/	[skɛti]
5. computer	/kəmpjutɚ/	[fʷu.tɑ]
6. mosquito	/məskito/	[ski.to]
7. butterflies	/bʌtɚflaɪz/	[bʌ.fwaɪz]
8. caterpillars	/kætəˑpɪləˑz/	[kæʔ.pɪʔ.wəs]
9. television	/telɪvɪʒən/	[te.bɪs]
10. hippopotamus	/hɪpəpɑtəməs/	[hɪ.tɜ.pɑt.nəs]

Source: 10 of 50 words from Gozzard, Baker, and McCabe (2004). Used with permission.

◼ Intervention studies of children who have CAS

CAS is a rare type of SSD. Children who have CAS can also present with comorbid medical and/or developmental issues. Unless you are involved in a systematic program of research on CAS or working in a specialized clinic for children with SSD, children with CAS will not be common on a generalist clinician's pediatric caseload. You might therefore find the 10 case study reports listed in Table 16-16 helpful when you manage a child with CAS for the first time.

LIAN (14;2 YEARS): CHILDHOOD DYSARTHRIA

Lian has childhood dysarthria associated with cerebral palsy. Cerebral palsy is evident in approximately 2 per 1,000 births (Anderson, Mjoen, & Vik, 2010), with approximately 35% of these children having a speech difficulty (Parks, Hill, Platt, & Donnelly, 2010).

◼ Lian: Case history

Lian (14;2 years) is the youngest of two daughters. Like her family, she speaks both Cantonese and General American English. Lian is second-generation American Chinese. Following an unremarkable pregnancy, Lian was born via an emergency caesarean section at 39 weeks. At 5.1 lbs (2,313 g), Lian's birth weight was low. Lian was diagnosed with congenital cerebral palsy (specifically, right-sided spastic hemiplegia) at 22 months. The cause is unknown. Lian also has epilepsy, controlled with medication. Lian received therapy (physical, occupational, and speech) regularly throughout infancy and early childhood.

Lian sat unaided by 11 months, and crawled at 16 months. She used a walking frame followed by forearm crutches until around 6 years. She now functions at Level II on the Gross Motor Function Classification System (GMFCS) (Palisano et al., 1997). This means that she walks independently both indoors and outdoors, although slowly and with a limp. Uneven surfaces and crowds can be difficult for her to navigate. Lian can climb stairs with a railing for support. Jumping is difficult for Lian. With regards to hand function, Lian functions at Level II of the Manual Ability Classification System (MACS) (Eliasson et al., 2006). She can handle most objects, although with reduced speed and quality of achievement in her left hand. Lian is right-handed. On the Communication Function Classification System (CFCS) (Hidecker et al., 2011), Lian functions at Level II. She is able to use speech to communicate with familiar and unfamiliar partners, given extra time. Lian's speech intelligibility is adequate despite obvious spastic dysarthria. With background noise, however, Lian's familiar and unfamiliar communication partners can have difficulty understanding her.

Lian's hearing and vision are normal. Although she experienced some difficulties with eating and drinking as a toddler, she now manages a varied diet. Occasionally she experiences fatigue with foods that require considerable chewing. On the Wechsler Intelligence Scale for Children—Fourth Edition (WISC-IV) (Wechsler, 2003), Lian's full-scale intelligence quotient (FSIQ) score (at 12;2 years) was 95 (equivalent to 37th percentile). Lian's performance on the verbal comprehension, perceptual reasoning, working memory, and processing speed indexes were in the average range for her age.

◼ Lian: Assessment results

Lian received early intervention followed by local school-based services from SLPs through to the middle-school years. Over this period, a systems approach to intervention (Pennington, Smallman, & Farrier, 2006) was used to increase Lian's speech intelligibility. This intervention targeted Lian's respiration (particularly speech breathing), phonation (particularly loudness), resonance, and articulation. By the end of middle school, Lian's speech was generally intelligible. The need for further speech-language pathology services was reviewed when Lian started high school at age 14;2 years. Table 16-17 provides a summary of the results of that review assessment.

TABLE 16-16　Intervention studies of children who have CAS

Authors (year)	Child(ren), gender, age, characteristics	Languages and/or dialects	Intervention approach	Why is this study interesting?
Ballard et al. (2010)	M1: male (10;10 years) F1: female (9;2 years) M2: male (7;8 years)	Australian English	Rapid Syllable Transition Treatment (ReST)	Single-case experimental study about three siblings with CAS (two mild and one mild-moderate). Intervention targeted prosody in three- and four-syllable nonwords guided by principles of motor learning.
Edeal & Gildersleeve-Neumann (2011)	Jamie: male (6;2 years) Felix: male (3;4 years)	American English	Integral stimulation with focus on effect of production frequency	Detailed case descriptions of two boys who received integral stimulation intervention for CAS. Focus of study was on the benefit of high (100+) versus moderate (30–40) production frequency or dose per target per session.
Hall, Hardy, & Lavelle (1990)	TB: female (7 years)	American English	Palatal lift	Case report of a girl (TB) with severe CAS that included "excessive nasal resonance and nasal emission of air due to velopharyngeal port dysfunction" (Hall et al., 1990, p. 454). TB had concomitant language and learning difficulties. First words appeared at 4 years, with two-word combinations by 7 years. Hall et al. describe how a palatal lift was used to manage TB's disordered resonance.
Lundeborg & McAllister (2007)	R: female (5;1 years)	Swedish	Intra-oral sensory stimulation and electropalatography (EPG) and a Swedish version of the Nuffield Dyspraxia Programme (NDP-3) (Williams & Stephens, 2004)	Overview of two approaches for treatment CAS, including intra-oral sensory stimulation and EPG feedback targeting lingual consonants. The child's electropalatograms provide insight into the difficulty the child had in achieving accurate placement of articulation for /s/ before intervention. (Note: Child's dysprosodic features not described).
Martikainen & Korpilahti (2011)	SS: female (4;7 years)	Finnish	Melodic intonation therapy (MIT) and touch-cue method (TCM)	Detailed case study of two different approaches to intervention.
McNeill, Gillon, & Dodd (2009a)	12 children (4–7 years)	New Zealand English	Integrated phonological awareness	Helpful study for understanding the role of literacy in intervention for children with CAS. The intervention targeted speech production, phonological awareness, and letter knowledge. Measures of word decoding and spelling were also reported before and after intervention.
Strand & Debertine (2000)	Child: female (5;9 years)	American English	Integral stimulation intervention	Informative case example of integral stimulation intervention, guided by principles of motor learning.
Strand, Stoeckel, & Baas (2006)	LH: male (5;7 years) CK: male (5;8 years) CD: male (5;5 years) BS: male (6;1 years)	American English	Dynamic Temporal and Tactile Cueing (DTTC)	Valuable intervention study of four children with severe CAS who were nonverbal prior to the study (despite receiving between 2 to 4 years of therapy). Two of the four children also had mild dysarthria. The children developed "a number of functional intelligible utterances in 6 weeks" (Strand et al., 2006, p. 305).
Zaretsky, Velleman, & Curro (2010)	LH: female (6;0) years	American English	Integrated speech and literacy intervention	Longitudinal case study of a child with severe CAS and borderline IQ, who received intervention between 6;0–11;6 years targeting "speech sounds, oral sequencing, phonological awareness (PA), speech-print connections, syllabic structure, and real and non-word decoding" (Zaretsky et al., 2010, p. 58).

TABLE 16-17 Lian (14;2 years): Summary speech-language pathology assessment results

Skill area	Assessment	Measure and/or observation	Result
Receptive and expressive language	Clinical Evaluation of Language Fundamentals-4 (CELF-4) (Semel, Wiig, & Secord, 2004) Core Language Subtests	Core language standard score = 95 (Receptive language index = 101) (Expressive language index = 92)	Receptive ✓ Expressive ✓
Oral structure and non-speech function	Informal assessment of the speech mechanism in non-speech functions based on Duffy (2013)	Informal observation of Lian's face, lips, jaw, tongue, palate, and respiration were conducted in two contexts: at rest and during non-speech movements. Although direction of movement was adequate, her rate of movement was a little slow, and range of movement reduced. Excessive muscle tone was also evident. Lian's mother reported that Lian has a sensitive gag reflex: often gagging when brushing her rear molars. Additional information is provided in the background text about Lian's case.	✗
Speech production: perceptual characteristics	Informal assessment of deviant speech characteristics associated with motor speech disorders (Duffy, 2013) using a single-word speech sample, a sample of connected speech during reading, and conversational speech	Pitch: low and monopitch (mild-moderate) Loudness: reduced loudness and loudness decay evident during conversational speech (mild-moderate) Voice quality: transient breathy voice, with slight strained-strangled quality (mild) Resonance: hypernasality (mild) Respiration: mild audible inspiration intermittent breathiness/air wastage during conversational speech. Lian took three breaths when counting to 20. Prosody: Slow speech rate, with excess and equal stress particularly for polysyllabic words (mild-moderate). Articulation: Imprecise articulation for lingual consonants, particularly contrasting alveolar/velar plosive cognates, and postalveolar fricative/affricate cognates. Vowel distortion was evident.	✗
Speech production: maximum performance tasks, and speech motion rates	Maximum performance tasks, based on Wit, Maassen, Gabreels, and Thoonen (1993)	■ Maximum sound prolongation (MSP) in seconds: [a] = 9.4, [f] = 8.9, [z] = 10.2 [s] = 11.8 ■ Maximum repetition duration for [ma] in seconds = 11.4 ■ [s:z] ratio = 1.12	✗
	Informal observation of DDK or alternating motion rates (AMRs) and sequential motion rates (SMRs), based on Duffy (2013)	There was relatively little difference between Lian's AMRs (e.g., [pʌ pʌ pʌ pʌ pʌ] and [tʌ tʌ tʌ tʌ tʌ]) and SMRs (e.g., [pʌ tʌ kʌ pʌ tʌ kʌ]). All attempts were quite slow and effortful. The faster her attempt, the less precise her articulation. Her production of /t/ was closer to [c].	
Speech production: intelligibility	Children's Speech Intelligibility Measure (CSIM) (Wilcox & Morris, 1999). Single-words and connected speech in phrases and sentences.	■ Single-word percentage intelligibility based on closed-set identification = 82% (Unfamiliar listener 78%, familiar listener 86%) ■ Connected speech intelligibility based on open-set identification = 72% (Unfamiliar listener 78%, familiar listener 86%)	✗
	Conversational speech sample (in English and Cantonese) (2 × 5 minutes)	During conversational speech, Lian was rated (in English and Cantonese) as mostly intelligible by familiar listeners. Lian's mother commented that people unfamiliar with Lian find her speech somewhat intelligible. Various factors (e.g., hypernasality, slow rate of speech, monotone pitch, imprecise articulation) had a negative impact on Lian's speech intelligibility. Lian commented that she uses English more often than Cantonese.	

(continued)

TABLE 16-17	*Continued*		
Skill area	**Assessment**	**Measure and/or observation**	**Result**
Speech production: strategic sampling	Informal probe of postalveolar fricatives and affricates in minimal pair words	Lian's articulation of /tʃ, ʤ, ʃ/ consonants in minimal pair words (e.g., *shoe* versus *chew*; *jeep* versus *sheep*) was imprecise, making it difficult to identify which word she had said. Often /tʃ/ and /ʤ/ were produced as /ʃ/. When Lian slowed her speech, intelligibility and consonant accuracy improved.	✗
Quality of life, including activity and participation	Lian completed the Quality of Life Questionnaire for Adolescents (CP QOL-Teen): Adolescent Questionnaire, and Lian's mother completed the Quality of Life Questionnaire for Adolescents (CP QOL-Teen): Primary Caregiver Questionnaire (Davis, Davern, et al., 2013)	Lian was considered generally healthy. Epilepsy was controlled with medication. On the "communication" related questions, Lian rated being happiest (7 out of 9) about using technology (specifically social media) to communicate, followed by communicating with familiar family and friends. She was somewhat unhappy (4/9) about communication with people she did not know well. Lian indicated that she was happy at middle school and enjoyed participating in social events with her close friends. She was anxious about starting high school and developing new relationships with peers and teachers. She was particularly concerned about being misunderstood and people not including her in conversation. Lian enjoys caring for her pet cat, learning how to cook, and spending time with friends.	✓✗

✓ = acceptable, ✗ = problematic.

Further observations about Lian's oral structure and non-speech function are provided below.

- **Facial symmetry:** Lian's face was generally symmetrical. There was slight lip asymmetry at rest, which was more noticeable when Lian smiled or rounded or retracted her lips. Lian could seal her lips. Alternating spread/round lip movements were somewhat slow.
- **Jaw:** There was slight asymmetry on jaw opening. Efforts to rapidly open and close the mouth were a little slow.
- **Tongue:** Lian could protrude her tongue. Muscle weakness was apparent when she was asked to resist the pressure of a tongue blade pushing against her tongue. Although the direction of her alternating lateral tongue movement was normal, the rate of movement was slow and the range was reduced.
- **Velopharynx:** At rest, Lian's palate appeared normal in color and shape. During vowel prolongation, her palate elevated, slowly.
- **Larynx:** Lian's cough on command was a little weak and breathy.
- **Respiration:** At rest, Lian showed signs of shallow breathing, with noticeable inhalation and exhalation.
- **Oral movement control and sequencing:** Lian could complete a range of non-speech oral movements both separately and in sequence, although slowly (e.g., bite bottom lip, puff out her cheeks). Some movements were also reduced in range (e.g., licking her lips).

Lian: Speech production skills

During assessment interview with Lian and her family, Lian commented that she wanted to work on her pronunciation of /ʃ, tʃ, ʤ/, as she had noticed that words containing these sounds were a source of confusion with unfamiliar listeners. Although there were other factors that impacted on her overall intelligibility (e.g., hypernasality, monotone pitch, reduced loudness), part of the assessment focused on Lian's articulation of sibilant consonants, to better understand the problem underlying her motivation for wanting to work on these sounds. Table 16-18 shows Lian's pronunciation of a selection of words important to her.

TABLE 16-18	Lian (14;2 years): Single-word sample of words important to Lian

Target word	Adult pronunciation	Child's production
1. chocolate	/tʃɑklət/	[tsɑ.kələ̰ʔ]
2. chips	/tʃɪps/	[tsɪːps]
3. choose	/tʃuz/	[ʃy̆ːs]
4. teacher	/titʃɚ/	[ti.ʃɝ]
5. Jenny	/dʒɛni/	[tsɛ̃ni̥]
6. Rachel	/retʃəl/	[reʔ.tsy̆l]

COMMENT: *Lian's difficulty with affricates*

Lian speaks both English and Cantonese. Her difficulty with affricates was thought to be associated with both childhood dysarthria and Cantonese. Cantonese contains two affricates: voiceless alveolar plosive /ts/ and voiceless aspirated alveolar plosive /tsʰ/ (Chan, 2010). Lian produced the words *Jenny* and *Rachel* with the alveolar affricate [ts]. Other errors (e.g., /tʃ/ as /ʃ/) were also consistent with common errors identified in Cantonese speakers learning English (Chan, 2010).

■ Intervention studies of children who have childhood dysarthria

Lian presented with spastic dysarthria. Table 16-19 provides a brief overview of a selection of intervention studies of children with different types of dysarthria, including children with acquired dysarthria following traumatic brain injury.

TABLE 16-19	Intervention studies of children who have childhood dysarthria

Authors (year)	Child(ren), gender, age, characteristics	Languages and/or dialects	Intervention approach	Why is this study interesting?
Levy, Ramig, & Camarata (2012)	P1: 8;10 years P2: 3;3 years P3: 9;7 years	American English	Lee Silverman Voice Treatment (LSVT LOUD) compared with traditional intervention	Two children (P1 and P2) were provided with LSVT LOUD (based on Fox and Boliek, 2012) in 60-minute sessions 4 times per week for 4 weeks while the third child received traditional intervention in 50-minute sessions 2 times per week for 4 weeks. All three children showed improvements in speech function.
Marchant, McAuliffe, & Huckabee (2008)	CB: female (13 years)	New Zealand English	Phonetic placement therapy (PPT) and sEMG-facilitated biofeedback relaxation therapy	This case provides insight into choices and challenges of intervention for teenagers with spastic dysarthria. Two different interventions are described.

(continued)

TABLE 16-19	*Continued*

Authors (year)	Child(ren), gender, age, characteristics	Languages and/or dialects	Intervention approach	Why is this study interesting?
Morgan, Liégeois, & Occomore (2007)	Male (15;0 years) Male (14;10 years) Female (15;1 years)	British English	EPG feedback	EPG intervention study of three adolescents with acquired dysarthria following traumatic brain injury. Participants improved their articulatory precision of phonemes in words and sentences; however, minimal change was detected in overall speech intelligibility.
Fox & Boliek (2012)	P1: male (7;10 years) P2: female (5;10 years) P3: male (6;1 years) P4: male (7;7 years) P5: female (6;7 years) (served as the control participant)	American English	Lee Silverman Voice Treatment (LSVT LOUD)	Using a non-concurrent multiple baseline design across participants, Fox and Boliek (2012) report of an intensive intervention (LSVT LOUD) (traditionally used with adults who have Parkinson's disease or dysarthria) with children with spastic cerebral palsy and dysarthria. Intervention was delivery (1 hr, 4 times per week for 4 weeks). An improvement in vocal loudness was evident immediately post-treatment, with maintenance 6 weeks post varying across participants.
Pennington et al., (2013)	15 children with dysarthria and cerebral palsy, ranging from 5 to 11 years.	British English	Systems approach	Pennington et al. (2013) reported that speech intelligibility improved given 35- to 40-minute sessions 3 times per week for 6 weeks using a systemic approach to intervention based on Pennington et al. (2010).
Gibbon & Wood (2003)	D: male (9;3)	British English	EPG	Detailed case study (including progress notes) about a 12-week block of intervention for a child with mild cerebral palsy. Intervention focused on the child learning alveolar-velar contrasts using EPG.
Ward, Strauss, & Leitão (2013)	F (11;9 years) F (8;5 years) F (5;4 years) M (5;2 years) M (3;0 years) M (3;6 years)	Australian English	Prompts for Restructuring Oral Muscular Phonetic Targets (PROMPT)	Ward et al. (2013) examined the kinematic movements of the jaw and lips before, during, and following PROMPT intervention for children with dyskinetic (n = 1) or spastic (n = 5) cerebral palsy.
Trabacca et al. (2012)	Male (12 years)	Italian	ICF-CY-based neurorehabilitation program	Comprehensive case study describing improvements in functional independence and activity and participation in a 12-year-old boy with dyskinetic (athetoid-dystonic subtype) cerebral palsy. This paper illustrates the value and importance of a multidisciplinary and interdisciplinary approach when working with children and their families.

Chapter summary

In this chapter we have provided an overview of the case history and assessment results for five children who have SSD—Luke, Susie, Jarrod, Michael, and Lian. Unlike previous chapters, the main purpose of this chapter was to provide you with useful case-based infor-

mation for completing the clinical exercises throughout the book. We hope that the cases both encouraged you and reminded you that all children are different, and that they require individualized, evidence-based approaches to management.

Suggested reading

- Chabon, S. W., & Cohn, E. R. (2011). *The communication disorders casebook: Learning by example.* Upper Saddle River, NJ: Pearson Education.

- Oller, J. W., Oller, S. D., & Bandon, L. C. (2010). *Cases: Introducing communication disorders across the lifespan.* San Diego, CA: Plural Publishing.

- Tanner, D. C. (2006). *Case studies in communication sciences and disorders.* Upper Saddle River, NJ: Pearson/Merrill Prentice Hall.

Application of knowledge from Chapter 16

Throughout this chapter we referred to published intervention studies of children who have SSD. Many of the studies are detailed case descriptions. While it is important that your clinical decisions are guided by experimental research associated with the most, the best quality, and the highest level of evidence, detailed case studies have an important role to play in the conduct of evidence-based practice. As a student, case studies can help you develop your critical thinking and clinical decision-making skills. They allow you to reflect on the decisions made by others. They offer a window into the expertise of the authors. The final clinical exercise of this book is our attempt to nurture your clinical expertise and spur you on towards lifelong learning.

1. Search your relevant library databases for a recently published intervention case study about:

- a preschool-age child diagnosed with a phonological impairment;
- a school-age child who has an articulation impairment;
- a child diagnosed with inconsistent speech disorder;
- a child diagnosed with CAS; and
- a preschooler, school-age child, or adolescent diagnosed with childhood dysarthria.

2. Compare, contrast, and critique the case study reports you identify. Consider the case history information, assessment, and intervention procedures.

3. With a small group of peers, present a verbal summary and critique of one of the intervention case studies you identified.

Acoustic nerve The major cranial nerve (VIII) involved in hearing.

Acoustic-phonetic representations Abstract mental representations of speech, based on the perception of speech sounds.

Acute otitis media (AOM) A painful middle ear infection often accompanied by fever and general malaise.

Addition error A type of speech production error, present when a speech sound has been added to a word (e.g., *see* /si/ → [sis]).

Additive segmentation A teaching technique used in pre-practice to help a child produce a targeted speech production skill. The technique involves dividing the skill along a temporal dimension into parts then practicing them in an additive manner, such as learning to say polysyllables by adding one syllable at a time until the word is pronounced fluently and with normal prosody.

Affricate A consonant produced by briefly stopping then releasing the oral airflow as a fricative.

Affrication Phonological process where fricatives are replaced by affricates.

Allophone Language-specific phonetic realizations of a phoneme.

Alveolar consonants Speech sounds articulated with the tongue tip against or near the alveolar ridge (e.g., /t, d, n/).

Alveolarization (apicalization) A type of phonological process where labiodental or interdental consonants are replaced with an alveolar consonant, such as /f/ → [s].

Ankyloglossia A condition where the lingual frenulum is short, resulting in reduced tongue mobility (also known as tongue-tie).

Approximants Consonants /w, j, ɹ/ produced when articulators in the mouth approach one another, but not closely enough to create turbulence (/w, j/ are also known as glides, and /ɹ/ is also known as a liquid). (Also see lateral approximant.)

Articulation Coordinated movement of body structures and systems involved in the production of speech sounds.

Articulation delay A type of articulation impairment where a child's speech production errors may be present in the speech of typically developing younger children (Also see articulation impairment).

Articulation disorder A type of articulation impairment where a child produces speech production errors not found in the speech of typically developing children (Also see articulation impairment).

Articulation impairment A motor speech difficulty involving the physical production (i.e., articulation) of specific speech sounds; usually the errors are limited to distortion or substitution errors involving sibilants (e.g., lateral lisp) and/or rhotics (e.g., [w] for /ɹ/).

Articulatory-phonetic representations Abstract mental representations of speech, based on the physical production of speech sounds.

Assimilation A type of phonological process where one speech sound is influenced by and becomes more like another speech sound in the same word. Assimilation can be progressive (the influencing speech sound is at or towards the beginning of a word) or regressive (the influencing speech sound is at or towards the end of a word).

Auditory Perceived by the sense of hearing.

Auditory discrimination The ability to discern that two speech sounds or two spoken words sound the same or different.

Auditory model A spoken example of targeted speech skill offered to a child to imitate.

Auditory ossicles The three small bones of the middle ear: the malleaus, incus, and stapes.

Augmented feedback Supplementary information from a person or technology about an attempt at a skill an individual is learning; the information or feedback helps a learner improve that skill.

Babbling Repetitions of consonant and vowel-like syllables (reduplicated or variegated) produced by infants in the pre-linguistics period of speech and language acquisition.

Back [± back] Speech sounds in which the tongue is retracted back, including vowels [u, ʊ, ɑ, ɒ, ɔ, ʌ, ə, a] and [k, g, ŋ].

Backing A phonological process referring to a consonant further forward in the mouth being substituted with a consonant further back the mouth; usually backing of velars (e.g., *two* /tu/ → [ku]).

Backward chaining A facilitating phonetic context designed to provide a child with a strategy for building a word from the final syllable to the first syllable.

Baseline data Information about a particular skill (identified as a problem during an assessment) that is collected *before* intervention is started.

Bifid tongue A cleft in the tongue, giving rise to a tongue with two points.

Bifid uvula A cleft in the uvula, giving the appearance of two uvulas. A bifid uvula can be a sign of a submucous cleft.

Bilabial consonant A speech sound articulated with both lips.

Binary feature A distinctive feature of a speech sound notated as either present [+] or absent [−].

Block scheduling Intervention targeting one goal for a period of time followed by intervention targeting other goals for a similar length of time.

Body function A component of the ICF-CY framework (WHO, 2007), focused on the physiological or psychological working of body systems.

Body structure A component of the ICF-CY framework (WHO, 2007), focused on anatomical or physical parts of the body.

Bunched /ɹ/ An approximant consonant produced with the tongue tip turned down, the tongue blade elevated towards the palate, and the sides of the tongue bracing against the upper teeth.

Cardinal vowels A set of eight reference vowels evenly spaced around the boundaries of the vowel quadrilateral.

Categorical perception The tendency to divide auditory or visual information on a continuum into distinct groups; categorical perception is evident when listeners perceive a range in voice onset time as a voiced consonant, and another range as the voiceless counterpart.

Central auditory processing deficits A difficulty interpreting (rather than detecting) speech sounds associated with problems with the structure or function of the auditory nerves, also known as retrocochlear pathology and central auditory processing deficits.

Childhood apraxia of speech (CAS) A neurological childhood motor speech disorder associated with a difficulty planning and programming movement sequences in the absence of neuromuscular deficits. CAS is typically characterized by inconsistent speech errors, dysprosody, and difficulty with coarticulatory transitions between sounds and syllables.

Childhood dysarthria A neurological childhood motor speech disorder characterized by difficulty with the ability to control and execute speech movements, impacting speech subsystems including respiration, phonation, resonance, and articulation.

Cleft lip and palate A congenital condition where there is an opening or division in the lip (cleft lip) and hard and/or soft palate (cleft palate); clefts may be unilateral or bilateral.

Cluster reduction A phonological process referring to a consonant (usually the marked consonant) being deleted from a consonant cluster.

Cluster simplification A phonological process referring to a consonant (usually the marked consonant) being simplified in a consonant cluster.

Coalescence A phonological process referring to features of two adjacent consonants (usually in a cluster) combining into a new consonant.

Collaborative consultation A type of service delivery model where professionals with different expertise work alongside one another on a particular goal, such as an SLP working with a teacher, coordinating and running lessons together in the classroom.

Complementary distribution When allophones of a phoneme do not occur in the same environment in a word (e.g., [kʰ] occurs syllable-initial word-initial position whereas [k˭] occurs in word-initial consonant clusters after [s]).

Complexity The idea that systems are made up of hierarchically organized parts that relate to one another; parts higher in the system implicate the existence of parts lower in the system.

Conductive hearing loss Hearing loss associated with problems with the structure or function of the outer or middle ear.

Consonant A speech sound produced with constriction in the vocal tract (in contrast to vowels).

Consonant cluster Two or more consonants occurring in the same syllable position in a word (e.g., in *blue*, /bl/ is a syllable-initial word-initial consonant cluster).

Consonantal A distinctive feature that separates true consonants [+ cons] (including plosives, affricates, fricatives, nasals, the lateral, and [ɹ]) from vowels and glides [w, j].

Constraint-based nonlinear phonology Theories that focus on the hierarchical organization and relationships within phonological systems (addressing prosodic and segmental components).

Constraint A theoretical concept in optimality theory that captures phonologically universal ways for pronouncing words; some constraints promote easier pronunciation (markedness constraints) whereas others promote pronunciation closer or matching the adult form (faithfulness constraints).

Constricted glottis [± c.g.] A distinctive feature that differentiates speech sounds in which the vocal folds are pulled tight and drawn together (such as the glottal plosive [ʔ]) from those in which they are not.

Context sensitive voicing (CSV) A phonological process referring to a loss of phonemic contrast between voiced and voiceless consonants in syllable-initial and/or syllable-final positions.

Continuant [± cont] A distinctive feature differentiating speech sounds in which air moves uninterrupted or freely through the oral cavity (vowels, glides, liquids, and fricatives) from those that block the airflow (plosives, affricates, and nasals).

Continuous schedule Reinforcement given immediately following every response.

Contrastive intervention Phonological intervention that uses minimal pair words.

Control data Information gathered outside treatment conditions on a behavior that is unrelated to the behavior(s) being targeted in intervention.

Core vocabulary therapy An intervention approach targeting lexical inconsistency; suitable for children with inconsistent speech disorder.

Coronal Speech sounds produced with the tongue tip or blade.

Cumulative intervention intensity A quantitative measure of intervention intensity based on the product of the amount of practice in a session (dose), session frequency, and total intervention duration (e.g., 100 trials × 2 sessions per week × 10 weeks).

Cycles approach A phonological intervention approach for children with severe or profound phonological impairment that targets phonological patterns in cycles.

Cyclical goal attack strategy A strategy for scheduling intervention targets, where several targets are addressed within a specified period of time, independent of accuracy.

Deaffrication A phonological process referring to the substitution of an affricate consonant with a fricative.

Default A speech sound that a child uses for many other speech sounds.

Denasalization A phonological process referring to a nasal consonant being substituted with a homorganic plosive.

Dental lisp A type of speech production error involving sibilants, typically dentalization of /s, z/ → [s̪, z̪] (frontal lisp; addental lisp) or the substitution of dental fricatives /s, z/ → [θ, ð] (interdental lisp).

Dentalization Speech sounds produced with the tongue tip articulated against the maxillary central incisors, noted by the dental diacritic (e.g., [s̪, z̪]).

Diacritics Small phonetic marks added to consonants or vowels that denote different allophones of a phoneme, different phonemes, or unique variations in speakers' articulation of speech sounds.

Diaphragm Dome-shaped muscle that sits below the lungs but above the abdominal cavity. The diaphragm and intercostal muscles are used to inhale and exhale air.

Diminutization A phonological process referring to the addition of the vowel /i/ or /ɪ/ to the end of a word (e.g., *dog* → *doggy*).

Directions into velocities of articulators (DIVA) model A neurocomputational model designed to capture what goes on in specific regions of the brain when we speak; focused on the motor control processes involved in articulation.

Distinctive features Articulatory and acoustic characteristics of speech sounds that may be present or absent; they are useful for distinguishing one phoneme from another, and for describing the similarities and differences between groups of phonemes.

Distortion Change in the production of a speech sound such that a listener perceives the target phoneme as unclear or imprecise rather than another phoneme (i.e., the phonemic contrast is preserved).

Distributed [± distr] A distinctive feature involving coronal speech sounds produced with a wide area of contact between the tip or blade of the tongue and the roof of the mouth or the teeth.

Disyllabic/disyllable A word containing two syllables.

Dorsal Speech sounds articulated with the back of the tongue.

Dorsum Surface area of the tongue comprising two parts: body and root.

Dose The number of teaching episodes in a single intervention session, such as the number of times a targeted speech skill is practiced in words, in one session.

Dose form The type of activity where teaching and learning moments are provided, such as adult-directed drill play or child-directed play.

Dose frequency How often intervention sessions are scheduled per unit of time, such as once or twice weekly.

Drill A dose form characterized by a high dose or rate of practice and minimal play.

Drill play A dose form or intervention activity characterized by a relatively high dose or rate of practice conducted within a simple game or play activity.

Dysarthria A neurological childhood motor speech disorder characterized by difficulty with the ability to control and execute speech movements, impacting speech subsystems including respiration, phonation, resonance, and articulation. (Also see childhood dysarthria.)

Dysprosody When prosodic aspects of speech (e.g., intonation, lexical and phrasal stress, intensity) are disturbed, such as weak syllables being produced as strong syllables, and pauses being evident between syllables.

Egressive airflow Speech that is produced during exhalation.

Electropalatography (EPG) An instrumental method that uses an artificial palate containing electrodes linked to a computer; the computer displays contact between the tongue and hard palate during speech, in real time (also known as palatometry).

Epenthesis A phonological process where a schwa is inserted between two consonants comprising a consonant cluster.

Esophageal speech Vibration of the sphincter of the esophagus to produce speech.

Esophagus Muscular tube through which food and drink travels from the pharynx to the stomach.

Eustachian tube A tube extending from the middle ear to the nasopharynx that allows pressure in the middle ear to equalize with the atmosphere, and serves to drain secretions from the middle ear into the nasopharynx.

Evidence-based practice (EBP) A decision-making framework incorporating the best available research evidence, evidence from clinical practice, and client values and preferences to guide clinical decisions.

Exosystem Settings that do not include the child as an active participant, but have an impact on the child.

External evidence Published literature on assessment tools, diagnostic criteria, and/or intervention approaches for guiding clinical decisions within an evidence-based practice framework.

Facial nerve The major cranial nerve (VII) involved in the sensation and movement of the face.

Family-centered practice A model of clinical practice that considers the family to be the client, not just the child; the family has the primary decision-making role.

Family-friendly practice A combination of therapist- and family-centered practice where families are the client (rather than the child) and are involved in intervention planning; however, in contrast to family-centered practice, the professional is the primary decision-maker.

Faucial pillars Column-like structures in the oropharynx containing connective tissue and muscles that link the soft palate to the sides of the tongue.

Final consonant deletion A phonological process referring to the deletion of a consonant in syllable-final, word-final position.

Fixed interval Reinforcement is given after a predetermined period of time.

Fixed ratio Reinforcement is given after a predetermined number of responses.

Foot In phonology, a foot refers to an element consisting one stressed syllable and any associated unstressed or weak syllables.

Fractionation Dividing simultaneously produced movements in a skill into independent components, then practicing each movement.

Free variation When different allophones occur in the same phonetic environment to produce subtly different pronunciations of the same word (e.g., [lʊkˀ] and [lʊkʰ]).

Frenulectomy Surgical alteration of the lingua frenulum to increase tongue mobility (also known as fraenectomy, frenectomy, frenulotomy, or frenotomy).

Fricative A manner class of consonants characterized by constriction of (but not stopping) the airflow, with the constriction creating turbulence or friction.

Fricative simplification A phonological process referring to the substitution of an interdental fricative with a labiodental fricative.

Frontal lisp A type of dental lisp where sibilants (typically /s, z/) are dentalized [s̪, z̪] or articulated further forward in the mouth towards the teeth, also known as addental lisp. The sibilants sound distorted because the tongue tip is articulated close to or against rather than between the maxillary central incisors, as occurs in the interdental lisp.

Fronting A phonological process referring to the substitution of a consonant further back in the mouth with a consonant produced further forward, typically velar fronting.

Frozen form When a child pronounces a word using a less mature pronunciation, despite the child's phonological system being more advanced.

Ganong effect To adjust perception of an ambiguous or acoustically unclear segment towards a word that is already known.

Generalization The phenomenon where intervention on one behavior in one intervention context facilitates change in the same behavior in other non-treatment contexts, and in related behaviors.

Generalization data Information gathered once intervention has started but is outside of intervention conditions.

Generalized motor program (GMP) An abstract motor program that can be expressed in different ways, depending on the parameters supplied to the program.

Generative phonology A derivational phonological theory that proposes that underlying phonemes are transformed into allophones through the application of rules.

Glide An approximant consonant (/w, j/) produced by articulators approaching one another but not close enough to produce turbulence; also known as a semivowel.

Gliding of liquids A phonological process involving the substitution of a liquid /l, ɹ/ with a glide [w, j].

Glottal insertion A phonological process involving the substitution of a consonant with a glottal stop.

Glottis The space between the vocal folds.

Goal An ambition that an individual aspires to achieve.

Grooved [± grooved] A distinctive feature that distinguishes speech sounds produced with a narrow midline groove in the tongue /s, z, ʃ, ʒ, ʧ, ʤ/ from those produced with a flatter tongue /θ, ð, j/ or block in the airflow /t, d/.

Guidance hypothesis Use of infrequent feedback to develop internal response evaluations and error correction mechanisms.

High [± high] Sounds in which the tongue body is raised above the neutral position (as in [ə]), including the vowels [i, ɪ, u, ʊ, ɛ] and consonants /k, g, ŋ, w, j/.

Homonyms Words with different meanings pronounced the same way.

Horizontal goal attack strategy Intervention targeting several targets within a session.

Hypernasal Speech that is perceived as excessively nasal because the velum does not have adequate closure (or the person has a cleft palate) and allows too much air to pass through the nasal cavity during speech.

Hyponasal Speech perceived as having limited nasality because air is blocked from passing through the nose.

Iambic stress A lexical stress pattern where unstressed syllables precede stressed syllables, that is, weak strong (wS).

Impairment Problems with a body structure or body function.

Implicational relationship A concept in phonology where the existence of a marked trait in a phonological system assumes the existence of the unmarked counterpart, with the relationship being unidirectional.

Impressionistic transcription The type of transcription used when the transcriber does not know the pronunciation patterns of the person speaking, such as when transcribing the speech of children with SSD. Impressionistic transcription can be simple (broad) or detailed (narrow).

Incisors Teeth with a sharp cutting edge.

Inconsistent speech disorder A type of phonologically based speech difficulty involving phonological planning, with the disorder characterized by inconsistency productions of the same lexical item in the absence of prosodic disturbance.

Individual Education Program (IEP) A management plan for a child with a diagnosed disability.

Individual Family Service Plan (IFSP) A management plan for a younger child (birth to under 3 years of age) receiving early intervention services.

Ingressive consonant Consonant produced during inhalation (ingressive air).

Initial consonant deletion A phonological process involving the deletion of the initial consonant in syllable-initial word-initial position.

Intelligibility The degree to which a listener understands a person's speech.

Intensity The loudness of sound.

Interdental lisp A type of dental lisp where sibilants (typically /s, z/) are substituted with dental fricatives [θ, ð].

Interdisciplinary When professionals work interdependently; they maintain their discipline-specific identities but have a coordinated organizational structure to identify children's areas of need, and they share responsibility for children's outcomes across the team.

Internal clinical evidence Data from clinicians' clinical practice (e.g., assessment, baseline, treatment, generalization, control data), gathered from the children and families they work with.

Internal patient/client evidence Information about the factors, values, and informed preferences of the children and families with whom clinicians work; it is used to guide clinical decisions within an evidence-based practice framework.

Intervention A goal-directed activity based on plans and procedures designed to improve a presenting problem.

Intervention approach A specific method of intervention developed by a researcher or team of researchers designed to improve children's speech, usually specifying the types of goals, service delivery, and/or intervention procedures used to address a particular type of SSD.

Intervention goals Aims of intervention based on an impairment, social, and biopsychosocial perspective designed to improve a child's well-being; speech goals are typically referred to as intervention targets.

Intervention plan A proposal outlining what needs to be done, when, and how it should be done in order to achieve a predetermined goal.

Intervention principle A statement about a condition that promotes learning.

Intervention procedure A teaching instruction or action performed by an intervention agent (e.g., clinician, parent, computer) designed to elicit learning in a child.

Intonation The rise and fall in the pitch of the voice.

Knowledge of performance (KP) Feedback regarding why a specific response was correct or incorrect.

Knowledge of results (KR) Feedback regarding whether a response was correct or incorrect.

Labial Speech sounds produced with one or both lips.

Labialization Substitution of a non-labial consonant with a labial (bilabial or labiodental) consonant.

Lack of invariance Absence of clear, consistent acoustic cues corresponding to a speech sound within and across speakers, speaking contexts, and phonetic contexts.

Lateral [± lat] A distinctive feature that distinguishes speech sounds in which one or both sides of the tongue are lowered (while the tongue tip is in contact with the alveolar ridge) allowing air to flow over the sides of the tongue, from those that do not.

Lateral approximant The consonants produced with lateral airflow around the sides of the tongue. There are four lateral approximants across the world's languages; the only lateral approximant in English is /l/.

Lateral fricative A fricative produce with airflow around the sides of the tongue.

Lateral lisp A type of lisp where sibilants (typically /s, z/) are replaced by lateral fricatives [ɬ, ɮ].

Least knowledge Having relatively little or no information about a phonological construct such as a distinctive feature or class of consonants.

Letter-sound knowledge Understanding of the names and sounds associated with individual letters comprising an alphabet.

Lexical representation Abstract store about what a child knows about a word, such as the phonological information comprising the word (i.e., phonological representation) and what the word means (i.e., semantic representation).

Lexical (word) stress Stress patterns in words such as strong weak (Sw, e.g., *paper*), weak strong (wS, e.g., *giraffe*).

Lingual frenulum The small fold of mucous membrane that extends from the underside of the tongue to the floor of the mouth.

Linguistic universal Something that is common across the world's languages.

Linking-r The inclusion of /ɹ/ in non-rhotic dialects when words that are spelled with a final 'r' are followed by a word commencing with a vowel.

Liquid A type of approximant produced by the articulators approaching one another but not coming so close as to create turbulence, including /ɹ, l/.

Long-term goal The overall goal a child and his or her family aspire to; when it is reached, the child may no longer require intervention services.

Low [± low] Sounds in which the bunched tongue body is lower than the neutral position, including the vowels [æ, ɔ, ɒ, ɑ, a].

Macroglossia The medical term for an overly large (macro) tongue.

Manner The way consonants are articulated, such as stopping, constricting, or redirecting airflow.

Manual guidance/ motokinesthetic cue A type of phonetic cue where a child is given physical assistance (from a tool or clinician) to articulate speech.

Marked features Phonetically more complex, universally less common, and later developing features of phonological systems.

Markedness constraints In optimality theory, output constraints that are as simple as possible or phonologically less marked.

Maximal oppositions intervention A contrastive approach to phonological intervention using minimal pair words that contrast one phoneme known to a child with a maximally different unknown phoneme.

McGurk effect A phenomenon where hearing one speech sound and seeing another results in perception of a third speech sound, such as hearing [ba], seeing [ga], then perceiving [da].

Metacommunication Knowing or being aware of what is involved in successful and unsuccessful communication.

Metaphonology Knowing or having an awareness of the phonological system of a language.

Metaphor A figure of speech where one thing is likened to another, such as /h/ being likened to the sound of a panting dog.

Metathesis Phonological process where two consonants in a word swap positions with one another.

Migration Phonological process where a speech sound moves from one position to another in a word.

Minimal pairs Word pairs that differ by a single phoneme.

Minimally opposing features Phonemes that have one or few feature differences.

Minimally opposing minimal pairs Word pairs that differ by a single phoneme, with the differing phonemes having one or few feature differences.

Mixed hearing loss A hearing loss that is both conductive and sensorineural.

Mnemonic method The use of a memory stimulator or mnemonic for addressing syllable-based speech production problems.

Molars The largest teeth, useful for crushing and grinding food.

Monolingual Speaking one language only.

Monosyllabic Words comprising one syllable.

Mora The timing unit of a syllable, denoted by the Greek letter mu, symbolized as μ.

Morphophonemic The expression of morphemes through phonemes; words can be monomorphemic (e.g., *cat*) or bimorphemic through the addition of grammatical markers (e.g., *cats*).

Most knowledge When an aspect of a child's phonological system is nearest to or identical to the adult system; most knowledge contrasts with least knowledge.

Motokinesthetic A type of phonetic cue involving physical touch and/or manual manipulation of the articulators.

Motor equivalence The idea that different movements of the articulators can produce the same acoustic result.

Motor execution The physical production of programmed motor movements.

Motor learning When practice of a motor skill leads to permanent changes in the ability to produce that skill.

Motor planning The process of formulating a strategy to determine which articulators will be used and when, in order to produce a word or utterance.

Motor program See motor programming.

Motor programming The process of specifying which muscles will be used, when, and how (including tone, speed, direction, and range of movement) to realize a motor plan.

Motor speech disorders Speech sound disorders characterized by difficulty with the coordination and production of precise mouth movements, respiration, and phonation required for fluent and rapid speech.

Multidisciplinary When professionals from different disciplines work independently or in parallel with a child and his or her family.

Multilingual Speaking and understanding more than one language.

Multiple oppositions A contrastive approach to phonological intervention using sets of minimal and near minimal pair words (produced as homonyms by a child) that differ by selected phonemes from a child's phoneme collapse.

Nasal Consonants produced with nasal (rather than oral) airflow.

Nasal cavity The space behind the nose, above the palate.

Nasal emission When air flows through the nasal cavity rather than solely through the oral cavity.

Nasal septum An anatomical structure that divides the nose vertically into two nostrils.

Nasopharynx The back of the nasal cavity comprising the upper part of the pharynx and the space above the soft palate.

Natural class Groups of phonemes that share particular distinctive features, such as nasals and fricatives.

Natural features Distinctive features of speech sounds thought to be more common within and across languages, learned earlier by children, and easier to produce.

Naturalistic speech intelligibility training (NSIT) An intervention approach designed to improve children's speech intelligibility in naturalistic child-directed play-based contexts; the approach is characterized by conversational recasts.

Near minimal pairs Word pairs that differ only by the presence or absence of a phoneme (e.g., *ski*, *key*).

Neighborhood density A lexical measure of a word based on its number of neighbors or words differing by one phoneme.

Non-contrastive approaches Intervention approaches in which minimal pair words are an optional component.

Non-default Marked elements of a phonological system that need to be learned.

Non-randomized controlled trial A type of research design where participants are assigned (rather than randomly allocated) to a group.

Non-rhotic English dialects that only use /ɹ/ in syllable-initial and word-initial position and do not have r-colored vowels.

Nonlinear approach An approach to phonological analysis, target selection, and intervention adopting nonlinear phonological theories.

Normative studies Large-scale cross-sectional studies designed to gather information about the typical way a population does something, such as the age when most children acquire specific speech sounds.

Obstruents Consonants that impede or obstruct airflow through the vocal tract.

Onset-rime tier A tier in nonlinear phonology comprising onsets (i.e., consonants to the left of a vowel) and a rime (i.e., a vowel and any consonants to the right of a vowel).

Operant conditioning A theory about how behaviors can be trained through consequences.

Oropharynx The middle region of the pharynx from the soft palate through the hyoid bone.

Orthographic cues The use of written words corresponding to a spoken phoneme or word to elicit speech and/or facilitate letter-sound knowledge and phonological awareness.

Otitis media with effusion (OME) A buildup of fluid in the middle ear cavity, without signs of infection.

Palatal The place of articulation involving the tongue body being raised up against the hard palate.

Palatal fronting (depalatalization) Phonological process where a postalveolar consonant is substituted with an alveolar consonant.

Parent-as-therapist aide A method of service delivery in which a family helps provide but not necessarily plan intervention.

Parents and Children Together (PACT) A family-centered assessment and intervention approach for children with speech sound disorders.

Partial assimilation A phonological process where a feature of a sound rather than an entire sound is copied or assimilated onto another sound in a word.

Participation An individual's involvement in different life situations.

Personal factors Characteristics about a person (e.g., race, gender, age).

Pharynx The pharynx is an oval-shaped chamber or tube at the back of the throat divided into three parts: the nasopharynx, oropharynx, and laryngopharynx.

Philtrum The vertical groove extending from the upper lip to the nasal septum.

Phonation The process of vocal fold vibration that results in voice.

Phone A single speech sound.

Phoneme A speech sound that contrasts meaning between minimal pair words in a language.

Phoneme awareness See phonemic awareness.

Phoneme input frequency How often a phoneme occurs in a language.

Phoneme level A level or stage of a task focused on phonemes, in contrast with conversation, sentences, phrases, words, syllables, or rhymes.

Phoneme restoration effect Using established representations of words to help perceive spoken words when they have omitted or replaced acoustic information.

Phonemic awareness An awareness of and the ability to detect, categorize, match, isolate, blend, segment, or manipulate phonemes in words.

Phonemic repertoire The range or inventory of phonemes in an individual's phonological system.

Phonetic/articulatory complexity The degree to which a phone is difficult to articulate.

Phonetic awareness An awareness of what the articulators are doing as you speak (e.g., when saying /m/ the lips come together).

Phonetic cues Instructional information (using one or more modalities) about how a particular speech sound or word is physically articulated.

Phonetic transcription Transcription in square brackets [ ] that captures subtle differences within phones that do not change the meaning of a word, but provide a more thorough description of the pronunciation (also known as allophonic transcription).

Phonological awareness The ability to detect, categorize, match, isolate, blend, segment, or manipulate phonological elements (e.g., syllables, rhyme, phonemes) of an oral language.

Phonological competence A child's knowledge of the lexical representation of morphemes in addition to the application of phonological rules in a phonological system.

Phonological delay When a child's speech contains phonological processes or errors that are typical in the speech of younger children but should have been resolved.

Phonological disorder When a child's speech contains phonological processes or errors that are not typical in the speech of younger children.

Phonological idioms When a child pronounces a word in a more advanced form relative to the rest of his or her phonological system.

Phonological impairment A cognitive-linguistic difficulty with learning the phonological system of a language characterized by pattern-based speech errors.

Phonological knowledge A child's multilayered knowledge of several types of representations of speech (acoustic-phonetic, articulatory-phonetic, phonological) and the relationship between the different representations. (Also see productive phonological knowledge.)

Phonological performance A child's explicit (as opposed to tacit) knowledge of the phonological system being learned, as evidenced by phonetic and phonemic inventory and distributional properties of speech sounds.

Phonological processes Descriptive terms for phonological pattern-based errors in children's speech.

Phonological processing The way you mentally handle (i.e., perceive, create, store, retrieve) phonological information relevant to a language, in order to read, write, and speak that language.

Phonological recognition The process of determining whether the speech you hear belongs to a familiar phonological system or another system.

Phonological representation The abstract mental store of the phonological information about a spoken word.

Phonological representation accuracy judgment A task involving a listener making a judgment about the accuracy of a spoken word.

Phonological response generalization Improvement in a child's phonological system beyond the skill targeted in intervention; changes may be evident in non-treatment words, across word positions, within sound classes, across sound classes, or in linguistically more complex levels such as sentences or conversation.

Phonological working memory The part of working memory that temporarily stores spoken information for processing.

Phonology A branch of linguistics concerned with the study of the sound systems of languages.

Phonotactic probability The likelihood of a particular speech sound or sequence of speech sounds occurring in a language.

Phonotactic structure of words The length and syllabic structure of words.

Phonotactics Language-specific rules or constraints about how speech sounds are allowed to combine to form words in a phonological system.

Place The location where consonants and vowels are articulated in the vocal tract.

Plosive A class of consonants involving the articulators that stop then quickly release the airflow (also known as a **stop**).

Polysyllable A word containing three or more syllables.

Postvocalic devoicing Phonological process involving the substitution of a voiced consonant with the voiceless counterpart in syllable-final position in words.

Practice Repetitively engaging in a task to refine a skill.

Practice-based evidence Internal clinical evidence from a speech-language pathology service or a group of similar speech-language pathology services.

Pre-molar A type tooth (also known as bicuspid) useful for cutting and tearing food.

Pre-practice A period of time in intervention when a learner figures out what needs to be done and how in order to produce a targeted motor skill, before practicing that skill.

Prevocalic voicing Phonological process involving voiceless consonants being replaced by voiced counterparts in syllable-initial position in words.

Primary intervention An intervention designed to prevent a problem, in contrast with a secondary or tertiary intervention designed to address an existing problem.

Primary stress The syllable in a word with the most prominent stress.

Primary target patterns A set of phonological patterns targeted in the first cycle of the Cycles Phonological Remediation Approach to intervention.

Procedures Teaching cues, stimuli, resources, and activities that clinicians use to help children learn during intervention.

Productive phonological knowledge A speaker's competence and performance (i.e., tacit and explicit knowledge) about the phonological system of a language. (Also see phonological knowledge.)

Progressive assimilation Phonological process involving a sound earlier in a word replacing or influencing a sound later in a word.

Prompted self-correction A type of cue where a clinician unintentionally misunderstands a child's speech, which subsequently serves as a prompt for the child to reflect on and correct his or her own speech.

Prosodic awareness Awareness of prosodic characteristics in speech such as loudness, fluency, intonation, and stress.

Prosodic cues When a clinician provides a child with visual and/or verbal information about prosodic aspects of speech such as speech rate, loudness, stress, and fluency.

Prosodic tier A tier in nonlinear phonology comprised of all the phonological elements beyond the segment, such as phrases, words, feet, syllables, onsets and rimes, and timing units or mora.

Prosody Suprasegmental aspects of speech including stress, rhythm, intonation, and lexical and grammatical tones.

Psycholinguistic approach An assessment, target selection, and intervention approach for managing speech and literacy difficulties in children; the approach considers input and output speech processing skills in addition to the quality of children's underlying representation of speech.

Pull-out model When a clinician sees children for an assessment and/or intervention in the clinician's office or a clinical room set aside for that purpose.

Pulmonic A consonant is produced on air expelled from the lungs.

Push-in model When a clinician sees one or more children in a separate area of the classroom while the rest of the class completes other activities.

Randomized controlled trial An experimental research design where participants are randomly allocated (rather than assigned) to a group, usually an experimental or control group.

Rapid naming The ability to quickly retrieve spoken words from permanent or long-term memory.

Rate of change Trend and latency of change.

Rebus A series of pictures used to represent words or parts of words (sounds or syllables).

Recall schema A theoretical concept in the schema theory of motor learning that captures rules about relationships between initial conditions before conducting a movement, the parameters used to execute a movement, and the outcome.

Recognition schema A theoretical concept in the schema theory of motor learning that captures rules about relationships between initial conditions, the sensory consequences, and the outcome.

Reduplication (complete or partial) Phonological process involving the complete or partial repetition of a syllable in a disyllabic or polysyllabic word, replacing some or all other syllables in the word.

Regressive assimilation Phonological process involving a sound later in a word replacing or influencing a sound earlier in a word.

Reinforcement schedule A schedule that describes how often or when reinforcement is provided during intervention.

Reinforcing activity An activity that a child enjoys doing.

Repair processes From a nonlinear phonological perspective, strategies that a child uses (such the addition or deletion of a phonological element or an association line) to address constraints in the child's phonological system.

Representation See phonological representation.

Requests for self-monitoring A type of auditory cue provided by a clinician to a child encouraging the child to monitor and correct his or her own speech. A request may be elicited (intentional) or prompted (unintentional).

Residual articulation errors Common clinical distortions that continue beyond 9 years of age, usually /s/ produced as a lateral [ɬ] or interdental lisp [θ] and /ɹ/ produced as [w] or a derhotacized consonant [ʋ].

Resonance The quality of a child's speech with respect to airflow through the oral and nasal cavities.

Resources The supplies used in intervention, such as pictures, objects, equipment, and/or toys.

Respiration The process of breathing or movement of air (including oxygen and carbon dioxide) through the respiratory system.

Response generalization Improvement or carryover change in a non-targeted goal that is related to the targeted intervention goal. (Also see phonological response generalization.)

Response to intervention A three-tiered process through which children can be provided with intervention before receiving an assessment to determine if they are eligible for special education services.

Retroflex A manner of articulation where the tongue tip is up and the tongue body is in the mid-central position.

Rhotic dialect An English dialect that pronounces /ɹ/ in syllable-initial, syllable-final, word-initial, and word-final positions, and has r-colored vowels (e.g., /ɜ˞, ə˞/).

Round A distinctive feature where the lips are rounded during articulation, evident in [w, ɹ] and the rounded vowels [u, ʊ, ɒ, ɔ] in English.

Rugae The wrinkled membranous covering across the slope of the alveolar arch.

Schema theory A theory proposed to account for motor learning.

Schemas Sets of rules that guide decisions about how motor movements will be achieved under particular conditions.

Secondary stress The syllable(s) in a word that are stressed, but not as prominently as the syllable with primary stress.

Secondary target patterns A set of phonological patterns targeted only once primary patterns have been targeted, as part of the Cycles Phonological Remediation Approach to intervention.

Secondary/tertiary intervention An intervention designed to address an existing problem, in contrast with a primary intervention designed to prevent a problem.

Segmental tier A tier in nonlinear phonology comprising the features that characterize consonants and vowels.

Segmentation The process of dividing a skill along a temporal dimension into parts then practicing the parts in an additive manner.

Self-awareness/self-reflection The ability to reflect on your own beliefs, culture, perspectives, communication styles, skills, and biases and their impact on your professional practice.

Self-correction The ability to reflect on, then correct, one's own speech error.

Self-monitoring and self-evaluation The ability to consciously monitor and evaluate the accuracy of one's own speech.

Self-reinforcement Taking pleasure in one's own improved performance.

Semantic representation Abstract store of information about the meaning of a word.

Sensorineural hearing loss A type of hearing loss associated with problems with the structure or function of the inner ear.

Sentence stress The strategic emphasis on selected words in a sentence.

Sequential language learner Sequential language learners learn additional languages once their first language(s) are established, typically after the age of 3 years, and often at the commencement of schooling.

Seriation Ordering objects along a continuum from smallest to largest.

Service delivery plan A service delivery plan describes the intervention setting, intervention agent, session duration, session frequency, intervention format, and intervention continuity.

Session duration The period of time taken to run a session.

Session goals The behaviors, skills, or knowledge taught through intervention procedures within an activity during intervention sessions with an intervention agent.

Severity Severity adjectives (e.g., mild, moderate, severe) capture the degree or severity of involvement of a problem.

Short-term goals The specific behaviors or skills being targeted to achieve the long-term goal.

Sibilant Sibilants are consonants that sound like a hiss and are produced by creating a groove along the midline of the tongue to channel the air.

Side-by-side model A traditional model of assessment and intervention where the SLP and child are in the same room. This is contrasted with a telehealth model of intervention where the SLP and child are in different locations.

Simplification Modifying a skill to make it easier.

Simultaneous language learners Simultaneous language learners learn more than one language during the first years of life.

Simultaneous scheduling Intervention targeting goals across two or more domains within each session.

Single-case experimental design An experimental research design that examines change over time for a participant or cluster of participants (e.g., a classroom). The research involves a comparison of a behavior between the baseline phase and the experimental/intervention phase(s).

Social construction Knowledge gained by interacting with others in cooperative activities.

Social model The personal and environmental contexts that contribute to and impact a child's life.

Social reinforcers Verbal or nonverbal social responses that a child would find pleasant.

Socioeconomic status Stratification of an individual or group based on measures of education, income, occupation, and access to resources.

SODA analysis A speech analysis that calculates the presence of substitutions, omissions, distortions, and additions.

Sonorant [± son] Distinguishes sounds that allow airflow to be relatively unimpeded through the oral or nasal cavity [+ son] from sounds that either block or constrict the airflow [– son].

Sonority The amount of sound present in a speech segment.

Sonority difference A calculation of the difference between the sonority hierarchy score of the second sound (consonant or vowel) from the first sound.

Sonority hierarchy A numerical hierarchy, with more sonorous sounds being lower in the hierarchy (e.g., vowels) and the less sonorous sounds higher in the hierarchy (e.g., voiceless plosives).

Sonority profile The natural tendency to sequence speech sounds in words from less to more sound.

Sonority scale The hierarchical organization of speech sounds according to their sonority.

Sonority sequencing principle A principle that outlines the sonority structure of a syllable. Onsets tend to rise towards the vowel and rimes tend to fall after the vowel.

Sound-referenced rebuses The use of a rebus, or pictures representing sounds or parts of sounds in words (also known as pictograms), to make the sounds and syllables visually more salient for children.

Speaker normalization A strategy to manage acoustic variance among speakers by the perceptual reduction of differences between speakers before identification of linguistic categories.

Specificity The ability of an assessment tool to accurately identify absence of difficulty in children who do not have difficulty (i.e., are typically developing).

Spectral moment analysis An acoustic measure for quantifying and distinguishing elements of the speech signal that may or may not be perceptible to the ear. For example, to distinguish between stops and fricatives by considering the concentration (centroid), spread, tilt, and peakedness of the spectrum.

Spectrography A technique for dispersing sound waves into a spectrum to quantify and distinguish elements of the speech signal.

Speech difference Speech that may not be acceptable or intelligible to a particular community. Speech difference may be due to pronunciation differences from the ambient language (e.g., as a result of learning English as a second language), but is not because of a speech sound disorder.

Speech processing model A model designed to capture processes involved in the perception (input), storage, and production of speech (output).

Speech rate The rate of spoken speech (often measured in syllables per minute).

Speech sound disorders (SSD) An overarching term to describe difficulties with speech production and perception that are not typical of the person's age, cognitive ability, and language background. SSD includes phonological impairment, articulation impairment, inconsistent speech disorder, childhood apraxia of speech (CAS), and childhood dysarthria.

Speech-related mouth movement Mouth movements that relate to a speech sound in response to a model, verbal instruction, or visual information.

Spoken word recognition Recognition of a spoken word (e.g., by pointing to a picture of the word).

Spontaneous production Production of a word without requiring a model to imitate.

Spread glottis [± s.g.] A sound in which the vocal folds are spread wide and accompanied by frication or turbulent airflow at the glottis (including [h] and the aspirated plosives [pʰ, tʰ, kʰ]).

Standardized assessment An assessment that uses consistent test materials, consistent procedures for test administration, and consistent scoring rules.

Statistical learning Discovering patterns in spoken language to support learning of new words.

Stepping down Changing and/or increasing cues so that a task becomes easier.

Stepping up Changing and/or reducing cues so that a task becomes more challenging.

Stimulus Something that elicits a response.

Stimulus generalization When a trained behavior is evoked with different stimuli.

Stop A class of consonants involving the articulators that stop then quickly release the airflow (also known as a plosive).

Stopping of affricates Substitution of an affricate consonant with a plosive consonant that has a similar place of articulation, such as /tʃ/ → [t] and /dʒ/ → [d] (e.g., *chew* /tʃu/→ [tu]; *jam* /dʒæm/ → [dæm]).

Stopping of fricatives Substitution of a fricative consonant with a plosive consonant that has a similar place of articulation, such as /s/ → [t] and /z/ → [d] (e.g., *Sue* /su/→ [tu]; *zap* /zæp/ → [dæp]).

Stopping of liquids Substitution of a liquid consonant with a plosive consonant that has a similar place of articulation, such as /l/ → [d] and /ɹ/ → [d] (e.g., *run* /ɹʌn/→ [dʌn]; *lamb* /læm/ → [dæm]).

Stress Emphasis of a syllable within a word, or a word within a sentence. Stress may be indicated by increasing loudness or by lengthening of a vowel.

Stridency deletion A process similar to stopping of fricatives to describe the substitution of a strident phoneme with a non-strident phoneme (e.g., the substitution of strident fricatives with plosives /s/ → [t]).

Strident [± strid] Speech sounds that force air quickly through a small constriction creating a noisy or hissing airflow, including [f, v, s, z, ʃ, ʒ, tʃ, dʒ].

Structure of practice A description of the amount, distribution, variability, and schedule of practice.

Structured play An enjoyable activity or craft designed to elicit responses during intervention.

Stuttering An involuntary repetition of sounds, syllables, words, or sentences that disrupts the rhythm of flow of speech.

Submucosal cleft An anatomical abnormality along the midline of the posterior hard palate and musculature that can be associated with a bifid uvula.

Substitution One speech sound replaced by another speech sound (e.g., *see* /si/ → *tee* [ti]).

Successive approximation/shaping Gradually shaping the production of a sound or word towards the target with the intent to gradually build up task complexity and naturalness.

Successive repetition Imitation of a model several times successively.

Suprasegmental features Suprasegmental features, or prosody, include stress, rhythm, intonation, and lexical and grammatical tones.

Surface prompts Tactile information about the place, timing, or transition of an articulator.

Syllable A segment of speech typically containing a vowel. A syllable may also contain consonants.

Syllable prompts A combination of parameter and surface prompts that shape syllables.

Syllable segregation Brief pausing between syllables. Syllable segregation is considered another characteristic of CAS.

Symbolic function of language Use of language to represent objects and thoughts.

Systematic sound preference Substitution of one speech sound for a range of other speech sounds (e.g., using [f] for all fricatives and affricates).

Systematic transcriptions Systematic transcriptions primarily are used by linguists and phoneticians to transcribe typical, standard, or common realizations of speech.

Systemic approach The function of sounds within children's phonological systems as opposed to the characteristics of individual sounds.

Tactile Perceived by the sense of touch.

Tactile-phonetic cue Provision of spoken information about what it should feel like in the mouth when articulating particular speech sounds.

Tangible reward A concrete and pleasant reinforcer.

Tap/flap A consonant produced by the tongue tapping the alveolar ridge.

Telepractice Telepractice (also known as telehealth, telemedicine, telerehabilitation, telespeech, or speech teletherapy) uses telecommunication technology to provide speech-language pathology services with the speech-language pathologist and client in different locations.

Temporal Relating to time.

Temporomandibular joint The joint connecting the mandible to the temporal bone.

Tense [± tense] The distinction between long vowels such as [i, e, a, o, u, ɔ] (considered [+ tense]) from short vowels such as [ɪ, ɛ, ɒ, ʌ, ə, ʊ] (considered [− tense]).

Therapist-centered practice Practice where the professional is considered the expert who directs and controls the planning and delivery of intervention, as well as how parents may or may not be involved in the therapeutic process.

Tier one Involves universal screening for all children and the provision of short-term monitoring programs for children at risk within a general education setting.

Tier two Involves targeted small-group, school-based interventions that are validated and standardized and includes assessment to determine children's response to this intervention.

Tier three Involves multidisciplinary interventions (including from speech-language pathologists) with individualized intervention and regular assessment and monitoring of progress.

Tiers Separate levels of representation, with tiers higher up in the hierarchy dominating lower tiers.

Time-based criterion Specification of a time during which a particular skill is worked on.

Token Something that can be exchanged for another positive reinforcer.

Tones Pitch patterns associated with syllables or words. Some languages differentiate word meanings using different tones (e.g., Burmese, Cantonese, Putonghua (Mandarin), Thai, Vietnamese).

Tongue-tie A short, tight lingual frenulum (membrane extending from the underside of the tongue to the floor of the mouth) can result in a tongue-tie (also known as ankyloglossia).

Total intervention duration The period of time during which intervention is provided.

Traditional developmental approach Intervention targeting early developing, stimulable speech sounds derived from a SODA analysis, and worked through developmentally, sound by sound.

Training deep Using a vertical goal attack strategy in intervention.

Training wide Using a horizontal goal attack strategy in intervention.

Transdisciplinary Professionals within transdisciplinary teams share aims, information, tasks, and responsibilities. While transdisciplinary team members are the authoritative resource about their discipline, all team members have to expand their traditional roles.

Transitivity Using logic to determine relationships between objects.

Transverse The transverse plane is an imaginary plane that divides a person horizontally.

Treatment data Information collected during an intervention session that provides a measure of a child's response to teaching procedures.

Treatment of the empty set A contrastive approach to phonological intervention using minimal pair words that contrast two maximally opposing phonemes, both unknown by a child.

Trill A consonant produced by vibrating the articulators to interrupt the airstream.

Trochaic Stress patterns that occur when a strong syllable is followed by a weak syllable (i.e., Sw) (e.g., *mushroom* /ˈmʌʃˌɹum/). Trochees are the primary stress pattern in English disyllabic words.

Ultrasound A technique that bounces sound waves off organs and tissues to view internal body structures.

Undifferentiated lingual gesture Using the whole tongue body to cover the whole palate.

Univalent feature A superordinate term or umbrella feature (e.g., LABIAL) for a group of binary features (e.g., ± round) associated with the univalent feature.

Unstructured play Child-directed, rather than clinician-directed, activities.

Variable interval Reinforcement given after an average period of time.

Variable random practice Practicing skills in different ways and contexts.

Variable ratio Reinforcement given after an average number of responses.

Velar fronting Substitution of a velar consonant with an alveolar, such as /k/ → [t]; /g/ → [d]; /ŋ/ → [n].

Velocity The speed and direction of movement of the articulators.

Velopharyngeal insufficiency Inability to prevent the airstream from escaping through the nose (i.e., to block the nasal cavity in order to produce oral consonants and vowels).

Verbal-phonetic cue The clinician provides a child with spoken information and/or instruction about how to articulate speech sounds.

Verbal-prosodic cue The clinician provides verbal information about prosodic aspects of speech.

Vertical goal attack strategy Targeting one or two speech targets (e.g., phonemes, phonological processes, word shapes, stress patterns, prosodic pattern) at a time.

Visual-phonetic cue The clinician provides visual information about what the articulators need to do (and in particular where they need to be placed) to articulate speech.

Visual-prosodic cue The clinician provides visual information about a prosodic aspect of speech.

Visually reinforced head-turn procedure A behavioral technique where babies learn to turn their head to look at new stimuli when they hear a new sound.

Vocal folds Shelf-like structures in the larynx made of muscles and connective tissue that are lined with mucous membrane.

Vocal nodules A non-cancerous mass of tissue that grows on the vocal folds. Vocal nodules are the most common impairment of the larynx, typically as a result of vocal abuse (e.g., excessive shouting).

Vocalis muscle A muscle in the larynx that vibrates during phonation.

Vocalization Substitution of a syllabic consonant with a vowel (e.g., /l/ → [ʊ] in the word *apple*).

Voice Whether vocal fold vibration is present (voiced consonant) or absent (voiceless consonant).

Voice [± voice] Speech sounds involving vibration of the vocal folds (vowels and voiced consonants). Voiced consonants are [+ voice] and voiceless consonants are [– voice].

Voice onset time (VOT) The time (in milliseconds) between the release of a stop consonant and the vibration of the vocal folds.

Vowel quadrilateral A depiction of the vowels of the world's languages that bears a general relationship to the tongue position during the production of the vowels.

Weak syllable deletion Omission of an unstressed syllable in a disyllabic or polysyllabic word.

Word A distinct element of a language.

Word frequency The frequency (high versus low) that words occur in languages.

Word shapes Consonant and vowel sequences that form words (e.g., CV, CVC, CCVCC).

Word stress patterns Stress patterns within words of more than one syllable (also known as lexical stress patterns).

Zone of proximal development (ZPD) The distance between the level that the child can attain without assistance and the level that the child can attain with assistance from others.

References

Abercrombie, D. (1967). *Elements of general phonetics*. Edinburgh, UK: Edinburgh University Press.

Adegbola, A. A., Cox, G. F., Bradshaw, E. M., Hafler, D. A., Gimelbrant, A., & Chess, A. (2015). Monoallelic expression of the human FOXP2 speech gene. *Proceedings of the National Academy of Sciences, 112*(22), 6848–6854.

Adler-Bock, M., Bernhardt, B. M., Gick, B., & Bacsfalvi, P. (2007). The use of ultrasound in remediation of north American English /r/ in 2 adolescents. *American Journal of Speech-Language Pathology, 16*(2), 128–139.

Aguilar-Mediavilla, E. M., Sanz-Torrent, M., & Serra-Raventos, M. (2002). A comparative study of the phonology of pre-school children with specific language impairment (SLI), language delay (LD) and normal acquisition. *Clinical Linguistics and Phonetics, 16*(8), 573–596.

Aitken, N. T., & Fisher, J. P. (1996). *Articulation survey*. Melbourne, Australia: Royal Children's Hospital.

Al-Tamimi, F., Khamaiseh, Z., & Howell, P. (2013). Phonetic complexity and stuttering in Arabic. *Clinical Linguistics and Phonetics, 27*(12), 874–887.

Allard, E. R., & Williams, D. F. (2008). Listeners' perceptions of speech and language disorders. *Journal of Communication Disorders, 41*(2), 108–123.

Allen, C. M., Nikolopoulos, T. P., Dyar, D., & O'Donoghue, G. M. (2001). Reliability of a rating scale for measuring speech intelligibility after pediatric cochlear implantation. *Otology and Neurotology, 22*(5), 631–633.

Allen, G., & Hawkins, S. (1980). Phonological rhythm: Definition and development. In G. Yeni-Komshian, J. Kavanagh, & C. Ferguson (Eds.), *Child phonology* (Vol. 1, pp. 227–256). New York, NY: Academic Press.

Allen, M. M. (2013). Intervention efficacy and intensity for children with speech sound disorders. *Journal of Speech, Language, and Hearing Research, 56*, 865–877.

Almost, D., & Rosenbaum, P. (1998). Effectiveness of speech intervention for phonological disorders: A randomised controlled trial. *Developmental Medicine and Child Neurology, 40*, 319–325.

Amayreh, M. M., & Dyson, A. T. (2000). Phonetic inventories of young Arabic-speaking children. *Clinical Linguistics and Phonetics, 14*, 193–215.

American Educational Research Association [AERA], American Psychological Association [APA], & National Council on Measurement in Education [NCME]. (1985). *Standards for educational and psychological testing*. Washington, DC: American Psychological Association.

American Educational Research Association, American Psychological Association, & National Council on Measurement in Education. (1999). *Standards for educational and psychological testing*. Washington, DC: American Educational Research Association.

American Psychiatric Association. (2000). *Diagnostic and statistical manual of mental disorders (DSM IV-TR)*. Washington, DC: Author.

American Psychiatric Association. (2013). *Diagnostic and statistical manual of mental disorders (DSM-5)* (5th ed.). Arlington, VA: Author. (Chapter 1 list, page 5: Reprinted with permission from *Diagnostic and statistical manual of mental disorders (DSM-5)* (5th ed.). Copyright © 2013. American Psychiatric Association. All Rights Reserved.)

American Speech-Language-Hearing Association. (n.d.). *Bilingual service delivery*. Retrieved from http://www.asha.org/Practice-Portal/Professional-Issues/Bilingual-Service-Delivery.

American Speech-Language-Hearing Association. (1998). *Provision of instruction in English as a second language by speech-language pathologists in school settings*. Retrieved from http://www.asha.org/docs/html/PS1998-00102.html.

American Speech-Language-Hearing Association. (2000). *Guidelines for the roles and responsibilities of the school-based speech-language pathologist*. Retrieved from http://www.asha.org/policy.

American Speech-Language-Hearing Association. (2003). *National Outcomes Measurement System (NOMS): K–12 speech-language pathology user's guide*. Rockville, MD: Author.

American Speech-Language-Hearing Association (2004a). *Evidence-based practice in communication disorders: An introduction*. Retrieved from http://www.asha.org/policy/TR2004-00001/.

American Speech-Language-Hearing Association (2004b). *Knowledge and skills needed by speech-language pathologists and audiologists to provide culturally and linguistically appropriate services*. Retrieved from http://www.asha.org/policy.

American Speech-Language-Hearing Association (2004c). *Preferred practice patterns for the profession of speech-language pathology*. Retrieved from http://www.asha.org/policy/PP2004-00191/.

American Speech-Language-Hearing Association. (2005). *Cultural competence*. Retrieved from http://www.asha.org/docs/pdf/ET2005-00174.pdf.

American Speech-Language-Hearing Association. (2007a). *Scope of practice in speech-language pathology*. Retrieved from http://www.asha.org/policy.

American Speech-Language-Hearing Association. (2007b). *Childhood apraxia of speech*. Retrieved from http://www.asha.org/policy. doi: 10.1044/policy.PS2007-00277. (Chapter 2 excerpts, page 44: Used by permission from American Speech-Language-Hearing Association [ASHA].)

American Speech-Language-Hearing Association. (2010a). *Code of ethics*. Retrieved from www.asha.org/policy. (Chapter 15 quote, page 534: Used by permission from American Speech-Language-Hearing Association [ASHA].)

American Speech-Language-Hearing Association. (2010b). *Cultural competence checklist: Personal reflection*. Retrieved from http://www.asha.org/uploadedFiles/Cultural-Competence-Checklist-Personal-Reflection.pdf

American Speech-Language-Hearing Association. (2010c). *Cultural competence in professional service delivery*. Retrieved from http://www.asha.org.

American Speech-Language-Hearing Association. (2010d). *Professional issues in telepractice for speech-language pathologists*. Retrieved from http://www.asha.org/policy.

American Speech-Language-Hearing Association. (2011). *Pre-kindergarten NOMS fact sheet: Does service delivery model influence SLP outcomes in preschoolers?* Rockville, MD: American Speech-Language-Hearing Association.

American Speech-Language-Hearing Association. (2016). *National outcome measurement system*. Retrieved from http://www.asha.org/NOMS/.

Anderson, C., & Cohen, W. (2012). Measuring word complexity in speech screening: Single-word sampling to identify phonological delay/disorder in preschool children. *International Journal of Language and Communication Disorders, 47*(5), 534–541.

Anderson, G., Mjoen, T. R., & Vik, T. (2010). Prevalence of speech problems and the use of augmentative and alternative communication in children with cerebral palsy: A registry-based study in Norway. *Perspectives in Augmentative and Alternative Communication, 19*, 12–20.

Anderson, J. D., & Byrd, C. T. (2008). Phonotactic probability effects in children who stutter. *Journal of Speech, Language, and Hearing Research, 51*(4), 851–866.

Andrews, N., & Fey, M. (1986). Analysis of the speech of phonologically impaired children in two sampling conditions. *Language, Speech, and Hearing Services in Schools, 17*, 187–198.

Angle, E. H. (1899). Classification of malocclusion. *Dental Cosmos 899, 41*(18), 248–264.

Angle, E. H. (1907). *Treatment of malocclusion of the teeth.* Philadelphia, PA: White Dental Manufacturing.

Anthony, A., Bogle, D., Ingram, T. T. S., & McIsaac, M. W. (1971). *The Edinburgh Articulation Test.* Edinburgh: E. and S. Livingstone.

Anthony, J. L., Greenblatt, R., Aghara, R., Dunkelburger, M., Anthony, T. I., Williams, J. M., & Zhanga, Z. (2011). What factors place children with speech sound disorders at risk for reading problems? *American Journal of Speech-Language Pathology, 20*, 146–160.

Anthony, J. L., Lonigan, C. J., Driscoll, K., Phillips, B. M., & Burgess, S. R. (2003). Phonological sensitivity: A quasi-parallel progression of word structure units and cognitive operations. *Reading Research Quarterly, 38*, 470–487.

Anthony, J. L., Williams, J. M., Aghara, R., Dunkelberger, M., & Novak, B. (2010). Assessment of individual differences in phonological representation. *Reading and Writing: An Interdisciplinary Journal, 23*, 969–994.

Archangeli, D. (1988). Aspects of underspecification theory. *Phonology, 5*, 183–208.

Archibald, L. M. D., & Gathercole, S. E. (2006). Nonword repetition: A comparison of tests. *Journal of Speech, Language, and Hearing Research, 49*, 970–983.

Arlt, P. B., & Goodban, M. T. (1976). A comparative study of articulation acquisition as based on a study of 240 normals, aged three to six. *Language, Speech, and Hearing Services in Schools, 7*, 173–180.

Armstrong, S., & Ainley, M. (1988). *South Tyneside Assessment of Phonology (STAP).* Ponteland, UK: STASS Publications.

Arndt, J., & Healey, E. C. (2001). Concomitant disorders in school-age children who stutter. *Language, Speech, and Hearing Services in Schools, 32*, 68–78.

Arndt, W. B., Elbert, M., & Shelton, R. L. (1971). Prediction of articulation improvement with therapy from early lesson sound production task scores. *Journal of Speech, Language, and Hearing Research, 14*(1), 149–153.

Aronson, J. (2009). When I use a word ... Words misheard: Medical mondegreens. *QJM: An International Journal of Medicine, 102*(4), 301–302.

Ashby, P. (2005). *Speech sounds* (2nd ed.). Abingdon, UK: Routledge.

Austin, D., & Shriberg, L. D. (1997). *Lifespan reference data for ten measures of articulation competence using the speech disorders classification system (SDCS).* Madison, WI: Phonology Project, Waisman Center, University of Wisconsin-Madison.

Australian Council for Educational Research. (2013). *Tests of Reading Comprehension (TORCH)* (3rd ed.). Camberwell, Australia: ACER Press.

Ayyad, H., & Bernhardt, B. M. H. (2007, June 22–23). *Phonological patterns in the speech of an Arabic-speaking Kuwaiti child with hearing impairment compared with a bilingual Arabic-English 2-year-old.* Paper presented at the Child Phonology Conference, Seattle, WA.

Baarda, D., de Boer-Jongsma, N., & Haasjes-Jongsma, W. (2005). *Logo-Art Articulatieonderzoek* [Logo-Art Articulation Assessment], Ternat/Axel, The Netherlands: Baert.

Baas, B. S., Strand, E. A., Elmer, L. M., & Barbaresi, W. J. (2008). Treatment of severe childhood apraxia of speech in a 12-year-old male with CHARGE association. *Journal of Medical Speech-Language Pathology, 16*, 181–190.

Baayen, R. H., Piepenbrock, R., & Gulikers, L. (1995). *The CELEX lexical database* (Release 2). Philadelphia, PA: University of Pennsylvania, Linguistic Data Consortium.

Bacon, C., & Rappold, G. A. (2012). The distinct and overlapping phenotypic spectra of FOXP1 and FOXP2 in cognitive disorders. *Human Genetics, 131*, 1687–1698.

Bacsfalvi, P. (2010). Attaining the lingual components of /r/ with ultrasound for three adolescents with cochlear implants. *Canadian Journal of Speech-Language Pathology and Audiology, 34,* 206–217.

Bacsfalvi, P., & Bernhardt B. M. (2011). Long-term outcomes of speech therapy for seven adolescents with visual feedback technologies: Ultrasound and electropalatography. *Clinical Linguistics and Phonetics, 25*, 1034–1043.

Bagnall, A. K., Al-Muhaizea, M. A., & Manzur, A. Y. (2006). Feeding and speech difficulties in typical congenital Nemaline Myopathy. *International Journal of Speech-Language Pathology, 8*(1), 7–16.

Bai, P. M., & Vaz, A. C. (2014). Ankyloglossia among children of regular and special schools in Karnataka, India: A prevalence study. *Journal of Clinical and Diagnostic Research, 6*, ZC36–ZC38.

Baker, E. (2010a). The experience of discharging children from phonological intervention. *International Journal of Speech-Language Pathology, 12*(4), 325–328.

Baker, E. (2010b). Minimal pair intervention. In A. L. Williams, S. McLeod & R. J. McCauley (Eds.), *Interventions for speech sound disorders in children* (pp. 41–72). Baltimore, MD: Paul H. Brookes.

Baker, E. (2010c). *Toddler Polysyllable Test (T-POT).* Sydney: Author.

Baker, E. (2012a). Optimal intervention intensity. *International Journal of Speech-Language Pathology, 14*(5), 401–409.

Baker, E. (2012b). Optimal intervention intensity in speech-language pathology: Discoveries, challenges, and unchartered territories. *International Journal of Speech-Language Pathology, 14*(5), 478–485.

Baker, E. (2013). *Polysyllable Preschool Test (POP).* Sydney: Author.

Baker, E. (2015). The why and how of prioritizing complex targets for intervention. In C. Bowen (Ed.), *Children's speech sound disorders* (2nd ed., pp. 28–31). Oxford, UK: Wiley-Blackwell.

Baker, E. (2016). *Children's independent and relational phonological analysis (CHIRPA): General American English.* Sydney, Australia: Author.

Baker, E., & Bernhardt, B. (2004). From hindsight to foresight: Working around barriers to success in phonological intervention. *Child Language Teaching and Therapy, 20*(3), 287–318.

Baker, E., Croot, K., McLeod, S., & Paul, R. (2001). Psycholinguistic models of speech development and their application to clinical practice. *Journal of Speech, Language, and Hearing Research, 44*, 685–702.

Baker, E., & McLeod, S. (2004). Evidence-based management of phonological impairment in children. *Child Language Teaching and Therapy, 20*(3), 261–285.

Baker, E., & McLeod, S. (2011a). Evidence-based practice for children with speech sound disorders: Part 1 narrative review. *Language, Speech, and Hearing Services in Schools, 42*(2), 102–139.

Baker, E., & McLeod, S. (2011b). Evidence-based practice for children with speech sound disorders: Part 2 application to clinical practice. *Language, Speech, and Hearing Services in Schools, 42*(2), 140–151.

Ball, M. J. (2001). On the status of diacritics. *Journal of the International Phonetic Association, 31*(2), 259–264.

Ball, M. J. (2012). Vowels and consonants of the world's languages. In S. McLeod & B. A. Goldstein (Eds.), *Multilingual aspects of speech sound disorders in children* (pp. 32–41). Bristol, UK: Multilingual Matters.

Ball, M. J., & Code, C. (Eds.). (1997). *Instrumental clinical phonetics.* London, UK: Whurr.

Ball, M. J., Esling, J. & Dickson, C. (1995). The VoQS System for the transcription of voice quality. *Journal of the International Phonetic Association, 25*, 61–70.

Ball, M. J., & Gibbon, F. (2012). *Handbook of vowels and vowel disorders.* New York, NY: Psychology Press.

Ball, M., Manuel, R., & Müller, N. (2004). An atypical articulatory setting as learned behaviour: A videofluorographic study. *Child Language Teaching and Therapy, 20*, 153–162.

Ball, M. J., Müller, N., & Granese, A. (2013). Towards an evidence-base for /r/-therapy in English. *Journal of Clinical Speech and Language Studies, 20*, 1–23.

Ball, M. J., Müller, N., Klopfenstein, M., & Rutter, B. (2009). The importance of narrow phonetic transcription for highly unintelligible speech: Some examples. *Logopedics Phoniatrics Vocology, 34*, 84–90.

Ball, M. J., Müller, N., Klopfenstein, M., & Rutter, B. (2010). My client is using non-English sounds! A tutorial in advanced phonetic transcription, Part II: Vowels and diacritics. *Contemporary Issues in Communication Sciences and Disorders, 37*, 103–110.

Ball, M. J., Müller, N., & Rutter, B. (2010). *Phonology for communication disorders.* New York, NY: Psychology Press.

Ball, M. J., Müller, N., Rutter, B., & Klopfenstein, M. (2009). My client's using non-English sounds! A tutorial in advanced phonetic transcription. Part I: Consonants. *Contemporary Issues in Communication Sciences and Disorders, 36*, 133–141.

Ball, M. J., Rahilly, J., & Tench, P. (1996). *The phonetic transcription of disordered speech.* San Diego, CA: Singular.

Ballard, E., & Farao, S. (2008). The phonological skills of Samoan speaking 4-year-olds. *International Journal of Speech-Language Pathology*, *10*(6), 379–391.

Ballard, E., Wilson, J., Campbell, S., Purdy, S. C., & Yee, T. (2011). Phonological development: Establishing norms for New Zealand-English speaking children aged 5;0 to 5;11 years. *New Zealand Journal of Speech-Language Therapy*, *66*, 66–77.

Ballard, J. L., Auer, C. E., & Khoury, J. C. (2002). Ankyloglossia: Assessment, incidence, and effect of frenuloplasty on the breastfeeding dyad. *Pediatrics*, *110*(5), e63.

Ballard, K. J., Djaja, D., Arciuli, J., James, D. G. H., & van Doorn, J. (2012). Developmental trajectory for production of prosody: Lexical stress contrastivity in children 3 to 7 years and adults. *Journal of Speech, Language, and Hearing Research*, *55*(6), 1822–1835.

Ballard, K. J., Robin, D. A., McCabe, P., & McDonald, J. (2010). A treatment for dysprosody in childhood apraxia of speech. *Journal of Speech, Language, and Hearing Research*, *53*(5), 1227–1245.

Bankson, N. W., & Bernthal, J. E. (1982). A comparison of phonological processes identified through word and sentence imitation tasks of the PPA. *Language, Speech, and Hearing Services in Schools*, *13*, 96–99.

Bankson, N. W., & Bernthal, J. E. (1990). *Bankson-Bernthal Test of Phonology (BBTOP)*. San Antonio, TX: Special Press.

Barbosa, C., Vasquez, S., Parada, M. A., Carlos, J., Gonzalez, V., Jackson, C., . . . Fitzpatrick, A. L. (2009). The relationship of bottle feeding and other sucking behaviors with speech disorder in Patagonian preschoolers. *BMC Pediatrics*, *9*(66), 1–8.

Barlow, J. A., & Gierut, J. A. (1999). Optimality theory in phonological acquisition. *Journal of Speech, Language, and Hearing Research*, *42*, 1482–1498.

Barlow, J. A., & Gierut, J. A. (2002). Minimal pair approaches to phonological remediation. *Seminars in Speech and Language*, *23*(1), 57–67.

Barnes, E., Roberts, J., Long, S. H., Martin, G. E., Berni, M. C., Mandulak, K. C., & Sideris, J. (2009). Phonological accuracy and intelligibility in connected speech of boys with Fragile X syndrome or Down syndrome. *Journal of Speech, Language, and Hearing Research*, *52*(4), 1048–1061.

Barr, J., & McLeod, S. (2010). They never see how hard it is to be me: Siblings' observations of strangers, peers and family. *International Journal of Speech-Language Pathology*, *12*(2), 162–171.

Barr, J., McLeod, S., & Daniel, G. (2008). Siblings of children with speech impairment: Cavalry on the hill. *Language, Speech, and Hearing Services in Schools*, *39*(1), 21–32. (Chapter 1 quotes, pages 25 and 26: Used by permission from American Speech-Language-Hearing Association [ASHA].)

Barrow, I. M., Holbert, D., & Rastatter, M. P. (2000). Effect of color on developmental picture-vocabulary naming of 4-, 6-, and 8-year-old children. *American Journal of Speech-Language Pathology*, *9*(4), 310–318.

Barton, D. (1980). Phonemic perception in children. In G. H. Yeni-Komshian, J. F. Kavanagh & C. A. Ferguson (Eds.), *Child phonology: Perception* (Vol. 2, pp. 97–116). New York, NY: Academic Press.

Bashir, A. S., Grahamjones, F., & Bostwick, R. Y. (1984). A touch-cue method of therapy for developmental verbal apraxia. *Seminars in Speech and Language*, *5*, 127–137.

Bates, S., & Watson, J. (2012). *Phonetic and Phonological Systems Analysis (PPSA)*. Retrieved from http://www.qmu.ac.uk/ppsa/.

Baudonck, N. L. H., Buekers, R., Gillebert, S., & Lierde, K. M. V. (2009). Speech intelligibility of Flemish children as judged by their parents. *Folia Phoniatrica et Logopaedica*, *61*, 288–295.

Bauer, L. & Warren, P. (2004). New Zealand English: Phonology. In E. Schneider, K. Burridge, B. Kortmann, R. Mesthrie, & C. Upton (Eds.), *A handbook of varieties of English: Vol. 1, Phonology* (pp. 580–602). Berlin, Germany: Mouton de Gruyer.

Bauman-Waengler, J. (2014). *Articulatory and phonological impairments: A clinical focus* (4th ed.). Essex, UK: Pearson Education.

Bax, M., Tydeman, C., & Flodmark, O. (2006). Clinical and MRI correlates of cerebral palsy: The European Cerebral Palsy Study. *Journal of the American Medical Association*, *296*, 1602–1608.

Beauchamp, T., & Childress, J. (2012). *Principles of biomedical ethics* (7th ed.). Oxford, UK: Oxford University Press.

Bebout, L., & Arthur, B. (1992). Cross-cultural attitudes toward speech disorders. *Journal of Speech and Hearing Research*, *35*(1), 45–52.

Beckman, M. E., & Edwards, J. (2010). Generalizing over lexicons to predict consonant mastery. *Laboratory Phonology*, *1*(2), 319–343.

Bedore, L., Leonard, L., & Gandour, J. (1994). The substitution of a click for sibilants: A case study. *Clinical Linguistics and Phonetics*, *8*, 283–293.

Beitchman, J., Brownlie, E., Inglis, A., Wild, J., Mathews, R., Schachter, D., . . . Lancee, W. (1994). Seven-year follow-up of speech/language impaired and control children: Speech stability and outcome. *Journal of the American Academy of Child and Adolescent Psychiatry*, *33*, 1322–1330.

Beitchman, J. H., Hood, J., & Inglis, A. (1990). Psychiatric risk in children with speech and language disorders. *Journal of Abnormal Child Psychology*, *18*(3), 283–296.

Beitchman, J. H., Nair, R., Clegg, M., & Patel, P. G. (1986a). Prevalence of speech and language disorders in 5-year-old kindergarten children in the Ottawa-Carleton region. *Journal of Speech and Hearing Disorders*, *51*(2), 98–110.

Beitchman, J. H., Nair, R., Clegg, M., Patel, P. G., Ferguson, B., Pressman, E., & Smith, A. (1986b). Prevalence of psychiatric disorders in children with speech and language disorders. *Journal of the American Academy of Child Psychiatry*, *25*(2), 528–535.

Beitchman, J. H., Wilson, B., Brownlie, E. B., Walters, H., & Lancee, W. (1996a). Long-term consistency in speech/language profiles: I. Developmental and academic outcomes. *Journal of the American Academy of Child and Adolescent Psychiatry*, *35*(6), 804–814.

Beitchman, J. H., Wilson, B., Brownlie, E. B., Walters, H., Inglis, A., & Lancee, W. (1996b). Long-term consistency in speech/language profiles: II. Behavioral, emotional, and social outcomes. *Journal of the American Academy of Child and Adolescent Psychiatry*, *35*, 815–825.

Beitchman, J. H., Wilson, B., Johnson, C. J., Atkinson, L., Young, A., Adlaf, E., & Douglas, L. (2001). Fourteen-year follow-up of speech/language impaired and control children: Psychiatric outcome. *Journal of the American Academy of Child and Adolescent Psychiatry*, *40*, 75–82.

Bellon-Harn, M. L., Credeur-Pampolina, M. E., & LeBoeuf, L. (2013). Scaffolded-language intervention: Speech production outcomes. *Communication Disorders Quarterly*, *34*(2), 120–132.

Belton, E. (2006). *Evaluation of the effectiveness of the Nuffield Dyspraxia Programme as a treatment approach for children with severe speech disorders*. Unpublished master's dissertation, University College London, London, UK.

Ben-David, A. (2001). *Language acquisition and phonological theory: Universal and variable processes across children and across languages* [in Hebrew]. Unpublished doctoral dissertation, Tel Aviv University, Israel.

Ben-David, A., & Berman, R. A. (2007). Israeli Hebrew speech acquisition. In S. McLeod (Ed.), *The international guide to speech acquisition* (pp. 437–456). Clifton Park, NY: Thomson Delmar Learning.

Bennett, C. W., & Runyan, C. M. (1982). Educators' perceptions of the effects of communication disorders upon educational performance. *Language, Speech, and Hearing Services in Schools*, *13*(4), 260–263.

Bercow, J. (2008). *The Bercow report: A review of services for children and young people (0–19) with speech, language and communication needs*. London, UK: Department for Children, Schools and Families. Retrieved from http://webarchive.nationalarchives.gov.uk/20130401151715/http://www.education.gov.uk/publications/standard/publicationdetail/page1/DCSF-00632-2008.

Bergan, C. (2010). Motor learning principles and voice pedagogy: Theory and practice. *Journal of Singing*, *66*(4), 457–468.

Berk, L. (2007). *Development through the lifespan*. Boston, MA: Pearson Education.

Bernhardt, B. (1992). The application of nonlinear phonological theory to intervention with one phonologically disordered child. *Clinical Linguistics and Phonetics*, *6*, 283–316.

Bernhardt, B. (1994). Phonological intervention techniques for syllable and word structure development. *Clinics in Communication Disorders*, *4*(1), 54–65.

Bernhardt, B. H. (2003). Nonlinear phonology: Application and outcomes evaluation. *Perspectives on Language Learning and Education*, *10*(1), 26–30.

Bernhardt, B. H. (2005). Selection of phonological goals and targets. In A. G. Kamhi & K. E. Pollock (Eds.), *Phonological disorders in children: Clinical decision making in assessment and intervention* (pp. 109–120). Baltimore, MD: Paul H. Brookes.

Bernhardt, B. H., Bopp, K. E., Daudlin, B., Edwards, S. M., & Wastie, S. E. (2010). Nonlinear phonological intervention. In A. L. Williams, S. McLeod, & R. J. McCauley (Eds.), *Interventions for speech sound disorders in children* (pp. 315–331). Baltimore, MD: Paul H. Brookes.

Bernhardt, B. M. H., & Deby, J. (2007). Canadian English speech acquisition. In S. McLeod (Ed.), *The international guide to speech acquisition* (pp. 177–187). Clifton Park, NY: Thomson Delmar Learning.

Bernhardt, B. H., Gick, N., Bacsfalvi, P., & Alder-Bock, M. (2005). Ultrasound in speech therapy with adolescents and adults. *Clinical Linguistics and Phonetics, 19*, 605–617.

Bernhardt, B., Gick, B., Bacsfalvi, P., & Ashdown, J. (2003). Speech habilitation of hard of hearing adolescents using electropalatography and ultrasound as elevated by trained listeners. *Clinical Linguistics and Phonetics, 17*, 199–216.

Bernhardt, B. H., & Holdgrafer, G. (2001a). Beyond the basics I: The need for strategic sampling for in-depth phonological analysis. *Language, Speech, and Hearing Services in Schools, 32*, 18–27.

Bernhardt, B. H., & Holdgrafer, G. (2001b). Beyond the basics II: Supplemental sampling for in-depth phonological analysis. *Language, Speech, and Hearing Services in Schools, 32*, 27–36.

Bernhardt, B. H., & Major, E. (2005). Speech, language and literacy skills 3 years later: A follow-up study of early phonological and metaphonological intervention. *International Journal of Language and Communication Disorders, 40*(1), 1–27.

Bernhardt, B. M., Másdóttir, T., Stemberger, J. P., Leonhardt, L., & Hansson, G. Ó. (2015). Fricative acquisition in English- and Icelandic-speaking preschoolers with protracted phonological development. *Clinical Linguistics and Phonetics, 29*(8–10), 642–665.

Bernhardt, B. H., & Stemberger, J. P. (1998). *Handbook of phonological development from the perspective of constraint-based nonlinear phonology.* San Diego, CA: Academic Press.

Bernhardt, B. H., & Stemberger, J. P. (2000). *Workbook in nonlinear phonology for clinical application.* Austin, TX: Pro-Ed.

Bernhardt, B. M., Stemberger, J., & Bacsfalvi, P. (2010). Vowel intervention. In A. L. Williams, S. McLeod, & R. McCauley (Eds.), *Interventions for speech sound disorders in children* (pp. 537–555). Baltimore, MD: Paul H. Brookes.

Bernhardt, B. H., Stemberger, J. P., & Major, E. (2006). General and nonlinear phonological intervention perspectives for a child with a resistant phonological impairment. *International Journal of Speech-Language Pathology, 8*(3), 190–206.

Bernhardt, B., & Stoel-Gammon, C. (1994). Nonlinear phonology: Introduction and clinical application. *Journal of Speech and Hearing Research, 37*, 123–143.

Bernhardt, B. H., & Stoel-Gammon, C. (1996). Underspecification and markedness in normal and disordered phonological development. In C. E. Johnson & J. H. V. Gilbert (Eds.), *Children's language* (Vol. 9, pp. 33–54). Mahwah, NJ: Lawrence Erlbaum Associates.

Bernhardt, M. B., Bacsfalvi, P., Adler-Bock, M., Shimizu, R., Cheney, A., Giesbrecht, N., Radanov, B. (2008). Ultrasound as visual feedback in speech habilitation: Exploring consultative use in rural British Columbia, Canada. *Clinical Linguistics and Phonetics, 22*, 149–162.

Bernthal, J. E., Bankson, N. W., & Flipsen, P., Jr. (Eds.). (2009). *Articulation and phonological disorders: Speech sound disorders in children* (6th ed). Boston, MA: Pearson Education.

Bernthal, J. E., Bankson, N. W., & Flipsen, P., Jr. (Eds.). (2013). *Articulation and phonological disorders* (7th ed.). Needham Heights, MA: Allyn & Bacon.

Betancourt, J. R., Green, A. R., Carrillo, J. E., & Ananeh-Firempong, O. (2003). Defining cultural competence: A practical framework for addressing racial/ethnic disparities in health and health care. *Public Health Reports, 118*(4), 293–302.

Bhandari, M., Richards, R. R., Sprague, S., & Schemitsch, E. H. (2001). Quality in the reporting of randomized trials in surgery: Is the Jadad scale reliable? *Controlled Clinical Trials, 22*, 687–688.

Bhatnager, S. C., & Andy, O. J. (1995). *Neuroscience for the study of communicative disorders.* Baltimore, MD: Williams & Wilkins.

Binger, C. (2007). Aided AAC intervention for children with suspected childhood apraxia of speech. *SIG 12 Perspectives on Augmentative and Alternative Communication, 16*(1), 10–12.

Bird, J., Bishop, D. V. M., & Freeman, N. H. (1995). Phonological awareness and literacy development in children with expressive phonological impairments. *Journal of Speech and Hearing Research, 38*, 446–462.

Bishop, D. V. M., & Adams, C. (1990). A prospective study of the relationship between Specific Language Impairment, phonological disorders and reading retardation. *Journal of Child Psychology and Psychiatry, 31*(7), 1027–1050.

Bishop, D. V. M., & Clarkson, B. (2003). Written language as a window into residual language deficits: A study of children with persistent and residual speech and language impairments. *Cortex, 39*, 215–237.

Bishop, D. V. M., Maybery, M., Wong, D., Maley, A., Hill, W., & Hallmayer, J. (2004). Are phonological processing deficits part of the broad Autism phenotype? *American Journal of Medical Genetics Part B (Neuropsychiatric Genetics), 128B*, 54–60.

Blache, S. E., Parsons, C. L., & Humphreys, J. M. (1981). A minimal-word-pair model for teaching the linguistic significant difference of distinctive feature properties. *Journal of Speech and Hearing Disorders, 46*, 291–296.

Blakeley, R. W. (2001). *Screening Test for Developmental Apraxia of Speech —Second Edition* (STDAS-2). Austin, TX: Pro-Ed.

Blamey, P. (1997). *Computer Aided Speech and Language Assessment: Version Student 2.0.* Melbourne, Australia: University of Melbourne.

Blanton, M. G., & Blanton, S. (1919). *Speech training for children: The hygiene of speech.* New York, NY: The Century Company.

Bleile, K. M. (1995). *Manual of articulation and phonological disorders.* San Diego, CA: Singular.

Bleile, K. M. (1996). *Articulation and phonological disorders: A book of exercises.* (2nd ed.). San Diego, CA: Singular Publishing.

Bleile, K. (2002). Evaluating articulation and phonological disorders when the clock is running. *American Journal of Speech-Language Pathology, 11*(3), 243–249.

Bleile, K. M. (2004). *Manual of articulation and phonological disorders: Infancy through adulthood* (2nd ed.). Clifton Park, NY: Delmar Learning.

Bleile, K. (2006a). *International directory of communicative disorders.* Retrieved from http://www.comdisinternational.com/agreement.html.

Bleile, K. M. (2006b). *The late eight.* San Diego, CA: Plural Publishing.

Bleile, K. M. (2014). *The late eight* (2nd ed.). San Diego, CA: Plural Publishing.

Bleile, K., & Wallach, H. (1992). A sociolinguistic investigation of the speech of African-American preschoolers. *American Journal of Speech-Language Pathology, 1*, 54–62.

Blood, G. W., Ridenour, V. J., Qualls, C. D., & Hammer, C. S. (2003). Co-occurring disorders in children who stutter. *Journal of Communication Disorders, 36*(6), 427–448.

Blount, R. L., & Stokes, T. F. (1984). Self-reinforcement by children. In M. Hersen, R. Eisler, & P. Miller (Eds.), *Progress in behavior modification* (pp. 195–225). New York, NY: Academic Press.

Body, R., & McAllister, L. (Eds.). (2009). *Ethics in speech and language therapy.* Chichester, UK: Wiley-Blackwell.

Boersma, P. & Weenink, D. (2013). *Praat: Doing phonetics by computer* [Computer program]. Version 5.3.42, Retrieved from http://www.praat.org/.

Bohland, J. W., Bullock, D., & Guenther, F. H. (2009). Neural representations and mechanisms for the performance of simple speech sequences. *Journal of Cognitive Neuroscience, 22*(7), 1504–1529.

Boliek, C. A., & Fox, C. M. (2014). Individual and environmental contributions to treatment outcomes following a neuroplasticity-principled speech treatment (LSVT LOUD) in children with dysarthria secondary to cerebral palsy: A case study review. *International Journal of Speech-Language Pathology, 16*(4), 372–385.

Booth, T., & Ainscow, M. (2002). *Index for inclusion: Developing learning and participation in schools.* London, UK: Centre for Studies on Inclusive Education. Retrieved from http://www.eenet.org.uk/resources/docs/Index%20English.pdf.

Bowen, C. (1996). *The quick screener.* Retrieved from http://www.speech-language-therapy.com/tx-a-quickscreener.html.

Bowen, C. (1998). *Development phonological disorders: A practical guide for families and teachers.* Melbourne, Victoria: ACER Press.

Bowen, C. (2009). *Children's speech sound disorders.* Chichester, UK: Wiley-Blackwell.

Bowen, C. (2010). Parents and children together (PACT) intervention. In A. L. Williams, S. McLeod, & R. J. McCauley (Eds.), *Interventions for speech sound disorders in children* (pp. 407–426). Baltimore, MD: Paul H. Brookes.

Bowen, C. (2015). *Children's speech sound disorders* (2nd ed.). Oxford, UK: Wiley Blackwell.

Bowen, C., & Cupples, L. (1998). A tested phonology therapy in practice. *Child Language, Teaching and Therapy, 14*(1), 29–50.

Bowen, C., & Cupples, L. (1999a). Parents and children together (PACT): A collaborative approach to phonological therapy. *International Journal of Language and Communication Disorders, 34*(1), 35–56.

Bowen, C., & Cupples, L. (1999b). A phonological therapy in depth: A reply to commentaries. *International Journal of Language and Communication Disorders, 34*, 65–83.

Bowen, C., & Cupples, L. (2006). PACT: Parents and children together in phonological therapy. *International Journal of Speech-Language Pathology, 8*(3), 245–260.

Boyce, S., & Espy-Wilson, C. Y. (1997). Coarticulatory stability in American English /r/. *Journal of the Acoustical Society of America, 101,* 3741–3753.

Boyle, J., McCartney, E., Forbes, J., & O'Hare, A. (2007). A randomised controlled trial and economic evaluation of direct versus indirect and individual versus group modes of speech and language therapy for children with primary language impairment. *Health Technology Assessment, 11*(25), 1–139.

Brackenbury, T., Burroughs, E., & Hewitt, L. E. (2008). A qualitative examination of current guidelines for evidence-based practice in child language intervention *Language, Speech, and Hearing Services in Schools, 39,* 78–88.

Braddock, B. A., Farmer, J. E., Deidrick, K. M., Iverson, J. M., & Maria, B. L. (2006). Oromotor and communication findings in Joubert syndrome: Further evidence of multisystem apraxia. *Journal of Child Neurology, 21*(2), 160–163.

Bradford, A., & Dodd, B. (1996). Do all speech-disordered children have motor deficits? *Clinical Linguistics and Phonetics, 10,* 77–101.

Bradford, A., & Dodd, B. (1997). A treatment case study of inconsistent speech disorder. *Australian Communication Quarterly, Autumn,* 24–28.

Bradford-Heit, A., & Dodd, B. (1998). Learning new words using imitation and additional cues: Differences between children with disordered speech. *Child Language Teaching and Therapy, 14*(2), 159–179.

Bradlow, A. R., & Bent, T. (2008). Perceptual adaptation to non-native speech. *Cognition, 106,* 707–729.

Bralley, R. C., & Stoudt, R. J. (1977). A five year longitudinal study of development of articulation. *Language, Speech, and Hearing Services in Schools, 8,* 176–180.

Bressmann, T. (2006). Speech adaptation to a self-inflicted cosmetic tongue split: Perceptual and ultrasonographic analysis. *Clinical Linguistics and Phonetics, 20,* 205–210.

Bressmann, T., Thind, P., Uy, C., Bollig, C., Gilbert, R., & Irish, J. (2005). Quantitative three-dimensional ultrasound analysis of tongue protrusion, grooving and symmetry: Data from 12 normal speakers and a partial glossectomee. *Clinical Linguistics and Phonetics, 19*(6–7), 573–588.

Bridgeman, E., & Snowling, M. (1988). The perception of phoneme sequence: A comparison of dyspraxic and normal children. *British Journal of Disorders of Communication, 23,* 245–252.

Briggs, M. H. (1997). *Building early intervention teams: Working together for children and families.* Gaithersburg, MD: Aspen Publishers.

Brinton, L., & Fee, M. (2001). Canadian English. In J. Algeo (Ed.), *The Cambridge history of the English Language: Volume VI, English in North America* (pp. 422–440). Cambridge, UK: Cambridge University Press.

Briscoe, J., Bishop, D. V. M., & Norbury, C. F. (2001). Phonological processing, language, and literacy: A comparison of children with mild-to-moderate sensorineural hearing loss and those with specific language impairment. *Journal of Child Psychology and Psychiatry, 42*(3), 329–340.

Broen, P. A., Strange, W., Doyle, S. S., & Heller, J. H. (1983). Perception and production of approximant consonants by normal and articulation delayed preschool children. *Journal of Speech and Hearing Research, 26,* 601–608.

Broen, P. A., & Westman, M. J. (1990). Project parent: A preschool speech program implemented through parents. *Journal of Speech and Hearing Disorders, 55,* 495–502.

Bronfenbrenner, U. (1979). *The ecology of human development.* Cambridge, MA: Harvard University Press.

Bronfenbrenner, U. (1994). Ecological models of human development. In T. N. Postlethwaite & T. Husen (Eds.), *International encyclopaedia of education* (Vol. 3, 2nd ed., pp. 1643–1647). Oxford: Elsevier.

Broomfield, J., & Dodd, B. (2004a). Children with speech and language disability: Caseload characteristics. *International Journal of Language and Communication Disorders, 39*(3), 303–324.

Broomfield, J., & Dodd, B. (2004b). The nature of referred subtypes of primary speech disability. *Child Language Teaching and Therapy, 20*(2), 135–151.

Broomfield, J., & Dodd, B. (2011). Is speech and language therapy effective for children with primary speech and language impairment? Report of a randomized control trial. *International Journal of Language and Communication Disorders, 46*(6), 628–640.

Brosseau-Lapré, F., & Rvachew, S. (2014). Cross-linguistic comparison of speech errors produced by English- and French-speaking preschool-age children with developmental phonological disorders. *International Journal of Speech-Language Pathology, 16*(2), 98–108.

Browman, C. P., & Goldstein, L. (1986). Towards an articulatory phonology. *Phonology Yearbook 3,* 219–252.

Browman, C. P., & Goldstein, L. (1992). Articulatory phonology: An overview. *Phonetica, 49,* 155–180.

Brown, R. (1973). *A first language: The early stages.* Cambridge, MA: MIT Press.

Brumbaugh, K. M., & Smit, A. B. (2013). Treating children ages 3–6 who have speech sound disorder: A survey. *Language, Speech, and Hearing Services in Schools, 44*(3), 306–319.

Brunnegård, K., Lohmander, A., & van Doorn, J. (2012). Comparison between perceptual assessments of nasality and nasalance scores. *International Journal of Language and Communication Disorders, 47*(5), 556–566.

Brutten, G. J., & Dunham, S. L. (1989). The communication attitude test: A normative study of grade school children. *Journal of Fluency Disorders, 14,* 71–77.

Buccino, G., Binkofski, F., & Riggio, L. (2004). The mirror neuron system and action recognition. *Brain and Language, 89*(2), 370–376.

Bunton, K., Kent, R. D., Kent, J. F., & Rosenbek, J. C. (2000). Perceptuo-acoustic assessment of prosodic impairment in dysarthria. *Clinical Linguistics and Phonetics, 14*(1), 13–24.

Burke, P. (2004). *Brothers and sisters of disabled children.* London, UK: Jessica Kingsley Publishers.

Burkholder-Juhasz, R. A., Levi, S. V., Dillon, C. M., & Pisoni, D. B. (2007). Nonword repetition with spectrally reduced speech: Some developmental and clinical findings from pediatric cochlear implantation. *Journal of Deaf Studies and Deaf Education, 12*(4), 472–485.

Burnham, D., & Dodd, B. (2004). Auditory-visual speech integration by prelinguistic infants: Perception of an emergent consonant in the McGurk effect. *Developmental Psychobiology, 45,* 204–220.

Burt, L., Holm, A., & Dodd, B. (1999). Phonological awareness skills of 4-year-old British children: An assesment and developmental data. *International Journal of Language and Communication Disorders, 34*(3), 311–335.

Buryk, M., Bloom, D., & Shope, T. (2011). Efficacy of neonatal release of ankyloglossia: A Randomized trial. *Pediatrics, 128*(2), 280–288.

Bybee, J. (2001). *Phonology and language use.* Cambridge, UK: Cambridge University Press.

Byng, S. (2001). Integrating therapies. *International Journal of Speech-Language Pathology, 3*(1), 67–71.

Cabell, S. Q., Justice, L. M., Kaderavek, J. N., Pence Turnbull, K., & Breit-Smith, A. (2009). *Emergent literacy: Lessons for success.* San Diego, CA: Plural Publishing.

Calabrese, A. (2012). Auditory representations and phonological illusions: A linguist's perspective on the neuropsychological bases of speech perception. *Journal of Neurolinguistics, 25*(5), 355–381.

Camarata, S. M. (1993). The application of naturalistic conversation taining to speech production in children with speech disabilities. *Journal of Applied Behaviour Analysis, 26*, 173–182.

Camarata, S. M. (1995). A rationale for naturalistic speech intelligibility training. In M. E. Fey, J. Windsor, & S. F. Warren (Eds.), *Language intervention: Preschool through the elementary years* (pp. 63–84). Baltimore, MD: Paul H. Brookes.

Camarata, S. M. (2010). Naturalistic intervention for speech intelligibility and speech accuracy. In A. L. Williams, S. McLeod, & R. J. McCauley (Eds.) *Interventions for speech sound disorders in children* (pp. 381–405). Baltimore, MD: Paul H. Brookes.

Camarata, S. (2014). Validity of early identification and early intervention in autism spectrum disorders: Future directions. *International Journal of Speech-Language Pathology, 16*(1), 61–68.

Camargo, Z. A., Marchesan, I. Q., Oliveira, L. R., Svicero, M. A. F., Pereira, L. C. K., & Madureira, S. (2013). Lingual frenectomy and alveolar tap production: An acoustic and perceptual study. *Logopedics Phoniatrics Vocology, 38*(4), 157–166.

Cambra, C. (1996). A comparative study of personality descriptors attributed to the deaf, the blind, and individuals with no sensory disability. *American Annals of the Deaf, 141*(1), 24–28.

Campbell, T. F., Dollaghan, C., Janosky, J., Rusiewicz, H. L., Small, S. L., Dick, F., . . . Adelson, P. D. (2013). Consonant accuracy after severe pediatric traumatic brain injury: A prospective cohort study. *Journal of Speech, Language, and Hearing Research, 56*(3), 1023–1034.

Campbell, T. F., Dollaghan, C. A., Rockette, H. E., Paradise, J. L., Feldman, H. M., Shriberg, L. D., . . . Kurs-Lasky, M. (2003). Risk factors for speech delay of unknown origin in 3-year-old children. *Child Development, 74*, 346–357.

Canadian Association of Speech-Language Pathologists and Audiologists (1997). *Position paper on speech-language pathology and audiology in the multicultural, multilingual context.* Retrieved from http://sac-oac.ca/professional-resources/resource-library/sac-position-paper-speech-language-pathology-and-audiology.

Carahaly, L. (2010). *The Speech-EZ apraxia program.* Gilbert, AZ: Foundations Developmental House.

Carbajal, R., Chauvet, X., Couderc, S., & Olivier-Martin, M. (1999). Randomised trial of analgesic effects of sucrose, glucose, and pacifiers in term neonates. *BMJ: British Medical Journal, 319*(7222), 1393–1397.

Cardon, G., Campbell, J., & Sharma, A. (2012). Plasticity in the developing auditory cortex: Evidence from children with sensorineural hearing loss and auditory neuropathy spectrum disorder. *Journal of the American Academy of Audiology, 23*(6), 396–411.

Carrier, J. J. K. (1970). A program of articulation therapy administered by mothers. *Journal of Speech and Hearing Disorders, 35*(4), 344–353.

Carrigg, B., Baker, E., Parry, L., & Ballard, K. J. (2015). Persistent speech sound disorder in a 22-year-old male: Communication, educational, socio-emotional, and vocational outcomes. *SIG 16 Perspectives on School-Based Issues, 16*(2), 37–49.

Carroll, J. M., Snowling, M. J., Stevenson, J., & Hulme, C. (2003). The development of phonological awareness in preschool children. *Developmental Psychology, 39*, 913–923.

Carruth, B. R., & Skinner, J. D. (2002). Feeding behaviors and other motor development in healthy children (2–24 months). *Journal of the American College of Nutrition, 21*(2), 88–96.

Cartwright, J. (2002). *Determinants of animal behaviour.* East Sussex, UK: Routledge.

Caruso, A. J., & Strand, E. A. (1999). Motor speech disorders in children: Definitions, backgrounds, and a theoretical framework. In A. J. Caruso & E. A. Strand (Eds.), *Clinical management of motor speech disorders in children* (pp. 1–27). New York, NY: Thieme.

Case, R. (2000). Conceptual structures. In M. Bennett (Ed.), *Developmental psychology.* Philadelphia, PA: Psychology Press.

Cash, J. C., & Glass, C. A. (2010). *Family practice guidelines* (2nd ed.). New York, NY: Springer.

Caspari, S. S., Strand, E. A., Kotagal, S., & Bergqvist, C. (2008). Obstructive sleep apnea, seizures, and childhood apraxia of speech. *Pediatric Neurology, 38*(6), 422–425.

Cassidy, S., & Harrington, J. (2010). *The EMU speech database system.* Munich, Germany: Institute of Phonetics and Speech Processing.

Catlin, F. I. (1971). Tongue-tie. *Archives of Otolaryngology-Head and Neck Surgery, 94*(6), 548–557.

Ceron, M. I., & Keske-Soares, M. (2012). Analysis of the therapeutic progress of children with phonological disorders after the application of the multiple oppositions approach. *Jornal da Sociedade Brasileira de Fonoaudiologia, 24*(1), 91–95.

Chabon, S. W., & Cohn, E. R. (2011). *The communication disorders casebook: Learning by example.* Upper Saddle River, NJ: Pearson Education.

Chan, A. Y. W. (2010). Advanced Cantonese ESL learners' production of English speech sounds: Problems and strategies. *System, 38*(2), 316–328.

Chan, R. K. K., McPherson, B., & Whitehill, T. L. (2006). Chinese attitudes toward cleft lip and palate: Effects of personal contact. *The Cleft Palate-Craniofacial Journal, 43*(6), 731–739.

Chang, S.-E., Ohde, R. N., & Conture, E. G. (2002). Coarticulation and formant transition rate in young children who stutter. *Journal of Speech, Language, and Hearing Research, 45*(4), 676–688.

Chapman, K. L., Hardin-Jones M., & Halter K. A. (2003). The relationship between early speech and later speech and language performance for children with cleft lip and palate. *Clinical Linguistics and Phonetics, 17*, 173–197.

Chen, K.-L., Wang, H.-Y., Tseng, M.-H., Shieh, J.-Y., Lu, L., Yao, K.-P. G., & Huang, C.-Y. (2013). The cerebral palsy quality of life for children (CP QOL-Child): Evidence of construct validity. *Research in Developmental Disabilities, 34*(3), 994–1000.

Cheng, H. Y., Murdoch, B. E., Goozée, J. V., & Scott, D. (2007). Physiologic development of tongue-jaw coordination from childhood to adulthood. *Journal of Speech, Language, and Hearing Research, 50*(2), 352–360.

Cheng, L.-R. L. (1999). Moving beyond accent: Social and cultural realities of living with many tongues. *Topics in Language Disorders, 19*(4), 1–10.

Cheour, M., Korpilahti, P., Martynova, O., & Lang, A.-H. (2001). Mismatch negativity and late discriminative negativity in investigating speech perception and learning in children and infants. *Audiology and Neurotology, 6*, 2–11.

Cheung, P. S. P., Ng, A., & To, C. K. S. (2006). *Hong Kong Cantonese Articulation Test.* Hong Kong, China SAR: Language Information Sciences Research Centre, City University of Hong Kong.

Chin, S. (2002). Aspects of stop consonant product by pediatric users of cochlear implants. *Language, Speech, and Hearing Services in Schools, 33*, 38–51.

Ching, A. B. (2008). For all "intensive" purposes: A primer on malapropisms, eggcorns, and other rogue elements of the English language. *The Army Lawyer, December*, 66–72.

Ching, T. Y. C., & Hill, M. (2007). The parent's evaluation of aural/oral performance of children (PEACH) scale: Normative data. *Journal of the American Academy of Audiology, 18*(3), 220–235.

Ching, T. Y. C., Hill, M., & Dillon, H. (2008). Effect of variations in hearing-aid frequency response on real-life functional performance of children with severe or profound hearing loss. *International Journal of Audiology, 47*(8), 461–475.

Chirlian, N. S., & Sharpley, C. F. (1982). Children's articulation development: Some regional differences. *Australian Journal of Human Communication Disorders, 10*, 23–30.

Chomsky, N., & Halle, M. (1968). *The sound pattern of English (SPE).* New York, NY: Harper and Row.

Chumpelik, D. (1984). The PROMPT system of therapy: Theoretical framework and application for developmental apraxia in speech. *Seminars in Speech and Language, 5*(2), 139–156.

Cirrin, F. M., Schooling, T. L., Nelson, N. W., Diehl, S. F., Flynn, P. F., Staskowski, M., . . . Adamczyk, D. F. (2010). Evidence-based systematic review: Effects of different service delivery models on communication outcomes for elementary school-age children. *Language, Speech, and Hearing Services in Schools, 41*(3), 233–264.

Clark, C. E., Conture, E. G., Walden, T. A., & Lambert, W. E. (2013). Speech sound articulation abilities of preschool-age children who stutter. *Journal of Fluency Disorders, 38*(4), 325–341.

Cleland, J., Gibbon, F. E., Peppé, S. J. E., O'Hare, A., & Rutherford, M. (2010). Phonetic and phonological errors in children with high functioning autism and Asperger syndrome. *International Journal of Speech-Language Pathology, 12*(1), 69–76.

Cleland, J., Scobbie, J. M., & Wrench, A. A. (2015). Using ultrasound visual biofeedback to treat persistent primary speech sound disorders. *Clinical Linguistics and Phonetics, 29*(8–10), 575–597.

Cleland, J., Wood , S., Hardcastle, W., Wishart, J., & Timmins, C. (2010). Relationship between speech, oromotor, language and cognitive abilities in children with Down's syndrome. *International Journal of Language and Communication Disorders, 45*, 83–95.

Coady, J. A., & Evans, J. L. (2008). Uses and interpretations of non-word repetition tasks in children with and without specific language impairments (SLI). *International Journal of Language and Communication Disorders, 43*(1), 1–40.

Cockerill, H., Elbourne, D., Allen, E., Scrutton, D., Will, E., McNee, A., . . . Baird, G. (2014). Speech, communication and use of augmentative communication in young people with cerebral palsy: The SH&PE population study. *Child: Care, Health and Development, 40*(2), 149–157.

Cohen, W., & Anderson, C. (2011). Identification of phonological processes in preschool children's single-word productions. *International Journal of Language and Communication Disorders, 46*(4), 481–488.

Coleman, L. M. (1997). Stigma: An enigma demystified. In L. J. Davis (Ed.), *The disabilities studies reader* (pp. 216–231). New York, NY: Routledge.

Collicut McGrath, J. (2007). *Ethical practice in brain injury rehabilitation.* Oxford, UK: Oxford University Press.

Comina, E., Marion, K., Renaud, F. N., Dore, J., Bergeron, E., & Freney, J. (2006). Pacifiers: A microbial reservoir. *Nursing and Health Sciences, 8*(4), 216–223.

Commonwealth of Australia. (2014). *Senate Community Affairs References Committee: Prevalence of different types of speech, language and communication disorders and speech pathology services in Australia.* Canberra, Australia: Commonwealth of Australia.

Connery, V. (1985). *Nuffield Dyspraxia Programme (NDP).* London, UK: The Miracle Factory.

Constable, A., Stackhouse, J., & Wells, B. (1997). Developmental word-finding difficulties and phonological processing: The case of the missing handcuffs. *Applied Psycholinguistics, 18*, 507–536.

Conture, E. G., Kelly, E. M., & Walden, T. A. (2013). Temperament, speech and language: An overview. *Journal of Communication Disorders, 46*(2), 125–142.

Conture, E. G., Louko, L. J., & Edwards, M. L. (1993). Simultaneously treating stuttering and disordered phonology in children. *American Journal of Speech-Language Pathology, 2*(3), 72–81.

Corsaro, W. A. (1976). The clarification request as a feature of adult interactive styles with young children. *Language in Society, 6*, 183–207.

Costello, J. (1975). Articulation instruction based on distinctive features theory. *Language, Speech, and Hearing Services in Schools, 6*, 61–71.

Costello, J., & Schoen, J. (1978). The effectiveness of paraprofessionals and a speech clinician as agents of articulation intervention using programmed instruction. *Language, Speech, and Hearing Services in Schools, 9*(2), 118–128.

Cox, F. (2008). Vowel transcription systems: An Australian perspective. *International Journal of Speech-Language Pathology, 10*(5), 327–333.

Cox, F. (2012). *Australian English pronunciation and transcription.* Melbourne, Australia: Cambridge University Press.

Crais, E. R. (2009). Working with families of young children with communication and language impairments: Identification and assessment. In N. Watts Pappas & S. McLeod (Eds.), *Working with families in speech-language pathology* (pp. 112–129). San Diego, CA: Plural Publishing.

Crais, E. R. (2011). Testing and beyond: Strategies and tools for evaluating and assessing infants and toddlers. *Language, Speech, and Hearing Services in Schools, 42*, 341–364.

Crais, E. R., Roy, V. P., & Free, K. (2006). Parents' and professionals' perceptions of the implementation of family-centered practices in child assessments. *American Journal of Speech-Language Pathology, 15*, 365–377.

Crary, M. A. (1983). Phonological process analysis from spontaneous speech: The influence of sample size. *Journal of Communication Disorders, 16*, 133–141.

Creel, S. C., & Jimenez, S. R. (2012). Differences in talker recognition by preschoolers and adults. *Journal of Experimental Child Psychology, 113*(4), 487–509.

Creel, S. C., & Tumlin, M. A. (2011). On-line acoustic and semantic interpretation of talker information. *Journal of Memory and Language, 65*(3), 264–285.

Crosbie, S., Holm, A., & Dodd, B. (2005). Intervention for children with severe speech disorder: A comparison of two approaches. *International Journal of Language and Communication Disorders, 40*(4), 467–491.

Crosbie, S., Holm, A., & Dodd, B. (2009). Cognitive flexibility in children with and without speech disorder. *Child Language Teaching and Therapy, 25*(2), 250–270.

Crosbie, S., Pine, C., Holm, A., & Dodd, B. (2006). Treating Jarrod: A core vocabulary approach. *International Journal of Speech-Language Pathology, 8*(3), 316–321.

Cross, I. (2009). Communicative development: Neonate crying reflects patterns of native-language speech. *Current Biology, 19*(23), R1078–R1079.

Crow, G., & Pounder, D. (2000). Interdisciplinary teacher teams: Context, design, and process. *Educational Administration Quarterly, 36*, 216–254.

Crowe, K., & McLeod, S. (2014). A systematic review of cross-linguistic and multilingual speech and language outcomes for children with hearing loss. *International Journal of Bilingual Education and Bilingualism, 17*(3), 287–309.

Crowe, K., McLeod, S., & Ching, T. Y. C. (2012). The cultural and linguistic diversity of 3-year-old children with hearing loss. *Journal of Deaf Studies and Deaf Education, 17*(4), 421–438.

Crowe, K., McLeod, S., McKinnon, D. H., & Ching, T. Y. C. (2014). Speech, sign, or multilingualism for children with hearing loss: Quantitative insights into caregivers' decision-making. *Language, Speech, and Hearing Services in Schools, 45*(3), 234–247.

Crumrine, L. & Lonegan, H. (1999). *Pre-literacy skills screening.* Austin, TX: Pro-Ed.

Cruttenden, A. (1982). How long does intonation acquisition take? *Papers and Reports on Child Language Development, 21*, 112–118.

Cruttenden, A. (2014). *Gimson's pronunciation of English* (8th ed.). London, UK: Routledge.

Crystal, D. (1982). *Profiling linguistic disability.* London, UK: Edward Arnold.

Crystal, D. (1987a). Towards a "bucket" theory of language disability: Taking account of interaction between linguistic levels. *Child Language Teaching and Therapy, 1*, 7–22.

Crystal, D. (1987b). Meeting the need for case studies. *Child Language Teaching and Therapy, 3*, 305–310.

Culatta, B., Setzer, L. A., & Horn, D. (2005). Meaning-based intervention for a child with speech and language disorders. *Topics in Language Disorders, 25*(4), 388–401.

Cummings, A. E., & Barlow, J. A. (2011). A comparison of word lexicality in the treatment of speech sound disorders. *Clinical Linguistics and Phonetics, 25*(4), 265–286.

Curtin, S. (2010). Young infants encode lexical stress in newly encountered words. *Journal of Experimental Child Psychology, 105*, 376–385.

Czarnik, K. (2010). *Treatment program for childhood apraxia of speech.* East Moline, IL: LinguaSystems.

Dagenais, P. A. (1995). Electropalatography in the treatment of articulation/phonological disorders. *Journal of Communication Disorders, 28*, 303–329.

Dagenais, P. A., Critz-Crosby, P., & Adams, J. B. (1994). Defining and remediating persistent lateral lisps in children using electropalatography: Preliminary findings. *American Journal of Speech-Language Pathology, 3*(3), 67–76.

Dale, P., & Fenson, L. (1996). Lexical development norms for young children. *Behavior Research Methods, Instruments, and Computers, 28*(1), 125–127.

Dale, P. S., & Hayden, D. A. (2013). Treating speech subsystems in childhood apraxia of speech with tactual input: The PROMPT approach. *American Journal of Speech-Language Pathology, 22*(4), 644–661.

Daly, G. H. (1999). *Scissors, glue, and phonological processes, too!* East Moline, IL: LinguaSystems.

Darwin, E. (1803). *The temple of nature.* London, UK: Jones & Co.

Davenport, M., & Hannahs, S. J. (2010). *Introducing phonetics and phonology* (3rd ed.). London, UK: Hodder Education.

Davis, B. (2005). Goal and target selection for developmental speech disorders. In A. G. Kamhi & K. E. Pollock (Eds.), *Phonological disorders in children: Assessment and intervention* (pp. 89–100). Baltimore, MD: Paul. H. Brookes.

Davis, B. L. (2007). Applications of typical acquisition information to understanding of speech impairment. In S. McLeod (Ed.), *The international guide to speech acquisition* (pp. 50–54). Clifton Park, NY: Thomson Delmar Learning.

Davis, B. L., & MacNeilage, P. F. (1995). The articulatory basis of babbling. *Journal of Speech and Hearing Research, 38*(6), 1199–1211.

Davis, B. L., MacNeilage, P. F., Matyear, C. L., & Powell, J. K. (2000). Prosodic correlates of stress in babbling: An acoustical study. *Child Development, 71*, 1258–1270.

Davis, E., Davern, M., Waters, E., Boyd, R., Reddihough, D., Mackinnon, A., & Graham, H. K. (2013). *Cerebral palsy quality of life questionnaire for adolescents (CP QOL-Teen) manual*. Melbourne, Australia: University of Melbourne.

Davis, E., Mackinnon, A., Davern, M., Boyd, R., Bohanna, I., Waters, E., . . . Reddihough, D. (2013). Description and psychometric properties of the CP QOL-Teen: A quality of life questionnaire for adolescents with cerebral palsy. *Research in Developmental Disabilities, 34*(1), 344–352.

Davison, P. M., Razzell, R. E., & Watson, A. C. H. (1990). The role of pharyngoplasty in congenital neurogenic speech disorders. *British Journal of Plastic Surgery, 43*(2), 187–196.

Dawson, J., Stout, C., Eyer, J., Tattersall, P., Foukalsrud, J., & Croley, K. (2005). *Structured Photographic Expressive Language Test – Preschool 2 (SPELT-P2)*. Dekalb, IL: Janelle.

Dawson, J. I., & Tattersall, P. J. (2001). *Structured Photographic Articulation Test II: Featuring Dudsberry (SPAT-D II)*. Austin, TX: Pro-Ed.

de Bree, E., Rispens, J., & Gerrits, E. (2007). Non-word repetition in Dutch children with (a risk of) dyslexia and SLI. *Clinical Linguistics and Phonetics, 21*(11–12), 935–944.

De la Fuenta, M. T. (1985). *The order of acquisition of Spanish consonant phonemes by monolingual Spanish speaking children between the ages of 2.0 and 6.5*. Washington, DC: Georgetown University.

De Lamo White, C., & Jin, L. (2011). Evaluation of speech and language assessment approaches with bilingual children. *International Journal of Language and Communication Disorders, 46*(6), 613–627.

de Marco, S., & Harrell, R. M. (1995). Perception of word junctures by children. *Perceptual and Motor Skills, 80*, 1075–1082.

De Nil, L. F., & Brutten, G. J. (1990). Speech-associated attitudes: Stuttering, voice disordered, articulation disordered, and normal speaking children. *Journal of Fluency Disorders, 15*(2), 127–134.

Dean, E. C., Howell, J., Hill, A., & Waters, D. (1990). *Metaphon resource pack*. Windsor, UK: NFER Nelson.

Dean, E. C., Howell, J., Reid, J., Grieve, R., & Donaldson, M. (1996). Evaluating therapy for child phonological disorder: A group study of Metaphon therapy. In T. W. Powell (Ed.), *Pathologies of speech and language: Contributions of clinical phonetics and linguistics* (pp. 279–285). New Orleans, LA: International Clinical Phonetics and Linguistics Association.

Dean, E. C., Howell, J., Waters, D., & Reid, J. (1995). Metaphon: A metalinguistic approach to the treatment of phonological disorder in children. *Clinical Linguistics and Phonetics, 9*, 1–19.

Deeley, S. (2002). Professional ideology and learning disability: An analysis of internal conflict. *Disability and Society, 17*, 19–33.

Dehaene-Lambertz, G., Dehaene, S., & Hertz-Pannier, L. (2002). Functional neuroimaging of speech perception in infants. *Science, 298*(5600), 2013–2015.

Dehaene-Lambertz, G., & Gliga, T. (2004). Common neural basis for phoneme processing in infants and adults. *Journal of Cognitive Neuroscience, 16*(8), 1375–1387.

Department for Children, Schools and Families (2008). *Every child a talker*. Retrieved from http://www.foundationyears.org.uk/2011/10/every-child-a-talker-guidance-for-early-language-lead-practitioners/.

Desai, S. S. (1997). Down syndrome: A review of the literature. *Oral Surgery, Oral Medicine, Oral Pathology, Oral Radiology, and Endodontics, 84*(3), 279–285.

DeThorne, L. S., Johnson, C. J., Walder, L., & Mahurin-Smith, J. (2009). When "Simon says" doesn't work: Alternatives to imitation for facilitating early speech development. *American Journal of Speech-Language Pathology, 18*, 133–145.

Dinnsen, D. A., Barlow, J. A., & Morrisette, M. L. (1997). Long-distance place assimilation with an interacting error pattern in phonological acquisition. *Clinical Linguistics and Phonetics, 11*, 319–338.

Dinnsen, D. A., Chin, S. B., Elbert, M., & Powell, T. W. (1990). Some constraints on functionally disordered phonologies: Phonetic inventories and phonotactics. *Journal of Speech and Hearing Research, 33*, 28–37.

Dinnsen, D. A., & Elbert, M. A. (1984). On the relationship between phonology and learning. In M. Elbert, D. A. Dinnsen, & G. Weismer (Eds.), *Phonological theory and the misarticulating child* (pp. 59–68). Rockville Pike, MD: American Speech-Language-Hearing Association.

Dinnsen, D. A., & Gierut, J. A. (Eds.). (2008). *Optimality theory, phonological acquisition and disorders*. London, UK: Equinox Publishing.

Dispaldro, M., Leonard, L. B., & Deevy, P. (2013). Real-word and non-word repetition in Italian-speaking children with specific language impairment: A study of diagnostic accuracy. *Journal of Speech, Language, and Hearing Research, 56*(1), 323–336.

Dobinson, C., & Wren, Y. (Eds.). (2013). *Creating practice-based evidence: A guide for SLTs*. London, UK: J&R Press.

Dockrell, J., Lindsay, G., Roulstone, S., & Law, J. (2014). Supporting children with speech, language and communication needs: An overview of the results of the Better Communication Research Programme. *International Journal of Language and Communication Disorders, 49*(5), 543–557.

Dodd, B. (Ed.). (1995a). *Differential diagnosis and treatment of young children with speech disorder*. London, UK: Whurr.

Dodd, B. (1995b). Children's acquisition of phonology. In B. Dodd (Ed.), *Differential diagnosis and treatment of speech disordered children* (pp. 21–48). London, UK: Whurr.

Dodd, B. (2005). *Differential diagnosis and treatment of speech disordered children* (2nd ed.). London, UK: Whurr.

Dodd, B. (2013). *Differential diagnosis and treatment of speech disordered children* (3rd ed.). Hoboken, NJ: Wiley.

Dodd, B. (2014). Differential diagnosis of pediatric speech sound disorder. *Current Developmental Disorders Reports, 1*(3), 189–196.

Dodd, B., & Bradford, A. (2000). A comparison of three therapy methods for children with different types of developmental phonological disorder. *International Journal of Language and Communication Disorders, 35*(2), 189–209.

Dodd, B., & Carr, A. (2003). Young children's letter-sound knowledge. *Language, Speech, and Hearing Services in Schools, 34*(2), 128–137.

Dodd, B., Crosbie, S., McIntosh, B., Holm, A., Harvey, C., Liddy, M., . . . Rigby, H. (2008). The impact of selecting different contrasts in phonological therapy. *International Journal of Speech-Language Pathology, 10*(5), 334–345.

Dodd, B., Crosbie, S., McIntosh, B., Teitzel, T., & Ozanne, A. (2000). *PIPA: Preschool and Primary Inventory of Phonological Awareness*. London, UK: Psychological Corporation.

Dodd, B., Crosbie, S., McIntosh, B., Teitzel, T., & Ozanne, A. (2003). *Pre-Reading Inventory of Phonological Awareness* (PIPA). San Antonio, TX: Harcourt Assessment.

Dodd, B., & Gillon, G. (2001). Exploring the relationship between phonological awareness, speech impairment and literacy. *International Journal of Speech-Language Pathology, 3*, 139–147.

Dodd, B., Holm, A., Crosbie, S., & McIntosh, B. (2006). A core vocabulary approach for management of inconsistent speech disorder. *International Journal of Speech-Language Pathology, 8*(3), 220–230.

Dodd, B., Holm, A., Crosbie, S., & McIntosh, B. (2010). Core vocabulary intervention. In A. L. Williams, S. McLeod, & R. J. McCauley (Eds.), *Interventions for speech sound disorders in children* (pp. 117–136). Baltimore, MD: Paul H. Brookes.

Dodd, B., Holm, A., Hua, Z., & Crosbie, S. (2003). Phonological development: A normative study of British English-speaking children. *Clinical Linguistics and Phonetics, 17*(8), 617–643.

Dodd, B., Hua, Z., Crosbie, S., Holm, A., & Ozanne, A. (2002). *Diagnostic Evaluation of Articulation and Phonology* (DEAP). London, UK: Psychological Cooporation.

Dodd, B., Hua, Z., Crosbie, S., Holm, A., & Ozanne, A. (2006). *Diagnostic Evaluation of Articulation and Phonology* (DEAP, US Edition). San Antonio, TX: Harcourt Assessment.

Dodd, B., & Iacano, T. (1989). Phonological disorders in children: Changes in phonological process use during treatment. *British Journal of Disorders of Communication, 24*, 333–351.

Dodd, B., & McIntosh, B. (2008). The input processing, cognitive linguistic and oro-motor skills of children with speech difficulty. *International Journal of Speech-Language Pathology, 10*(3), 169–178.

Dodd, B., Oerlemans, M., MacCormack, M., & Holm, A. (1996). *The Queensland University Inventory of Literacy*. Brisbane, Australia: University of Queensland.

D'Odorico, L., Majorano, M., Fasolo, M., Salerni, N., & Suttora, C. (2011). Characteristics of phonological development as a risk factor for language development in Italian-speaking pre-term children: A longitudinal study. *Clinical Linguistics and Phonetics, 25*(1), 53–65.

Doidge, N. (2010). *The brain that changes itself* (Revised ed.). Carlton North, Australia: Scribe Publications.

Dollaghan, C. A. (2007). *The handbook for evidence-based practice in communication disorders*. Baltimore, MD: Paul H. Brookes.

Dollaghan, C., & Campbell, T. F. (1998). Nonword repetition and child language impairment. *Journal of Speech, Language, and Hearing Research, 41*, 1136–1146.

Dollaghan, C. A., Campbell, T. F., Paradise, J. L., Feldman, H. M., Janosky, J. E., Pitcairn, D. N., & Kurs-Lasky, M. (1999). Maternal education and measures of early speech and language. *Journal of Speech, Language, and Hearing Research, 42*, 1432–1443.

Domjan, M. (2015). *The principles of learning and behaviour* (7th ed.). Stamford, CT: Cengage Learning.

Donegan, P. (2002). Normal vowel development. In M. J. Ball, & F. E. Gibbon (Eds.), *Vowel disorders* (pp. 1–35). Woburn, MA: Butterworth-Heinemann.

Donicht, G., Pagliarin, K. C., Mota, H. B., & Keske-Soares, M. (2011). The treatment with rothics and generalization obtained in two models of phonological therapy. *Jornal da Sociedade Brasileira de Fonoaudiologia, 23*(1), 71–76.

Dowden, P. (1997). Augmentative and alternative communication decision making for children with severely unintelligible speech. *Augmentative and Alternative Communication, 13*(1), 48–59.

Drane, D. (1996). The effect of use of dummies and teats on orofacial development. *Breastfeeding Review, 4*, 59–64.

DuBois, E., & Bernthal, J. (1978). A comparison of three methods for obtaining articulatory responses. *Journal of Speech and Hearing Disorders, 43*, 295–305.

Duchan, J. F. (2001). Impairment and social views of speech-language pathology: Clinical practices re-examined. *International Journal of Speech-Language Pathology, 3*(1), 37–45.

Duchan, J. F. (2010). The early years of language, speech, and hearing services in U.S. schools. *Language, Speech, and Hearing Services in Schools, 41*(2), 152–160.

Duckworth, M., Allen, G., Hardcastle, W., & Ball, M. (1990). Extensions to the International Phonetic Alphabet for the transcription of atypical speech. *Clinical Linguistics and Phonetics, 4*, 273–280.

Duffy, J. R. (2013). *Motor speech disorders: Substrates, differential diagnosis, and management* (3rd ed.). St. Louis, MO: Elsevier.

Dunn, A. L., & Fox Tree, J. E. (2009). A quick, gradient Bilingual Dominance Scale. *Bilingualism: Language and Cognition, 12*(03), 273–289.

Dunn, L. M., & Dunn, D. M. (2007). *The Peabody Picture Vocabulary Test: Fourth Edition (PPVT-4)*. Bloomington, MN: NCS Pearson.

Dunst, C. J. (2002). Family-centred practices: Birth through high school. *The Journal of Special Education, 36*(3), 139–147.

Dworzynski, K., & Howell, P. (2004). Predicting stuttering from phonetic complexity in German. *Journal of Fluency Disorders, 29*(2), 149–173.

Dyer, J. A. (2003). Multidisciplinary, interdisciplinary, and transdisciplinary educational models and nursing education. *Nursing Education Perspectives, 24*(4), 186–188.

Dyson, A. T. (1988). Phonetic inventories of 2- and 3- year old children. *Journal of Speech and Hearing Disorders, 53*, 89–93.

Dyson, A. T., & Amayreh, M. M. (2007). Jordanian Arabic speech acquisition In S. McLeod (Ed.), *The international guide to speech acquisition* (pp. 288–299). Clifton Park, NY: Thomson Delmar Learning.

Dyson, A. T., & Paden, E. P. (1983). Some phonological acquisition strategies used by two-year olds. *Journal of Childhood Communication Disorders, 7*, 6–18.

Dyson, A. T., & Robinson, T. W. (1987). The effect of phonological analysis procedure on the selection of potential remediation targets. *Language, Speech, and Hearing Services in Schools, 18*, 364–377.

Eadie, P., Morgan, A., Ukoumunne, O. C., Ttofari Eecen, K., Wake, M., & Reilly, S. (2015). Speech sound disorder at 4 years: Prevalence, comorbidities, and predictors in a community cohort of children. *Developmental Medicine and Child Neurology, 57*(6), 578–584.

Ebert, K. A., & Prelock, P. A. (1994). Teachers' perceptions of their students with communication disorders. *Language, Speech, and Hearing Services in Schools, 25*(4), 211–214.

Ebert, K. D., Kalanek, J., Cordero, K. N., & Kohnert, K. (2008). Spanish nonword repetition: Stimuli development and preliminary results. *Communication Disorders Quarterly, 29*, 69–74.

Edeal, D. M., & Gildersleeve-Neumann, C. E. (2011). The importance of production frequency in therapy for childhood apraxia of speech. *American Journal of Speech-Language Pathology, 20*(2), 95–110.

Edelman, G. (1987). *Neural Darwinism: The theory of neuronal group selection*. New York, NY: Basic Books.

Edwards, J., & Beckman, M. E. (2008a). Some cross-linguistic evidence for modulation of implicational universals by language-specific frequency effects in phonological development. *Language Learning and Development, 4*(2), 122–156.

Edwards, J., & Beckman, M. E. (2008b). Methodological questions in studying consonant acquisition. *Clinical Linguistics and Phonetics, 22*(12), 937–956.

Edwards, J., Fourakis, M., Beckman, M. E., & Fox, R. A. (1999). Characterizing knowledge deficits in phonological disorders. *Journal of Speech, Language, and Hearing Research, 42*(1), 169–186.

Edwards, J., Munson, B., & Beckman, M. E. (2011). Lexicon-phonology relationships and dynamics of early language development. *Journal of Child Language, 38*, 35–40.

Edwards, M. L., & Shriberg, L. D. (1983). *Phonology: Applications in communicative disorders*. San Diego, CA: College-Hill.

Ehrler, D. J., & McGhee, R. L. (2008). *Primary Test of Nonverbal Intelligence (PTONI)*. Austin, TX: Pro-Ed.

Eimas, P. D., Siqueland, E. R., Jusczyk, P. W., & Vigorito, J. (1971). Speech perception in infants. *Science, 171*, 303–306.

Eisenberg, S. L., & Hitchcock, E. R. (2010). Using standardized tests to inventory consonant and vowel production: A comparison of 11 tests of articulation and phonology. *Language, Speech, and Hearing Services in Schools, 41*(4), 488–503.

Eiserman, W. D., McCoun, M., & Escobar, C. M. (1990). A cost-effectiveness analysis of two alternative program models for serving speech-disordered preschoolers. *Journal of Early Intervention, 14*(4), 297–317.

Elbers, L., & Ton, J. (1985). Play pen monologues: The interplay of words and babbles in the first words period. *Journal of Child Language, 12*, 551–565.

Elbert, M. (1989). Generalisation in treatment of phonological disorders. In L. McReynolds & J. Spradlin (Eds.), *Generalisation strategies in the treatment of communication disorders* (pp. 31–43). Toronto, Canada: B. C. Decker.

Elbert, M., Dinnsen, D. A., Swartzlander, P., & Chin, S. B. (1990). Generalization to conversational speech. *Journal of Speech and Hearing Research, 55*, 694–699.

Elbert, M., Dinnsen, D., & Powell, T. (1984). On the prediction of phonological generalization learning pattern. *Journal of Speech and Hearing Disorders, 49*, 309–317.

Elbert, M., & Gierut, J. A. (1986). *Handbook of clinical phonology: Approaches to assessment and treatment*. San Diego, CA: College-Hill Press.

Elbert, M., & McReynolds, L. (1975). Transfer of /r/ across contexts. *Journal of Speech and Hearing Disorders, 40*, 380–387.

Elbert, M., & McReynolds, L. V. (1979). Aspects of phonological acquisition during articulation training. *Journal of Speech and Hearing Disorders, 64*, 459–471.

Elbert, M., Powell, T. W., & Swartzlander, P. (1991). Toward a technology of generalisation: How many exemplars are sufficient? *Journal of Speech and Hearing Research, 34*, 81–87.

Elbert, M., Rockman, B., & Saltzman, D. (1980). *Contrasts: The use of minimal pairs in articulation training*. Austin, TX: Exceptional Resources.

Elbro, C., Borstrøm, I., & Petersen, D. K. (1998). Predicting dyslexia from kindergarten: The importance of distinctness of phonological representations of lexical items. *Reading Research Quarterly, 33*(1), 36–60.

Eliasson, A.-C., Krumlinde-Sundholm, L., Rösblad, B., Beckung, E., Arner, M., Öhrvall, A.-M., & Rosenbaum, P. (2006). The Manual Ability Classification System (MACS) for children with cerebral palsy: Scale development and evidence of validity and reliability. *Developmental Medicine and Child Neurology, 48*(07), 549–554.

Ellis, C. M., & Hodson, B. W. (2013). Treatment design and implementation. In B. Peter & A. A. N. MacLeod (Eds.), *Comprehensive perspectives on speech sound development and disorders: Pathways from linguistic theory to clinical practice* (pp. 519–557). New York, NY: Nova Publishers.

Emond, A., Ingram, J., Johnson, D., Blair, P., Whitelaw, A., Copeland, M., & Sutcliffe, A. (2014). Randomised controlled trial of early frenotomy in breastfed infants with mild–moderate tongue-tie. *Archives of Disease in Childhood—Fetal and Neonatal Edition, 99*(3), F189–F195.

Enderby, P. (2014). Use of the extended therapy outcome measure for children with dysarthria. *International Journal of Speech-Language Pathology, 16*(4), 436–444.

Enderby, P., & John, A. (1997). *Therapy outcome measures: Speech-language pathology technical manual*. London, UK: Singular.

Enderby, P., & John, A. (2015). *Therapy outcome measures for rehabilitation professionals* (3rd ed.). London, UK: J&R Press.

Engel, D. C., & Groth, L. R. (1976). Case studies of the effect on carry-over of reinforcing postarticulation responses based on feedback. *Language, Speech, and Hearing Services in Schools, 7*(2), 93–101.

Engel, G. L. (1977). The need for a new medical model: A challenge for biomedicine. *Science, 196*, 129–136.

Ertmer, D. J. (2011). Assessing speech intelligibility in children with hearing loss: Toward revitalizing a valuable clinical tool. *Language, Speech, and Hearing Services in Schools, 42*(1), 52–58.

Ertmer, D. J., & Ertmer, P. A. (1998). Constructivist strategies in phonological intervention facilitating self-regulation for carryover. *Language, Speech, and Hearing Services in Schools, 29*(2), 67–75. (Chapter 12 list, page 432: Used by permission from American Speech-Language-Hearing Association [ASHA].)

Evans, C., Connell, J., Barkham, M., Marshall, C., & Mellor-Clark, J. (2003). Practice-based evidence: benchmarking NHS primary care counseling services at national and local levels. *Clinical Psychology and Psychotherapy, 10*(6), 374–388.

Fabiano-Smith, L., & Goldstein, B. A. (2010a). Phonological acquisition in bilingual Spanish-English speaking children. *Journal of Speech, Language, and Hearing Research, 53*(1), 160–178.

Fabiano-Smith, L., & Goldstein, B. A. (2010b). Early-, middle-, and late-developing sounds in monolingual and bilingual children: An exploratory investigation. *American Journal of Speech-Language Pathology, 19*(1), 66–77.

Faircloth, M., & Faircloth, S. (1970). An analysis of the articulatory behaviour of a speech defective child in connected speech and in isolated word responses. *Journal of Speech and Hearing Disorders, 35*, 51–61.

Falconer, E. K., Geffen, G. M., Olsen, S. L., & McFarland, K. (2006). The rapid screen of concussion: An evaluation of the non-word repetition test for use in mTBI research. *Brain Injury, 20*(12), 1251–1263.

Fawcett, S., Bacsfalvi, P., & Bernhardt, B. M. (2008). Ultrasound as visual feedback in speech therapy for /r/ with adults with Down syndrome. *Down Syndrome Quarterly, 10*, 4–12.

Fehrenbach, M. J., & Herring, S. W. (2007). *Anatomy of the head and neck*. St. Louis, MO: Saunders Elsevier.

Fekkes, M., Theunissen, N. C., Brugman, E., Veen, S., Verrips, E. G., Koopman, H. M., . . . Verloove-Vanhorick, S. P. (2000). Development and psychometric evaluation of the TAPQOL: A health-related quality of life instrument for 1-5-year-old children. *Quality of Life Research, 9*(8), 961–972.

Felsenfeld, S., Broen, P. A., & McGue, M. (1992). A 28-year follow-up of adults with a history of moderate phonological disorder: Linguistic and personality results. *Journal of Speech and Hearing Research, 35*(5), 1114–1125.

Felsenfeld, S., Broen, P. A., & McGue, M. (1994). A 28-year follow up of adults with a history of moderate phonological disorder: Educational and occupational results. *Journal of Speech and Hearing Research, 37*, 1341–1353.

Felsenfeld, S., McGue, M., & Broen, P. A. (1995). Familial aggregation of phonological disorders: Results from a 28-year follow-up. *Journal of Speech and Hearing Research, 38*(5), 1091–1107.

Felsenfeld, S., & Plomin, R. (1997). Epidemiological and offspring analysis of developmental speech disorders using data from the Colorado Adoption Project. *Journal of Speech, Language, and Hearing Research, 40*, 778–791.

Fernando, C. (2000). The commonly ignored side effects of tongue tie. *ACQuiring Knowledge in Speech, Language and Hearing, 2*(2), 62–64.

Fey, M. E. (1986). *Language intervention with young children*. Boston, MA: College-Hill Press.

Fey, M. E., & Finestack, L. H. (2009). Research and development in child language intervention: A 5-phase model. In R. G. Schwartz (Ed.), *Handbook of child language disorders* (pp. 513–529). New York, NY: Psychology Press.

Fish, M. (2011). *Here's how to treat childhood apraxia of speech*. San Diego, CA: Plural Publishing.

Fisher, H. B., & Logemann, J. A. (1971). *Fisher-Logemann Test of Articulation Competence*. Chicago, IL: The Riverside Publishing Company.

Fitts, P. M. (1964). Perceptual-motor skills learning. In A. W. Melton (Ed.), *Categories of human learning* (pp. 254–285). New York, NY: Academic Press.

Fitzsimons, D. A., Jones, D. L., Barton, B., & North, K. N. (2012). A procedure for the computerized analysis of cleft palate speech transcription. *Clinical Linguistics and Phonetics, 26*(1), 18–38.

Flahive, L. K., & Lanza, J. R. (1998). *Just for kids: Phonological processing*. East Moline, IL: LinguaSystems.

Flasher, L. V., & Fogle, P. T. (2012). *Counseling skills for speech-language pathologists and audiologists* (2nd ed.). Clifton Park, NY: Delmar Cengage Learning.

Fleming, P. S., & Flood, T. R. (2005). Bifid tongue: A complication of tongue piercing. *British Dental Journal, 198*(5), 265–266.

Fletcher, S. G., McCutcheon, M. J., & Wolf, M. B. (1975). Dynamic palatometry. *Journal of Speech and Hearing Research, 18*, 812–819.

Flipsen, P., Jr. (1995). Speaker-listener familiarity: Parents as judges of delayed speech intelligibility. *Journal of Communication Disorders, 28*, 3–19.

Flipsen, P., Jr. (2006a). Syllables per word in typical and delayed speech acquisition. *Clinical Linguistics and Phonetics, 20*(4), 293–301.

Flipsen, P., Jr. (2006b). Measuring the intelligibility of conversational speech in children. *Clinical Linguistics and Phonetics, 20*(4), 303–312.

Flipsen, P., Jr., & Ogiela, D. A. (2015). Psychometric characteristics of single-word tests of children's speech sound production. *Language, Speech, and Hearing Services in Schools, 46*(2), 166–178.

Fluharty, N. B. (2001). *Fluharty Preschool Speech and Language Screen Test: Second Edition* (Fluharty-2). Austin, TX: Pro-Ed.

Forrest, K. (2002). Are oral-motor exercises useful in the treatment of phonological/articulatory disorders? *Seminars in Speech and Language, 23*(1), 14–25.

Forrest, K., & Iuzzini, J. (2008). A comparison of oral motor and production training for children with speech sound disorders. *Seminars in Speech and Language, 29*, 304–311.

Foss, M., Whitehead, B., Paterson, M., & Whitehead, R. (1990). Ultrasound as a visual feedback aid for the hearing-impaired. *Journal of Diagnostic Medical Sonography, 6*, 80–86.

Foster, B., & Gold, H. (2002). *The giant book of phonology*. Greenville, SC: SuperDuper Publications.

Foulkes, P., & Docherty, G. (2000). Another chapter in the story of /r/: "Labiodental" variants in British English. *Journal of Sociolinguistics, 4*, 30–59.

Fox, A. V. (2007). German speech acquisition. In S. McLeod (Ed.), *The international guide to speech acquisition* (pp. 386–397). Clifton Park, NY: Thomson Delmar Learning.

Fox, A. V., & Dodd, B. J. (1999). Der Erwerb des phonologischen Systems in der deutschen Sprache. *Sprache-Stimme-Gehör, 23*, 183–191.

Fox, A. V., Dodd, B., & Howard, D. (2002). Risk factors for speech disorders in children. *International Journal of Language and Communication Disorders, 37*, 117–132.

Fox, C. M., & Boliek, C. A. (2012). Intensive voice treatment (LSVT LOUD) for children with spastic cerebral palsy and dysarthria. *Journal of Speech, Language, and Hearing Research, 55*(3), 930–945.

Fox, C. M., Boliek, C., Namdaran, N., Nickerson, C., Gardner, B., Piccott, C., . . . Archibald, E. (2008). Intensive voice treatment (LSVT LOUD) for children with spastic cerebral palsy. *Movement Disorders, 23*(Suppl. 1), s378.

Foy, J. G., & Mann, V. A. (2012). Speech production deficits in early readers: Predictors of risk. *Reading and Writing: An Interdisciplinary Journal, 25*(4), 799–830.

Frederick, M. (2005). *Webber Spanish phonology cards*. Greenville, SC: Super Duper Publications.

Freeman, G. G., & Sonnega, J. A. (1956). Peer evaluation of children in speech correction class. *Journal of Speech and Hearing Disorders, 21*(2), 179–182.

French, A. (1989). The systematic acquisition of word forms by a child during the first fifty word stage. *Journal of Child Language, 16,* 69–90.

Friberg, J. C. (2010). Considerations for test selection: How do validity and reliability impact diagnostic decisions? *Child Language Teaching and Therapy, 26*(1), 77–92.

Friel, S. (1998). When is a /k/ not a [k]? EPG as a diagnostic and therapeutic tool for abnormal velar stops. *International Journal of Language and Communication Disorders, 33*(suppl), 439–444.

Froeschels, E. (1952). *Dysarthric speech*. Magnolia, MA: Expression.

Fromkin, V., Rodman, R., & Hyams, N. (2013). *An introduction to language* (10th ed.). Boston, MA: Wadsworth.

Fromkin, V., Rodman, R., Hyams, N., Collins, P., Amberber, M., & Cox, F. (2012). *An introduction to language: Australia and New Zealand* (7th ed.). South Melbourne, Australia: Cengage Learning Australia.

Fuchs, L. S., & Fuchs , D. F. (2007). A model for implementing responsiveness to intervention. *Council for Exceptional Children, 39,* 14–20.

Fudala, J. B. (2000). *Arizona Articulation Proficiency Scale-Third Edition* (*Arizona-3*). Los Angeles, CA: Western Psychological Services.

Fujiwara, Y. (2007). Electropalatography home training using a portable training unit for Japanese children with cleft palate. *International Journal of Speech-Language Pathology, 9*(1), 65–72.

Fulcher, A., Baker, E., Purcell, A., & Munro, N. (2014). Typical consonant cluster acquisition in auditory-verbal children with early-identified severe/profound hearing loss. *International Journal of Speech-Language Pathology, 16*(1), 69–81.

Fulcher, A. N., Purcell, A., Baker, E., & Munro, N. (2015). Factors influencing speech and language outcomes of children with early identified severe/profound hearing loss: Clinician-identified facilitators and barriers. *International Journal of Speech-Language Pathology, 17*(3), 325–333.

Fulcher, A., Purcell, A. A., Baker, E., & Munro, N. (2012). Listen up: Children with early identified hearing loss achieve age-appropriate speech/language outcomes by 3 years-of-age. *International Journal of Pediatric Otorhinolaryngology, 76,* 1785–1794.

Fuller, D. R., Pimentel, J. T., & Peregoy, B. M. (2012). *Applied anatomy and physiology for speech-language pathology and audiology*. Baltimore, MD: Lippincott Williams & Wilkins.

Galantucci, B., Fowler, C., & Turvey, M. T. (2006). The motor theory of speech perception reviewed. *Psychonomic Bulletin and Review, 13*(3), 361–377.

Gallagher, T. M. (1977). Revision behaviours in the speech of normal children developing language. *Journal of Speech and Hearing Research, 20,* 303–318.

Galloway, J. H. F., & Blue, C. M. (1975). Paraprofessional personnel in articulation therapy. *Language, Speech, and Hearing Services in Schools, 6*(3), 125–130.

Ganong, W. F. (1980). Phonetic categorization in auditory perception. *Journal of Experimental Psychology and Human Performance, 6,* 110–125.

Gardner, H. (1989). An investigation of maternal interaction with phonologically disordered children as compared to two groups of normally developing children. *British Journal of Disorders of Communication, 24,* 41–59.

Garn-Nunn, P. G., & Lynn, J. M. (2004). *Calvert's descriptive phonetics* (3rd ed.). New York, NY: Theime.

Garner, H. (1995). *Teamwork models and experience in education*. Boston, MA: Allyn & Bacon.

Gathercole, S., & Baddeley, A. (1996). *Children's Test of Nonword Repetition (CNRep)*. London, UK: Psychological Corporation.

Gibbon, F. E. (1999). Undifferentiated lingual gestures in children with articulation/phonological disorders. *Journal of Speech, Language, and Hearing Research, 42,* 382–397.

Gibbon, F. E. (2003). Using articulatory data to inform speech pathology theory and clinical practice. *Proceedings of the 15th International Congress of Phonetic Sciences* (pp. 261–264). Barcelona, Spain: Causal Productions.

Gibbon, F., Dent, H., & Hardcastle, W. (1993). Diagnosis and therapy of abnormal alveolar stops in a speech-disordered child using EPG. *Clinical Linguistics and Phonetics, 7,* 247–268.

Gibbon, F., & Hardcastle, W. (1987). Articulatory description and treatment of "lateral /s/" using electropalatography: A case study. *British Journal of Disorders of Communication, 22,* 203–217.

Gibbon, F. E., & Smyth, H. (2013). Preschool children's performance on Profiling Elements of Prosody in Speech-Communication (PEPS-C). *Clinical Linguistics and Phonetics, 27*(6–7), 428–434.

Gibbon, F. E., & Wood, S. E. (2003). Using electropalatography (EPG) to diagnose and treat articulation disorders associated with mild cerebral palsy: A case study. *Clinical Linguistics and Phonetics, 17,* 365–374.

Gibbon, F., & Wood, S. (2010). Visual feedback therapy with electropalatography. In A. L. Williams, S. McLeod & R. J. McCauley (Eds.), *Interventions for speech sound disorders in children* (pp. 509–536). Baltimore, MD: Paul H. Brookes.

Gierut, J. A. (1985). *On the relationship between phonological knowledge and generalization learning in misarticulating children*. Unpublished doctoral dissertation, Indiana University, Bloomington, IL.

Gierut, J. A. (1989). Maximal opposition approach to phonological treatment. *Journal of Speech and Hearing Disorders, 54,* 9–19.

Gierut, J. A. (1990). Differential learning of phonological oppositions. *Journal of Speech and Hearing Research, 33,* 540–549.

Gierut, J. A. (1991). Homonymy in phonological change. *Clinical Linguistics and Phonetics, 5,* 119–137.

Gierut, J. A. (1992). The conditions and course of clinically induced phonological change. *Journal of Speech and Hearing Research, 35,* 1049–1063.

Gierut, J. A. (1998). Natural domains of cyclicity in phonological acquisition. *Clinical Linguisitic and Phonetics, 12*(6), 481–499.

Gierut, J. A. (1999). Syllable onsets: Clusters and adjuncts in acquisition. *Journal of Speech, Language, and Hearing Research, 42,* 708–726.

Gierut, J. (2001). Complexity in phonological treatment: Clinical factors. *Language, Speech, and Hearing Services in Schools, 32,* 229–241.

Gierut, J. (2005). Phonological intervention: The how or the what? In A. G. Kamhi & K. E. Pollock (Eds.), *Phonological disorders in children: Clinical decision making in assessment and intervention* (pp. 201–210). Baltimore, MD: Paul H. Brookes.

Gierut, J. (2007). Phonological complexity and language learnability. *American Journal of Speech-Language Pathology, 16*(1), 6–17.

Gierut, J. A. (2008). Fundamentals of experimental design and treatment. In D. A. Dinnsen & J. A. Gierut (Eds.), *Optimality theory, phonological acquisition and disorders* (pp. 93–118). London, UK: Equinox.

Gierut, J. A., & Champion, A. H. (2000). Ingressive substitutions: Typical or atypical phonological pattern? *Clinical Linguistics and Phonetics, 14*(8), 603–617.

Gierut, J. A., & Champion, A. H. (2001). Syllable onsets II: Three-element clusters in phonological treatment. *Journal of Speech, Language, and Hearing Research, 44,* 886–904.

Gierut, J., Elbert, M., & Dinnsen, D. (1987). A functional analysis of phonological knowledge and generalization learning in misarticulating children. *Journal of Speech and Hearing Research, 30,* 462–479.

Gierut, J. A., & Hulse, L. E. (2010). Evidence-based practice: A matrix for predicting phonological generalization. *Clinical Linguistics and Phonetics, 24*(4–5), 323–334.

Gierut, J. A., & Morrisette, M. L. (2005). The clinical significance of optimality theory for phonological disorders. *Topics in Language Disorders, 25*(3), 266–280.

Gierut, J. A., & Morrisette, M. L. (2010). Phonological learning and lexicality of treated stimuli. *Clinical Linguistics and Phonetics, 24*(2), 122–140.

Gierut, J. A., & Morrisette, M. L. (2012a). Age of word acquisition effects in treatment of children with phonological delays. *Applied Psycholinguistics, 33*(1), 121–144.

Gierut, J. A., & Morrisette, M. L. (2012b). Density, frequency and the expressive phonology of children with phonological delay. *Journal of Child Language, 39*(04), 804–834.

Gierut, J. A., Morrisette, M. L., & Champion, A. H. (1999). Lexical constraints in phonological acquisition. *Journal of Child Language, 26,* 261–294.

Gierut, J. A., Morrisette, M. L., Hughes, M. T., & Rowland, S. (1996). Phonological treatment efficacy and developmental norms. *Language, Speech, and Hearing Services in Schools, 27,* 215–230.

Gierut, J. A., Morrisette, M. L., & Ziemer, S. M. (2010). Nonwords and generalization in children with phonological disorders. *American Journal of Speech-Language Pathology, 19*(2), 167–177.

Gierut, J. A., & Neumann, H. J. (1992). Teaching and learning /t/: A non-confound. *Clinical Linguistics and Phonetics, 6*(3), 191–200.

Gierut, J. A., & O'Connor, K. M. (2002). Precursors to onset clusters in acquisition. *Journal of Child Language, 29,* 495–517.

Gierut, J. A., Simmerman, C. L., & Neumann, H. J. (1994). Phonemic structures of delayed phonological systems. *Journal of Child Language, 21,* 291–316.

Gildersleeve-Neumann, C., & Goldstein, B. (2012). Intervention for multilingual children with speech sound disorder. In S. McLeod & B. Goldstein (Eds.), *Multilingual aspects of speech sound disorder in children* (pp. 214–227). Clevedon, UK: Multilingual Matters.

Gildersleeve-Neumann, C., & Goldstein, B. A. (2015). Cross-linguistic generalization in the treatment of two sequential Spanish–English bilingual children with speech sound disorders. *International Journal of Speech-Language Pathology, 17*(1), 26–40.

Gillam, S. L., & Gillam, R. B. (2006). Making evidence-based decisions about child language intervention in schools. *Language, Speech, and Hearing Services in Schools, 37*(4), 304–315.

Gillham, B. (2000). *Early literacy test.* London, UK: Hodder & Stoughton.

Gillon, G. (2000). The efficacy of phonological awareness intervention for children with spoken language impairments. *Language, Speech, and Hearing Services in Schools, 31,* 26–41.

Gillon, G. (2004). *Phonological awareness: From research to practice.* New York, NY: Guildford Press.

Gillon, G. T. (2005). Facilitating phoneme awareness development in 3- and 4-year-old children with speech impairment. *Language, Speech, and Hearing Services in Schools, 36,* 308–324.

Gillon, G., & McNeill, B. (2007). *An integrated phonological awareness programme for preschool children with speech disorder.* Unpublished manuscript. Christchurch, New Zealand: University of Canterbury.

Gillon, G. T., & Moriarty, B. (2007). Childhood apraxia of speech: Children at risk for persistent reading and spelling disorder. *Seminars in Speech and Language, 28*(1), 48–57.

Gillon, G. T., & Schwarz, I. E. (2001). Screening New Zealand children's spoken language skills for academic success. In L. Wilson & S. Hewat (Eds.), *Proceedings of the 2001 Speech Pathology Australia National Conference* (pp. 207–214). Melbourne: Speech Pathology Australia.

Gimson, A. C., & Cruttenden, A. (1994). *Gimson's pronunciation of English* (5th ed.). London, UK: Arnold.

Girolametto, L., Pearse, P., & Weitzman, E. (1997). Effects of lexical intervention on the phonology of late talkers. *Journal of Speech, Language, and Hearing Research, 40,* 338–348.

Glascoe, F. P. (2000). *Parents' Evaluation of Developmental Status: Authorized Australian Version.* Parkville, Victoria: Centre for Community Child Health.

Glaspey, A. M., & MacLeod, A. A. N. (2010). A multi-dimensional approach to gradient change in phonological acquisition: A case study of disordered speech development. *Clinical Linguistics and Phonetics, 24*(4–5), 283–299.

Glaspey, A., & Stoel-Gammon, C. (2005). Dynamic assessment in phonological disorders: The Scaffolding Scale of Stimulability. *Topics in Language Disorders, 25*(3), 220–230.

Glaspey, A., & Stoel-Gammon, C. (2007). A dynamic approach to phonological assessment. *International Journal of Speech-Language Pathology, 9*(4), 286–296.

Glogowska, M., Roulstone, S., Enderby, P., & Peters, T. J. (2000). Randomised controlled trial of community based speech and language therapy in preschool children. *British Medical Journal, 321,* 1–5.

Goldberg, L. R. (2015). The importance of interprofessional education for students in communication sciences and disorders. *Communication Disorders Quarterly, 36*(2), 121–125.

Goldman, R., & Fristoe, M. (2000). *Goldman-Fristoe Test of Articulation-2 (GFTA-2).* Circle Pines, MN: American Guidance Service.

Goldstein, B. (2007). Spanish-influenced English speech acquisition. In S. McLeod (Ed.), *The international guide to speech acquisition* (pp. 277–287). Clifton Park, NY: Thomson Delmar Learning.

Goldstein, B. A. (2007). Spanish speech acquisition. In S. McLeod (Ed.), *The international guide to speech acquisition* (pp. 539–553). Clifton Park, NY: Thomson Delmar Learning.

Goldstein, B. A., & Bunta, F. (2012). Positive and negative transfer in the phonological systems of bilingual speakers. *International Journal of Bilingualism, 16*(4), 388–401.

Goldstein, B. A., Bunta, F., Lange, J., Rodriguez, J., & Burrows, L. (2010). The effects of measures of language experience and language ability on segmental accuracy in bilingual children. *American Journal of Speech-Language Pathology, 19*(3), 238–247.

Goldstein, B., & Cintrón, P. (2001). An investigation of phonological skills in Puerto Rican Spanish-speaking 2-year-olds. *Clinical Linguistics and Phonetics, 15,* 343–361.

Goldstein, B. A., Fabiano, L., & Iglesias, A. (2004). Spontaneous and imitated productions in Spanish-speaking children with phonological disorders. *Language, Speech, and Hearing Services in Schools, 35*(1), 5–15.

Goldstein, B. A., Fabiano, L., & Washington, P. S. (2005). Phonological skills in predominantly English-speaking, predominantly Spanish-speaking, and Spanish-English bilingual children. *Language, Speech, and Hearing Services in Schools, 36,* 201–218.

Goldstein, B., & Iglesias, A. (2006). *CPAC-S: Contextual Probes of Articulation Competence: Spanish.* Greenville, SC: Super Duper.

Goldstein, B., & Iglesias, A. (2009). *Contextual Probes of Articulation Competence: Spanish. Normative Data Manual.* Greenville, SC: Super Duper.

Goldstein, B. A., & McLeod, S. (2012). Typical and atypical multilingual speech acquisition. In S. McLeod & B. A. Goldstein (Eds.), *Multilingual aspects of speech sound disorders in children* (pp. 84–100). Bristol, UK: Multilingual Matters.

Gollin, E. S. (1981). Development and plasticity. In E. S. Gollin (Ed.), *Developmental plasticity* (pp. 231–251). New York, NY: Academic Press.

Good, R. H., & Kaminski, R. A. (Eds.). (2011). *DIBELS Next assessment manual.* Eugene, OR: Dynamic Measurement Group. Retrieved from https://dibels.org/dibelsnext.html.

Goodman, R. (1997). The Strengths and Difficulties Questionnaire: A research note. *Journal of Child Psychology and Psychiatry, 38*(5), 581–586.

Gordon-Brannan, M. (1994). Assessing intelligibility: Children's expressive phonologies. *Topics in Language Disorders, 14,* 17–25.

Gordon-Brannan, M., Hodson, B. W., & Wynne, M. K. (1992). Remediating unintelligible utterances of a child with a mild hearing loss. *American Journal of Speech-Language Pathology, 1*(4), 28–38.

Gordon-Brannan, M. E., & Weiss, C. E. (2007). *Clinical management of articulatory and phonologic disorders* (3rd ed.). Baltimore, MD: Lippincott Williams & Wilkins.

Gozzard, H., Baker, E., & McCabe, P. (2004). *Single Word Test of Polysyllables.* Sydney, Australia: Authors.

Gozzard, H., Baker, E., & McCabe, P. (2008). Requests for clarification and children's speech responses: Changing "pasghetti" to "spaghetti." *Child Language Teaching and Therapy, 24*(3), 249–263.

Gray, B. B. (1974). A field study on programmed articulation therapy. *Language, Speech, and Hearing Services in Schools, 5*(3), 119–131.

Gray, S. I., & Shelton, R. L. (1992). Self-monitoring effects on articulation carryover in school-age children. *Language, Speech, and Hearing Services in Schools, 23*(4), 334–342.

Grech, H. (1998). *Phonological development of normal Maltese speaking children.* Unpublished doctoral dissertation, University of Manchester, Manchester, UK.

Grech, H. (2007). Maltese speech acquisition. In S. McLeod (Ed.), *The international guide to speech acquisition* (pp. 483–494). Clifton Park, NY: Thomson Delmar Learning.

Green, B., & Kostogriz, A. (2002). Learning difficulties and the new literacy studies: A socially cricical perspective. In J. Soler, J. Wearmouth, & G. Reid (Eds.), *Contextualising difficulties in literacy development: Exploring politics, culture ethnicity and ethics* (pp. 102–114). Milton Keynes: The Open University.

Green, J. R., Moore, C. A., & Reilly, K. J. (2002). The sequential development of jaw and lip control for speech. *Journal of Speech, Language, and Hearing Research, 45*(1), 66–79.

Greenfield, P., & Smith, J. (1976). *Communication and the beginnings of language: The development of semantic structure in one-word speech and beyond.* New York, NY: Academic Press.

Gregg, B., & Yairi, E. (2007). Phonological skills and disfluency levels in preschool children who stutter. *Journal of Communication Disorders*, *40*, 97–115.

Gresham, F. M., & Elliott, S. N. (1990). *Social Skills Rating System manual*. Circle Pines, MN: American Guidance Service.

Greven, A. J., Meijer, M. F., & Tiwari, R. M. (1994). Articulation after total glossectomy: A clinical study of speech in six patients. *International Journal of Language and Communication Disorders*, *29*, 85–93.

Grigos, M. I., Hayden, D., & Eigen, J. (2010). Perceptual and articulatory changes in speech production following PROMPT treatment. *Journal of Medical Speech-Language Pathology 18*(4), 46–53.

Grogan-Johnson, S., Gabel, R. M., Taylor, J., Rowan, L. E., Alvares, R., & Schenker, J. (2011). A pilot exploration of speech sound disorder intervention delivered bytelehealth to school-age children. *International Journal of Telerehabilitation*, *3*(1), 31–41.

Grogan-Johnson, S., Schmidt, A. M., Schenker, J., Alvares, R., Rowan, L. E., & Taylor, J. (2013). A comparison of speech sound intervention delivered by telepractice and side-by-side service delivery models. *Communication Disorders Quarterly*, *34*(4), 210–220.

Grosjean, F. (1982). *Life with two languages: An introduction to bilingualism*. Cambridge, MA: Harvard University Press.

Grossman, R. B., Bemis, R. H., Plesa Skwerer, D., & Tager-Flusberg, H. (2010). Lexical and affective prosody in children with high-functioning autism. *Journal of Speech, Language, and Hearing Research*, *53*(3), 778–793.

Gruber, F. A. (1999). Probability estimates and paths to consonant normalization in children with speech delay. *Journal of Speech, Language, and Hearing Research*, *42*, 448–459.

Grunwell, P. (1981). The development of phonology: A descriptive profile. *First Language*, *3*, 161–191.

Grunwell, P. (1982). *Clinical phonology*. Rockville, MD: Aspen Systems.

Grunwell, P. (1983, August). *Phonological therapy: premises, principles and procedures*. Paper presented at the XIX Congress of International Association of Logopedics and Phoniatrics, University of Edinburgh.

Grunwell, P. (1985). *Phonological Assessment of Child Speech (PACS)*. Windsor, UK: NFER-Nelson.

Grunwell, P. (1987). *Clinical phonology* (2nd ed.). London, UK: Chapman and Hall.

Grunwell, P. (1997). Developmental phonological disorders: Order in disorder. In B. W. Hodson & M. L. Edwards (Eds.), *Perspectives in applied phonology* (pp. 61–104). Gaithersburg, MD: Aspen.

Guadagnoli, M. A., & Lee, T. D. (2004). Challenge point: A framework for conceptualizing the effects of various practice conditions in motor learning. *Journal of Motor Behavior*, *36*(2), 212–224.

Guenther, F. H. (1995). Speech sound acquisition, coarticulation, and rate effects in a neural network model of speech production. *Psychological Review*, *102*, 594–621.

Guimaraes, C., Donnelly, L., Shott, S., Amin, R., & Kalra, M. (2008). Relative rather than absolute macroglossia in patients with Down syndrome: implications for treatment of obstructive sleep apnea. *Pediatric Radiology*, *38*(10), 1062–1067.

Guimarães, I . & Grilo, M. (1996). *Curso teorico-pratico sobre articulacao verbal [A course in articulation]*. Lisboa, Portugal: Fisiopraxis.

Günther, T., & Hautvast, S. (2010). Addition of contingency management to increase home practice in young children with a speech sound disorder. *International Journal of Language & Communication Disorders*, *45*(3), 345–353.

Gussenhoven, C., & Jacobs, H. (2011). *Understanding phonology* (3rd ed.). London, UK: Hodder Education.

Gutiérrez-Clellen, V. F., & Kreiter, J. (2003). Understanding child bilingual acquisition using parent and teacher reports. *Applied Psycholinguistics*, *24*(2), 267–288.

Gutiérrez-Clellen, V. F., & Peña, E. (2001). Dynamic assessment of diverse children: A tutorial. *Language, Speech, and Hearing Services in Schools*, *32*(4), 212–224.

Hack, J., Marinova-Todd, S. H., & Bernhardt, B. M. (2012). Speech assessment of Chinese-English bilingual children: Accent versus developmental level. *International Journal of Speech-Language Pathology*, *14*(6), 509–519.

Haelsig, P. C., & Madison, C. L. (1986). A study of phonological processes exhibited by 3, 4, and 5-year-old children. *Language, Speech, and Hearing Services in Schools*, *17*, 107–114.

Hageman, C. (2014). Motor learning guided therapy. In K. M. Bleile (Ed.), *The late eight* (pp. 317–335). San Diego, CA: Plural Publishing.

Hakim, H. B., & Ratner, N. B. (2004). Nonword repetition abilities of children who stutter: An exploratory study. *Journal of Fluency Disorders*, *29*(3), 179–199.

Hall, A. (2006). *Have you ever . . .? Eight interactive books for phonological processes*. Greenville, SC: Super Duper Publications.

Hall, B. J. C. (1991). Attitudes of fourth and sixth graders toward peers with mild articulation disorders. *Language, Speech, and Hearing Services in Schools*, *22*(1), 334–340.

Hall, P. K. (1992). At the centre of controversy: Developmental dyspraxia. *American Journal of Speech-Language Pathology, May*, 23–25.

Hall, P. K., Hardy, J. C., & Lavelle, W. E. (1990). A child with signs of developmental apraxia of speech with whom a palatal lift prosthesis was used to manage palatal dysfunction. *Journal of Speech and Hearing Disorders*, *55*(3), 454–460.

Hall, P. K., & Tomblin, J. B. (1975). Case study: Therapy procedures for remediation of a nasal lisp. *Language, Speech, and Hearing Services in Schools*, *6*(1), 29–32.

Hambly, H., Wren, Y., McLeod, S., & Roulstone, S. (2013). The influence of bilingualism on speech production: A systematic review. *International Journal of Language and Communication Disorders*, *48*(1), 1–24.

Hanson, E. K. (2014). My client talks! Do I still need to consider AAC in my treatment planning? Speech supplementation strategies: AAC for clients who talk! *Perspectives on Augmentative and Alternative Communication*, *23*(3), 124–131.

Harasty, J., & Reed, V. A. (1994). The prevalence of speech and language impairment in two Sydney metropolitan schools. *Australian Journal of Human Communication Disorders*, *22*, 1–23.

Harbers, H. M., Paden, E. P., & Halle, J. W. (1999). Phonological awareness and production: Changes during intervention. *Language, Speech, and Hearing Services in Schools*, *30*, 50–60.

Harcourt, D. (2011). An encounter with children: Seeking meaning and understanding about childhood. *European Early Childhood Education Research Journal*, *19*(3), 331–343.

Hardcastle, W. (1976). *Physiology of speech production*. London, UK: Academic Press.

Hardcastle, W. J. (1972). The use of electropalatography in phonetic research. *Phonetica*, *25*, 197–215.

Harding, A., & Grunwell, P. (1998). Active versus passive cleft-type speech characteristics. *International Journal of Language and Communication Disorders*, *33*, 329–352.

Harrington, J., Cox, F., & Evans, Z. (1997). An acoustic phonetic study of broad, general, and cultivated Australian English vowels. *Australian Journal of Linguistics*, *17*, 155–184.

Harrison, L. J., & McLeod, S. (2010). Risk and protective factors associated with speech and language impairment in a nationally representative sample of 4- to 5-year-old children. *Journal of Speech, Language, and Hearing Research*, *53*(2), 508–529.

Harrison, L. J., McLeod, S., Berthelsen, D., & Walker, S. (2009). Literacy, numeracy and learning in school-aged children identified as having speech and language impairment in early childhood. *International Journal of Speech-Language Pathology*, *11*(5), 392–403.

Hart, B. (1991). Input frequency and children's first words. *First Language*, *11*, 289–300.

Haskill, A. A. M., Tyler, A. A., & Tolbert, L. C. (2001). *Months of morphemes: A theme-based cycles approach*. Eau Claire, WI: Thinking Publications.

Haskill, A. M., & Tyler, A. A. (2007). A comparison of linguistic profiles in subgroups of children with specific language impairment. *American Journal of Speech-Language Pathology*, *16*(3), 209–221.

Hasson, N., Camilleri, B., Jones, C., Smith, J., & Dodd, B. (2013). Discriminating disorder from difference using dynamic assessment with bilingual children. *Child Language Teaching and Therapy*, *29*(1), 57–75.

Hasson, N., & Joffe, V. (2007). The case for dynamic assessment in speech and language therapy. *Child Language Teaching and Therapy*, *23*(1), 9–25.

Hauner, K. K. Y., Shriberg, L. D., Kwiatkowski, J., & Allen, C. T. (2005). A subtype of speech delay associated with developmental psychosocial involvement. *Journal of Speech, Language, and Hearing Research*, *48*(3), 635–650.

Havstam, C., Sandberg, A. D., & Lohmander, A. (2011). Communication attitude and speech in 10-year-old children with cleft (lip and) palate: An ICF perspective. *International Journal of Speech-Language Pathology, 13*(2), 156–164.

Hayden, D. (2006). The PROMPT model: Use and application for children with mixed phonological-motor impairment. *International Journal of Speech-Language Pathology, 8*(3), 265–281.

Hayden, D., Eigen, J., Walker, A., & Olsen, L. (2010). PROMPT: A tactually grounded model for the treatment of childhood speech production disorders. In A. L. Williams, S. McLeod, & R. J. McCauley (Eds.), *Interventions for speech sound disorders in children* (pp. 453–474). Baltimore, MD: Paul H. Brookes.

Hayden, D., & Square, P. (1999). *VMPAC: Verbal Motor Production Assessment for Children*. San Antonio, TX: Psychological Coorporation.

Healy, T. J., & Madison, C. L. (1987). Articulation error migration: A comparison of single word and connected speech samples. *Journal of Communication Disorders, 20*, 129–136.

Hedlund, M. (2000). Disability as a phenomenon: A discourse of social and biological understanding. *Disability and Society, 15*, 765–780.

Hegde, M. N. (1985). *Treatment procedures in communicative disorders*. London, UK: Taylor & Francis.

Hegde, M. N., & Davis, D. (2010). *Clinical methods and practicum in speech-language pathology* (5th ed.). Clifton Park, NY: Delmar Learning.

Helfrich-Miller, K. R. (1994). A clinical perspective: Melodic intonation therapy for developmental apraxia. *Clinics in Communication Disorders, 4*, 175–182.

Heller, J., Gabbay, J., O'Hara, C., Heller, M., & Bradley, J. P. (2005). Improved ankyloglossia correction with four-flap z-frenuloplasty. *Annals of Plastic Surgery, 54*(6), 623–628.

Henningsson, G., Kuehn, D. P., Sell, D., Sweeney, T., Trost-Cardamone, J. E., & Whitehill, T. L. (2008). Universal parameters for reporting speech outcomes in individuals with cleft palate. *Cleft Palate-Craniofacial Journal, 45*(1), 1–17.

Henrich, J., Heine, S. J., & Norenzayan, A. (2010). The weirdest people in the world? *Behavioral and Brain Sciences, 33*(2–3), 61–83.

Herbert, R., Moseley, A., & Sherrington, C. (1998/99). PEDro: A database of RCTs in physiotherapy. *Health Information Management, 28*, 186–188.

Hesketh, A. (2010). Metaphonological intervention: Phonological awareness. In A. L. Williams, S. McLeod, & R. J. McCauley (Eds.), *Interventions for speech sound disorders in children* (pp. 247–274). Baltimore, MD: Paul H. Brookes.

Hesketh, A., Adams, C., Nightingale, C., & Hall, R. (2000). Phonological awareness therapy and articulatory training approaches for children with phonological disorders: a comparative outcome study. *International Journal of Language and Communication Disorders, 35*(3), 337–354.

Hewlett, N. (1985). Phonological versus phonetic disorders: Some suggested modifications to the current use of the distinction. *British Journal of Disorders of Communication, 20*, 155–164.

Hickey, J. (1992). The treatment of lateral fricatives and affricates using electropalatography: A case study of a 10 year old girl. *Clinical Speech and Language Studies, 1*, 80–87.

Hickman, L. (1997). *Apraxia Profile*. San Antonio, TX: The Psychological Corporation.

Hickok, G. (2010). The role of mirror neurons in speech and language processing. *Brain and Language, 112*(1), 1–2.

Hidecker, M. J. C., Paneth, N., Rosenbaum, P. L., Kent, R. D., Lillie, J., Eulenberg, J. B., . . . Taylor, K. (2011). Developing and validating the Communication Function Classification System for individuals with cerebral palsy. *Developmental Medicine and Child Neurology, 53*(8), 704–710.

Hillenbrand, J., Getty, L., Clark, M., & Wheeler, L. (1995). Acoustic characteristics of American English vowels. *Journal of the Acoustical Society of America, 97*, 3099–3111.

Hirschberg, J., & Van Demark, D.-R. (1997). A proposal for standardization of speech and hearing evaluations to assess velopharyngeal function. *Folia Phoniatrica et Logopaedica, 49*, 158–167.

Hitchcock, E. R., & McAllister Byun, T. (2015). Enhancing generalisation in biofeedback intervention using the challenge point framework: A case study. *Clinical Linguistics and Phonetics, 29*(1), 59–75.

Hobbs, N. (1975). *The futures of children: Categories, labels, and their consequences* (Report of the project on classification of exceptional children). San Francisco, CA: Jossey-Bass.

Hodge, M. M. (2010). Developmental dysarthria interventions. In A. L. Williams, S. McLeod & R. J. McCauley (Eds.), *Interventions for children with speech sound disorder* (pp. 557–578). Baltimore, MD: Paul H. Brookes.

Hodge, M., Daniels, J., & Gotzke, C. L. (2009). *Test of Children's Speech Plus* TOCS+ intelligibility measures (version 5.3) [computer software]. Edmonton, AB: University of Alberta. Retrieved from http://www.tocs.plus.ualberta.ca.

Hodge, M., & Gotzke, C. (2007). Preliminary results of an intelligibility measure for English-speaking children with cleft palate. *Cleft Palate-Craniofacial Journal, 44*, 163–174.

Hodge, M. M., & Gotzke, C. L. (2014). Construct-related validity of the TOCS measures: Comparison of intelligibility and speaking rate scores in children with and without speech disorders. *Journal of Communication Disorders, 51*(0), 51–63.

Hodge, M., & Wellman, L. (1999). Management of children with dysarthria. In A. Caruso & E. A. Strand (Eds.), *Clinical management of motor speech disorders in children* (pp. 209–280). New York, NY: Thieme.

Hodson, B. W. (1978). A preliminary hierarchical model for phonological remediation. *Language, Speech, and Hearing Services in Schools, 9*(4), 236–240.

Hodson, B. W. (1982). Remediation of speech patterns associated with low levels of phonological performance. In M. Crary (Ed.), *Phonological intervention: Concepts and procedures* (pp. 97–115). San Diego, CA: College-Hill Press.

Hodson, B. W. (1989). From articulation to phonology: Remediating unintelligible speech patterns. *Seminars in Speech and Language, 10*, 153–161.

Hodson, B. W. (1992). Applied phonology: Constructs, contributions, and issues. *Language, Speech, and Hearing Services in Schools, 23*, 247–253.

Hodson, B. W. (1994). Helping individuals become intelligible, literate, and articulate: The role of phonology. *Topics in Language Disorders, 14*, 1–16.

Hodson, B. W. (1997). Disordered phonologies: What have we learned about assessment and treatment? In B. W. Hodson & M. L. Edwards (Eds.), *Perspectives in applied phonology* (pp. 43–60). Frederick, MD: Aspen.

Hodson, B. W. (1998). Research and practice: Applied phonology. *Topics in Language Disorders, 18*(2), 58–70.

Hodson, B. W. (2003). *Hodson Computerized Analysis of Phonological Patterns* (HCAPP). Wichita, KS: Phonocomp Publishers.

Hodson, B. W. (2004). *Hodson Assessment of Phonological Patterns: Third Edition*. Austin, TX: Pro-Ed.

Hodson, B. W. (2006). Identifying phonological patterns and projecting remediation cycles: Expediting intelligibility gains of a 7 year old Australian child. *International Journal of Speech-Language Pathology, 8*(3), 257–264.

Hodson, B. W. (2007). *Evaluation and enhancing children's phonological systems: Research and theory to practice*. Greenville, SC: Thinking Publications.

Hodson, B. W. (2011). Enhancing phonological patterns of young children with highly unintelligible speech. *The ASHA Leader, 16*(4), 16–19.

Hodson, B. W., Chin, L., Redmond, B., & Simpson, R. (1983). Phonological evaluation and remediation of speech deviations of a child with a repaired cleft palate: A case study. *Journal of Speech and Hearing Disorders, 48*(1), 93–98.

Hodson, B. W., Nonomura, C. W., & Zappia, M. J. (1989). Phonological disorders: Impact on academic performance? *Seminars in Speech and Language, 10*(3), 252–259.

Hodson, B. W., & Paden, E. P. (1981). Phonological processes which characterize unintelligible and intelligible speech in early childhood. *Journal of Speech and Hearing Disorders, 46*, 369–373.

Hodson, B. W., & Paden, E. P. (1983). *Targeting intelligible speech: A phonological approach to remediation*. San Diego, CA: College-Hill.

Hodson, B. W., & Paden, E. P. (1991). *Targeting intelligible speech: A phonological approach to remediation* (2nd ed.). Austin, TX: Pro-Ed.

Hodson, B. W. & Prezas, R. F. (2010). *Hodson-Prezas Assessment of Spanish Phonological Patterns.* Unpublished manuscript, Wichita State University.

Hodson, B. W., & Scudder, R. R. (1990). Phonological disorders in children. *Seminars in Speech and Language, 11*(03), 192–199.

Hodson, S. L., & Jardine, B. R. (2009). Revisiting Jarrod: Applications of gestural phonology theory to the assessment and treatment of speech sound disorder. *International Journal of Speech-Language Pathology, 11*(2), 122–134.

Hoeman, S. (1996). *Rehabilitation nursing: Process and application.* St. Louis, MO: Mosby Year Book.

Hoffman, P. R. (1983). Interallophonic generalization of /r/ training. *Journal of Speech and Hearing Disorders, 48*(2), 215–221.

Hoffman, P. R., & Norris, J. A. (2010). Dynamic systems and whole language intervention. In A. L. Williams, S. McLeod, & R. J. McCauley (Eds.), *Interventions for speech sound disorders in children* (pp. 333–354). Baltimore, MD: Paul. H. Brookes.

Hoffman, P. R., Norris, J. A., & Monjure, J. (1990). Comparison of process targeting and whole language treatments for phonologically delayed preschool children. *Language, Speech, and Hearing Services in Schools, 21*, 102–109.

Hogan, M., Westcott, C., & Griffiths, M. (2005). Randomized, controlled trial of division of tongue-tie in infants with feeding problems. *Journal of Paediatrics and Child Health, 41*(5–6), 246–250.

Holley, L. R., Hamby, G. R., & Taylor, P. P. (1973). Palatal lift for velopharyngeal incompetence. *Journal of Dentistry for Children, 40*, 476–470.

Holliday, E. L., Harrison, L. J., & McLeod, S. (2009). Listening to children with communication impairment talking through their drawings. *Journal of Early Childhood Research, 7*(3), 244–263.

Holm, A., & Crosbie, S. (2006). Introducing Jarrod: A child with a phonological impairment. *International Journal of Speech-Language Pathology, 8*(3), 164–175.

Holm, A., Crosbie, S., & Dodd, B. (2007). Differentiating normal variability from inconsistency in children's speech: Normative data. *International Journal of Language and Communication Disorders, 42*(4), 467–486.

Holm, A., Crosbie, S., & Dodd, B. (2013). Treating inconsistent speech disorders. In B. Dodd (Ed.), *Differential diagnosis and treatment of children with speech disorder* (pp. 182–201). Hoboken, NJ: Wiley.

Holm, A., & Dodd, B. (1999). An intervention case study of a bilingual child with phonological disorder. *Child Language Teaching and Therapy, 15*, 139–158.

Holm, A., & Dodd, B. (2001). Comparison of cross-language generalisation following speech therapy. *Folia Phoniatrica et Logopaedica, 53*, 166–172.

Holm, A., Dodd, B., & Ozanne, A. (1997). Efficacy of intervention for a bilingual child making articulation and phonological errors. *International Journal of Bilingualism, 1*(1), 55–69.

Honorof, D. N., McCullough, J. & Somerville, B. (2000). *Comma gets a cure: A diagnostic passage for accent study.* New Haven, CT: Haskins Laboratories.

Horn, D., Kapeller, J., Rivera-Brugués, N., Moog, U., Lorenz-Depiereux, B., Eck, S., Strom, T. M. (2010). Identification of *FOXP1* deletions in three unrelated patients with mental retardation and significant speech and language deficits. *Human Mutation, 31*, E1851-1860.

Horne, R. S. C., Hauck, F. R., Moon, R. Y., L'Hoir, M. P., Blair, P. S., Physiology, . . . Infant, D. (2014). Dummy (pacifier) use and sudden infant death syndrome: Potential advantages and disadvantages. *Journal of Paediatrics and Child Health, 50*(3), 170–174.

Hourcade, J., Everhart Pilotte, T., West, E., & Parette, P. (2004). A history of augmentative and alternative communication for individuals with severe and profound disabilities. *Focus on Autism and Other Developmental Disabilities, 19*(4), 235–244.

Howard, S. (1993). Articulatory constraints on a phonological system: A case study of cleft palate speech. *Clinical Linguistics and Phonetics, 7*, 299–317.

Howard, S. (2007a). English speech acquisition. In S. McLeod (Ed.), *The international guide to speech acquisition* (pp. 188–203). Clifton Park, NY: Thomson Delmar Learning.

Howard, S. (2007b). The interplay between articulation and prosody in children with impaired speech: Observations from electropalatographic and perceptual analysis. *International Journal of Speech-Language Pathology, 9*(1), 20–35.

Howell, J., & Dean, E. C. (1987). "I think that's a noisy sound." Reflection on learning in the therapeutic situation. *Child Language Teaching and Therapy, 3*, 259–266.

Howell, J., & Dean, E. (1994). *Treating phonological disorders in children: Metaphon: Theory to practice* (2nd ed.). London, UK: Whurr.

Howell, P., Au-Yeung, J., Yaruss, S. J., & Eldridge, K. (2006). Phonetic difficulty and stuttering in English. *Clinical Linguistics and Phonetics, 20*(9), 703–716.

Hua, Z. (2002). *Phonological development in specific contexts: Studies of Chinese-speaking children.* Clevedon, UK: Multilingual Matters.

Hua, Z. & Dodd, B. (Eds.). (2006). *Phonological development and disorders in children: A multilingual perspective.* Clevedon, UK: Multilingual Matters.

Huckvale, M. (2009). *Speech filing system* [Computer program]. London, UK: University College London.

Hugo, G. (2010). Circularity, reciprocity, and return: An important dimension of contemporary transnationalism. *ISSBD Bulletin, 58*(2), 2–5.

Hulterstam, I., & Nettelbladt, U. (2002). Clinician elicitation strategies and child participation. Comparing two methods of phonological intervention. *Logopedics Phoniatrics Vocology, 27*(4), 155–168.

Hurley, J. C., & Underwood, M. K. (2002). Children's understanding of their research rights before and after debriefing: Informed assent, confidentiality and stopping participation. *Child Development, 73*, 132–143.

Hustad, K. C. (2010). Childhood dysarthria: Cerebral palsy. In K. M. Yorkston, D. R. Beukelman, E. A. Strand, & M. Hakel (Eds.), *Management of motor speech disorders in children and adults* (3rd ed., pp. 359–384). Austin, TX: Pro-Ed.

Hustad, K. C. (2012). Speech intelligibility in children with speech disorders. *Perspectives on Language Learning and Education, 19*(1), 7–11.

Hustad, K. C., Gorton, K., & Lee, J. (2010). Classification of speech and language profiles in 4-year-old children with cerebral palsy: A prospective preliminary study. *Journal of Speech, Language, and Hearing Research, 53*(6), 1496–1513.

Hustad, K. C., Schueler, B., Schultz, L., & DuHadway, C. (2012). Intelligibility of 4-year-old children with and without cerebral palsy. *Journal of Speech, Language, and Hearing Research, 55*, 1177–1189.

Hyde, J. S. & Linn, M. C. (1988). Sex differences in verbal ability: A meta-analysis. *Psychological Bulletin, 104*, 53–69.

Hyman, L. M. (1975). *Phonology: theory and analysis.* New York, NY: Holt, Rinehart & Winston.

Icht, M., & Ben-David, B. M. (2015). Oral-diadochokinetic rates for Hebrew-speaking school-age children: Real words vs. non-words repetition. *Clinical Linguistics and Phonetics, 29*(2), 102–114.

Imada, T., Zhang, Y., Cheour, M., Taulu, S., Ahonen, A., & Kuhl, P. K. (2006). Infant speech perception activates Broca's area: A developmental magnetoencephalography study. *NeuroReport, 17*(10), 957–962.

Indefrey, P., & Levelt, W. J. M. (2004). The spatial and temporal signatures of word production components. *Cognition, 92*(1–2), 101–144.

Individuals with Disabilities Education Improvement Act (2004). PL 108-466, *20* U.S.C. §§ 1400 *et. seq.* C.F.R.

Ingram, D. (1976). *Phonological disability in children.* New York, NY: American Elsevier Publishing.

Ingram, D. (1981). *Procedures for the phonological analysis of children's language.* Baltimore, MD: University Park Press.

Ingram, D. (2002). The measurement of whole-word productions. *Journal of Child Language, 29*, 713–733.

Ingram, D. (2012). Cross-linguistic and multilingual aspects of speech sound disorders in children. In S. McLeod & B. A. Goldstein (Eds.), *Multilingual aspects of speech sound disorders in children* (pp. 3–12). Bristol, UK: Multilingual Matters.

Ingram, D., & Ingram, K. D. (2001). A whole-word approach to phonological analysis and intervention. *Language, Speech, and Hearing Services in Schools, 32*(4), 271–283.

International Association of Logopedics and Phoniatrics (IALP) (2012). *About us.* Retrieved from http://www.ialp.info.

International Expert Panel on Multilingual Children's Speech (2012). *Multilingual children with speech sound disorders: Position paper.* Bathurst, Australia: Research Institute for Professional

Practice, Learning and Education (RIPPLE), Charles Sturt University. Retrieved from http://www.csu.edu.au/research/multi-lingual-speech/position-paper. (Chapter 15 feature box, page 539: Copyright © Sharynne McLeod.)

International Phonetic Association. (1999). *Handbook of the International Phonetic Association: A guide to the use of the International Phonetic Alphabet*. Cambridge, UK: Cambridge University Press.

International Phonetic Association. (2005). *International Phonetic Alphabet chart*. Retrieved from https://www.internationalphoneticassociation.org/content/ipa-chart.

Iuzzini, J., & Forrest, K. (2010). Evaluation of a combined treatment approach for childhood apraxia of speech. *Clinical Linguistics and Phonetics, 24*(4–5), 335–345.

Jaafar, S. H., Jahanfar, S., Angolkar, M., & Ho, J. J. (2012). Effect of restricted pacifier use in breastfeeding term infants for increasing duration of breastfeeding. *Cochrane Database of Systematic Reviews, 7*, Cd007202.

Jacoby, G., Lee, L., Kummer, A., Levin, K., & Creaghead, N. (2002). The number of individual treatment units necessary to facilitate functional communication to improvements in the speech and language of young children. *American Journal of Speech-Language Pathology, 11*, 370–380.

Jakielski, K. J. (2011). Sarah: Childhood apraxia of speech: Differential diagnosis and evidence-based intervention. In S. S. Cabon & E. R. Cohn (Eds.), *The communication disorders casebook: Learning by example.* (pp. 173–184). Upper Saddle River, NJ: Pearson Education.

Jakobson, R. (1941/1968). *Child language, aphasia and phonological universals*. Transl. by A. R. Keiler. Kindersprache, Aphasie und allgemeine Lautgesetze (1941). The Hague, The Netherlands: Mouton.

James, D. G. H. (2001a). The use of phonological processes in Australian children aged 2 to 7:11 years. *International Journal of Speech-Language Pathology, 3*, 109–128.

James, D. G. H. (2001b). An item analysis of Australian English words for an articulation and phonological test for children aged 2 to 7 years. *Clinical Linguistics and Phonetics, 15*, 457–485.

James, D. G. H. (2006). *Hippopotamus is so hard to say:Children's acquisition of polysyllabic words*. Unpublished PhD thesis, University of Sydney, Sydney. Retrieved from http://ses.library.usyd.edu.au/handle/2123/1638.

James, D. G. H. (2009). The relationship between the underlying representation and surface form of long words. In C. Bowen (Ed.), *Children's speech sound disorders* (pp. 329–334). Oxford, UK: Wiley-Blackwell.

James, D., McCormack, P., & Butcher, A. (1999). Children's use of phonological processes in the age range of five to seven years. In S. McLeod & L. McAllister (Eds.), *Proceedings of the 1999 Speech Pathology Australia National Conference* (pp. 48–57). Melbourne, Australia: Speech Pathology Australia.

James, D., van Doorn, J. & McLeod, S. (2001). Vowel production in mono-, di-and poly-syllabic words in children 3;0 to 7;11 years. In L. Wilson & S. Hewat (Eds.). *Proceedings of the Speech Pathology Australia Conference.* (pp. 127–136). Melbourne, Australia: Speech Pathology Australia.

James, D., van Doorn, J., McLeod, S. (2002). Segment production in mono-, di- and polysyllabic words in children aged 3–7 years. In F. Windsor, L. Kelly & N. Hewlett (Eds.) *Themes in clinical phonetics and linguistics* (pp. 287–298), Hillsdale, NJ: Lawrence Erlbaum.

James, D. G. H., van Doorn, J., & McLeod, S. (2008). The contribution of polysyllabic words in clinical decision making about children's speech. *Clinical Linguistics and Phonetics, 22*(4), 345–353.

James, D. G. H., van Doorn, J., McLeod, S., & Esterman, A. (2008). Patterns of consonant deletion in typically developing children aged 3 to 7 years. *International Journal of Speech-Language Pathology, 10*(3), 179–192.

James, S. L. (1990). *Normal language acquisition*. Boston, MA: Allyn & Bacon.

Jamieson, G. (2004). *Children's attention on tabletop versus computer administered phonology therapy*. Unpublished dissertation, College of St Mark & St John, Plymouth, UK.

Jamieson, D. G., & Rvachew, S. (1992). Remediating speech production errors with sound identification training. *Journal of Speech-Language Pathology and Audiology, 16*, 201–210.

Jarvis, J. (1989). Taking a Metaphon approach to phonological development: A case study. *Child Language Teaching and Therapy, 5*(1), 16–32.

Jelm, J. M. (2001). *Verbal Dyspraxia Profile*. DeKalb, IL: Janelle.

Jessup, B., Ward, E., Cahill, L., & Keating, D. (2008). Prevalence of speech and/or language impairment in preparatory students in northern Tasmania. *International Journal of Speech-Language Pathology, 10*(5), 364–377.

Jimenez, B. C. (1987). Acquisition of Spanish consonants in children aged 3–5 years, 7 months. *Language, Speech, and Hearing Services in Schools, 18*, 357–363.

Joffe, V., & Pring, T. (2008). Children with phonological problems: A survey of clinical practice. *International Journal of Language and Communication Disorders, 43*(2), 154–164.

Johannisson, T. B., Lohmander, A., & Persson, C. (2014). Assessing intelligibility by single words, sentences and spontaneous speech: A methodological study of the speech production of 10-year-olds. *Logopedics Phoniatrics Vocology, 39*(4), 159–168.

Johannisson, T. B., Wennerfeldt, S., Havstam, C., Naeslund, M., Jacobson, K., & Lohmander, A. (2009). The Communication Attitude Test (CAT-S): Normative values for 220 Swedish children. *International Journal of Language and Communication Disorders, 44*(6), 813–825.

Johnson, C. J. (2006). Getting started in evidence-based practice for childhood speech-language disorders. *American Journal of Speech-Language Pathology, 15*(1), 20–35.

Johnson, C. J., Beitchman, J. H., & Brownlie, E. B. (2010). Twenty-year follow-up of children with and without speech-language impairments: Family, educational, occupational, and quality of life outcomes. *American Journal of Speech-Language Pathology, 19*(1), 51–65.

Johnson, C. J., Beitchman, J. H., Young, A., Escobar, M., Atkinson, L., Wilson, B., . . . Wang, M. (1999). Fourteen-year follow-up of children with and without speech/language impairments: Speech/language stability and outcomes. *Journal of Speech, Language, and Hearing Research, 42*(3), 744–760.

Johnson, K. (1997). Speech perception without speaker normalization: An exemplar model. In K. Johnson & J. W. Mullennix (Eds.), *Talker variability in speech processing* (pp. 145–165). San Diego, CA: Academic Press.

Johnson, K. (2005). Speaker normalization in speech perception. In D. B. Pisoni & R. Remez (Eds.), *The handbook of speech perception* (pp. 363–389). Oxford, UK: Blackwell Publishers.

Johnson, S., & Somers, H. (1978). Spontaneous and imitated responses in articulation testing. *British Journal of Disorders of Communication, 13*, 107–116.

Johnson, W., & Reimers, P. (2010). *Patterns in child phonology*. Edinburgh, UK: Edinburgh University Press.

Jones, C. E., Chapman K.L., & Hardin-Jones M.A. (2003). Speech development of children with cleft palate before and after palatal surgery. *Cleft Palate-Craniofacial Journal, 40*, 19–31.

Jongman, A., Fourakis, M., & Sereno, J. A. (1989). The acoustic vowels space of Modern Greek and German. *Language and Speech, 32*, 221–248.

Jordaan, H. (2008). Clinical intervention for bilingual children: An international survey. *Folia Phoniatrica et Logopaedica, 60*, 97–105.

Juliena, H. M., & Munson, B. (2012). Modifying speech to children based on their perceived phonetic accuracy. *Journal of Speech, Language, and Hearing Research, 55*, 1836–1849.

Jusczyk, P. (1999). How infants begin to extract words from speech. *Trends in Cognitive Science, 3*, 323–328.

Jusczyk, P. W., Houston, D. M., & Newsome, M. (1999). The beginnings of word segmentation in English-learning infants. *Cognitive Psychology, 39*, 159–207.

Justice, L. M. (2006). Emergent literacy: Development, domains, and intervention approaches. In L. M. Justice (Ed.), *Clinical approaches to emergent literacy intervention* (pp. 3–28). San Diego, CA: Plural Publishing.

Justice, L. M. (2010). When craft and science collide: Improving therapeutic practices in schools through evidence-based innovations, *International Journal of Speech-Language Pathology, 12*(2), 79–88.

Justice, L. M., & Ezell, H. K. (2001). Word and print awareness in 4-year-old children. *Child Language Teaching and Therapy, 17*(3), 207–225.

Kachru, B. B. (1985). Standards, codification and sociolinguistic realism: The English language in the outer circle. In R. Quirk & H. G. Widdowson (Eds.), *English in the world: Teaching and learning the language and literatures* (pp. 11–30). Cambridge, UK: Cambridge University Press.

Kachru, B. B. (1997). World Englishes and English-using communities. *Annual Review of Applied Linguistics, 17,* 66–87.

Kadis, D., Goshulak, D., Namasivayam, A., Pukonen, M., Kroll, R., De Nil, L., . . . Lerch, J. (2014). Cortical thickness in children receiving intensive therapy for idiopathic apraxia of speech. *Brain Topography, 27*(2), 240–247.

Kaipa, R., Robb, M. P., O'Beirne, G. A., & Allison, R. S. (2012). Recovery of speech following total glossectomy: An acoustic and perceptual appraisal. *International Journal of Speech-Language Pathology, 14*(1), 24–34.

Kame'enui, E. J., Simmons, D. C., Baker, S., Chard, D. J., Dickson, S. V., Gunn, B., Smith, S. B., Sprick, M., & Lin, S. J. (1997). Effective strategies for teaching beginning reading. In E. J. Kame'enui & D. W. Carnine (Eds.), *Effective teaching strategies that accommodate diverse learners.* Columbus, OH: Merrill.

Kamhi, A. G. (1994). Research to practice: Toward a theory of clinical expertise in speech-language pathology. *Language, Speech, and Hearing Services in Schools, 25,* 115–118.

Kamhi, A. G. (1995). Research to practice: Defining, developing and maintaining clinical expertise. *Language, Speech, and Hearing Services in Schools, 26,* 353–356.

Kamhi, A. G. (2011). Balancing certainty and uncertainty in clinical practice. *Language, Speech, and Hearing Services in Schools, 42*(1), 59–64.

Kamhi, A. G., & Pollock, K. E. (Eds.). (2005). *Phonological disorders in children: Clinical decision making in assessment and intervention.* Baltimore, MD: Paul H. Brookes.

Kantor, P. T., Wagner, R. K., Torgesen, J. K., & Rashotte, C. A. (2011). Comparing two forms of dynamic assessment and traditional assessment of preschool phonological awareness. *Journal of Learning Disabilities, 44*(4), 313–321.

Karlsson, H. B., Shriberg, L. D., Flipsen, P., Jr., & McSweeny, J. L. (2002). Acoustic phenotypes for speech-genetics studies: Towards an acoustic marker for residual /s/ distortions. *Clinical Linguistics and Phonetics, 16*(6), 403–424.

Karnell, M. P. (2011). Instrumental assessment of velopharyngeal closure for speech. *Seminars in Speech and Language, 32*(02), 168–178.

Katz, W., McNeil, M., & Garst, D. (2010). Treating apraxia of speech (AOS) with EMA-supplied visual augmented feedback. *Aphasiology, 24,* 826–837.

Kaufman, N. (1995). *Kaufman Speech Praxis Test for Children.* Detroit, MI: Wayne State University Press.

Kaufman, N. (1998). *Kaufman speech praxis treatment kit for children: Basic level.* Gaylord, MI: Northern Speech Services.

Kazdin, A. E. (1982). *Single-case research designs: Methods for clinical and applied settings.* New York, NY: Oxford University Press.

Keating, D., Turrell, G., & Ozanne, A. (2001). Childhood speech disorders: Reported prevalence, comorbidity and socioeconomic profile. *Journal of Paediatrics and Child Health, 37*(5), 431–436.

Kehoe, M. (1997). Stress error patterns in English-speaking children's word productions. *Clinical Linguistics and Phonetics, 11,* 389–409.

Kehoe, M. M. (2001). Prosodic patterns in children's multisyllabic word productions. *Language, Speech, and Hearing Services in Schools, 32,* 284–294.

Keilmann, A., Kluesener, P., Freude, C., & Schramm, B. (2011). Manifestation of speech and language disorders in children with hearing impairment compared with children with specific language disorders. *Logopedics Phoniatrics Vocology, 36*(1), 12–20.

Kenney, K. W., & Prather, E. M. (1986). Articulation development in preschool children: Consistency of productions. *Journal of Speech and Hearing Research, 29,* 29–36.

Kenney, K. W., Prather, E. M., Mooney, M. A., & Jeruzal, N. C. (1984). Comparisons among three articulation sampling procedures with preschool children. *Journal of Speech and Hearing Research, 27,* 226–231.

Kent, R. D. (1992). The biology of phonological development. In C. A. Ferguson, L. Menn, & C. Stoel-Gammon (Eds.), *Phonological development: Models, research, implications* (pp. 65–90). Timonium, MD: York Press.

Kent, R. D. (2000). Research on speech motor control and its disorders: A review and prospective. *Journal of Communication Disorders, 33,* 391–428.

Kent, R. D. (2006). Evidence-based practice in communication disorders: Progress not perfection. *Language, Speech, and Hearing Services in Schools, 37,* 268–270.

Kent, R. D., Miolo, G., & Bloedel, S. (1994). The intelligibility of children's speech: A review of evaluation procedures. *American Journal of Speech-Language Pathology, 3,* 81–95.

Kent, R. D., & Read, C. (2002). *Acoustic analysis of speech* (2nd ed.). Albany, NY: Singular Thomson Learning.

Kent, R. D., & Tilkens, C. (2007). Oromotor foundations of speech acquisition. In S. McLeod (Ed.), *The international guide to speech acquisition* (pp. 8–13). Clifton Park, NY: Thomson Delmar Learning.

Kent, R. D., & Vorperian, H. K. (2013). Speech impairment in Down syndrome: A review. *Journal of Speech, Language, and Hearing Research, 56*(1), 178–210.

The KIDSCREEN Group Europe (2006). *The KIDSCREEN Questionnaires—Quality of life questionnaires for children and adolescents.* Lengerich, Germany: Pabst Science Publishers. Retrieved from http://www.kidscreen.org/english/.

Kier, W. M., & Smith, K. K. (1985). Tongues, tentacles and trunks: The biomechanics of movement in muscular-hydrostats. *Zoological Journal of the Linnean Society, 83*(4), 307–324.

Kilminster, M. G. E., & Laird, E. M. (1978). Articulation development in children aged three to nine years. *Australian Journal of Human Communication Disorders, 6,* 23–30.

Kim, D., Stephens, J. D. W., & Pitt, M. A. (2012). How does context play a part in splitting words apart? Production and perception of word boundaries in casual speech. *Journal of Memory and Language, 66*(4), 509–529.

Kim, M., & Pae, S. (2007). Korean speech acquisition. In S. McLeod (Ed.), *The international guide to speech acquisition* (pp. 472–482). Clifton Park, NY: Thomson Delmar Learning.

Kim, M., & Stoel-Gammon, C. (2010). Segmental timing of young children and adults. *International Journal of Speech-Language Pathology, 12,* 221–229.

King, A. M., Hengst, J. A., & DeThorne, L. S. (2013). Severe speech sound disorders: An integrated multimodal intervention. *Language, Speech, and Hearing Services in Schools, 44*(2), 195–210.

King, G., Rosenbaum, P., & King, S. (1997). Evaluating family-centred service using a measure of parents' perceptions. *Child: Care, Health and Development, 23*(1), 47–62.

Kirk, C., & Gillon, G. T. (2007). Longitudinal effects of phonological awareness intervention on morphological awareness in children with speech impairment. *Language, Speech, and Hearing Services in Schools, 38*(4), 342–352.

Kirk, C., & Vigeland, L. (2014). A psychometric review of norm-referenced tests used to assess phonological error patterns. *Language, Speech, and Hearing Services in Schools, 45*(4), 365–377.

Kirkpatrick, E., & Ward, J. (1984). Prevalence of articulation errors in New South Wales primary school pupils. *Australian Journal of Human Communication Disorders, 12,* 55–62.

Kisilevsky, B. S., Hains, S. M. J., Brown, C. A., Lee, C. T., Cowperthwaite, B., Stutzman, S. S., . . . Wang, Z. (2009). Fetal sensitivity to properties of maternal speech and language. *Infant Behavior and Development, 32*(1), 59–71.

Kjelgaard, M. M., & Tager-Flusberg, H. (2001). An investigation of language impairment in autism: Implications for genetic subgroups. *Language and Cognitive Processes, 16,* 287–308.

Klajman, S., Huber, W., Neumann, H., Wein, B., & Bockler, R. (1988). Ultrasonographische Unterstuetzung der Artikulationsanbahnumg bei gehoerlosen Kindern. *Sprache-Stimme-Gehoer, 12,* 117–120.

Kleim, J. A., & Jones, T. A. (2008). Principles of experience-dependent neural plasticity: Implications for rehabilitation after brain damage. *Journal of Speech, Language, and Hearing Research, 51*(1), S225–S239.

Klein, E. S. (1996a). *Clinical phonology: Assessment and treatment of articulation disorders in children and adults.* San Diego, CA: Singular.

Klein, E. S. (1996b). Phonological/traditional approaches to articulation therapy: A retrospective group comparison. *Language, Speech, and Hearing Services in Schools, 27,* 314–323.

Klein, H. B., & Moses, N. (1999). *Intervention planning for children with communication disorders: A guide for clinical practicum and professional practice.* (2nd ed.). Needham Heights, MA: Allyn & Bacon.

Kluender, K. R., & Kiefte, M. (2006). Speech perception within a biologically realistic information-theoretic framework. In M. A. Gernsbacher & M. Traxler (Eds.), *Handbook of psycholinguistics* (2nd ed., pp. 153–199). London, UK: Elsevier.

Koegel, L., Koegel, R., & Ingham, J. (1986). Programming rapid generalization of correct articulation through self-monitoring procedures. *Journal of Speech and Hearing Disorders, 51,* 24–32.

Koegel, R. L., Koegel, L. K., Ingham, J. C., & Van Voy, K. (1988). Within-clinic versus outside-of-clinic self-monitoring of articulation to promote generalization. *Journal of Speech and Hearing Disorders, 53*(4), 392–399.

Kogovšek, D., & Ozbič, M. (2013). Lestvica razumljivosti govora v vsakdanjem življenju: slovenščina [Intelligibility in Context Scale: Slovenian]. *Komunikacija, 2*(3), 28–34.

Kohler, K. (1999). German. In International Phonetic Association (Ed.), *Handbook of the International Phonetic Association* (pp. 86–89). Cambridge, UK: Cambridge University Press.

Kohnert, K. (2013). *Language disorders in bilingual children and adults* (2nd ed.). San Diego, CA: Plural Publishing.

Korczak, J. (1929, republished in English 2009). *Prawo Dziecka do Szacunku [The child's right to respect]* (E. P. Kulawiec, Trans.). Strasbourg, France: Council of Europe.

Krauss, T., & Galloway, H. (1982). Melodic intonation therapy with language delayed apraxic children. *Journal of Music Therapy, 19,* 102–113.

Kresheck, J., & Socolofsky, G. (1972). Imitative and spontaneous articulation assessment of 4-year-old children. *Journal of Speech and Hearing Research, 15,* 729–733.

Kristoffersen, K. E. (2007). Norwegian speech acquisition. In S. McLeod (Ed.), *The international guide to speech acquisition* (pp. 495–504). Clifton Park, NY: Thomson Delmar Learning.

Kristoffersen, K. E. (2008). Speech and language development in cri du chat syndrome: A critical review. *Clinical Linguistics and Phonetics, 22*(6), 443–457.

Kristoffersen, K. E., Garmann, N. G., & Simonsen, H. G. (2014). Consonant production and intelligibility in cri du chat syndrome. *Clinical Linguistics and Phonetics, 28*(10), 769–784.

Krupa, L. (1995). *Minimal contrast stories.* Greenville, SC: Super Duper Publications.

Kuhl, P. K. (2009). Early language acquisition: Phonetic and word learning, neural substrates, and a theoretical model. In B. Moore, L. Tyler, & W. Marslen-Wilson (Eds.), *The perception of speech: From sound to meaning* (pp. 103–131). Oxford, UK: Oxford University Press.

Kuhn, D. (2006). Speedy speech: Efficient service delivery for articulation errors. *SIG 16 Perspectives on School-Based Issues, 7*(4), 11–14.

Kummer, A. W. (2011). Speech therapy for errors secondary to cleft palate and velopharyngeal dysfunction. *Seminars in Speech and Language, 32*(2), 191–198.

Kummer, A. W. (2014). *Cleft palate and craniofacial anomalies: Effects on speech and resonance* (3rd ed.). Clifton Park, NY: Cengage.

Kunnari, S., & Savinainen-Makkonen, T. (2007). Finnish speech acquisition. In S. McLeod (Ed.), *The international guide to speech acquisition* (pp. 351–363). Clifton Park, NY: Thomson Delmar Learning.

Kwiatkowski, J., & Shriberg, L. D. (1992). Intelligibility assessment in developmental phonological disorders: Accuracy of caregiver gloss. *Journal of Speech and Hearing Research, 35,* 1095–1104.

Kwiatkowski, J., & Shriberg, L. D. (1998). The capability focus treatment framework for child speech disorders. *American Journal of Speech-Language Pathology, 7,* 27–38.

Ladefoged, P. (1971). *Preliminaries to linguistics phonetics.* Chicago, IL: University of Chicago Press.

Ladefoged, P. (1975). *A course in phonetics.* New York, NY: Harcourt, Brace, Jovanovich.

Ladefoged, P. (2001a). *A course in phonetics* (4th ed.). Orlando, FL: Harcourt College Publishers.

Ladefoged, P. (2001b). *Vowels and consonants: An introduction to the sounds of languages.* Oxford: Blackwell.

Ladefoged, P. (2005). *Vowels and consonants* (2nd ed.). Oxford, UK: Blackwell.

Lagerberg, T. B., Åsberg, J., Hartelius, L., & Persson, C. (2014). Assessment of intelligibility using children's spontaneous speech: Methodological aspects. *International Journal of Language and Communication Disorders, 49*(2), 228–239.

Lagerberg, T. B., Hartelius, L., Johnels, J. Å., Ahlman, A.-K., Börjesson, A., & Persson, C. (2015). Swedish Test of Intelligibility for Children (STI-CH): Validity and reliability of a computer-mediated single word intelligibility test for children. *Clinical Linguistics and Phonetics, 29*(3), 201–215.

Lai, C. S. L., Fisher, S. E., Hurst, J. A., Vargha-Khadem, F., & Monaco, A. P. (2001). A forkhead-domain gene is mutated in severe speech and language disorder. *Nature, 413,* 519–523.

Lai, K. Y., Skuse, D., Stanhope, R., & Hindmarsh, P. (1994). Cognitive abilities associated with the Silver-Russell syndrome. *Archives of Disease in Childhood, 71*(6), 490–496.

Lancaster, G., Keusch, S., Levin, A., Pring, T., & Martin, S. (2010). Treating children with phonological problems: does an eclectic approach to therapy work? *International Journal of Language and Communication Disorders, 45*(2), 174–181.

Larrivee, L. S., & Catts, H. W. (1999). Early reading achievement in children with expressive phonological disorders. *American Journal of Speech-Language Pathology, 8,* 118–128.

Law, J., Boyle, J., Harris, F., Harkness, A., & Nye, C. (1998). Screening for speech and language delay: A systematic review of the literature. *Health Technology and Assessment, 2*(9), 1–183.

Law, J., Boyle, J., Harris, F., Harkness, A., & Nye, C. (2000). Prevalence and natural history of primary speech and language delay: Findings from a systematic review of the literature. *International Journal of Language and Communication Disorders, 35*(2), 165–188.

Law, J., Garrett, Z., & Nye, C. (2003). Speech and language therapy interventions for children with primary speech and language delay or disorder. *Cochrane Database of Systematic Reviews, 3,* CD004110.

Law, J., Garrett, Z., & Nye, C. (2010). Speech and language therapy interventions for children with primary speech and language delay or disorder (Review). *Cochrane Database of Systematic Reviews, 5.* doi: 10.1002/14651858.CD004110

Law, J., Garrett, Z., Nye, C., & Dennis, J. A. (2012). Speech and language therapy interventions for children with primary speech and language delay or disorder: Update. *Cochrane Database of Systematic Reviews 2003, 3,* CD004110.

Law, N. C. W., & So, L. K. H. (2006). The relationship of phonological development and language dominance in bilingual Cantonese-Putonghua children. *International Journal of Bilingualism, 10*(4), 405–427.

Lawson, E., Scobbie, J. M., & Stuart-Smith, J. (2013). Bunched /r/ promotes vowel merger to schwar: An ultrasound tongue imaging study of Scottish sociophonetic variation. *Journal of Phonetics, 41*(3–4), 198–210.

Lawson, E., Stuart-Smith, J., Scobbie, J. M., Nakai, S., Beavan, D., Edmonds, F., Edmonds, I., Turk, A., Timmins, C., Beck, J., Esling, J., Leplatre, G., Cowen S., Barras, W., & Durham, M. (2015). *Seeing speech: An articulatory web resource for the study of phonetics.* Glasgow, Scotland: University of Glasgow. Retrieved from http://www.seeingspeech.ac.uk/.

Lee, A.-Y., & Gibbon, F. (2015). Non-speech oral motor treatment for children with developmental speech sound disorders. *Cochrane Database of Systematic Reviews, 3,* CD009383.

Lee, K. Y. S. (2006). *Cantonese Basic Speech Perception Test.* Hong Kong, SAR China: The Chinese University of Hong Kong.

Lee, K. Y. S. (2010). *Hong Kong Cantonese Tone Identification Test.* Hong Kong, SAR China: Department of Otorhinolaryngology, Head and Neck Surgery, The Chinese University of Hong Kong.

Leitão, S., & Fletcher, J. (2004). Literacy outcomes for students with speech impairment: Long-term follow-up. *International Journal of Language and Communication Disorders, 39,* 245–256.

Lenden, J. M., & Flipsen, P., Jr. (2007). Prosody and voice characteristics of children with cochlear implants. *Journal of Communication Disorders, 40*(1), 66–81.

Leonard, L. B., & McGregor, K. K. (1991). Unusual phonological patterns and their underlying representations: A case study. *Journal of Child Language, 18*, 261–271.

Leonard, L. B., Schwartz, R. G., Folger, M. K., & Wilcox, M. J. (1978). Some aspects of child phonology in imitative and spontaneous speech. *Journal of Child Language, 5*, 403–415.

Leopold, W. (1947). *Speech development of a bilingual child: A linguist's record. Vol. 2: Sound learning in the first two years*. Evanstown, IL: Northwestern University Press.

Levelt, W. J. M., Roelofs, A., & Meyer, A. S. (1999). A theory of lexical access in speech production. *Behavioral and Brain Sciences, 22*, 1–75.

Levy, E. S. (2014). Implementing two treatment approaches to childhood dysarthria. *International Journal of Speech-Language Pathology, 16*(4), 344–354.

Levy, E. S., Ramig, L. O., & Camarata, S. (2012). The effects of two speech interventions on speech function in pediatric dysarthria. *Journal of Medical Speech-Language Pathology, 20*(4), 82–87.

Lewis, B. A., Ekelman, B. L., & Aram, D. M. (1989). A familial study of severe phonological disorders. *Journal of Speech and Hearing Research, 32*, 713–724.

Lewis, B. A., & Freebairn, L. (1992). Residual effects of preschool phonology disorders in grade school, adolescence, and adulthood. *Journal of Speech and Hearing Research, 35*, 819–831.

Lewis, B. A., & Freebairn, L. (1993). A clinical tool for evaluating the familial basis of speech and language disorders. *American Journal of Speech-Language Pathology, 2*, 38–43.

Lewis, B. A., Freebairn, L. A., Hansen, A. J., Miscimarra, L., Iyengar, S. K., & Taylor, H. G. (2007). Speech and language skills of parents of children with speech sound disorders. *American Journal of Speech-Language Pathology, 16*, 108–118.

Lewis, B. A., Freebairn, L. A., Hansen, A. J., Stein, C. M., Shriberg, L. D., Iyengar, S. K., & Taylor, H. G. (2006). Dimensions of early speech sound disorders: A factor analytic study. *Journal of Communication Disorders, 39*(2), 139–157.

Lewis, B. A., Freebairn, L., Tag, J., Ciesla, A. A., Iyengar, S. K., Stein, C. M., & Taylor, H. G. (2015). Adolescent outcomes of children with early speech sound disorders with and without language impairment. *American Journal of Speech-Language Pathology, 24*(2), 150–163.

Lewis, B. A., Freebairn, L. A., & Taylor, H. G. (2000a). Academic outcomes in children with histories of speech sound disorders. *Journal of Communication Disorders, 33*(1), 11–30.

Lewis, B. A., Freebairn, L. A., & Taylor, H. G. (2000b). Follow-up of children with early expressive phonology disorders. *Journal of Learning Disabilities, 33*, 433–444.

Lewis, B. A., Freebairn, L. A., & Taylor, H. G. (2000c). Predicting school-age outcomes for children with histories of speech sound disorders. *Journal of Communication Disorders, 33*, 11–30.

Lewis, B. A., Freebairn, L. A., & Taylor, H. G. (2002). Correlates of spelling abilities in children with early speech sound disorders. *Reading and Writing: An Interdisciplinary Journal, 15*, 389–407.

Lewis, B. A., Short, E. J., Iyengar, S. K., Taylor, H. G., Freebairn, L., Tag, J., . . . Stein, C. M. (2012). Speech-sound disorders and attention-deficit/hyperactivity disorder symptoms. *Topics in Language Disorders, 32*(3), 247–263.

Lewis, B. A., Shriberg, L. D., Freebairn, L. A., Hansen, A. J., Stein, C. M., Taylor, H. G., & Iyengar, S. K. (2006). The genetic bases of speech sound disorders: Evidence from spoken and written language. *Journal of Speech, Language, and Hearing Research, 49*(6), 1294–1312.

Lewis, M. P., Simons, G. F., & Fennig, C. D. (Eds.). (2016). *Ethnologue: Languages of the world* (19th ed.). Dallas, TX: SIL International. Online version: http://www.ethnologue.com.

Leydekker-Brinkman, W. J. M., & Bast, A. (2002). *Manual translated from Metaphon Resource Pack*. Leiden, The Netherlands: Swets & Zeitlinger.

Liberman, A. M., Cooper, F. S., Harris, K. S., & MacNeilage, P. F. (1962). *A motor theory of speech perception*. Proceedings of the Speech Communication Seminar, Stockholm, Sweden.

Liberman, A. M., Cooper, F. S., Shankweiler, D. P., & Studdert-Kennedy, M. (1967). Perception of the speech code. *Psychological Review, 74*(6), 431–461.

Liégeois, F., Morgan, A. T., Stewart, L. H., Helen Cross, J., Vogel, A. P., & Vargha-Khadem, F. (2010). Speech and oral motor profile after childhood hemispherectomy. *Brain and Language, 114*(2), 126–134.

Lillvik, M., Allemark, E., Karlström, P., & Hartelius, L. (1999). Intelligibility of dysarthric speech in words and sentences: Development of a computerised assessment procedure in Swedish. *Logopedics Phoniatrics Vocology, 24*(3), 107–119.

Lim, V. P. C., Liow, S. J. R., Lincoln, M., Chan, Y. H., & Onslow, M. (2008). Determining language dominance in English-Mandarin bilinguals: Development of a self-report classification tool for clinical use. *Applied Psycholinguistics, 29*, 389–412.

Limbrick, N., McCormack, J., & McLeod, S. (2013). Designs and decisions: The creation of informal measures for assessing speech production in children. *International Journal of Speech-Language Pathology, 15*(3), 296–311.

Linares, T. A. (1981). Articulation skills in Spanish-speaking children. In R. Padilla (Ed.), *Ethnoperspectives in bilingual education research: Bilingual education technology* (pp. 363–367). Ypsilanti, MI: Eastern Michigan University Press.

Ling, D. (1976). *Speech and the hearing-impaired child: Theory and practice*. Washington, DC: Alexander Graham Bell Association for the Deaf.

Ling, D. (1989). *Foundations of spoken language for the hearing-impaired child*. Washington, DC: Alexander Graham Bell Association for the Deaf.

LinguiSystems. (2007). *Preschool phonology cards*. East Moline, IL: LinguiSystems.

Lipetz, H. M., & Bernhardt, B. M. (2013). A multi-modal approach to intervention for one adolescent's frontal lisp. *Clinical Linguistics and Phonetics, 27*(1), 1–17.

Lippke, B. A., Dickey, S. E., Selmar, J. W., & Soder, A. L. (1997). *Photo Articulation Test* (3rd ed.). Austin, TX: Pro-Ed.

Lisman, A. L., & Sadagopan, N. (2013). Focus of attention and speech motor performance. *Journal of Communication Disorders, 46*(3), 281–293.

Lively, S. E., Logan, J. S., & Pisoni, D. B. (1993). Training Japanese listeners to identify English /r/ and /l/ II: The role of phonetic environment and talker variability in learning new perceptual categories. *Journal of the Acoustical Society of America, 94*(3), 1242–1255.

Lleó, C. (1990). Homonymy and reduplication: On the extended availability of two strategies in phonological acquisition. *Journal of Child Language, 17*, 267–278.

Lleó, C., & Prinz, M. (1996). Consonant clusters in child phonology and the directionality of syllable structure assignment. *Journal of Child Language, 23*, 31–56.

Lockart, R., & McLeod, S. (2013). Factors that enhance English-speaking speech-language pathologists' transcription of Cantonese-speaking children's consonants. *American Journal of Speech-Language Pathology, 22*(3), 523–539.

Locke, J. L. (1980a). The inference of speech perception in the phonologically disorder child. Part I: A rationale, some criteria, the conventional tests. *Journal of Speech and Hearing Disorders, 4*, 431–444.

Locke, J. L. (1980b). The inference of speech perception in the phonologically disordered child. Part II: Some clinically novel procedures, their use, some findings. *Journal of Speech and Hearing Disorders, 45*(4), 445–468.

Locke, J. L. (1983). *Phonological acquisition and change*. New York, NY: Academic Press.

Lof, G. L. (2003). Oral motor exercises and treatment outcomes. *Perspectives on Language Learning and Education, 10*(1), 7–11.

Lof, G. L. (2011). Science-based practice and the speech-language pathologist. *International Journal of Speech-Language Pathology, 13*(3), 189–196.

Lof, G. L. (2015). The nonspeech-oral motor exercise phenomenon in speech pathology practice. In C. Bowen (Ed.), *Children's speech sound disorders* (2nd ed.). Oxford, UK: Wiley-Blackwell.

Lohmander, A., Borell, E., Henningsson, G., Havstam, C., Lundeborg, I., & Persson, C. (2005). *SVANTE- Svenskt artikulations-och Nasalittets Test (Swedish Articulation and Nasality Test) [in Swedish]*. Skivarp, Sweden: Pedagogisk Design.

Lollar, D. J., & Simeonsson, R. J. (2005). Diagnosis to function: Classification for children and youths. *Journal of Developmental and Behavioral Pediatrics, 26*(4), 323–330.

Long, S. H. (2001). About time: A comparison of computerised and manual procedures for grammatical and phonological analysis. *Clinical Linguistics and Phonetics, 15*(5), 399–426.

Long, S. (2008). *Computerized profiling* (version 9.7.0) [Computer program]. Retrieved from http://computerizedprofiling.org/.

Lonigan, C. J., Burgess, S. R., Anthony, J. L., & Barker, T. A. (1998). Development of phonological sensitivity in 2- to 5-year-old children. *Journal of Educational Psychology, 90*, 294–311.

Lonigan, C. J., Wagner, R. K., Torgesen, J. K., & Rashotte, C. (2002). *Preschool Comprehensive Test of Phonological and Print Processing.* Austin, TX: Pro-Ed.

Lorwatanapongsa, P., & Maroonroge, S. (2007). Thai speech acquisition. In S. McLeod (Ed.), *The international guide to speech acquisition* (pp. 554–565). Clifton Park, NY: Thomson Delmar Learning.

Lotto, A. J., Hickok, G. S., & Holt, L. L. (2009). Reflections on mirror neurons and speech perception. *Trends in Cognitive Sciences, 13*(3), 110–114.

Lousada, M., Jesus, L. M. T., Capelas, S., Margaça, C., Simões, D., Valente, A., . . . Joffe, V. L. (2013). Phonological and articulation treatment approaches in Portuguese children with speech and language impairments: A randomized controlled intervention study. *International Journal of Language and Communication Disorders, 48*(2), 172–187.

Lousada, M., Jesus, L. M. T., Hall, A., & Joffe, V. (2014). Intelligibility as a clinical outcome measure following intervention with children with phonologically based speech–sound disorders. *International Journal of Language and Communication Disorders, 49*(5), 584–601.

Love, R. J. (1992). *Childhood motor speech disability.* Needham Heights, MA: Allyn & Bacon.

Love, R. J. (2000). *Childhood motor speech disability* (2nd ed.). Needham Heights, MA: Allyn & Bacon.

Low, E. L., Grabe, E., & Nolan, F. (2000). Quantitative characterizations of speech rhythm: Syllable-timing in Singapore English. *Language and Speech, 43*, 377–401.

Lowe, R. J. (1994). *Phonology: Assessment and intervention application in speech pathology.* Baltimore, MD: Williams and Wilkins.

Lowe, R. J., Knutson, P. J., & Monson, M. A. (1985). Incidence of fronting in preschool children. *Language, Speech, and Hearing Services in Schools, 16*, 119–123.

Lundeborg, I., & McAllister, A. (2007). Treatment with a combination of intra-oral sensory stimulation and electropalatography in a child with severe developmental dyspraxia. *Logopedics Phoniatrics Vocology, 32*, 71–79.

Luotonen, M. (1998). *Factors associated with linguistic development and school performance: The role of early otitis media, gender, and day care.* Acta Universitatis Ouluensis, series D Medica, *453*, Oulu, Finland: University of Oulu.

Lyytinen, H., Ahonen, T., Eklund, K., Guttorm, T. K., Laakso, M.-L., Leinonen, S., . . . Viholainen, H. (2001). Developmental pathways of children with and without familial risk for dyslexia during the first years of life. *Developmental Neuropsychology, 20*(2), 535–554.

Maas, E., Butalla, C. E., & Farinella, K. A. (2012). Feedback frequency in treatment for childhood apraxia of speech. *American Journal of Speech-Language Pathology, 21*(3), 239–257.

Maas, E., & Farinella, K. A. (2012). Random versus blocked practice in treatment for childhood apraxia of speech. *Journal of Speech, Language, and Hearing Research, 55*(2), 561–578.

Maas, E., Robin, D. A., Hula, S. N. A., Freedman, S. E., Wulf, G., Ballard, K. J., & Schmidt, R. A. (2008). Principles of motor learning in treatment of motor speech disorders. *American Journal of Speech-Language Pathology, 17*, 277–298.

Maassen, B. (2002). Issues contrasting adult acquired versus developmental apraxia of speech. *Seminars in Speech and Language, 23*, 257–266.

Maassen, B., & van Lieshout, P. (Eds.). (2010). *Speech motor control: New developments in basic and applied research.* New York, NY: Oxford University Press.

Macharey, G., & von Suchodoletz, W. (2008). Perceived stigmatization of children with speech-language impairment and their parents. *Folia Phoniatrica et Logopaedica, 60*(5), 256-263.

Macken, M. A., & Barton, D. (1980). The acquisition of the voicing contrast in English: A study of voice onset time in word-initial stop consonants. *Journal of Child Language, 7*, 41–74.

Maclagan, M. (2009). Reflecting connections with the local language: New Zealand English. *International Journal of Speech-Language Pathology, 11*(2), 113–121.

Maclagan, M., & Gillon, G. T. (2007). New Zealand English speech acquisition In S. McLeod (Ed.), *The international guide to speech acquisition* (pp. 257–268). Clifton Park, NY: Thomson Delmar Learning.

MacLean, M., Bryant, P., & Bradley, L. (1987). Rhymes, nursery rhymes, and reading in early childhood. *Merrill-Palmer Quarterly, 33*, 255–282.

MacLeod, A. A. N., & Glaspey, A. M. (2014). A multidimensional view of gradient change in velar acquisition in three-year-olds receiving phonological treatment. *Clinical Linguistics and Phonetics, 28*(9), 664–681.

MacLeod, A. A. N., Sutton, A., Trudeau, N., & Thordardottir, E. (2011). The acquisition of consonants in Quebecois French: A cross-sectional study of pre-school aged children. *International Journal of Speech-Language Pathology, 13*(2), 93–109.

Macrae, T., & Tyler, A. A. (2014). Speech abilities in preschool children with speech sound disorder with and without co-occurring language impairment. *Language, Speech, and Hearing Services in Schools, 45*(4), 302–313.

Maddieson, I. (2008a). Consonant inventories. In M. Haspelmath, M. S. Dryer, D. Gil, & B. Comrie (Eds.), *The world atlas of language structures online.* Munich, Germany: Max Planck Digital Library. Retrieved from http://wals.info/chapter/1.

Maddieson, I. (2008b). Presence of uncommon consonants. In M. Haspelmath, M. S. Dryer, D. Gil, & B. Comrie (Eds.), *The world atlas of language structures online.* Munich, Germany: Max Planck Digital Library. Retrieved from http://wals.info/feature/19.

Maddieson, I. (2008c). Vowel quality inventories. In M. Haspelmath, M. S. Dryer, D. Gil, & B. Comrie (Eds.), *The world atlas of language structures online.* Munich, Germany: Max Planck Digital Library. Retrieved from http://wals.info/chapter/2.

Maher, C. G., Sherrington, C., Herbert, R. D., Mosley, A., & Elkins, M. (2003). Reliability of the PEDro Scale for rating quality of randomized controlled trials. *Physical Therapy, 83*, 713–721.

Major, E. M., & Bernhardt, B. H. (1998). Metaphonological skills of children with phonological disorders before and after phonological and metaphonological intervention. *International Journal of Language and Communication Disorders, 33*(4), 413–444.

Mampe, B., Friederici, A. D., Christophe, A., & Wermke, K. (2009). Newborns' cry melody is shaped by their native language. *Current Biology, 19*, 1994–1997.

Marchant, J., McAuliffe, M. J., & Huckabee, M.-L. (2008). Treatment of articulatory impairment in a child with spastic dysarthria associated with cerebral palsy. *Developmental Neurorehabilitation, 11*(1), 81–90.

Marian, V., Blumenfeld, H. K., & Kaushanskaya, M. (2007). The Language Experience and Proficiency Questionnaire (LEAP-Q): Assessing language profiles in bilinguals and multilinguals. *Journal of Speech, Language, and Hearing Research, 50*(4), 940–967.

Markham, C., & Dean, T. (2006). Parents' and professionals' perceptions of quality of life in children with speech and language difficulty. *International Journal of Language and Communication Disorders, 41*(2), 189–212.

Markham, C., van Laar, D., Gibbard, D., & Dean, T. (2009). Children with speech, language and communication needs: Their perceptions of their quality of life. *International Journal of Language and Communication Disorders, 44*(5), 748–768.

Marshall, C. R., Harcourt-Brown, S., Ramus, F., & van der Lely, H. K. J. (2009). The link between prosody and language skills in children with specific language impairment (SLI) and/or dyslexia. *International Journal of Language and Communication Disorders, 44*(4), 466–488.

Marshalla, P. (2007). *Frontal lisp, lateral lisp: Articulation and oro-motor procedures for diagnosis and treatment.* Mill Creek, WA: Marshalla Speech and Language.

Marshalla, P. (2010). *Carryover techniques in articulation and phonological therapy.* Mill Creek, WA: Marshalla Speech and Language.

Martikainen, A., & Korpilahti, P. (2011). Intervention for childhood apraxia of speech: A single-case study. *Child Language Teaching and Therapy, 27*(1), 9–20.

Martin, K. L., Hirson, A., Herman, R., Thomas, J., & Pring, T. (2007). The efficacy of speech intervention using electropalatography with an 18-year-old deaf client: A single case study. *International Journal of Speech-Language Pathology, 9*(1), 46–56.

Martin, N., & Brownell, R. (2005). *Test of Auditory Processing Skills: Third Edition (TAPS-3)*. Novato, CA: Academic Therapy Publications.

Martínez-Castilla, P., & Peppé, S. (2008). Intonation features of the expression of emotions in Spanish: Preliminary study for a prosody assessment procedure. *Clinical Linguistics and Phonetics, 22*(4), 363–370.

Masso, S., McCabe, P., & Baker, E. (2014). How do children with phonological impairment respond to requests for clarification containing polysyllables? *Child Language Teaching and Therapy, 30*(3), 367–382.

Masso, S., McLeod, S., Baker, E., & McCormack, J. (2016). Polysyllable productions in preschool children with speech and sound disorders: Error categories and the Framework of Polysyllable Maturity. *International Journal of Speech-Language Pathology.* doi: 10.3109/17549507.2016.1168483.

Masterson, J. J. (1993). Classroom-based phonological intervention. *American Journal of Speech-Language Pathology, 2*(1), 5–9.

Masterson, J., & Bernhardt, B. H. (2001). *Computerized Articulation and Phonology Evaluation System (CAPES)*. San Antonio, TX: The Psychological Corporation.

Masterson, J., & Daniels, D. (1991). Motoric versus contrastive approaches to phonology therapy: A case study. *Child Language Teaching and Therapy, 7*(2), 127–140.

Mattes, L. J. (1995). *Spanish Articulation Measures: Revised edition*. Oceanside, CA: Academic Communication Associates.

McAllister Byun, T., & Hitchcock, E. R. (2012). Investigating the use of traditional and spectral biofeedback approaches to intervention for /r/ misarticulation. *American Journal of Speech-Language Pathology, 21*(3), 207–221.

McAllister Byun, T., Hitchcock, E. R., & Swartz, M. T. (2014). Retroflex versus bunched in treatment for rhotic misarticulation: Evidence from ultrasound biofeedback intervention. *Journal of Speech, Language, and Hearing Research, 57*(6), 2116–2130.

McAuliffe, M. J., & Cornwell, P. L. (2008). Intervention for lateral /s/ using electropalatography (EPG) biofeedback and an intensive motor learning approach: A case report. *International Journal of Language and Communication Disorders, 43*(2), 219–229.

McCabe, P., & Ballard, K. (2015). ReST program. In C. Bowen (Ed.), *Children's speech sound disorders* (2nd ed.). Oxford, UK: Wiley-Blackwell.

McCabe, P., Macdonald-D'Silva, A. G., van Rees, L. J., Ballard, K. J., & Arciuli, J. (2014). Orthographically sensitive treatment for dysprosody in children with childhood apraxia of speech using ReST intervention. *Developmental Neurorehabilitation, 17*(2), 137–145.

McCabe, P., Rosenthal, J., & McLeod, S. (1998). Features of developmental dyspraxia in the speech-impaired population? *Clinical Linguistics and Phonetics, 12*, 105–126.

McCabe, R. B., & Bradley, D. P. (1973). Pre- and post-articulation therapy assessment. *Language, Speech, and Hearing Services in Schools, 4*, 13–22.

McCabe, R., & Bradley, D. P. (1975). Systematic multiple phonemic approach to articulation therapy. *Acta Symbolica, 61*, 1–18.

McCann, J., Peppé, S., Gibbon, F. E., O'Hare, A., & Rutherford, M. (2007). Prosody and its relationship to language in school-aged children with high-functioning autism. *International Journal of Language and Communication Disorders, 42*(6), 682–702.

McCarty, C., & Ruttle, K. (2012). *Phonics and early reading assessment*. Oxon, UK: Hodder Education.

McCauley, R. J., & Strand, E. A. (2008). A review of standardized tests of nonverbal oral and speech motor performance in children. *American Journal of Speech-Language Pathology, 17*(1), 81–91.

McCauley, R. J., Strand, E., Lof, G. L., Schooling, T., & Frymark, T. (2009). Evidence-based systematic review: Effects of nonspeech oral motor exercises on speech. *American Journal of Speech-Language Pathology, 18*(4), 343–360.

McCauley, R. J., & Swisher, L. (1984a). Psychometric review of language and articulation tests for preschool children. *Journal of Speech and Hearing Disorders, 49*(1), 34–42.

McCauley, R. J., & Swisher, L. (1984b). Use and misuse of norm referenced tests in clinical assessment: A hypothetical case. *Journal of Speech and Hearing Disorders, 49*, 338–348.

McClowry, S. G. (1995). The development of the School-Age Temperament Inventory. *Merrill-Palmer Quarterly, 41*(3), 271–285.

McCormack, J., Harrison, L. J., McLeod, S., & McAllister, L. (2011). A nationally representative study of the association between communication impairment at 4–5 years and children's life activities at 7–9 years. *Journal of Speech, Language, and Hearing Research, 54*(5), 1328–1348.

McCormack, J., McAllister, L. McLeod, S. & Harrison, L. J., (2012). Knowing, having, doing: The battles of childhood speech impairment. *Child Language Teaching and Therapy, 28*, 141–157.

McCormack, J., McLeod, S., Harrison, L. J., & McAllister, L. (2010). The impact of speech impairment in early childhood: Investigating parents' and speech-language pathologists' perspectives using the ICF-CY. *Journal of Communication Disorders, 43*(5), 378–396.

McCormack, J., McLeod, S., McAllister, L., & Harrison, L. J. (2009). A systematic review of the association between childhood speech impairment and participation across the lifespan. *International Journal of Speech-Language Pathology, 11*(2), 155–170.

McCormack, J., McLeod, S., McAllister, L., & Harrison, L. J. (2010). My speech problem, your listening problem, and my frustration: The experience of living with childhood speech impairment. *Language, Speech, and Hearing Services in Schools, 41*(4), 379–392.

McDermott, R. P. (1993). The acquisition of a child by a learning disability. In S. Chaiklin & J. Love (Eds.), *Understanding practice: Perspectives on activity and context* (pp. 269–305). Cambridge, UK: Cambridge University Press.

McDonagh, S. H. (2015). Literacy: Reading. In S. McLeod & J. McCormack (Eds), *Introduction to speech, language and literacy* (pp. 349–397). Melbourne, Australia: Oxford University Press.

McDowell, K. B., Lonigan, K. J., & Goldstein, H. (2007). Relations among socio-economic status, age, and predictors of phonological awareness. *Journal of Speech, Language, and Hearing Research, 50*, 1079–1092.

McGlaughlin, A., & Grayson, A. (2003). A cross sectional and prospective study of crying in the first year of life. In S. P. Sohov (Ed.), *Advances in psychology research* (Vol. 22, pp. 37–58). New York, NY: Nova Science.

McGowan, R. W., McGowan, R. S., Denny, M., & Nittrouer, S. (2014). A longitudinal study of very young children's vowel production. *Journal of Speech, Language, and Hearing Research, 57*(1), 1–15.

McGrath, L. M., Hutaff-Lee, C., Scott, A., Boada, R., Shriberg, L. D., & Pennington, B. F. (2008). Children with comorbid speech sound disorder and specific language impairment are at increased risk for attention-deficit/hyperactivity disorder. *Journal of Abnormal Child Psychology, 36*, 151–163.

McGregor, K. K. (2008). Gesture supports children's word learning. *International Journal of Speech-Language Pathology, 10*(3), 112–117.

McGregor, K. K., & Johnson, A. C. (1997). Trochaic template use in early words and phrases. *Journal of Speech, Language, and Hearing Research, 40*(6), 1220–1231.

McGregor, K. K., & Schwartz, R. G. (1992). Converging evidence for underlying phonological representation in a child who misarticulates. *Journal of Speech and Hearing Research, 35*(3), 596–603.

McGurk, H., & MacDonald, J. (1976). Hearing lips and seeing voices. *Nature, 264*, 746–748.

McHugh, M. (2003). *Special siblings: Growing up with someone with a disability* (revised ed.). Baltimore, MD: Paul H. Brookes.

McIntosh, B., & Dodd, B. (2008). Two-year-olds' phonological acquisition: Normative data. *International Journal of Speech-Language Pathology, 10*(6), 460–469.

McIntosh, B., & Dodd, B. (2009). Evaluation of core vocabulary intervention for treatment of inconsistent phonological disorder: Three treatment case studies. *Child Language Teaching and Therapy, 25*(1), 9–24.

McIntosh, B., & Dodd, B. (2011). *Toddler Phonology Test* (TPT). Austin, TX: Pearson.

McKercher, M., McFarlane, L., & Schneider, P. (1995). Phonological treatment dismissal: Optimal criteria. *Journal of Speech-Language Pathology and Audiology, 19*, 115–123.

McKinnon, D. H., McLeod, S., & Reilly, S. (2007). The prevalence of stuttering, voice and speech-sound disorders in primary school students in Australia. *Language, Speech, and Hearing Services in Schools, 38*(1), 5–15.

McKinnon, S. L., Hess, C. W., & Landry, R. G. (1986). Reactions of college students to speech disorders. *Journal of Communication Disorders, 19*(1), 75–82.

McLeod, S. (1997). Sampling consonant clusters: Four procedures designed for Australian children. *Australian Communication Quarterly, Autumn,* 9–12.

McLeod, S. (2004). Speech pathologists' application of the ICF to children with speech impairment. *International Journal of Speech-Language Pathology, 6*(1), 75–81.

McLeod, S. (2006a). Perspectives on a child with unintelligible speech. *International Journal of Speech-Language Pathology, 8*(3), 153–155.

McLeod, S. (2006b). An holistic view of a child with unintelligible speech: Insights from the ICF and ICF-CY. *International Journal of Speech-Language Pathology, 8*(3), 293–315.

McLeod, S. (Ed). (2007a). *The international guide to speech acquisition.* Clifton Park, NY: Thomson Delmar Learning.

McLeod, S. (2007b). Australian English speech acquisition. In S. McLeod (Ed.), *The international guide to speech acquisition* (pp. 241–256). Clifton Park, NY: Thomson Delmar Learning.

McLeod, S. (2010). Laying the foundations for multilingual acquisition: An international overview of speech acquisition. In M. Cruz-Ferreira (Ed.), *Multilingual norms* (pp. 53–71). Frankfurt, Germany: Peter Lang Publishing.

McLeod, S. (2011). Speech-language pathologists' knowledge of tongue/palate contact for consonants. *Clinical Linguistics and Phonetics, 25*(11–12), 1004–1013.

McLeod, S. (2012a). Multilingual speech assessment. In S. McLeod & B. A. Goldstein (Eds.), *Multilingual aspects of speech sound disorders in children* (pp. 113–143). Bristol, UK: Multilingual Matters.

McLeod, S. (2012b). *Multilingual children's speech.* Bathurst, Australia: Charles Sturt University. Retrieved from http://www.csu.edu.au/research/multilingual-speech/

McLeod, S., & Arciuli, J. (2009). School-aged children's production of /s/ and /r/ consonant clusters. *Folia Phoniatrica et Logopaedica, 61*(6), 336–341.

McLeod, S., & Baker, E. (2014). Speech-language pathologists' practices regarding assessment, analysis, target selection, intervention, and service delivery for children with speech sound disorders. *Clinical Linguistics and Phonetics, 28*(7–8), 508–531.

McLeod, S., & Bleile, K. M. (2004). The ICF: A framework for setting goals for children with speech impairment. *Child Language Teaching and Therapy, 20*(3), 199–219.

McLeod, S., Crowe, K., & Shahaeian, A. (2015). Intelligibility in Context Scale: Normative and validation data for English-speaking preschoolers. *Language, Speech, and Hearing Services in Schools, 46*(3), 266–276.

McLeod, S., Crowe, K., McCormack, J., White, P., Wren, Y., Baker, E., Masso, S., & Roulstone, S. (2015). *Preschool children's communication, motor and social development: What concerns parents and educators?* Manuscript in submission.

McLeod, S., Daniel, G., & Barr, J. (2006). Using children's drawings to listen to how children feel about their speech. In C. Heine & L. Brown (Eds.), *Proceedings of the 2006 Speech Pathology Australia National Conference* (pp. 38–45). Melbourne, Australia: Speech Pathology Australia.

McLeod, S., Daniel, G., & Barr, J. (2013). "When he's around his brothers . . . he's not so quiet": The private and public worlds of school-aged children with speech sound disorder. *Journal of Communication Disorders, 46*(1), 70–83.

McLeod, S., Hand, L., Rosenthal, J. B., & Hayes, B. (1994). The effect of sampling condition on children's productions of consonant clusters. *Journal of Speech and Hearing Research, 37,* 868–882.

McLeod, S., & Harrison, L. J. (2009). Epidemiology of speech and language impairment in a nationally representative sample of 4- to 5-year-old children. *Journal of Speech, Language, and Hearing Research, 52*(5), 1213–1229.

McLeod, S., Harrison, L. J., Holliday, E. L., McCormack, J., & McAllister, L. (2010, June). *Children draw talking: Art exhibition* [Invited address and art exhibition]. *International Clinical Phonetics and Linguistics Association,* Oslo, Norway.

McLeod, S., Harrison, L. J., McAllister, L., & McCormack, J. (2013). Speech sound disorders in a community study of preschool children. *American Journal of Speech-Language Pathology, 22*(3), 503–522.

McLeod, S., Harrison, L. J., & McCormack, J. (2012a). *Intelligibility in Context Scale.* Bathurst, Australia: Charles Sturt University. Retrieved from http://www.csu.edu.au/research/multilingual-speech/ics.

McLeod, S., Harrison, L. J., & McCormack, J. (2012b). Intelligibility in Context Scale: Validity and reliability of a subjective rating measure. *Journal of Speech, Language, and Hearing Research, 55*(2), 648–656.

McLeod, S., Harrison, L. J., & McCormack, J. (2012c). *Escala de Inteligibilidad en Contexto* [Intelligibility in Context Scale: Spanish] (R. Prezas, R. Rojas, & B. A. Goldstein, Trans.). Bathurst, NSW, Australia: Charles Sturt University. Retrieved from http://www.csu.edu.au/research/multilingual-speech/ics.

McLeod, S., Harrison, L. J., Whiteford, C., & Walker, S. (2016). Multilingualism and speech-language competence in early childhood: Impact on academic and social-emotional outcomes at school. *Early Childhood Research Quarterly, 34,* 53–66.

McLeod, S., & Hewett, S. R. (2008). Variability in the production of words containing consonant clusters by typical two- and three-year-old children. *Folia Phoniatrica et Logopaedica, 60,* 163–172.

McLeod, S., & Isaac, K. (1995). Use of spectrographic analyses to evaluate the efficacy of phonological intervention. *Clinical Linguistics and Phonetics, 9,* 229–234.

McLeod, S., McAllister, L., McCormack, J., & Harrison, L. J. (2014). Applying the World Report on Disability to children's communication. *Disability and Rehabilitation, 36*(18), 1518–1528.

McLeod, S., & McCormack, J. (2007). Application of the ICF and ICF-Children and Youth in children with speech impairment. *Seminars in Speech and Language, 28,* 254–264.

McLeod, S., & McCormack, J. (Eds.). (2015). *Introduction to speech, language and literacy.* Melbourne, Australia: Oxford University Press.

McLeod, S., McCormack, J., McAllister, L., Harrison, L. J., & Holliday, E. L. (2011). Listening to 4- to 5-year-old children with speech impairment using drawings, interviews and questionnaires. In S. Roulstone & S. McLeod (Eds.), *Listening to children and young people with speech, language and communication needs* (pp. 179–186). London, UK: J&R Press.

McLeod, S., & McKinnon, D. H. (2007). The prevalence of communication disorders compared with other learning needs in 14,500 primary and secondary school students. *International Journal of Language and Communication Disorders, 42*(S1), 37–59.

McLeod, S., & McKinnon, D. H. (2010). Required support for primary and secondary students with communication disorders and/or other learning needs. *Child Language Teaching and Therapy, 26*(2), 123–143.

McLeod, S., Press, F., & Phelan, C. (2010). The (in)visibility of children with communication impairment in Australian health, education, and disability legislation and policies. *Asia Pacific Journal of Speech, Language, and Hearing, 13*(1), 67–75.

McLeod, S., & Singh, S. (2009a). *Speech sounds: A pictorial guide to typical and atypical speech.* San Diego, CA: Plural Publishing.

McLeod, S., & Singh, S. (2009b). *Seeing speech: A quick guide to speech sounds.* San Diego, CA: Plural Publishing.

McLeod, S., & Threats, T. T. (2008). The ICF-CY and children with communication disabilities. *International Journal of Speech-Language Pathology, 10*(1), 92–109.

McLeod, S., van Doorn, J., & Reed, V. (1996). Homonyms and cluster reduction in the normal development of children's speech. In P. McCormack & A. Russell (Eds.), *Proceedings of the Sixth Australian International Conference on Speech Science and Technology* (pp. 331–336). Adelaide, Australia: Australian Speech Science and Technology Association.

McLeod, S., van Doorn, J., & Reed, V.A. (1998). Homonyms in children's productions of consonant clusters. In W. Zeigler & K. Deger (Eds.), *Clinical Phonetics and Linguistics* (pp. 108–116). London, UK: Whurr.

McLeod, S., van Doorn, J., & Reed, V. A. (2001a). Normal acquisition of consonant clusters. *American Journal of Speech-Language Pathology*, *10*, 99–110.

McLeod, S., van Doorn, J., & Reed, V. A. (2001b). Consonant cluster development in two-year-olds: General trends and individual difference. *Journal of Speech, Language, Hearing Research, 44*, 1144–1171.

McLeod, S., van Doorn, J., & Reed, V. A. (2002). Typological description of the normal acquisition of consonant clusters. In F. Windsor, L. Kelly, & N. Hewlett (Eds.), *Themes in Clinical Phonetics and Linguistics* (pp. 185–200). Hillsdale, NJ: Lawrence Erlbaum.

McLeod, S., & Verdon, S. (2014). A review of 30 speech assessments in 19 languages other than English. *American Journal of Speech-Language Pathology, 23*(4), 708–723.

McLeod, S., & Wrench, A. (2008). Protocol for restricting head movement when recording ultrasound images of speech. *Asia Pacific Journal of Speech, Language, and Hearing, 11*(1), 23–29.

McNamara, J. A., Jr. (1981). Components of class II malocclusion in children 8 to 10 years of age. *The Angle Orthodontist, 51*(2), 177–202.

McNeill, B. C., Gillon, G. T., & Dodd, B. (2009a). Effectiveness of an integrated phonological awareness approach for children with childhood apraxia of speech (CAS). *Child Language Teaching and Therapy, 25*(3), 341–366.

McNeill, B. C., Gillon, G. T., & Dodd, B. (2009b). A longitudinal case study of the effects of an integrated phonological awareness program for identical twin boys with childhood apraxia of speech (CAS). *International Journal of Speech-Language Pathology, 11*(6), 482–495.

McNeill, B. C., Gillon, G. T., & Dodd, B. (2010). The longer term effects of an integrated phonological awareness intervention for children with childhood apraxia of speech. *Asia Pacific Journal of Speech, Language, and Hearing, 13*(3), 145–161.

McReynolds, L. V., & Huston, K. (1971). A distinctive feature analysis of children's misarticulations. *Journal of Speech and Hearing Disorders, 36*, 156–166.

McReynolds, L., & Jetzke, E. (1986). Articulation generalization of voiced-voiceless sounds in hearing-impaired children. *Journal of Speech and Hearing Disorders, 51*, 348–355.

Mendes, A,. Afonso, M., Lousada, M., & Andrade, F. (2013). *Teste fonetico-fonologico ALPE (TFF-ALPE)[Phonetic–phonological Test ALPE (TFF-ALPE)]*. Aveiro, Portugal: Edubox.

Menn, L. (1971). Phonotactic rules in beginning speech. *Lingua, 26*, 225–241.

Menn, L. (1983). Development of articulatory, phonetic and phonological capabilities. In B. Butterworth (Ed.), *Language production* (Vol. 2, pp. 3–50). London, UK: Academic Press.

Menn, L., & Matthei, E. (1992). The "two-lexicon" account of child phonology looking back, looking ahead. In C. A. Ferguson, L. Menn, & C. Stoel-Gammon (Eds.), *Phonological development: Models, research, implications* (pp. 211–247). Timonium, MD: York Press.

Mennen, I., Levelt, C., & Gerrits, E. (2007). Dutch speech acquisition. In S. McLeod (Ed.), *The international guide to speech acquisition* (pp. 327–339). Clifton Park, NY: Thomson Delmar Learning.

Mennen, I., & Okalidou, A. (2007). Greek speech acquisition. In S. McLeod (Ed.), *The international guide to speech acquisition* (pp. 398–411). Clifton Park, NY: Thomson Delmar Learning.

Merrick, R. (2011). Ethics, consent and assent when listening to children with speech, language and communication needs. In S. Roulstone & S. McLeod (Eds.), *Listening to children and young people with speech, language and communication needs* (pp. 63–72). London, UK: J&R Press.

Merrick, R., & Roulstone, S. (2011). Children's views of communication and speech-language pathology. *International Journal of Speech-Language Pathology, 13*(4), 281–290.

Messner, A. H., & Lalakea, M. L. (2000). Ankyloglossia: Controversies in management. *International Journal of Pediatric Otorhinolaryngology, 54*(2–3), 123–131.

Mestala, J. L., & Walley, A. C. (1998). Spoken vocabulary growth and the segmental restructuring of lexical representations: Precursors to phonemic awareness and early reading ability. In J. L. Mestala & L. C. Ehri (Eds.), *Word recognition in beginning literacy*. New York, NY: Erlbaum.

Miccio, A. W. (2002). Clinical problem solving: Assessment of phonological disorders. *American Journal of Speech-Language Pathology, 11*(3), 221–229.

Miccio, A. W. (2005). A treatment program for enhancing stimulability. In A. G. Kamhi & K. E. Pollock (Eds.), *Phonological disorders in children: Clinical decision making in assessment and intervention.* (pp. 163–174). Baltimore, MD: Paul H. Brookes.

Miccio, A. W. (2009). First things first: Stimulability therapy for children with small phonetic repertoires. In C. Bowen (Ed.), *Children's speech sound disorders* (pp. 96–101). Oxford, UK: Wiley-Blackwell.

Miccio, A. W. (2015). First things first: Stimulability therapy for children with small phonetic repertoires. In C. Bowen (Ed.), *Children's speech sound disorders* (pp. 177–182). Oxford, UK: Wiley-Blackwell.

Miccio, A. W., & Elbert, M. (1996). Enhancing stimulability: A treatment program. *Journal of Communication Disorders, 29*(4), 335–351.

Miccio, A. W., Gallagher, E., Grossman, C. B., Yont, K. M., & Vernon-Feagans, L. (2001). Influence of chronic otitis media on phonological acquisition. *Clinical Linguistics and Phonetics, 15*(1–2), 47–51.

Miccio, A. W., & Ingrisano, D. R. (2000). The acquisition of fricatives and affricates: Evidence from a disordered phonological system. *American Journal of Speech-Language Pathology, 9*(3), 214–229.

Miccio, A. W., & Williams, A. L. (2010). Stimulability intervention. In A. L. Williams, S. McLeod, & R. J. McCauley (Eds.), *Interventions for speech sound disorders in children* (pp. 179–202). Baltimore, MD: Paul H. Brookes.

Middleton, E. L., & Schwartz, M. F. (2012). Errorless learning in cognitive rehabilitation: A critical review. *Neuropsychological Rehabilitation, 22*(2), 138–168.

Milenkovic, P. (2001). *Time-frequency analysis for 32-bit windows*. Madison, WI: University of Wisconsin-Madison.

Milisen, R. (1954). The disorder of articulation: A systematic clinical and experimental approach. *Journal of Speech and Hearing Disorders, Monograph Supplement, 4*, 5–17.

Miller, N. (2013). Measuring up to speech intelligibility. *International Journal of Language and Communication Disorders, 48*(6), 601–612.

Mills, L., Gosling, A., & Sell, D. (2006). Extending the communication phenotype associated with 22q11.2 microdeletion syndrome. *International Journal of Speech-Language Pathology, 8*(1), 17–27.

Miltenberger, R. G. (2016). *Behavior modification: Principles and procedures* (2nd ed.). Boston, MA: Cengage.

Mire, S. P., & Montgomery, J. K. (2009). Early intervening for students with speech sound disorders: Lessons from a school district. *Communication Disorders Quarterly, 30*(3), 155–166.

Miscimarra, L., Stein, C., Millard, C., Kluge, A., Cartier, K., Freebairn, L., Iyengar, S. K. (2007). Further evidence of pleiotropy influencing speech and language: Analysis of the DYX8 region. *Human Heredity, 63*, 47–58.

Mitchell, A. (1946). *The pronunciation of English in Australia*. Sydney: Angus & Robertson.

Mitchell, P. R. (1995). A dynamic interactive developmental view of early speech and language production: Application to clinical practice in motor speech disorders. *Seminars in Speech and Language, 16*, 100–109.

Mitchell, P. R. (1997). Prelinguistic vocal development: A clinical primer. *Contemporary Issues in Communication Science and Disorders, 24*, 87–92.

Mitchell, P. R., McMahon, B. T., & McKee, D. (2005). Speech impairment and workplace discrimination: The national EEOC ADA research project. *Journal of Vocational Rehabilitation, 23*(3), 163–169.

Modha, G., Bernhardt, B. M., Church, R., & Bacsfalvi, P. (2008). Case study using ultrasound to treat [ɹ]. *International Journal of Language and Communication Disorders, 43*, 323–329.

Moimaz, S. A., Garbin, A. J., Lima, A. M., Lolli, L. F., Saliba, O., & Garbin, C. A. (2014). Longitudinal study of habits leading to malocclusion development in childhood. *BMC Oral Health, 14*, 96.

Monsen, R., Moog, J. S., & Geers, A. E. (1988). *Picture Speech Intelligibility Evaluation*. St. Louis, MO: Central Institute for the Deaf.

Montgomery, J. K., & Bonderman, R. I. (1989). Serving preschool children with severe phonological disorders. *Language, Speech, and Hearing Services in Schools, 20*, 76–84.

Moore, B. C. J., Tyler, L. K., & Marslen-Wilson, W. D. (Eds.). (2009). *The perception of speech: From sound to meaning.* New York, NY: Oxford University Press.

Moore, M. L., Howard, V. F., & McLaughlin, T. F. (2002). Siblings of children with disabilities: A review and analysis. *International Journal of Special Education, 17,* 49–64.

Morgan, A. (2013). Speech-language pathology insights into genetics and neuroscience: Beyond surface behaviour. *International Journal of Speech-Language Pathology, 15*(3), 245–254.

Morgan, A. T., Liégeois, F., & Occomore, L. (2007). Electropalatography treatment for articulation impairment in children with dysarthria post-traumatic brain injury. *Brain Injury, 21*(11), 1183–1193.

Morgan, A. T., & Vogel, A. P. (2008a). Intervention for childhood apraxia of speech. *Cochrane Database of Systematic Reviews, CD006278*(3).

Morgan, A. T., & Vogel, A. P. (2008b). Intervention for dysarthria associated with acquired brain injury in children and adolescents. *Cochrane Database Systematic Review*(3), CD006279.

Morgan, D. L., & Morgan, R. K. (2009). *Single-case research methods for the behavioral and health sciences.* Thousand Oaks, CA: Sage.

Moriarty, B. C., & Gillon, G. T. (2006). Phonological awareness intervention for children with childhood apraxia of speech. *International Journal of Language and Communication Disorders, 41*(6), 713–734.

Morris, P. S., & Leach, A. J. (2009). Acute and chronic otitis media. *Pediatric Clinics of North America, 56*(6), 1383–99.

Morris, S. R., Wilcox, K. A., & Schooling, T. L. (1995). The Preschool Speech Intelligibility Measure. *American Journal of Speech-Language Pathology, 4*(4), 22–28.

Morrisette, M. L., Dinnsen, D. A., & Gierut, J. A. (2003). Markedness and context effects in the acquisition of place features. *Canadian Journal of Linguistics, 48,* 329–355.

Morrisette, M. L., Farris, A. W., & Gierut, J. A. (2006). Applications of learnability theory to clinical phonology. *International Journal of Speech-Language Pathology, 8*(3), 207–219.

Morrisette, M. L., & Gierut, J. (2002). Lexical organisation and phonological change in treatment. *Journal of Speech, Language, and Hearing Research, 45,* 143–159.

Morrisette, M. L., & Gierut, J. A. (2003). Unified treatment recommendations: A response to Rvachew and Nowak. *Journal of Speech, Language, and Hearing Research, 46*(2), 382–385.

Morrison, J. A., & Shriberg, L. D. (1992). Articulation testing versus conversational speech sampling. *Journal of Speech and Hearing Research, 35,* 259–273.

Moses, E. R., Jr. (1939). Palatography and speech improvement. *Journal of Speech Disorders, 4*(2), 103–114.

Moskowitz, A. (1973). The acquisition of phonology and syntax: A preliminary study. In K. Hintikka, J. Moravcsik, & P. Suppes (Eds.), *Approaches to natural language* (pp. 48–84). Dordrecht, The Netherlands: Reidel.

Mota, H. B., Bagetti, T., Keske-Soares, M., & Pereira, L. F. (2005). Generalization based on implicational relationships in subjects treated with phonological therapy. *Pro-Fono Revista de Atualizacao Cientifica, Barucri (SP), 17*(1), 99–110.

Mota, H. B., Keske-Soares, M., Bagetti, T., Ceron, M. I., & Melo Filha, M. G. C. (2007). Comparative analyses of the effectiveness of three different phonological therapy models. *Pro-Fono Revista de Atualizacao Cientifica, Barucri (SP), 19*(1), 67–74.

Mowrer, D. E. (1968). *S-Pack.* Palos Verdes Estates, CA: California Education Psychological Research Association.

Mowrer, D. E. (1989). The behavioral approach to treatment. In N. Creaghead, P. W. Newman, & W. A. Secord (Eds.), *Assessment and remediation of articulatory and phonological disorders* (pp. 159–192). New York, NY: Macmillian.

Mowrer, D., & Burger, S. (1991). A comparative analysis of phonological acquisition of consonants in the speech of 2 ½ – 6-year Xhosa- and English-speaking children. *Clinical Linguistics and Phonetics, 5,* 139–164.

Mowrer, D. E., Wahl, P., & Doolan, S. J. (1978). Effect of lisping on audience evaluation of male speakers. *Journal of Speech and Hearing Disorders, 43*(2), 140–148.

Moxley, A. (2003, February 18). What's your multicultural IQ? Take this quiz and find out. *The ASHA Leader.* Retrieved from http://leader.pubs.asha.org/article.aspx?articleid=2293384.

Moyle, J. (2004). *The New Zealand Articulation Test.* Lower Hutt, New Zealand: Special Education Services.

Mullen, R., & Schooling, T. (2010). The National Outcomes Measurement System for pediatric speech-language pathology. *Language, Speech, and Hearing Services in Schools, 41,* 44–60.

Müller, N., Ball, M. J., & Rutter, B. (2006). A profiling approach to intelligibility problems. *International Journal of Speech-Language Pathology, 8*(3), 176–189.

Munro, M. J., & Derwing, T. M. (1995). Foreign accent, comprehensibility, and intelligibility in the speech of second language learners. *Language Learning, 45*(1), 73–97.

Munro, N., Lee, K., & Baker, E. (2008). Building vocabulary knowledge and phonological awareness skills in children with specific language impairment through hybrid language intervention: A feasibility study. *International Journal of Language and Communication Disorders, 43*(6), 662–682.

Munro, S. M., Ball, M. J., & Müller, N. (2007). Welsh speech acquisition. In S. McLeod (Ed.), *The international guide to speech acquisition* (pp. 592–607). Clifton Park, NY: Thomson Delmar Learning.

Munson, B., Baylis, A. L., Krause, M. O., & Yim, D. (2010). Representation and access in phonological impairment. In C. Fougeron, B. Kühnert, M. D'Imperio, & N. Vallée (Eds.), *Laboratory Phonology 10* (pp. 381–404). Berlin, Germany: Mouton de Gruyter.

Munson, B., Bjorum, E. M., & Windsor, J. (2003). Acoustic and perceptual correlates of stress in nonwords produced by children with suspected developmental apraxia of speech and children with phonological disorder. *Journal of Speech, Language, and Hearing Research, 46*(1), 189–202.

Munson, B., Edwards, J., & Beckman, M. E. (2005a). Relationships between nonword repetition accuracy and other measures of linguistic development in children with phonological disorders. *Journal of Speech, Language, and Hearing Research, 48,* 61–78.

Munson, B., Edwards, J., & Beckman, M. E. (2005b). Phonological knowledge in typical and atypical speech-sound development. *Topics in Language Disorders, 25,* 190–206.

Munson, B., Edwards, J., & Beckman, M. E. (2011). Phonological representations in language acquisition: Climbing the ladder of abstraction. In A. C. Cohn, C. Fougeron, & M. K. Huffman (Eds.), *The Oxford handbook of laboratory phonology* (pp. 288–309). Oxford, UK: Oxford University Press.

Munson, B., Edwards, J., Schellinger, S. K., Beckman, M. E., & Meyer, M. K. (2010). Deconstructing phonetic transcription: Covert contrast, perceptual bias, and an extraterrestrial view of vox humana. *Clinical Linguistics and Phonetics, 24,* 245–260.

Munson, B., Schellinger, S. K., & Urberg Carlson, K. U. (2012). Measuring speech-sound learning using visual analog scaling. *SIG 1 Perspectives on Language Learning and Education, 19*(1), 19–30.

Murdoch, B. E. (1998). *Dysarthria: A physiological approach to assessment and treatment.* Cheltenham, UK: Stanley Thornes.

Murdoch, B. E., & Goozée, J. V. (2003). EMA analysis of tongue function in children with dysarthria following traumatic brain injury. *Brain Injury, 17*(1), 79–93.

Murray, E., McCabe, P., & Ballard, K. (2012). A comparison of two treatments for childhood apraxia of speech: Methods and treatment protocol for a parallel group randomized control trial. *BMC Pediatrics, 12*(1), 1–9.

Murray, E., McCabe, P., & Ballard, K. J. (2014). A systematic review of treatment outcomes for children with childhood apraxia of speech. *American Journal of Speech-Language Pathology, 23*(3), 486–504.

Murray, E., McCabe, P., & Ballard, K. J. (2015). A randomized controlled trial for children with childhood apraxia of speech comparing rapid syllable transition treatment and the Nuffield Dyspraxia Programme–Third Edition. *Journal of Speech, Language, and Hearing Research, 58*(3), 669–686.

Murray, E., McCabe, P., Heard, R., & Ballard, K. J. (2015). Differential diagnosis of children with suspected childhood apraxia of speech. *Journal of Speech, Language, and Hearing Research, 58*(1), 43–60.

Murray, J. C. (2002). Gene/environment causes of cleft lip and/or palate. *Clinical Genetics, 61*(4), 248–256.

Nagy, J. (1980). 5-6 éves gyermekeink iskolakészültsége [Preparedness for school of five- to six-year-old children]. Budapest, Hungary: Akadémiai Kiadó.

Nagy, N., & Roberts, J. (2004). New England phonology. In E. Schneider, K. Burridge, B. Kortmann, R. Mesthrie, & C. Upton (Eds.), *A handbook of varieties of English. Volume 1: Phonology* (pp. 270–281). Berlin, Germany: Mouton de Gruyter.

Nakanishi, Y., Owada, K., & Fujita, N. (1972). Kōonkensa to sono kekka ni kansuru kōsatsu. *Tokyo Gakugei Daigaku Tokushu Kyoiku Shisetsu Hokoku, 1*, 1–19.

Namasivayam, A. K., Pukonen, M., Goshulak, D., Hard, J., Rudzicz, F., Rietveld, T., . . . van Lieshout, P. (2015). Treatment intensity and childhood apraxia of speech. *International Journal of Language and Communication Disorders, 50*(4), 529–546.

Nath, A. R., Fava, E. E., & Beauchamp, M. S. (2011). Neural correlates of interindividual differences in children's audiovisual speech perception. *Journal of Neuroscience, 31*(39), 13963–13971.

Nathan, L., Stackhouse, J., Goulandris, N., & Snowling, M. J. (2004a). The development of early literacy skills among children with speech difficulties: A test of the "critical age hypothesis." *Journal of Speech, Language, and Hearing Research, 47*(2), 377–391.

Nathan, L., Stackhouse, J., Goulandris, N., & Snowling, M. J. (2004b). Educational consequences of developmental speech disorder: Key Stage 1 National Curriculum assessment results in English and mathematics. *British Journal of Educational Psychology, 74*, 173–186.

National Center for Education Statistics. (2002). Early Childhood Longitudinal Study—Kindergarten Class of 1998–99 (ECLS-K). *Psychometric report for kindergarten through first grade, NCES 2002–2005.* Washington, DC: US Department of Education.

National Human Genome Research Institute (2012). *An overview of the Human Genome Project.* Retrieved from http://www.genome.gov/12011238.

National Reading Panel (2000). *Teaching children to read: An evidenced-based assessment of the scientific research literature on reading and its implications for reading instruction.* Washington, DC: National Institute of Child Health and Human Development/ National Institutes of Health.

Naylor, A., & Prescott, P. (2004). Invisible children? The need for support groups for siblings of disabled children. *British Journal of Special Education, 31*, 199–206.

Neale, M. D. (1999). *Neale Analysis of Reading Ability–Third Edition.* Camberwell, Australia: ACER Press.

Neilson, R. (2003). *Sutherland Phonological Awareness Test–Revised.* NSW, Australia: Author.

Nelson, H. D., Nygren, P., Walker, M., & Panoscha, R. (2006). Screening for speech and language delay in preschool children: Systematic evidence review for the U.S. Preventive Services Task Force. *Pediatrics, 117*, e298–e319.

Nelson, K. E. (1989). Strategies for first language teaching. In M. Rice & R. Schiefelbusch (Eds.), *The teachability of language* (pp. 263–310). Baltimore, MD: Paul H. Brookes.

Nelson, N., Plante, E., Helm-Estabrooks, N., & Hotz, G. (2015). *Test of Integrated Language and Literacy Skills (TILLS).* Baltimore, MD: Paul H. Brookes.

Neumann, S., & Romonath, R. (2012). Application of the International Classification of Functioning, Disability, and Health–Children and Youth Version (ICF-CY) to cleft lip and palate. *The Cleft Palate-Craniofacial Journal, 49*(3), 325–346.

Newbold, E. J., Stackhouse, J., & Wells, B. (2013). Tracking change in children with severe and persisting speech difficulties. *Clinical Linguisitcs and Phonetics, 27*(6–7), 521–539.

Newcomer, P., & Barenbaum, E. (2003). *Test of Phonological Awareness Skills* (TOPAS). Austin, TX: Pro-Ed.

Newcomer, P., & Hammill, D. (1988). *Test of Language Development–2 Primary.* Austin, TX: Pro-Ed.

Newcomer, P. L., & Hammill, D. D. (2008) *Test of Language Development–Primary: Fourth Edition* (TOLD-P 4). Austin, TX: Pro-Ed.

Ng, K. Y. M., To, C. K. S., & McLeod, S. (2014). Validation of the Intelligibility in Context Scale as a screening tool for preschoolers in Hong Kong. *Clinical Linguistics and Phonetics, 28*(5), 316–328.

Ng, S. B., Turner, E. H., Robertson, P. D., Flygare, S. D., Bigham, A. W., Lee, C., . . . Shendure, J. (2009). Targeted capture and massively parallel sequencing of 12 human exomes. *Nature, 461*, 272–276.

Niedenthal, P. M., Augustinova, M., Rychlowska, M., Droit-Volet, S., Zinner, L., Knafo, A., & Brauer, M. (2012). Negative relations between pacifier use and emotional competence. *Basic and Applied Social Psychology, 34*(5), 387–394.

Nippold, M. A. (2002). Stuttering and phonology: Is there an interaction? *American Journal of Speech-Language Pathology, 11*(May), 99–110.

Nippold, M. A. (2004). Phonological and language disorders in children who stutter: impact on treatment recommendations. *Clinical Linguistics and Phonetics, 18*, 145–160.

Nittrouer, S. (2002). From ear to cortex: A perspective on what clinicians need to understand about speech perception and language processing. *Language, Speech, and Hearing Services in Schools, 33*(4), 237–252.

Nordberg, A., Carlsson, G., & Lohmander, A. (2011). Electropalatography in the description and treatment of speech disorders in five children with cerebral palsy. *Clinical Linguistics and Phonetics, 25*(10), 831–852.

Nordness, A. S., & Beukelman, D. R. (2010). Speech practice patterns of children with speech sound disorders: The impact of parental record keeping and computer-led practice. *Journal of Medical Speech-Language Pathology, 18*(4), 104–108.

Norris, J. A., & Hoffman, P. R. (2005). Goals and targets: Facilitating the self-organizing nature of a neuro-network. In A. G. Kamhi & K. E. Pollock (Eds.), *Phonological disorders in children: Clinical decision making in assessment and intervention* (pp. 77–100). Baltimore, MD: Paul H. Brookes.

Northern, J. L., & Downs, M. P. (2002). *Hearing in children* (5th ed.). Baltimore, MD: Lippincott, Williams & Wilkins.

O'Connor, S., & Pettigrew, C. M. (2009). The barriers perceived to prevent the successful implementation of evidence-based practice by speech and language therapists. *International Journal of Language and Communication Disorders, 44*(6), 1018–1035.

Odell, K. H., & Shriberg, L. D. (2001). Prosody-voice characteristics of children and adults with apraxia of speech. *Clinical Linguistics and Phonetics, 15*(4), 275–307.

O'Grady, W., Archibald, J., Aronoff, M., & Rees-Miller, J. (2005). *Contemporary linguistics: An introduction* (5th ed.). Boston, MA: Bedford/St. Martin's.

Oliveira, C., Lousada, M., & Jesus, L. M. (2015). The clinical practice of speech and language therapists with children with phonologically based speech sound disorders. *Child Language Teaching and Therapy, 31*(2), 173–194.

Oller, D. K., Eilers, R. E., Neal, A. R., & Schwartz, H. K. (1999). Precursors to speech in infancy: The prediction of speech and language disorders. *Journal of Communication Disorders, 32*, 223–245.

Oller, J. W., Oller, S. D., & Bandon, L. C. (2010). *Cases: Introducing communication disorders across the lifespan.* San Diego, CA: Plural Publishing.

Olswang, L., & Bain, B. (1985). Monitoring phoneme acquisition for making treatment withdrawal decisions. *Applied Psycholinguistics, 6*, 17–37.

Olswang, L., & Bain, B. (1994). Data collection: Monitoring children's treatment progress. *American Journal of Speech-Language Pathology, 3*, 55–66.

Oommen, E. R., & McCarthy, J. W. (2014). Natural speech and AAC intervention in childhood motor speech disorders: Not an either/or situation. *Perspectives on Augmentative and Alternative Communication, 23*(3), 117–123.

Orimadegun, A. E., & Obokon, G. O. (2015). Prevalence of non-nutritive sucking habits and potential influencing factors among children in urban communities in Nigeria. *Frontiers in Pediatrics, 3*, 30.

Osberger, M. J., Robbins, A. M., Todd, S. L., & Riley, A. (1994). Speech intelligibility of children with cochlear implants. *Volta Review, 96*, 169–180.

Ota, M., & Ueda, I. (2007). Japanese speech acquisition. In S. McLeod (Ed.), *The international guide to speech acquisition* (pp. 457–471). Clifton Park, NY: Thomson Delmar Learning.

Otomo, K., & Stoel-Gammon, C. (1992). The acquisition of unrounded vowels in English. *Journal of Speech and Hearing Research, 35*, 604–616.

Overby, M., Carrell, T., & Bernthal, J. (2007). Teachers' perceptions of students with speech sound disorders: A quantitative and qualitative analysis. *Language, Speech, and Hearing Services in Schools, 38*(4), 327–341.

Owen, R., Hayett, L., & Roulstone, S. (2004). Children's views of speech and language therapy in school: Consulting children with communication difficulties. *Child Language Teaching and Therapy, 20*(1), 55–73.

Owens, R. E. (1996). *Language development: An introduction* (4th ed.). Boston, MA: Allyn & Bacon.

Oxley, J., Buckingham, H., Roussel, N., & Daniloff, R. (2006). Metrical/syllabic factors in English allophony: Dark /l/. *Clinical Linguistics and Phonetics, 20*(2–3), 109–117.

Ozanne, A. (2013). Childhood apraxia of speech. In B. Dodd (Ed.), *Differential diagnosis and treatment of speech disordered children* (3rd ed., pp. 71–82). Hoboken, NJ: Wiley.

Özçalışkan, Ş., & Goldin-Meadow, S. (2005). Gesture is at the cutting edge of early language development. *Cognition, 96*(3), B101–B113.

Paden, E. (1970). *A history of the American Speech and Hearing Association 1925–1958.* Rockville, MD: American Speech and Hearing Association.

Paden, E. (2007). Foreword. In B. W. Hodson (Ed.), *Evaluating and enhancing children's phonological systems: Research and theory to practice* (pp. vii–ix). Greenville, SC: Thinking Publications.

Paden, E. P., & Moss, S. A. (1985). Comparison of three phonological analysis procedures. *Language, Speech, and Hearing Services in Schools, 16*, 103–109.

Pagliarin, K. C., Mota, H. B., & Keske-Soares, M. (2009). Therapeutic efficacy analysis of three contrastive approach phonological models. *Pró-Fono Revista de Atualização Científica, 21*(4), 297–302.

Palisano, R., Rosenbaum, P., Walter, S., Russell, D., Wood, E., & Galuppi, B. (1997). Development and reliability of a system to classify gross motor function in children with cerebral palsy. *Developmental Medicine and Child Neurology, 39*(4), 214–223.

Palle, N., Berntsson, A., Miniscalco, C., & Persson, C. (2014). The effectiveness of phonological intervention in preschool children: A single-subject design study. *Logopedics Phoniatrics Vocology, 39*(1), 19–29.

Palmer, J. M. (1993). *Anatomy for speech and hearing* (4th ed.). Baltimore, MD: Williams & Wilkins.

Pamplona, M. C., Ysunza, A., & Espinosa, J. (1999). A comparative trial of two modalities of speech intervention for compensatory articulation in cleft palate children, phonologic approach versus articulatory approach. *International Journal of Pediatric Otorhinolaryngology, 49*, 21–26.

Paradis, J. (2007). Bilingual children with specific language impairment: Theoretical and applied issues. *Applied Psycholinguistics, 28*(3), 551–564.

Paradis, J., Emmerzael, K., & Duncan, T. S. (2010). Assessment of English language learners: Using parent report on first language development. *Journal of Communication Disorders, 43*(6), 474–497.

Paradis, J., Genesee, F., & Crago, M. (Eds.). (2011). *Dual language development and disorders: A handbook on bilingualism and second language learning* (2nd ed.). Baltimore, MD: Paul H. Brookes.

Paradis, M. (1987). *The Assessment of Bilingual Aphasia.* Mahwah, NJ: Erlbaum.

Paradise, J. L., Dollaghan, C. A., Campbell, T. F., Feldman, H. M., Bernard, B. S., Colborn, D. K., . . . Smith, C. G. (2000). Language, speech sound production, and cognition in three-year-old children in relation to otitis media in their first three years of life. *Pediatrics, 105*(5), 1119–1130.

Paradise, J. L., Feldman, H. M., Campbell, T. F., Dollaghan, C. A., Colborn, D. K., Bernard, B. S., . . . Smith, C. G. (2001). Effect of early or delayed insertion of tympanostomy tubes for persistent otitis media on developmental outcomes at the age of three years. *New England Journal of Medicine, 344*(16), 1179–1187.

Parham, D. F. (2013). Speech-related breathing in infants: how much do we really know? *Perspectives on Speech Science and Orofacial Disorders, 23*(1), 27–33.

Pariani, M. J., Spencer, A., Graham, J. M., & Rimoin, D. L. (2009). A 785kb deletion of 3p14.1p13, including the FOXP1 gene, associated with speech delay, contractures, hypertonia and blepharophimosis. *European Journal of Medical Genetics, 52*, 123–127.

Parks, J., Hill, N., Platt, M. J., & Donnelly, C. (2010). Oromotor dysfunction and communication impairments in children with cerebral palsy: A register study. *Developmental Medical Child Neurology, 52*, 1113–1119.

Pascoe, M., Stackhouse, J. & Wells, B. (2006). *Persisting speech difficulties in children: Children's speech and literacy difficulties. Book 3.* Chichester, UK: Wiley.

Patel, R., Connaghan, K., Franco, D., Edsall, E., Forgit, D., Olsen, L., . . . Russell, S. (2013). "The Caterpillar": A novel reading passage for assessment of motor speech disorders. *American Journal of Speech-Language Pathology, 22*(1), 1–9.

Paul, R. (Ed.). (2014). *Introduction to clinical methods in communication disorders* (3rd ed.). Baltimore, MD: Paul H. Brookes.

Paul, R., & Flipsen, P., Jr. (Eds.). (2010). *Speech sound disorders in children: In honor of Lawrence D. Shriberg.* San Diego, CA: Plural Publishing.

Paul, T. J., Desai, P., & Thorburn, M. J. (1992). The prevalence of childhood disability and related medical diagnoses in Clarendon, Jamaica. *West Indian Medical Journal, 41*(1), 8–11.

Paulson, L. H., Kelly, K. L., Jepson, S., van den Pol, R., Ashmore, R., Farrier, M., & Guilfoyle, S. (2003). The effects of an early reading curriculum on language and literacy development of Head Start children. *Journal of Research in Childhood Education, 18*, 169–178.

Paynter, E. T., & Petty, N. A. (1974). Articulatory sound acquisition of two-year-old children. *Perceptual and Motor Skills, 39*, 1079–1085.

Pearson. (2014). *Speech and language:Diagnostic Evaluation of Articulation and Phonology.* Retrieved from http://www.pearsonclinical.com/language/products/100000295/diagnostic-evaluation-of-articulation-and-phonology-deap.html.

Pearson, B. Z., Velleman, S. L., Bryant, T. J., & Charko, T. (2009). Phonological milestones for African American English-speaking children learning mainstream American English as a second dialect. *Language, Speech, and Hearing Services in Schools, 40*(3), 229–244.

Peckham, C. S. (1973). Speech defects in a national sample of children aged seven years. *British Journal of Disorders of Communication, 8*(1), 2–8.

Peña-Brooks, A., & Hegde, M. N. (2007). *Articulation and phonological disorders: Assessment and treatment resource manual.* Austin, TX: Pro-Ed.

Peña-Brooks, A., & Hegde, M. N. (2015). *Assessment and treatment of speech sound disorders in children: A dual-level text.* Austin, TX: PRO-ED.

Peña, E. D., Gutiérrez-Clellen, V. F., Iglesias, A., Goldstein, B. A., & Bedore, L. M. (2014). *BESA: Bilingual English-Spanish Assessment.* San Rafael, CA: AR-Clinical Publications.

Peña, E., Iglesias, A., & Lidz, C. S. (2001). Reducing test bias through dynamic assessment of children's word learning ability. *American Journal of Speech-Language Pathology, 10*(2), 138–154.

Peña, E. D., Spaulding, T. J., & Plante, E. (2006). The composition of normative groups and diagnostic decision making: Shooting ourselves in the foot. *American Journal of Speech-Language Pathology, 15*, 247–254.

Pendergast, K., Dickey, S., Selmar, T., & Soder, A. (1969). *Photo Articulation Test.* Danville, IL: Interstate Press.

Pennington, L. (2012). Speech and communication in cerebral palsy. *Eastern Journal of Medicine, 17*(4), 171–177.

Pennington, L., Miller, N., & Robson, S. (2009). Speech therapy for children with dysarthria acquired before three years of age. *Cochrane Database of Systematic Reviews,* doi: 10.1002/14651858.CD006937.pub2

Pennington, L., Miller, N., Robson, S., & Steen, N. (2010). Intensive speech and language therapy for older children with cerebral palsy: A systems approach. *Developmental Medicine and Child Neurology, 52*(4), 337–344.

Pennington, L., Roelant, E., Thompson, V., Robson, S., Steen, N., & Miller, N. (2013). Intensive dysarthria therapy for younger children with cerebral palsy. *Developmental Medicine and Child Neurology, 55*(5), 464–471.

Pennington, L., Smallman, C., & Farrier, F. (2006). Intensive dysarthria therapy for older children with cerebral palsy: Findings from six cases. *Child Language Teaching and Therapy, 22*(3), 255–273.

Peppé, S. J. E. (2009). Why is prosody in speech-language pathology so difficult? *International Journal of Speech-Language Pathology, 11*(4), 258–271.

Peppé, S. (2012). Prosody in the world's languages. In S. McLeod & B. A. Goldstein (Eds.), *Multilingual aspects of speech sound disorders in children* (pp. 42–52). Bristol, UK: Multilingual Matters.

Peppé, S., Coene, M., Hesling, I., Martínez-Castilla, P., & Moen, I. (2012). Translation to practice: Prosody in five European languages. In S. McLeod & B. A. Goldstein (Eds.), *Multilingual aspects of speech sound disorders in children* (pp. 53–56). Bristol, UK: Multilingual Matters.

Peppé, S. (2015). *Profiling Elements of Prosody in Speech-Communication (PEPS-C), 2015 edition.* Tynron, Scotland: Author. Retrieved from http://www.peps-c.com/index.html.

Peppé, S., & McCann, J. (2003). Assessing intonation and prosody in children with atypical language development: The PEPS-C test and the revised version. *Clinical Linguistics and Phonetics, 17,* 345–354.

Peter, B., & Stoel-Gammon, C. (2005). Timing errors in two children with suspected childhood apraxia of speech (sCAS) during speech and music-related tasks. *Clinical Linguistics and Phonetics, 19*(2), 67–87.

Peters, S. (2000). Is there a disability culture? A syncretisation of three possible world views. *Disability and Society, 15,* 583–601.

Peterson, G. E., & Barney, H. L. (1952). Control methods used in a study of the vowels. *The Journal of the Acoustical Society of America, 24,* 175–184.

Peterson, G. E., & Lehiste, I. (1960). Duration of syllable nuclei in English. *The Journal of the Acoustical Society of America, 32*(6), 693–703.

Peterson, R. L., Pennington, B. F., Shriberg, L. D., & Boada, R. (2009). What influences literacy outcome in children with speech sound disorder? *Journal of Speech, Language, and Hearing Research, 52*(5), 1175–1188.

Peterson-Falzone, S. J., Hardin-Jones, M. A., & Karnell, M. P. (2010). *Cleft palate speech* (4th ed.). St Louis, MO: Mosby Elsevier.

Phạm, B. & McLeod, S. (2016). Consonants, vowels, and tones across Vietnamese dialects. *International Journal of Speech-Language Pathology, 18*(2), 122–134.

Phoon, H. S., Abdullah, A. C., & Maclagan, M. (2012). The effect of dialect on the phonological analysis of Chinese-influenced Malaysian English speaking children. *International Journal of Speech-Language Pathology, 14*(6), 487–498.

Piaget, J. (1952). *The origins of intelligence in children.* New York, NY: International Universities Press.

Pinborough-Zimmerman, J., Satterfield, R., Miller, J., Bilder, D., Hossain, S., & McMahon, W. (2007). Communication disorders: Prevalence and comorbid intellectual disability, autism, and emotional/behavioral disorders. *American Journal of Speech-Language Pathology, 16*(4), 359–367.

Pit-ten Cate, I. M., & Loots, G. M. P. (2000). Experiences of siblings of children with physical disabilities: An empirical investigation. *Disability and Rehabilitation, 22,* 399–408.

Plant, G., & Moore, A. (1993). *The PLOTT screening test and PLOTT sentence test.* Sydney, Australia: National Acoustic Laboratories.

Plant, G., & Westcott, S. (1983). *The PLOTT test.* Sydney, Australia: National Acoustic Laboratories.

Plante, E., & Vance, R. (1994). Selection of preschool language tests: A data-based approach. *Language, Speech, and Hearing Services in Schools, 25*(1), 15–24.

Polka, L., & Bohn, O.-S. (2011). Natural Referent Vowel (NRV) framework: An emerging view of early phonetic development. *Journal of Phonetics, 39*(4), 467–478.

Polka, L., Rvachew, S., & Mattock, K. (2007). Experiential influences on speech perception and speech production in infancy. In E. Hoff & M. Shatz (Eds.), *Blackwell handbook of language development.* Oxford, UK: Blackwell.

Pollock, K. E. (1991). The identification of vowel errors using traditional articulation or phonological process test stimuli. *Language, Speech, and Hearing Services in Schools, 22*(2), 39–50.

Pollock, K. E. (2002). Identification of vowel errors: Methodological issues and preliminary data from the Memphis Vowel Project. In M. J. Ball & F. E. Gibbon (Eds.), *Vowel disorders* (pp. 83–113). Boston, MA: Butterworth Heinemann.

Pollock, K. E., & Berni, M. C. (2003). Incidence of non-rhotic vowel errors in children: Data from the Memphis Vowel Project. *Clinical Linguistics and Phonetics, 17,* 393–401.

Pollock, K. E., & Keiser, N. (1990). An examination of vowel errors in phonologically disordered children. *Clinical Linguistics and Phonetics, 4*(2), 161–178.

Poole, E. (1934). Genetic development of articulation of consonant sounds in speech. *Elementary English Review, 11,* 159–161.

Porter, J. H., & Hodson, B. W. (2001). Collaborating to obtain phonological acquisition data for local schools. *Language, Speech, and Hearing Services in Schools, 32,* 165–171.

Potter, N. L., Nievergelt, Y., & Shriberg, L. D. (2013). Motor and speech disorders in classic galactosemia. In J. Zschocke, K. M. Gibson, G. Brown, E. Morava, & V. Peters (Eds.), *JIMD Reports: Volume 11* (pp. 31–41). Berlin, Germany: Springer.

Powell, T. W. (1991). Planning for phonological generalization: An approach to treatment target selection. *American Journal of Speech-Language Pathology, September,* 21–27.

Powell, T. W. (1995). A clinical screening procedure for assessing consonant cluster production. *American Journal of Speech-Language Pathology, 4,* 59–65.

Powell, T. W. (1996). Stimulability considerations in the phonological treatment of a child with a persistent disorder of speech-sound production. *Journal of Communications Disorders, 29,* 315–333.

Powell, T. W. (1997). Assessing consonant cluster production under imitative and more spontaneous conditions. *Perceptual and Motor Skills, 84, 1134.*

Powell, T. W. (2002). *Phonological generalisation.* Paper presented at the School of Communication Sciences and Disorders Research Seminar Series, University of Sydney, Australia.

Powell, T. W., Elbert, M., & Dinnsen, D. A. (1991). Stimulability as a factor in the phonological generalization of misarticulating preschool children. *Journal of Speech and Hearing Research, 14,* 1318–1328.

Powell, T. W., Elbert, M., Miccio, A. W., Strike-Roussos, C., & Brasseur, J. (1998). Facilitating [s] production in young children: An experimental evaluation of motoric and conceptual treatment approaches. *Clinical Linguistics and Phonetics, 12*(2), 127–146.

Powell, T. W., & Miccio, A. W. (1996). Stimulability: A useful clinical tool. *Journal of Communication Disorders, 29,* 237–253.

Powell, T. W., Müller, N., & Ball, M. J. (2003). Electronic publishing: Opportunities and challenges for clinical linguistics and phonetics. *Clinical Linguistics and Phonetics, 17*(4–5), 421–426.

Power-de Fur, L. (2011). Special education eligibility: When is a speech-language impairment also a disability? *ASHA Leader, 16*(4), 12–15.

Prather, E. M., Hedrick, D. L., & Kern, C. A. (1975). Articulation development in children aged two to four years. *Journal of Speech and Hearing Disorders, 60,* 179–191.

Preisser, D. A., Hodson, B. W., & Paden, E. P. (1988). Developmental phonology: 18–29 months. *Journal of Speech and Hearing Disorders, 53,* 125–130.

Preston, J. L., Brick, N., & Landi, N. (2013). Ultrasound biofeedback treatment for persisting childhood apraxia of speech. *American Journal of Speech-Language Pathology, 22*(4), 627–643.

Preston, J., & Edwards, M. L. (2010). Phonological awareness and types of sound errors in preschoolers with speech sound disorders. *Journal of Speech, Language, and Hearing Research, 53*(1), 44–60.

Preston, J. L., McCabe, P., Rivera-Campos, A., Whittle, J. L., Landry, E., & Maas, E. (2014). Ultrasound visual feedback treatment and practice variability for residual speech sound errors. *Journal of Speech, Language, and Hearing Research, 57*(6), 2102–2115.

Prezas, R. F., & Hodson, B. W. (2010). The cycles phonological remediation approach. In A. L. Williams, S. McLeod, & R. J. McCauley (Eds.), *Interventions for speech sound disorders in children* (pp. 137–157). Baltimore, MD: Paul. H. Brookes.

Priester, G. H., Post, W. J., & Goorhuis-Brouwer, S. M. (2009). Problems in speech sound production in young children: An inventory study of the opinions of speech therapists. *International Journal of Pediatric Otorhinolaryngology, 73*(8), 1100–1104.

Prince, A., & Smolensky, P. (1993). *Optimality theory: Constraint interaction in generative grammar.* Technical Report CU-CS-696-93. Department of Computer Science, University of Colorado at Boulder, and Technical Report TR-2, New Brunswick, NJ: Rutgers Center for Cognitive Science, Rutgers University.

Pukui, M. K., & Elbert, S. H. (1992). *New pocket Hawaiian dictionary.* Honolulu, HI: University of Hawai'i Press.

Raitano, N. A., Pennington, B. F., Tunick, R. A., Boada, R., & Shriberg, L. D. (2004). Pre-literacy skills of subgroups of children with speech sound disorders. *Journal of Child Psychology and Psychiatry, 45*(4), 821–835.

Rance, G., Barker, E. J., Mok, M., Dowell, R., Rincon, A., & Garratt, R. (2007). Speech perception in noise for children with auditory neuropathy/dys-synchrony type hearing loss. *Ear and Hearing, 28*(3), 351–360.

Rapin, I., Dunn, M., Allen, D., Stevens, M., & Fein, D. (2009). Subtypes of language disorders in school-age children with autism. *Developmental Neuropsychology, 34*, 66–84.

Rappaport, J. M., & Provencal, C. (2002). Neuro-otology for audiologists. In J. Katz (Ed.), *Handbook of clinical audiology* (5th ed., pp. 9–32). Baltimore, MD: Lippincott, Williams & Wilkins.

Rauscher, F. H., Krauss, R. M., & Chen, Y. (1996). Gesture, speech, and lexical access: The role of lexical movements in speech production. *Psychological Science, 7*(4), 226–231.

Ray, J. (2002). Treating phonological disorders in a multilingual child: A case study. *American Journal of Speech-Language Pathology, 11*(3), 305–315.

Recasens, D. (2004). Darkness in [l] as a scalar phonetic property: Implications for phonology and articulatory control. *Clinical Linguistics and Phonetics, 18*(6–8), 593–603.

Reed, S. K. (2013). *Cognition: Theories and applications* (9th ed.). Belmont, CA: Wadsworth, Cengage Learning.

Reid, J. (2003). The vowel house: A cognitive approach to vowels for literacy and speech. *Child Language Teaching and Therapy, 19*(2), 152–180.

Reilly, O. (2012). Managing children individually or in groups. In M. Kersner & J. A. Wright (Eds.), *Speech and language therapy: The decision-making process when working with children* (2nd ed., pp. 67–78). Abingdon, UK: Routledge.

Renfrew, C. E., & Geary, L. (1973). Prediction of persisting speech deficit. *British Journal of Disorders of Communication, 8*, 37–41.

Rice, M. L., Sell, M. A., & Hadley, P. A. (1991). Social interactions of speech, and language-impaired children. *Journal of Speech and Hearing Research, 34*(6), 1299–1307.

Rice, M. L., & Wexler, K. (1996). Toward tense as a clinical marker of specific language impairment in English-speaking children. *Journal of Speech, Language, and Hearing Research, 39*(6), 1239–1257.

Rice, M. L., & Wexler, K. (2001). *Rice/Wexler Test of Early Grammatical Impairment (RWTEGI)*. San Antonio, TX: Pearson.

Rickard Liow, S. J., & Poon, K. K. L. (1998). Phonological awareness in multilingual Chinese children. *Applied Psycholinguistics, 19*, 339–362.

Ricke, L. A., Baker, N. J., Madlon-Kay, D. J., & DeFor, T. A. (2005). Newborn tongue-tie: Prevalence and effect on breast-feeding. *Journal of the American Board of Family Practice, 18*(1), 1–7.

Rigby, M. J., & Chesham, I. (1981). A trial speech screening test for school entrants. *British Medical Journal, 282*(6262), 449–451.

Ripich, D., & Panagos, J. (1985). Accessing children's knowledge of sociolinguistic rules for speech therapy lessons. *Journal of Speech and Hearing Disorders, 50*, 335–346.

Rizzolatti, G., & Craighero, L. (2004). The mirror-neuron system. *Annual Review of Neuroscience, 27*, 169–192.

Robb, M. P., & Bleile, K. M. (1994). Consonant inventories of young children from 8 to 25 months. *Clinical Linguistics and Phonetics, 8*, 295–320.

Robb, M. P., Bleile, K. M., & Yee, S. S. L. (1999). A phonetic analysis of vowel errors during the course of treatment. *Clinical Linguistics and Phonetics, 13*(4), 309–321.

Robb, M. P., & Gillon, G. T. (2007). Speech rates of New Zealand English- and American English-speaking children. *Advances in Speech-Language Pathology, 9*(2), 173–180.

Robb, P. J., & Williamson, I. (2011). Otitis media with effusion in children: Current management. *Paediatrics and Child Health, 22*(1), 10–12.

Robbins, A. M., & Osberger, M. J. (1990). *Meaningful Use of Speech Scale.* Retrieved from https://medicine.iu.edu/oto/index.php/download_file/view/254/267/.

Robbins, A. M., Renshaw, J. J., & Berry, S. W. (1991). Evaluating meaningful auditory integration in profoundly hearing-impaired children. *American Journal of Otolaryngology, 12*(Suppl.), 144–150.

Robbins, J., & Klee, T. (1987). Clinical assessment of oropharyngeal motor developement in young children. *Journal of Speech and Hearing Disorders, 52*, 271–277.

Roberts, J. E., Burchinal, M., & Footo, M. M. (1990). Phonological process decline from 2;6 to 8 years. *Journal of Communication Disorders, 23*, 205–217.

Roberts, J. E., Rosenfeld, R. M., & Zeisel, S. A. (2004). Otitis media and speech and language: A meta-analysis of prospective studies. *Pediatrics, 113*(3), e238–e248.

Robertson, C., & Salter, W. (1997). *The Phonological Awareness Test.* East Moline, IL: LinguiSystems.

Robertson, L. M., Harding, M. S., & Morrison, G. M. (1998). A comparison of resilience indicators among Latino/a students: Differences between students identified as at-risk, learning disabled, speech impaired and not at-risk. *Education and Treatment of Children, 21*(3), 333–354.

Robinson, B. F., Mervis, C. B., & Robinson, B. W. (2003). The roles of verbal short-term memory and working memory in the acquisition of grammar by children with Williams syndrome. *Developmental Neuropsychology, 23*, 12–31.

Roca, I., & Johnson, W. (1999). *A course in phonology.* Oxford, UK: Blackwell Publishers.

Romberg, A. R., & Saffran, J. R. (2010). Statistical learning and language acquisition. *Wiley Interdisciplinary Reviews: Cognitive Science, 1*(6), 906–914.

Rose, Y., & MacWhinney, B., (2014). The PhonBank project: Data and software-assisted methods for the study of phonology and phonological development. In J. Durand, U. Gut, & G. Kristoffersen (Eds.), *The Oxford handbook of corpus phonology* (pp. 308–401). Oxford, UK: Oxford University Press.

Rose, Y., MacWhinney, B., Byrne, R., Hedlund, G., Maddocks, K., O'Brien P., & Wareham, T. (2006). Introducing Phon: A software solution for the study of phonological acquisition. In D. Bamman, T. Magnitskaia, & C. Zaller (Eds.), *Proceedings of the 30th Annual Boston University Conference on Language Development* (pp. 489–500). Somerville, MA: Cascadilla Press.

Rose, Y., & Wauquier-Gravelines, S. (2007). French speech acquisition. In S. McLeod (Ed.), *The international guide to speech acquisition* (pp. 364–385). Clifton Park, NY: Thomson Delmar Learning.

Rosenbaum, P. (2007). The environment and childhood disability: Opportunities to expand our horizons. *Developmental Medicine and Child Neurology, 49*(9), 643.

Rosenbek, J. C., Lemme, M. L., Ahern, M. B., Harris, E. H., & Wertz, R. T. (1973). A treatment for apraxia of speech in adults. *Journal of Speech and Hearing Disorders, 38*(4), 462–472.

Rosenthal, J. (1984). Rate control therapy for developmental apraxia of speech. *Clinics in Communication Disorders, 4*(3), 190–200.

Rosner, J. (1999). *Test of Auditory Analysis (TAAS).* New York, NY: Academic Therapy.

Rotten, D., Levaillant, J. M., Martinez, H., le Pointe, H. D., & Vicaut, É. (2002). The fetal mandible: A 2D and 3D sonographic approach to the diagnosis of retrognathia and micrognathia. *Ultrasound in Obstetrics and Gynecology, 19*(2), 122–130.

Roulstone, S., Loader, S., Northstone, K., Beveridge, M., & the ALSPAC team. (2002). The speech and language of children aged 25 months: Descriptive data from the Avon Longitudinal Study of Parents and Children. *Early Child Development and Care, 172*(3), 259–268.

Roulstone, S., & McLeod, S. (Eds.). (2011). *Listening to children and young people with speech, language and communication needs.* London, UK: J&R Press.

Roulstone, S., Miller, L. L., Wren, Y., & Peters, T. J. (2009). The natural history of speech impairment of 8-year-old children in the Avon Longitudinal Study of Parents and Children: Error rates at 2 and 5 years. *International Journal of Speech-Language Pathology, 11*(5), 381–391.

Roulstone, S., Peters, T. J., Glogowska, M., & Enderby, P. (2003). A 12 month follow-up of preschool children investigating the natural history of speech and language delay. *Child: Care, Health and Development, 29*(4), 245–255.

Roush, P.A. (2011). Children with auditory neuropathy spectrum disorder. In R. Seewald & A. M. Tharpe (Eds.), *Comprehensive handbook of pediatric audiology* (pp. 731–750). San Diego, CA: Plural Publishing.

Rousseau, I., Packman, A., Onslow, M., Harrison, E., & Jones, M. (2007). An investigation of language and phonological development and the responsiveness of preschool age children to the Lidcombe Program. *Journal of Communication Disorders, 40*(5), 382–397.

Rovers, M. M., Numans, M. E., Langenbach, E., Grobbee, D. E., Verheij, T. J., & Schilder, A. G. (2008). Is pacifier use a risk factor for acute otitis media? A dynamic cohort study. *Family Practice, 25*(4), 233–236.

Royal College of Speech and Language Therapists. (2011a). *Communicating quality*. Retrieved from http://www.rcslt.org/members/professional_standards/communicating_quality_live

Royal College of Speech and Language Therapists. (2011b). *Policy statement on developmental verbal dyspraxia (DVD)*. London, UK: Author.

Ruben, R. J. (1997). A time frame of critical/sensitive periods of language development. *Acta Otolaryngology, 117*, 202–205.

Ruben, R. J. (2000). Redefining the survival of the fittest: Communication disorders in the 21st century. *Laryngoscope, 110*(2 part 1), 241–245.

Rudolph, M., Kummer, P., Eysholdt, U., & Rosanowski, F. (2005). Quality of life in mothers of speech impaired children. *Logopedics Phoniatrics Vocology, 30*, 3–8.

Ruggero, L., McCabe, P., Ballard, K. J., & Munro, N. (2012). Paediatric speech-language pathology service delivery: An exploratory survey of Australian parents. *International Journal of Speech-Language Pathology, 14*(4), 338–350.

Ruscello, D. M. (1975). The importance of word position in articulation therapy. *Language, Speech, and Hearing Services in Schools, 6*(4), 190–196.

Ruscello, D. M. (2008). *Treating articulation and phonological disorders in children*. St. Louis, MO: Mosby Elsevier.

Ruscello, D. M., Cartwright, L. R., Haines, K. B., & Shuster, L. I. (1993). The use of different service delivery models for children with phonological disorders. *Journal of Communication Disorders, 26*, 193–203.

Ruscello, D., Toth, D., & Stutler, S. (1983). Classroom teachers' attitudes toward children with articulatory disorders. *Perceptual and Motor Skills, 57*, 527–530.

Rutter, B. (2011). Acoustic analysis of a sound change in progress: The consonant cluster /str/ in English. *Journal of the International Phonetic Association, 41*, 27–40.

Rutter, B., Klopfenstein, M., Ball, M. J., & Müller, N. (2010). My client is using non-English sounds! A tutorial in advanced phonetic transcription, Part III: Prosody and unattested sounds. *Contemporary Issues in Communication Sciences and Disorders, 37*, 111–122.

Rvachew, S. (1994). Speech perception training can facilitate sound production learning. *Journal of Speech and Hearing Research, 37*, 347–357.

Rvachew, S. (2009). *Speech Assessment and Interactive Learning System* (Version 2). Montréal, Québec, Canada: Author.

Rvachew, S., & Andrews, E. (2002). The influence of syllable position on children's production of consonants. *Clinical Linguistics and Phonetics, 16*, 183–198.

Rvachew, S., & Bernhardt, B. M. (2010). Clinical implications of dynamic systems theory for phonological development. *American Journal of Speech-Language Pathology, 19*(1), 34–50.

Rvachew, S., & Brosseau-Lapré, F. (2010). Speech perception intervention. In A. L. Williams, S. McLeod, & R. J. McCauley (Eds.), *Interventions for speech sound disorders in children* (pp. 295–314). Baltimore, MD: Paul H. Brookes.

Rvachew, S., & Brosseau-Lapré, F. (2012). *Developmental phonological disorders: Foundations of clinical practice*. San Diego, CA: Plural Publishing.

Rvachew, S., Chiang, P., & Evans, N. (2007). Characteristics of speech errors produced by children with and without delayed phonological awareness skills. *Language, Speech, and Hearing Services in Schools, 38*, 60–71.

Rvachew, S., & Grawburg, M. (2006). Correlates of phonological awareness in preschoolers with speech sound disorders. *Journal of Speech, Language, and Hearing Research, 49*(1), 74–87.

Rvachew, S., Hodge, M., & Ohberg, A. (2005). Obtaining and interpreting maximum performance tasks from children: A tutorial. *Journal of Speech-Language Pathology and Audiology, 29*(4), 146–157.

Rvachew, S., & Jamieson, D. G. (1989). Perception of voiceless fricatives by children with a functional articulation disorder. *Journal of Speech and Hearing Disorders, 54*, 193–208.

Rvachew, S., & Nowak, M. (2001). The effect of target-selection strategy of phonological learning. *Journal of Speech, Language, and Hearing Research, 44*, 610–623.

Rvachew, S., Nowak, M., & Cloutier, G. A. (2004). Effect of phonemic perception training on the speech production and phonological awareness skills of children with expressive phonological delay. *American Journal of Speech-Language Pathology, 13*(3), 250–263.

Rvachew, S., Rafaat, S., & Martin, M. (1999). Stimulability, speech perception skills, and treatment of phonological disorders. *American Journal of Speech-Language Pathology, 8*, 33–43.

Sackett, D. L., Rosenberg, W. M. C., Muir Gray, J. A., Hayes, R. B., & Richardson, W. S. (1996). Evidence-based medicine: What it is and what is isn't. *British Medical Journal, 312*, 71–72.

Sackett, D. L., Straus, S. E., Richardson, W. S., Rosenberg, W., & Haynes, R. B. (2000). *Evidence-based medicine: How to practice and teach EBM*. Edinburgh, Scotland: Churchill Livingstone.

Sadler, J. (2005). Knowledge, attitudes and beliefs of the mainstream teachers of children with a preschool diagnosis of speech/language impairment. *Child Language Teaching and Therapy, 21*(2), 147–163.

Sagey, E. (1986). *The representation of features and relations in nonlinear phonology*. Cambridge, MA: Massachusetts Institute of Technology.

Saiegh-Haddad, E. (2007). Linguistic constraints on children's ability to isolate phonemes in Arabic. *Applied Psycholinguistics, 28*(4), 607–625.

Salidis, S. J., & Johnson, J. S. (1997). The production of minimal words: A longitudinal case study of phonological development. *Language Acquisition, 6*(1), 1–36.

Salmoni, A. W., Schmidt, R. A., & Walter, C. B. (1984). Knowledge of results and motor learning: A review and critical appraisal. *Psychological Bulletin, 95*(3), 355–386.

Samuel, A. G. (2011). Speech perception. *Annual Review of Psychology, 62*(1), 49–72.

Sanetti, L. M. H., & Kratochwill, T. R. (2009). Toward developing a science of treatment integrity: Introduction to the special series. *School Psychology Review, 38*(4), 445–459.

Sanger, D., Mohling, S., & Stremlau, A. (2011). Speech-language pathologists' opinions on response to intervention. *Communication Disorders Quarterly, 34*, 3–16.

Sanson, A., Prior, M., Garino, E., Oberklaid, F., & Sewell, J. (1987). The structure of infant temperament: Factor analysis of the Revised Infant Temperament Questionnaire. *Infant Behavior and Development, 10*, 97–104.

Santos, F. H., & Bueno, O. F. A. (2003). Validation of the Brazilian Children's Test of Pseudoword Repetition in Portuguese speakers aged 4 to 10 years. *Brazilian Journal of Medical and Biological Research, 36*(11), 1533–1547.

Santrock, J. W. (2004). *Educational psychology*. Boston, MA: McGraw Hill.

Sasisekaran, J., & Byrd, C. (2013). Nonword repetition and phoneme elision skills in school-age children who do and do not stutter. *International Journal of Language and Communication Disorders, 48*(6), 625–639.

Scherer, N. J., Boyce, S., & Martin, G. (2013). Pre-linguistic children with cleft palate: Growth of gesture, vocalization, and word use. *International Journal of Speech-Language Pathology, 15*(6), 586–592.

Scherer, N. J., & Chapman, K. (2014, November). *Early assessment and intervention for children with cleft palate*. Seminar presented at the American Speech-Language-Hearing Association convention, Orlando, FL.

Scherer, N. J., D'Antonio, L. L., & Kalbfleisch, J. H. (1999). Early speech and language development in children with velocardiofacial syndrome. *American Journal of Medical Genetics, 88*(6), 714–723.

Scherer, N. J., & Kaiser, A. P. (2010). Enhanced milieu teaching with phonological emphasis for children with cleft lip and palate. In A. L. Williams, S. McLeod, & R. J. McCauley (Eds.), *Interventions for speech sound disorders in children* (pp. 427–452). Baltimore, MD: Paul H. Brookes.

Scherer, N. J., Williams, L. A., & Proctor-Williams, K. (2008). Early and later vocalisation skills in children with and without cleft palate. *International Journal of Pediatric Otorhinolaryngology, 72*, 827–840.

Scherer, N. J., Williams, L., Stoel-Gammon, C., & Kaiser, A. (2012). Assessment of single-word production for children under three years of age: Comparison of children with and without cleft palate. *International Journal of Otolaryngology, 2012,* 1–8.

Scheuerle, J., Guilford, A., & Garcia, S. (1982). Employee bias associated with cleft lip/palate. *Journal of Applied Rehabilitation Counseling, 13*(20), 6–8, 45.

Schlosser, R. W., & Sigafoos, J. (2008). Identifying "evidence-based practice" versus "empirically supported treatment." *Evidence-Based Communication Assessment and Intervention, 2*(2), 61–62.

Schmidt, A. M., & Meyers, K. A. (1995). Traditional and phonological treatment for teaching English fricatives and affricates to Koreans. *Journal of Speech and Hearing Research, 38,* 828–838.

Schmidt, R. A. (1975). *Motor skills.* New York, NY: Harper and Row.

Schmidt, R. A., & Bjork, R.A. (1992). New conceptualizations of practice: Common principles in three paradigms suggest new concepts for training. *Psychological Science, 3,* 207–217.

Schmidt, R. A., & Lee, T. D. (2005). *Motor control and learning: A behavioral emphasis* (4th ed.). Champaign, IL: Human Kinetics.

Schmitt, L. S., Howard, B. H., & Schmitt, J. F. (1983). Conversational speech sampling in the assessment of articulation proficiency. *Language, Speech, and Hearing Services in Schools, 14,* 210–214.

Schneider, P., Rivard, R., & Debreuil, B. (2011). Does colour affect the quality or quantity of children's stories elicited by pictures? *Child Language Teaching and Therapy, 27*(3), 371–378.

Schneider, S., & Frens, R. (2005). Training four-syllable CV patterns in individuals with acquired apraxia of speech: Theoretical implications. *Aphasiology, 19*(3–5), 451–471.

Schwartz, R. G., & Leonard, L. B. (1982). Do children pick and choose? An examination of phonological selection and avoidance in early lexical acquisition. *Journal of Child Language, 9,* 319–336.

Scripture, M. K., & Jackson, E. (1919). *A manual of exercises for the correction of speech disorders.* Philadelphia, PA: F. A. Davis.

Secord, W. A. (1989). The traditional approach to treatment. In N. Creaghead, P. W. Newman, & W. A. Secord (Eds.), *Assessment and remediation of articulatory and phonological disorders* (pp. 129–158). New York, NY: Macmillan.

Secord, W., Boyce, S. E., Donohue, J. S., Fox, F. A., & Shine, S. E. (2007). *Eliciting sounds: Techniques and strategies for clinicians* (2nd ed.). Clifton Park: NY: Thomson Delmar Learning.

Secord, W. A., & Donohue, J. S. (2002). *Clinical Assessment of Articulation and Phonology.* Greenville, SC: Super Duper Publications.

Secord, W. A., & Shine, R. E. (1997). *Secord Contextual Articulation Test (S-CAT).* Greenville, SC: Super Duper.

Sedaris, D. (2000). *Me talk pretty one day.* New York, NY: Little, Brown and Company.

Seedhouse, D. (1998). *Ethics: The heart of healthcare* (2nd ed.). Chichester, UK: Wiley.

Segal, L. M., Stephenson, R., Dawes, M., & Feldman, P. (2007). Prevalence, diagnosis, and treatment of ankyloglossia: Methodologic review. *Canadian Family Physician, 53*(6), 1027–1033.

Seikel, J. A., Drumright, D. G., & Seikel, P. (2014). *Essentials of anatomy and physiology for communication disorders* (2nd ed.). Clifton Park, NY: Cengage Learning.

Selby, J. C., Robb, M. P., & Gilbert, H. R. (2000). Normal vowel articulations between 15 and 36 months of age. *Clinical Linguistics and Phonetics, 14,* 255–266.

Sell, D., Harding, A., & Grunwell, P. (1999). Revised GOS.SP.ASS(98): Speech assessment for children with cleft palate and/or velopharyngeal dysfunction. *International Journal of Language and Communication Disorders, 34*(1), 7–33.

Semel, E., Wiig, E., & Secord, W. (2004). *Clinical Evaluation of Language Fundamentals—Fourth Edition, Screening Test (CELF-4 Screener).* Austin, TX: Pearson.

Semel, E., Wiig, E. H., & Secord, W. A. (2013). *Clinical Evaluation of Language Fundamentals—Fifth Edition (CELF-5).* San Antonio, TX: Pearson.

Service, E., Maury, S., & Luotoniemi, E. (2007). Individual differences in phonological learning and verbal STM span. *Memory and Cognition, 35*(5), 1122–1135.

Setter, J., Stojanovik, V., Van Ewijk, L., & Moreland, M. (2007). Affective prosody in children with Williams syndrome. *Clinical Linguistics and Phonetics, 21*(9), 659–672.

Shaughnessy, A., Netsell, R., & Farrage, J. (1983). Treatment of a four-year-old with a palatal lift prosthesis. In W. R. Berry (Ed.), *Clinical dysarthria* (pp. 217–230). San Diego, CA: College-Hill Press.

Shawker, T. H., & Sonies, B. C. (1985). Ultrasound biofeedback for speech training. Instrumentation and preliminary results. *Investigative Radiology, 20,* 90–93.

Shea, R. L., & Tyler, A. A. (2001). The effectiveness of a prosodic intervention on children's metrical patterns. *Child Language Teaching and Therapy, 17*(1), 55–76.

Shibata, S. (1968). A study of dynamic palatography. *Annual Bulletin, Research Institute of Logopedics and Phoniatrics, University of Tokyo, 2,* 28–36.

Shibata, S., Ino, A., & Yamashita, S. (1979). *Teaching articulation by use of electro-palatograph.* Tokyo, Japan: Rion.

Shiller, D. M., Rvachew, S., & Brosseau-Lapré, F. (2010). Importance of the auditory perceptual target to the achievement of speech production accuracy. *Canadian Journal of Speech-Language Pathology and Audiology, 34*(3), 181–192.

Shine, R. E. (2007). An elicitation strategy for clients who lisp. In W. Secord, S. E. Boyce, J. S. Donohue, R. A. Fox, & R. E. Shine (Eds.), *Eliciting sounds: Techniques and strategies for clinicians* (2nd ed., pp. 175–184). Clifton Park, NY: Thomson Delmar Learning.

Shipster, C., Oliver, B., & Morgan, A. (2006). Speech and oral motor skills in children with Beckwith Wiedemann Syndrome: Pre- and post-tongue reduction surgery. *International Journal of Speech-Language Pathology, 8*(1), 45–55.

Shohara, H. H., & Hanson, C. (1941). Palatography as an aid to the improvement of articulatory movements. *Journal of Speech Disorders, 6,* 115–124.

Shotts, L. L., McDaniel, D. M., & Neeley, R. A. (2008). The impact of prolonged pacifier use on speech articulation: A preliminary investigation. *Contemporary Issues in Communication Science and Disorders, 53,* 72–75.

Shriberg, L. D. (1975). A response evocation program for /ɝ/. *Journal of Speech and Hearing Disorders, 40*(1), 92–105.

Shriberg, L. D. (1980). Developmental phonological disorders. In T. J. Hixon, L. D. Shriberg, & J. S. Saxman (Eds.), *Introduction to communicative disorders* (pp. 262–309). Englewood Cliffs, NJ: Prentice-Hall.

Shriberg, L. D. (1993). Four new speech and prosody-voice measures for genetics research and other studies in developmental phonological disorders. *Journal of Speech and Hearing Research, 36,* 105–140.

Shriberg, L. D. (2010a). Childhood speech sound disorders: From postbehaviourism to the postgenomic era. In R. Paul & P. Flipsen Jr. (Eds.), *Speech sound disorders in children: In honour of Lawrence D. Shriberg* (pp. 1–33). San Diego, CA: Plural Publishing.

Shriberg, L. D. (2010b). A neurodevelopmental framework for research in childhood apraxia of speech. In B. Maassen & P. van Lieshout (Eds.), *Speech motor control: New developments in basic and applied research* (pp. 259–270). Oxford, UK: Oxford University Press.

Shriberg, L., Aram, D. M., & Kwiatkowski, J. (1997a). Developmental apraxia of speech: I Descriptive and theoretical perspectives. *Journal of Speech, Language, and Hearing Research, 40,* 273–285.

Shriberg, L. D., Aram, D. M., & Kwiatkowski, J. (1997b). Developmental apraxia of speech: III. A subtype marked by inappropriate stress. *Journal of Speech, Language, and Hearing Research, 40*(2), 313–337.

Shriberg, L. D., Austin, D., Lewis, B. A., McSweeny, J. L., & Wilson, D. L. (1997a). The percentage of consonants correct (PCC) metric: Extensions and reliability data. *Journal of Speech, Language, and Hearing Research, 40,* 708–722.

Shriberg, L. D., Austin, D., Lewis, B. A., McSweeny, J. L., & Wilson, D. L. (1997b). The speech disorders classification system (SDCS): Extensions and lifespan reference data. *Journal of Speech, Language, and Hearing Research, 40,* 723–740.

Shriberg, L. D., Ballard, K. J., Tomblin, J. B., Duffy, J. R., Odell, K. H., & Williams, C. A. (2006). Speech, prosody, and voice characteristics of a mother and daughter with a 7;13 translocation affecting FOXP2. *Journal of Speech, Language, and Hearing Research, 49*(3), 500–525.

Shriberg, L. D., Flipsen, P., Jr., Karlsson, H. B., & McSweeny, J. L. (2001). Acoustic phenotypes for speech-genetics studies: An acoustic marker for residual /ɝ/ distortions. *Clinical Linguistics and Phonetics, 15*(8), 631–650.

Shriberg, L. D., Flipsen, P., Jr., Thielke, H., Kwiatkowski, J., Kertoy, M. K., Katcher, M. L., . . . Block, M. G. (2000). Risk for speech disorder associated with early recurrent otitis media with effusion: Two retrospective studies. *Journal of Speech, Language, and Hearing Research, 43,* 79–99.

Shriberg, L. D., Fourakis, M., Hall, S. D., Karlsson, H. B., Lohmeier, H. L., McSweeny, J. L., ... Wilson, D. L. (2010a). Extensions to the Speech Disorders Classification System (SDCS). *Clinical Linguistics and Phonetics, 24*(10), 795–824. (Chapter 2, Figure 2-2, Speech Disorders Classification System: Used with permission.)

Shriberg, L. D., Fourakis, M., Hall, S. D., Karlsson, H. B., Lohmeier, H. L., McSweeney, J. L., ... Wilson, D. L. (2010b). Perceptual and acoustic reliability estimates for the speech disorders classification system (SDCS). *Clinical Linguistics and Phonetics, 24*(10), 825–846.

Shriberg, L. D., Friel-Patti, S., Flipsen, P., Jr., & Brown, R. L. (2000). Otitis media, fluctuant hearing loss, and speech-language outcomes: A preliminary structural equation model. *Journal Speech, Language, and Hearing Research, 43,* 100–120.

Shriberg, L. D., Gruber, F. A., & Kwiatkowski, J. (1994). Developmental phonological disorders III: Long-term speech-sound normalisation. *Journal of Speech and Hearing Research, 37,* 1151–1177.

Shriberg, L. D., & Kent, R. D. (2003). *Clinical phonetics* (3rd ed.). Boston, MA: Allyn & Bacon.

Shriberg, L. D., & Kent, R. D. (2013). *Clinical phonetics* (4th ed.). Boston, MA: Pearson.

Shriberg, L., & Kwiatkowski, J. (1980). *Natural process analysis.* New York, NY: Wiley.

Shriberg, L. D., & Kwiatkowski, J. (1982a). Phonological disorders I: A diagnostic classification system. *Journal of Speech and Hearing Disorders, 47,* 226–241.

Shriberg, L. D., & Kwiatkowski, J. (1982b). Phonological disorders II: A conceptual framework of management. *Journal of Speech and Hearing Disorders, 42,* 242–256.

Shriberg, L. D., & Kwiatkowski, J. (1982c). Phonological disorders III: A procedure for assessing severity of involvement. *Journal of Speech and Hearing Disorders, 47,* 256–270.

Shriberg, L. D., & Kwiatkowski, J. (1990). Self-monitoring and generalization in preschool speech-delayed children. *Language, Speech, and Hearing Services in Schools, 21,* 157–170.

Shriberg, L. D., & Kwiatkowski, J. (1994). Developmental phonological disorders I: A clinical profile. *Journal of Speech and Hearing Research, 37,* 1100–1126.

Shriberg, L. D., Kwiatkowski, J., Best, S., Hengst, J., & Terselic-Weber, B. (1986). Characteristics of children with phonologic disorders of unknown origin. *Journal of Speech and Hearing Disorders, 51,* 140–161.

Shriberg, L. D., Kwiatkowski, J., & Gruber, F. A. (1992, November). *Short-term and long-term normalization in developmental phonological disorders.* Paper presented at the American Speech Language-Hearing Association Convention, San Antonio, TX.

Shriberg, L. D., Kwiatkowski, J., & Rasmussen, J. (1990). *Prosody-Voice Screening Profile.* Tucson, AZ: Communication Skill Builders.

Shriberg, L. D., Lewis, B. A., Tomblin, J. B., McSweeny, J. L., Karlsson, H. B., & Scheer, A. R. (2005). Toward diagnostic and phenotype markers for genetically transmitted speech delay. *Journal of Speech, Language, and Hearing Research, 48*(4), 834–852.

Shriberg, L. D., Lohmeier, H. L., Campbell, T. F., Dollaghan, C. A., Green, J. R., & Moore, C. A. (2009). A nonword repetition task for speakers with misarticulations: The Syllable Repetition Task (SRT). *Journal of Speech, Language, and Hearing Research, 52*(5), 1189–1212.

Shriberg, L. D., Lohmeier, H. L., Strand, E. A., & Jakielski, K. J. (2012). Encoding, memory, and transcoding deficits in Childhood Apraxia of Speech. *Clinical Linguistics and Phonetics, 26*(5), 445–482.

Shriberg, L. D., Paul, R., McSweeny, J. L., Klin, A., Cohen, D. J., & Volkmar, F. R. (2001). Speech and prosody characteristics of adolescents and adults with high-functioning autism and Asperger syndrome. *Journal of Speech, Language, and Hearing Research, 44*(5), 1097–1115.

Shriberg, L. D., Potter, N. L., & Strand, E. A. (2011). Prevalence and phenotype of childhood apraxia of speech in youth with galactosemia. *Journal of Speech, Language, and Hearing Research, 54*(2), 487–519.

Shriberg, L. D., Tomblin, J. B., & McSweeny, J. L. (1999). Prevalence of speech delay in 6-year-old children and comorbidity with language impairment. *Journal of Speech, Language, and Hearing Research, 42,* 1461–1481.

Shriberg, L. D., & Widder, C. J. (1990). Speech and prosody characteristics of adults with mental retardation. *Journal of Speech, Language, and Hearing Research, 33*(4), 627–653.

Shuster, L. I. (1998). The perception of correctly and incorrectly produced /r/. *Journal of Speech, Language, and Hearing Research, 41*(4), 941–950.

Shuster, L. I., Ruscello, D. M., & Smith, K. D. (1992). Evoking [r] using visual feedback. *American Journal of Speech-Language Pathology, May,* 39–24.

Shuster, L. I., Ruscello, D. M., & Toth, A. R. (1995). The use of visual feedback to elicit correct /r/. *American Journal of Speech-Language Pathology, 4*(2), 37–44.

Sices, L., Taylor, G., Freebairn, L., Hansen, A., & Lewis, B. (2007). Relationship between speech-sound disorders and early literacy skills in preschool-age children: Impact of comorbid language impairment. *Journal of Developmental and Behavioral Pediatrics, 28*(6), 438–447.

Silverman, F. H. (1995). *Communication for the speechless.* Boston, MA: Allyn & Bacon.

Silverman, F. H., & Falk, S. M. (1992). Attitudes of teenagers toward peers who have a single articulation error. *Language, Speech, and Hearing Services in Schools, 23,* 187.

Silverman, F. H., & Paulus, P. G. (1989). Peer reactions to teenagers who substitute /w/ for /r/. *Language, Speech, and Hearing Services in Schools, 20,* 219–221.

Sjölander, K., & Beskow, J. (2006). *WaveSurfer* [Computer program]. Stockhom, Sweden: Karolinska Institute.

Skahan, S. M., Watson, M., & Lof, G. L. (2007). Speech-language pathologists' assessment practices for children with suspected speech sound disorders: Results of a national survey. *American Journal of Speech-Language Pathology, 16*(3), 246–259.

Skelton, S. L. (2004a). Concurrent task sequencing in single-phoneme phonologic treatment and generalization. *Journal of Communication Disorders, 37*(2), 131–155.

Skelton, S. L. (2004b). Motor skill learning approaches to the treatment of speech sound disorders. *California Speech Hearing Association Magazine, Summer,* 8–9.

Skelton, S. L., & Funk, T. E. (2004). Teaching speech sounds to young children using randomly ordered, variably complex task sequences. *Perceptual and Motor Skills, 99*(2), 602–604.

Skelton, S. L., & Hagopian, A. L. (2014). Using randomized variable practice in the treatment of childhood apraxia of speech. *American Journal of Speech-Language Pathology, 23*(4), 599–611.

Skelton, S. L., & Kerber, J. R. (2005, November). *Using concurrent treatment to teach multiple phonemes to phonologically-disordered children.* Presentation to the American Speech-Language Hearing Association Convention, San Diego, CA.

Skelton, S. L., & Resciniti, D. N. (2009, November). *Using a motor learning treatment with phonologically-disordered children.* Presentation to the the American Speech-Language Hearing Association Convention, New Orleans, LA.

Skelton, S. L., & Taps, J. (2008, November). *Concurrent treatment in the speech improvement class: A motor-skill-based treatment for speech sound disorders.* Presentation to the American Speech-Language-Hearing Association Convention, Chicago, IL.

Skinner, B. F. (1936). The effect on the amount of conditioning of an interval of time before reinforcement. *Journal of General Psychology, 14,* 279–295.

Skinner, B., F. (1938). *The behavior of organisms: An experimental analysis.* New York, NY: Appleton-Century-Crofts.

Smit, A. B. (1993a). Phonologic error distributions in the Iowa-Nebraska articulation norms project: Consonant singletons. *Journal of Speech and Hearing Research, 36,* 533–547.

Smit, A. B. (1993b). Phonologic error distributions in the Iowa-Nebraska articulation norms project: Word-initial consonant clusters. *Journal of Speech and Hearing Research, 36,* 931–947.

Smit, A. B. (2004). *Articulation and phonology: Resource guide for school-age children and adults.* Clifton Park, NY: Thomson Delmar Learning.

Smit, A. B. (2007). General American English speech acquisition. In S. McLeod (Ed.), *The international guide to speech acquisition* (pp. 128–147). Clifton Park, NY: Thomson Delmar Learning.

Smit, A. B., & Hand, L. (1997). *Smit-Hand Articulation and Phonology Evaluation (SHAPE)*. Los Angeles, CA: Western Psychological Services.

Smit, A. B., Hand, L., Freilinger, J. J., Bernthal, J. E., & Bird, A. (1990). The Iowa articulation norms project and its Nebraska replication. *Journal of Speech and Hearing Disorders, 55*, 779–798.

Smith, B. L., McGregor, K. K., & Demille, D. (2006). Phonological development in lexically precocious 2-year-olds. *Applied Psycholinguistics, 27*, 355–375.

Smith, N. (1973). *The acquisition of phonology: A case study*. New York, NY: Cambridge University Press.

Smith, N. V. (1978). Lexical representation and the acquisition of phonology. *Studies in the Linguistic Sciences, 8*, 259–273.

Smith, S. D., Pennington, B. F., Boada, R., & Shriberg, L. D. (2005). Linkage of speech sound disorder to reading disability loci. *Journal of Child Psychology and Psychiatry, 46*, 1057–1066.

Smyth, A. (2014). Clinical grading system for submucous cleft palate. *British Journal of Oral and Maxillofacial Surgery, 52*(3), 275–276.

Snow, D. (1994). Phrase-final syllable lengthening and intonation in early child speech. *Journal of Speech and Hearing Research, 37*, 831–840.

Snow, P. C., Sanger, D. D., Childers, C., Pankonin, C., & Wright, S. (2013). Response to intervention in secondary settings: Speech-language pathologists' perspectives. *International Journal of Speech-Language Pathology, 15*(5), 463–470.

Snowling, M. J., Adams, J. W., Bishop, D. V. M., & Stothard, S. E. (2001). Educational attainments of school leavers with a preschool history of speech-language impairments. *International Journal of Language and Communication Disorders, 36*(2), 173–183.

So, L. K. H. (1993). *Cantonese Segmental Phonology Test*. Hong Kong, SAR China: Bradford Publishing.

So, L. K. H. (2007). Cantonese speech acquisition. In S. McLeod (Ed.), *The international guide to speech acquisition* (pp. 313–326). Clifton Park, NY: Thomson Delmar Learning.

So, L. K. H., & Dodd, B. J. (1994). Phonologically disordered Cantonese-speaking children. *Clinical Linguistics and Phonetics, 8*, 235–255.

So, L. K. H., & Jing, Z. (2000). *Putonghua Segmental Phonology Test (PSPT)*. Nanjing, China: Nanjing Normal University Press.

Sodoro, J., Allinder, R. M., & Rankin-Erickson, J. L. (2002). Assessment of phonological awareness: Review of methods and tools. *Educational Psychology Review, 14*(3), 223–260.

Sokol, S. B., & Fey, M. E. (2013). Consonant and syllable complexity of toddlers with Down syndrome and mixed-aetiology developmental delays. *International Journal of Speech-Language Pathology, 15*(6), 575–585.

Sommerlad, B. C., Fenn, C., Harland, K., Sell, D., Birch, M. J., Dave, R., . . . Barnett, A. (2004). Submucous cleft palate: A grading system and review of 40 consecutive submucous cleft palate repairs. *The Cleft Palate-Craniofacial Journal, 41*(2), 114–123.

Sommers, M. S. (n.d.). *Speech and Hearing Lab Neighborhood Database*. St Louis, MO: Washington University. Retrieved from http://128.252.27.56/Neighborhood/Home.asp.

Sommers, R. K., Leiss, R. H., Fundrella, D., Manning, W., Johnson, R., Oerther, P., . . . Siegel, M. (1970). Factors in the effectiveness of articulation therapy with educable retarded children. *Journal of Speech, Language, and Hearing Research, 13*(2), 304–316.

Sommers, R. K., Schaeffer, M. H., Leiss, R. H., Gerber, A. J., Bray, M. A., Fundrella, D., . . . Tomkins, E. R. (1966). The effectiveness of group and individual therapy. *Journal of Speech, Language, and Hearing Research, 9*(2), 219–225.

Sosa, A. V., & Stoel-Gammon, C. (2012). Lexical and phonological effects in early word production. *Journal of Speech, Language, and Hearing Research, 55*(2), 596–608.

Speake, J., Howard, S., & Vance, M. (2011). Intelligibility in children with persisting speech disorders: A case study. *Journal of Interactional Research in Communication Disorders, 2*(1), 131–151.

Speake, J., Stackhouse, J., & Pascoe, M. (2012). Vowel targeted intervention for children with persisting speech difficulties: Impact on intelligibility. *Child Language Teaching and Therapy, 28*(3), 277–295.

Speech Pathology Association of Australia (2009a). *Position statement: Transdisciplinary practice*. Melbourne, Australia: Speech Pathology Association of Australia.

Speech Pathology Australia (2016a). Working in a culturally and linguistically diverse society: Position paper. Melbourne, Australia: Author.

Retrieved from http://www.speechpathologyaustralia.org.au/library/position_statements/Working%20in%20a%20Culturally%20And%20Linguistically%20Diverse%20Society.pdf

Speech Pathology Australia (2016b). Working in a culturally and linguistically diverse society: Clinical guidelines. Melbourne, Australia: Author. Retrieved from http://www.speechpathologyaustralia.org.au/library/Clinical_Guidelines/Working_in_a_CALD_Society.pdf

Speech Pathology Association of Australia. (2011). *Competency-based occupational standards (C-BOS) for speech pathologists: Entry level*. Melbourne, Australia: Speech Pathology Association of Australia.

Square, P. A., Namasivayam, A. K., Bose, A., Goshulak, D., & Hayden, D. (2014). Multi-sensory treatment for children with developmental motor speech disorders. *International Journal of Language and Communication Disorders, 49*(5), 527–542.

St. Louis, K. O., & Ruscello, D. (2000). *Oral Speech Mechanism Screening Examination-Third Edition*. Austin, TX: Pro-Ed.

Stackhouse, J. (1992). Developmental verbal dyspraxia I: A review and critique. *European Journal of Disorders of Communication, 27*, 19–34.

Stackhouse, J., Pascoe, M., & Gardner, H. (2006). Intervention for a child with persisting speech and literacy difficulties: A psycholinguistic approach. *International Journal of Speech-Language Pathology, 8*(3), 231–244.

Stackhouse, J., & Snowling, M. (1992a). Barriers to literacy development in two case of developmental verbal dyspraxia. *Cognitive Neuropsychology, 9*, 273–299.

Stackhouse, J., & Snowling, M. (1992b). Developmental verbal dyspraxia II: A developmental perspective on two case studies. *International Journal of Language and Communication Disorders, 27*, 35–54.

Stackhouse, J., Vance, M., Pascoe, M., & Wells, B. (2007). *Compendium of auditory and speech tasks. Children's speech and literacy difficulties 4*. Chichester, UK: Wiley.

Stackhouse, J., & Wells, B. (1997). *Children's speech and literacy difficulties: A psycholinguistic framework*. London, UK: Whurr.

Stackhouse, J., & Wells, B. (2001). *Children's speech and literacy difficulties: Book 2, Identification and intervention*. London, UK: Whurr.

Stampe, D. L. (1969). *The acquisition of phonetic representation*. Paper presented at the Fifth Regional Meeting of the Chicago Linguistic Society, Chicago, IL.

Stampe, D. L. (1979). *A dissertation on natural phonology*. New York, NY: Garland.

Stark, R. E., Bernstein, L. E., & Demorest, M. E. (1993). Vocal communication in the first 18 months of life. *Journal of Speech and Hearing Research, 36*, 548–558.

Stark, R. E., & Blackwell, P. B. (1997). Oral volitional movements in children with language impairments. *Child Neuropsychology, 3*(2), 81–97.

Stein, C. M., Schick, J. H., Gerry Taylor, H., Shriberg, L. D., Millard, C., Kundtz-Kluge, A., Russo, K., Minich, N., Hansen, A., Freebairn, L. A., Elston, R. C., Lewis, B. A., & Iyengar, S. K. (2004). Pleiotropic effects of a chromosome 3 locus on speech-sound disorder and reading. *American Journal of Human Genetics, 74*(2), 283–297.

Stemberger, J. P. (1988). Between-word processes in child phonology. *Journal of Child Language, 15*, 39–61.

Stemberger, J. P. (1989). Speech errors in early child language production. *Journal of Memory and Language, 28*, 164–188.

Steppling, M., Quattlebaum, P., & Brady, D. E. (2007). Toward a discussion of issues associated with speech-language pathologists' dismissal practices in public school settings. *Communication Disorders Quarterly, 28*(3), 179–187.

Steriade, D. (1990). *Greek prosodies and the nature of syllabification (Doctoral dissertation, Massachuesetts Instituted of Technology, 1982)*. New York, NY: Garland Press.

Stetson, R. H. (1928). *Motor phonetics: A study of speech movements in action*. [Archives néerlandaises de phonétique expérimentale, Tome 3].

Stewart, J. M., & Taylor, O. L. (1986). Prevalence of language, speech, and hearing disorders in an urban preschool black population. *Communication Disorders Quarterly, 9*(2), 107–123.

Stewart Keck, C., & Doarn, C. R. (2014). Telehealth technology applications in speech-language pathology. *Telemedicine and e-Health, 20*(7), 653–659.

Stinchfield-Hawk, S., & Young, E. H. (1938). *Children with delayed or defective speech*. Stanford, CA: Stanford University Press.

Stockman, I. J. (2007). African American English speech acquisition. In S. McLeod (Ed.), *The international guide to speech acquisition* (pp. 148–160). Clifton Park, NY: Thomson Delmar Learning.

Stoel-Gammon, C. (1985). Phonetic inventories, 15–24 months: A longitudinal study. *Journal of Speech and Hearing Research, 28*, 505–512.

Stoel-Gammon, C. (1987). Phonological skills of 2-year-olds. *Language, Speech, and Hearing Services in Schools, 18*, 323–329.

Stoel-Gammon, C. (2011). Relationships between lexical and phonological development in young children. *Journal of Child Language, 38*(1), 1–34.

Stoel-Gammon, C., & Cooper, J. (1984). Patterns of early lexical and phonological development. *Journal of Child Language, 11*, 247–271.

Stoel-Gammon, C., & Dunn, C. (1985). *Normal and disordered phonology in children*. Baltimore, MD: University Park Press.

Stoel-Gammon, C., & Herrington, P. B. (1990). Vowel systems of normally developing and phonologically disordered children. *Clinical Linguistics and Phonetics, 4*(2), 145–160.

Stoel-Gammon, C., & Peter, B. (2008). Syllables, segments, and sequences: Phonological patterns in the words of young children acquiring American English. In B. Davis & K. Zajdo (Eds.), *Syllable development: The frame/content theory and beyond* (pp. 293–323). Mahwah, NJ: Lawrence Erlbaum.

Stoel-Gammon, C., & Williams, A. L. (2013). Early phonological development: Creating an assessment test. *Clinical Linguistics and Phonetics, 27*(4), 278–286.

Stokes, S. F., & Klee, T. (2009). The diagnostic accuracy of a new test of early nonword repetition for differentiating late talking and typically developing children. *Journal of Speech, Language, and Hearing Research, 52*(4), 872–882.

Stokes, S. F., & Surendran, D. (2005). Articulatory complexity, ambient frequency, and functional load as predictors of consonant development in children. *Journal of Speech, Language, and Hearing Research, 48*(3), 577–591.

Stokes, S. F., Whitehill, T. L., Tsui, A. M. Y., & Yuen, K. C. P. (1996). EPG treatment of sibilants in two Cantonese speaking children with cleft palate. *Clinical Linguistics and Phonetics, 10*, 265–280.

Stokes, T. F., & Baer, D. M. (1977). An implicit technology of generalization. *Journal of Applied Behavior Analysis, 10*(2), 349–367.

Stone, M. (2005). A guide to analyzing tongue motion from ultrasound images. *Clinical Linguistics and Phonetics, 19*, 455–501.

Storkel, H. L., Maekawa, J., & Hoover, J. R. (2010). Differentiating the effects of phonotactic probability and neighborhood density on vocabulary comprehension and production: A comparison of preschool children with versus without phonological delays. *Journal of Speech, Language, and Hearing Research, 53*, 933–949.

Storkel, H. L., & Morrisette, M. L. (2002). The lexicon and phonology: Interactions in language acquisition. *Language, Speech, and Hearing Services in Schools, 33*, 24–37.

Stow, C., & Dodd, B. (2003). Providing an equitable service to bilingual children in the UK: A review. *International Journal of Language and Communication Disorders, 38*(4), 351–377.

Stow, C., & Pert, S. (2006). *Bilingual Speech Sound Screen: Pakistani Heritage Languages*. Bicester, UK: Speechmark.

Strand, E. (1998). Treatment of developmental apraxia of speech: Application of motor learning principles. *Perspectives in Language, Learning and Education, 5*, 16–21.

Strand, E. A. (2003). Clinical and professional ethics in the management of motor speech disorders. *Seminars in Speech and Language, 24*(4), 301–311.

Strand, E. (2010). *An overview of dynamic temporal and tactile cueing for childhood apraxia of speech and other motor speech disorders [DVD]*. Pittsburgh, PA: Childhood Apraxia of Speech Association of North America (CASANA).

Strand, E. (2012, May). *Treatment of childhood apraxia of speech*. Presentation to the California Speech-Language-Hearing Association Conference, San Jose, CA.

Strand, E. A., & Debertine, P. (2000). The efficacy of integral stimulation intervention with developmental apraxia of speech. *Journal of Medical Speech-Language Pathology, 8*(4), 295–300.

Strand, E. A., McCauley, R. J., Weigand, S. D., Stoeckel, R. E., & Baas, B. S. (2013). A motor speech assessment for children with severe speech disorders: Reliability and validity evidence. *Journal of Speech, Language, and Hearing Research, 56*(2), 505–520.

Strand, E. A., & Skinder, A. (1999). Treatment of developmental apraxia of speech: Integral stimulation methods. In A. Caruso & E. A. Strand (Eds.), *Clinical management of motor speech disorders in children* (pp. 109–148). New York, NY: Thieme.

Strand, E. A., Stoeckel, R., & Baas, B. (2006). Treatment of severe childhood apraxia of speech: A treatment efficacy study. *Journal of Medical Speech-Language Pathology, 14*(4), 297–307.

Straus, S. E., & Sackett, D. L. (1998). Getting research findings into practice: Using research findings in clinical practice. *British Medical Journal, 317*, 339–342.

Stredler-Brown, A., & Johnson, D. C. (2003). *Functional auditory performance indicators: An integrated approach to auditory development*. Retrieved from http://www.tsbvi.edu/attachments/FunctionalAuditoryPerformanceIndicators.pdf.

Sturner, R. A., Layton, T. L., Evans, A. W., Heller, J. H., Funk, S. G., & Machon, M. W. (1994). Preschool speech and language screening: A review of currently available tests. *American Journal of Speech-Language Pathology, January*, 25–36.

Sullivan, S. R., Vasudavan, S., Marrinan, E. M., & Mulliken, J. B. (2010). Submucous cleft palate and velopharyngeal insufficiency: Comparison of speech outcomes using three operative techniques by one surgeon. *The Cleft Palate-Craniofacial Journal, 48*(5), 561–570.

Sunderland, L. C. (2004). Speech, language and audiology services in public schools. *Intervention in School and Clinic, 39*(4), 209–217.

Sutherland, D., & Gillon, G. T. (2005). Assessment of phonological representations in children with speech impairment. *Language, Speech, and Hearing Services in Schools, 36*(4), 294–307.

Sweeney, T., & Sell, D. (2008). Relationship between perceptual ratings of nasality and nasometry in children/adolescents with cleft palate and/or velopharyngeal dysfunction. *International Journal of Language and Communication Disorders, 43*(3), 265–282.

Sweeting, H., & West, P. (2001). Being different: Correlates of the experience of teasing and bullying at age 11. *Research Papers in Education, 16*(3), 225–246.

Swillen, A., Glorieux, N., Peeters, M., & Fryns, J.-P. (1995). The Coffin-Siris syndrome: Data on mental development, language, behavior and social skills in 12 children. *Clinical Genetics, 48*(4), 177–182.

Tanner, D. C. (2006). *Case studies in communication sciences and disorders*. Upper Saddle River, NJ: Pearson/Merrill Prentice Hall.

Tanner, D., & Culbertson, W. (1999). *Quick Assessment for Dysarthria*. Oceanside, CA: Academic Communication Associates.

Taps, J. (2006). An innovative educational approach for addressing articulation differences. *Perspectives on School-Based Issues, 7*(4), 7–11.

Taps, J. (2008). RTI Services for children with mild articulation needs: Four years of data. *Perspectives on School-Based Issues, 9*(3), 104–110.

Tate, R. L., McDonald, S., Perdices, M., Togher, L., Schultz, R., & Savage, S. (2008). Rating the methodological quality of single-subject designs and no-of-1 trials: Introducing the Single-Case Experimental Design (SCED) Scale. *Neuropsychological Rehabilitation, 18*, 385–401.

Taylor, D. (1996). The Valsalva manoeuvre: A critical review. *South Pacific Underwater Medicine Society Journal, 26*(1), 8–13.

Teal, J. (2005). *An investigation into classification approaches and therapy outcomes for a child with a severe persisting speech difficulty*. Unpublished master's dissertation, University of Sheffield, Sheffield, UK.

Templin, M. (1957). *Certain language skills in children (Monograph Series No. 26)*. Minneapolis, MN: University of Minnesota, Institute of Child Welfare.

Templin, M. (1966). A study of articulation and language development during early school years. In F. Smith & G. Millers (Eds.), *The genesis of language* (pp. 173–186). Cambridge, MA: MIT Press.

Templin, M. C., & Darley, F. L. (1969). *Templin-Darley Tests of Articulation* (2nd ed.). Iowa City, IO: Bureau of Educational Research and Service, Division of Extension and University Services, University of Iowa.

Terband, H., Maassen, B., Guenther, F. H., & Brumberg, J. (2014). Auditory–motor interactions in pediatric motor speech disorders: Neurocomputational modeling of disordered development. *Journal of Communication Disorders, 47*, 17–33.

Teverovsky, E. G., Bickel, J. O., & Feldman, H. M. (2009). Functional characteristics of children diagnosed with childhood apraxia of speech. *Disability and Rehabilitation, 31*(2), 94–102.

Thelen, E., & Smith, L. B. (1994). *A dynamic systems approach to the development of cognition and action.* Cambridge, MA: Bradford Books/ MIT Press.

Thomas, D. C., McCabe, P., & Ballard, K. J. (2014). Rapid Syllable Transitions (ReST) treatment for childhood apraxia of speech: The effect of lower dose-frequency. *Journal of Communication Disorders, 51*, 29–42.

Thomas, R. M. (2000). *Comparing theories of child development* (5th ed.). Belmont, CA: Wadsworth.

Thomas-Stonell, N. L., Oddson, B., Robertson, B., & Rosenbaum, P. L. (2010). Development of the FOCUS (Focus on the Outcomes of Communication Under Six), a communication outcome measure for preschool children. *Developmental Medicine and Child Neurology, 52*(1), 47–53.

Thomas-Stonell, N., Oddson, B., Robertson, B., & Rosenbaum, P. (2013). Validation of the FOCUS (Focus on the Outcomes of Communication Under Six) outcome measure. *Developmental Medicine and Child Neurology, 55*(6), 546–552.

Thomas-Stonell, N., Robertson, B., Walker, J., Oddson, B., Washington, K., & Rosenbaum, P. (2012). *FOCUS: Focus on the Outcomes of Communication Under Six.* Toronto, Canada: Holland Bloorview Kids Rehabilitation Hospital.

Thoonen, G., Maassen, B., Gabreels, F., & Schreuder, R. (1999). Validity of maximum performance tasks to diagnose motor speech disorders in children. *Clinical Linguistics and Phonetics, 13*, 1–23.

Thoonen, G., Maassen, B., Wit, J., Gabreels, F., & Schreuder, R. (1996). The integrated use of maximum performance tasks in differential diagnostic evaluations among children with motor speech disorders. *Clinical Linguistics and Phonetics, 10*, 311–336.

Tian, W., Yin, H., Redett, R. J., Shi, B., Shi, J., Zhang, R., & Zheng, Q. (2010). Magnetic resonance imaging assessment of the velopharyngeal mechanism at rest and during speech in Chinese adults and children. *Journal of Speech, Language, and Hearing Research, 53*(6), 1595–1615.

To, C. K. S., & Cheung, P. S. P. (2012). Translation to practice: Assessment of children's speech sound production in Hong Kong. In S. McLeod & B. A. Goldstein (Eds.), *Multilingual aspects of speech sound disorders in children* (pp. 165–169). Bristol, UK: Multilingual Matters.

To, C. K. S., Cheung, P. S. P., & McLeod, S. (2013a). A population study of children's acquisition of Hong Kong Cantonese consonants, vowels, and tones. *Journal of Speech, Language, and Hearing Research, 56*(1), 103–122.

To, C. K. S., Cheung, P. S. P., & McLeod, S. (2013b). The impact of extrinsic demographic factors on Cantonese speech acquisition. *Clinical Linguistics and Phonetics, 27*(5), 323–338.

To, C. K. S., McLeod, S., & Cheung, P. S. P. (2015). Phonetic variations and sound changes in Hong Kong Cantonese: Diachronic review, synchronic study and implications for speech sound assessment. *Clinical Linguistics and Phonetics, 29*(5), 333–353.

Toll, E. C., & Nunez, D. A. (2012). Diagnosis and treatment of acute otitis media: Review. *The Journal of Laryngology and Otology, 126*, 976–983.

Tomasello, M., & Stahl, D. (2004). Sampling children's spontaneous speech: How much is enough? *Journal of Child Language, 31*, 101–121.

Tomblin, B. (2011). Co-morbidity of autism and SLI: Kinds, kin and complexity. *International Journal of Language and Communication Disorders, 46*(2), 127–137.

Tomblin, J. B. (2010). The EpiSLI Database: A publicly available database on speech and language. *Language, Speech, and Hearing Services in Schools, 41*(1), 108–117.

Tomblin, J. B., & Christiansen, M. H. (2010). Explaining developmental communication disorders. In R. Paul & P. Flipsen Jr. (Ed.), *Speech sound disorders in children: In Honor of Lawrence D. Shriberg* (pp. 35–49). San Diego, CA: Plural Publishing.

Tomblin, J. B., Hardy, J. C., & Hein, H. A. (1991). Predicting poor-communication status in preschool children using risk factors present at birth. *Journal of Speech and Hearing Research, 34*(5), 1096–1105.

Tomblin, J. B., Smith, E., & Zhang, X. (1997). Epidemiology of specific language impairment: Prenatal and perinatal risk factors. *Journal of Communication Disorders, 30*(4), 325–344.

Tomić, D. & Mildner, V. (2014, June). *Validation of Croatian Intelligibility in Context Scale.* Paper presented at ICPLA Symposium, Stockholm, Sweden.

Toohill, B. J., McLeod, S., & McCormack, J. (2012). Effect of dialect on identification and severity of speech impairment in Indigenous Australian children. *Clinical Linguistics and Phonetics, 26*(2), 101–119.

Topbaş, S. (2005). *Türkçe Sesletim-Sesbilgisi Testi [Turkish Articulation and Phonology Test].* Ankara, Turkey: Milli EğitimYayınevi 4. Akşam Sanat Okulu.

Topbaş, S. (2007). Turkish speech acquisition. In S. McLeod (Ed.), *The international guide to speech acquisition* (pp. 566–579). Clifton Park, NY: Thomson Delmar Learning.

Topbaş, S., Kaçar-Kütükçü, D., & Kopkalli-Yavuz, H. (2014). Performance of children on the Turkish Nonword Repetition Test: Effect of word similarity, word length, and scoring. *Clinical Linguistics and Phonetics, 28*(7–8), 602–616.

Topbaş, S., & Ünal, Ö. (2010). An alternating treatment comparison of minimal and maximal opposition sound selection in Turkish phonological disorders. *Clinical Linguistics and Phonetics, 24*(8), 646–668.

Torgeson, J. K., & Bryant, B. R. (2004). *Test of Phonological Awareness-Second Edition: PLUS* (TOPA-2+). Austin, TX: Pro-Ed.

Torgesen, J., Wagner, R., & Rashotte, C. (1994). Longitudinal studies of phonological processing and reading. *Journal of Learning Disabilities, 27*, 276–286.

Torgesen, J. K., Wagner, R. K., & Rashotte, C. A. (2012). *Test of Word Reading Efficiency (TOWRE) - 2.* Austin, TX: Pro-Ed.

Tourville, J. A., & Guenther, F. H. (2011). The DIVA model: A neural theory of speech acquisition and production. *Language and Cognitive Processes, 26*(7), 952–981.

Trabacca, A., Russo, L., Losito, L., Rinaldis, M. D., Moro, G., Cacudi, M., & Gennaro, L. (2012). The ICF-CY perspective on the neurorehabilitation of cerebral palsy: A single case study. *Journal of Child Neurology, 27*(2), 183–190.

Trubetzkoy, N. S. (1939). *Grundzüge der Phonologie. Travaux du Cercle Linguistique de Prague 7*, Reprinted 1958, Göttingen: Vandenhoek & Ruprecht. Translated into English by C. A. M. Baltaxe 1969 as *Principles of phonology.* Berkeley, CA: University of California Press.

Tsao, F.-M., Liu, H.-M., & Kuhl, P. K. (2004). Speech perception in infancy predicts language development in the second year of life: A longitudinal study. *Child Development, 75*(4), 1067–1084.

Ttofari Eecen, K., Reilly, S., & Eadie, P. (2007, May). *Parent concern and parent report of speech sound development at 12 months of age.* Paper presented at the Speech Pathology Australia National Conference, Sydney, Australia.

Tucker, G. R. (1998). A global perspective on multilingualism and multilingual education. In J. Cenoz & F. Genesee (Eds.), *Beyond bilinguals: Multilingualism and multilingual education* (pp. 3–15). Clevedon, UK: Multilingual Matters.

Tuomi, S., & Ivanoff, P. (1977). Incidence of speech and hearing disorders among kindergarten and grade 1 children. *Special Education in Canada, 51*, 5–8.

Tyler, A. A. (1995). Durational analysis of stridency errors in children with phonological impairment. *Clinical Linguistics and Phonetics, 9*, 211–228.

Tyler, A. A. (2002). Language-based intervention for phonological disorders. *Topics in Language Disorders, 23*(1), 69–81.

Tyler, A. A. (2005a). Planning and monitoring intervention programs. In A. G. Kamhi & K. E. Pollock (Eds.), *Phonological disorders in children: Clinical decision making in assessment and intervention* (pp. 123–137). Baltimore, MD: Paul H. Brookes.

Tyler, A. A. (2005b). Promoting and generalization: Selecting, scheduling, and integrating goals. In A. G. Kamhi & K. E. Pollock (Eds.), *Phonological disorders in children: Clinical decision making in assessment and intervention* (pp. 67–75). Baltimore, MD: Paul H. Brookes.

Tyler, A. A. (2006). Commentary on "Treatment decisions for children with speech-sound disorders": Revisiting the past in EBP. *Language, Speech, and Hearing Services in Schools, 37*(4), 280–283.

Tyler, A. A. (2008). What works: Evidence-based intervention for children with speech sound disorders. *Seminars in Speech and Language, 29*, 320–330.

Tyler, A. A., & Edwards, M. L. (1993). Lexical acquisition and acquisition of initial voiceless stops. *Journal of Child Language, 20,* 253–273.

Tyler, A. A., Edwards, M. L., & Saxman, J. H. (1987). Clinical application of two phonologically based treatment procedures. *Journal of Speech and Hearing Disorders, 52,* 393–409.

Tyler, A. A., Edwards, M. L., & Saxman, J. H. (1990). Acoustic validation of phonological knowledge and its relationship to treatment. *Journal of Speech and Hearing Disorders, 55,* 251–261.

Tyler, A. A., & Figurski, G. R. (1994). Phonetic inventory changes after treating distinctions along an implicational hierarchy. *Clinical Linguistics and Phonetics, 8*(2), 91–107.

Tyler, A. A., Figurski, G. R., & Lansdale, T. (1993). Relationships between acoustically determined knowledge of stop place and voicing contrasts and phonological treatment progress. *Journal of Speech and Hearing Research, 36,* 746–759.

Tyler, A. A., Gillon, G., Macrae, T., & Johnson, R. L. (2011). Direct and indirect effects of stimulating phoneme awareness vs. other linguistic skills in preschoolers with co-occurring speech and language impairments. *Topics in Language Disorders, 31*(2), 128–144.

Tyler, A. A., & Haskill, A. (2010). Morphosyntax intervention. In A. L. Williams, S. McLeod, & R. J. McCauley (Eds.), *Interventions for speech sound disorders in children* (pp. 355–380). Baltimore, MD: Paul H. Brookes.

Tyler, A. A., & Lewis, K. E. (2005). Relationships among consistency/variability and other phonological measures over time. *Topics in Language Disorders, 25*(3), 243–253.

Tyler, A. A., Lewis, K. E., Haskill, A., & Tolbert, L. C. (2002). Efficacy and cross-domain effects of a morpho-syntax and a phonology intervention. *Language, Speech, and Hearing Services in Schools, 33,* 52–66.

Tyler, A. A., Lewis, K. E., Haskill, A., & Tolbert, L. C. (2003). Outcomes of different speech and language goal attack strategies. *Journal of Speech, Language, and Hearing Research, 46,* 1077–1094.

Tyler, A. A., Lewis, K. E., & Welch, C. M. (2003). Predictors of phonological change following intervention. *American Journal of Speech-Language Pathology, 12*(3), 289–298.

Tyler, A. A., & Tolbert, L. C. (2002). Speech-language assessment in the clinical setting. *American Journal of Speech-Language Pathology, 11*(3), 215–220.

Tyler, A. A., & Watterson, K. H. (1991). Effects of phonological versus language intervention in preschoolers with both phonological and language impairment. *Child Language Teaching and Therapy, 7*(2), 141–160.

Tyler, A. A., Williams, M. J., & Lewis, K. E. (2006). Error consistency and the evaluation of treatment outcomes. *Clinical Linguistics and Phonetics, 20*(6), 411–422.

UK and Ireland Specialists in Specific Speech Impairment Network. (2013). *Good practice guidelines for transcription of children's speech samples in clinical practice and research.* London, UK: Royal College of Speech and Language Therapists. Retrieved from http://www.rcslt.org/members/publications/transcriptionguidelines.

Ullrich, A., Stemberger, J. P., & Bernhardt, B. M. (2008). Variability in a German-speaking child as viewed from a constraint-based nonlinear phonology perspective. *Asia Pacific Journal of Speech, Language, and Hearing, 11*(4), 221–238.

UNICEF. (1989). *The United Nations Convention on the Rights of the Child* (UNCRC). Retrieved from http://www.unicef.org/crc.

Unicomb, R., Hewat, S., Spencer, E., & Harrison, E. (2013). Clinicians' management of young children with co-occurring stuttering and speech sound disorder. *International Journal of Speech-Language Pathology, 15*(4), 441–452.

United Nations. (2011). *United Nations Convention on the Rights of Persons with Disability* Retrieved from http://www.un.org/disabilities/convention/conventionfull.shtml.

University of Melbourne. (2013). *Quality of Life Questionnaire for Children* (CP QOL-Child). Retrieved from http://cpqol.org.au/index.html.

Usdan, V. L. (1978). Utilization of the "straw technique" for correction of the lateral lisp. *Language, Speech, and Hearing Services in Schools, 9*(1), 5–7.

U.S. Department of Education. (2005). *To assure the free appropriate public education of all Americans: Twenty-seventh annual report to Congress on the implementation of the Individuals with Disabilities Education Act.* Retrieved from http://www.ed.gov/about/reports/annual/osep/2005/index.html.

UT Dallas. (2014). *Automated transcription.* Retrieved from http://www.utdallas.edu/ctech/projects-overview/automated-transcription/.

Utley, A., & Astill, S. (2008). *Motor control, learning and development* (Vol. 32). Portland, OR: Book News.

Vallino, L. D., Peterson-Falzone, S. J., & Napoli, J. A. (2006). The syndromes of Treacher Collins and Nager. *International Journal of Speech-Language Pathology, 8*(1), 34–44.

Van Borsel, J., Van Rentergem, S., & Verhaeghe, L. (2007). The prevalence of lisping in young adults. *Journal of Communication Disorders, 40*(6), 493–502.

Van Borsel, J., Van Snick, K., & Leroy, J. (1999). Macroglossia and speech in Beckwith-Wiedemann syndrome: A sample survey study. *International Journal of Language and Communication Disorders, 34*(2), 209–221.

van Bysterveldt, A. K., Gillon, G., & Foster-Cohen, S. (2010). Integrated speech and phonological awareness intervention for pre-school children with Down syndrome. *International Journal of Language and Communication Disorders, 45*(3), 320–335.

Van Demark, D. R. (1997). Diagnostic value of articulation tests with individuals having clefts. *Folia Phoniatrica et Logopaedica, 49,* 147–157.

Van den Elzen, A. P. M., Semmekrot, B. A., Bongers, E. M. H. F., Huygen, P. L. M., & Marres, H. A. M. (2001). Diagnosis and treatment of the Pierre Robin sequence: Results of a retrospective clinical study and review of the literature. *European Journal of Pediatrics, 160*(1), 47–53.

van der Merwe, A. (2007). Self-correction in apraxia of speech: The effect of treatment. *Aphasiology, 21,* 658–669.

van der Merwe, A. (2009). A theoretical framework for the characterization of pathological speech sensorimotor control. In M. R. McNeil (Ed.), *Clinical management of sensorimotor speech disorders* (pp. 3–18). New York, NY: Thieme.

Van Lierde, K. M., Vinck, B. M., Baudonck, N., De Vel, E., & Dhooge, I. (2005). Comparison of the overall intelligibility, articulation, resonance, and voice characteristics between children using cochlear implants and those using bilateral hearing aids: A pilot study. *International Journal of Audiology, 44*(8), 452–465.

Van Riper, C. (1939). *Speech correction: Principles and methods.* Englewood Cliffs, NJ: Prentice-Hall.

Van Riper, C. (1947). *Speech correction: Principles and methods* (2nd ed.). Englewood Cliffs, NJ: Prentice-Hall.

Van Riper, C. (1954). *Speech correction: Principles and methods* (3rd ed.). Englewood Cliffs, NJ: Prentice-Hall.

Van Riper, C. (1963). *Speech correction: Principles and methods* (4th ed.). Englewood Cliffs, NJ: Prentice-Hall.

Van Riper, C. (1972). *Speech correction: Principles and methods* (5th ed.). Englewood Cliffs, NJ: Prentice-Hall.

Van Riper, C. (1978). *Speech correction: Principles and methods* (6th ed.). Englewood Cliffs, NJ: Prentice-Hall.

Van Riper, C., & Emerick, L. (1984). *Speech correction: An introduction to speech pathology and audiology* (7th ed.). Englewood Cliffs, NJ: Prentice-Hall.

Van Riper, C., & Emerick, L. (1990). *Speech correction: An introduction to speech pathology and audiology* (8th ed.). Englewood Cliffs, NJ: Prentice-Hall.

Van Riper, C., & Erickson, R. L. (1996). *Speech correction: An introduction to speech pathology and audiology* (9th ed.). Needham Heights, MA: Allyn & Bacon.

Van Severen, L., Van Den Berg, R., Molemans, I., & Gillis, S. (2012). Consonant inventories in the spontaneous speech of young children: A bootstrapping procedure. *Clinical Linguistics and Phonetics, 26*(2), 164–187.

Van Zaalen-op't Hof, Y., Wijnen, F., & De Jonckere, P. H. (2009). Differential diagnostic characteristics between cluttering and stuttering: Part one. *Journal of Fluency Disorders, 34*(3), 137–154.

Vance, M., & Clegg, J. (2012). Use of single case study research in child speech, language and communication interventions. *Child Language Teaching and Therapy, 28*(3), 255–258.

Vanryckeghem, M., & Brutten, G. J. (2006). *KiddyCat: Communication attitude test for preschool and kindergarten children who stutter.* San Diego, CA: Plural Publishing.

Vanryckeghem, M., Brutten, G., & Hernandez, L. (2005). The KiddyCAT: A normative investigation of stuttering and nonstuttering preschoolers' speech-associated attitude. *Journal of Fluency Disorders, 30*, 307–318.

Vargha-Khadem, F., Carr, L. J., Isaacs, E., Brett, E., Adams, C., & Mishkin, M. (1997). Onset of speech after left hemispherectomy in a nine-year-old boy. *Brain, 120*(1), 159–182.

Velleman, S. L. (1998). *Making phonology functional: What do I do first?* Boston, MA: Butterworth-Heinemann.

Velleman, S. (2002). Phonotactic therapy. *Seminars in Speech and Language, 23*(1), 43–55.

Velleman, S. (2003). *Childhood apraxia of speech: Resource guide.* Clifton Park, NY: Thomson Delmar Learning.

Velleman, S. L., & Shriberg, L. D. (1999). Metrical analysis of the speech of children with suspected developmental apraxia of speech. *Journal of Speech, Language, and Hearing Research, 42*, 1444–1460.

Velten, H. (1943). The growth of phonemic and lexical patterns in infant language. *Language, 19*, 281–292.

Verdon, S. (2015). Enhancing practice with culturally and linguistically diverse families: Six key principles from the field. *Journal of Clinical Practice in Speech-Language Pathology, 17*(1), 2–6.

Verdon, S., McLeod, S., & Wong, S. (2015). Supporting culturally and linguistically diverse children with speech, language and communication needs: Overarching principles, individual approaches. *Journal of Communication Disorders, 58*, 74–90.

Verhagen, A. P., de Vet, H. C. W., de Bie, R. A., Kessels, A. G. H., Boers, M., Bouter, L. M., & Knipschild, G. (1998). The Delphi list: A criteria list for quality assessment of randomised clinical trials for conducting systematic reviews developed by Delphi consensus. *Journal of Clinical Epidemiology, 51*(12), 1235–1241.

Veríssimo, A., van Borsel, J., & de Britto Pereira, M. (2012). Residual /s/ and /r/ distortions: The perspective of the speaker. *International Journal of Speech-Language Pathology, 14*(2), 183–186.

Vernes, S. C., Newbury, D. F., Abrahams, B. S., Winchester, L., Nicod, J., Groszer, M., . . . Fisher, S. E. (2008). A functional genetic link between distinct developmental language disorders. *New England Journal of Medicine, 359*, 2337–2345.

Vick, J. C., Campbell, T. F., Shriberg, L. D., Green, J. R., Truemper, K., Rusiewicz, H. L., & Moore, C. A. (2014). Data-driven subclassification of speech sound disorders in preschool children. *Journal of Speech, Language, and Hearing Research, 57*(6), 2033–2050.

Vihman, M. M. (1981). Phonology and the development of the lexicon: Evidence from children's errors. *Journal of Child Language, 8*, 239–264.

Vihman, M. M., & Croft, W. (2007). Phonological development: Toward a "radical" templatic phonology. *Linguistics, 45*, 683–725.

Vogel, A. P., & Maruff, P. (2014). Monitoring change requires a rethink of assessment practices in voice and speech. *Logopedics Phoniatrics Vocology, 39*(2), 56–61.

Vogel, A. P., & Morgan, A. T. (2009). Factors affecting the quality of sound recording for speech and voice analysis. *International Journal of Speech-Language Pathology, 11*(6), 431–437.

Vygotsky, L. (1978). *Mind in society: The development of higher psychological processes.* (M. Cole, V. John-Steiner, S. Scribner, & E. Souberman, Eds. Trans.). Cambridge, MA: Harvard University Press.

Wagner, R. K., & Torgesen, J., K. (1987). The nature of phonological processing and its causal role in the acquisition of reading skills. *Psychological Bulletin, 101*(2), 191–212.

Wagner, R. K., Torgesen, J. K., Rashotte, C. A., Hecht, S. A., Barker, T. A., Burgess, S. R., . . . Garon, T. (1997). Changing relations between phonological processing abilities and word-level reading as children develop from beginning to skilled readers: A 5-year longitudinal study. *Developmental Psychology, 33*(3), 468–479.

Wagner, R. K., Torgesen, J. K., Rashotte, C. A., & Pearson, N. A. (2013). *Comprehensive Test of Phonological Processing: Second Edition (CTOPP-2).* Austin, TX: Pro-Ed.

Walsh, B., & Smith, A. (2002). Articulatory movements in adolescents: Evidence for protracted development of speech motor control processes. *Journal of Speech, Language, and Hearing Research, 45*(6), 1119–1133.

Walters, B. (1970). *How to talk with practically anybody about practically anything.* Garden City, NY: Doubleday.

Ward, R., Leitão, S., & Strauss, G. (2014). An evaluation of the effectiveness of PROMPT therapy in improving speech production accuracy in six children with cerebral palsy. *International Journal of Speech-Language Pathology, 16*(4), 355–371.

Ward, R., Strauss, G., & Leitão, S. (2013). Kinematic changes in jaw and lip control of children with cerebral palsy following participation in a motor-speech (PROMPT) intervention. *International Journal of Speech-Language Pathology, 15*(2), 136–155.

Waring, R., Fisher, J., & Aitken, N. (2001). The articulation survey: Putting numbers to it. In L. Wilson & S. Hewat (Eds.), *Proceedings of the 2001 Speech Pathology Australia national conference: Evidence and innovation* (pp. 145–151). Melbourne, Australia: Speech Pathology Australia.

Waring, R., & Knight, R. (2013). How should children with speech sound disorders be classified? A review and critical evaluation of current classification systems. *International Journal of Language and Communication Disorders, 48*(1), 25–40.

Warr-Leeper, G. A., McShea, R. S., & Leeper, J. H. A. (1979). The incidence of voice and speech deviations in a middle school population. *Language, Speech, and Hearing Services in Schools, 10*(1), 14–20.

Warren, R. M. (1970). Perceptual restoration of missing speech sounds. *Science, 167*, 392–393.

Warren, S. F., Fey, M. E., & Yoder, P. J. (2007). Differential treatment intensity research: A missing link to creating optimally effective communication interventions. *Mental Retardation and Developmental Disabilities Research Reviews, 13*, 70–77.

Washington, K. N., McDonald, M. M., McLeod, S., Crowe, K., & Devonish, H. (2015). *Validation of the Intelligibility in Context Scale for Jamaican Creole-speaking preschoolers.* Manuscript in submission.

Washington, K., Thomas-Stonell, N., Oddson, B., McLeod, S., Warr-Leeper, G., & Rosenbaum, P. (2013). Construct validity of the FOCUS (Focus on the Outcomes of Communication Under Six): A functional communication outcome measure for preschool children. *Child Care Health and Development, 39*(4), 481–489.

Waterlow, J. C., Buzina, R., Keller, W., Lane, J. M., Nichaman, M. Z., & Tanner, J. M. (1977). The presentation and use of height and weight data for comparing the nutritional status of groups of children under the age of 10 years. *Bulletin of the World Health Organization, 55*(4), 489–498.

Waterson, N. (1971). Child phonology: A prosodic view. *Journal of Linguistics, 7*, 179–211.

Watson, D., Townsley, R., & Abbott, D. (2002). Exploring multi-agency working in services to disabled children with complex healthcare needs and their families. *Journal of Clinical Nursing, 11*, 367–375.

Watson, M. M., & Scukanec, G. P. (1997a). Phonological changes in the speech of two-year olds: A longitudinal investigation. *Infant-Toddler Intervention, 7*, 67–77.

Watson, M. M., & Scukanec, G. P. (1997b). Profiling the phonological abilities of 2-year-olds: A longitudinal investigation. *Child Language Teaching and Therapy, 13*, 3–14.

Watson, M. M., & Terrell, P. (2012). Longitudinal changes in phonological whole-word measures in 2-year-olds. *International Journal of Speech-Language Pathology, 14*(4), 351–362.

Watts Pappas, N. (2010). Family-friendly intervention. In A. L. Williams, S. McLeod, & R. J. McCauley (Eds.), *Interventions for speech sound disorders in children* (pp. 475–496). Baltimore, MD: Paul H. Brookes.

Watts Pappas, N., & McLeod, S. (2009). Working with families of children with speech impairment. In N. Watts Pappas & S. McLeod (Eds.), *Working with families in speech-language pathology* (pp. 189–228). San Diego, CA: Plural Publishing.

Watts Pappas, N., McLeod, S., McAllister, L., & McKinnon, D. H. (2008). Parental involvement in speech intervention: A national survey. *Clinical Linguistics and Phonetics, 22*(4), 335–344.

Webb, A. N., Hao, W., & Hong, P. (2013). The effect of tongue-tie division on breastfeeding and speech articulation: A systematic review. *International Journal of Pediatric Otorhinolaryngology, 77*(5), 635–646.

Webb, M.-Y. L., & Lederberg, A. R. (2014). Measuring phonological awareness in deaf and hard-of-hearing children. *Journal of Speech, Language, and Hearing Research, 57*(1), 131–142.

Webber, S. G. (2005). *Webber photo phonology minimal pair cards.* Greenville, SC: Super Duper Publications.

Wechsler, D. (2002). *The Wechsler Preschool and Primary Scale of Intelligence—Third Edition (WPPSI-III)*. San Antonio, TX: The Psychological Corporation.

Wechsler, D. (2003). *Wechsler Intelligence Scale for Children—Fourth Edition (WISC-IV)*. San Antonio, TX: The Psychological Corporation.

Wedel, A., Kaplan, A., & Jackson, S. (2013). High functional load inhibits phonological contrast loss: A corpus study. *Cognition, 128*(2), 179–186.

Weigl, V., Rudolph, M., Eysholdt, U., & Rosanowski, F. (2005). Anxiety, depression, and quality of life in mothers of children with cleft lip/palate. *Folia Phoniatrica et Logopaedica, 57,* 20–27.

Wein, B., Böckler, R., Klajman, S., & Obrebowski, A. (1991). Ultrasonography of the tongue in the rehabilitation of speech articulation disorders. *Otolaryngologia Polska [The Polish Otolaryngology], 45,* 133–140.

Weindrich, D., Jennen-Steinmetz, C., Laucht, M., Esser, G., & Schmidt, M. H. (2000). Epidemiology and prognosis of specific disorders of language and scholastic skills. *European Child and Adolescent Psychiatry, 9*(3), 186–194.

Weiner, F. F. (1979). *Phonological process analysis*. Baltimore, MD: University Park Press.

Weiner, F. F. (1981). Treatment of phonological disability using the method of meaningful minimal contrast: Two case studies. *Journal of Speech and Hearing Disorders, 46,* 97–103.

Weiner, F. F. (1984). A phonologic approach to assessment and treatment. In J. Costello (Ed.), *Speech disorders in children* (pp. 75–91). San Diego, CA: College-Hill Press.

Weismer, G. (2006). Philosophy of research in motor speech disorders. *Clinical Linguistics and Phonetics, 20*(5), 315–349.

Weiss, C. E. (1980). *Weiss Comprehensive Articulation Test (WCAT)*. Austin, TX: Pro-Ed.

Weiss, C. E. (1982). *Weiss Intelligibility Test*. Tigard, OR: C. C. Publications.

Wells, B. (1994). Junction in developmental speech disorder: A case study. *Clinical Linguistics and Phonetics, 8*(1), 1–25.

Wells, B., & Peppé, S. (2001). Intonation within a psycholinguistic framework. In J. Stackhouse & B. Wells (Eds.), *Children's speech and literacy difficulties 2: Identification and intervention* (pp. 366–395). London, UK: Whurr.

Wells, B., Peppé, S., & Goulandris, N. (2004). Intonation development from five to thirteen. *Journal of Child Language, 31*(4), 749–778.

Wells, J. C. (1982). *Accents of English*. Cambridge, UK: Cambridge University Press.

Wells, J. C. (2006). Phonetic transcription and analysis. In K. Brown (Ed.), *Encyclopedia of language and linguistics* (2nd ed., pp. 386–396). Oxford, UK: Elsevier.

Wepman, J. M., & Reynolds, W. M. (1987). *The Wepman Auditory Discrimination Test: Second Edition*. Los Angeles, CA: Western Psychological Services.

Werker, J. F., & Tees, R. C. (1992). The organization and reorganization of human speech perception. *Annual Review of Neuroscience, 15*(1), 377–402.

Wertzner, H. F., Alves, R. R., & de Oliveira Ramos, A. C. (2008). Análise do desenvolvimento das habilidades diadococinéticas orais em crianças normais e com transtorno fonológico [Development of oral diadochokinetic abilities in normal and phonologically disordered children]. *Revista da Sociedade Brasileira de Fonoaudiologia, 31*(2).

Westerveld, M. F., & Claessen, M. (2014). Clinician survey of language sampling practices in Australia. *International Journal of Speech-Language Pathology, 16*(3), 242–249.

Weston, A. D., & Shriberg, L. D. (1992). Contextual and linguistic correlates of intelligibility in children with developmental phonological disorders. *Journal of Speech, Language, and Hearing Research, 35*(6), 1316–1332.

Weston, A. J., & Harber, S. K. (1975). The effects of scheduling on progress in paired-stimuli articulation therapy. *Language, Speech, and Hearing Services in Schools, 6*(2), 96–101.

Wetherby, A., & Prizant, B. (1993). *Communication and symbolic behavior scales*. Baltimore, MD: Paul H. Brookes.

Whelan, D. T., Feldman, W., & Dost, I. (1975). The oro-facial-digital syndrome. *Clinical Genetics, 8*(3), 205–212.

Whitehill, T. (2002). Assessing intelligibility in speakers with cleft palate: A critical review of the literature. *Folio Phoniatrica et Logopaedica, 54,* 50–58.

Whitney, W. D. (1865). The relation of vowel and consonant. *Journal of the American Oriental Society, Vol. 8.* Reprinted in W. D. Whitney (1874) *Oriental and Linguistic Studies,* Second Series, New York, NY: Charles Scribner's Sons.

Widgerow, A. D. (1990). Klippel-Feil anomaly, cleft palate, and bifid tongue. *Annals of Plastic Surgery, 25*(3), 216–222.

Wightman, D., & Lintern, G. (1985). Part-task training for tracking and manual control. *Human Factors, 27,* 267–283.

Wiig, E., Secord, W. A., & Semel, E. (2004). *Clinical Evaluation of Language Fundamentals: Preschool-2 (CELF-P2)* (2nd ed.). San Antonio, TX: Psychological Corporation.

Wilcox, K., & Morris, S. (1999). *Children's Speech Intelligibility Measure*. San Antonio, TX: Harcourt Assessment.

Williams, A. L. (1991). Generalisation patterns associated with least knowledge. *Journal of Speech and Hearing Research, 34,* 722–733.

Williams, A. L. (1993). Phonological reorganization: A qualitative measure of phonological improvement. *American Journal of Speech-Language Pathology, May,* 44–51.

Williams, A. L. (2000a). Multiple oppositions: Case studies of variables in phonological intervention. *American Journal of Speech-Language Pathology, 9,* 289–299.

Williams, A. L. (2000b). Multiple oppositions: Theoretical foundations for an alternative contrastive intervention approach. *American Journal of Speech-Language Pathology, 9,* 282–288.

Williams, A. L. (2002). Prologue: Perspectives in the assessment of children's speech. *American Journal of Speech-Language Pathology, 11*(3), 211–212.

Williams, A. L. (2003). *Speech disorders resource guide for preschool children*. Clifton Park, NY: Delmar Learning.

Williams, A. L. (2005a). Assessment, target selection, and intervention: Dynamic interactions within a systemic perspective. *Topics in Language Disorders, 25*(3), 231–242.

Williams, A. L. (2005b). From developmental norms to distance metics: Past, present, and future directions for target selection practices. In A. G. Kamhi & K. E. Pollock (Eds.), *Phonological disorders in children: Clinical decision making in assessment and intervention* (pp. 101–108). Baltimore: MD: Paul H. Brookes.

Williams, A. L. (2005c). A model and structure for phonological intervention. In A. G. Kamhi & K. E. Pollock (Eds.), *Phonological disorders in children: Clinical decision making in assessment and intervention* (pp. 189–199). Baltimore, MD: Paul H. Brookes.

Williams, A. L. (2006). *SCIP—Sound Contrasts in Phonology: Evidence-based treatment program*. Greenville, SC: Super Duper Publications.

Williams, A. L. (2010). Multiple oppositions. In A. L. Williams, S. McLeod, & R. J. McCauley (Eds.), *Interventions for speech sound disorders in children* (pp. 73–93). Baltimore, MD: Paul H. Brookes.

Williams, A. L. (2012). Intensity in phonological intervention: Is there a prescribed amount? *International Journal of Speech-Language Pathology, 14*(5), 456–461.

Williams, A. L., & Elbert, M. (2003). A prospective longitudinal study of phonological development in late talkers. *Language, Speech, and Hearing Services in Schools, 34,* 138–153.

Williams, A. L., McLeod, S., & McCauley, R. J. (Eds.). (2010). *Interventions for speech sound disorders in children*. Baltimore, MD: Paul H. Brookes.

Williams, A. L., & Stoel-Gammon, C. (in preparation). *Profiles of Early Expressive Phonological Skills* (PEEPS). Johnson City, TN: Author.

Williams, C., & McLeod, S. (2012). Speech-language pathologists' assessment and intervention practices with multilingual children. *International Journal of Speech-Language Pathology, 14*(3), 292–305.

Williams, D. F., & Dietrich, S. (1996). Effects of speech and language disorders on raters' perceptions. *Journal of Communication Disorders, 29*(1), 1–12.

Williams, K. T. (2007). *Expressive Vocabulary Test: Second Edition*. Circle Pines, MN: AGS Publishing.

Williams, P., & Stackhouse, J. (2000). Rate, accuracy and consistency: Diadochokinetic performance of young, normally developing children. *Clinical Linguistics and Phonetics, 14,* 267–293.

Williams, P., & Stephens, H. (2004). *Nuffield Centre Dyspraxia Programme: Third Edition* (NDP-3). Windsor, UK: The Miracle Factory.

Williams, P., & Stephens, H. (2010). The Nuffield Centre Dyspraxia Programme. In A. L. Williams, S. McLeod, & R. J. McCauley (Eds.), *Interventions for speech sound disorders in children* (pp. 159–177). Baltimore, MD: Paul H. Brookes.

Williamson, I. (2007). Otitis media with effusion in children. *Clinical Evidence, 8,* 1–15.

Windsor, J., Kohnert, K., Lobitz, K. F., & Pham, G. T. (2010). Cross-language nonword repetition by bilingual and monolingual children. *American Journal of Speech-Language Pathology, 19*(4), 298–310.

Winitz, H., & Bellerose, B. (1962). Sound discrimination as a function of pretraining conditions. *Journal of Speech, Language, and Hearing Research, 5*(4), 340–348.

Wit, J., Maassen, B., Gabreels, F. J. M., & Thoonen, G. (1993). Maximum performance tests in children with developmental spastic dysarthria. *Journal of Speech and Hearing Research, 36*(3), 452–459.

Wolfe, V., Presley, C., & Mesaris, J. (2003). The importance of sound identification training in phonological intervention. *American Journal of Speech-Language Pathology, 12,* 282–288.

Wolk, L., Edwards, M. L., & Conture, E. G. (1993). Coexistence of stuttering and disordered phonology in young children. *Journal of Speech, Language, and Hearing Research, 36*(5), 906–917.

Wood, K. S. (1946). Parental maladjustment and functional articulatory defects in children. *Journal of Speech Disorders, 11,* 255–275.

Woodcock, R. W., Mather, N., & Schrank, F. A. (2004). *Woodcock-Johnson III diagnostic reading battery.* Itasca, IL: Riverside.

Woodyatt, G., & Ozanne, A. (1992). Communication abilities and Rett syndrome. *Journal of Autism and Developmental Disorders, 22*(2), 155–173.

World Health Organization. (2001). ICF: *International classification of functioning, disability and health.* Geneva, Switzerland: World Health Organization.

World Health Organization (WHO Workgroup for development of version of ICF for Children & Youth). (2007). *International classification of functioning, disability and health: Children and youth version: ICF-CY.* Geneva, Switzerland: World Health Organization. (Chapter 2 list, page 50: Reprinted from World Health Organization (WHO), Copyright 2007.)

World Health Organization (2015a). *ICD-11 Beta Draft 7A10 developmental speech sound disorder.* Retrieved from http://apps.who.int/classifications/icd11/browse/l-m/en#/http%3a%2f%2fid.who.int%2ficd%2fentity%2f551966778.

World Health Organization (2015b). *ICD-10 2015: Disorders of psychological development (F80–F89).* Retrieved from http://apps.who.int/classifications/icd10/browse/2015/en#/F80.0.

World Health Organization and the World Bank (2011). *World report on disability.* Geneva, Switzerland: World Health Organization. (Chapter 15 list recommendations, page 535: Reprinted from World Health Organization (WHO), *World report on disability.* Copyright 2011.)

Wren, Y. (2015). "He'll grow out of it soon—won't he?" The characteristics of older children's speech when they do—and don't—grow out of it. *SIG 16 Perspectives on School-Based Issues, 16*(2), 25–36.

Wren, Y., Hughes, T., & Roulstone, S. (2006). *Phoneme Factory Phonology Screener.* London, UK: NFER Nelson.

Wren, Y., McLeod, S., White, P., Miller, L. L., & Roulstone, S. (2013). Speech characteristics of 8-year-old children: Findings from a prospective population study. *Journal of Communication Disorders, 46*(1), 53–69.

Wren, Y., & Roulstone, S. (2006). *Phoneme Factory Sound Sorter* [Computer software]. London, UK: GL Assessment.

Wren, Y., & Roulstone, S. E. (2013). *Phoneme Factory Sound Sorter* (version 2, Australian adapation) [Computer software]. Bristol, UK: Bristol Speech and Language Therapy Research Unit, North Bristol NHS Trust.

Wren, Y. E., Roulstone, S. E., & Miller, L. L. (2012). Distinguishing groups of children with persistent speech disorder: Findings from a prospective population study. *Logopedics Phoniatrics Vocology, 37*(1), 1–10.

Wrench, A. A. (2007). Advances in EPG palate design. *International Journal of Speech-Language Pathology, 9*(1), 3–12.

Wrench, A. (2013). *Articulate Assistant Advanced (AAA)* [Computer software]. Edinburgh: Articulate Instruments.

Wright, J. E. (1995). Review article: Tongue-tie. *Journal of Paediatrics and Child Health, 31*(4), 276–278.

Wulf, G., McNevin, N., & Shea, C. H. (2001). The automaticity of complex motor skill learning as a function of attentional focus. *The Quarterly Journal of Experimental Psychology, 54*(4), 1143–1154.

Wyllie-Smith, L., McLeod, S., & Ball, M. J. (2006). Typically developing and speech-impaired children's adherence to the sonority hypothesis. *Clinical Linguistics and Phonetics, 20*(4), 271–291.

Xu, D., Richards, J. A., & Gilkerson, J. (2014). Automated analysis of child phonetic production using naturalistic recordings. *Journal of Speech, Language, and Hearing Research, 57*(5), 1638–1650.

Yavaş, M., Ben-David, A., Gerrits, E., Kristoffersen, K. E., & Simonsen, H. G. (2008). Sonority and cross-linguistic acquisition of initial s-clusters. *Clinical Linguistics and Phonetics, 22*(6), 421–441.

Yavaş, M., & Mota, H. B. (2007). Portuguese speech acquisition. In S. McLeod (Ed.), *The international guide to speech acquisition* (pp. 505–515). Clifton Park, NY: Thomson Delmar Learning.

Yildiz, A., & Arikan, D. (2012). The effects of giving pacifiers to premature infants and making them listen to lullabies on their transition period for total oral feeding and sucking success. *Journal of Clinical Nursing, 21*(5–6), 644–656.

Yliherva, A., Olsén, P., Mäki-Torkko, E., Koiranen, M., & Järvelin, M. R. (2001). Linguistic and motor abilities of low-birthweight children as assessed by parents and teachers at 8 years of age. *Acta Paediatrica, 90*(12), 1440–1449.

Yorkston, K. M., & Beukelman, D. R. (1978). A comparison of techniques for measuring intelligibility of dysarthric speech. *Journal of Communication Disorders, 11*(6), 499–512.

Yorkston, K. M., Beukelman, D. R., Strand, E. A., & Hakel, M. (2010). *Management of motor speech disorders in children and adults* (3rd ed.). Austin, TX: Pro-Ed.

Yorkston, K. M., Strand, E. A., & Kennedy, M. R. T. (1996). Comprehensibility of dysarthric speech: Implications for assessment and treatment planning. *American Journal of Speech-Language Pathology, 5*(1), 55–66.

Yoshinaga-Itano, C., Sedey, A. L., Coulter, D. K., & Mehl, A. L. (1998). Language of early- and later-identified children with hearing loss. *Pediatrics, 102*(5), 1161–1171.

Young, E. C. (1987). The effects of treatment on consonant cluster and weak syllable reduction processes in misarticulating children. *Language, Speech, and Hearing Services in Schools, 18,* 23–33.

Young, E. C. (1995). An analysis of a treatment approach for phonological errors in polysyllabic words. *Clinical Linguistics and Phonetics, 9,* 59–77.

Young, E. C., & Thompson, C. K. (1987). An experimental analysis of treatment effects on consonant clusters and ambisyllabic consonants in two adults with developmental phonological problems. *Journal of Communication Disorders, 20,* 137–149.

Young, E. H., & Stinchfield-Hawk, S. (1955). *Moto-kinesthetic speech training.* Stanford, CA: Stanford University Press.

youthinmind. (2012). *SDQ.* Retrieved from http://www.sdqinfo.org/.

Zajac, D. J. (2013). Nasalance scores of children with repaired cleft palate who exhibit normal velopharyngeal closure during aerodynamic testing. *American Journal of Speech-Language Pathology, 22*(3), 572–576.

Zajac, D. J., Plante, C., Lloyd, A., & Haley, K. L. (2011). Reliability and validity of a computer-mediated, single-word intelligibility test: Preliminary findings for children with repaired cleft lip and palate. *The Cleft Palate-Craniofacial Journal, 48*(5), 538–549.

Zajdó, K. (2007). Hungarian speech acquisition. In S. McLeod (Ed.), *The international guide to speech acquisition* (pp. 412–436). Clifton Park, NY: Thomson Delmar Learning.

Zampini, L., Fasolo, M., Spinelli, M., Zanchi, P., Suttora, C., & Salerni, N. (2016). Prosodic skills in children with Down syndrome and in typically developing children. *International Journal of Language and Communication Disorders. 51*(1), 74–83.

Zaretsky, E., Velleman, S. L., & Curro, K. (2010). Through the magnifying glass: Underlying literacy deficits and remediation potential in childhood apraxia of speech. *International Journal of Speech-Language Pathology, 12*(1), 58–68.

Zee, E. (1999). Chinese (Hong Kong Cantonese). In International Phonetic Association (Ed.), *Handbook of the International Phonetic Association* (pp. 58–60). Cambridge, UK: Cambridge University Press.

Zemlin, W. R. (1998). *Speech and hearing science: Anatomy and physiology* (4th ed.). Boston, MA: Allyn & Bacon.

Zhichao, W., & Jing, Y. (2006). The development and primary analysis of the test of nonword repetition. *Psychological Science, 29*(2), 401–405.

Zimmerman, E., & Thompson, K. (2015). Clarifying nipple confusion. *Journal of Perinatology, 35*(11), 895–899.

Zimmerman, I. L., Steiner, V. G., & Pond, R. E. (2012). *PLS-5: Preschool Language Scales, Fifth Edition, Spanish edition*. Bloomington, MN: Pearson.

Zimmerman, S., Osberger, M. J., & McConkey Robbins, A. (2000). *Infant-Toddler Meaningful Auditory Integration Scale*. Retrieved from http://c324175.r75.cf1.rackcdn.com/IT-MAS_20brochure_20_2.pdf.

Note: 'f' and 't' followed by page numbers indicate figures and tables.

A

absolute linguistic universals, 145
ABX task, 267
acceptability, assessment of, 249
acceptable speech acquisition, 178–185
accommodation, 185
acoustic analysis
    of children's speech, 326–329, 326f
    high-quality sound recording for, 328
    software, 327
acoustic feature of speech sounds, 141
acoustic nerve, 81
acoustic-phonetic, 165, 457
Activities
    as component of ICF-CY, 50, 50f
    defined, 420–422
    and Participation, 342
acute otitis media (AOM), 80
adaptation of services, 224–225
adenoid pad, 75
adolescence, manifestation of SSD in, 16–17
adulthood, manifestation of SSD in, 16–17
affricate pair, 444
affricates, 94, 124, 124f
    voiced postalveolar, 124
    voiceless postalveolar, 124
affrication, 158
Afrikaans, 127–131
age
    of acquisition of consonant clusters, 196, 202, 204t, 210
    of acquisition of consonants, 196, 197t, 202, 203t, 210
    of acquisition of tones, 214t
    of acquisition of vowels, 196, 205, 210
    of acquisition of words, 182
    typical speech acquisition and, 180
Agency for Healthcare Research and Quality (AHRQ) National Guideline Clearinghouse, 524
Alberta Language and Development Questionnaire (ALDeQ), 231–232
allophones, 136–138, 137
allophonic transcription, 87. *See also* phonetic transcription
alternating sequencing, 369
alveolar, 93, 444
alveolar approximant, 121–122, 122f
    bunched, 121
    retroflex, 121
alveolar fricatives, 117–120, 118f
alveolarization (apicalization), 155

alveolar lateral approximant, 123, 123f
alveolar plosives, 111–113, 113f
    voiced, 111–113
    voiceless, 111–113
alveoli, 77
American Psychiatric Association, 5
American Speech-Language-Hearing Association (ASHA), 5, 9, 44, 51, 224, 400, 402, 524, 529, 538
ankyloglossia, 66
antecedent stimulus, 387
anterior faucial pillars, 73
approximant, 139
approximant consonant articulation, 90, 94
approximant pair, 444
Arabic
    intervention approaches, 472t
    Jordanian, 96, 107, 127–131
    Lebanese, 107, 127–131
Articulate Instruments, 497, 499
    Articulate Assistant Advanced (AAA), 327
articulation, 4, 5, 38
    schematic sagittal section of the head showing, 64f
    of speech sounds, 42, 258
articulation competence index (ACI), 319
articulation disorders, 9. *See also* articulation impairment
articulation errors, terminology for, 43
articulation impairment, 38, 42–43, 279
    for children, with goal setting, 363–367
    intervention for, 486–499
    lateral lisp, 554–555
    vs. phonological impairment, 292
    traditional articulation intervention for, 486–493
articulation intervention
    based on principles of motor learning, 493–496
    historical perspective on, 485
    traditional, 486–493
    using instrumental feedback, 496–499
articulatory abilities, 361
articulatory-phonetic, 165, 457
arytenoid cartilages, 76
assessment contexts, 227–228
assessment data, 423, 424f
assessment(s)
    of acceptability and comprehensibility, 249
    child-friendly, 225–226
    of children's communicative participation, 273–275

of children's views of their speech within educational and social contexts, 273–275
for children with suspected articulation impairment, 279
for children with suspected CAS, 279–280
for children with suspected childhood dysarthria, 280–281
for children with suspected inconsistent speech disorder, 279
for children with suspected phonological impairment, 278
components of children's speech, 245
connected speech, 261–263
of conventional literacy skills, 271–272
criterion-referenced, 238
descriptive, 234–235
diagnostic, 235
dynamic, 241–242
of early literacy skills, 271–272
of emergent literacy skills, 271–272
face-to-face, 221
family-centered, 227
family-friendly, 227
of fluency, 275–276
of hearing, 269
of inconsistency and variability, 265
informal, 237–238
of intelligibility, 245–249
of language, 275–276
norm-referenced, 238
of oral structure and function, 265–267
of phonological processing, 269–271
of psychosocial aspects, 272–273
screening, 239–240
single-word speech, 258–260
of speech perception, 267–268
of speech production, 250–265
of SSD for child with craniofacial anomalies, 281–282
of SSD for child with hearing loss, 282–283
of stimulability, 264–265
standardized, 236–237
static, 240
of voice, 275–276
assimilation, 185
assimilation processes (consonant harmony), 155–156
association lines, 161
associations
    national and international professional, 537t

supporting children with SSD, 537t
supporting clinical practice of SLPs, 536–539
supporting continuing education of SLPs, 536–539
audiologists, 228
auditory and visual models, DTTC and, 501
auditory cues, 414–415
    auditory detection of a target sound or prosodic characteristics, 414
    auditory discrimination, 414
    auditory identification of target sound or prosodic characteristic, 414
    auditory judgment of correctness tasks, 414
    focused auditory input/auditory stimulation, 414
    metaphonological input tasks, 415
    phonological awareness input tasks, 415
    self-monitoring requests, 414–415
auditory discrimination, 414
    tasks, 267–268
auditory input/auditory stimulation, 414
auditory judgment of correctness tasks, 414
    judgment of others' speech, 414
    judgment of own speech, 414
auditory lexical discrimination tasks, 268
auditory model for imitation, 415
    delayed imitation, 415
    immediate imitation, 415
    mimed imitation, 415
    simultaneous imitation, 415
    successive repetition, 415
auditory ossicles, 78
auditory transcription
    understanding English consonants using, 108–125
augmentative or alternative communication (AAC), 516–518
auricle (pinna), 78
Australian English diphthongs, 101
Australian English vowels, 101
autism spectrum disorders, 56

B

babbling, 70, 193–194
back, tongue, 63
backing
    of fricatives, 158
    of velars, 158
baseline data, 423–424, 424f

basic movement sequences, 365–366
Beckwith-Wiedemann syndrome, 67
behavioral learning, 387–390
    operant conditioning, 387
    pleasant consequence, 388
    positive reinforcement, 388–390
    unpleasant consequence, 388
behavior control, 426
Bercow Report of Services
    for Children with
    Speech, Language and
    Communication Needs, 536
Bernhardt, May, 467
Better Communication: An Action
    Plan to Improve Services for
    Children and Young People
    with Speech, Language and
    Communication Needs, 536
bifid tongue, 67
bifid uvula, 74
bilabial consonants, 90
bilabial places, 93
bilabial plosives, 110–111, 113f
Bilingual English-Spanish
    Assessment (BESA), 232
binary features, 138
biopsychosocial model, 46
blade, tongue, 63
blocked practice, 380–381
block formats intervention, 400
block scheduling, 369
body, tongue, 63
Body Function, 342
    as component of ICF-CY, 50, 50f
Body Structure, 342
    as component of ICF-CY, 50, 50f
Bowen, Caroline, 440, 455
bridge, of nose, 75
Bronfenbrenner, Urie, 186–187
bunched alveolar approximant, 121
butterfly imagery, 489

C

Camarata, Stephen, 467
Campbell Collaboration, 524
Canadian Association of Speech-
    Language Pathologists and
    Audiologists (CASLPA), 51
Canadian English diphthongs,
    101
Canadian English vowels, 101
canine, 68
Cantonese
    consonants, acquisition of, 214t
    diphthongs, acquisition of, 214t
    core vocabulary words, 479
    intervention approaches, 472t
    minimal pairs, 441–442t
    names, 230
    syllables, 108
    tones, 105, 105f
    tones, age of acquisition of, 214t
    transcription of, 474f
    vowels, age of acquisition of, 214t
capacity
    in assessment contexts, 227
    dynamic assessments and, 241
    static assessments and, 240
cardinal vowels, 98
carryover, 432

cartilage, 75
case history information, 229
case studies, 439
    articulation impairment—
        lateral lisp, 554–555
    childhood apraxia of speech
        (CAS), 559–563
    childhood dysarthria, 563–568
    inconsistent speech disorder,
        555–559
    phonological impairment,
        542–553
categorical perception, 166
central auditory processing
    deficits, 81
centration, 186
cerebral palsy, children with,
    55–56
challenge point framework, 377
child development, theories of,
    185–187
child-friendly assessments,
    225–226
childhood apraxia of speech
    (CAS), 38, 41, 43–44, 83,
    279–280, 559–563
    assessment results, 560–562,
        561t–562t
    case history, 560
    childhood dysarthria and, 45
    goal setting, 364–367
    commercial intervention
        programs for, 505, 505t
    inconsistent speech disorder
        and, 45
    integrated phonological
        awareness intervention for,
        511–513, 512t
    intervention for, 500–513
    intervention for dysprosody in,
        506–509
    intervention goals for young
        children with, 365–366
    intervention studies for, 563,
        564t
    intervention targets for
        children with, 364–365
    obstructive sleep apnea and,
        506
    speech production skills, 562,
        562t
childhood dysarthria, 38, 41,
    44–45, 280–281, 563–568
    assessment results, 563,
        565t–566t
    augmentative or alternative
        communication (AAC),
        516–518
    CAS and, 45
    case history, 563
    goal setting for children with,
        367
    inconsistent speech disorder
        and, 45
    intervention for, 513–518
    intervention studies for, 567,
        567t–568t
    single-word speech sample,
        567t
    speech production skills, 566
    systems approach, 513–516
Children Act 2004, 536

Children and Youth Version of the
    International Classification
    of Functioning, Disability
    and Health (ICF-CY), 50–51
    Activities, 50, 50f
    Body Function, 50, 50f
    Body Structure, 50, 50f
    Environmental Factors, 50, 50f
    interactions between the
        components of, 50f
    Participation, 50, 50f
    Personal Factors, 50, 50f
Children's Independent and
    Relational Phonological
    Analysis (CHIRPA), 295–296.
    See also independent
    phonological analysis;
    relational phonological
    analysis
children's responses (teaching and
    learning moment), 418–420
    gesture, 419
    imitating or spontaneously
        producing speech, 419
    listening, 418–419
    metalinguistic comment
        (solicited or unsolicited), 420
    phonological awareness, 420
    pragmatic response, 419–420
    reading, 420
    self-correction, 420
    speech-related mouth
        movement, 419
    visual information, 419
children's speech. See also speech
    acoustic analysis of, 326–329,
        326f
    electropalatography (EPG),
        329–330, 330f
    independent and relational
        phonological analyses,
        292–318
    instrumental analyses of,
        324–332
    phonemic (phonological)
        vs. phonetic (articulation)
        errors, 292
    speech measures, 319–324
    traditional articulation
        analysis, 289–291
    ultrasound, 331, 331f
children with suspected SSD
    typical assessments for, 221
chronic suppurative otitis media
    (CSOM), 80
chronosystem, 187
CINAHL (Cumulative Index to
    Nursing and Allied Health
    Literature), 524
circular migration, 231
classic theories of phonology,
    148–165
    contemporary theories of
        phonology, 159–164
    generative phonology,
        representations, and rules,
        148–151
    natural phonology and
        phonological processes,
        151–159
    representation-based accounts
        of SSD, 164–165

Class I malocclusion, 71, 71f
Class I occlusion, 70–71, 71f
Class II malocclusion, 71, 71f
Class III malocclusion, 71, 71f
cleft, 74
cleft lip, 68
cleft palate, 72
Cleft Palate and Craniofacial
    Anomalies (Kummer), 52
Cleft Palate Speech (Peterson-
    Falzone, Hardin-Jones, &
    Karnell), 52
Cleveland Family Speech and
    Language Study, 19
clinical case-based evidence,
    528–529
Clinical Evaluation of Language
    Fundamentals (CELF-4)
    Screening Test, 554
clinical expertise, 531–532
Clinical Linguistics and Phonetics,
    107
clinical practice
    ethical guidelines for, 533
    international conventions and
        frameworks, 534–535
    national policies and laws, 536
    policies affecting, 533–536
cluster reduction, 153, 308
cluster simplification, 153
coalescence, 153
cochlea, 78
Cochrane Collaboration, 524
cognition, 385–386
cognitive/intellectual
    impairment, 54
cognitive-linguistic abilities, 361
collaborative consultation, 397
collapse of contrast, 313
combination intervention,
    400–402
communication
    components of, 4f
    disorders, prevalence of, 10–14
    impairment, 56–59
communication difficulties
    documenting family history of,
        229–230
Communication Function
    Classification System (CFCS),
    563
communicative participation,
    assessment of, 273–275
comparative studies, 189–190
complementary distribution, 149
complete assimilation, 155
complete noncontiguous
    regressive alveolar
    assimilation, 159
CompleteSpeech, 497, 499
complexity, concept of, 352
complexity approach to target
    selection, 351–356
    complexity, 352
    learnability, 352–353
    phonological intervention
        research supporting,
        354t–355t
    suitable children for, 356
complex learning, 381
complex onsets, 457
complex prompt, 510

complex syllables, 184
comprehensibility, assessment of, 249
Computerized Speech Lab (CSL), 327
concomitant phonology intervention for, 459–462
concurrent treatment, 493–496
  children suited to, 496
  evidence, 495–496
  historical background, 493
  procedure, 494–495
  resources for conducting, 496
  theoretical background, 494
conditioned reinforcers, 388
conditions of feedback, motor learning, 383–385
  feedback frequency, 384
  feedback timing, 384–385
  feedback type, 383–384
conditions of practice, motor learning, 377–383, 378f
  attentional focus, 383
  practice accuracy, 381–383
  practice amount, 378
  practice distribution, 378–379
  practice fraction, 381
  practice schedule, 380–381
  practice task, 381
  practice variability, 379–380
conductive hearing loss, 79
connected speech assessments, 261–263
conscious attention, 502–503
consequences
  in intervention, 388
  pleasant, 388
  unpleasant, 388
conservation, 186
consonantal, 139
consonantal misarticulations, 290
consonant cluster error analysis, 308, 309f
consonant clusters, 106–107, 296–297, 297f
  age of acquisition of, 196
  assessment of, 252–253
  phonetic inventory of, 195
  sampling, 546, 548t
  simplification, 155
consonants, 88
  age of acquisition of, 196
  assessment of, 250–251
  mastery of, 214
  nasal, 115f
  phonetic inventory of, 194–195
  sonorant, 85
  voiced, 85
  voiceless, 85
consonants correct, 301–302, 301f
constant practice, 379–380
constraint-based nonlinear approach to target selection, 360–362
  constraint-based nonlinear phonology, 360
  suitable children for, 362
constraint-based nonlinear phonology, 360
  intervention, 467
constraints, 162
  optimality theory, 162

constricted glottis, 140
constructivist approach, 432
contemporary theories of phonology, 159–164
  nonlinear phonology, 159–162
  optimality theory, 162–164
context sensitive voicing (CSV), 155
  postvocalic devoicing, 155
  prevocalic, 155
contiguous assimilation, 155
continuous schedule reinforcement, 390
contrastive approaches, 435
contrastive minimal pairs, 268
control data, 426–427
conventional literacy skills assessment of, 271–272
conversational speech sample, 546
core vocabulary intervention, 464–467
CORONAL sounds, 141
  anterior, 141
  distributed, 141
  grooved, 141
cortical lobes, 81
cranial nerves, 82t
craniofacial anomalies, 53–54
credibility, of evidence, 526–527
  research design, 526–527
  scientific quality of intervention research, 526–527
cricoid cartilage, 76
criterion-referenced assessments, 238
critical age hypothesis, 57, 208
cross-sectional studies, 188–189
crying, 193–194
cultural competence, 223–225
cultural humility, 224
culture, knowledge of, 224
cycles approach to target selection, 356–358
  advanced patterns, 357, 357t
  primary patterns, 357, 357t
  secondary patterns, 357, 357t
  suitable children for, 358
Cycles Phonological Remediation Approach
  children suited to, 454
  evidence, 454–455
  historical background, 453
  procedure, 453–454
  resources for conducting, 455–456
  theoretical background, 453
cyclical goal attack strategy, 368

D

data collection, 422
  plans, 427
data evaluation plans, for children with SSD, 427t
data types, 423–427
deaffrication, 154
Dean, Elizabeth, 450–451, 452
default consonants, 111
default elements, 161
denasalization, 158
dental fricatives, 93, 116–117, 117f
dentalization, 119

dental lisp, 118
dentists, 71
descriptive assessments, 234–235
detailed impressionistic transcription, 88
developmental SSD, 302
diacritics, 88
diacritics chart, 97–98
diadochokinesis (DDK), 192, 192t, 201, 201t, 209
Diagnostic and Statistical Manual of Mental Disorders (DSM-5), 5
diagnostic assessments, 235
Diagnostic Evaluation of Articulation and Phonology (DEAP): Phonology Assessment, 545, 546
diaphragm, 77
diary studies, 188
differential diagnosis, 283
Differential Diagnosis System (DDS), 48
diminutization, 154
diphthongs
  assessment of, 253–254
  English vowels and, 100
direct intervention, 397–399
directions, 170
directions into velocities of articulators (DIVA) model, 170
disordered SSD, 302
distinctive features, 138
distributed practice, 378–379
disyllabic words, 106, 107
  conceptualization of word and syllable positions for, 108f
DIVA models of speech acquisition, 170–171, 171f, 462
Dodd, Barbara, 464
DORSAL sounds, 142
  tense, 142
  tongue-body feature, 142
dorsum, 63
Down syndrome, 54, 67
drill, 421
drill play, 421–422
drill-play format, 445
Dutch, 107, 127–131
  intervention approaches, 472t
dynamic assessments, 241–242
dynamic cues of DTTC, 501
dynamic systems and whole-language intervention, 468
Dynamic Temporal and Tactile Cueing (DTTC), 500–504
  attention and motivation, 503
  auditory and visual models, 501
  children suited to, 504
  conscious attention, 502–503
  evidence, 504
  general overview of, 501
  historical background, 500
  intense production practice, 503
  movement sequences, 502
  procedures, 501–503
  resources for conducting, 504
  speech rate, 502
  stimuli used in, 503
  supporting cues, 501–502
  theoretical background, 500
dysarthria, 44, 81

E

early efficacy studies, 526
early intervening services (EIS), 395
early literacy skills, assessment of, 271–272
ears, 78–81
  external, 80f
  function of, 78
  structural impairments of, 79–81
  structure of, 78–79, 79f
education, maternal, 180
effectiveness study, 526
effective parent training, home practice and, 398
egocentric, 186
egressive air, 77
Eight-Step Continuum, 501
electropalatography (EPG), 329–330, 330f
  articulation intervention using, 496–499
  children suited to articulation intervention using, 499
  diagram and electrode placement, 110f
  evidence, 498
  historical background, 497
  intervention procedure, 498
  theoretical background, 497
elicited production activities, 460
eliciting consonantal and rhotic vowels, 490–491
eliciting /s/, cues for, 489
Embase, 524
emergent literacy intervention, 477
emergent literacy skills, assessment of, 271–272
empirically supported practice *vs.* evidence-based practice (EBP), 521
EMU, 327
English consonants, 108–125, 127–131
  features for, 143t
  place and features of tongue/palate contact for, 111t
  sagittal diagrams of, 109
  transverse diagrams of, 109–110
  typology of the manner of articulation of, 94f
  understanding using knowledge of anatomy and auditory transcription, 108–125
English diphthongs, 100
English pulmonic consonants, 91–92
English-speaking children
  rare or atypical processes produced by, 157–158
  typical speech acquisition for, 191
English-speaking infants
  speech acquisition for, 191–200
English vowels, 100
  typology of the manner of articulation of, 94f
Environmental Factors, as component of ICF-CY, 50, 50f
epenthesis, 153
ERIC (Education Resources Information Center), 524
Erickson, R. L., 487, 488
errorful learning, 381–383

errorless learning, 381–383
esophageal speech, 77
esophagus, 75
ethics
  clinical practice and, 533
  defined, 533
  ethical practice principles, 533
Eustachian tube, 75, 78
*Evaluating and Enhancing
  Children's Phonological
  Systems: Research and Theory
  to Practice* (Hodson), 453
evaluation
  credibility of evidence, 526–527
  intervention, 422–429
  nature of evidence, 526
  of research evidence, 525–527,
    528t
Evaluator (EVAL), optimality
  theory, 162
event-related potentials (ERPs), 193
Every Child a Talker, 536
Every Child Matters, 536
evidence
  associated with traditional
    articulation intervention, 492
  clinical case-based, 528–529
  credibility, 526–527
  external research, 523–525
  integration of, 531–532
  internal, evaluation of, 528–530
  levels of, 526–527, 527t
  nature of, 526
  practice-based, 529–530
evidence-based practice (EBP)
  client values and preferences,
    33–34, 34f
  clinical expertise, 33–34, 34f
  decision-making process for
    engaging in, 522–532, 522t
  described, 521
  vs. empirically supported
    practice, 521
  importance of, 532
  research evidence, 33–34, 34f
execution, 45
exosystem, 187
experience-dependent neural
  plasticity, 391, 392
external auditory meatus (ear
  canal), 78
external research evidence, 523–525
  critical evaluation of, 525–527,
    528t
extrinsic feedback, 383–384
extrinsic muscles, 63

F
face-to-face assessments, 221
facial nerve, 81
faithfulness constraints, 163
family-centered
  assessments, 227
  practice, 393
family-friendly
  assessments, 227
  practice, 393
feasibility study, 526
feature geometry, 161
feedback
  extrinsic, 383–384
  frequency, 384

  intrinsic, 383
  motor learning and, 383–385
  timing, 384–385
Felsenfeld, Susan, 17
Filipino, 107
final consonant deletion, 153
finite morpheme composite
  (FMC), 461
Finnish, 96, 102, 127–131
  intervention approaches, 472t
fixed interval reinforcement, 390
fixed ratio reinforcement, 390
flexible criteria, 402
focus stimulation activities, 460
foot, 161
foundational knowledge and
  skills, 222–223
fractionation, speech production,
  382
fraenectomy. *See* frenulectomy
free variation, 149
French, 96, 107, 127–131
  intervention approaches, 472t
  speech acquisition, 184, 189
frenulectomy, 67 (frenectomy,
  frenectomy, frenotomy,
  frenulotomy)
fricative consonant articulation,
  90, 94
fricative simplification, 117, 155
front, tongue, 63
fronting
  palatal, 154
  velar, 154
full-scale intelligence quotient
  (FSIQ) score, 563
function, of phonemes, 447
functional communication
  measures (FCM), 529
functional magnetic resonance
  imaging (fMRI), 193

G
Ganong effect, 166
General American English (GAE)
  diphthongs, 100–101
General American English (GAE)
  vowels, 100–101
  pronunciation of, 102t
  transcription conventions of,
    100t
General British diphthongs, 101
General British English (GBE)
  vowels
  pronunciation of, 102t
generalization
  concept of, 341
  data, 424, 424f
  response, 348–349, 349f
  stimulus, 348, 349f
generalized motor program
  (GMP), 380
generative phonology, 148
Generator (GEN), optimality
  theory, 162
German, 96, 102, 107, 127–131
  intervention approaches, 472t
gestural cues, 417
  iconic, 417
  metaphoric, 417
Gierut, Judith, 444–445, 457
Gillon, Gail, 511

Glaspey Dynamic Assessment of
  Phonology (GDAP), 241, 241f
glide consonant articulation, 94
gliding, 123
  of fricatives, 158
  of liquids, 154–155
GlobalMed, 499
glossectomy, 67
glottal consonants, 90
glottal fricative, 121, 121f
glottal insertion, 158
glottal places, 93
glottis, 76
glue ear, 80
goal attack strategies, 368–369
  for children with SSD and
    expressive language
    impairment, 369
  cyclical goal attack strategy, 368
  horizontal goal attack strategy,
    368
  vertical goal attack strategy, 368
goals
  frameworks and hierarchies,
    346–347
  identifying, for children with
    SSD, 341–344
  intervention, 341
  operationally defined, 344–346
goal setting
  for children with articulation
    impairment, 363–367
  for children with CAS, 364–367
  for children with childhood
    dysarthria, 367
  for children with inconsistent
    speech disorder, 364
  for children with phonological
    impairment, 350–363
  considerations for children
    with highly unintelligible
    speech, 367–368
  goal frameworks and
    hierarchies, 346–347
  intervention goals, 341
  operationally defined goals,
    344–346
  overview, 341
GODIVA models of speech
  acquisition, 170–171
Goldman-Fristoe Test of
  Articulation, 13, 59, 554
gradient order DIVA (GODIVA), 170
grandparents, 232–233
Greek, 107, 127–131
  intervention approaches, 472t
groove, 94
Gross Motor Function
  Classification System
  (GMFCS), 563
group intervention, 400–402, 401t
guidance hypothesis, 384

H
hard palate, 71–73
  function of, 72
  structural impairments of, 72–73
  structure of, 72
Hawai'ian, 96, 102
Hayden, Deborah, 509–510
healthy loudness, 515–516
hearing, assessment of, 269

hearing loss, 54–55
  children with, 54–55
  SSD and, 29
Hebrew, Israeli, 107, 127–131
  intervention approaches, 472t
hemispherectomy, 392
hierarchies, 346–347
high amplitude sucking
  technique, 193
Hodson, Barbara, 453
Hoffman, Paul, 468
homographs, 104
homonyms words, 136
homonymy, 444
horizontal goal attack strategy, 368
Howell, Janet, 450–451, 452
*How to Talk with Practically
  Anybody About Practically
  Anything* (Walters), 17
Hungarian, 107, 127–131
  speech acquisition, 189
hybrid telepractice, 397
hyoid bone, 76
hypernasality, 515
hypernasal speech, 75
hypoglossal nerve, 81
hyponasal speech, 75, 115
hypothetical-deductive reasoning,
  186

I
iambic stress pattern, 104
iambic stress patterns, 305
Icelandic, 127–131
  few minimal pairs, 441
ICF-CY framework, 342–344
identified genetic causes, 52–53
illegal nonwords, 267
imitation
  delayed, 415
  DTTC and, 502
  immediate, 415
  mimed, 415
  simultaneous, 415
  verbal imitation hierarchy, 502
implicational relationships, 145
impressionistic transcriptions,
  87–88
  detailed (narrow), 88
  simple (broad), 88
incisors, 68
inconsistent speech disorder, 38,
  41, 279, 435, 555–559
  assessment results, 555–559, 557t
  CAS and, 45
  case history, 555
  childhood dysarthria and, 45
  for children, with goal setting,
    364
  children suited to, 466
  evidence, 466
  historical background, 464
  intervention for, 464–467
  intervention studies for, 559, 559t
  procedure, 465–466
  resources for conducting, 466
  single-word speech sample,
    555–558, 558f, 559t
  theoretical background, 464–465
incremental production practice,
  487
incus, 78

independent phonological analysis, 292–318. *See also* relational phonological analysis
  components, 294t
  consonant clusters, 296–297, 297f
  singleton consonants, 296, 296f
  syllable shape inventory, 298–299, 299f
  syllable stress inventory, 299–300, 300f
  vowels, 297–298, 297f
  word length inventory, 299, 300f
indirect intervention, 397–399
Individual Education Program (IEP), 395
Individual Family Service Plan (IFPS), 395
individual intervention, 400–402, 401t
Individuals with Disabilities Education Act (IDEA), 536
informal assessments, 237–238
informative reinforcer, 389
Ingram, David, 152
ingressive air, 77
initial consonant deletion, 158
inner ear, 78
in-person model, 397
instrumental feedback. *See* electropalatography (EPG); spectrography; ultrasound
integrated phonological awareness intervention, 511–513
  children suited to, 513
  evidence, 512–513
  historical background, 511
  intervention targets and stimuli, 511
  letter knowledge tasks, 511, 512t
  phonemic awareness, 511, 512t
  procedure, 511–512
  resources for conducting, 513
  service delivery, 512
  speech production practice, 511–512
  theoretical background, 511
intelligibility, 4, 194, 201, 210, 212–213
  assessments of, 245–249
  rating scales that quantify perceptions of, 246
Intelligibility in Context Scale (ICS), 246, 247t, 543t
intelligible phonetic contrasts, single-word measures quantifying, 247–248
intercostal muscles, 77
interdental lisp, 118, 290
interdisciplinary teams, 228
internal auditory meatus, 78
internal clinical evidence
  clinical case-based evidence, 528–529
  evaluation, 530–531
  evaluation of, 528–530
  practice-based evidence, 529–530
Internal Metronome Hypothesis, 506
International Association of Logopedics and Phoniatrics (IALP), 51, 536, 538

International Classification of Functioning, Disability and Health – Children and Youth Version (ICF-CY), 276–277, 535
International Expert Panel on Multilingual Children's Speech, 4, 538
International Journal of Speech-Language Pathology, 535, 555, 556
International Phonetic Alphabet (IPA), 16, 88–90
  chart, 89f
  diacritics chart from, 98f
  extensions to, 105–106
  features of English pulmonic consonants as labeled in, 93t
  non-pulmonic consonant chart and other symbols chart from, 95f
  pulmonic consonant chart from, 91f
  suprasegmentals chart and the tones and word accent chart from, 103f
  vowel chart from, 99f
International Phonetic Association, 90
International Statistical Classification of Diseases and Related Health Problems 11th Revision (ICD-11), 5
intervention
  for articulation impairment, 486–499
  for childhood apraxia of speech (CAS), 500–513
  for childhood dysarthria, 513–518
  defined, 373
  for dysprosody in childhood apraxia of speech (CAS), 506–509
  evaluating, 422–429
  goals, 341
  management plans, 393–395, 394f
  for motor speech disorders, 509–510
  planning, 235
  plans, 392–402
  practice models, 393
  principles of, 373–374, 374f, 375–392
  service delivery options, 396–402
  session plans, 395–396, 396f
  speech acquisition and, 375, 375f
  speech perception, 456–459
  stimulability, 462–464
  targeting complex onsets, 457
intervention intensity
  cumulative intervention intensity, 400
  dose, 399
  dose form, 399
  dose frequency, 399
  session duration, 399
  total intervention duration, 399
intervention procedures
  activities, 420–422

  described, 413
  materials, 420–422
  resources, 420–422
  stimuli, 420–422
  teaching and learning moment, 413–420
intervention research, scientific quality evaluation, 527, 528t
intervention studies
  for articulation impairment—lateral lisp, 554–555, 555t, 556t
  for childhood apraxia of speech (CAS), 563, 564t
  for childhood dysarthria, 567, 567t–568t
  for inconsistent speech disorder, 559, 559t
  for phonological impairment, 547, 553t
intonation, 104–105, 200, 366
intrinsic feedback, 383
intrinsic muscles, 63
intuitive thought, 186
inventory constraints, 146

J
Jackson, Eugene, 485–486
Japanese, 127–131
joint activity dyads, 187

K
Kay Elemetrics Sonograph, 497
Kay-Pentax CSL Sona-Match, 497
Klippel-Feil syndrome, 67
knowledge of anatomy English consonants and, 108–125
knowledge of culture and language, 224
knowledge of performance (KP), 497
  feedback, 383–384
knowledge of results (KR) feedback, 383–384
Korczak, Janusz, 21
Korean, 127–131
  intervention approaches, 472t

L
labialization, 155
labial-velar places, 93
labiodental fricatives, 116, 116f
labiodental places, 93
labiovelar approximant, 123–124, 123f
lack of invariance, 166
language impairment, SSD and, 57
language intervention
  effectiveness study, 526
  early efficacy study, 526
  effectiveness study, 526
  feasibility study, 526
  later efficacy study, 526
  pre-trial study, 526
language(s)
  assessment of, 275–276
  documenting family history of, 229–230
  knowledge of, 224
  SSD and, 30–31
  typical speech acquisition and, 180

laryngectomy, 77
laryngopharynx, 75
larynx, 76–77
  function of, 76
  structural impairments of, 77
  structure of, 76–77
lateral approximant consonant articulation, 90, 94
lateral fricative consonant articulation, 90
lateral lisp, 118, 119, 290, 554–555
  assessment results, 554
  case history, 554
  intervention studies for, 554–555, 555t, 556t
later efficacy study, 526
late talkers, and phonological intervention approaches, 469–471t
learnability, 352–353
least knowledge, 151
left lateralized, 81
legal nonwords, 267
letter knowledge tasks, 511, 512t
letter-sound knowledge, 476
level of evidence (LOE), 526–527, 527t
lexical representations, 165, 457
lexical stress, 366
lingual frenulum (lingual frenum), 66
linguistic universals, 145
lips, 67–68
  function of, 68
  structural impairments of, 68
  structure of, 68
liquid consonant articulation, 94
Listening to Children and Young People With Speech, Language and Communication Needs (Roulstone & McLeod), 19
literacy difficulties, SSD and, 57
Locke, John, 456
longitudinal studies, 189
  Cleveland Family Speech and Language Study, 19
  Ottawa Language Study, 18–19
  Templin Longitudinal Study, 17–18
long-term goals, 346
LSVT LOUD (Lee Silverman Voice Treatment), 515–516
lungs, 77

M
macroglossia (large tongue), 67
macrosystem, 187
Madison Speech Assessment Protocol (MSAP), 47
magnitude of change (behavior control), 426
malleus, 78
Maltese, 107, 127–131
  intervention approaches, 472t
management plans
  Individual Education Program (IEP), 395
  Individual Family Service Plan (IFPS), 395
  intervention, 393–395, 394f
  response to intervention (RTI), 395

mandible, 70–71
  function of, 70
  structural impairments of, 70–71
  structure of, 70
manner, 90, 192
  pulmonic consonants, 93–94
Manual Ability Classification
    System (MACS), 563
*Manual of Exercises for the
    Correction of Speech Disorders*
    (Scripture and Jackson), 485
marked features, 145
markedness, 145
markedness constraints, 163
Martinez, Francesca, 17
massed practice, 378–379
materials, described, 420–422
maternal education, typical
    speech acquisition and, 180
maximally opposing features, of
    phonemes, 437
maximal oppositions approach,
    437
  children suited to, 446
  evidence, 445–446
  historical background, 444
  vs. minimal pair approach, 446
  procedure, 444–445
  theoretical background, 444
maximum phonation time, 192,
    201, 209
McGurk effect, 167
meaningful minimal pair
    approach, 437–438
  familiarization, 438
  listen and pick up, 438
  production of minimal pair
    words, 438
medical model, 46
MEDLINE, 524
mesosystem, 187
meta-awareness, 385–386
metacognition, 385
metacognitive control, 432
metacognitive knowledge, 432
metacommunication, 450
  metaphonological awareness
    and, 451–452
metalinguistic awareness, 385
metalinguistic skills, 200
Me Talk Pretty One Day (Sedaris), 17
Metaphon approach, 437
  children suited to, 452
  evidence, 452
  historical background, 450
  procedure, 451–452
  resources for conducting, 452
  theoretical background, 450
metaphonological awareness
  listening and developing, 451
  metacommunication and,
    451–452
  speech production and,
    451–452
metaphonological cues, 417
metaphonological input tasks, 415
metaphonology, 385, 450
metaphors, 385, 417, 418t
metathesis, 153
methodological issues, in speech
    acquisition, 187–191
  comparative studies, 189–190

cross-sectional studies, 188–189
  diary studies, 188
  longitudinal studies, 189
microsystem, 187
midline raphe, 72
migration of sound, 154
minimally opposing features, of
    phonemes, 437
minimally opposing minimal
    pairs, 136
minimal pair approach, 437–443
  children suited to, 440
  for children who speak
    languages other than
    English, 440–443, 441t
  evidence, 439–440
  historical background, 437
  vs. maximal opposition
    approach, 446
  procedure, 437–439
  resources for conducting, 440
  theoretical background, 437
  for tonal languages, 442–443
minimal pairs, 136–138
minimal pair words sampling, 546
mixed hearing loss, 81
mnemonic method, 468
model, 387
Moebius syndrome, 55
molars, 68
monolingual children, 472
monosyllabic words, 106
Months of Morphemes (Haskill), 462
mora, 161
morphophonemic consonant
    clusters, 107
morphosyntactic approach
  children suited to, 461
  evidence, 461–462
  historical background, 459
  procedure, 460–461
  resources for conducting, 462
  theoretical background, 460
morphosyntax difficulties,
    intervention for, 459–462
most knowledge, 151
Mota, Helena, 446
motivation
  DTTC and, 503
  home practice and, 398
  intervention outcomes and, 530
motor equivalence, 170
motor execution, 81, 170
  speech production and,
    168–170
motor impairment, 55–56
motor learning, 376–385
  conditions of feedback,
    383–385
  conditions of practice, 377–383,
    378f
  defined, 377
  phases of, 377
  principles, articulation
    intervention based on,
    493–496
  schema theory of, 171–172
motor planning, 45, 169
  speech production and,
    168–170
motor production, 4, 38
motor program, 172

motor programming, 45, 169
  speech production and, 168–170
motor speech, 41–45
motor speech disorders
  augmentative or alternative
    communication and, 516–517
  intervention approaches for
    different types of, 485f
  intervention for, 509–510
motor speech interventions
  historical perspective on, 485
motor theory of speech
    perception, 168
movement sequences, 500, 502
multidisciplinary teams, 228
multilingual children,
    phonological intervention
    approaches for, 472–475, 474t
multiple oppositions approach,
    437, 447–450
  children suited to, 449
  evidence, 449
  historical background, 447
  procedure, 447–449
  resources for conducting, 449
  theoretical background, 447
multiple phonological processes,
    158–159
muscular hydrostats, 63

N

nasal cavity, 75
nasal consonant articulation, 90, 93
nasal consonants, 115–116, 115f
nasal emission, 121
nasal septum, 75
nasopharynx, 75
National Center for Evidence-Based
    Practice in Communication
    Disorders (N-CEP), 524
National Outcome Measurement
    System (NOMS), 400, 402, 529
national policies and laws, 536
natural class, 138
natural features, 145
naturalistic intervention
  for speech accuracy, 467
  for speech intelligibility, 467
naturalness, 145
natural phonology, 151–159
near minimal pairs, 136
  of phonemes, 437
negative punishers, 388
negative reinforcers, 388
neighborhood density
  typical speech acquisition and,
    183
neurological system, 81–83
  function of, 81
  impairments of, 81–83
  structure of, 81
neuro-network approach to target
    selection, 362–363
New Zealand English
  diphthongs, 101
  vowels, 101
Nijmegen model and the
    importance of syllables, 170
No Child Left Behind (NCLB) Act,
    521, 536
noncontiguous assimilation, 155
non-contrastive approaches, 435

non-default elements, 161
nonlinear phonological hierarchy,
    160f
nonlinear phonology, 159–162, 329
  central concepts in, 161–162
  prosodic tier, 161
  segmental tier, 161
non-pulmonic consonant chart,
    95–96
  pulmonic and non-pulmonic
    consonants in the world's
    languages, 95–96
non-pulmonic consonants, 95–96
nonword repetition tasks, 270
normative studies, 188
norm-referenced assessments, 238
Norris, Janet, 468
Norwegian, 107, 127–131
  intervention approaches, 472t
nose, 74–75
  bridge of, 75
  function of, 74–75
  structural impairments of, 75
  structure of, 75
nostrils (nares), 75
novel word, 444

O

object permanence, 185
observational dyads, 187
obstructive sleep apnea,
    childhood apraxia of speech
    (CAS) and, 506
obstruents, 93, 139, 444
olfactory nerve, 75
ongoing intervention, 400
onset-rime tier, 161
operant conditioning, 387
optimality theory, 162–164
  Constraints (CON), 162
  conventional tableau used in,
    163f
  Evaluator (EVAL), 162
  Generator (GEN), 162
oral mechanism, 192, 200–201,
    208–209
oral sucking habits, SSD and, 29
orbicularis oris muscle, 68
organization, 185
organ of Corti (spiral organ), 78
orientation training, 494, 495t
oromotor difficulties, SSD and,
    57–58
oropharynx, 75
orthodontists, 71
orthographic cues, 416
orthographic representation, 165
otitis media with effusion (OME),
    55, 80
  children with, 55
otoscope, 78
Ottawa Language Study, 18–19
outcome measurement, 235–236
oval windows, 78

P

Paden, Elaine Pagel, 453
palatal approximant, 122f, 123
palatal fronting (depalatalization),
    154
palatal places, 93

palatine and alveolar processes, 72
palatine tonsils, 74, 74f
parameter prompt, 510
parameters, 380
parent-as-therapist aide, 393
parents, 232–233
Parents and Children Together (PACT)
    approach, 393
    intervention, 437, 455
Parents' Evaluation of Developmental Status (PEDS), 239
partial assimilation, 155
Participation, as component of ICF-CY, 50, 50f
parts of the whole movement (motor skill), 381
Patient, Intervention, Comparison, Outcome (PICO) clinical question, 522–523
    intervention questions, 523
patterns, 40
perceiving errors, 488
percentage
    of consonant clusters, correct (PCCC) 196–198, 198t, 205, 211, 214–215
percentage of consonants correct (PCC), 196–198, 198t, 205, 211, 214–215, 319
    guidelines and rules for calculating, 320t
    variations on, 319
percentage of consonants in the inventory (PCI), 319
percentage of vowels correct (PVC), 196–198, 198t, 205, 211, 214–215
perception, 4, 38, 192–193
    anatomical structures for, 61, 81–83
perception-production minimal pair intervention, 439
    familiarization and perception training, 439
    production involving independent naming, 439
    production involving word imitation, 439
    production of minimal pair words, 439
perceptual abilities, 361
performance
    in assessment contexts, 227
    dynamic assessments and, 241
    static assessments and, 240
performance-based criteria, 402
peripheral auditory system, 172
Personal Factors, as component of ICF-CY, 50, 50f
personal-social abilities, 361
pharynx, 75
    function of, 75
    structural impairments of, 75
    structure of, 75
philtrum, 68
phone, 136
phoneme awareness, 476
phoneme input frequency
    typical speech acquisition and, 184

phoneme restoration effect, 166
phonemes, 136–138, 137
    functional load of, 184
phonemic awareness, 476, 511, 512t
phonemic contrast, loss of, 311–314, 313f
phonemic impairment
    vs. phonetic impairment, 292, 292f
phonemic repertoire, 136
phonemic transcription, 87, 88. See also phonological transcription
phones, 136–138, 137
phonetic/articulatory complexity
    typical speech acquisition and, 184
phonetic awareness, 385, 386
phonetic contexts or key environments, 417
phonetic cues, 415–416
    manual guidance/ motokinesthetic cue, 416
    tactile-phonetic cue, 416
    verbal-phonetic cue, 416
    visual-phonetic cue, 415–416
phonetic impairment
    vs. phonemic impairment, 292, 292f
phonetic inventory, 194–195, 201–202, 210, 213, 365–366
    of consonant clusters, 195, 202
    of consonants, 194–195, 201
    of vowels, 195, 202
phonetic symbols, 90
phonetic transcription, 87. See also allophonic transcription
phonological access, 269–270
phonological awareness, 165, 208, 212, 270–271, 385
phonological awareness input tasks, 415
phonological competence, 151
phonological deficiencies, 152
phonological delay, 5–6, 40
Phonological Disability in Children (Ingram), 152
phonological disorder, 9, 40
phonological impairment, 38, 40–41, 278, 435, 542–553
    vs. articulation impairment, 292
    assessment results, 543–546, 543t–545t
    case history, 542–543
    consonant clusters sampling, 546, 548t
    conversational speech sample, 546
    goal setting for children with, 350–363
    intervention studies for, 547, 553t
    management approaches (See phonological intervention approaches)
    minimal pair words sampling, 546
    polysyllabic words sampling, 546
    risk of literacy difficulties in preschoolers with, 476–477

single-word speech sample, 545, 549t, 550t–552t
phonological intervention, principles of, 436
phonological intervention approaches
    for children who are late talkers, 469–471t
    constraint-based nonlinear phonology intervention, 467
    Cycles Phonological Remediation Approach, 454–456
    dynamic systems and whole-language intervention, 468
    maximal oppositions approach, 437, 444–446
    meaningful minimal pair approach, 437–438
    Metaphon approach, 437, 450–452
    minimal pair approach, 437–443
    mnemonic method, 468
    morphosyntactic approach, 459–462
    for multilingual children, 472–475
    multiple oppositions approach, 437, 447–450
    naturalistic intervention, 467
    phonological target selection approaches and, 468–469, 469f
    phonotactic therapy, 468
    psycholinguistic approach, 467
    schematic timeline of, 435f
    speech perception intervention, 456–459
    stimulability intervention, 462–464
phonological knowledge, 165
phonological literacy, 212
phonological mean length of utterance (pMLU), 322, 323t
phonological naming (rapid naming), 165
phonological organization, 38
phonological patterns, 152
phonological performance, 151
phonological planning, 45, 169
    speech production and, 168–170
phonological processes, 40, 151–159, 152, 165, 199, 206–207, 215, 308–311, 310f
    assessment of, 269–271
    assimilation processes (consonant harmony), 155–156
    defined, 151
    developing children's speech, 157t
    multiple, 158–159
    rare or atypical processes produced by English-speaking children, 157–158
    substitution (systemic) processes, 154–155
    syllable structure processes, 152–154
phonological recognition, 172
phonological representation,

165, 172
phonological representation accuracy judgment, 268
phonological representation of consonants, 4
phonological representation of vowels, 4
phonological targets, 152
phonological target selection approaches
    phonological intervention approaches and, 468–469, 469f
phonological theories, 148
phonological transcription, 87. See also phonemic transcription
phonological working memory, 165, 270
phonology, 40–41, 135–148, 258, 375–376
    allophones, 136–138
    contemporary theories of, 159–164
    features, 138–144
    implicational relationships, 145
    inconsistent speech disorder, 41
    laryngeal features, 139–140
    major class features, 139
    manner features, 140
    markedness, 145
    minimal pairs, 136–138
    naturalness, 145
    phonemes, 136–138
    phones, 136–138
    phonological impairment, 40–41
    phonotactics, 145–146
    place features, 140–144
    sonority, 146–148
phonotactic probability
    typical speech acquisition and, 183
phonotactics, 4, 106–108, 145–146
    consonant clusters, 106–107
    syllable shapes and word positions, 107–108
phonotactic therapy, 468
Photo Articulation Test, 13
Piaget, Jean, 185–186
Piaget's theory of child development, 185–186
    concrete operational stage, 186
    formal operational stage, 186
    preoperational stage, 185–186
Pierre Robin syndrome, 71
place, 90, 192
    pulmonic consonants, 93
pleasant consequences, 388
plosives
    alveolar, 111–113, 113f
    bilabial, 110–111, 113f
    consonant articulation, 90, 93
    velar, 114–115, 114f
polysyllabic words, 106
polysyllabic words sampling, 546
polysyllables, assessment of, 255
Portuguese, 107, 127–131
    Brazilian Portuguese intervention approaches, 472t
    Portuguese intervention approaches, 472t
positional constraints, 146

position papers
  about working with children with childhood apraxia of speech, 538
  about working with children with SSD, 538
  about working with multilingual children, 538–539
positive punishers, 388
positive reinforcement, 388–390
positive reinforcers, 388
postalveolar fricatives, 120, 120f
postalveolar pair, 444
postalveolar places, 93
post-assessment tasks, 221
posterior faucial pillars, 73
postvocalic devoicing, 155
Praat, 85f, 86f, 327
practice-based evidence (PBE), 529–530
practicing, traditional articulation intervention, 489–491
  concurrent treatment, 494–495
  isolation, 489
  nonsense syllables, 489
  sentences, 491
  words, 491
pragmatic/communication awareness, 385
pragmatic cues, 417
pre-assessment tasks, 221
prediction, of errors, 488
predictive validity, 237
premolars, 68
pre-practice instruction, 487, 488–489, 494, 508
preschoolers
  emergent literacy intervention, 477
  with phonological impairment, 476–477
pre-trial study, 526
prevocalic voicing, 155
primary dyads, 187
primary prevention approach, 476
primary reinforcers, 388
primary stress, 103
principles of intervention, 373–374, 374f, 375–392
  behavioral learning, 387–390
  cognition and meta-awareness, 385–386
  defined, 374
  motor learning, 376–385
  neurological experience, 391–392
  phonology, 375–376
  speech perception, 376
problem-solving slow progress, framework for, 429–431t
production cues
  auditory model for imitation, 415
  facilitating phonetic contexts or key environments, 417
  gestural cues, 417
  metaphonological cues, 417
  metaphors, 417, 418t
  orthographic cues, 416
  phonetic cues, 415–416
  pragmatic cues, 417
  prosodic cues, 416

sound-referenced rebuses, 416–417
successive approximation/shaping, 417
production-perception loop, 164
productive phonological knowledge, 150
professional knowledge and skills, 223
prognostic statements, 283
progress and discharge planning
  long-term goals, 402–403
  short-term goal criteria, 402
progressive assimilation, 155
Prompts for Restructuring Oral Muscular Phonetic Targets (PROMPT) program, 509–510
  children suited to, 510
  evidence, 510
  historical background, 509
  procedure, 510
  resources for conducting, 510
  theoretical background, 509–510
proportion of whole-word proximity (PWP), 322, 323t
proportion of whole-word variability (PWV), 324, 324t
prosodic awareness, 385
prosodic cues, 416
  manual guidance/motokinesthetic cue, 416
  verbal-prosodic cue, 416
  visual-prosodic cue, 416
prosodic tier, 161, 360
  nonlinear phonology, 161
prosody, 103, 199–200, 207–208, 212, 215–216
  assessment of, 256–257
prosody-voice profile, 257f
pseudo-word stimuli, 507
psycholinguistic approach, for SSD in children, 467
Psycholinguistic Framework, 48–49
psycholinguistics, 329
psycholinguistic speech processing model, 49f, 172–173, 172f
psychologists, 228
psychosocial aspects, assessment of, 272–273
psychosocial behaviors SSD and, 29–30
PsycINFO, 524
PubMed, 524
pull-out model, 396
pulmonic consonant chart, 90–94
pulmonic consonants, 90
  English, 91–92
  features of, 92–94
  manner, 93–94
  place, 93
  voice, 92–93
  in the world's languages, 95–96
Punjabi-English intervention approaches, 472t
push-in model, 396
Putonghua (Mandarin), 127–131

R
r, sound of, 121
race, SSD and, 30–31
randomized controlled trials, 439

random practice, 380–381
Rapid Syllable Transition Treatment (ReST), 506–509
  children suited to, 509
  evidence, 508–509
  generalization probes, 508
  historical background, 506
  practice, 508
  pre-practice, 508
  procedure, 507
  pseudo-word stimuli, 507
  resources for conducting, 509
  service delivery, 508
  skills, 507–508
  theoretical background, 506
rare or atypical processes
  produced by English-speaking children, 157–158
rate of change (behavior control), 426
Reading/WinEPG, 497
real time service, 397
recall, 488
recall schema, 380
recognition schema, 380
reduplication
  complete, 153
  partial, 153
referral and background information, 228–233
  case history information, 229
  children's language use and proficiency, 230–232
  family history of speech, language, and communication difficulties, 229–230
  learning from parents, grandparents, teachers, siblings, and friends, 232–233
regressive assimilation, 156
reinforcement
  positive, 388–389
  schedules of, 389–390
reinforcing activity, 388–389
relational phonological analysis, 292–318. See also independent phonological analysis
  components, 294t
  consonant cluster error analysis, 308, 309f
  consonants correct, 301–302, 301f
  loss of phonemic contrast, 311–314, 313f
  phonological processes, 308–311, 310f
  sampling constraints, 317–318, 317f
  singleton consonant error analysis, 306–308, 306f
  speech ratings, 316–317, 316f
  suprasegmentals, 314–316, 314f
  syllable shapes correct, 304, 304f
  syllable stress patterns correct, 305, 305f
  vowels correct, 302–304, 303f
  word lengths correct, 304–305, 304f
relative distortion index (RDI), 319

repair processes, 162
representation-based accounts of SSD in children, 164–165
residual articulation errors, 43
resources, 420–422
respiratory system, 77–78
  function of, 77
  impairments of, 78
  structure of, 77–78
response generalization, 348–349, 349f
response to intervention (RTI), 395
retrocochlear pathology, 81
retroflex alveolar approximant, 121
rhythm, 104
Robin, Donald A., 506
root, tongue, 63
Ross, Jonathan, 17
round windows, 78
Royal College of Speech and Language Therapists (RCSLT), 51, 538
rugae, 72
Rvachew, Susan, 456, 458

S
sagittal diagrams of English consonants, 109
sampling constraints, 317–318, 317f
scaffolding, 186
schemas, 185, 380
schema theory of motor learning, 171–172
Scopus, 524
screening assessments, 239–240
Scripture, May, 485–486
secondary intervention, 476
secondary stress, 103
Sedaris, David, 17
segmental tier, 360
  nonlinear phonology, 161
segmentation, speech production, 382
self-awareness, 224
self-evaluation, 385
self-monitoring, 385
self-monitoring requests, 414–415
  elicited self-correction, 414
  prompted self-correction, 415
self-reflection, 224
self-reinforcement, 389
semantic representation, 165, 172
semicircular canals, 78, 79
sensitivity, defined, 237
sensorineural hearing loss, 81
sensory-perceptual (ear) training, 487–488
  discrimination, 488
  identifying, 487
  locating, 487
  stimulation, 488
sequential constraints, 146
sequential language, 231
seriation, 186
service delivery options, 396–402
  continuity, 400
  intervention agents, 397–399
  intervention format, 400–402
  intervention intensity, 399–400
  intervention settings, 396–397

services, adaptation of, 224–225
session goals, 347
session plans, 395–396, 396f
sex
  SSD and, 28
  typical speech acquisition and, 180
Short Temperament Scale for Children (STSC), 543
short-term goals, 346–347
sibilant (hissing) sound, 118
siblings, 232–233
side-by-side model, 397
simple impressionistic transcription, 88
simple learning, 381
simple transcription, 88
simplification, speech production, 382
simultaneous language, 231
simultaneous scheduling, 369
single-case experimental design (SCED)
  methodology, 529
  and SSD intervention, 428–429
  studies, 439
singleton consonant error analysis, 306–308, 306f
singleton consonants, 296, 296f
single-word speech assessments, 258–260
single-word speech sample
  articulation impairment, 279
  childhood apraxia of speech, 279, 562t
  childhood dysarthria, 280, 567t
  inconsistent speech disorder, 555–558, 558f, 559t
  phonological impairment, 278, 545, 549t, 550t–552t
single-word testing for young children, 260–261
Skelton, Steve, 493
skills
  foundational knowledge and, 222–223
  professional knowledge and, 223
social construction, 186
social model, 46
social reinforcers, 388
socioeconomic status
  typical speech acquisition and, 180
socioeconomic status (SES)
  SSD and, 32
SODA taxonomy, 290
  consonantal misarticulations, 290
  interdental lisp, 290
  lateral lisp, 290
  vocalic misarticulations, 290
soft palate (velum), 73–74
  function of, 73
  structural impairments of, 74
  structure of, 73–74
sonorant, 444
sonorant consonants, 85
sonorants, 93, 139
sonorant vowels, 85
sonority, 146–148
  difference, 147
  hierarchy, 146, 147f

sonority sequencing principle (SSP), 147
The Sound Pattern of English (Chomsky and Halle), 138
sound-referenced rebuses, 416–417
Spanish, 127–131
  consonants, 96
  consonants, acquisition of, 213
  core vocabulary words, 482
  Intelligibility in Context Scale, 247t
  intervention approaches, 472t
  intervention, 473
  intonation, 105
  minimal pairs, 441–442t
  stress, 104
  vowels, 101
speaker normalization, 166–167
specificity, defined, 237
spectral moment analysis, 329
spectrography
  articulation intervention using, 496–499
  children suited to articulation intervention using, 499
  evidence, 498
  historical background, 497
  intervention procedure, 498
  theoretical background, 497
speech. *See also* children's speech
  augmentative or alternative communication and, 516–517
  documenting family history of, 229–230
  intelligibility, and targeting articulation, 515
  measures, 319–324
  perception, 376
  rate, 502
  ratings, 316–317, 316f
  representation of, 38
  respiratory support and breath control for, 514–515
  transcription of, 85–105
speech acquisition
  areas of clinical practice, 177f
  comparative studies, 189–190
  cross-sectional studies, 188–189
  diary studies, 188
  DIVA models of, 170–171, 171f
  for English-speaking infants and toddlers, 191–200
  for English-speaking preschoolers, 200–208
  for English-speaking school-aged children, 208–212
  GODIVA models of, 170–171
  important issues when considering children's, 177
  longitudinal studies, 189
  methodological issues in studying, 187–191
  phonetic, phonological, and lexical factors, 182f
  theories of child development, 185–187
  typical, for all children, 212–216
  typical, for English-speaking children, 191
  typical *vs.* acceptable, 178–185

Speech Assessment and Interactive Learning System (SAILS), 458–459
speech assessments
  communicative participation, 273–275
  components of, 245
  conventional literacy skills, 271–272
  differential diagnosis and prognostic statements, 283
  early literacy skills, 271–272
  emergent literacy skills, 271–272
  hearing, 269
  intelligibility, 245–249
  language, voice, and fluency, 275–276
  oral structure and function, 265–267
  overview, 245
  phonological processing, 269–271
  psychosocial aspects, 272–273
  single-word *vs.* connected, 264
  speech perception, 267–268
  speech production, 250–265
  using the ICF-CY framework to scaffold assessment planning, 276–277
speechBITE (Speech Best Interventions in Treatment Efficacy), 524, 526–527
Speech Correction: Principles and Methods (van Riper), 486
speech delay, 5–6
speech detection
  structures involved in, 78–81
speech difference, 39
Speech Disorders Classification System (SDCS), 46–48, 47f
Speech Filing System, 327
Speech-Language and Audiology Canada, 51, 538
speech-language pathologists (SLPs), 225–226
  associations supporting clinical practice of, 536–539
  associations supporting continuing education of, 536–539
  code of ethics for, 533t
  cultural competence, 223–225
  foundational knowledge and skills, 222–223
  preparation, 221–228
  professional knowledge and skills, 223
speech measures, 319–324
  speech segments, 319–320t
  whole words measures, 320–324, 323t, 324t
speech/non-speech discrimination, 172
Speech Participation and Activity Assessment of Children (SPAA-C), 549f
Speech Pathology Australia (SPA), 51, 538
speech perception, 165–168, 193
  assessment of, 267–268
  categorical perception, 166

event-related potentials (ERPs), 193
functional magnetic resonance imaging (fMRI), 193
the Ganong effect, 166
high amplitude sucking technique, 193
indexical cues and, 167
lack of invariance, 166
phoneme restoration effect, 166
speaker normalization, 166–167
statistical learning, 166
theoretical relevance for children with SSD, 167–168
visually reinforced head-turn procedure, 193
speech perception intervention, 456–459
  children suited to, 458
  evidence, 458
  historical background, 456
  procedure, 458
  resources for, 459
  theoretical background, 457–458
speech processing model, 49f, 170, 172f
speech production, 168–173
  anatomical structures for, 61, 61f, 62f, 81–83
  assessment of, 250–265
  DIVA and GODIVA models of, 170–171
  DIVA models of, 170–171, 171f
  elements and methods, 250t
  GODIVA models of, 170–171
  imitated *vs.* spontaneous, 259–260
  motor execution, 168–170
  motor planning, 168–170
  motor programming, 168–170
  Nijmegen model and the importance of syllables, 170
  phonological planning, 168–170
  psycholinguistic model, 172–173
  schema theory of motor learning, 171–172
  structures involved in, 61–78
  theories and models of, 170–173
speech production skills
  childhood apraxia of speech, 562, 562t
  childhood dysarthria, 566
speech sound disorders (SSD), 9
  articulation impairment, 38
  articulation impairment-lateral lisp, 554–555
  CAS, 38
  child factors, 28–31
  childhood dysarthria, 38
  classification systems of, 46–51
  classification systems of children with, 46–51
  conceptualization of, 39f
  co-occurrence of, 56–59, 57
  defining, 4–9
  educational impact of, 20–21
  evidence-based practice, 33–36, 34f
  family factors, 32–33
  family history of speech and language problems and, 31

family size and birth order, 33
goal setting for children with, 350
hearing loss and, 29
identifying goals for children with, 341–344
impact and outcomes of childhood, 17–26
impact on children's families, 23–26
impact on children's lives, 19–20
impact on parents' lives, 23–24
impact on siblings' lives, 24–26
inconsistent speech disorder, 38, 555–559
intervention strategies for infants at risk of, 470, 470t
intervention strategies for toddlers at risk of, 470, 470t
of known and unknown origins, 51–56
language impairment and, 57
and literacy difficulties, 57
longitudinal studies of the impact and outcomes of, 17–19
manifestation in adolescence and adulthood, 16–17
manifestation in late childhood, 15–16
maternal and paternal education level and, 32
minority status, race, and languages spoken and, 30–31
motor speech, 41–45
natural history and long-term manifestation of, 14–17
natural history of, 15
occupational impact of, 23
oral sucking habits and, 29
and oromotor difficulties, 57–58
parent factors, 31–32
phonological impairment, 38, 542–553
phonology, 40–41
pre- and postnatal factors for, 28–29
prevalence and impact, 9
prevalence of children with, 10–13
prevalence of subtypes of, 48
proportion of children with, on SLPs' caseloads, 13–14
psychosocial behaviors and temperament, 29–30
reasons for knowing about children with, 3
referral scenarios for different types of, 277t
representation-based accounts of, 164–165
representation of, 6
risk and protective factors for, 26–33, 27t
sex and, 28
social impact of, 21–22
socioeconomic status and, 32
steps involved in clinical decision-making in, 35–36
strategic assessments suited to, 277–283
studies examining prevalence

of children with, 11t–12t
and stuttering, 58–59
terminology, 7t–8t
theoretical relevance of speech perception for, 167–168
types of, 38–45
types of, in children, 38–45
typical characteristics of children referred for, 28
and voice difficulties, 58
speech sound errors, examples of, 39t
spondees, 104
spread glottis, 139
SSD of known origins, 52–56
children with autism spectrum disorders, 56
children with cognitive/ intellectual impairment, 54
children with craniofacial anomalies, 53–54
children with hearing loss, 54–55
children with identified genetic causes, 52–53
children with motor impairment, 55–56
children with otitis media with effusion (OME), 55
Stackhouse, Joy, 467
Stampe, David, 152
standardized assessments, 236–237
standardized speech assessment, 554
stapes, 78
static assessments, 240
statistical learning, 166
Stemberger, Joe, 467
stepping down (teaching and learning moment), 420
stepping up (teaching and learning moment), 420
stimulability assessment of, 264–265
stimulability intervention, 462–464
children suited to, 463
evidence, 463–464
historical background, 462
procedure, 463
resources for conducting, 464
theoretical background, 462–463
stimuli, 420–422
color vs. black and white, 260
pictures vs. written, 260
used in DTTC, 503
stimulus generalization, 348, 349f
stop consonant articulation, 93
stopping, 118
of affricates, 154
of fricatives, 120, 154
of liquids, 155
store-and-forward manner, 397
strategic speech assessment, 554
straw technique, 489
stress, 103–104, 200
primary, 103
secondary, 103
stridency deletion, 154
structure, of phonemes, 447
structured play, 422

stuttering, SSD and, 58–59
submucosal cleft, 72
substitution, omission, distortion, and addition (SODA) analysis, 289–291, 350
how to use, 291
when to use, 291
substitution (systemic) processes, 154–155
successive approximation/ shaping, 417
suprasegmental features, 88
suprasegmentals, 314–316, 314f
articulation of words, 315
intonation, 315
phonation, 315
resonance, 315
respiration, 315–316
speech rate, 315
stress, 314–315
syllable segregation, 315
suprasegmentals chart, 103–105
intonation, 104–105
rhythm, 104
stress, 103–104
surface phonetic representation, 149
surface prompt, 510
Swedish
intelligibility assessments, 248
minimal pairs intervention, 440
syllable and word shape inventory, 195, 202, 210, 213–214
syllable prompt, 510
syllables, 161
syllable shape inventory, 298–299, 299f
syllable shapes, 107–108
syllable shapes correct, 304, 304f
syllable stress inventory, 299–300, 300f
syllable stress patterns correct, 305, 305f
syllable structure, 199
syllable structure processes, 152–154
symbolic function, 185
symbols chart, 96–97
systematic sound preference, 158
systematic transcriptions, 87
phonemic, 87
phonetic, 87
systemic (functional) approach to target selection, 358–359
Systemic Phonological Analysis of Child Speech (SPACS), 447
systems approach
children suited to, 516
evidence, 516
historical background, 513–514
procedure, 514–516
resources for conducting, 516
theoretical background, 514

T
tableau, 163
tactile cues of DTTC, 501
tangible reward, 388
tap/flap consonant articulation, 90
Targeting Intelligible Speech (Hodson and Paden), 453

target sound or prosodic characteristic
auditory detection, 414
auditory identification, 414
teachers, 232–233
technological transcriptions, 263
teeth, 68–70, 69f, 70f, 72f
canine, 68
function of, 68
incisors, 68
molars, 68
premolars, 68
structural impairments of, 69–70
structure of, 68–69
telepractice, 397
temperament, SSD and, 29–30
Templin, Mildred, 17
Templin Longitudinal Study, 17–18
temporal cues of DTTC, 501
temporomandibular joint, 70
tendency, 145
terminology
for the transcription of speech, 88f
tertiary intervention, 476
TF32, 327
Thai, 127–131
theories of child development, 185–187
Jean Piaget, 185–186
Lev Vygotsky, 186
Urie Bronfenbrenner, 186–187
therapist-centered practice, 393
thoracic cage (ribs), 77
thyroarytenoid muscle, 77
thyroid cartilage, 76
tier one, RTI, 242
tiers, 161
tier three, RTI, 242
tier two, RTI, 242
time-based criteria, 402
tip, tongue, 63
toddlers
speech acquisition for, 191–200
token, 389
tonal languages, and minimal pair approach, 442–443
tones
and accents, 88
assessment of, 257
and word accents chart, 105
Cantonese, 105f
Vietnamese, 105
tongue, 63–67, 64f–65f, 66f, 66t
back, 63
blade, 63
body, 63
dorsum of, 63
extrinsic muscles, 63
front, 63
function of, 63
intrinsic muscles, 63
regions, 63
root, 63
structural impairments of, 66–67
structure of, 63–66
tip, 63
tongue-tie, 66
trachea (windpipe), 76, 77
traditional articulation analysis, 289–291

traditional articulation
    intervention, 486–493, 488f
    children suited to, 492
    evidence associated with, 492
    historical background, 486
    phonetic errors and, 493t
    practice, 489–491
    procedure, 487–491
    resources for conducting, 493
    theoretical background, 486
traditional developmental
    approach, 350–351
    suitable children for, 351
    target selection, 351
training deep strategy, 368
training wide strategy, 368
transcription of speech, 85–105
    diacritics chart, 97–98
    impressionistic, 87–88
    International Phonetic
        Alphabet (IPA), 88–90
    non-pulmonic consonant chart,
        95–96
    other symbols chart, 96–97
    pulmonic consonant chart,
        90–94
    suprasegmentals chart, 103–105
    systematic, 87
    terminology for, 88f
    tones and word accents chart,
        105
    vowel chart, 98–103
transdisciplinary teams, 228
transitivity, 186
transverse diagrams of English
    consonants, 109–110
transverse plane, 109
Treacher Collins syndrome, 71
treatment data, 424, 424f, 504
    intervention and, 425
treatment of the empty set
    approach, 437
    children suited to, 446
    evidence, 445–446
    historical background, 444
    procedure, 444–445
    theoretical background, 444
trigeminal nerve, 70, 81
trill consonant articulation, 90
trochaic stress pattern, 104
trochaic stress patterns, 305
Trubetzkoy, Nikolai, 138
Turkish, 107, 127–131
    intervention approaches, 472t
    minimal pairs versus maximal
        pairs, 446
tympanic membrane (eardrum),
    78
typical, defined, 178
typical assessments for SSD, 221
    assessment contexts, 227–228
    child-friendly assessments,
        225–226
    collaboration with other
        professionals, 228
    face-to-face assessments, 221
    family-centered and family-
        friendly assessments, 227
    post-assessment tasks, 221
    pre-assessment tasks, 221

purposes of, 233–236
    referral and background
        information, 228–233
    types of, 236–242
typical speech acquisition,
    178–185
    for children, 212–216
    factors influencing, 179–185
typical speech acquisition, factors
    influencing, 179–185
    age, 180
    age of acquisition of words, 182
    between child factors, 179–180
    within child factors, 181
    elicitation factors, 181
    functional load of phonemes,
        184
    language ability, 180
    maternal education, 180
    neighborhood density, 183
    personal factors, 181
    phoneme input frequency, 184
    phonetic, phonological, and
        lexical factors, 181–185
    phonetic/articulatory
        complexity, 184
    phonotactic probability, 183
    phonotactic structure of words,
        183–184
    pragmatic factors, 181
    sex, 180
    socioeconomic status, 180
    vocabulary size, 182
    word frequency, 181–182

U
ultrasound, 331, 331f
    articulation intervention using,
        496–499
    children suited to articulation
        intervention using, 498–499
    evidence, 498
    historical background, 496–497
    intervention procedure, 498
    theoretical background, 497
underlying phonological
    representation, 148
undifferentiated lingual gestures,
    113, 114f
undifferentiated tongue
    movements, 42
unintelligible speech
    goal setting considerations for
        children with, 367–368
United Nations conventions,
    534–535
United Nations Conventions
    on the Rights of the Child
    (UNCRC), 21, 521, 534
univalent feature, 140
unpleasant consequences, 388
unstructured play, 422
uvula, 73

V
vagus nerve, 81
Valsalva maneuver, 80
van Riper, Charles, 290, 486, 487,
    488

variable interval reinforcement,
    390
variable practice, 379–380
variable ratio reinforcement, 390
velar fronting, 115, 154, 159
velar places, 93
velar plosives, 114–115, 114f
    voiced, 114–115
    voiceless, 114–115
Velleman, Shelley, 468
velocity, 170
velopharyngeal insufficiency, 115
verbal imitation hierarchy, 502
vertical goal attack strategy, 368
vestibular labyrinth, 78, 79
Vietnamese, 127–131
    core vocabulary words, 480–481
    minimal pairs, 441–442t, 443
    names, 230
    syllables, 108
    tones, 105
violation, 164
visual biofeedback, 497
vocabulary size
    typical speech acquisition and,
        182
vocal folds, 76
vocalic misarticulations, 290
vocalis muscle, 77
vocalization, 155, 193–194
vocal nodules, 77
voice, 90, 139
    assessment of, 275–276
    pulmonic consonants, 92–93
voiced alveolar approximant,
    121–122
voiced alveolar fricative, 117–120
voiced alveolar nasal consonants,
    115–116
voiced alveolar plosive, d, 111–113
voiced bilabial nasal consonants,
    115–116
voiced consonants, 85
voiced dental fricative, 116–117
voiced labiodental fricative, 116
voiced lateral approximant, 123
voiced pair, 444
voiced palatal approximant, 123
voiced postalveolar affricate, 124
voiced postalveolar fricative, 120
voiced velar nasal consonants,
    115–116
voiced velar plosive, 114–115
voiceless alveolar fricative,
    117–120
voiceless alveolar plosive, 111–113
voiceless consonants, 85
voiceless dental fricative, 116–117
voiceless glottal fricative, 121
voiceless labiodental fricative, 116
voiceless pair, 444
voiceless postalveolar affricate,
    124
voiceless postalveolar fricative,
    120
voiceless velar plosive, 114–115
voice onset time (VOT), 329
vowel chart, 98–103
vowel quadrilateral, 98
vowels, 88, 297–298, 297f

age of acquisition of, 196
assessment of, 253–254
mastery of, 214
phonetic inventory of, 195
in world's languages, 101–103
vowels correct, 302–304, 303f
Vygotsky, Lev, 186

W
Walters, Barbara, 17
WaveSurfer (X waves), 327
weak syllable deletion (post-
    tonic and pre-tonic),
    152–153
Web of Science, 524
Wechsler Intelligence Scale for
    Children—Fourth Edition
    (WISC-IV), 563
Wells, Bill, 467
Welsh, 107, 127–131
    intervention approaches, 472t
What Works Clearinghouse
    (WWC), 524
whole movement (motor skill),
    381
whole-word correctness (PWC),
    322
whole words measurement,
    320–324, 323t, 324t
    phonological mean length of
        utterance (pMLU), 322, 323t
    proportion of whole-word
        proximity (PWP), 322, 323t
    proportion of whole-word
        variability (PWV), 324, 324t
    whole-word correctness (PWC),
        322
Williams, A. Lynn, 447, 449
within-group design, 439
word frequency
    typical speech acquisition and,
        181–182
word length inventory, 299, 300f
word lengths correct, 304–305,
    304f
word perception, areas of brain
    activation during, 82t
word positions, 107–108
word production
    areas of brain activation during,
        82t
words
    age of acquisition of, 182
    connected speech measures
        quantifying identification of,
        248–249
    phonotactic structure of,
        183–184
World Health Organization, 5
    publications, 535
World Report on Disability, 535

Y
Young, Edna Carter, 468

Z
zone of proximal development,
    186, 241